IAN Textbook of
Neurology

IAN Textbook of Neurology

SECOND EDITION

VOLUME 1

Editors

Satish V Khadilkar MD DM DNB FIAN FICP FAMS FRCP (London)
Dean
Bombay Hospital Institute of Medical Sciences
Mumbai, Maharashtra, India

Gagandeep Singh MD DM (Neurology) FAMS FRCP (London) FIAN FICP
Professor and Head
Department of Neurology
Dayanand Medical College and Hospital
Ludhiana, Punjab, India
and
Honorary Senior Research Fellow
Department of Clinical and Experimental Epilepsy
Institute of Neurology
Queen Square
London, United Kingdom

Foreword

Wolfgang Grisold

JAYPEE BROTHERS MEDICAL PUBLISHERS
The Health Sciences Publisher
New Delhi | London

Jaypee Brothers Medical Publishers (P) Ltd

Headquarters
EMCA House
23/23-B, Ansari Road, Daryaganj
New Delhi 110 002, India
Landline: +91-11-23272143, +91-11-23272703
+91-11-23282021, +91-11-23245672
E-mail: jaypee@jaypeebrothers.com

Corporate Office
4838/24, Ansari Road, Daryaganj
New Delhi 110 002, India
Phone: +91-11-43574357
Fax: +91-11-43574314
E-mail: jaypee@jaypeebrothers.com

Overseas Office
J.P. Medical Ltd
83 Victoria Street, London
SW1H 0HW (UK)
Phone: +44 20 3170 8910
E-mail: info@jpmedpub.com

EU GPSR Authorised Representative
Logos Europe, 9 rue Nicolas Poussin
17000, La Rochelle, France
Phone: +33 (0) 6 67 93 73 78
E-mail: contact@logoseurope.eu

Website: www.jaypeebrothers.com
Website: www.jaypeedigital.com

Inquiries for bulk sales may be solicited at: jaypee@jaypeebrothers.com

IAN Textbook of Neurology (Volume 1) / Satish V Khadilkar, Gagandeep Singh

First Edition: 2018

Second Edition: 2024

Reprint: 2026

ISBN: 978-93-5465-682-8

Printed in India

CONTRIBUTORS

Editors

Satish V Khadilkar MD DM DNB FIAN FICP FAMS FRCP (London)
Dean
Bombay Hospital Institute of Medical Sciences
Mumbai, Maharashtra, India

Gagandeep Singh MD DM (Neurology) FAMS FRCP (London) FIAN FICP
Professor and Head
Department of Neurology
Dayanand Medical College and Hospital
Ludhiana, Punjab, India
and
Honorary Senior Research Fellow
Department of Clinical and Experimental Epilepsy
Institute of Neurology
Queen Square
London, United Kingdom

Contributing Authors

Aamna Maniyar MD (Medicine)
Resident (DM Neurology)
Department of Neurology
Sir JJ Hospital
Mumbai, Maharashtra, India

Aarti Sarwal MD FCCM FNCS FAAN RPNI
Professor
Department of Neurology
Atrium Wake Forest School of Medicine
Winston Salem, North Carolina, USA

Aastha Takkar DM
Associate Professor
Department of Neurology
Postgraduate Institute of Medical Education and Research (PGIMER)
Chandigarh, India

Abhinay M Huchche MD (Medicine) DM (Neurology)
Consultant Neurologist
KIMS Hospitals, Hyderabad
Managing Director
Intero Speciality Clinics and Neuro Centre
Hyderabad, Telangana, India

Abhishek Srivastava MD DNB PhD
Neurorehabilitation Specialist and Director
Centre for Physical Medicine and Rehabilitation
Kokilaben Dhirubhai Ambani Hospital
Mumbai, Maharashtra, India

AB Taly MD (Internal Medicine) DM (Neurology)
Formerly Senior Professor of Neurology and Emeritus Medical Scientist (ICMR)
National Institute of Mental Health and Neurosciences (NIMHANS)
Bengaluru, Karnataka, India

Achal Kumar Srivastava MD (Medicine) DM (Neurology) FRCP (London) FAAN FANA FIAN FICP FAMS FNASc
Professor, Department of Neurology
All India Institute of Medical Sciences
New Delhi, India

Aditya Aundhakar DNB (Neurology)
Neurologist, Hiranandani Hospital
Navi Mumbai, Maharashtra, India

Aditya Vijayakrishnan Nair MD DM
Associate Professor of Neurology
Department of Neurological Sciences
Christian Medical College
Vellore, Tamil Nadu, India

Afshan Jabeen DM
Professor and Head
Department of Neurology
Nizam's Institute of Medical Sciences
Hyderabad, Telangana, India

Ajay Chavan MD (Pediatrics)
Senior Resident
Department of Neurology
Sanjay Gandhi Postgraduate Institute of Medical Sciences
Lucknow, Uttar Pradesh, India

Ajith Sivadasan MD DM DNB PDF (Neuromuscular Disorders)
Professor of Neurology
Department of Neurological Sciences
Christian Medical College
Vellore, Tamil Nadu, India

Alika Sharma MD
Associate Consultant
Department of Clinical Neurophysiology (EMG and EP)
Bombay Hospital
Mumbai, Maharashtra, India

Ambar Chakravarty MD FRCPC FRCP FRCPE FICP FIAN
Honorary Professor and Emeritus Consultant
Department of Neurology
Vivekananda Institute of Medical Science
Kolkata, West Bengal, India

Amit Halder MD DM
Associate Professor
Department of Neurology
Vivekananda Institute of Medical Science
Kolkata, West Bengal, India

Anandkumar Anandakuttan MD (General Medicine) DM (Neurology)
Professor and Head
Department of Neurology
Amrita Institute of Medical Sciences
Kochi, Kerala, India

Anirban Biswas MBBS DLO
Consultant Neurotologist and Director of Neurotology
Institute of Neurosciences, Kolkata
Founder Proprietor
Vertigo and Deafness Clinic
Kolkata, West Bengal, India

Anjana Munshi MPhil PhD
Professor
Department of Human Genetics and Molecular Medicine
Central University of Punjab
Bathinda, Punjab, India

Anna Grisold MD PhD
Consultant
Department of Neurology
Medical University of Vienna
Vienna, Austria, Europe

Annamma Mathai MSc PhD
Research Scientist
Department of Neurology
Amrita Institute of Medical Sciences
Kochi, Kerala, India

Anuja Patil MD DM
Consultant Neurologist
Department of Neurology
Krishna Institute of Medical Sciences
Secunderabad, Telangana, India

Apoorva Pauranik MD DM
Director
Pauranik Academy of Medical Education
Ex-Professor
Department of Medicine/Neurology
MGM Medical College and MY Hospital
Indore, Madhya Pradesh, India

Aralikatte Onkarappa Saroja MD DM
Professor
Department of Neurology
Jawaharlal Nehru Medical College
Belagavi, Karnataka, India

Archana B Netto MD (Internal Medicine) DM (Neurology)
Professor
Department of Neurology
Bangalore Medical College and Research Institute
Bengaluru, Karnataka, India

Lt Col (Dr) Arindam Mukherjee MD (Medicine) DNB (Neurology)
Assistant Professor
Armed Forces Medical College
Pune, Maharashtra, India

Arjun Shah DM (Neurology)
Assistant Professor
Department of Neurology
Sir JJ Hospital
Mumbai, Maharashtra, India

Arvind Sharma DM (Neurology)
Head
Department of Neurology
Zydus Hospitals
Ahmedabad, Gujarat, India

Ashish Kumar Duggal MD DM (Neurology)
Professor
Department of Neurology
Atal Bihari Vajpayee Institute of Medical Sciences and Dr RML Hospital
New Delhi, India

Ashok Verma MD DM MBA FAAN FANA
Professor
Department of Neurology
Director
Neuromuscular Medicine Fellowship Training Program
Medical Director
Bruce W Carter Veterans ALS Clinic
University of Miami
Miami, Florida, USA

Atchayaram Nalini DM PhD
Professor, Department of Neurology
National Institute of Mental Health and Neurosciences (NIMHANS)
Bengaluru, Karnataka, India

Avni Anand B-BMED (Bachelor of Biomedicine)
Research Intern, Genomics and Molecular Medicine, CSIR-Institute of Genomics and Integrative Biology
Civil Lines, Delhi, India

Ayush Agarwal MD DM DNB MNAMS AsFAMS
Assistant Professor
Department of Neurology
All India Institute of Medical Sciences
New Delhi, India

Bhagyadhan Patel MD DM
Consultant Neurologist and Neuromuscular Disorder Specialist
Brain & Nerve Clinic
Ahmedabad, Gujarat, India

Bhawna Sharma MD (Medicine) DM (Neurology)
Professor and Head
Department of Neurology
SMS Medical College
Jaipur, Rajasthan, India

Bhushan Mishal MD DNB (Neurology) Fellowship in Movement Disorders
Associate Consultant
Department of Neurology
Deenanath Mangeshkar Hospital
Pune, Maharashtra, India

Bidisha Banerjee MD (Pediatrics) DM (Pediatric Neurology)
Consultant Pediatric Neurologist
Manipal Hospital HAL
Bengaluru, Karnataka, India

Bijoy Jose MD (General Medicine) DM (Neurology)
Senior Resident
Department of Neurology
Amrita Institute of Medical Sciences
Kochi, Kerala, India

Bindu Menon MD (Medicine) DM (Neurology) DNB (Neurology) PGDCN (Neurology) (London) FRCP (Edinburgh) MNAMS FICP FIAN FWSO FAAN
Professor and Head
Department of Neurology
Apollo Specialty Hospitals
Nellore, Andhra Pradesh, India

Birinder Singh Paul MD DM (Neurology)
Professor, Department of Neurology
Dayanand Medical College and Hospital
Ludhiana, Punjab, India

Boby Varkey Maramattom DM FRCP (London, Edinburgh)
Neurologist, Department of Neurology
Aster Medcity
Kochi, Kerala, India

Chamanjot Kaur MD
Senior Resident, Department of Neurology
Postgraduate Institute of Medical Education and Research (PGIMER)
Chandigarh, India

Chandan Mohanty MS MCh
Consultant Neurosurgeon
Department of Neurosurgery
Bombay Hospital Institute of Medical Sciences
Mumbai, Maharashtra, India

Chandrashekhar E Deopujari MS MCh MSc FAMS
Professor and Head
Department of Neurosurgery
Bombay Hospital Institute of Medical Sciences
Mumbai, Maharashtra, India

Chandrashekhar Meshram MD DM (Neurology)
Director and Consultant Neurologist
Brain and Mind Institute
Nagpur, Maharashtra, India

Charulata Savant Sankhla MD DNB
Neurophysician
Department of Neurology
PD Hinduja National Hospital and Medical Research Centre
Mumbai, Maharashtra, India

Chaturbhuj Rathore MD DM PDF (Epilepsy)
Senior Consultant
Department of Neurosciences
Zydus Hospital
Vadodara, Gujarat, India

Debashish Chowdhury DTCD MD (Medicine) DM (Neurology) FIAN FRCP (Edinburgh) Commonwealth Fellow in Stroke Medicine (Edinburgh)
Director Professor and Head
Department of Neurology
GB Pant Institute of Postgraduate Medical Education and Research
New Delhi, India

Debasish Hota DM (Neurology)
Clinical Stroke Fellow
Zydus Hospitals
Ahmedabad, Gujarat, India

Deepak Menon MD (Medicine) DM (Neurology) Postdoctoral Fellowship Neuromuscular Disorders
Associate Professor
Department of Neurology
National Institute of Mental Health and Neurosciences (NIMHANS)
Bengaluru, Karnataka, India

Devangi Desai MD (Medicine)
Professor
Department of Medicine
Shree Krishna Hospital, Pramukhswami Medical College
Bhaikaka University, Karamsad
Anand, Gujarat, India

Devashish Ruikar MD (General Medicine) DrNB (Neurology)
Assistant Professor
Department of Medicine
Maharashtra Institute of Medical Sciences and Research Medical College
Latur, Maharashtra, India

Dhananjay Duberakar DM (Neurology)
Consultant Neurologist
Nine Pearls Hospital
Nashik, Maharashtra, India

Dhananjay Gupta MD DM FINR
Assistant Professor
Department of Neurology
Dayanand Medical College
Ludhiana, Punjab, India

Dharshini Sathishkumar MD DDVL Fellowship in Pediatric Dermatology (United Kingdom)
Professor
Department of Dermatology
Christian Medical College
Vellore, Tamil Nadu, India

Dheeraj Khurana MD DM
Incharge Stroke Program and Professor
Department of Neurology
Postgraduate Institute of Medical Sciences
Chandigarh, India

Divya M Radhakrishnan MD DM
Assistant Professor
Department of Neurology
All India Institute of Medical Sciences
New Delhi, India

Divyani Garg MD (Internal Medicine) DM (Neurology)
Assistant Professor, Department of Neurology, Vardhaman Mahavir Medical College and Safdarjung Hospital
Ansari Nagar West, New Delhi, India

Dulari Gupta MD (Pediatrics) DNB (Pediatrics) DM (Neurology) DNB (Neurology)
Assistant Professor
Department of Neurology
Bharati Vidyapeeth Deemed University Medical College
Pune, Maharashtra, India

Durgam Sathya Tejaswini MD
Resident, Department of Neurology
Institute of Neurology
Madras Medical College
Chennai, Tamil Nadu, India

DV Seshagiri DM
Associate Professor
Department of Neurology
National Institute of Mental Health and Neurosciences (NIMHANS)
Bengaluru, Karnataka, India

Easwer HV MS MCh
Professor and Head
Department of Neurosurgery
Sree Chitra Tirunal Institute for Medical Sciences and Technology
Thiruvananthapuram, Kerala, India

Elizabeth W Choi PhD
Neuropsychology Postdoctoral Fellow
University of California, San Francisco
Zuckerberg San Francisco General Hospital and Trauma Center
San Francisco, California, USA

Faheem Arshad MD DM (Neurology)
Assistant Professor
Department of Neurology
National Institute of Mental health and Neurosciences (NIMHANS)
Bengaluru, Karnataka, India

Ganesh Divakar MS MCh
Assistant Professor
Department of Neurosurgery
Sree Chitra Tirunal Institute for Medical Sciences and Technology
Thiruvananthapuram, Kerala, India

Gargi Kar MBBS MS (ENT)
Junior Consultant Neurotologist
Vertigo and Deafness Clinic
Kolkata, West Bengal, India

Gagandeep Singh MD DM (Neurology) FAMS FRCP (London) FIAN FICP
Professor and Head
Department of Neurology
Dayanand Medical College and Hospital
Ludhiana, Punjab, India
and
Honorary Senior Research Fellow
Department of Clinical and Experimental Epilepsy
Institute of Neurology
Queen Square
London, United Kingdom

Gautam Kamila MD DNB DM (Pediatric Neurology)
Centre of Excellence and
Advanced Research for Childhood Neurodevelopmental Disorders
Child Neurology Division
Department of Pediatrics
All India Institute of Medical Sciences
New Delhi, India

George C Vilanilam MS MCH
Professor
Department of Neurosurgery
Sree Chitra Tirunal Institute for Medical Sciences and Technology
Thiruvananthapuram, Kerala, India

Girish Soni MD (Medicine) DM (Neurology)
Associate Professor
Sir JJ Hospital and GGMC
Cosultant Neurologist
Lilavati Hospital and Research Centre
Wockhardt Hospital Mumbai Centre
Mumbai, Maharashtra, India

Guhan Ramamurthy MD DM DrNB FEBN FSM
Consultant Neurologist
BG Institute of Neurosciences and Neurorehabilitation
BG Hospital
Tiruchendur, Tamil Nadu, India

Gunchan Paul MD (Anesthesia) IDCCM
Professor
Department of Critical Care Medicine
Dayanand Medical College and Hospital
Ludhiana, Punjab, India

Guruprasad Hosurkar MD DNB (Neurology)
Senior Consultant Neurologist
Manipal Hospitals, Yeshwanthpur
Bengaluru, Karnataka, India

Hansashree Padmanabha MD (Pediatrics) DM (Pediatric Neurology)
Associate Professor
Department of Neurology
National Institute of Mental Health and Neurosciences (NIMHANS)
Bengaluru, Karnataka, India

Harish Jayakumar MD MRCP (United Kingdom) DM (Neurology) DNB (Neurology) FEBN PDF (Epilepsy) FRCP (Edinburgh) FACP (USA)
Consultant Neurologist and Epileptologist
JK Institute of Neurology
Madurai, Tamilnadu, India

Harisuthan T MD DM
Assistant Professor
Department of Neurology
Jubilee Mission Medical College
Thrissur, Kerala, India

Heli Shah MD DM (Neurology)
Consultant Neurologist
Department of Neurosciences
Sterling Hospital
Jivraj Mehta Hospital
Ahmedabad, Gujarat, India

Himmatrao Saluba Bawaskar MD
Chairman
Bawaskar Hospital and Clinical Research Centre
Mahad, Maharashtra, India

Hiral Halani DM (Neurology)
Associate Consultant
Department of Neurology
Bombay Hospital Institute of Medical Sciences
Mumbai, Maharashtra, India

Hrishikesh Kumar MD DM (Neurology) PDF (Movement Disorders)
Director, Movement Disorders Program
Vice Chairman
Institute of Neurosciences Kolkata
Kolkata, West Bengal, India

HV Srinivas MD (General Medicine) DM (Neurology)
Senior Consultant Neurologist
Sagar Hospital and Agadi Hospital
Former Associate Professor
Department of Neurology
National Institute of Mental Health and Neurosciences (NIMHANS)
Bengaluru, Karnataka, India

Idha Sood MBBS
Demonstrator
Department of Neurology
Christian Medical College and Hospital
Ludhiana, Punjab, India

Imtiyaz Khan MD (Radio Diagnosis and Imaging) FRCR FTIR (AIIMS)
Fellow in Interventional Neurosurgery and Stroke
Artemis Hospital
Gurugram, Haryana, India

Inder MS Sawhney MD DM FRCP MNAMS (Neurology) FIAN
Consultant Neurologist
Morriston Hospital
Clinical Director Neurosciences Swansea Bay University Health Board
Honorary Professor of Neurology
Swansea University
Swansea, Wales, United Kingdom

Jacky Ganguly MD DM (Neurology) PDF (Movement Disorders)
Consultant Movement Disorders
Institute of Neurosciences Kolkata
Kolkata, West Bengal, India

Jagadish Annapureddy DM (Neurology)
Consultant Neurologist
Department of Neurovascular Intervention
Breach Candy Hospital Trust
Mumbai, Maharashtra, India

Jagarlapudi MK Murthy MD DM FAMS FAAN FIAN
Clinical Director and Chair
Department of Neurology
CARE Hospitals, Banjara Hills
Hyderabad, Telangana, India

Jain RS MD DM FRCP (London, Edinburgh) FIAN
Senior Professor and Head
Neurology Unit
University SMS Medical College
Jaipur, Rajasthan, India

James Jose MD DM (Neurology)
Head
Department of Neurology
Calicut Medical College
Kozhikode, Kerala, India

Jasmine Parihar MD DM
Assistant Professor
Department of Neurology
All India Institute of Medical Sciences
National Cancer Institute
Jhajjar, Haryana and New Delhi, India

Jayakumar Vaikundam MD DCH DM (Neurology)
Founder Chairman and Director
JK Institute of Neurology
Madurai, Tamil Nadu, India

Jayantee Kalita MD DM FIAN FANA FAMS
Professor and Neurologist
Department of Neurology
Sanjay Gandhi Postgraduate Institute of Medical Sciences
Lucknow, Uttar Pradesh, India

Jeyaraj Durai Pandian MD (Internal Medicine) DM (Neurology) FRACP FRCP FESO FWSO FNAMS
Professor and Principal
Department of Neurology
Christian Medical College
Ludhiana, Punjab, India

Jino Vincent MD (General Medicine) DM (Neurology)
Senior Resident
Department of Neurology
Amrita Institute of Medical Sciences
Kochi, Kerala, India

Jitesh Agrawal MD DM
Senior Resident
Department of Neurology
University SMS Medical College
Jaipur, Rajasthan, India

Joe James MD DM MRCP (United Kingdom)
Consultant Neurologist
Department of Neurology
Malabar Hospital
Kozhikode, Kerala, India

John C Klick MD
Associate Professor
Department of Anesthesiology
University of Vermont Medical Center
Burlington, Vermont, USA

Joy D Desai MD DNB
Director Neurology
The Jaslok Hospital and Research Centre
Mumbai, Maharashtra, India

Joydeep Biswas MD DNB (Neurology)
Consultant Neurologist
Ruby General Hospital
Kolkata, West Bengal, India

Junling Dong DO
PGY-5, Neurology
Washington University in St Louis
Barnes-Jewish Hospital
St Louis, Missouri, USA

Kalyan B Bhattacharyya MD DM MAMS FIAN FRCP (Edinburgh)
Adviser and Senior Consultant
Department of Neurology
Medica Superspecialty Hospital
Kolkata, West Bengal, India

Kamakshi Dhamija MD DM (Neurology) PDF (Fellowship in CNS Demyelinating Disorders)
Senior Resident
Department of Neurology
National Institute of Mental Health and Neurosciences (NIMHANS)
Bengaluru, Karnataka, India

Karan Desai MD DM
Consultant Neurologist
Prashanti Clinic
Surat, Gujarat, India

Karan Sharma MBBS
Medical Officer
Department of Stroke and Neurointervention
Artemis Hospitals
Gurugram, Haryana, India

Karkal Ravishankar Naik DM
Professor and Head
Department of Neurology
Jawaharlal Nehru Medical College
Belagavi, Karnataka, India

Karthik Vinay Mahesh DM
Assistant Professor
Department of Neurology
Postgraduate Institute of Medical Education and Research (PGIMER)
Chandigarh, India

Kaumil Kothari MD (Medicine) DM (Neurology) FSNVI
Consultant Intervention Neurologist
Divyam Advanced Neurology Clinic
Rajkot, Gujarat, India

Khushnuma Mansukhani MBBS
Head, Department of Clinical Neurophysiology (EMG and EP)
Bombay Hospital
Mumbai, Maharashtra, India

Kiran Katoch MD
Ex Director
National JALMA Institute for Leprosy and Other Mycobacterial Diseases (ICMR)
Agra, Uttar Pradesh, India

Kiran Preet Malhotra MD DNB PDCC
Professor, Department of Pathology
Dr Ram Manohar Lohia Institute of Medical Sciences
Lucknow, Uttar Pradesh, India

Koustubh Bavdhankar DM (Neurology)
Third Year Resident
Department of Neurology
Seth GS Medical College and KEM Hospital
Mumbai, Maharashtra, India

KP Vinayan MD DNB DM
Professor and Head
Department of Pediatric Neurology
Amrita Institute of Medical Sciences
Kochi, Kerala, India

K Ravishankar MD
Consultant In-Charge
The Headache and Migraine Clinic
Jaslok Hospital and Research Centre
Lilavati Hospital and Research Centre
Mumbai, Maharashtra, India

K Srinivasa Babu PhD
Senior Scientist and Head
Neurophysiological Laboratory
Department of Neurological Sciences
Christian Medical College
Vellore, Tamil Nadu, India

Kurupath Radhakrishnan MD DM FAMS FAAN FANA
Senior Consultant Neurologist
Department of Neurosciences
Avitis Institute of Medical Sciences
Palakkad, Kerala, India

Lajita Balakrishnan MD
Consultant
Department of Clinical Neurophysiology
Apollo Hospital
Navi Mumbai, Maharashtra, India

Lakshmi Narasimhan Ranganathan
MD DNB DM DNB FEBN FRCP (London, Glasgow) FAAN FACP FIAN PhD
Director and Professor
Department of Neurology
Madras Medical College
Chennai, Tamil Nadu, India

Lekha Pandit MD DM PhD
Professor of Neurology and Director
Center for Advanced Neurological Research
KS Hegde Medical Academy Nitte (Deemed to be University)
Mangaluru, Karnataka, India

Madhu Nagappa MD DM
Professor
Department of Neurology
National Institute of Mental Health and Neurosciences (NIMHANS)
Bengaluru, Karnataka, India

Mahadevan Kumar MD (Microbiology)
Professor
Department of Microbiology
Bharati Vidyapeeth Deemed University Medical College
Pune, Maharashtra, India

Mahesh P Kate MD DM FRCP
Associate Professor
Division of Neurology
Department of Medicine
Member, Neurosciences and Mental Health Sciences
Member, Cardiovascular Research Institute
University of Alberta
Edmonton, Alberta, Canada

Manish Modi MD DM (Neurology)
Professor
Department of Neurology
Postgraduate Institute of Medical Education and Research (PGIMER)
Chandigarh, India

Manjari Tripathi DM (Neurology) FNASc FRCP (Edinburgh)
Professor and Unit Head
Department of Neurology
NIH Fellow (UCLA)
Neurosciences Centre
All India Institute of Medical Sciences
New Delhi, India

Manju Netto MBBS MRCOG BSc International Health PG Diploma Medical Education
Specialist Registrar
Barnet General Hospital,
Royal Free NHS Trust, Wellhouse Lane, Barnet
Clinical Fellow
The London and Kent, Surrey and Sussex Supported Return to Training (SuppoRTT)
Health Education
England, United Kingdom

Man Mohan Mehndiratta MD (Medicine) DNB (Medicine) DM (Neurology) FAAN FANA FAMS MNAMS FRCP (London, Edinburgh, Glasgow) FICP FIAN
Senior Director and Senior Consultant
Department of Neurology
Dr BL Kapur Memorial (BLK-MAX) Hospital
MAX Healthcare
Rajendra Place, New Delhi, India

Maya Bhat DM (Neuroradiology)
Professor
Department of Neuroimaging and Interventional Neuroradiology (NIIR)
National Institute of Mental Health and Neurosciences (NIMHANS)
Bengaluru, Karnataka, India

Mayank Kumar Shrivastava MD DM
Assistant Professor
Department of Neurology
ESIC Medical College and Hospital
Faridabad, Haryana, India

Maya Thomas DCH MD (Pediatrics) DM (Neurology)
Professor and Head
Department of Pediatric Neurology
Christian Medical College
Vellore, Tamil Nadu, India

Meenakshisundaram Umaiorubahan MD DM FAAN FIAN FRCP (Edinburgh, Glasgow)
Director of Neurology
SRM Institutes for Medical Science
Chennai, Tamil Nadu, India

Megha S Uppin MD FICP
Additional Professor
Department of Pathology
Nizam's Institute of Medical Sciences
Hyderabad, Telangana, India

Megha Varshney MD DM
Senior Resident
Department of Neurology
Postgraduate Institute of Medical Sciences
Chandigarh, India

Milind Deogaonkar MD
Neurosurgeon
Department of Neurosurgery
West Virginia University Medical Center
West Virginia University
Morgantown, West Virginia, USA

Minu George MD (General Medicine) DM (Neurology)
Consultant Neurologist
Department of Neurology
Renai Medicity Hospital
Kochi, Kerala, India

Mohammed Faruq MBBS PhD
Senior Principal Scientist
Genomics and Molecular Medicine
CSIR-Institute of Genomics and Integrative Biology
Civil Lines, Delhi, India

Monika Singla DM
Professor (Grade)
Department of Neurology
Dayanand Medical College and Hospital
Ludhiana, Punjab, India

Morris Freedman MD FRCPC
Professor
Department of Medicine
Division of Neurology
University of Toronto;
Head
Division of Neurology
Department of Medicine
Baycrest Health Sciences;
Scientist
Rotman Research Institute of Baycrest Centre
Staff Neurologist
Department of Medicine (Neurology)
Mount Sinai Hospital
Toronto, Ontario, Canada

Mrinal Acharya MD DM
Assistant Professor
Dr BC Roy Multi Speciality Medical Research Centre
IIT Kharagpur, West Bengal, India

MV Padma Srivastava MD DM FRCP (Edinburgh) FAMS FNASc FIAN FNA
Professor and Head
Department of Neurology
Chief – Neurosciences Center
All India Institute of Medical Sciences
New Delhi, India

Nadir E Bharucha MD FAMS (India) FRCP (London) FRCP(C) Diplomate American Board of Neurology and Psychiatry
Former Professor and Head
Department of Neurology
Head
Department of Neuroepidemiology
Bombay Hospital Institute of Medical Sciences
Mumbai, Maharashtra, India

Nagalaxmi Patnala MD DNB FIPM BMJ Certified Fellow in Palliative Care
Senior Consultant Pain Physician
Adi's Libero Neuro and Pain Care Center
KIMS and Sunshine Hospitals
Hyderabad, Telangana, India

Nagaraj AR MD DM (Neurology) DNB (Neurology)
Senior Resident
Postdoctoral Fellow in Pediatric Neurology
National Institute of Mental Health and Neurosciences (NIMHANS)
Bengaluru, Karnataka, India

Nahush Roop Bansal MBBS
Resident, Department of Cardiology
Hero Dayanand Medical College Heart Institute
Ludhiana, Punjab, India

Narayan Deshmukh MD DM (Neurology)
Consultant Neurologist
Department of Neurovascular Intervention, Breach Candy Hospital Trust
Mumbai, Maharashtra, India

Natalia Gonzalez Caldito MD
MS and Neuroimmunology Fellow
Department of Neurology
Northwestern Medicine
Chicago, Illinois, USA

Neena Baby MD DM FIPN
Consultant Neurologist
Renai Medicity Multisuperspeciality Hospital
Kochi, Kerala, India

Neera Chaudhry MD (Medicine) DM (Neurology)
Director Professor and Head
Department of Neurology
Vardhaman Mahavir Medical College and Safdarjung Hospital
New Delhi, India

Neeraj Jain DM (Neurology)
Head
Department of Neurology
Seth GS Medical College and KEM Hospital
Mumbai, Maharashtra, India

Netravathi M DM (Neurology)
Professor
Department of Neurology
National Institute of Mental Health and Neurosciences (NIMHANS)
Bengaluru, Karnataka, India

Ninad Desai MD
Consultant Neurologist
St. Vincent's Medical Center
Bridgeport, Connecticut, USA

Nirmal Surya MD DNB (Neurology) FIAN MNAMS FRCP (London)
Chairman
Surya Neuro Centre
Assistant Professor
Bombay Hospital Institute of Medical Sciences
Mumbai, Maharashtra, India

Nitin Chandak MD DM (Neurology)
Senior Consultant Neurologist
Department of Neurology
GM Taori Central India Institute of Medical Sciences
Nagpur, Maharashtra, India

Nitin K Sethi MD FAAN
Professor
Department of Neurology
New York-Presbyterian Hospital
Weill Cornell Medical Center
New York, USA

Padma Youron MD
Senior Resident
Department of Neurology
Postgraduate Institute of Medical Education
and Research (PGIMER)
Chandigarh, India

Pankaj A Agarwal MD DNB DM
Honorary Teaching Faculty
Movement Disorders Clinic
Department of Neurology
Seth GS Medical College and KEM Hospital
Senior Consultant Neurologist and Head
Movement Disorders and Deep Brain Stimulation Clinic
Global Hospitals
Mumbai, Maharashtra, India

Parag Himmatrao Bawaskar DM (Card)
Postdoctoral Research Associate
University of Minnesota
Minneapolis, Minnesota, USA

Paramjeet Singh MD FICR CCST (United Kingdom)
Professor
Department of Radiodiagnosis
Postgraduate Institute of Medical Education and Research (PGIMER)
Chandigarh, India

Parthvi Ravat MD DrNB (Neurology)
Assistant Professor
Department of Neurology
Seth GS Medical College and KEM Hospital
Mumbai, Maharashtra, India

Parul Dubey MD (Medicine) DM (Neurology)
Consultant Neurologist
Manipal Hospital
Panaji, Goa, India

Parveen Goel PhD
Neuropsychologist
Department of Neurology
Dayanand Medical College and Hospital
Ludhiana, Punjab, India

Pawan Ojha DM (Neurology) DNB (Neurology)
Associate Professor
Department of Neurology
Sir JJ Hospital
Mumbai, Maharashtra, India

PC Gilvaz MD DM (Neurology) FRCP FAAN
Professor and Head
Department of Neurology
Jubilee Mission Medical College
Thrissur, Kerala, India

Pettarusp M Wadia MD DNB (Medicine) DM DNB (Neurology)
Clinical Fellowship in Movement Disorders
University of Toronto
Consultant Neurologist
Movement Disorders Specialist
Department of Neurology
Jaslok Hospital and Research Centre
Mumbai, Maharashtra, India

PN Sylaja MD DM FRCP (Edinburgh) FESO FIAN
Professor and Head
In-Charge, Comprehensive Stroke Care Program
Department of Neurology
Sree Chitra Tirunal Institute for Medical Sciences and Technology
Thiruvananthapuram, Kerala, India

Porrselvi AP PhD
Founder and Cognitive Neuropsychologist
Unified Brain Health Care
Chennai, Tamil Nadu, India
Clinical Psychologist
King's College Hospital
London, United Kingdom

Prachi P Barvalia MD (Medicine) DM (Neurology)
Assistant Professor
TNMC and Nair Hospital
Mumbai, Maharashtra, India

Prachi Sahu MSc
Research Scholar
Department of Human Genetics and Molecular Medicine
Central University of Punjab
Bathinda, Punjab, India

Prafulla Shembalkar MD DM (Neurology) FAAN
Consultant Neurologist and Director
Getwell Hospital and Research Institute
Nagpur, Maharashtra, India

Pragya Chaturvedi MSc
Research Scholar
Department of Human Genetics and Molecular Medicine
Central University of Punjab
Bathinda, Punjab, India

Prahlad K Sethi MD FAAN
Professor, Department of Neurology
Sir Ganga Ram Hospital
New Delhi, India

Prakash Nair MS MCH
Additional Professor
Department of Neurosurgery
Sree Chitra Tirunal Institute for Medical Sciences and Technology
Thiruvananthapuram, Kerala, India

Pramodinin Himmatrao Bawaskar MBBS
Medical Officer
Bawaskar Hospital and Clinical Research Centre
Mahad, Maharashtra, India

Pramod Kumar Pal MD DNB DM FIAN FRCP (London)
Professor, Department of Neurology
National Institute of Mental Health and Neurosciences (NIMHANS)
Bengaluru, Karnataka, India

Priyanka Sehrawat MD DM
Consultant Neurologist
Department of Neurology
Aarvy Healthcare Super Speciality Hospital
Gurugram, Haryana, India

Priya Thomas PhD
Additional Professor
Department of Psychiatric Social Work
National Institute of Mental Health and Neurosciences (NIMHANS)
Bengaluru, Karnataka, India

Puneet Talwar PhD
Senior Research Associate
Department of Neurology
Institute of Human Behaviour and Allied Sciences (IHBAS)
Dilshad Garden, New Delhi, India

Radhika Nair MD DM FCSC-S
Division of Neurology
Department of Medicine
University of Alberta
Edmonton, Alberta, Canada

Raghunandan Nadig MD DNB
Professor, Department of Neurology
St John's Medical College Hospital
Bengaluru, Karnataka, India

Rahul Khan MSc
Research Scholar
Department of Human Genetics and Molecular Medicine
Central University of Punjab
Bathinda, Punjab, India

Rajesh Benny DM (Neurology)
Professor and Senior Consultant Neurologist
Department of Neurology
Fortis Hospital, Mulund
Mumbai, Maharashtra, India

Rajeswari Aghoram DM (Neurology)
Associate Professor
Department of Neurology
Jawaharlal Institute of Postgraduate Medical Education and Research (JIPMER)
Gorimedu, Puducherry, India

Rajinder K Dhamija MD DNB (Neurology) FRACP
Professor of Neurology and Director
Institute of Human Behaviour and Allied Sciences (IHBAS)
Dilshad Garden, New Delhi, India

Rajsrinivas Parthasarathy CCT (United Kingdom) Neurology
Head Stroke and Senior Consultant Neurointerventional Surgery
Artemis Hospital
Gurugram, Haryana, India

Rakesh Singh MD DM (Neurology)
Consultant and Interventional Neurologist
Department of Neurology
Bombay Hospital and Institute of Medical Sciences
Mumbai, Maharashtra, India

Rakhil S Yadav MD DM (Neurology)
Consultant Neurologist
Suyog Neurology Center
Ahmedabad, Gujarat, India

Rama Shankari Padmanabhan MD (Anesthesia) PDF (Neurology and Ortho Anesthesia)
Consultant Neuroanesthesiologist
JK Institute of Neurology
Madurai, Tamil Nadu, India

Ratnav Singh MBBS
Junior Resident
Department of Pharmacology
All India Institute of Medical Sciences
New Delhi, India

Raviteja Kakarla MD DM (Neurology)
Fellow in Interventional Neurosurgery and Stroke
Artemis Hospital
Gurugram, Haryana, India

Riddhi Patel MD DM (Neurology)
Consultant Neurologist
Department of Neurovascular Intervention
Breach Candy Hospital Trust
Mumbai, Maharashtra, India

Rohan R Mahale DM (Neurology) PDF (Movement Disorders)
Additional Professor
Department of Neurology
National Institute of Mental Health and Neurosciences (NIMHANS)
Bengaluru, Karnataka, India

Roopa Rajan MD DM
Associate Professor
Department of Neurology
All India Institute of Medical Sciences
New Delhi, India

Roop Gursahani MD DM FAAN
Consultant Neurologist
PD Hinduja National Hospital
Mumbai, Maharashtra, India

R Sureshkumar MD (General Medicine) DM (Neurology)
Senior Consultant Neurologist
Renai Medicity Hospital
Former Professor
Department of Neurology
Amrita Institute of Medical Sciences
Kochi, Kerala, India

Ruchika Tandon DM (Neurology)
Associate Professor
Department of Neurology
Sanjay Gandhi Postgraduate Institute of Medical Sciences
Lucknow, Uttar Pradesh, India

Ruta Savaj MD
Senior Resident
Department of Neurology
PD Hinduja National Hospital and Medical Research Centre
Mumbai, Maharashtra, India

Sadanandavalli Retnaswami Chandra MD (General Medicine) DM (Neurology) FIAN
Retired Professor
Department of Neurology
National Institute of Mental Health and Neurosciences (NIMHANS)
Bengaluru, Karnataka, India

Sahil Patel MD
Senior Resident, Department of Neurology
PD Hinduja National Hospital and Medical Research Centre,
Mumbai, Maharashtra, India

Sajad Ahmad Tak MD
Senior Resident, Super Speciality Hospital
Government Medical College
Srinagar, Jammu and Kashmir, India

Salman Bhai MD
Director
Neuromuscular Center
Institute for Exercise and Environmental Medicine
Texas Health Presbyterian
Assistant Professor
Department of Neurology
University of Texas Southwestern Medical Center
Dallas, Texas, USA

Samim MM DM
Senior Resident
Department of Neurology
National Institute of Mental Health and Neurosciences (NIMHANS)
Bengaluru, Karnataka, India

Sandeep Kaushal MD FRCP (Edinburgh) FCP (ACCP) FIMSA MBPhS MAMS
Dean Academics
Professor and Head
Department of Pharmacology
Dayanand Medical College and Hospital
Ludhiana, Punjab, India

Sandeep Kumar MD DM
Postdoctoral Fellow
Cognitive Neurosciences
Department of Neurology
National Institute of Mental Health and Neurosciences (NIMHANS)
Bengaluru, Karnataka, India

Sangeeta H Ravat MD DM
Dean and Head
Department of Neurology
Seth GS Medical College and KEM Hospital
Mumbai, Maharashtra, India

Sangeetha Yoganathan MD (Pediatrics) DNB (Pediatrics) DM (Pediatric Neurology)
Professor
Department of Pediatric Neurology
Christian Medical College
Vellore, Tamil Nadu, India

Sanjay Behari MS MCh DNB FAMS
Director
Department of Neurosurgery
Sree Chitra Tirunal Institute for Medical Sciences and Technology
Thiruvananthapuram, Kerala, India

Sanjay Prakash DM (Neurology)
Professor and Head
Department of Neurology
Smt BK Shah Medical Institute and Research Centre
Vadodara, Gujarat, India

Sanjeeda PGDRP PhD
Centre of Excellence and Advanced Research for Childhood Neurodevelopmental Disorders
Child Neurology Division
Department of Pediatrics
All India Institute of Medical Sciences
New Delhi, India

Sanjeev Jha DM (Neurology)
Professor and Head
Department of Neurology
Sanjay Gandhi Postgraduate Institute of Medical Sciences
Lucknow, Uttar Pradesh, India

Sanjeev V Thomas MD DM FANA FAAN FAMS FIAN
Professor, Department of Neurology
Director
Institute for Communicative and Cognitive Neurosciences
Thiruvananthapuram, Kerala, India

Sanjib Sinha MD DM FIAN FAMS
Professor, Department of Neurology
National Institute of Mental Health and Neurosciences (NIMHANS)
Bengaluru, Karnataka, India

Sapna Erat Sreedharan MD DM
Professor
Comprehensive Stroke Care Program
Department of Neurology
Sree Chitra Tirunal Institute for Medical Sciences and Technology
Thiruvananthapuram, Kerala, India

Saraswati Nashi DM Postdoctoral Fellowship Neuromuscular Disorders
Associate Professor
Department of Neurology
National Institute of Mental Health and Neurosciences (NIMHANS)
Bengaluru, Karnataka, India

Sarika Patil MD (Medicine) DM (Neurology) FMDS
Consultant Neurologist and Movement Disorders Specialist
Department of Neuroscience
Sterling Hospital
Rajkot, Gujarat, India

Sarosh M Katrak MD DM
Professor Emeritus
Department of Neurology
Grant Medical College and
Sir JJ Group of Hospitals, Mumbai
Emeritus Director
Department of Neurology
Jaslok Hospital and Research Centre
Mumbai, Maharashtra, India

Satish V Khadilkar MD DM DNB FIAN FICP FAMS FRCP (London)
Dean
Bombay Hospital Institute of Medical Sciences
Mumbai, Maharashtra, India

Saurabh Nigam MD (Medicine)
Senior Resident
Department of Neurology
Sanjay Gandhi Postgraduate Institute of Medical Sciences
Lucknow, Uttar Pradesh, India

Seena Vengalil MD DM Postdoctoral Fellowship Neuromuscular Disorders
Associate Professor
Department of Neurology
National Institute of Mental Health and Neurosciences (NIMHANS)
Bengaluru, Karnataka, India

Senthil Amudhan MD (Community Medicine)
Additional Professor
Department of Epidemiology
National Institute of Mental Health and Neurosciences (NIMHANS)
Bengaluru, Karnataka, India

Shalini Arora MD
Professor
Department of Pharmacology
Dayanand Medical College and Hospital
Ludhiana, Punjab, India

Sharath Kumar GG MD DM
Consultant Neuroradiology
St John's Medical College Hospital and Apollo Hospitals
Bengaluru, Karnataka, India

Sheffali Gulati FRCPCH (United Kingdom) FAMS FIAP FIMSA
Professor and Coordinator
DM Pediatric Neurology Program
Faculty I/C, Centre of Excellence and Advanced Research for Childhood Neurodevelopmental Disorders
Chief, Child Neurology Division
Department of Pediatrics
All India Institute of Medical Sciences
New Delhi, India

Shivani Sharma PhD
PhD Scholar
Department of Neuropathology
National Institute of Mental Health and Neurosciences (NIMHANS)
Bengaluru, Karnataka, India

Shlok Patel MBBS
Student, BJ Medical College
Ahmedabad, Gujarat, India

Shruti Agrawal DM (Neurology)
Assistant Professor
Department of Neurology
Seth GS Medical College and KEM Hospital
Mumbai, Maharashtra, India

Shweta Prasad MBBS PhD
DBT/ Wellcome Trust India Alliance Early Career Fellow
Department of Neuroimaging and Interventional Radiology
National Institute of Mental Health and Neurosciences (NIMHANS)
Bengaluru, Karnataka, India

Sinjan Ghosh MD DM
Behavioural Neurology Fellow
Division of Neurology
Department of Medicine
Baycrest Health Sciences and University of Toronto
Toronto, Ontario, Canada

Sita Jayalakshmi MD DM
Consultant Neurologist
Department of Neurology
Krishna Institute of Medical Sciences
Secunderabad, Telangana, India

Soaham Desai MD DM (Neurology)
Senior Consultant Neurologist, Professor and Head
Department of Neurology
Shree Krishna Hospital, Pramukhswami Medical College
Bhaikaka University, Karamsad
Anand, Gujarat, India

Sonali Singh MD DNB DM (Pediatric Neurology)
Centre of Excellence and Advanced Research for Childhood Neurodevelopmental Disorders
Child Neurology Division
Department of Pediatrics
All India Institute of Medical Sciences
New Delhi, India

Soumya Sucharita Pattnaik MSc (Medical Pharmacology)
PhD Scholar, Department of Pharmacology
All India Institute of Medical Sciences
New Delhi, India

Soumya Sundaram MD DM
Additional Professor
Department of Neurology
Sree Chitra Tirunal Institute for Medical Sciences and Technology
Thiruvananthapuram, Kerala, India

SP Gorthi DM (Neurology) FAAN (USA) SCE (Neurology, United Kingdom)
Professor and Head
Department of Neurology
Bharati Hospital and Research Centre
Pune, Maharashtra, India

Sreenivas U Meenakshisundaram MD DM SCE FEBN
Consultant in Neurology and Stroke
King's College Hospital
London, United Kingdom

Srividhya S MD
Resident, Department of Neurology
Institute of Neurology
Madras Medical College
Chennai, Tamil Nadu, India

Steven L Lewis MD
Secretary General, World Federation of Neurology
Physician-in-Chief, Lehigh Valley Fleming Neuroscience Institute
Pennsylvania, USA

Stuti Shah MBBS
Student, BJ Medical College
Ahmedabad, Gujarat, India

Sudheeran Kannoth MD (General Medicine) DM (Neurology)
Clinical Associate Professor
Neuroimmunology Laboratory
Department of Neurology
Amrita Institute of Medical Sciences
Kochi, Kerala, India

Sudhir Chandra Sarangi MD DM (Clinical Pharmacology)
Additional Professor
Department of Pharmacology
All India Institution of Medical Sciences
New Delhi, India

Sudhir Kothari DM (Neurology)
Professor, HOD and Senior Consultant Neurologist
Department of Neurology
Poona Hospital and Research Centre
Pune, Maharashtra, India

Sudhir V Shah MD DM (Neurology) FRCP (London) FAAN FIAN
Head and Professor
Department of Neurology
Smt NHL Municipal Medical College and
Sardar Vallabhbhai Patel Institute of Medical
Sciences and Research
Director of Neurosciences
Sterling Hospital
Ahmedabad, Gujarat, India

Sujit Kumar MD DM
Senior Consultant Neurologist and Epileptologist
Department of Neurology
Apollo Hospitals, Seshadripuram
Bengaluru, Karnataka, India

Suman Kushwaha DM (Neurology)
Professor and Head
Department of Neurology
Institute of Human Behaviour and Allied Sciences (IHBAS)
Dilshad Garden, New Delhi, India

Sureshkumar Kamalakannan BOT MPH PhD
Associate Professor
Department of Social Work, Education, and
Community Well-Being
Northumbria University
United Kingdom
and Co-Director – Cochrane Affiliate for Public Health and Disability
Indian Institute of Public Health, Hyderabad
Public Health Foundation of India

Suvarna Alladi DM (Neurology)
Professor
Department of Neurology
National Institute of Mental Health and Neurosciences (NIMHANS)
Bengaluru, Karnataka, India

Swati H Shah MD (Neurology)
Fellow-Neuromuscular Disorders
Neuro Clinic and EMG Centre
Ahmedabad, Gujarat, India

Tanish Modi MBBS
Clinical Trainee, Department of Neurology
Postgraduate Institute of Medical Education and Research (PGIMER)
Chandigarh, India

Tapas Kumar Banerjee MD FRCP (London) FRCP (Edinburgh) FAAN FIAN
Medical Director and Chief Consultant Neurologist
National Neurosciences Centre Calcutta
Peerless Hospital Campus
Kolkata, West Bengal, India

Tejaswini Shanubhogue MD DrNB (Neurology)
Consultant Neurologist
Shree Krishna Hospital
Pramukhswami Medical College
Bhaikaka University, Karamsad
Anand, Gujarat, India

Thomas Mathew MD DM
Professor and Head
Department of Neurology
St John's Medical College Hospital
Bengaluru, Karnataka, India

Tobin George MS MCh
Assistant Professor
Department of Neurosurgery
Sree Chitra Tirunal Institute for Medical Sciences and Technology
Thiruvananthapuram, Kerala, India

UK Misra MD DM FRCP (Edinburgh, London) FNA FNASc FAMS FAAN
Director Neuroscience and Head of Neurology
Apollomedics Super Speciality Hospital
Lucknow, Uttar Pradesh, India

Vaibhav Mathur MD (Medicine) DM (Neurology) DrNB (Neurology)
Consultant Neurologist and Movement Disorders Specialist
Narayana Hospital
Jaipur, Rajasthan, India

Vaibhav Wadwekar DM (Neurology) PDF (Neuromuscular Disorders)
Professor, Department of Neurology
Jawaharlal Institute of Postgraduate Medical Education and Research (JIPMER)
Gorimedu, Puducherry, India

Vaishakh Anand MD DM
Associate Professor
Department of Pediatric Neurology
Amrita Institute of Medical Sciences
Kochi, Kerala, India

Vanessa Baute MD
Associate Professor
Department of Neurology
Atrium Wake Forest School of Medicine
Winston Salem, North Carolina, USA

Varsha A Patil MD DM (Neurology)
Consultant Neurologist
Department of Neurology
Bombay Hospital and Medical Research Centre
Mumbai, Maharashtra, India

Vedantam Rajshekhar MCh (Neurosurgery)
Professor of Neurosurgery
Department of Neurological Sciences
Christian Medical College
Vellore, Tamil Nadu, India

Venugopalan Y Vishnu MD DM
Associate Professor
Department of Neurology
All India Institute of Medical Sciences
New Delhi, India

Vikas Bhatia MD DM
Associate Professor
Section of Neuroimaging and Intervention Neuroradiology
Department of Radiodiagnosis and Imaging
Postgraduate Institute of Medical Education and Research (PGIMER)
Chandigarh, India

Col (Dr) Vikram Asturkar MD (Medicine) DNB (Neurology)
Associate Professor
Armed Forces Medical College,
Pune, Maharashtra, India

Vikram V Holla MD DM
Associate Professor
Department of Neurology
National Institute of Mental Health and Neurosciences (NIMHANS)
Bengaluru, Karnataka, India

Vinay Goyal MD DM FIAN
Director Neurology
Neurosciences Institute
Medanta – The Medicity
Gurugram, Haryana, India

Vineeth Jaison MD DM
Professor of Neurology
Lead Consultant, Neuromuscular Center of Excellence
Christian Medical College and Hospital
Ludhiana, Punjab, India

Surg Capt (Dr) Vinny Wilson MD (Medicine) DM (Neurology)
Professor, Armed Forces Medical College
Pune, Maharashtra, India

Vinod Puri MD DM
Senior Consultant and Head
Department of Neurology
National Heart Institute
East of Kailash, New Delhi, India

Vipul Gupta MD
Director – Neurointerventional Surgery and Co-Director – Stroke Unit
Artemis Agrim of Institute of Neurosciences
Artemis Hospital
Gurugram, Haryana, India

Viraj Sanghi MD DNB (Neurology)
Fellowship Pediatric Neurology (Toronto, Canada)
Senior Pediatric Neurologist
Division of Pediatric Neurology
SRCC Children's Hospital
KEM Hospital and Seth GS Medical College
Mumbai, Maharashtra, India

Vivek Lal MD (Medicine) DM (Neurology) FIAN FRCP (Edinburgh)
Director, PGIMER
Professor and Head
Department of Neurology
Postgraduate Institute of Medical Education
and Research (PGIMER)
Chandigarh, India

V Preethish Kumar MRCP PhD (Clinical Neurosciences) FRCP
Consultant in Neurology and Clinical Neurophysiology
Swansea Bay University Health Board
Swansea, Wales, United Kingdom

William Owen Pickrell MEng MA MB BChir PhD MRCP
Consultant Neurologist
Swansea Bay University Health Board
Honorary Associate Clinical Professor
Swansea University Medical School
Swansea University
Swansea, Wales, United Kingdom

Wolfgang Grisold MD FAAN
Professor
Department of Neurology
Ludwig Boltzmann Institute for Experimental and Clinical Traumatology
Vienna, Austria, Europe
President, World Federation of Neurology

FOREWORD

The "*IAN Textbook of Neurology*" edited by Satish V Khadilkar and Gagandeep Singh is based on classical neurological principles, which takes into account the history and neurological examinations, finds the correlates in anatomy, neurophysiology, and molecular levels, and is a large compendium on common neurological symptoms and signs.

The book contains a list of diseases of the brain that start from frequent types, such as stroke, toward rare diseases, such as diseases of the spinal cord as well as functional disorders.

The chapter on investigations explains the importance of imaging, neurophysiology, and testing with various other methods including genetics. Drug therapies are increasingly important and equally important to counselling and doctor–patient relationship.

The *IAN Textbook of Neurology* is a comprehensive textbook and will be useful for all physicians concerned in the treatment of neurology from trainees to practicing neurologists. In one of the countries with the world's second largest population, the impact will be meaningful.

The ongoing development of electronic media, availability of easy-access knowledge, and recent research as well as other electronic apps as libraries, blended learning apps have instigated an ongoing discussion of the value of textbooks.

Textbooks in neurology are essential and often the basis for training curricula and also individual studies and therapies. They are used in many scientific fields, and not only medicine, and are considered to be a legitimized and institutional knowledge. Textbooks are based on a broad width of knowledge, which cannot be provided in a single article, which is usually topic specific.

They thus have an impact on summarizing the current knowledge and at present remain the best expert platform, which must receive timely additional update from easily available media, and definitely case- and problem-specific additional research is necessary to be updated on the latest developments.

I hope that this tremendous work will be used for the care of patients and once a book of this dimension is released, the editors will start planning the next edition. The effort of the editors to collect such a large spectrum of sections and chapters is enormous and will benefit trainees and practicing neurologists. On behalf of the World Federation of Neurology whose mission is to foster neurology and education, this will be an important contribution.

Wolfgang Grisold MD FAAN
Professor
Department of Neurology
Ludwig Boltzmann Institute for
Experimental and Clinical Traumatology
Vienna, Austria, Europe
President, World Federation of Neurology

PREFACE TO THE SECOND EDITION

The second edition of the "*IAN Textbook of Neurology*" has been prepared for clinicians who participate in the care of neurological patients, including those who are in training to become neurologists, internists, neurosurgeons, and neuroscientists.

The basic structure of this second edition has changed. The book is divided into seven parts. Section 1 discusses the History-taking and the Neurological Examination, inclusive of the systemic examination that helps the neurological diagnoses. Section 2 covers the Applied Neuroanatomy and Neurophysiology aspects that are important to clinicians. Section 3 discusses the clinical Approach to various Common Neurological Symptoms. Section 4 describes Diseases of the Nervous System. Section 5 discusses Investigations, Section 6 the Principles of Management, and Section 7 is about the Counseling and Doctor–Patient Relationship.

Thus, in some ways, this edition has tried to make the book comprehensive. Conventionally, textbooks carrying information regarding neurological examination have been separate from those that discuss diseases of the nervous system. This book covers both aspects. In the section on diseases of the nervous system, peculiarities and points relevant to the Indian setting have been highlighted for the practitioners working with Indian patients. Diagrams and flowcharts have been used for the ease of assimilation and chapters are extensively referenced.

The hard copy of the book will have access to online materials like multiple-choice questions which can be utilized for self-assessment and illustrative videos.

The chapters are written by authorities in their field, mainly from India and some overseas. Their expositions of the subjects reflect the ever-expanding extent of accumulated information and how it applies directly to the clinicians caring for their patients. The standard templates have ensured uniformity of the style and content. As many of the authors for this edition are newly inducted to this edition, the coordination was challenging to an extent, but all the authors responded with precision and we would like to thank them.

Collaboration with many individuals has been the backbone of the preparation of this edition. Jaypee Brothers Medical Publishers, Shri Jitendar P Vij (Group Chairman), and his team, namely, Ms Chetna Malhotra (Senior Director—Professional Publishing, Marketing and Business Development), Ms Nedup Bhutia Pillai (Team Leader—Print Publishing) and entire production team have worked systematically for many months and we thank them. Deepak Sharma from the office of Dr Gagandeep Singh has been instrumental in the early and continuing electronic communication with the authors for the past whole year and we thank him.

Medicine is an ever-changing science and the information pool changes at a phenomenal speed. We do hope that the readers keep themselves updated with the emerging information, using the base that this edition provides.

Satish V Khadilkar
Gagandeep Singh

PREFACE TO THE FIRST EDITION

Neurology is a field in medical sciences which has made phenomenal progress over the last two decades. Advancement in technology has changed our understanding of many diseases leading to improvement of patient care. Textbooks provide rapid access to the current status of the diseases and serve as ready reference for the physicians. There are many textbooks in neurology available in print and electronic versions. They are comprehensive, well-written, and serve as important source of information to the practicing and trainee neurologists. However, majority of them are contributed by authors from the Western world and are based on their research and clinical experience in Western countries. It is well documented that prevalence, presentations, genetics, and treatment response of various neurological diseases have significant regional variation. In order to overcome this, Indian Academy of Neurology envisaged bringing out a textbook of neurology to be planned and written by neurologists and neuroscientists who are researching, teaching, and practicing in India. It is impossible to capture the entire spectrum of neurological disorders in one volume of a textbook. In fact, literature concerning each subspecialty of neurology would constitute an enormous compendium of information. The chapters are, therefore, designed to give broad overview with recent advances in the designated field.

The book has 12 sections. Each section is dedicated to one subspecialty of neurology. Each section is edited by a senior member of the society with special interest in the specialty. The authors are chosen based on their experience and contributions in the specialized areas. The book chapters are comprehensive, well-written, and carry information with special emphasis on Indian scenario. The references quoted are extensive and will guide interested readers for further reading.

Thus, the book will be an important addition to already existing books in neurology with the unique feature of being contributed by neuroscientists of India who have extensive experience in the field of neurological diseases prevalent in India.

Arabinda Mukherjee

CONTENTS

VOLUME 1

Section 1: History and Clinical Neurological Examination

Section 2: Applied Neuroanatomy and Neurophysiology

Section 3: Approach to Common Neurological Symptoms

VOLUME 2

Part 4F: Cognitive Decline

Part 4G: Diseases of the Lower Motor Neuron

Part 4H: Ataxias

Part 4I: Miscellaneous

Section 5: Investigations

Section 6: Principles of Management

Section 7: Counseling and Doctor–Patient Relationship

VIDEO CONTENT

Chapter 66: Psychogenic Nonepileptic Seizures

Video 1: Swoon. This nonepileptic attack disorder (NEAD) video shows the neurologist giving a "suggestion" to the patient using the tuning fork as an induction protocol. This is a swoon as described in our text. This patient had no postictal confusion and a very rapid recovery.

Video 2: This nonepileptic attack disorder (NEAD) video shows the posturing of opisthotonus, also called "arc de cercle" as seen in NEAD. This nonepileptic spell also stopped when suggested to the patient.

Video 3: This nonepileptic attack disorder (NEAD) episode shows ictal biting, bipedaling movements, side-to-side head movements. His electroencephalogram (EEG) during this record was also without any epileptiform discharges. The patient's ictus stopped on giving suggestion.

Chapter 71: Parkinson's Disease

Video 1: Bradykinesia: Video demonstrates bradykinesia in the form of an asymmetric reduction (right>left) in amplitude of finger tapping, hand movement, rapid alternating movement and leg agility. The patient also has a stooped posture with reduced arm swing while walking, slowness of gait with freezing and a positive pull test.

Video 2: Tremor dominant Parkinson's disease (PD): Video demonstrates the tremor dominant phenotype of PD wherein the patient has a severe rest and action tremor of bilateral upper and lower limbs (left>right).

Video 3: Choreiform peak dose dyskinesia occurring post comsumption of dopaminergic medication (levodopa–carbidopa). Segment 1: Mild choreiform dyskinesia. Segment 2: Severe choreiform dyskinesia.

Video 4: Freezing of gait: The patient has significant gait freezing with improves significantly with visual cues.

Video 5: Effect of bilateral STN DBS in a patient with akinetic rigid variant of PD: In the Pre DBS, OFF state, the patient has significant bradykinesia and freezing of gait. In the post DBS. OFF state, the patient has no evident bradykinesia and gait is normal.

Chapter 109: Functional Neurological Disorders

Video 1: A boy with functional imbalance falls to either side when doing the Romberg test with his feet close and eyes closed.

Video 2: Now when the boy is asked to stand the same way with feet close, but instructed to focus on doing rapid alternating movements with the hands (dysdiadochokinesia), he no longer loses balance, even when his eyes are closed as in the earlier Romberg test. This shows the effect of distraction on the Romberg test.

Video 3: La belle indifference seen in a lady with focal "dystonic" movements of the left lower face.

Video 4: A man with functional tremor first affecting the whole hand. When the thumb is plugged into the ear, preventing it from moving, only the hand moves. When the thumb is removed, only the thumb moves. When the hands are placed on a pillow the hands tremble again, and finally when the feet are placed against each other they get the same tremor immediately. This is the whack-a-mole sign where movement (tremor) suppression of one body part is followed by immediate reemergence of movement (tremor) in another.

Video 5: An irregular tremor in the outstretched left hand, which slows down and almost stops when the person is asked to do tapping movements with the normal right thumb and finger.

Video 6: This video shows how suggestion using a tuning fork could induce the dystonia of the lips and jaw that the patient came for. On reminding, even her eyes close, like in her "spontaneous attacks." In the later part of the video, just pressing on the cheeks abruptly ends this dystonia.

Video 7: A lady showing functional hemifacial movements of the left face involving only the left lower face, with rhythmic movements unlike the irregular jerks of hemifacial spasm. The movements abruptly cease when she is asked to show her teeth. When she holds her hands outstretched, there emerges the tremor of the right hand on suggestion.

Video 8: A person with functional imbalance of gait demonstrates exquisite balance when doing tandem walking. The wild, flailing movements actually show excellent balance.

Video 9: A boy with functional ataxic gait suddenly veers and takes support of the wall, both when walking toward us and walking away from us and also when standing.

Video 10: A girl with functional hemiplegia dragging the right leg like a stick without circumduction, as would be expected in hemiplegic gait.

Video 11: A man with functional hemiplegia dragging the right leg very slowly like a stick without circumduction.

Video 12: This lady with shrug-like jerking of her shoulders while walking and standing later starts getting a tremor of her feet when she lies down in bed. This is also akin to whack-a-mole sign.

Video 13: A lady with a functional gait disorder shows her suddenly coming backward without losing balance, every time she takes a few steps ahead.

Video 14: A lady with a functional gait disorder shows wild swinging and swaying, as well as giving way at the knees without actually losing balance or falling.

Video 15: This girl with functional drop attacks shows how she walks quite normally, and then gets some sort of warning in her head and falls down without any injury.

Video 16: A girl with functional seizures shows a dystonic posture of the right hand, neck, face, and body as she holds her breath and keeps her eyes clenched tightly and resists opening. The attack stops suddenly when the doctor speaks to her, and she takes a breath again without any postictal confusion.

Video 17: This boy with functional seizure shows the gradual buildup of asynchronous limb and body movements. The video also demonstrates preserved consciousness as shown by him showing the tongue when asked to.

Video 18: A boy with a functional seizure, which is induced by suggestion with the use of a tuning fork. The attack shows typical asynchronous limb movements as well as arching of the back. It also shows how suggestion abruptly stops the attack, and there is no postictal confusion.

Video 19: A girl with functional loss of vision who also shows convergence spasm.

Video 20: Preserved optokinetic nystagmus in a lady who is functionally blind.

Video 21A: A lady able to touch her fingers to each other accurately when the "blind eye" is patched and she can see with the other one.

Video 21B: The same lady with functional blindness missing her fingers, when asked to touch both her index fingers to each other, when her seeing eye is patched. The ability to touch fingers to each other is not dependent on vision but on proprioception.

Video 22: Radio tactical shows a boy with functional voice order showing irregular stammering speech with hyperventilation and tremor of the body toward the end of the video.

Video 23: A person with an acute onset of whispering voice. He can make a sound when coughing though.

Free Online Resources

You can access following content on https://learn.ejaypee.com/login/ by redeeming the scratch code given on the front-in of the cover.

1. **E-version of the book:** All the chapters in the printed version can be accessed online.
2. **MCQs:** Each section is followed by 5–10 MCQs. These MCQs have 4–5 options and one correct answer. They are from the contents of the chapter. You are advised to solve these after reading the whole chapter.
3. **Videos:** Some of the chapters have videos and these videos can be accessed online.

1

SECTION

History and Clinical Neurological Examination

1

CHAPTER

History Taking in Neurology

Satish V Khadilkar

INTRODUCTION

History is an important part of the diagnostic process in medicine and neurology. It has often been stated that the diagnosis is revealed in the patient's narration of the illness, and "Listen to your patient; he is telling you the diagnosis" is a clinical truism. A good history can go further than the medical diagnosis of the patient's ailment and gather information about his fears, worries, ideas, and expectations as well. The patient's perspective of the problem is as much the central theme of management as diagnostic labeling, and listening before systematic questioning is the best way forward. Listening is the heart of history taking.

The basis of an informative history is good communication. Patients share experiences with the doctor while narrating their history. When invited to tell account of their ailments, patients get an opportunity to unburden themselves and may therefore put in bits and pieces of information about a variety of emotions emerging from the difficulties that they faced and the resulting frustrations. Communication skills come into play here, as reaching a point of relaxed interaction with the patient takes practice, patience, understanding, and concentration. It also relates to faith and trust, which builds over time. If a true representative account of what has happened over time and how it affects the individual can be gathered during the history taking, further examination, investigations, and management steps can be effectively executed.

ESTABLISHING THE CONNECTION

The setting of the consultation is important. The place should have enough privacy, and the arrangements should be organized such that the seating is on the same level as the doctor. It provides a sense of equality and helps establish good eye contact. A bright ambiance is desirable. A warm and friendly greeting as the patient and the relatives come in can start the ball rolling in the right direction. In the current times, documentation has moved to electronic media, and computers tend to be placed between the patient and the doctor. While this is inescapable, these machines should be unobtrusive and sidestep the "distance" between the patient and his doctor. Patients like to interact while narrating their stories and if the doctor is busy typing as they talk, a little disappointment can creep in. If time permits, information can be filled in after the consultation is over. In many situations in India, the arrangements for the consultation tend to be suboptimal, and the available time is short, affecting the output. Bridging strategies need to be individually evolved as per the limitations of the setups that individuals are working in.

SCHEME

- Let the patient tell his narrative and listen to it. The listening should be active, with expressions of interest, for it to be most informative.

  In the beginning, the patient is encouraged to describe his symptoms. Lots of variations can be encountered in the way patients narrate their symptoms. Some individuals can talk about their problem accurately and construct a logical sequence leading the doctor to the diagnosis. Some other patients fill in information and details which are unclear and do not focus on what they are suffering from. Patients have the desire to tell the doctor about the various medical opinions that they have been through and the variety of tests that have been carried out, before arriving for the present consultation. In the present times, many investigations are ordered to elucidate the patient's problem, and some patients think that the answer will come from these investigations; therefore, they want you to see the investigations first and then, if required, talk about their problem. Such patients need to be gently reoriented to the fact that listening to their problems is the first and the most important part of the consultation. Patients who have been searching the web have a certain disadvantage, as the reading can potentially influence their thinking process.

The abovementioned caveats make it necessary to interrupt some patients to inform them of what you are hoping to hear from them and direct talk to them about the unadulterated version of their problems. At this stage, the doctor can make notes about the facts what he thinks are important in the patient's narrative, which can be used later while constructing the diagnosis and marking the areas where he needs to subsequently get into, for clarifying some of the details.

In the initial stages of listening to the historical account, mental notes can also be made regarding the structure of the family, the important individuals who will need to be part of the discussion, and more importantly, the patient's reactions to what has been happening to him. This is significant in the total management of the patient, and we must remember that we are not only treating the disease but also a person having the disease.

A patient's "experience" of his illness is a completely different perspective from the medical perspective of the disease. While we as medical practitioners concentrate on systematically achieving the diagnosis and planning therapy, patients' perspective needs to be considered. History can potentially provide this information. For example, a patient who has suffered an adverse effect from a certain medication in the past will need a much longer discussion while prescribing the new medication at the end of the current consultation. Remember that it is the patient's perspective that you are aiming to improve, by working on the medical diagnosis.

- Patient's narrative may not be clear enough in some parts, and these will need clarification. As the patient is explaining his symptoms, such emerging areas can be noted down by the doctor and after the patient has finished speaking, these are taken up for analysis. Examples are words such as giddiness and heaviness. Patients use the word giddiness to imply a variety of sensations ranging from rotation to subjective imbalance and blackouts. Similarly, heaviness could mean weakness, fatigue, or various sensory phenomena. In India, there is a lot of regional diversity in the dialects and the way in which patients narrate their symptoms. Expressions like *"uper ka sans upper aur neeche ka sans neeche"* or *"pindlian phooti hai"* are specific to certain regions of the country and while working in a part of the country where the doctor has not resided previously, this can pose special challenges.
- Personal history and family history are best discussed after the initial interactions have set the tone and when rapport has been established. The patient is more likely to inform of the true extent of his addictions and sexual history only after a certain trust is perceived. Relatives' presence may be a deterrent, and privacy can be the key. Some patients may come back alone after the consultation to tell things that they could not tell earlier; same is the case with relatives, and the practitioner should keep space for these additional bits of time for information.

  Family history can be a sensitive part and needs to be handled tactfully. Many individuals are not comfortable with the fact that the disease can be genetic, particularly if they have been recently married or if they have young children to whom they could have passed on the condition. In cases of maternally transmitted diseases, the young mother may face an impediment in her new family. In India, the maternal side of history is not always provided, as that part of the family is considered separate. It is hence important to ask about both sides of the family while remembering that diseases coming from the maternal side can pose social issues, and maturity on part of the consultant goes a long way toward smooth interactions.

  Similarly, special care is necessary when there are functional and psychosomatic connotations to the situation. Doctors are likely to develop a dismissive approach to this realization. However, it pays to remember that these individuals are also suffering just like those having "organic" issues, and in fact, handing out a "cure" for the so-called nonorganic disorders is often more difficult.
- Some "direct" questions may have to be asked to demarcate the localization and the etiology. These can be divided into two sets: firstly, to get leads to the extent of the disease and secondly, to possible clues toward the pathophysiology. It is an often mentioned fact that examination tells you where the lesion would be and history tells you what the lesion is likely to be.
- Special points that need to be checked in various areas of neurological involvement are as follows. In cases of cognitive concerns, a relative who knows about the patient's problems and preferably lives with the patient, and the caregiver, should be interviewed. When the patient is a child, the mother's interview is often the most informative. In cases of extrapyramidal dysfunctions and peripheral neuropathies, it is important to check all the available prescriptions and tablets, as the offending agent may be discovered by this inquiry. The chronicity of a disease needs to be "dug out" by asking questions relating to activities in childhood, sports capabilities, early milestones, etc. In diseases that have pleomorphic manifestations, the family may not associate the bits and pieces and direct inquiry becomes necessary, e.g., cataracts, baldness, diabetes mellitus, infertility, and cardiac diseases in the family of a patient presenting with myotonic dystrophy.

HISTORY LEADS TO A TAILORED EXAMINATION

The neurological examination can be conducted in various ways. One approach is "take the history, keep it aside, and perform a complete neurological examination." In this approach, the neurological examination is performed as an independent task, in all its completeness. This approach can yield findings that have not emerged from history, e.g., unearthing a lateral popliteal nerve paresis in a patient with motor neuron disease. While desirable, this approach takes time. Another approach is to have the historical information with you, formulate a differential diagnosis, and conduct the examination in line with your thoughts. This approach runs the risk of confirmation and anchoring biases. A middle path would be a combination of the above two methods. Have your differential diagnosis from the history, and use the examination in an unbiased manner. The doctor can line out the areas that need special attention. For example, when history points to demyelinating myelopathy, more time can be spent on the examination of the visual system, or in the case of wrist drop, the manual muscle testing will need to be checked fully, along with the sensory system, to localize the lesion.

COGNITIVE BIAS IN HISTORY TAKING

Doctors are human and are open to a variety of biases. Each one of us is unique in his ways of thinking and reacting and so is every patient. Hence, the dynamics of each interaction are highly individualized and fluid. Some of the common biases experienced by doctors as they take histories are discussed below.

- *Confirmation and anchoring bias*: "I see what I want to see." The doctor is acting according to his beliefs and gathering information that supports his thinking on priority. After the first few pieces of information are given by the patient (the 18-second rule),[1] the doctor makes up his mind as to what he is likely to be dealing with and then takes charge of the questioning, asking and probing areas where the information supporting his diagnosis lies. He then clings to that information and makes light of the contrary information coming in the further course of discussion. The doctor, who is giving in to his belief and not considering contrary information, runs the risk of making an incorrect diagnosis. To counter this bias, one could make a habit of asking oneself why it could not be the diagnosis that initially came to his mind and would there be another diagnosis.
- *Affect heuristics*: This bias is based on the emotion-related aspects of the interaction during history taking, again a very individualized phenomenon on the part of the patient, the doctor, and the timing and circumstances of the consultation. The doctor's reactions and assessments are swayed by the emotional contents of the consultation rather than the facts being presented to the intellect. For example, a patient enters the room and declares, "doctor, I decided to see you because you are new and less busy, and I thought you will give me more time." This would immediately start a chain of negative emotions for the doctor, and the interview will not remain unbiased. It is indeed difficult to keep this bias aside and get an impartial evaluation.
- *Outcome bias*: Human intellect associates decisions with outcomes intuitively and logistically. This is likely to assume pessimistic or unduly optimistic judgments at the end of history. For example, features of motor neuron disease start the thoughts of the futility of the situation. It is important not to give in to this bias and to persist with best efforts to reduce the suffering of the ailing patient.

The following case studies make some useful points regarding the aspects of history taking.

CASE STUDIES

- A 57-year-old teacher came for the first consultation. As he sat down, he mentioned how difficult it was for him to get my appointment and how he had travelled and stayed in a hotel. He wanted to make the most of the consultation. We started off well with his account of the illness, and I began making my notes. After 15 minutes passed and he was determined to tell me about all the details of the previous consultations and the trivia associated with them, and he had a notepad full of events that he was keen to show and discuss. As he saw things, details could be important, and he should not skip any, so he had them all well compiled and insisted that I see each of the papers. He had been told that serum sodium was important for the causation of some of his symptoms, and hence he had taken it upon himself to get the electrolytes done every 15 days and had a chart of how his symptoms fluctuated with the serum sodium levels.

  This is a common situation in clinical practice. The patient does not know which points will be relevant to the doctor and hence chooses to recite all. This can make the consultation very lengthy. Also, the previous consultations make an impact on the doctor's thinking process and that can be an issue when discussing the relativity of these.

  In this patient, the information provided by his wife was very important as she discussed changes in his personality and habits. Cognitive testing showed features of the behavioral variant of frontotemporal dysfunction.
- A 27-year-old girl who lived in the United States of America came for a consultation while she was in India. After we went through the pleasantries, she started by telling me that she has multiple sclerosis and is on therapy for it, and has come to me to "go over things" and make suggestions if need be. Since I was seeing her for

the first time, I thought we should start with the history and build the situation afresh. She was reluctant as she was tired of telling the facts again and again and that she already had tests done, the diagnosis established, and was carrying the relevant documentary support. She said that her younger brother also did not like telling every new doctor about his condition and that he also had multiple sclerosis but was not improving. On further investigations of the brother and sister, a diagnosis of Krabbe disease was established.

When the patient begins with the diagnosis, he "corrupts" your thinking in a certain way and introduces a bias. It is important to be aware and circumvent it by adhering to the principles of history taking as mentioned previously in this chapter.

- A 36-year-old man working in the information technology (IT) sector saw me for the progressive weakness of limbs and recent difficulty in swallowing. He had been worked up by a neurologist, his serum creatine kinase (CK) was elevated, muscle membranes were irritable on electrophysiology, and the vastus lateralis muscle biopsy had shown inflammatory exudates and de- and regenerating fibers. A diagnosis of idiopathic inflammatory myopathy (IIM) seemed secure, and he had begun to improve after corticosteroids were used. He had a sheaf of papers downloaded from the Web and had multiple doubts and fears about the outlook, which had brought him to see me.

  In the present times, this situation is common. The patient accumulates information available to him on the Web. Such information can help the patient to understand his illness and the problems thereof. However, excess information and descriptions of unusual happenings can make the patient fearful. Some patients doubt whether the therapy given to them is appropriate, as there are various ways of treating a condition, and only one can be chosen by the patient and his doctor.

  It is important to understand the patient's mindset and his fears based on his new knowledge while going ahead with the history and the subsequent examination and discussions. In modern times, the real difference between the patient and his doctor is not "the uninformed and the informed," but that the patient is facing the situation for the first time, and the practitioner has guided many patients who have been in that position. The discussion around the point of having dealt with the situation many times before puts the patient at ease. In many ways, the doctor–patient relationship has evolved from "I will tell you what to do" to "I give you facts and help you find your preferences."[2]
- A 23-year-old man walked into my room with a severe gait ataxia and as he spoke, there was slurring of his speech and I noticed the head thrust due to slow eye movements. In my mind, the diagnostic process had moved on and I knew that I was dealing with spinocerebellar ataxia. I asked him whether anyone in the family had it and he mentioned that his brother, father, and grandfather had also been like this, but at later ages, the anticipation. I asked him to walk to the examination table and made sure of the slow eye movements and ataxia and found an absence of ankle jerks. I sat down to discuss the situation with him when he said, "Doctor, I know I have this condition and it is in the family, but today I have come for my headaches".

  I had made a mistake. We are tuned to the process of reaching the diagnosis and are looking for threads to reach there. In this case, the leads were obvious, and hence my mind focused on them quickly, ignoring the history taking. The diagnostic process is of course one of the aims, but what is worrying the patient supersedes it and this was an example to learn from. Many times, what bothers the patient may not be directly linked to the diagnosis and may go unaddressed.
- A 56-year-old lady was seen for visual disturbances for 2 months. When she looked at objects, they would jump. Clinical examination showed oscillopsia, the cause of which was not clear when she was sent to me. She had been investigated and a positron emission tomography–computed tomography (PET–CT) scan and magnetic resonance imaging (MRI) brain were normal, and the hematological parameters showed a mild rise of creatinine, at 1.9. Details of the medications revealed that she was taking lithium for many years. As she was taking it for a long time, and this symptom was new, she did not think that the two were related and did not mention it. The recent changes in renal functions probably led to this toxicity. Reducing the doses reduced the symptoms.

  This case underlines the importance of drug history in neurology, and examining the drug box is important. We cannot expect our patients to relate the symptoms to the medicines particularly when they are prescribed by different specialists. A common example is levosulpiride, given by the gastrointestinal (GI) doctor and showing its unwanted effects in the neurologist's review.
- A 33-year-old lady had taken an appointment to discuss her medical issues. As she and her husband sat down and the consultation began, she mentioned that she has Wilson's disease and is being treated for it. As is the practice, I told her to keep the medical details aside for the time being, and to tell me about the symptoms from the beginning. She described the tremors and gait changes and liver issues. Going over the medical reports and the doctor's notes, it was clear that she was being treated in a very good center and was receiving all the medical help that could be provided.

  So, I had to shift my line of discussion, and I asked her what made her arrange this consultation. Which answers was she seeking? She said, I do not think I have Wilson's disease but I may have Parkinson's disease. We then had a productive interaction about the differences in the tremors of the two diseases and the coexistence of symptoms. She had another question. If I stop tablets for a week or so, nothing happens, so are the tablets working? She had seen parkinsonian patients who miss a dose and know it.

Enquiring what made the patient arrange for the consultation oftentimes reveals the crux of the problem, particularly when certain medical attention has already been received, and focusing on this aspect can lead to a satisfactory outcome.

CONCLUSION

History taking is the initial and important part of achieving the diagnosis and arriving at a therapy plan. Taking a good history is an art, and practice and experience hone the skills over time. The more information exchanged between the patient and his doctor, the easier it gets to manage the ill health. This initial part of the interview process also goes a long way in building a trusting relationship toward easing the suffering.

REFERENCES

1. Groopman JE, Hartzband P. Your Medical Mind: How to Decide What is Right for You. London: Penguin Books; 2012.
2. Emanuel EJ, Emanuel LL. Four models of the physician–patient relationship. JAMA. 1992;267(16):2221-6.

2

CHAPTER

Testing the Cognition

Amit Halder, Ambar Chakravarty

INTRODUCTION: TESTING COGNITION THROUGH THE AGES

Physicians in the 17th and 18th centuries first observed the notable dissociations of mental faculties that were impaired while others remained intact in various brain disorders. Carl Wernicke (1848–1905), a German physician, anatomist, psychiatrist, and neuropathologist, first began to develop procedures for assessing more specific components of mental functioning in the mid-19th century. Konrad Rieger (1855–1939), a German psychiatrist, and Theodor Ziehen (1862–1950), a German neurologist, developed the first neuropsychological test batteries. Kurt Goldstein (1878–1965), a student of Wernicke and Edinger, laid more importance on the way patients performed with the test batteries rather than how much they scored. Alexander Luria (1902–1977), the Soviet neuropsychologist who was considered the father of modern clinical neuropsychology, developed an extensive and original battery of neuropsychological tests during his clinical work with brain-injured victims of World War II. Soon thereafter, Alfred Binet (1857–1911), a French psychologist and a pupil of Charcot, along with another psychologist Théodore Simon (1873–1971), developed the intelligence testing battery. Later this was transformed into the Army Alpha and Army Beta tests for selecting soldiers. However, the basics of this battery of tests are still being used by modern-day neuropsychologists for assessing intelligence. The 20th century witnessed the contributions of two great neuropsychologists: Shepherd Ivory Franz (1874–1933), an American psychologist favoring a clinical approach, and Ward Halstead (1908–1968), another American who stimulated a strongly psychometric-based approach. Henry Charlton Bastian (1837–1915), a Queen Square neurologist, formulated the first comprehensive language battery tests. While in the 19th and first half of 20th centuries neurologists and psychiatrists had to depend solely on autopsy studies for clinico-anatomical correlation of different domains of cognition, advancements in neuroimaging techniques in the latter part of the 20th century and early 21st century greatly enriched our knowledge in regard to structure–function correlation.

The myth has been propagated through generations of medical practitioners that the mental status of an individual cannot be evaluated at the bedside and needs extensive standardized neuropsychological testing. This notion is impractical as in the hospital ward or intensive care unit, the real-life situation is entirely different. The clinician is often faced with the challenging job of evaluating a patient who has suddenly become confused and/or agitated. Time is of the essence, and bedside testing is the only way forward. The clinician is faced with a plethora of questions. Is it delirium? Or, is it preexisting cognitive impairment that has got unmasked? Or, is it some new-onset neurological disease that is manifesting with altered mentation?

"Bedside cognitive testing" denotes a flexible, goal-oriented evaluation of mental function by the clinician that uses prepared test material or ad hoc devised tests (depending on the clinical situation).[1-3] Impaired cognition generally denotes a deficiency in knowledge, thought process, or judgment. Bedside cognitive testing can diagnose major cognitive impairment (i.e., dementia), diagnose mild cognitive impairment (MCI), evaluate overall brain functions in traumatic brain injuries, help determine the decision-making capacity of an individual (needed for assessment for fitness to continue in a responsible job), and make an approximation of any significant intellectual dysfunction.[4-7]

According to the Diagnostic and Statistical Manual of Mental Disorders, 5th edition (DSM-5) (2014, updated 2018),[8] major neurocognitive disorder requires demonstration of significant cognitive decline in at least one of the following cognitive domains: complex attention, executive function, language, learning and memory, perceptual–motor, and social cognition. Recognition of minor neurocognitive disorder requires only modest cognitive decline that does not interfere with instrumental activities of daily living. Most of the features mentioned above can be assessed with reasonable accuracy at the bedside using well-standardized methods, and only cases with doubtful and difficult-to-make decisions can be the candidates for detailed neuropsychological testing.

ANATOMICAL BASIS OF COGNITIVE DEFICITS

Localization is the key to the diagnosis of neurological disorders. In the field of cognition, there is a dichotomy. Some cognitive functions can be localized, others cannot. The term "distributed" is used to describe brain functions that cannot be strictly localized to one lateralized brain region **(Table 1)**. The three main domains of cognition that are distributed include arousal/attention, memory, and executive functions. Abnormalities of distributed brain function thus arise only in bilateral extensive lesions. A localized thalamic lesion may be an exception. Localized functions, on the other hand, can be divided into those associated with the dominant (usually, left) or nondominant hemisphere.[3] This is summarized in **Table 1**. Brain regions affected by different forms of cognitive dysfunctions are schematically shown in **Figures 1A and B**. Some detailing of the anatomical basis of the different domains of cognition would be made later in this chapter.

TABLE 1: Localizations of cognitive functions.

Cognitive function	Probable localization
Arousal/attention/ concentration	Reticular activating system (RAS) and thalamic projections along with multimodal association areas (prefrontal and parietal) with right hemispheric bias
Memory	Limbic system (hippocampus and diencephalon)
Complex executive functions	Frontal lobes

Source: Adapted with modifications from Hodges (2018).[3]

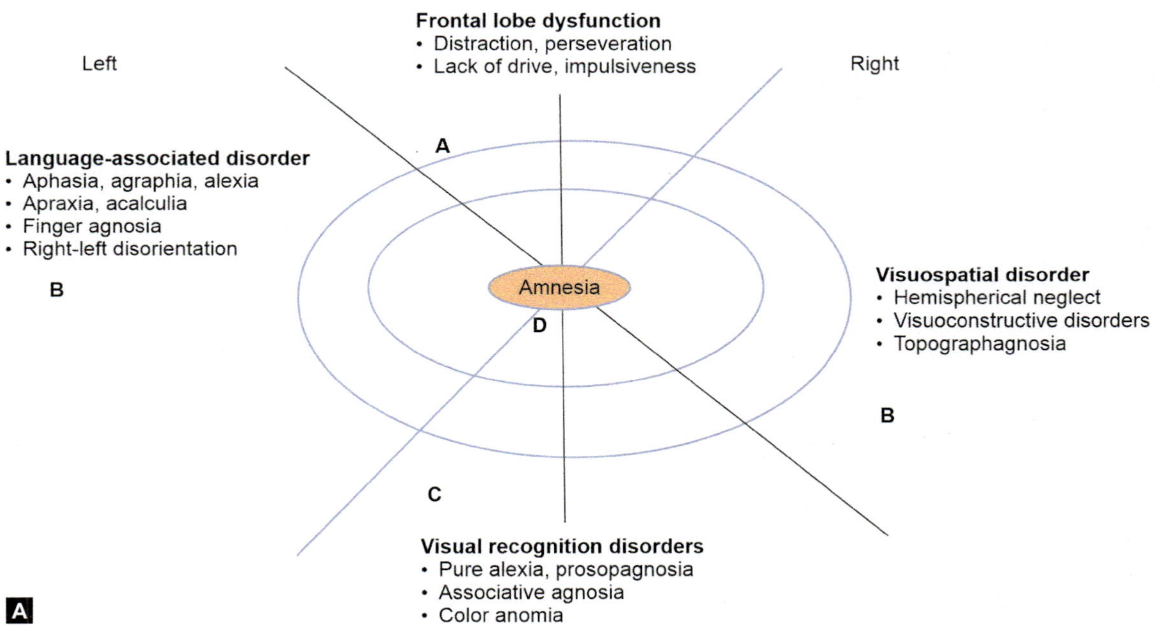

A

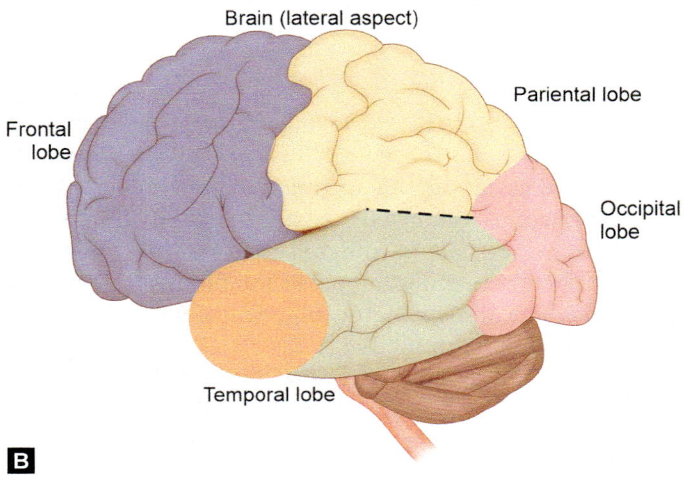

B

FIGS. 1A AND B: (A) Schematic representations of brain regions affected by different cognitive dysfunctions. *Index*: (a) Frontal lobe (blue as in **Fig. 1B**); (b) Parietal lobe (yellow as in **Fig. 1B**) and posterior temporal lobe (green as in **Fig. 1B**); (c) Occipital lobe (pink as in **Fig. 1B**); (d) Anterior temporal lobe (brown as in **Fig. 1B**). (B) Lobes of the brain (to be correlated with the index).

TESTING PROCESS

The classical scheme of history, observation, and examination is the key. The purpose of the clinical evaluation needs to be chalked out at the outset. Firstly, the presence or absence of well-defined behavioral/cognitive changes indicative of organic brain disease needs to be established. This has to be correlated with the patient's preexisting level of functioning. Knowing the educational and occupational status of the individual helps in this process. The possibility of adjustment disorder or functional psychiatric disorder needs to be looked into. The patient's general medical condition needs to be carefully ascertained. Endocrine diseases, hepatic or renal failure, alcohol or drug abuse, and systemic infection can all present with altered mental status.[2]

History

A detailed history relating to the presenting problem is of utmost importance. If the patient is unable to give a proper history, information should be obtained from an informant who stays with the patient. If both the patient and the informant are present, it is advisable to talk to the patient alone for some time. This may help the patient to reveal confidential information relevant to the illness to the examiner.

History taking is important as it helps in finding the precise complaints of the patient. Secondly, it helps in assessing the severity of the disorder and its impact on the patient's life. A person coming with a "memory complaint" and having difficulty in remembering names does not have the same severity of the illness as someone who has lost his way home. Thirdly, the premorbid cognitive abilities can be assessed from history. Lastly, the ease and precision of the patient's response can give the examiner an idea about the patient's language and memory functions. Behavioral abnormalities are sometimes more evident during history taking. A common but often overlooked entity is the " head-turning sign." Here, the patient looks to his accomplice for help when asked questions; this may be a useful sign in identifying a patient with major cognitive dysfunction.[3] The examiner must be capable of adjusting the examination process based on observations made during the elicitation of history.

Following pieces of information need to be obtained: (1) onset of the condition (insidious or acute), (2) presenting symptom, (3) course of the condition (gradually progressive, stepwise, fluctuating, or improving), and (4) duration of the symptoms.[2,3]

The establishment of rapport with the patient is the initial step. A few nonconfrontational questions about the patient's background including his/her hobbies and interests may go a long way in putting the patient at ease. If the patient is unable to engage in sensible conversation to answer coherently, the role of the informant becomes more important. The reason for referral to the clinic or admission to the hospital needs to be ascertained. Often, a cognitively impaired patient may not be able to provide correct answers.

Open-ended questions are preferred to obtain an unbiased narrative reply. The colloquial "phrases" used by the patient to describe his/her problems should be noted *ad verbatim* rather than using medical terms. A description of the principal symptoms along with their duration and progression is obtained. Alongside, questions need to be asked about any alteration or disturbance (unusual/inappropriate behavioral pattern). One should specifically ask for any history of poor judgment, difficulty in concentration, or language functions (not articulatory but inappropriate). Memory problems, history of losing way (even indoors), or trouble in carrying out activities of daily living (e.g., cooking or driving) may give important clues about the underlying domains affected.

The term "memory difficulty" used by the patient or the relatives may have various connotations—it may be the inability to concentrate while reading a book; it may be the inability to follow the conversation; there may be the inability to remember why they entered a room or also, remembering the proper sequence of mixing up ingredients during cooking. These are all examples of the inability to learn/retain new information.

Specific history for any psychiatric disorder such as depression, anxiety, or schizophrenia needs to be obtained. Any symptoms of delusion or hallucination must be recorded. Past medical history including any history of infection, head injury, stroke, or epilepsy may point to a possible underlying etiology for the cognitive decline. A history of intake of drugs or alcohol or exposure to toxins should not be missed (e.g., lead poisoning). A detailed birth and developmental history should be taken to account for any preexisting cognitive deficits. Educational history and academic records may corroborate this.

History is not complete without a detailed family history of neurological disorders or mental illness. For example, a family history of suicide may point to underlying Huntington's disease. Lastly, the dietetic history and sexual behavior need exploration (vitamin B12 deficiency and sexually transmitted diseases causing neurocognitive problems are not very uncommon).

Observing the Behavior

During the process of history taking, the general behavior of the patient should be observed. This can provide important clues regarding an organic or functional disorder. Several neurobehavioral syndromes (e.g., delirium and frontal lobe syndrome) can be diagnosed primarily based on their behavioral manifestations. Frontal lobe disinhibition may lead to a person being inappropriately jocular or making obscene comments. A delirious patient, on the other hand, can be noisy, restless, and easily distractible. This problem may also interfere with subsequent formal testing of specific domains such as memory.[4] Delirium (as defined in the DSM-5) is an acute and fluctuating neurological disorder that reflects a change from baseline cognition and is characterized by the cardinal features of inattention and disorganized thinking.[8] Several factors may predispose an elderly subject to develop this state. These include acute medical comorbidities (e.g., heart failure), disturbed sleep, sensory impairment, hospital isolation, lack of exposure to daylight, infections, drug/alcohol withdrawal, dehydration, blood loss, dyselectrolytemia, acid–base abnormalities, desaturation/hypoxemia, pyrexia, seizures, and endocrinologic dysfunction. A close lookout for these would be warranted. Observation of the general physical appearance of the subject is equally important. Unilateral neglect, both for body part and visual field, can be ascertained with ease at the bedside, and this can be confirmed later during physical examination. This would be of significant localizing value. Improper attire and lack of cleanliness suggest a lack of self-care and may be observed in both demented and severely depressed subjects.

The observed behavior of a subject in a specified situation is closely linked to the underlying emotion generated internally. While emotional responses are mostly generated in deep cortical and subcortical structures (hippocampus, amygdala, hypothalamus, and multiple regions in the brainstem), the final expression of the emotional response is largely modified by the prefrontal cortices. And here comes the role of inhibitory functions of the frontal lobes.

Anatomical Basis of Memory and Emotion

There exists an extensive network of regions in the frontal and temporal lobes involved in emotional and social processing. The well-known Papez circuit **(Fig. 2)** plays an important role.[9] The circuit involves such structures as the hippocampus, its efferent pathway through the fimbriae, posterior columns of the fornix, body of the fornix, and finally the anterior columns of the fornix, terminating in the mammillary bodies. The latter structures are connected to the anterior nucleus of the thalamus, which in turn project to the prefrontal and anterior cingulate cortices. Apart from generating emotional responses, many of the aforementioned structures are involved in the preservation of memory as well. Emotional responses to specified situations are indeed often governed by the memory of past experiences.

The inhibitory functions of the frontal lobes are often needed in the proper execution of our day-to-day activities as well as in determining our social responses. In daily life, it is sometimes necessary to suppress the impulse to perform certain tasks to reach our goals. The terms "utilization behavior" and "environmental dependency" were used by Lhermitte to describe the impaired inhibition seen in the daily activities of patients with frontal lobe injury.[10] Such patients lose the ability to inhibit motor programs (e.g., when given an empty cup, starts drinking from it), as the drive/desire to use an object overrides any logic whether such action is appropriate or not. Environmental dependency, on the other hand, relates to the tendency to passively follow the cues and gestures of others, even though that would not be socially appropriate (e.g., holding and shaking a guest's hand when the latter had only moved his hand to scratch his/her face). All these can be detected at the bedside in patients with frontal lobar lesions, with close observation, and also can be noted during detailed history elicitation.

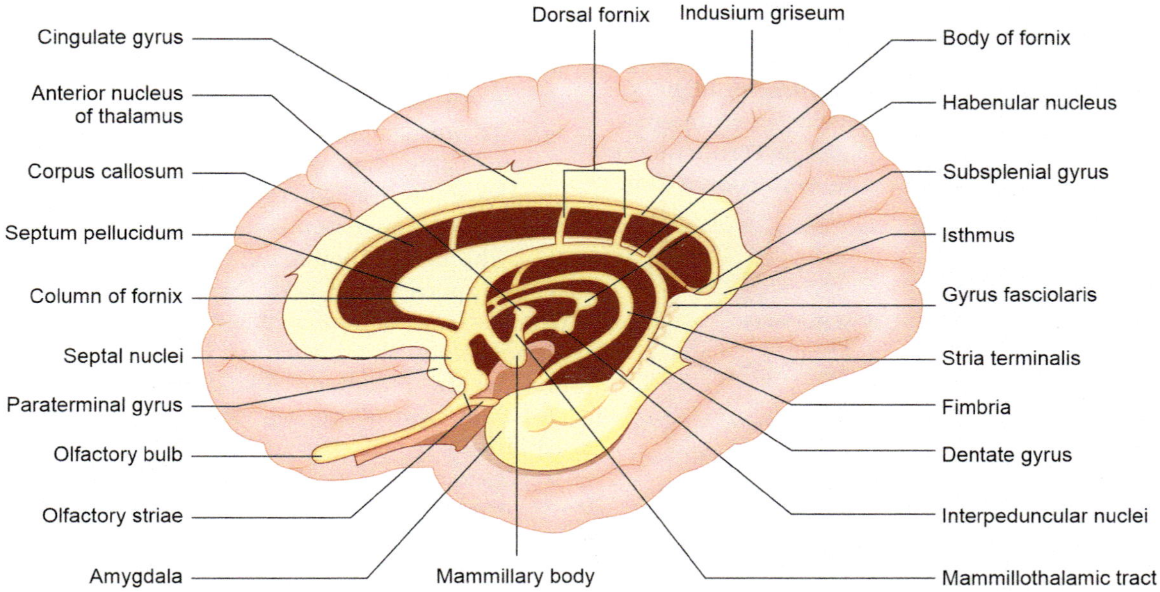

FIG. 2: The components of the Papez circuit and limbic system.

Physical Examination

Examination usually begins by testing the patient's alertness. Descriptive common-sense terms such as wakeful and cooperative are preferred to vague medical jargon such as stupor. A summary of the key deficits that can be elicited by testing the brain functions along with their localization are summarized in **Figures 1A and B**.

Testing Attention

Testing attention includes digit span, serial subtraction of sevens, and spelling familiar words backward. The problem with serial sevens is that the elderly and patients with left hemispheric dysfunction may not be able to perform the test even with intact attention.[11] The mini-mental state examination (MMSE) and Addenbrooke cognitive examination (ACE3)[12] have thus used spelling the word "WORLD" backward for those who are unable to perform the serial seven subtraction.[11] Ability to recite the months in a year backward is also a good test of sustained attention.

The normal digit span is 6 (±1). Reverse digit span is also an accurate measure of attention. It is usually one less than the forward digit span.[2,3] This depends on working memory, which is determined by frontal executive function and phonological processes. Subjects with predominant amnesic disorders such as Alzheimer's disease and Korsakoff's syndrome may have preserved digit span.

Orientation

Orientation is usually described in relation to time and place. This can be done practically as shown in **Table 2**. Date orientation is the least reliable test. Some clinicians would consider a date range of (±) 2 of the actual date to be a normal response. Hospital-admitted patients often do not have any clue as to the date (and often the time of the day); one needs to specifically ask for how long the patient has been admitted and whether it is daytime or night. The latter may be impossible for some staying in an intensive care ward with continuous artificial lighting. Disorientation in time is more prominent in acute confusional states (e.g., delirium) due to metabolic causes or diffuse brain injury. This may not be prominent in subjects with early dementia. Orientation to place is a less sensitive test of cognition than orientation to time.[13]

Even subjects with advanced dementia or acute confusional state are usually able to tell his or her name correctly. If a patient is unable to do that, the possibility of psychogenic amnesia needs to be considered. Subjects with motor aphasia may also be unable to utter their names, but can choose the right name if given options. Comprehension needs to be reasonably intact to understand the meaning of the question asked.

TABLE 2: Testing orientation.

Orientation	Time	Day of the week
		Date
		Month
		Season
		Year
	Place	Building
		Floor
		Town
		County/state (as applicable)
		Country

MEMORY

Memory can be divided into two main types: implicit or procedural memory and explicit or declarative memory. Explicit memory is again divided into two parts: episodic memory and semantic memory.[1]

Episodic memory is responsible for laying down of personally experienced and temporally specific events. Semantic memory, on the other hand, acts as a storehouse of facts and meanings about objects, concepts, and people.

Episodic memory can again be subdivided into anterograde and retrograde. Anterograde memory deals with the ability to learn new information while retrograde memory deals with the ability to recall old information.

The principal brain structures needed for the retention of episodic memory include the hippocampus (along with the subiculum), entorhinal cortex part of the parahippocampal gyrus, mammillary bodies, and thalamus.[14] Two major neural tracts, namely the septohippocampal and the mammillothalamic tracts, are needed for the maintenance of episodic memory. The former, a major cholinergic projection arising from the septal nuclei in the septum pellucidum, travels through the fornix and reaches the hippocampus and the entorhinal cortex in the parahippocampal cortex. The mammillothalamic tract is a part of the Papez circuit, and its course and projections have been discussed earlier in this chapter. The anterior cingulum, receiving the projection from the mammillothalamic tract, projects back to the hippocampus through anatomical continuity. Thus, the mammillothalamic system is connected to the septohippocampal tract. This intricate interconnecting pathway is needed for spatial processing controlled by the hippocampus. This organ can thus associate "what," "when," and "where" together.[15] Also, the limbic system links the pathways controlling memory functions and emotional expressions, which thus are interdependent.

A lesion anywhere along the septohippocampal pathway would lead to a severe loss of episodic memory. Such subjects would have anterograde amnesia with the inability to retain/memorize any new information. Memories that were established before (remote memories) would be relatively preserved. However, retrograde amnesia, going as far back as years, may be present. The extent of this retrograde memory loss would be dependent on the size of the lesion; with the healing of the lesion, the degree of memory loss tends to lessen. The most common cause of entorhinal cortical dysfunction is Alzheimer's disease; the entorhinal pathology subsequently involves the hippocampus. Hippocampal injury can also be caused by trauma, stroke, and encephalitis, commonly herpes simplex infection. Classical injury to the mammillary bodies leads to Korsakoff's syndrome, and a stroke involving the dorsomedial nucleus of the thalamus can cause severe amnesia.

Testing Anterograde Memory

Anterograde memory can be verbal or nonverbal.

There are formal and nonformal tests of anterograde verbal memory. Nonformal tests include asking the patient how he came to the hospital or what he had seen on television the previous weekend.

In ACE-3, the patient is asked to repeat seven-part name and address. This is repeated thrice, even if the response is correct on the first occasion. After a gap of about 10 minutes, when the rest of the test is completed, the patient is asked to recall the same name and address. A completely correct response virtually rules out a major amnesic deficit. Intermediate results are more difficult to judge. Recognition of the components that they have failed to recall will indicate anxiety, depression, or frontal lobe retrieval problems.[12]

Story recall and wordlist learning tasks can be employed for formal assessment. These are usually derived from the Wechsler memory scale.[16] The 15-item Rey auditory verbal learning test is frequently employed.[17] It consists of five learning trials of list A followed by an interfering list B. This is followed by a recall of list A and again after 20 minutes a delayed recall of list A.

Verbal memory relies disproportionately on the left (or dominant) hippocampus. With dominant side hippocampal lesions, the ability to learn new vocabulary is lost. Additionally, as much of day-to-day new learning requires intact verbal memory, it is not uncommon for such subjects to forget the time or place of appointments, the names of friends, or the content of the previous conversation. Dominant (mostly left) hippocampal lesions and dorsomedial thalamic lesions lead to more severe amnesia than damage to the other side.[18] Interestingly, damage to the right hippocampus seems to have a greater impact on memory for visual and spatial information than for verbal ones.

Anterograde Nonverbal Memory

The decline in nonverbal memory usually parallels the decline in verbal memory except in cases where there is selective damage to the nondominant medial temporal lobe (MTL). Unfortunately, there are no good bedside tests for nonverbal memory. Spatial learning can be tested by walking a route around the ward or clinic with the patient and then asking him/her to retrace the part. Tests of face memory using nonfamous face photographs from various magazines can also be employed.

A formal paired associate learning (PAL) from a computerized Cambridge neuropsychological test automated battery (CANTAB) and recognition memory test can be used.[19,20]

Retrograde Memory

Systematic questioning about past events from the preceding months, years, or decades can give a holistic picture. It must be correlated according to the patient's baseline performance. It is better to start with open-ended questions and then go to the details. A temporal gradient for retrograde memory loss may be present. They may be better for events of the distant past than for those of the recent past. This is known as Ribot's law of retrograde amnesia.[21,22] In Alzheimer's disease or Korsakoff's syndrome, memory loss is more extensive than in pure hippocampal damage.

Autobiographical or personal memory can be tested by asking the patient to sequence correctly and chronologically some specific events of his/her personal life, e.g., educational career or professional career.[23]

Semantic Memory

Semantic memory involves multiple domains of cognition. Hence, there is no single test. It may be both verbal and nonverbal. The common examples include:

- Category fluency (e.g., animals and fruits) is very sensitive, but is affected by executive functions.
- Naming pictures
- Tests of verbal knowledge
- Picture pointing in response to spoken name

Confrontation naming detects/semantic defects: Word-finding capacity and visual processing need to be intact for reliable testing.[24]

With semantic memory loss, the individual usually has no recollection of when or where the information was acquired. For example, when a subject is asked how many days are present in a month, most people would respond spontaneously with the answer "30 or 31." Retaining the knowledge that "30/31" days are present in a month is possible because the brain holds a complex set of constructs that include an abstract awareness of what a day represents, and how many of these abstract units of time are present in another abstract time concept, namely the month. The semantic memory system is capable of holding these ideas together. This system works independently of the septohippocampal and mammillothalamic memory systems (discussed earlier) and likely involves the anterior and lateral temporal lobes. Patients with MTL injury usually maintain their access to semantic knowledge, while patients with primarily anterior and lateral temporal lobe damage show intact episodic memory but impaired semantic memory.[25-27] In semantic dementia (a subtype of frontotemporal dementia) both simply naming an object and later knowledge about the identity of people and objects are lost. Such patients would tend to classify objects into increasingly superordinate categories (e.g., calling a "parrot" as just a "bird," and later with disease progression that "bird" becomes just an animal). It has been suggested that the hippocampus can store semantic memories for approximately 2 years and after that, these memories are transferred to the left temporal neocortex.[28] Hence, patients with semantic dementia can often remember current events as their hippocampi are spared, but they would reveal profound loss of remote memory, as their temporal neocortices are degenerated and dysfunctional. While bilateral (though at times asymmetrically) temporal lobar degeneration is a characteristic feature of semantic dementia, such a situation can also occur following herpes zoster encephalitis.

Working Memory

Working memory may be considered a form of episodic memory "that allowed the individual to hold and manipulate information for short periods: from seconds to minutes."[29] A simple way to test this would be to call an operator and ask for a telephone number. Working memory is needed to remember these numbers while they are being dialed into the telephone. Functional magnetic resonance imaging (fMRI) studies have shown that the dorsolateral frontal lobes, particularly Brodmann area 46, are critical for working memory. Working memory deficit may hamper the learning process in a subject and may affect daily life activities. Subjects with classic amnesic syndrome possess intact working memory but are unable to transfer information from working memory into a long-term store.[30,31]

FRONTAL EXECUTIVE FUNCTIONS

The frontal lobe is subdivided into several structurally and functionally specific regions for carrying out several important functions. These include motor planning, language, intelligence, working memory, generation/initiation of movements, inhibition of inappropriate social behavior, attention, abstraction, sequencing alternate tasks, drive, emotional expression, self-awareness, insight, and personality. All these functions (often grouped as frontal executive functions) are of higher order or executive processes that involve the organization of more basic cerebral processes to promote efficient and flawless task performance.[32,33] Current research casts some doubt about the sole role of the frontal cortex in executive memory functions as (1) executive processes involve links between different brain areas, not exclusively with the frontal cortex, (2) patients with no evidence of frontal damage present with executive deficits, and (3) patients with frontal lesions do not always show executive deficits. It is felt that it is time for a more dynamic and flexible view of the neural substrate of executive processes to be considered.[34]

History and observance of the patient's behavior may be more important than formal testing in assessing the executive functions. Nevertheless, there are several tests that can be useful for confirming the clinical impression. These include:

- Initiation
- Abstraction
- Problem-solving and decision-making
- Response inhibition and set-shifting

Initiation

Verbal fluency tests can range from words beginning with a particular letter (e.g., F, A, and S) to those from a common semantic category (e.g., fruits and animals). They depend on the coordinated functions of the frontal and temporal lobes. The patient is asked to generate as many words as possible in 1 minute, excluding proper nouns starting with the letters FAS. Normal young subjects should produce at least 15 words for each letter. A total of FAS of <30 words is abnormal. Patients with frontal lobe dysfunction, e.g., due to frontotemporal degeneration, produce few words and make rule breaks. Amnesic patients tend to repeat the same words several times in category fluency tests. The test is also a sensitive test for detecting speech disorders (discussed in detail elsewhere in this volume).[35,36]

In the category fluency test, subjects are asked to generate as many words as possible from semantic categories such as animals, fruits, and vegetables. 10 or below is usually considered abnormal.

It should be borne in mind that these tests are dependent on the age and baseline intellect of the subject.

Nonverbal drive and flexibility can be explored with the five-point test[37] in which subjects are asked to produce within 3 minutes simple designs by combining two-to-five points in a fixed array of five points. Normal subjects can produce at least 20 designs in 3 minutes. This is a sensitive test of right frontal dysfunction.

Abstraction: Proverbs, Similarities, and Cognitive Estimates

An idea about abstraction can be gained by proverb interpretation and similarities test. Subjects who lose this ability often have acquired frontal lobe lesions. Participation of multiple brain regions is needed in the process of abstraction, but the final pathway probably requires the proper functioning of the frontal lobes.

Test of Proverb Interpretation

While interpreting such common proverbs as *"a rolling stone gathers no moss,"* concrete interpretation with an inability to use analogies is a salient feature of patients with frontal lobe dysfunction. Again, this test is dependent on the educational and cultural backgrounds of the patient and is often language specific. Alternatives in regional languages need to be formulated beforehand.

Test of Similarities

Here subjects are asked in which way conceptually linked items are alike, for example, table and chair, apple and banana, and like that. Patients with frontal lobe dysfunction and dementia often fail to make proper associations or make wrong associations.

Cognitive Estimates Test

Here a subject is asked a range of questions that require common-sense judgment to answer correctly, e.g., *"what is the average height of a man?"* This would assess the subject's ability to conceptualize.

Response Inhibition and Set-shifting

These tests are designed to check a subject's ability to shift from one cognitive set to another and his/her ability to inhibit/suppress inappropriate responses.

Wisconsin Card Sorting Test

Wisconsin card sorting test is a formal test of set-shifting and also involves problem-solving and hypothesis testing.[38] The test involves sorting out cards containing geometric forms, which differ in number, shape, and color. After the correct sorting dimension asked for is made, subjects are required to shift to another dimension. Patients with frontal lobe impairment are unable to shift from one dimension to another. They make errors in way of repetitions. This phenomenon is called perseveration.

Go-no-go Test

Go-no-go test is also a test of response inhibition (impulsivity) and may be impaired in subjects with frontal lobe dysfunction.[39] Subjects respond to certain stimuli ("go" stimuli) and make no response for others ("no-go" stimuli). The examiner assesses the commission error rate (making a "go" response wrongly on a "no-go" task stimulus); fewer errors signify better response inhibition, signifying intact frontal inhibitory functions.

Trail-making Test

Trail-making test is a good measure of mental speed, attention shifting, and response inhibition.[40] Age and education can influence performance. There are two parts. In the first part, the patient is asked to draw a line connecting randomly arranged numbers in numerical sequence. In the second part, the numbers are intermixed with letters, and the subject is asked to connect the numbers and alphabets in an alternating sequence.

Motor Sequencing: The Luria Three-step Test and the Alternating Hand Movements Test

In Luria's three-step test, the examiner demonstrates a series of hand movements—fist, edge, palm—in sequence, five times without any verbal clues.[41] The subject is then asked to repeat the same series. Patients with frontal lobe dysfunction are unable to do the sequence correctly (even with verbal clues).[42] In the alternating hand movements test, the examiner again demonstrates a series of hand movements and asks the subject to repeat them.

Social Disinhibition and Changes in Emotional Reactivity

Good social behavior includes maintaining good judgment and honesty, understanding one's appropriate place in society, and shaping and modifying one's behavior and manners as required from time to time in response to social cues/needs.

Subjects with lesions in the orbitofrontal cortex (resulting from tumors, head trauma, anterior communicating artery aneurysms, and frontotemporal dementia) often present with selective deficits in social behavior (inappropriate behavior) but have relative sparing of drive and other neuropsychological functions.[43] The term "pseudopsychopathic personality disorder" had been used to describe such behavioral changes.[44] While these patients are socially disinhibited, inappropriately friendly, unreliable, and in constant trouble, they would rarely exhibit the systematic cruelty, or the careful planning of crimes, as noted in true psychopaths. These subjects have been noted to exhibit remorse, on occasions, after exhibiting some inappropriate social behavior.

Mood disorders such as depression and mania are often noted in subjects with lesions of the prefrontal cortex. Depression may be more common with left rather than right frontal lobe lesions.[45] Manic syndromes, on the other hand, are more likely to occur with right frontal pathologies. Frontal lobar dysfunction may lead to a lower threshold for crying, and occasionally for laughing (pseudobulbar affect).

The right hemisphere plays an important role in emotional processing, and hence subjects with right hemispheric pathology are at times emotionally flat, and exhibit difficulty in expressing the normal emotional signals in the voice with variations in pitch, speed, and loudness, designated as aprosody and amelody.[46] Although such subjects are emotionally flat, they would rarely complain of feeling depressed; the emotional blunting may make a true assessment of the affective disorder in these patients.

There cannot be any specific test to quantify the disinhibitory and emotional aberrations in patients with frontal lobar lesions; careful observation of patients' behavior during history elucidation and physical examination is essential to gauge the patient's mental and emotional status.

LOCALIZATION-RELATED CEREBRAL FUNCTIONS

The second part of cognitive assessment addresses the localizable functions of the cerebral cortex. Specific cognitive functions are divided by their localization in the dominant (usually left) and the nondominant (usually right) hemispheres. In almost 90% of people, the left hemisphere is the dominant hemisphere and houses the language functions.

Dominant Hemisphere Functions

The dominant hemisphere functions that are tested include speech and language, calculation, and praxis.

Language

Aphasia/dysphasia is defined as an impairment of language function caused by brain damage. This needs to be differentiated from dysarthria or anarthria, which are articulatory disorders without any affection of language. Since speech/language disorders would be discussed separately in this volume, only brief mention would be made of the neuroanatomical basis, classification, and bedside testing modalities.

Since the times of Paul Broca and Carl Wernicke,[47,48] it has been recognized that most aphasias occur with left hemispheric, particularly perisylvian, lesions. Broca's aphasia is characterized by the presence of nonfluent speech, phonemic paraphasias, and relatively intact language comprehension. Classically, this syndrome is associated with a lesion in the posterior portion of the left inferior frontal gyrus. On the other hand, lesions affecting the left parietal/posterior temporal region are associated with fluent, "gibberish" speech, comprehension difficulties, and semantic paraphasias. These are constituents of Wernicke's aphasia. A milder syndrome of relatively isolated anomia can occur as a result of any left-hemisphere lesion. Many aphasic patients evolve from a severe aphasic syndrome developing soon after the onset of the brain lesion to anomic aphasia on recovery. Global aphasia, where there is a complete inability to understand or produce language, results from large perisylvian lesions in the dominant hemisphere. In classical Broca's or Wernicke's aphasias, the ability to repeat words is impaired as much as the inability to speak spontaneously. A combination of features, such as speech pattern (fluent or nonfluent), word usage, comprehension, and repetition abilities, have been used to describe different aphasic syndromes with specific anatomical localizations.

The following language functions are commonly performed at the bedside: spontaneous speech, naming, comprehension, repetition, reading, and writing. While detailed testing procedures would be discussed elsewhere in this volume, based on the results obtained, speech disorders can be classified as follows:

- *Broca's aphasia*: Nonfluent speech, impaired naming, impaired repetition, intact comprehension
- *Wernicke's aphasia*: Fluent aphasia, intact naming, impaired repetition, impaired comprehension
- *Conduction aphasia*: Fluent speech, intact naming, impaired repetition, intact comprehension
- *Transcortical motor aphasia*: Nonfluent speech, impaired naming, intact repetition, intact comprehension
- *Transcortical sensory aphasia*: Fluent speech, intact naming, intact repetition, impaired comprehension (except auditory)
- *Global aphasia*: Nonfluent speech/mute, impaired naming, impaired repetition, impaired comprehension

Lesion localization of conduction aphasia is in the superior temporal lobe but without any significant damage to Wernicke's area, or it may involve the inferior parietal region. Conduction aphasia may be considered to be a form of "disconnection syndrome" wherein a lesion interrupting the arcuate fasciculus, connecting the anterior temporal lobe to the inferior frontal region, occurs. The site of lesion in transcortical motor aphasia may be anterior to Broca's area buried deep in the white matter; localization of transcortical sensory aphasia may also be close to Wernicke's area.[49]

Calculation

Calculation is tested if there are suggestions from the history of a suspected dementing illness, or if the patient is aphasic. The following sequence may be followed:

1. *Number reading and writing*:
   a. Subject is asked to read and write from a series of simple and complex numbers written by the examiner.
   b. Then the subject is asked to write numbers to dictation.
   c. If there are errors in the first two steps, copying the numbers and pointing to the numbers on command can also be done.
2. *Arithmetic operations*: After the basic reading and writing of numbers, the subject should be tested for basic arithmetic operations: addition, subtraction, multiplication, and division. This is followed by written calculations. At the bedside, often the serial subtraction ("100 - 7") test usually suffices, and this also tests the patient's ability for sustained attention.

Disorders of Calculation

Acalculia is a disturbance in the ability to comprehend or write numbers properly. It is common in patients with aphasia. Lesion localization is usually in the angular gyrus of the left hemisphere.[49] Some aphasic patients can perform calculations mentally and perform well with multiple choice answers.

Anarithmetria is characterized by the inability to perform numerical manipulations. These individuals can recognize and correctly reproduce numbers, but cannot perform simple arithmetic calculations (mental arithmetic).[50] This is common in patients with dementia like Alzheimer's disease. An occasional patient with an isolated left parietal lesion may have impaired calculating skills without producing any language disorder. This is the true syndrome of anarithmetria or loss of the concept of numbers. On the other hand, some patients with severe aphasia can play cards and look at business ledgers and accounting sheets.[50,51]

Spatial dyscalculia is a disorder of performing written calculations. These patients have difficulty aligning columns of figures and performing carrying tasks. They usually have right hemispherical damage and exhibit the phenomenon of neglect.

Gerstmann's syndrome is characterized by a constellation of clinical features that include:
- Agraphia
- Acalculia
- *Right-left disorientation*: Disorder in demonstrating the correct hand or body part on command
- *Finger agnosia*: Inability to name the fingers or point to/ move a finger when its name is given

The anatomical localization for this syndrome is in the angular gyrus. It is also known as the *angular gyrus syndrome*. In practice, often the full tetrad of Gerstmann's syndrome may not be obvious.[52,53] While the presence of at least three of the four features may suffice for an eponymous diagnosis, it is not uncommon to find additional features such as anomia, alexia, constructional apraxia, mild fluent dysphasia, and visual field defects. Some authorities would call the association of additional features the "angular gyrus syndrome" making a difference from classical Gerstmann's syndrome. The angular gyrus region, now designated as "heteromodal association cortices," coordinates information transfers among different sensory modalities.[49]

Apraxia: It is defined as "the inability to perform a skilled motor activity that is not explicable based on problems with basic motor function due to weakness, sensory loss, tremor, chorea, or other movement disorders, or due to deficits in attention, memory, or motivation."[54] The most common form is "ideomotor apraxia," where patients fail to perform skilled movements such as the use of a knife, toothbrush, or scissors, or learned limb movements not requiring the use of an object, such as waving goodbye or making the "OK," or "victory" sign, though it may be observed that they can perform these actions spontaneously. The other types of apraxia include limb kinetic apraxia, ideational apraxia (which needs differentiation from ideomotor apraxia; in the former, patients lack the very concept of using an object), constructional apraxia, dressing apraxia, and orobuccal apraxia.

Apraxia almost always results from a left hemispheric lesion, especially involving the left frontal or parietal lobe.[55,56] Corpus callosum lesions may cause apraxia limited to the left arm only. Loss of communication between the two hemispheres may be a cause.[57] It is possible that lesioning anywhere in the motor system in the dominant hemisphere may cause problems with skillful activities. Apraxia with the use of either limb can occur with lesions in the frontal lobar dorsomedial part, where complex motor movements are coordinated.[58]

Detailed discussion on apraxias would be made elsewhere in this volume.

Detection of Right (Nondominant) Hemispheric Lesions

Deficits produced by damage to the right hemisphere are more subtle and hence tougher to detect at the bedside. Close observation of the patient's behavior and movements is needed during elicitation of history and general physical examination. The following features may be noted.

Neglect

Neglect is a term used to describe deficits in spatially designed attention. It can again be of various types:
- Personal neglect
- Motor and sensory neglect
- Extrapersonal neglect

Personal Neglect

Some patients with left hemiplegia (right or nondominant hemispherical lesion) may not realize that they are paralyzed on one side and deny their deficit. There is a hierarchy in this denial.

Firstly, they may deny the existence of one side (the paretic side), along with somatic delusions.

Secondly, they accept the existence of the paretic side but refute the presence of hemiparesis. This is defined by the term *anosognosia*.

Thirdly, they accept they are hemiparetic, but underplay its severity and resultant disability *(anosodiaphoria)*.

Personal neglect may be evident in appearance when the patient fails to groom or shave one side.

Sensory Neglect

Persons with sensory neglect consistently ignore sensory inputs from the side contralateral to the side of their brain lesion. Commonly, there is left hemineglect as the causative lesion is generally on the nondominant right side. Neglect is particularly evident about the visual field; the subject ignores a person standing on the left side or fails to eat food lying on the left side of the plate. While drawing a clock face, the patient fails to put the numbers on the left side, and puts all numbers on the right **(Fig. 3)**. It is sometimes difficult to distinguish between visual hemineglect and hemianopic visual field loss. The line bisection test may be helpful in some of such cases.

Sensory extinction or perceptual rivalry is seen when patients respond to stimuli presented to each side, but fail to respond on the neglected side if the stimuli are presented on both sides simultaneously.[59] This, again, becomes more evident while testing visual field by confrontation.

Extrapersonal Neglect

This is tested by asking the patient to bisect lines of varying lengths, cancellation tasks, and drawing and copying figures.

A patient with a right hemispherical stroke is asked to copy a figure of a clock face. He draws the right half of the clock face, but misses out to copy the left half. This is an example of object-centered neglect. However, this could have

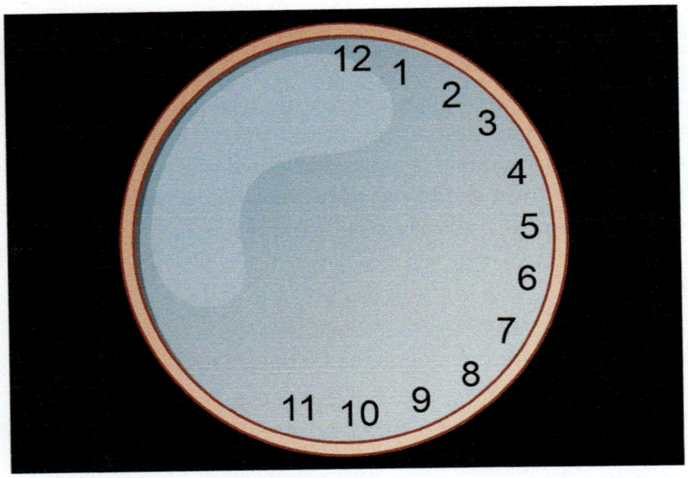

FIG. 3: Clock-face drawing in a patient with left visual hemineglect. All numbers are put on the right side, leaving the left side blank.

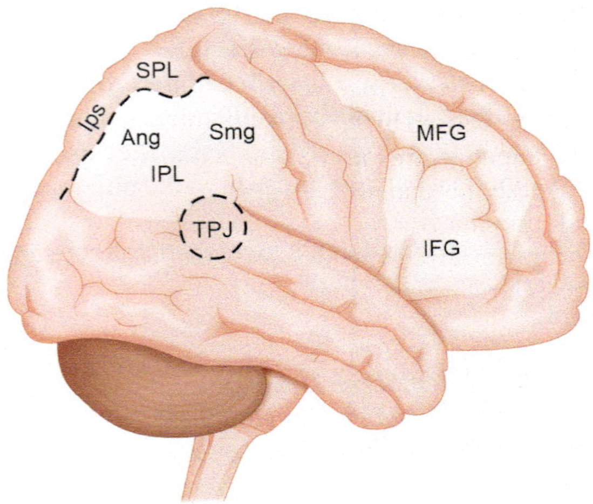

FIG. 4: Cortical areas in the nondominant hemisphere where lesions may produce visual hemineglect on the contralateral side.
(Ang: angular gyrus; IFG: inferior frontal gyrus; IPL: inferior parietal lobule; Ips: intraparietal sulcus; MFG: middle frontal gyrus; Smg: supramarginal gyrus; SPL: superior parietal lobule; TPJ: temporoparietal junction)

resulted from a left homonymous hemianopia as well as he would be unable to see the left half of his visual field. How to distinguish between the two—hemianopia or hemineglect? The line bisection test may help to differentiate between hemianopia on one side and a hemineglect on the same side due to a lesion in the contralateral parieto-occipital region.[60] Hemianopic patients tend to put the bisecting mark much beyond the actual central point, whereas patients with visual hemineglect on the same side would tend to put the bisecting mark much proximal to the actual midpoint. Visual hemineglect is usually more persistent in right hemispherical disorders, but can occur with lesions of either hemisphere. Lesions causing visual hemineglect need not necessarily be only in the visual association areas, but may be located much anteriorly in the nondominant hemisphere **(Fig. 4)**.

Dressing Apraxia

The term "apraxia" is a misnomer about dressing. The disturbance in the ability to dress is not a motor disorder. It is a deficit in the orientation of body parts about garments due to a disorder of the visuospatial mechanism. The site of the lesion is usually in the right posterior parietal area. Dressing apraxia may be evident when a subject is asked to wear a shirt or blouse after turning it inside out.

Testing Visuospatial and Constructional Ability

Disorders of constructional ability can be tested by asking the subject to draw 3D drawings or a complex 2D shape like the intersecting pentagons. For a more objective assessment, Rey-Osterrieth complex figure test is recommended.[61,62]

The clock setting/drawing test is not only a useful test of constructional ability but also tests the conceptualization of time and its abstract relation to the placement of hands. Patients with early dementia can usually draw the clock correctly, but have problems with placement of hands when asked to set a time. Some authorities have suggested that the patient should be asked to set a time when one arm of the clock should be placed on the right side and the other on the left (e.g., 10 minutes past 10 o'clock). This is useful in detecting unilateral neglect, as discussed earlier.[63]

Agnosias

Agnosias are disorders of recognition that cannot be attributed to general intellectual impairment, aphasia, or basic sensory dysfunction. They can be visual, tactile, or sensory.

A person with visual agnosia sees an object but is unable to recognize them. This can be so again for different categories of stimuli such as colors, objects, and faces.

The object recognition disorder can be categorized into two main types, depending on the stage at which visual perception breaks down.

Apperceptive Visual Agnosia

In this type of visual agnosia, patients have preserved elementary visual faculties such as acuity, simple shape, contour discrimination, and color perception, but fail to identify and name objects. They can sometimes name the objects by using tactile palpation. Common objects such as watches and pen can be used for testing. This may happen with bilateral posterior cortical lesions involving the visual association cortex (areas 18 and 19) and in carbon monoxide poisoning. When a person fails to name or identify a common object, differentiation needs to be made between anomia and visual agnosia. In the former case, the person would be able to choose the right name when given options and would explain the use of the object through gestures/pantomime. None of these would be possible for a person having apperceptive visual agnosia.

Associative Visual Agnosia

In this type of agnosia, a patient can demonstrate the use of an object, but is unable to recognize and name the object. It is believed to be caused by the disconnection of the visual area from the language area and the visual memory stores. The site of the lesion is usually in the bilateral inferior temporo-occipital junction or a lesion in the left occipital lobe and adjacent posterior corpus callosum. The same lesion can also cause alexia without agraphia.

Visual agnosias can be tested by:

- Visual object identification by inspecting shape, color, etc., but not feeling with hands
- Copying line drawings of common articles such as a house and bicycle
- *Visual matching tasks*: The ability to match pictures to objects

Some additional tests such as *object knowledge* (that is the ability to generate accurate verbal descriptions when given the name of objects) and *tactile naming* (the ability to name objects by touch) may help in detailed lesion localization. In cross-modal associative agnosia, there is generalized semantic memory impairment. These patients are unable to identify objects by any modality (visual, verbal, touch). They can identify the picture of an animal, but are unable to name the animal or describe its size or habitat. The site of the lesion is in the left anterior temporal lobe. This may be present in advanced Alzheimer's disease or patients with semantic dementia.[64]

Optic Aphasia

Optic aphasic subjects have a modality-specific (visual) recognition deficit but can recognize objects through both auditory and tactile modalities. This is similar to what is seen in patients with associative visual agnosias. As both groups of patients tend to display similarities in their deficits, one may argue for classification as a single syndrome, with varying degrees of severity. In both instances, lesion localization is suggestive of damage to the ventral visual stream.[65] Both types of patients retain the ability to copy presented line drawings.

Prosopagnosia

Prosopagnosia is a specific form of associative agnosia in which the subject has a disorder of face recognition and identification. The ability to describe and match faces is preserved. It is commonly tested by showing pictures of famous people, friends, and relatives. The site of the lesion is in the right posterior temporal lobe (fusiform gyrus), usually due to a stroke.

In semantic dementia, there is progressive atrophy of the right temporal lobe. These patients not only lose the ability to recognize people but also are unable to provide knowledge about the faces.[66]

LIMITATIONS OF BEDSIDE COGNITIVE TESTING

Bedside cognitive testing has got multiple limitations. Some of these, but not all, can be overcome by elaborate neuropsychological testing batteries.

First of all, most of these tools and test batteries have evolved in Western countries. Consequently, in non-English speaking populations like ours, these scales lack may lack reliability. Efforts are being made to develop reliable diagnostic tools and instruments that are culturally and linguistically valid for making an accurate diagnosis in the Indian population. The National Institute for Mental Health and Neurosciences (NIMHANS) neuropsychological battery[67] for the elderly and the Kolkata Cognitive Battery[68] are examples of this. But in a country like India, where there is so much linguistic and cultural diversity, the same scale may not have uniform utility everywhere. Another important limitation is the lack of normative data for different communities.

Secondly, it is tough to follow the hierarchy of assessment in bedside testing or a busy clinic. The clinician tries to use one or two tests to come to a quick diagnosis. The clock drawing test described above is one such example. It is a test for visuospatial (agnosia) and visual constructional (apraxia) abilities. Visual or hearing defects or lack of basic education can all impair the test results.

Thirdly, high-functioning individuals may perform well in the standard cognitive tests, even if they may be having major cognitive defects.

Last of all, abnormality of a single test does not signify impairment of a particular cognitive domain. For example, the serial subtraction seven test may be an attention test. But it can be impaired in patients with impaired calculative skills.

It should be remembered at the bedside that the way a subject performs a test may be more important than the absolute scores.

INDIVIDUALIZED TESTING VERSUS STANDARDIZED MENTAL TESTS

In this chapter, we have described a bedside testing scheme for cognition except those used for language and praxis assessment (discussed elsewhere in the volume). But time constraints may often prevent the examiner from utilizing all these tests. Standardized mental tests have evolved. Some of these are elaborate such as the dementia rating scale. Shorter scales such as the MMSE, Montreal cognitive assessment (MoCA),[69] and Addenbrooke's cognitive examination have been developed for use in the clinic or bedside.

The MMSE, devised by Folstein and colleagues in 1975,[70] had been the most popular bedside testing scale till a few years back. It was easy and standardized for testing the important domains of attention, language, memory, and visuospatial abilities. A person is scored out of 30. A score below 24 was considered abnormal. But it was not sensitive for detecting MCI, frontal lobe dysfunction, and focal cognitive deficits. Recently, it has been copyrighted (making it expensive), and this has contributed to its loss of popularity and usage. This is very disheartening.

Decline in the usage of MMSE has led to the rise in popularity of the MoCA. This is a 30-point test that can be administered in 10 minutes. The test is free and can be accessed by clinicians at http://www.mocatest.org. It has shown promise in detecting MCI and early Alzheimer's disease.[69]

The ACE has been modified to ACE3 (Indian English version).[12] It is more elaborate and time-consuming, but can help in separating frontotemporal dementia from Alzheimer's disease. The test toolkit can be accessed free at https://doi.org/10.1093/occmed/kqv041.

CONCLUSION

Cognitive neurology is a fascinating subject. It had been made more interesting and intriguing with the introduction of advanced functional neuroimaging modalities, which have made clinico-anatomical localizations more challenging. Accuracy of bedside lesion localization, in essence, depends on a very thorough knowledge of the clinical anatomy of the cerebral cortex. Testing without any attempt at lesion localization would have no value. Furthermore, as already stated, at the bedside, the way a subject performs a test may be more important than the absolute scores.

REFERENCES

1. Schnider A. Neuropsychologic testing: bedside approaches. In: Goldenberg G, Miller BL (Eds). Handbook of Clinical Neurology, Volume 88 (3rd series), Neuropsychology and behavioral neurology. Amsterdam: Elsevier; 2008. pp. 137-54.
2. Strub RL, Black FW. The Mental State Examination in Neurology, 4th edition. Delhi: Jaypee Brothers Medical Publishers; 2003.
3. Hodges RJ. Cognitive Assessment for Clinicians, 3rd edition. Oxford: Oxford University Press; 2018.
4. Sanford AM. Mild cognitive impairment. Clin Geriatr Med. 2017;33(3):325-37.
5. Petersen RC. Mild cognitive impairment. Continuum (Minneap Minn). 2016;22(2 Dementia):404-18.
6. Harmon KG, Drezner JA, Gammons M, Guskiewicz KM, Halstead M, Herring SA, et al. American Medical Society for Sports Medicine position statement: concussion in sport. Br J Sports Med. 2013;47(1):15-26.
7. Snyderman D, Rovner B. Mental status exam in primary care: a review. Am Fam Physician. 2009;80(8):809-14.
8. American Psychiatric Association. Diagnostic and Statistical Manual of Mental Disorders, 5th edition. Washington, DC: American Psychiatric Association; 2014 (updated 2018).
9. Papez JW. A proposed mechanism of emotion. Arch Neurol Psychiatry. 1937;387:25-38.
10. Lhermitte F. Human autonomy and the frontal lobes. Part II: Patient behavior in complex and social situations: the "environmental dependency syndrome." Ann Neurol. 1986;19:335-43.
11. Smith A. The series sevens subtraction test. Arch Neurol. 1976;17:18.
12. Noone P. (2015). Addenbrook's cognitive examination-III. [online] Available from https://doi.org/10.1093/occmed/kqv041. [Last accessed December, 2022].
13. Ettlin TM, Kischka U, Beckson M, Gaggiotti M, Rauchfleisch U, Benson DF. A frontal lobe score. Part I: construction of a mental status of frontal systems. Clin Rehabil. 2000;14:260-71.
14. Zola-Morgan S, Squire LR, Amaral DG. Human amnesia and the medial temporal region: enduring memory impairment following a bilateral lesion limited to the CA1 field of the hippocampus. J Neurosci. 1986;6:2950-67.
15. Rolls E. A theory of hippocampal function in memory. Hippocampus. 1996;6:601.
16. Wechsler D. Wechsler Memory Scale. Psychological Corporation; 1945.
17. Schoenberg MR, Dawson KA, Duff K, Patton D, Scott JG, Adams RL. Test performance and classification statistics for the Rey auditory verbal learning test in selected clinical samples. Arch Clin Neuropsychol. 2006;21(7):693-703.
18. Abrahams S, Pickering A, Polkey CE, Morris RG. Spatial memory deficits in patients with unilateral damage to the right hippocampal formation. Neuropsychologia. 1997;35:11-24.
19. Eling P. History of neuropsychological assessment. Front Neurol Neurosci. 2019;44:164-78.
20. Lenehan ME, Summers MJ, Saunders NL, Summers JJ, Vickers JC. Does the Cambridge automated neuropsychological test battery (CANTAB) distinguish between cognitive domains in healthy older adults? Assessment. 2016;23(2):163-72.
21. Wixted JT. On common ground: Jost's (1897) law of forgetting and Ribot's (1881) law of retrograde amnesia. Psychol Rev. 2004;111(4):864-79.
22. Pearce JM. A note on aphasia in bilingual patients: Pitres' and Ribot's laws. Eur Neurol. 2005;54(3):127-31.
23. Piolino P. Autobiographical memory in aging. Psychol Neuropsychiatr Vieil. 2003;1(1):25-35.
24. Hodges JR, Salmon DP, Butters N. Semantic memory impairment in Alzheimer's disease: failure of access or degraded knowledge? Neuropsychologia. 1992;30:301-14.
25. Hodges JR, Graham KS. A reversal of the temporal gradient for famous person knowledge in semantic dementia: implications for the neural organization of long-term memory. Neuropsychologia. 1998;36(8):803-25.
26. Viskontas IV, McAndrews MP, Moscovitch M. Remote episodic memory deficits in patients with unilateral temporal lobe epilepsy and excisions. J Neurosci. 2000;20(15):5853-7.
27. Estmacott RW, Moscovitch M. Temporally graded semantic memory loss in amnesia and semantic dementia: further evidence for opposite gradients. Cogn Neuropsychol. 2002;19(2):135-63.
28. Simons JS, Verfaellie M, Galton CJ, Miller BL, Hodges JR, Graham KS. Recollection-based memory in frontotemporal dementia: implications for theories of long-term memory. Brain. 2002;125 (Pt 11):2523-36.
29. Baddeley A, Della Sala S. Working memory and executive control. Philos Trans R Soc Lond B Biol Sci. 1996;351(1346):1397-403.
30. Moscovitch M. Multiple dissociations of function in amnesia. In: Cermak LS (Ed). Human Memory and Amnesia. Hillsdale, NJ: Lawrence Erlbaum Associates; 1982. pp. 337-70.

31. Milner B, Petrides M, Smith ML. Frontal lobes and the temporal organization of memory. Hum Neurobiol. 1985;4(3):137-42.
32. Luria AR. Human Brain and Psychological Processes. New York: Harper & Row; 1966.
33. Fuster J. The Prefrontal Cortex. New York: Raven Press; 1997.
34. Andrés P. Frontal cortex as the central executive of working memory: time to revise our view. Cortex. 2003;39(4-5):871-95.
35. Strauss E, Sherman EMS, Spreen O. A Compendium of Neuropsychological Tests: Administration, Norms, and Commentary, 3rd edition. New York: Oxford University Press; 2006.
36. Thurstone LL, Thurstone TG. Primary Mental Abilities (rev). Chicago: Science Research Associates; 1962.
37. Regard M, Strauss E, Knapp P. Children's production on verbal and nonverbal fluency tasks. Percept Mot Skills. 1982;55(3):839-44.
38. Miles S, Howlett CA, Berryman C, Nedeljkovic M, Moseley GL, Phillipou A. Considerations for using the Wisconsin card sorting test to assess cognitive flexibility. Behav Res Methods. 2021;53(5): 2083-91.
39. Wessels AM, Edgar CJ, Nathan PJ, Siemers ER, Maruff P, Harrison J. Cognitive go/no-go decision-making criteria in Alzheimer's disease drug development. Drug Discov Today. 2021;26(5):1330-6.
40. Llinàs-Reglà J, Vilalta-Franch J, López-Pousa S, Calvó-Perxas L, Torrents Rodas D, Garre-Olmo J. The trail-making test. Assessment. 2017;24(2):183-96.
41. Weiner MF, Hynan LS, Rossetti H, Falkowski. Luria's three-step test: what is it and what does it tell us? J Int Psychogeriatr. 2011;23(10):1602-6.
42. Luria AR. Higher Cortical Functions in Man, 2nd edition. New York: Basic Books; 1980.
43. Damasio AR, Graff-Radford NR, Damasio H. Transient partial amnesia. Arch Neurol. 1983;40:656-7.
44. Blumer D, Benson DF. Personality changes with frontal and temporal lobe lesions. In: Benson DF, Blumer D (Eds). Psychiatric Aspects of Neurologic Disease. New York: Grune & Stratton; 1975. pp. 151-69.
45. Robinson RG, Kubos KL, Starr LB, Rao K, Price TR. Mood disorders in stroke patients: importance of lesion location. Brain. 1984;107:81-93.
46. Ross ED. The aprosodias. In: TE Feinberg, MJ Farah (Eds). Behavioral Neurology and Neuropsychology. New York: McGraw Hill; 1997.
47. Broca P. Remarques Sur le siège de la faculté du langage articulé. suivies d'une observation d'aphémie. Bull Assoc Anat (Nancy). 1861;2:330-57.
48. Wernicke K. Der Aphasische Symtomen Complex. Breslau: Cohn & Weigert; 1874.
49. Kirshner HS. Speech and language disorders. Behavioral Neurology: Practical Science of Mind and Brain, 2nd edition. Oxford: Butterworth–Heinemann; 2002.
50. Mayer E, Reicherts M, Deloche G, Willadino-Braga L, Taussik I, Dordain M, et al. Number processing after stroke: anatomoclinical correlations in oral and written codes. J Int Neuropsychol Soc. 2003;9:899-912.
51. Pavlović D. Acalculia. Srp Arh Celok Lek. 1997;125(11-12):353-5.
52. Ardila A. Gerstmann syndrome. Curr Neurol Neurosci Rep. 2020;20(11):48.
53. Rusconi E. Gerstmann syndrome: historic and current perspectives. Handb Clin Neurol. 2018;151:395-411.
54. Rosen HJ, Viskontas IV. Cortical neuroanatomy and cognition. Handbook of Clinical Neurology, Vol. 88 (3rd series), Neuropsychology and behavioral neurology. Goldenberg G, Miller BL (Eds). Amsterdam: Elsevier; 2008. pp. 41-60.
55. Heilman KR, Valenstein E. Two forms of ideomotor apraxia. Neurology. 1982;32:342-6.
56. Rothi L, Heilman KM, Watson RT. Pantomime comprehension and ideomotor apraxia. J Neurol Neurosurg Psychiatry. 1985;48: 207-10.
57. Watson RT, Heilman KM. Callosal apraxia. Brain. 1983;106:391-403.
58. Watson RT, Fleet WS, Gonzalez-Rothi L, Heilman KM. Apraxia and the supplementary motor area. Arch Neurol. 1986;43:787-92.
59. Heilman KM, Watson RT, Valenstein E. Neglect and related disorders. In: Heilman KM, Valenstein E (Eds). Clinical Neuropsychology, 4th edition. New York: Oxford University Press; 2003. pp. 296-346.
60. Barton JJS, Black SE. Line bisection in hemianopia. J Neurol Neurosurg Psychiatry. 1998;64:660-2.
61. Spreen O, Strauss E. A Compendium of Neuropsychological Tests. Administration, Norms, and Commentary, 2nd edition. New York: Oxford University Press; 1998.
62. Zhang X, Lv L, Min G, Wang Q, Zhao Y, Li Y. Overview of the complex figure test and its clinical application in neuropsychiatric disorders, including copying and recall. Front Neurol. 2021;12:680474.
63. Freedman M, Leach L, Kaplan E, Winocur G, Shulman KI, Delis DC. Clock Drawing: A Neuropsychological Analysis. New York: Oxford University Press; 1994.
64. Grusser OJ, Landis T. Visual Agnosias and Other Disturbances of Visual Perception and Cognition. London: MacMillan; 1991.
65. Schnider A, Benson DF, Scharre DW. Visual agnosia and optic aphasia: are they anatomically distinct? Cortex. 1994;30(3): 445-57.
66. Meadows J. The anatomical basis of prosopagnosia. J Neurol Neurosurg Psychiatry. 1974;37:48.
67. Tripathi R, Kumar JK, Bharath S, Marimuthu P, Varghese M. Clinical validity of NIMHANS neuropsychological battery for elderly: a preliminary report. Indian J Psychiatry. 2013;55(3):279-82.
68. Das SK, Bose P, Biswas A, Dutt A, Banerjee TK, Hazra AM, et al. An epidemiologic study of mild cognitive impairment in Kolkata, India. Neurology. 2007;68(23):2019-26.
69. Nasreddine ZS, Phillips NA, Bédirian V, Charbonneau S, Whitehead V, Collin I, et al. The Montreal cognitive assessment, MoCA: a brief screening tool for mild cognitive impairment. J Am Geriatr Soc. 2005;53(4):695-9.
70. Folstein MF, Folstein SE, McHugh PR. "Mini-mental state". A practical method for grading the cognitive state of patients for the clinician. J Psychiatr Res. 1975;12(3):189-98.

3 CHAPTER

Testing Agnosia and Apraxia

James Jose, Joe James

INTRODUCTION

Agnosia and apraxia are cognitive impairments where agnosia is a disorder of sensory-semantic integration and apraxia is a disorder of sensory-motor integration. Agnosia and apraxia cause substantial impairment of basic and instrumental activities of daily living. Basic knowledge of the symptoms resulting from these disorders and the examinations to bring out them are part of all cognitive examinations.

AGNOSIA

Agnosia is a perceptual disorder where sensations are preserved but the ability to recognize a stimulus or identify its meaning is lost.[1] Gnosis means knowledge and hence the term agnosia means "without knowledge". Patients with agnosia cannot understand or recognize what they see, hear, or feel. Agnosia results when lesions disconnect and isolate visual, auditory, and somatosensory inputs from higher-level processing. This results in a specific inability to access semantic knowledge of an object or other stimuli. The result will be a percept stripped of its meaning.

VISUAL AGNOSIA

In visual agnosia, a person cannot recognize and understand an object by sight even though it is previously known to him. The first description of visual agnosia can be traced to Lissauer in 1890.[2] He described the disorder as "Seelenblindheit" or soul blindness. He made a distinction between deficits in the ability to consciously perceive the attributes of a stimulus (called apperceptive agnosia) versus the inability to ascribe meaning to what is perceived (called associative agnosia). Even after more than 100 years, this classification and concept are still used for describing visual agnosia in cognitive neurology.

Types of Visual Agnosia

From the time of Lissauer onward, two types of agnosia were identified—(1) apperceptive and (2) associative. In apperceptive agnosia, there is a failure to achieve a structured description of the shape of the object. In associative agnosia, there is an inability to attribute a meaning to a correctly perceived stimulus. Perceptual categorization defect, a form of apperceptive agnosia, is characterized by difficulty in recognizing objects that are presented at unusual angles.

Apperceptive Visual Agnosia

Apperceptive visual agnosia is characterized by an intact basic sensory visual ability. A defect in early-stage visual processing prevents a correct percept of the stimulus from being formed. The patient is unable to access the structure and special properties of a visual stimulus. The object is not seen as a whole or in a meaningful way. Patients with apperceptive visual agnosia may say that they are blind as they cannot identify the forms of the objects. However, for the examiner, they do not appear blind as they may walk without bumping into objects.

Tests for Detecting Apperceptive Agnosia[1]

- *Matching*: Patients with apperceptive agnosia cannot match an item with an identical item from a collection of items.
- *Copying*: A patient with apperceptive agnosia cannot copy an object. However, they may be able to draw it from their memory.

Perceptual Categorization Defect

Perceptual categorization defect is considered a form of apperceptive agnosia. These patients have difficulty in recognizing scenes or objects that are presented in unusual angles, views, or illumination. The key features of an object may not be seen and the object, therefore, is not recognized.[3] Normally, there is a stored representation of objects with information about the volume and structure of familiar objects (object-centered representation). When this information cannot be accessed, the patient cannot identify degraded or rotated versions of familiar objects. This results in the misidentification of objects.

Tests for Detecting Perceptual Categorization Defect

Perceptual categorization defect type of apperceptive agnosia can be identified by:

- Incomplete letter test
- Silhouettes (shadow)
- Gollin figures
- Usual/unusual view test
- Foreshortened match

In an incomplete letter test, the patient is asked to identify letters degraded by 70% or 30%. Silhouettes are blackened shapes of objects and animals. The patient is asked to identify them. In the usual/unusual view test, patient is asked to identify objects kept at unusual angles. In the Gollin figure test, subjects are shown a series of drawings in a sequence, from least to most clear, and asked to identify the image. The object cannot possibly be identified in the first sketch, and most people must see several of the panels before they can identify it.

Associative Visual Agnosia

In associative visual agnosia, early stage perceptual processing is intact. Patients can process information and can develop a percept of an object. However, the percept is not able to access semantics or knowledge of the object. The object is perceived as an object but it has no meaning. Patients with apperceptive visual agnosia may say that they are blind whereas patients with associative agnosia may say that they do not understand anything. Usually, they will have excuses like "light is poor" or "I have not taken my glasses".

Tests for Detecting Associative Visual Agnosia

- *Questionnaire*: The patient is presented with pictures of animals, tools, and other objects and is asked about their properties, name, and use. Patients with agnosia will see the object, but cannot describe its properties, name, or use of the objects.
- Match objects that are visually dissimilar but have the same functions, e.g., keys, glasses, combs, etc.
- *Real and unreal objects*:[4] This test consists of configurations of objects that may or may not be encountered in the real world. Ask the patient to say whether these items are from the real world or not.
- *Pyramids and palm trees test*:[4] In this test, two perceptually and functionally different but conceptually related pictures are given and asked to match. The patient is presented with one picture above two others. He is asked to identify which among the bottom items matches best with the top item.

In its standard form, a picture of pyramids in a desert is given on the top and a palm tree, which is seen in the desert, and another tree, which is not seen in the desert, is given at the bottom. The patient is supposed to match the palm tree with the pyramids, which is not possible if he is having visual agnosia. In the informal test, the pyramids and the trees can be replaced with similar locally familiar objects.

PROSOPAGNOSIA

Prosopagnosia is an inability to identify faces. These patients can discriminate faces according to sex and race and can decode emotional expressions. There are two variants of prosopagnosia—"apperceptive" and "associative".[5] Impairment in the ability to see the differences between faces, or their structures, is considered apperceptive prosopagnosia. In associative (amnestic) prosopagnosia subjects can perceive the facial structures accurately but cannot recall the faces of familiar people.

Testing of Prosopagnosia

Face Perception Test

The face perception test measures the ability to accurately discriminate and match shaded black and white photographs of unfamiliar persons. This test will be abnormal in apperceptive prosopagnosia. Benton Facial Recognition Test, Cambridge Face Perception Test, or the Glasgow Face Matching Test can be used for this purpose.[5] In Benton Facial Recognition Test, subjects are presented with a target face above and six test faces below and they are asked to indicate which of the six images matches the target face. Male and female faces are used, and faces are closely cropped so that no clothing and little hair are visible. In the first display, one of the six test faces matches the target individual and the target image and test image are identical. In the next item, three of the test faces match the target face and the poses for the test images are different from the target image.

Face Identification Using Familiar Photographs

The formal test for face identification is *Cambridge Face Memory Test* which uses anonymous faces and the subjects have to memorize the test face and select the correct match from the samples given subsequently.[5] Face identification using photographs of familiar persons and celebrities ensuring that photographs are culturally appropriate can be used to assess associative prosopagnosia. An abnormal face identification in the presence of a normal face perception test indicates associative (amnestic) prosopagnosia.

COLOR AGNOSIA

Patients with color agnosia can see colors and discriminate colors. However, they cannot recognize the color, i.e., a red color cannot be identified as red. In visual object agnosia, the objects are stripped of their meaning. Similarly, in color agnosia the color is stripped of its meaning.

Patients with color agnosia can read Ishihara plates, and sort and match colors according to their hue. However, they cannot name colors or point to colors named by the examiner. They cannot select the appropriate color for painting objects.

TACTILE AGNOSIA

Tactile agnosia is defined as the inability to recognize objects after tactile exploration, in the presence of relatively intact sensory functions and adequate cognitive abilities. The deficit is modality-specific, as the same object is promptly recognized through other modalities.

Several distinct disorders have been identified, and many classifications of tactile agnosia have been offered. Hoffmann used the term "astereognosis" in 1885 to describe an inability to distinguish between different three-dimensional forms which he explained in terms of impairment of spatial discrimination.[6] Delay in 1935 postulated three mechanisms involved in impaired object recognition: (1) "Amorphognosia", the inability to recognize the size and shape of objects, (2) "Anosognosia", the failure to discriminate distinctive qualities of objects such as weight, texture, and thermal properties, and (3) "Tactile asymboly", a form of impaired object recognition in the absence of ahylognosia and amorphognosia.[7]

To test tactile object-recognition, four or five common objects are used (e.g., coin, button, key, screw, and rubber). The test is done in three steps.[6] First the subject is asked to manipulate and identify an object. If he fails to recognize a given object tactually, a tactile selection task is given where he is asked to select the unidentified object tactually from among four or five objects. Finally, tactile visual matching is tested in which the subject is instructed to explore an object tactually and is then shown a group of four or five objects including the tactually explored object and the subject has to identify which of the visually presented objects matched the tactually explored object.

AUDITORY AGNOSIA

Auditory agnosia refers to the defective recognition of auditory stimuli in the context of a preserved hearing. Whereas cortically deaf patients typically behave as if they were deaf (despite normal peripheral hearing and brainstem evoked potentials), patients with auditory agnosia are aware of sounds but have difficulty with sound identification. Auditory agnosia can be divided into four major categories—(1) general auditory agnosia; (2) agnosia for speech (verbal auditory agnosia or pure word deafness); (3) agnosia for environmental sounds; and (4) agnosia for music (amusia).[8]

General auditory agnosia is characterized by impaired recognition of all types of auditory stimuli, including speech, environmental sounds, and music. Agnosia specific to speech sounds is often called pure word deafness.[8] This is, critically, distinct from posterior (sensory) aphasia in that other domain of linguistic processing, including reading, writing, and speaking, are relatively intact. Patients with verbal auditory agnosia are aware of speech but describe it as sounding like a foreign language, cartoonlike or with descriptions like "voice comes but no words. Auditory agnosia occurs with (relatively) intact speech perception, but impairment in perceiving and/or comprehending nonspeech environmental sounds is designated as environmental sound agnosia.[8] Many cases of environmental sound agnosia also involve deficits in musical perception.

The different clinical syndromes resulting from lesions in the cortical auditory areas constitute a spectrum of related auditory processing disorders. The clinical course may reveal a pattern of improvement from a usually transient cortical deafness to generalized auditory agnosia; selective auditory agnosia, pure word deafness, and/or amusia.[9]

The *sound recognition test* assesses a patient's ability to recognize familiar, nonlinguistic environmental sounds, such as a dog bark or thunder. The stimulus sounds were tape-recorded and presented on a tape deck. Patients identified each sound by pointing to a drawing of its source, with four response choices on each test trial.[9,10] The *aural comprehension test* assesses a patient's ability to recognize familiar, linguistic sounds. It requires patients to point to drawings of objects named by the examiner. Four response choices are available in each of the test trials.[10]

FINGER AGNOSIA

Finger agnosia, as described by Gerstmann includes the inability to distinguish, name, or recognize the fingers not only in the patient's own hands but also in the examiner's hand or a drawing of a hand. Most evident errors are observed in the index, middle, and ring fingers.[11] Interestingly, finger agnosia may be associated with toe agnosia also. Finger agnosia is a type of autotopagnosia or somatotopagnosia. *Autotopagnosia* is the inability to orient and point to parts of one's own body, as seen with left parietal lobe lesions.[12] Unlike autotopagnosia, which refers only to one's body parts, *somatotopagnosia* includes the inability to orient and recognize the body parts of others also.

APRAXIA

Apraxia is a disorder of motor cognition, where there is an inability to perform a learned motor task, that cannot be adequately explained by weakness, sensory loss, or a lack of understanding.[13] Even though used nonspecifically for several clinical conditions, apraxia usually means limb apraxia which is a deficit of purposive limb movements. The left hemisphere is dominant for limb praxis and limb apraxia is conventionally considered a dysfunction of the left parietal lobe. Apraxia reflects an impairment of the storage and transformation of motor representations in the brain, either due to degradation of the knowledge of gestures and tool use or due to the inability to translate the neural representations of movement accurately into lower-level patterns of muscle activation and inhibition.

DIFFERENT TYPES OF APRAXIA

The anatomical substrate of praxis is a two-part system consisting of praxis conceptual and praxis production components. The conceptual system subserves praxis knowledge, whereas the production system subserves praxis generation.[14] The conceptual system has three types of knowledge relevant to limb praxis: (1) knowledge of objects and tools, (2) knowledge of actions, and (3) knowledge of the organization of actions in a sequence.[15] The production system translates the conceptual representations into motor commands.[16] It retrieves and activates the praxicon and then associates it via cortical projections with the relevant motor engrams in the premotor regions. From here the innervatory information passes to the primary motor cortex before being fed down the corticospinal tracts. Apraxia can occur due to the abnormalities of the praxis conceptual system or praxis production and executing systems.

Conceptual Apraxia

Conceptual apraxia denotes a loss of different types of tool-object-action knowledge. A tool is defined as that which is used to provide a mechanical advantage in action and object as the recipient of an action. Patients with conceptual apraxia are unable to associate tools and objects with the corresponding action. They also fail to describe the function of a tool or point to a tool when the function is described by the examiner.[17] They use tools/objects improperly, and misselect tools/objects for an intended activity.

Patients with conceptual apraxia may be unable to recall which tool is associated with an object. This is called loss of tool-object association knowledge.[17] For example, when a partially driven nail is shown, they may select a screwdriver instead of a hammer for hammering the nail. Patients with conceptual apraxia may also be unable to recall which tool is associated with an action. This is called loss of tool-object-action knowledge.[17] For example, when they are asked to pantomime the use of a screwdriver they may pantomime hammering. Patients with conceptual apraxia lose the mechanical advantage afforded by tools (loss of mechanical knowledge).[17] For example, when asked to complete an action and if the appropriate tool is not available (e.g., a hammer to drive a nail), they may not select the most suitable tool for that action (e.g., a spanner) but rather inadequate one (e.g., a screwdriver).

Ideational Apraxia

Ideational apraxia is characterized by the impairment in carrying out sequences of actions requiring the use of various objects in the correct order to achieve an intended purpose.[18] Patients with ideational apraxia recognize single objects well and name them correctly, but they may be unable to recognize correct and incorrect sequences of actions represented in photographs.

Ideomotor Apraxia

Ideomotor apraxia is a disorder of the action production system. Here, the knowledge and the space-time plans are intact. However, they can no longer guide the innervatory engrams in the premotor cortex to implement the movements.[19] The motor engrams in the premotor cortex are disconnected from the praxicons in the parietal lobe. The idea of the movement is intact but there is an inability to map this accurately onto the motor engrams in the frontal lobes. The patient knows what to do but not how to do it. Patients with ideomotor apraxia often perform poorly when asked to pantomime an action. The performance significantly improves if they are given the object they have just been asked to pantomime. This is because the visual and tactile feedback associated with the natural use of an object improves the selection of an appropriate limb posture and finger configuration.

Limb-kinetic Apraxia

Limb-kinetic apraxia appears when there is a disruption of the innervatory motor engrams in the premotor cortex. This interferes with the selection of the required muscle synergies to perform the skilled movement. The deficit is confined mainly to finger and hand movements contralateral to the lesion, regardless of its hemispheric side, with preservation of power. The characteristic feature is the loss of coordination between the fine, individuated finger movements that are required to perform a skilled task. Limb-kinetic apraxia is a higher-order motor disorder due to the disruption of the final stages of motor processing in the frontal regions before the information is relayed to the ipsilateral primary motor cortex.

Assessment of Limb Praxis[13]

Evaluation for Conceptual Apraxia

Various tests are designed for the evaluation of the praxis conceptual system. The common tests are tool selection tasks, alternative tool selection tasks, and gesture recognition tasks.

- *Tool selection tasks:*[20] In tool selection tasks, an object is shown to the participants and they have to choose, among several tools, the associated tool to execute the action, such as a hammer for a partially driven nail. This is a test for tool-object association knowledge. Before administering the test, the examinee is asked the name and attributes of the tools and object to rule out anomia and agnosia.

- *Alternative tool selection tasks*:[20] In the alternative tool selection task, the examinee has to select an alternative tool such as a spanner to complete a task such as pounding a nail, when the appropriate tool (e.g., hammer) is not available. An alternative tool selection task is a test for mechanical knowledge.
- *Gesture recognition tasks*:[21] To name gestures performed by the examiner or to match a gesture performed by the examiner with cards depicting the tool or object corresponding to the pantomime. This is a test for tool action knowledge.
- Describing the use of a tool, e.g., spoon/knife. This also tests the tool action knowledge.

Evaluation for Ideational Apraxia

The subject is instructed to prepare a letter for mailing and the incorrect sequence of action, if any, is evaluated.

Evaluation for Ideomotor Apraxia

Ideomotor apraxia can be assessed by instructing to carry out pantomimes, actual tool use, or intransitive movements.

- *Pantomime*: In pantomime, subjects have to pretend the use of a tool as instructed by the examiner (e.g., using a hammer or a screwdriver). The pantomime is usually performed on verbal command. The tool can also be placed in front of the participants (visual) and instructed to pantomime the associated action without holding the tool.[16]
- *Actual tool use*: Actual tool use involves the achievement of action with the tool in hand. The tool and the associated object (e.g., a hammer and a nail) are both provided and participants have to complete the action (driving a nail with the hammer).
- *Intransitive movements*: Intransitive movements may be tested with representational or nonrepresentational gestures. Waving goodbye is an example of representational intransitive movement, whereas touching the nose is a nonrepresentational gesture.
- Imitation of meaningful and meaningless movements, postures, and sequences can also be used for assessing ideomotor apraxia.

Evaluation for the Limb-kinetic Apraxia

- Ask the patient to oppose their thumb to their index, middle, ring, and little fingers rapidly in succession.
- Ask the patient to imitate some arbitrary hand position.
- Rotation of a coin between fingers.[22]

CONCLUSION

Apraxias and agnosias are important clinical findings and systematic approach of evaluation and continued practice is necessary to gain proficiency in the testing. The demonstration of these alterations has important role in the localization of the lesions.

REFERENCES

1. Jose J. Agnosia. In: Jose J (Ed). Cognitive Neurological Examination : A Clinico-Anatomical Approach, 2nd edition. Kerala: NAAM; 2020. p. 24.
2. Riddoch MJ, Humphreys GW. Visual agnosia. Neurol Clin. 2003;21(2):501-20.
3. Hoffmann M. Cognitive, Conative and Behavioral Neurology: An Evolutionary Perspective. Switzerland: Springer International Publishing; 2016.
4. Ghadiali E. Cognitive Primer—Agnosia. Adv Clin Neurosci Rehabil. 2004;4(5):18-20.
5. Corrow SL, Dalrymple KA, Barton JJS. Prosopagnosia: Current perspectives. Eye Brain. 2016;8:165-75.
6. Platz T. Tactile agnosia: Casuistic evidence and theoretical remarks on modality-specific meaning representations and sensorimotor integration. Brain. 1996;119(5):1565-74.
7. Bauer RM. The Agnosias. In: Snyder PJ, Nussbaum PD, Robins DL (Eds). Clinical Neuropsychology: A Pocket Handbook for Assessment, 2nd edition. Washington, DC: American Psychological Association; 2006. pp. 508-33.
8. Slevc LR, Shell AR. Auditory Agnosia. Handb Clin Neurol. 2015;129:573-87.
9. Mendez MF, Geehan GR. Cortical auditory disorders: Clinical and psychoacoustic features. J Neurol Neurosurg Psychiatry. 1988;51(1):1-9.
10. Varney NR. The Prognostic Significance of Sound Recognition in Receptive Aphasia. Arch Neurol. 1984;41(2):181-2.
11. Mendoza JE. Autotopagnosia. In: Kreutzer JS, DeLuca J, Caplan B (Eds). Encyclopedia of Clinical Neuropsychology. New York: Springer Science + Business Media, LLC; 2011. pp. 333-4.
12. Ogden JA. Autotopagnosia. Brain. 1985;108(4):1009-22.
13. Leiguarda RC, Marsden CD. Limb apraxias. Higher-order disorders of sensorimotor integration. Brain. 2000;123(5):860-79.
14. Heilman KM, Maher LM, Greenwald ML, Rothi LJG. Conceptual apraxia from lateralized lesions. Neurology. 1997;49(2):457-64.
15. Gonzalez Rothi LJ, Ochipa C, Heilman KM. A Cognitive Neuropsychological Model of Limb Praxis. Cogn Neuropsychol. 1991;8(6):443-58.
16. Lesourd M, Le Gall D, Baumard J, Croisile B, Jarry C, Osiurak F. Apraxia and Alzheimer's disease: Review and perspectives. Neuropsychol Rev. 2013;23(3):234-56.
17. Ochipa C, Rothi LJG, Heilman KM. Ideational apraxia: A deficit in tool selection and use. Ann Neurol. 1989;25(2):190-3.
18. Poeck K. Survey of progress Ideational apraxia. J Neurol. 1983;230: 1-5.
19. Heilman KM, Watson RT. The disconnection apraxias. Cortex. 2008;44(8):975-82.
20. Ochipa C, Rothi LJG, Heilman KM. Conceptual apraxia in Alzheimer's disease. Brain. 1992;115(4):1061-71.
21. Bartolo A, Cubelli R, Sala S Della. Cognitive Approach to the Assessment of Limb Apraxia. Clin Neuropsychol. 2008;22(1):27-45.
22. Leiguarda R, Clarens F, Amengual A, Drucaroff L, Hallett M. Short apraxia screening test. J Clin Exp Neuropsychol. 2014;36(8):867-74.

4

CHAPTER

Testing Aphasia

Apoorva Pauranik

INTRODUCTION

Why is this Subject Important?

Disorders of speech, communication, and language are many and heterogeneous **(Table 1)**. Aphasia is one of them and involves a deficit in expression (motor), comprehension (sensory), or both. The modes of communication affected could be verbal, written, or both, and other unusual ones such as sign language in deafmutes. At the core of aphasia lies a disturbance in language. The burden of aphasia is larger than the combined populations of individuals with multiple sclerosis, muscular dystrophy, cerebral palsy, and Parkinson's disease. Poststroke aphasia persists as a long-term disability in about 25% of survivors (range from 21 to 38%). A community-based study from Sweden reported an incidence of 4/100,000 per year. The prevalence is around 300 per million **(Table 2)**.[1] We do not yet have a clear picture of the epidemiology of aphasia in India. By rough estimates, the number of persons with aphasia (PWA) in the country will be about three million.

Neurologists and medical practitioners caring for a patient with aphasia should be more knowledgeable about

TABLE 1: Disorder of speech and communication.

Types of disorder	Comment
Disorders of phonation: • Aphonia • Dysphonia	Almost always due to laryngeal dysfunction (local, non-neurogenic, neurogenic paralysis of vocal cord muscles)
Disorders of articulation: • Anarthria • Dysarthria	• *Non-neurological local causes*: Glossitis, tonsillitis, laryngitis, pharyngitis, neoplasia • *Neurological causes*: ○ *Muscles*: Polymyositis ○ *Neuromuscular*: Myasthenia gravis ○ *Neuropathic*: GB syndrome ○ *Brainstem, cerebellum, basal ganglia, and cerebrum*: Many pathologies, CVA, neoplasia, infection, degeneration (Parkinsonism), trauma, developmental
Disorders of fluency: • Stammering (stuttering) • Cluttering	• Usually developmental • No discernible underlying pathology in most
Disorders of language: • Aphasia • Alexia/dyslexia • Agraphia	• In cortical speech areas and subcortical connections, among many pathologies stroke is the most common • *Other less common causes*: ○ *Developmental*: Mental retardation, cerebral palsy ○ *Degenerative*: – *Young age*: Autism, Rett syndrome, leuko- and poliodystrophies – *Old age*: Alzheimer's and other dementias

(CVA: cerebrovascular accident; GB: Guillain–Barré)

TABLE 2: Community burden of aphasia and other disorders of speech and communication.

Disease condition	Overall burden	Proportion with aphasia
Stroke	Prevalence 0.5%	25%
Head injury	Prevalence 1.2%	5–10%
Dementia	10% above the age of 60 years	Almost all have variable impairment of language functions, depending on severity
Mental retardation	• 5% (all) • 1% (severe)	Almost all have variable impairment of language function, depending on severity
Learning disabilities (e.g., dyslexia)	5%	All have a variable handicap in reading and writing skills
Fluency and articulation disorders: • *Stuttering*: Stammering, lisping, cluttering, lalling	1%	Variable handicap in all

BOX 1 Purposes of testing aphasia.

- To diagnose aphasia
- To differentiate it from mimics (differential diagnosis)
- To determine the overall severity of aphasia
- To make a diagnosis of aphasia syndromes
- To get a detailed profile of speech, language, and communication
- To get informed about the goal(s) and type of therapy to be provided
- To make comparative follow-up assessments for recovery and effect of treatment
- To assess psychosocial issues
- To assess associated cognitive functions
- For research purposes

and interested in the subject. They should be aware of the literature on the robust evidence base of the efficacy of speech–language therapy and be convinced that a good clinical assessment is essential for speech therapy to work.[2,3]

A neurologist should be aware of the many purposes of testing, which will guide the approach and scope of the examination **(Box 1)**. It is likely that, more often, the purpose(s) will be limited to a few of the above.

Evidence-based on History and Examination

It is indisputable that any medical treatment and intervention should be based upon robust and high-quality evidence, mainly randomized controlled trials. Similar standards apply to the validity of laboratory diagnostic tests. The clinical methods of history taking and physical examination should be judged on a similar rigorous criterion. Not much literature is available on the evidence-based validity of clinical testing for aphasia.[4]

CLINICAL HISTORY TAKING

The clinical history for probable aphasia and related speech and communication disorders starts right from initial greetings and pleasantries. Some PWA will try to sustain the conversation on their own or with the help of relatives and caregivers. Those with more severe grades of aphasia will mostly remain quiet or speak only a few words. A significant burden of narrating the illness's story will fall upon the caregiver. To begin with, we must urge to let the patient make more effort. Surprisingly, many PWA can convey helpful information despite their severe handicap. Ultimately, a complete history will be obtained with input from relatives.

Back-and-forth Relationship of History with the Physical Examination

It is well known in clinical medicine that history and physical examination are not always linear in that order. They keep shuffling back and forth. Many observations are made while listening to the story, clarifying some symptoms and asking leading questions. It is almost universal that during or at the end of the "examination," the neurologist will go back to questioning some unaddressed issues, which were not covered earlier, but now a need is felt based on some "signs" in the physical examination.

Listen and Encourage

The neurologist should be "all ears" while PWA and significant others (SOs) narrate the story. We must resist the temptations to interrupt on any pretext, be it a clarification, a leading question, or something unrelated. However, we must constantly be encouraging them by saying:
"Well, I understand. Oh, so", "How did it all start?", "What is/are your main problem now?", "I am sorry to learn that", "That was good", "Keep on telling", "What else?", "What next?", "Describe it in detail", "What do you mean by that?", "Is that all?", "Since when?"

While listening, you may scribble some rough notes. Detailed notes must be reserved for later, as they would distract your attention. Give the PWA and SOs ample time. There should not be any hurrying up.

Checklist Approach to Symptomatology of Aphasia

There is a saying about the clinical physical examination that "your eyes see only that which your mind knows." Paraphrasing it, we may say, "your ears listen to only that which your mind knows."

We must know in somewhat detail the symptomatology of aphasia. Signs will follow during the physical examination, yet that should not be an excuse not to probe them during history.

Symptoms related to speech and communication are many and should be open in the mind's eyes of a neurologist in the form of a checklist and adjoining checkbox. As the history taking proceeds, many boxes will be checked randomly. If you think that even after giving ample time and good encouragement PWA and SOs are not coming up with any more symptoms, then only is the time to start asking leading questions and filling up the remaining unchecked boxes **(Box 2)**.

FEW ISSUES ABOUT TEST BATTERIES

Which Type of Test Battery? Ad Hoc or Standardized and Validated?

What is the criterion of a good test for assessment of aphasia? It should be *standardized*, *reliable*, valid, and discriminatory. Only then will it have precision and accuracy of measurement, which are sine qua non of good science.[5]

A limited number of aphasia language tests exist in most of the world's commonly spoken languages, other than English, European languages, and a few more. Very few have been constructed or adapted into Indian languages with all the rigor of a good test. Only a few have been published, along with normative data. This situation is a serious challenge to clinical practice and research in aphasia. There are many pitfalls of translating an existing test into a new language versus creating a new test. Many factors are to be considered in determining test content. The selection of test items corresponding to different language functions

BOX 2 A list of possible symptoms which PWA and SOs may complain of.

- Not talking at all, "no speech output"—mutism
- Reduced speed of talking, speaking fewer words at a time, speaking fewer utterances, hesitating while trying to speak, having pauses while speaking, taking a longer time to initiate the speech act, failing to take a turn while in conversation—nonfluency
- Groping for words, not finding the words, getting stuck up with words—anomia
- Response word differs from target word in the sound structure—phonemic paraphasia
- Response word differs, though the meaning is related—semantic paraphasia
- Uttering a word different than the one intended and which is unrelated to the target word and meaningless in the context—semantic jargon
- Uttering an unrecognizable string of sounds, not a word or phrase—phonemic jargon
- Uttering words which do not exist in the dictionary of the language (*lexicon*) known and used daily by a person with aphasia—nonwords, neologism
- Speech output restricted to a repetitive, meaningless, irrelevant *monosyllable* CV pair (CV recurrent utterance)
- Correct but roundabout description for a target word—circumlocution
- Uttering the same word again in response to different questions and need—preservations
- Speaking correctly but with distorted pronunciations, which remains unchanged each time the given word or sound is uttered—dysarthria
- *Repeating the word* or phrase spoken by others instead of answering—echolalia
- *Distorted pronunciation,* which keeps changing for a given word—apraxia of speech
- *Speaking excessively,* without a sense of completion, but mostly nonunderstandable, jargon-like, talking irrelevantly—fluent aphasia, empty speech
- *Not paying attention to* what others are speaking, not listening properly, not understanding whatever is being said, not following the conversation—defective auditory comprehension. It may appear as if hearing acuity is reduced, but hearing is normal
- *Not being able to repeat a syllable* or word or phrase spoken by others, despite comprehending it well—conduction, Broca's, Wernicke's aphasia
- *Reduced interest and efficiency in reading.* PWA may be holding a newspaper in his hands, but SOs are unsure if he is grasping anything. Unable to read aloud or read with distortions such as phonemic and semantic paraphasia, jargon, and nonwords. It may appear as if vision is reduced, but visual acuity remains normal—acquired alexia
- *Reduced memory*? Maybe the memory is intact, but relatives and caregivers think so because of anomia and paraphasia
- *Total or partial failure of writing*—agraphia
- Difficulties in writing with either hand—distorted handwriting. A similar range of problems in written expression as in oral verbal expressions (nonfluency, anomia, paraphasias, circumlocutions, jargon etc.)

(CV: consonant-vowel; PWA: persons with aphasia; SO: significant other)

BOX 3	Some tips for a busy neurologist.

- Always carry cards with pictures of objects, actions, scenes, printed words, and sentences in the examination bag
- Better still, carry all the above and more variety of examples on desktop, laptop, or smartphone
- Verbatim records of assessments of aphasia are important. Hence, keep a scoring sheet ready to enter the patient's responses to various subtests. The target answers are preprinted in one column, and a parallel column is left blank to be filled verbatim immediately by the clinician
- Make a video or an audio recording of the clinical assessment to be saved on a computer. An assistant can transcribe it later
- If possible, train a clinical assistant in basic assessment to do the testing, recording, and later writing the notes
- Train a caregiver of PWA to help in follow-up assessments
- Team up with an SLP and clinical (neuro) psychologist long term

(PWA: persons with aphasia; SLP: speech–language pathologist)

with special emphasis on controlling healthy subjects is crucial. Statistical guidance is needed for establishing the psychometric properties of *standardized* assessment tools.[6,7]

Indian versions of a few test batteries have been published but may be difficult to procure as a fully commercial set.[8-16] Tools are also needed for assessing functional communication, caregiver burden, aphasia-related quality of life (QOL), discourse analysis, and pragmatics.

A general neurologist often uses *nonstandardized* and nonvalidated ad hoc assessment, which varies across clinicians, institutions, and occasions. It is not an ideal situation. Formal and published test batteries are essential for planning speech–language therapy, publication, and research.

However, ad hoc testing in outpatient department (OPD) and bedside is a practical necessity for busy general neurologists and residents in training. The methods of testing described in this chapter are *standardized* and validated but not published. A few tips are enumerated in **Box 3** for a busy neurologist.

How Brief, How Detailed?

While a neurologist is most suited for physical examination of a person suffering from a neurological disease, clinical aphasia testing is teamwork. A neurologist may be able to and is expected to conduct a relatively brief and informal assessment.

A full clinical assessment of speech and language communication in a PWA in an ideal condition is time- and labor-intensive and needs expertise and experience. Comprehensive *profiling* is essential for proper and complete diagnosis and therapeutic planning. Speech-language pathologists (SLPs) are primarily suited for this task, but neurologists, neurosurgeons, and internists should also contribute as much as possible. Input from clinical (neuro) psychologists also helps.

Comprehensive popular test batteries are helpful for proper diagnosis, syndromic classification, and labeling. Very elaborate and extensive protocols also exist to create fine-grained profiles about a few or many aspects of speech, language, reading, and writing with the help of many subtests. These test batteries need not be and cannot be administered in toto and certainly not in one go. Based on an initial briefer assessment, the neurologist or SLP must pick and choose which aspect of competence and performance he is interested in **(Box 4)**.

Role of Computers and Digital Technology in Aphasia Testing

Computers and smartphones are proving literally handy in testing aphasia. It has become easy and efficient for audio–video recording of testing and conversation, replay, transcription, and online and offline analysis by artificial intelligence. Clinicians have access to an unlimited number and variety of *stimuli* (pictures, images, graphics, audio, videos) for testing. Computerized testing for aphasia is helpful because it is portable, editable, expandable, interactive, transferable, and participatory, and can be individualized. It is easier to be modified as a *multilingual*, *multiscriptal*, and multimodal tool. Timekeeping and scoring are facilitated. Testing can be done anytime, anywhere. Neurologists should keep themselves updated with new digital tools becoming available.[17]

Screening Tests/Brief Tests

A neurologist/physician can perform a brief clinical assessment of aphasia in the office or at the bedside in 5–10 minutes. All significant aspects of evaluation (as described further) must be covered, at least briefly. It is advisable to follow a set sequence of testing.[18]

The Hindi Aphasia Screening Indore Test (HASIT) is a *standardized* and validated *test battery*, though unpublished, modeled after the Frenchay Aphasia Screening Test (FAST) from the UK.[19]

A more rigorous Indian *adaptation* of FAST was developed as a part of the Indian Council of Medical Research (ICMR) toolbox[20] for cognitive assessment across six languages and different educational levels.[21]

SOME POPULAR COMPREHENSIVE TEST BATTERIES (TABLE 3)[22]

Western Aphasia Battery

The western aphasia battery was designed to assess linguistic skills (writing, reading, *naming* and word finding, repetition, auditory comprehension, fluency, and *information content*) and primary nonlinguistic skills (praxis, calculation, block design, and drawing).[23]

BOX 4 Headings and subheadings in clinical examination of aphasia.

- *Auditory comprehension*:
  - Pointing to objects, pictures
  - Carrying outspoken commands, sentences
  - Answering questions based upon the spoken discourse, paragraphs
- *Articulation*:
  - Recitation, singing
  - Simple words
  - Complex words
  - Sentences
- *Fluency in verbal expression*:
  - *During the conversation, while describing a picture or comic strip*:
    - Phrase length
    - Number of words per minute
    - *Agrammatism*
    - Stereotyped utterance
    - Word-finding difficulty
    - Phonological paraphasias
    - Semantic paraphasias
    - Neologisms
    - Circumlocution
- *Repetition*:
  - *Syllable*
  - *Words*: High frequency and high imageability
  - *Words*: Low frequency, low imageability
  - *Phrases*
- *Naming*:
  - Body parts
  - Real objects
  - Pictures
  - Question-based
  - Effect of *cueing* (phonemic and semantic)
  - Rejection of wrong answers

Acceptance of correct answers

- *Reading*:
  - Matching letters, syllables, words, numerals
  - Pointing to letters, syllables, words, numerals
  - Reading aloud letters, syllables, words, numerals
  - Sorting words and nonwords
  - Word–picture matching
  - Word–sentence matching
  - Filling in the blanks in sentences
  - Reading a paragraph and answering questions
  - Carrying out written commands
- *Writing*:
  - Copying letters, syllables, numerals, words, sentences
  - *Writing to dictation*: Letters, syllables, numerals, words, sentences
  - Signature, name, address, automatic sequences
  - Written naming of objects, pictures
  - Written description of a picture scene

TABLE 3: Current popular tests and methods of aphasia assessment.

Clinical bedside examination	Unstructured variable, as described in various textbooks, including this chapter
Screening test	Frenchay aphasia screening test, 5–10 minutes. *Standardized* and validated
Comprehensive examination	• Boston diagnostic aphasia examination • Western aphasia battery
Tests of specific aspects of language behavior	• Boston *naming* test • Token test (syntactic comprehension) • Tests for reading and writing
Tests based on cognitive neuropsychological approach	• PALPA • PAL • CAT
Assessment for functional communication and quality of life	• ASHA functional assessment • Communication activities of daily living • Quality of life scale in stroke–aphasia
Tests for special population	Infants and children, traumatic brain injury, right-hemisphere lesions, elderly and dementia subjects, *multilingual* subjects

(ASHA: American Speech–Language–Hearing Association; CAT: comprehensive aphasia test; PAL: psycholinguistic abilities in language; PALPA: psycholinguistic assessment of language processing in aphasia)

The scoring provides two key totals besides the subscale scores. These are the cortical quotient (CQ) score and the aphasia quotient (AQ) score. While AQ measures language ability, CQ assesses intellectual ability and entails the subscales. The overall severity of language impairment is represented by the AQ and is the total score.

Boston Naming Test

The Boston naming test assesses confrontational word retrievals in people with aphasia with the help of 60 black-line drawings graded according to difficulty. The patient is shown a picture and asked to respond to each. Approximately 20 seconds are allotted per answer. The examiner then writes down the responses of the patient in detail using codes.[24]

Boston Diagnostic Aphasia Examination

The Boston Diagnostic Aphasia Examination (BDAE) assesses various perceptual modalities (gestural, visual, and auditory), processing functions (analysis, problem-solving, comprehension), and response modalities (manipulation, articulation, and writing). It is used by psychologists, neurologists, occupational therapists, and SLPs.[25]

AphasiaBank Test

The AphasiaBank test follows standard procedures during a video-recorded session. The steps are as follows:

1. *Free speech samples*, stroke story, and coping and important events
2. Picture descriptions (broken window, cat rescue, refused umbrella)
3. Story narrative (Cinderella)
4. Procedural discourse (peanut butter and jelly sandwich)

These procedures provide researchers with a *standardized* database for studying phonological, *lexical*, semantic, morphological, syntactic, temporal, prosodic, gestural, and discourse features.[26]

Verb Naming Test

The verb naming test examines verb *naming* by showing a picture to the participant, who then names the actions depicted in the picture.[27]

Complex Ideational Material

Complex ideational material is a sentence comprehension task designed to assess receptive language skills via yes/no questions that involve common knowledge information and facts in four short narratives.[28]

Famous People Protocol

The famous people protocol is used for assessing communication in severe aphasia in the case of individuals who cannot provide discourse data.[29]

Comprehensive Aphasia Test

The comprehensive aphasia test is designed to (1) screen for associated cognitive deficits, (2) assess language impairment in people with aphasia, (3) investigate the consequences of aphasia on the individual's lifestyle and emotional well-being, and (4) monitor changes in aphasia and its consequences over time.[30]

Psycholinguistic Assessment of Language Processing in Aphasia

Psycholinguistic assessment of language processing in aphasia (PALPA) is a resource for speech and language therapists and cognitive and clinical neuropsychologists who wish to assess language processing skills in great detail in PWA.[31]

CLINICAL TESTING OF SPEECH AND LANGUAGE FUNCTIONS IN A PERSON WITH APHASIA AND RELATED DISORDERS

Please refer to the link for appendices **(Box 5)** to access various *stimuli* and instructions about their administration and scoring as developed by the present author.[32]

BOX 5 List of appendices. These appendices are available in detail in http://neurogyan2.arth-dhwani.com/aphasia.

- *HASIT*: Hindi Aphasia Screening Indore Test
- *HRWIT*: Hindi Reading Writing Indore Test
- *LEAP-Q*: Language Experience and Proficiency Questionnaire
- Handedness questionnaire
- Images for nouns
- Images for verbs
- Scenes and comic strips for picture description and narrative discourse
- Word and nonword list for repetition, reading aloud, and lexicality judgment
- Word–picture matching exercise
- Sentence–picture matching exercise
- Yes–no questions for auditory and reading comprehension
- Short story-based questions for auditory and reading comprehension
- Question for responsive *naming* with a single unambiguous one-word answer
- Scoring proforma
- Glossary of aphasiological terms (italicized in the main text)

Note: The link leads to a website developed by the author for public education and patient education about neurology and other subjects in Hindi. The section on aphasia hosts additional information and tools in English for neurologists and speech–language pathologists.

Verbal Expression

Listen carefully to the patient and ask questions like "Tell me about your illness, your family, the work done by you at your job." Efforts are needed to make patients speak, not merely isolated words or gestures but longer *phrases* and sentences. The patient should be asked to describe the things and actions in a picture. The response should be recorded and transcribed verbatim. In many PWA, it may be incomplete, halting, and sparse, with a failure to grasp the totality of the scene despite repeated hints.

Articulation: Dysarthria and Apraxia of Speech

Defective articulation and phonation are recognized during a conversation, reading aloud, and repetition. A list of target *syllable*s, words, nonwords, and short *phrases* is needed for testing articulation. Instruct the patient, "I am going to say a few words and sentences; listen carefully and repeat them after me. Are you ready?"

The *stimuli* for repetition and reading aloud are chosen based on alphabets, sounds, and *syllable*s of Indian languages, which have a good scientific arrangement of vowels and consonants into different groups according to the place of production. Try to have an audio recording because transcription of dysarthric output may be complex. While listening to dysarthric speech, pay attention to the type of sound distortion (*phonemes*).

The repetition test should be performed twice with the same *stimuli*. In the case of dysarthria, the distortions will

TABLE 4: Types of dysarthria.

Site of lesion	Disease example	Type of speech	Label
Bilateral upper motor neuron	Bilateral strokes, tumors, primary lateral sclerosis	Harsh voice, slow rate, strain strangle, imprecise consonants	Spastic ++
Unilateral upper motor neuron	Stroke, tumor	Consonant imprecision, harsh voice quality, slow rate	Spastic ++
Lower motor neuron	Bulbar palsy, myasthenia gravis	Breathy, nasal voice, imprecise consonants	Flaccid
Upper and lower motor neurons	Amyotrophic lateral sclerosis, multiple strokes	Strain–strangle, hypernasality, harsh voice, slow rate, imprecise consonants	Spastic and flaccid
Basal ganglia: a	Parkinson's disease	Rapid rate, reduced loudness, monotonous and nonvariable amplitude	Hypokinetic
Basal ganglia: b	Dystonia, Huntington's disease	Prolonged *as*, inappropriate silence, variable rate, voice stoppage	Hyperkinetic
Cerebellum	Stroke, degenerative disease, multiple sclerosis	Irregular articulatory breakdowns are made apparent on rapid repetition of equal *stress*	Ataxic

be the same each time. However, in a condition known as apraxia of speech, the same *stimuli* will yield slightly altered output.

Dysarthria is common in nonfluent aphasias. Pure dysarthria can occur in many disorders other than aphasia **(Table 4)**.

Fluency of Speech

Even healthy people have a wide range of fluency in speech. Some are talkative, verbose, descriptive, and detailed, while others are persons with a few words, precise, and speaking in minimum words, only what is required. Think about how we can quantify verbal fluency.

Many measures have been used in clinical practice and research, e.g., the number of words per minute, the total number of words, the ratio of *content words* and *grammatical or function words*, informativeness of speech, *articulatory agility*, pauses, hesitancies, *prosody, intonation*, and others.

A PWA with nonfluent speech speaks in *monosyllables* or short sentences. Sometimes only a single utterance is repetitively used in every conversation. These verbal stereotypies [consonant–vowel (CV) recurring utterances] are sometimes intoned differently to convey some meaning, as in (yes!), (yes?), (y..y..es?).

There may be a delay in initiating a response, increased effort, apparent strain, pauses between words and sentences, and interruptions. Nonfluent speech, as in Broca aphasia, also exhibits *agrammatism* in which there is an absence or a scarcity of *function words*. The short *phrases* are composed of *content words* only, though the meaning is conveyed somehow in a manner resembling "telegraphic language" as if to economize on words.

The word-finding difficulty is also a measure of fluency. It is encountered in almost all PWA. It is manifested by repetition of determiners (a, an, the), prepositions (this, that, which, so), other functional or grammatical units (and, yes), vocal and gestural mannerisms ("uh", pointing toward something), circumlocution, paraphasia, neologism, and jargon.

Many PWA can fluently recite overlearned lists (automatized sequences) such as counting, alphabets, days of the week, and months of a year, while the rest of the verbal output may be very nonfluent. The same is true for singing and uttering curse words and swear words.

Category fluency test requires the patient to think and speak names or words belonging to one specific *semantic category* within 1 minute, e.g., animals, vegetables, fruits, sweets, instruments, and vehicles. We may ask PWA to alternate between categories, such as clothes and furniture, to make the task more complex.

Another fluency test is to ask the person to think and speak rapidly, words beginning with specific letters within 1 minute, e.g., F or A or S.

Fluent but empty speech: Suppose one listens to the speech of a person with fluent aphasia from a distance, ignoring the actual content; in that case, it appears effortless, with typical melody, *accent*, *prosody*, and mannerisms. However, on close observation, the content is empty and abnormal. *Phrases* and sentences are of average length or sometimes overly lengthy. The patient fails to know when to stop. They may speak excessively (logorrhea), unaware of the abnormality. There are many paraphasias, circumlocutions, and an abundance of function or grammar words whose information load is low. The *content words*, which carry information, are scarce and are used, flouting the rules of grammar. Jargon is common. Such patients have profound defects in auditory and reading comprehension. A classic example is Wernicke's aphasia.

Discourse Analysis

As per the Merriam-Webster Dictionary, "discourse (noun)" is defined as "the verbal interchange of ideas, especially during conversation, expression of thought on a subject, connected speech or writing."

Discourse is a linguistic unit (such as a conversation or a story) larger than a sentence. It is an intransitive verb, too, meaning "to express oneself, especially in oral discourse", *to talk and converse.*

Spoken discourse is a fundamental form of communication, often disrupted in PWA and other neurogenic communication disorders. Discourse analysis is important for understanding language, its impairments, and language recovery in these populations. However, it is beyond the scope of this chapter. A neurologist should help SLP colleagues with discourse analysis by audio recording testing and conversation.[33]

Discourse analysis is time-consuming with an overwhelming and wide range of measures for the clinicians, such as the number of *T-units* and total words produced or *pragmatic protocol checklists.*[34,35]

Auditory Comprehension

Some ideas about a PWA's capacity to understand whatever is being spoken around him could have been obtained during history taking.

Command Comprehension

If a patient merely shows the tongue on command, nods the head this or that way, or responds to a question, that does not mean normal auditory comprehension. Further testing is needed through several tasks. Each command must be stated only once, at a slow and regular rate and not repeated piecemeal.

While giving a command, the examiner and bystanders must not help by gestures.

At the sentence level, command comprehension can be complicated by involving more than one step, e.g., *"Fold this piece of paper and put it into your pocket", "Pick up the piece of cloth, put it into the glass, and then invert the glass on the table."*

Pointing Test of Auditory Comprehension at the One-word Level

The examiner speaks out the word and asks the patient to point to the corresponding picture, object, or body part. The clinician scores the patient's performance in terms of correct answers, taking into account all the help or *cue*s and time latency. Some patients may perform poorly at the single-word level (identification by pointing) but better in sentence comprehension during day-to-day life, as meanings may be discernible through the context and redundancy of words.

Yes–No Questions

"Does the stone sink in water?", "Is an elephant larger than an ant?" Not uncommonly, many patients performing reasonably well in daily household communication through gestures fail miserably in these formal testing modes.

Picture–Sentence Matching Tasks

Picture–Sentence matching tasks use one sentence, many picture choices, and vice versa.

Discourse Level Comprehension

The clinician narrates a short story and asks questions based on it.

Repetition

The examiner asks the patient to repeat words, *nonwords*, *phrases*, and sentences after him. Initial *stimuli* are simple, short, and *high frequency*; later, they are long, hard to pronounce, and *low frequency*. The errors may be sound distortions, incomplete responses, deletions, or paraphasias. Some patients may perform well on auditory comprehension tests and do well during daily life but fail miserably on repeating simple words or *phrases* (conduction aphasia). In contrast, patients with transcortical sensory and mixed aphasia repeat long, complex *phrases* mechanically or slavishly. Still, they do not follow or extract a bit of meaning from whatever they are listening to and repeating.

Naming

Naming is not just telling the names of family members and friends. It is a broad concept that entails the ability to generate authentic, correct, and well-pronounced words in response to needs in communication, expression, and writing in daily life.

One begins with *naming* objects, pictures, body parts, or persons. The images used during auditory comprehension serve the purpose again, with a reversal of roles. Now the examiner puts her finger on the object or picture and asks PWA to name it. "Responsive *naming*" involves simple questions with an unambiguous one-word answer like, *"what do we call a person who delivers a letter at home."* Some PWA may fail, or there may be a delay. Sometimes the *response word* may be altered yet related to the target word by sound (phonemic paraphasia) or meaning (semantic paraphasia). The *response word* may be phonemic jargon (nonword) or semantic jargon (dictionary word but unconnected). Some patients may describe the word in a roundabout way (circumlocution). The clinician should give *cue*s or hints. The phonemic *cue* means uttering the first one or two *phonemes* of the word or producing its rhythm. Semantic *cue* involves indicating synonyms or attributes of that word. In case of persistent failure, the examiner then offers the answer by (1) suggesting a wrong answer and asking if it is correct or not and (2) suggesting the correct answer and again looking if the patient accepts it or not.

Reading

The reading tests and, to some degree, those for writing in aphasic alexia and agraphia overlap with tests for developmental dyslexia.[36-38]

The clinician tests the patient's ability to recognize, match, and discriminate the graphic symbols of alphabets. She asks PWA to read aloud words, *phrases*, or paragraphs, not necessarily paying attention to the meaning. Reading comprehension involves word-picture or word-object matching and carrying out some commands printed on a piece of paper (e.g., *touch your hair* and *make a fist*). A somewhat difficult task is to fill in the blanks in progressively complex sentences from amongst a choice of detractors. The PWA reads lengthy paragraphs (unseen passages) and is asked to write answers to questions based on them. The patient can be asked to sort words and nonwords from a mixed list.

Writing

A PWA with reasonably good motor dexterity of a hand should be able to reproduce his premorbid handwriting, at least in such mechanical tasks as copying from written *stimuli*, writing to dictation, and serial writing of automatized sequences (such as name, address, numbers, alphabets, weekdays, and months). However, patients with nonfluent aphasia fail in written expression too. In addition to various aspects of verbal nonfluency (reduced output, laborious start, pauses, and *agrammatism*), the mechanics of writing and calligraphy are also distorted. The writing of persons with fluent aphasia may be legible and well-formed, but the written expression will exhibit deficits of emptiness, paraphasias, jargon, circumlocution, etc. Picture *naming*, object *naming*, and describing events in a painted or sketched scene are further tests of written expression.

WHAT ELSE OTHER THAN SPEECH AND LANGUAGE?

Patient's Educational and Working Status

It is important to document the educational status of the patient in terms of number of years, subjects, degrees, and academic excellence. Working status refers to the type(s) of part and current jobs and occupation or being retired. Such information is necessary to set the goals for therapy.

Language Proficiencies

We in India have an exceptional opportunity to explore the effect of the same lesions on persons who speak structurally distinct languages. Aphasia in *multilingual* speakers poses special challenges. It becomes imperative to assess all the languages used by PWA. The clinical profile of aphasia may vary in the two or more languages used by PWA. Cross-language codeshifting and code-switching (shifting between vocabulary and grammar of different languages) are very common in Indian bi and *multilinguals* with aphasia, making it difficult to compare the performance across languages. A *standardized* assessment in all the languages the PWA uses is an important requirement in its own right and is also crucial for theoretical aspects and therapeutic planning.[39,40] The *bilingual* aphasia test is available in nine Indian languages but is lengthy.[41] Language Experience and Proficiency Questionnaire (LEAP-Q) is an internationally acclaimed objective tool for assessing the efficiency and use of languages in bi- or *multilingual* persons.[42] A Hindi version by the present author has been acknowledged and added to the host website of LEAP-Q.

Handedness

A PWA's handedness affects cerebral dominance of language function between the right and the left hemispheres. Neurologists must use a standard and valid battery to determine right- versus left-handedness degrees.[43] The present author has created a Hindi-English *bilingual* questionnaire for scoring handedness.

Communication in Daily Life

The scores obtained on formal aphasia tests (as measured on popular test batteries) and the actual communicative performance in daily life often vary. To test for the latter, we use a different set of batteries.[44]

Quality of Life and Psychosocial Issues: Aphasia Assessment and the International Classification of Functioning, Disability, and Health

The international classification of functioning, disability, and health (ICF)—developed by the World Health Organization (WHO)—is a framework to address functioning and disability related to a health condition within the context of the individual's activities and participation in everyday life.[45]

Applying ICF to the assessment of PWA and their family/carers leads to addressing all domains of *functioning* and disability and defines the person-centered and family-centered functional goals. The goals identified by the PWA, in partnership with the clinician and family, allow participation in meaningful activities and roles. Person-centered functional goals help in maximizing the outcomes that lead to functional improvements that are important and meaningful to the individual.[46]

It is essential to measure "QOL" in PWA to identify patients' problems, determine treatment priorities, manage interventions, and monitor disease periods. Indian questionnaires have been developed and validated for this purpose and should be part of the assessment protocol for aphasia.[47,48]

Anxiety and depression are common in PWA and interfere with therapy and rehabilitation. Simple and valid tools for assessing these mental states should also be part of testing for aphasia.[49]

Caregiver Burden

Caregivers' burden in supporting PWA may sometimes appear trivial and mutually satisfying, particularly in cultures (like India) where family values are held high. However, in the long term, it may be unbearable. Aphasia QOL studies should include "caregiver burden" and "supportive communication strategies" used by SOs and report them separately.[2,50] Caregivers have to double up as facilitators for home-based therapy and during therapy in the clinic.[51] Clinical tales or patient stories written by patients, caregivers, and clinicians may be compiled and published.[52,53]

Cognitive Functions

Aphasia is not an exclusively language-related problem.[54] Other cognitive functions, such as working memory, short-term memory, recent memory, attention, executive skills, sensory perception, motor dexterity, apraxia, agnosia, and spatial orientation, are simultaneously affected.[55] Aphasic deficits may be seen as impairments to working memory. It is very challenging to assess impairments in various aspects of cognition in a person whose comprehension and expression are affected.[56]

APHASIA SYNDROMES, THEIR IRREVERENCE, AND NEWER METHODS OF ASSESSMENT

Syndromic classifications **(Flowchart 1)** have been helpful as a shorthand summary of a patient's language disorder. However, syndromes have lost their theoretical and practical relevance.[57] Newer classifications based on *neurolinguistics* and cognitive neuropsychology require modifications in methods of clinical examination. We must adopt a deficit-based approach instead of syndrome based. SLPs and researchers are using ingenious and experimental ways of testing the competence and performance of PWA based on the cognitive neuropsychological model of language **(Flowchart 2)**.

Aphasiologists can take a *cue* from epileptology, wherein the classification of seizures has been revised. More emphasis is on seizure semiology rather than pigeon-holing subjects into a straitjacket of categories. Something like video monitoring has happened in aphasiology. Data from single patients have become the basis for cognitive neuropsychological research and therapy.[58]

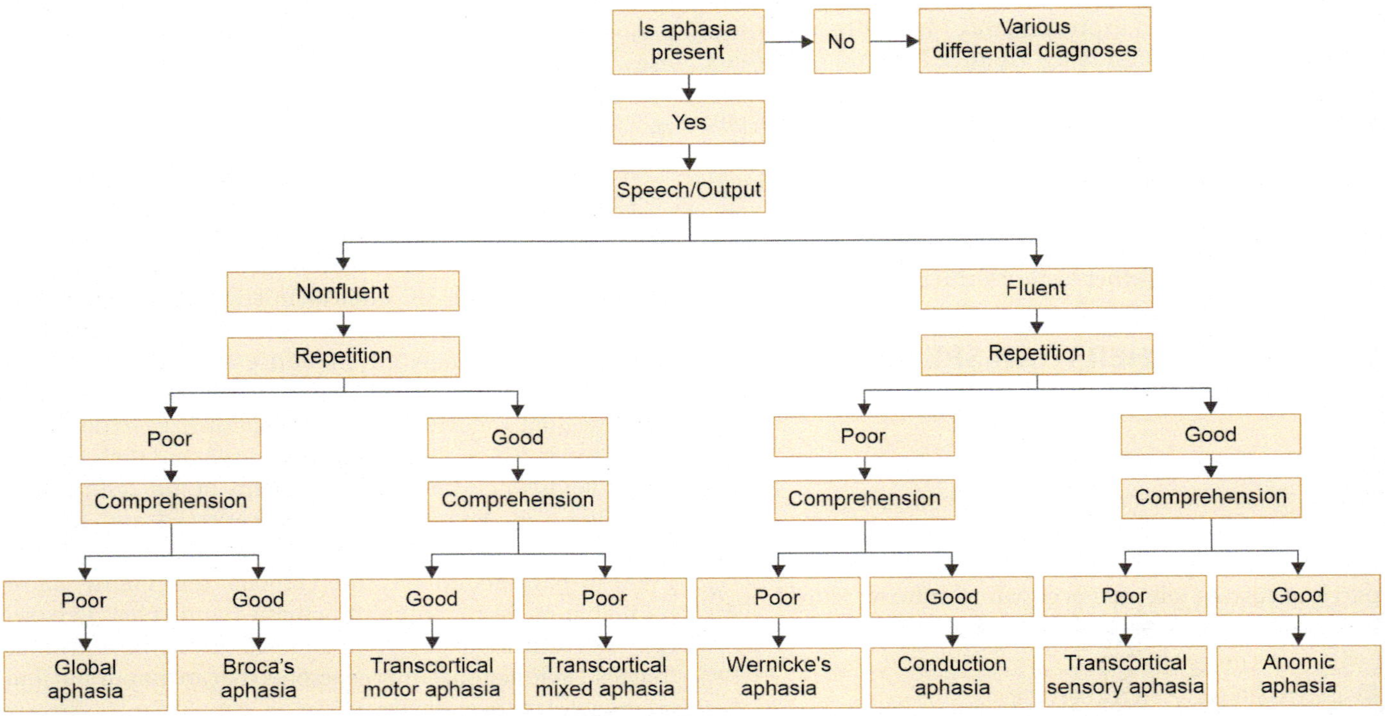

FLOWCHART 1: Aphasia syndrome diagnosis. Three dichotomous questions lead to the diagnosis of eight aphasia syndromes: (1) Is the speech fluent or nonfluent? (2) Is repetition good or poor? (3) Is auditory comprehension good or poor?

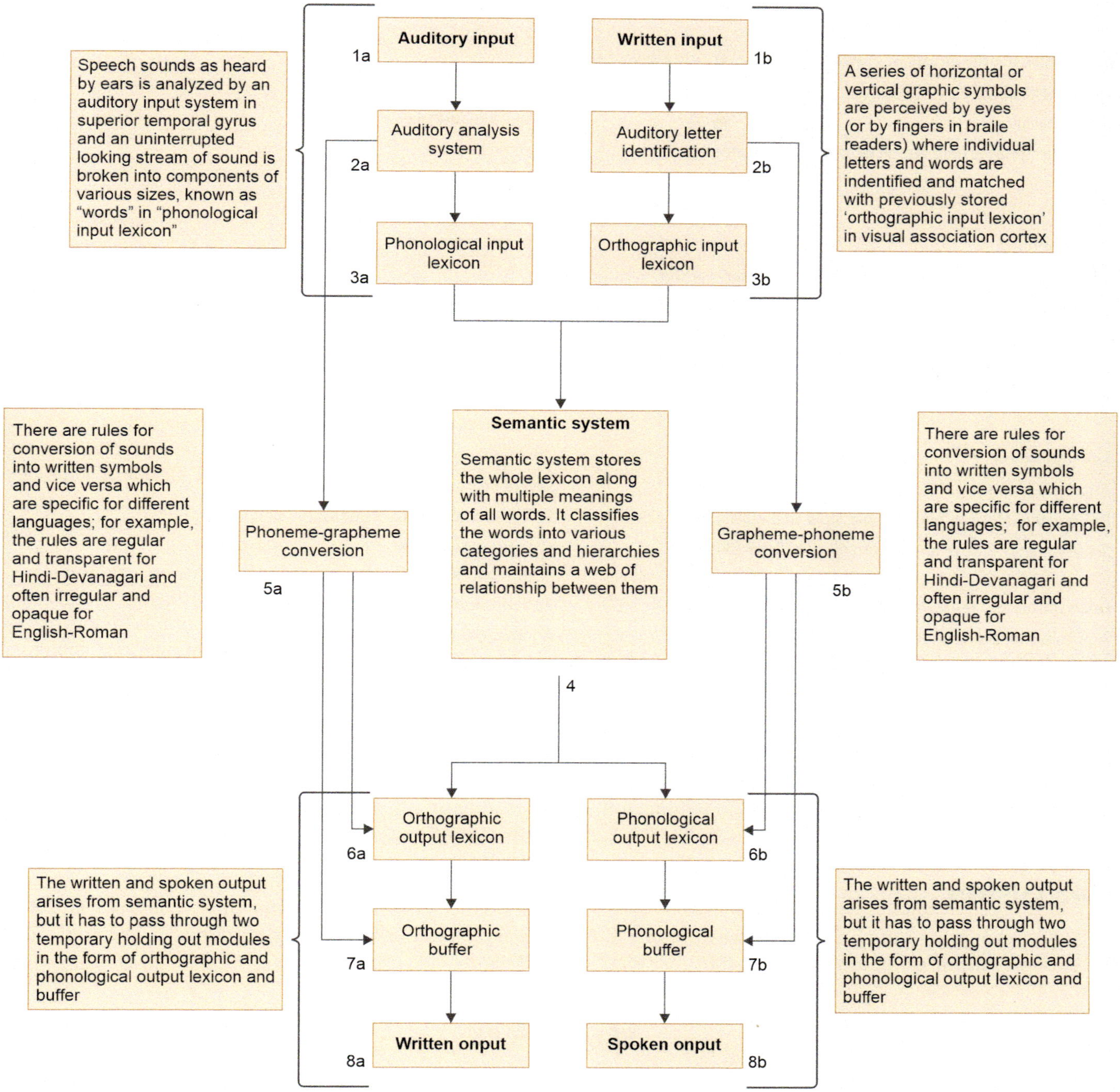

FLOWCHART 2: Cognitive neuropsychological model of language organization in the brain. A general neurologist need not memorize the model but should be aware that such frameworks lead to additional aphasia testing and *profiling* methods. It helps to localize the defect (not lesion on imaging) at one or more of the boxes and arrows in the model, leading to the choice of therapy.

DIFFERENTIAL DIAGNOSIS

It is beyond the scope of this chapter to discuss the differential diagnosis. However, it is necessary to emphasize that aphasia is a clinical diagnosis, and there are no laboratory tests. The differentiation relies on a more comprehensive and repeated examination and considering the overall picture. While clinically examining a PWA, the neurologist will tailor and modify the assessment methods so as not to make errors in diagnosis **(Table 5)**.

Psychogenic syndromes (conversion or dissociative states, catatonia) can also render a person speechless for a variable period. Impaired fluency during a conversation but not during formal verbal fluency tests following a minor cerebral concussion should raise suspicion about motivation and secondary gains. The same applies if

TABLE 5: Differential diagnosis.

Not to miss the diagnosis of aphasia when presenting a true diagnosis	
True diagnosis	**Mistaken for**
Mild aphasia	Normal variation
Receptive aphasia, mild Wernicke, pure word deafness	Impaired hearing
Anomia	Amnesia
Alexia	Visual impairment
Jargon aphasia	Delirium, psychosis
Not to make a false-positive diagnosis of aphasia when not present	
True diagnosis	**Mistaken for**
Developmental disorders of speech, learning disability	Aphasia, alexia
Developmental suppression of motor fluency, stuttering	Nonfluent aphasia
Hearing impairment, congenital deaf mutism	• Receptive aphasia • Global aphasia
Pure dysarthria	Nonfluent aphasia
Anarthria, mutism	Severe Broca's aphasia
Psychogenic: Mutism, hypophonia, slow speech, atypical halting	Severe Broca's or global aphasia
Schizophrenia: Bizarre and absurd speech, flight of ideas	• Jargon speech • Wernicke's (fluent) aphasia
Delirium, altered sensorium, muttering	Aphasia, anomia, jargon speech
Amnesia, Korsakoff syndrome	Anomia, paraphasia
Apraxia: Fails to comply with the command	Receptive aphasia

speech impairment develops many weeks or months after the event and if it keeps worsening. Another marker is the inconsistency of paraphasic errors for a particular sound. If a nearly mute person can express well in writing, it may indicate a functional disorder.

CONCLUSION

An expert group meeting on aphasia was organized by the present author on behalf of the Indian Academy of Neurology.[59] SLPs, clinical neuropsychologists, linguists, and imaging and computer professionals participated along with neurologists. It was realized that assessment or testing of aphasia in India needs much improvement and joint efforts. There are no shortcuts. It needs time, patience, experience, and commitment from neurologists and colleagues. Practice helps. Repeated drills enhance the quality of testing in lesser time. The PWA and SOs deserve a lot more from neurologists. We must not fail them.

REFERENCES

1. Engelter ST, Gostynski M, Papa S, Frei M, Born C, Ajdacic-Gross V, et al. Epidemiology of aphasia attributable to first ischemic stroke: incidence, severity, fluency, etiology, and thrombolysis. Stroke. 2006;37:1379-84.
2. Rehabilitation and Recovery of People With Aphasia After Stroke (RELEASE) Collaborators. Predictors of poststroke aphasia recovery: a systematic review-informed individual participant data meta-analysis. Stroke. 2021;52(5):1778-87.
3. Peitz D, Schumann-Werner B, Hussmann K, Chen H, Radermacher I, Binkofski F, et al. (2021). Predictors of therapy outcome after intensive treatment in post-acute and chronic aphasia. [online] Available from https://easychair.org/smart-program/AoA2021/2021-10-26.html. [Last accessed December, 2022].
4. Prasad K, Pauranik A, Neelakshi AB. An evidence-based clinical neurological examination. In: Banerjee D, Pauranik A (Eds). Progress in Clinical Neurosciences, volume 24. Delhi: Byword Books; 2010. pp. 3-17.
5. Ivanova MV, Hallowell B. A tutorial on aphasia test development in any language: key substantive and psychometric considerations. Aphasiology. 2013;27:891-920.
6. Rohde A, Worrall L, Godecke E, O'Halloran R, Farrell A, Massey M. Diagnosis of aphasia in stroke populations: a systematic review of language tests. PloS one. 2018;13(3):e0194143.
7. Wallace SJ, Worrall L, Le Dorze G, Brandenburg C, Foulkes J, Rose TA. Many ways of measuring: a scoping review of measurement instruments for use with people with aphasia. Aphasiology. 2022;36(4):401-66.
8. Keshree NK, Kumar S, Basu S, Chakrabarty M, Kishore T. Adaptation of the western aphasia battery in Bangla. Psychology of language and communication. 2013;17(2):189.

9. Chengappa SK, Kumar R. (2008). Normative and clinical data on the Kannada version of western aphasia battery (WAB-K). [online] Available from http://www.languageinindia.com/june2008/normativechengappa.pdf. [Last accessed December, 2022].
10. Kaur H, Bajpai S, Pershad D, Sreenivas V, Nehra A. Development and standardization of Indian aphasia battery. J Mental Health Hum Behav. 2017;22(2):116.
11. Bhatnagar S. Aphasia in the Indian context: An Indigenously Developed Aphasia Test Battery in Hindi. In: Continuing Medical Education Proceedings (Ed). Banaras: Neurological Society of India; 1984. pp. 183-219.
12. Nagendar K, Ravindra S. Adaptation of Mississippi aphasia screening test to Telugu language. J All India Inst Speech Hear. 2012;31:827.
13. Shah J, Karna SL, Verma H. Construction of western aphasia battery in Nepali: a pilot study. J Neurobehav Sci. 2020;7(2):47.
14. Nehra A, Pershad D, Sreenivas V. Indian aphasia battery: tool for specific diagnosis of language disorder post stroke. J Neurol Sci. 2013;333:e165.
15. Kumar S, Goswami SP. Development of syntax comprehension test in the Hindi language for persons with aphasia. Language In India. 2013;13(8):346.
16. Mazumdar B, Donovan NJ, Narang V. Sociolinguistic adaptation process of the Bangla Western aphasia battery-revised. J Indian Speech Lang Hear Assoc. 2018;32(1):23.
17. Lingraphica. Aphasia assessment tools. [online] Available from https://www.aphasia.com/clinical-guides/aphasia-assessment-tools/. [Last accessed December, 2022].
18. El Hachioui H, Visch-Brink EG, de Lau LM, van de Sandt-Koenderman MW, Nouwens F, Koudstaal PJ, et al. Screening tests for aphasia in patients with stroke: a systematic review. J Neurol. 2017;264: 211-20.
19. Enderby P, Crow E. Frenchay aphasia screening test: validity and comparability. Disabil Rehabil. 1996;18(5):238-40.
20. Paplikar A, Iyer GK, Varghese F, Alladi S, Pauranik A, Mekala S, et al. A screening tool to detect stroke aphasia: adaptation of Frenchay aphasia screening test (FAST) to the Indian context. Ann Indian Acad Neurol. 2020;23(Suppl 2):S143.
21. Iyer GK, Alladi S, Dutt A, Ellajosyula R, Ghosh A, Kaul S, et al; on behalf of the ICMR working group for the study of vascular cognitive impairment in India. Harmonizing cognitive assessment across six languages and different educational levels using the ICMR VCI neuropsychological test battery. 2014.
22. Spreen O, Risser AH. Assessment of Aphasia. Oxford: Oxford University Press; 2003.
23. Kertesz A. The western aphasia battery: a systematic review of research and clinical applications. Aphasiology. 2022;36(1):21-50.
24. Tombaugh TN, Hubiey AM. The 60-item Boston *naming* test: norms for cognitively intact adults aged 25 to 88 years. J Clin Exp Neuropsychol. 1997;19(6):922-32.
25. Fong MW, Van Patten R, Fucetola RP. The factor structure of the Boston diagnostic aphasia examination. J Int Neuropsychol Soc. 2019;25(7):772-6.
26. Forbes MM, Fromm D, MacWhinney B. AphasiaBank: a resource for clinicians. Seminars in speech and language. 2012;33(3):217-22.
27. Cho-Reyes S, Thompson CK. Verb and sentence production and comprehension in aphasia: northwestern assessment of verbs and sentences (NAVS). Aphasiology. 2012;26(10):1250-77.
28. Erdodi LA, Tyson BT, Abeare CA, Lichtenstein JD, Pelletier CL, Rai JK, et al. The BDAE complex ideational material—a measure of receptive language or performance validity. Psychol Inj Law. 2016;9(2):112-20.
29. Holland A, Forbes M, Fromm D, MacWhinney B. Communicative strengths in severe aphasia: the famous people protocol and its value in planning treatment. Am J Speech Lang Pathol. 2019;28(3):1010-8.
30. Swinburn K, Porter G, Howard D. Comprehensive Aphasia Test. Oxfordshire: Routledge; 2004.
31. Kay J, Lesser R, Coltheart M. Psycholinguistic assessments of language processing in aphasia (PALPA): an introduction. Aphasiology. 1996;10(2):159-80.
32. Neuroscience. Aphasia (aphasia, speech paralysis). [online] Available from http://neurogyan2.arth-dhwani.com/aphasia. [Last accessed December, 2022].
33. Pauranik A. Narrative discourse in healthy controls, aphasia, and dementia. Ann India Acad Neurol. 2008;11.
34. Dalton SG, Hubbard HI, Richardson JD. Moving toward non-transcription based discourse analysis in stable and progressive aphasia. Seminars in speech and language. 2020;41(01):032-44).
35. Kong AP. Analysis of Neurogenic Disordered Discourse Production: From Theory to Practice. Oxfordshire: Routledge; 2016.
36. Nelson HE. (1982). National adult reading test (NART): test manual for the assessment of premorbid intelligence in patients with dementia. [online] Available from https://www.academia.edu/2515150/National_Adult_Reading_Test_NART_test_manual_Part_1. [Last accessed December, 2022].
37. Karanth P. Analysis of acquired reading disorders in Kannada. J All India Inst Speech Hear. 1984;15:65-76.
38. Singh NC. DALI: Dyslexia Assessment for Languages in India. Manesar: National Brain Research Centre; 2015.
39. Sebastian D. Multilingual aphasia: an unresolved puzzle in the linguistic mosaic of India. Perspectives on global issues in communication sciences and related disorders. 2014;4(1):30-8.
40. Paradis M. Principles underlying the *bilingual* aphasia test (BAT) and its uses. Clin Linguist Phon. 2011;25:427-43.
41. Krishnan G, Mathew RE. A short version of the bilingual aphasia test in Malayalam. Ann Indian Acad Neurol. 2017;20:217-9.
42. Marian V, Blumenfeld HK, Kaushanskaya M. (2007). The language experience and proficiency questionnaire (LEAP-Q): assessing language profiles in bilinguals and multilinguals. [online] Available from https://pubs.asha.org/doi/10.1044/1092-4388%282007/067%29. [Last accessed December, 2022].
43. Gloning K. Handedness and aphasia. Neuropsychologia. 1977;15(2): 355-8.
44. Stahl B, Mohr B, Dreyer FR, Lucchese G, Pulvermüller F. Communicative–pragmatic assessment is sensitive and time effective in measuring the outcome of aphasia therapy. Front Hum Neurosci. 2017;11:223.
45. Worrall L, Sherratt S, Rogers P, Howe T, Hersh D, Ferguson A, et al. What people with aphasia want: their goals according to the ICF. Aphasiology. 2010;25:309-22.
46. Hersh D, Worrall L, Howe T, Sherratt S, Davidson B. SMARTER goal setting in aphasia rehabilitation. Aphasiology. 2012;26:220-33.
47. Hillari K, Byng S, Lamping DL, Smith SC. Stroke and aphasia quality of life scale–39 (SAQOL-39). Evaluation of acceptability, reliability, and validity. Stroke. 2003;34:1944-50.
48. Mitra IH, Krishnan G. Adaptation and validation of stroke–aphasia quality of life (SAQOL-39) scale to Hindi. Ann Indian Acad Neurol. 2015;18(1):29.
49. Kaur H, Chopra S, Pandey RM, Bhatia R, Nehra A. Translation and adaptation of stroke aphasia depression questionnaire-10 to Hindi. Ann Indian Acad Neurol. 2017;20(2):153.
50. Rombough RE, Howse EL, Bartfay WJ. Caregiver strain and caregiver burden of primary caregivers of stroke survivors with and without aphasia. Rehabil Nurs. 2006;31(5):199-209.
51. Singh P, Pauranik A. Supportive conversational strategies for persons with aphasia and their significant others. J Indian Speech Lang Hear Assoc. 2017;31:57.
52. Grawburg M, Howe T, Worrall L, Scarinci N. Third-party disability in family members of people with aphasia: a systematic review. Disabil Rehabil. 2013;35:1324-41.

53. Singh P, Pauranik A. The diversity of burden for significant others of a person with aphasia. J All India Inst Speech Hear. 2013;32: 167-72.
54. Fonseca J, Raposo A, Martins IP. Cognitive functioning in chronic poststroke aphasia. Appl Neuropsychol Adult. 2019;26(4):355-64.
55. Weintraub S, Dikmen SS, Heaton RK, Tulsky DS, Zelazo PD, Bauer PJ, et al. Cognition assessment using the NIH toolbox. Neurology. 2013;80:S54-64.
56. Wall KJ, Cumming TB, Copland AD. Determining the association between language and cognitive tests in poststroke aphasia. Front Neurol. 2017;8:149.
57. Kasselimis DS, Simos PG, Peppas C, Evdokimidis I, Potagas C. The unbridged gap between clinical diagnosis and contemporary research on aphasia: a short discussion on the validity and clinical utility of taxonomic categories. Brain Lang. 2017;164:63-7.
58. Whitworth A, Webster J, Howard D. A Cognitive Neuropsychological Approach to Assessment and Intervention in Aphasia: A Clinician's Guide. New York: Psychology Press; 2005.
59. Pauranik A, George A, Sahu A, Nehra A, Paplikar A, Bhat C, et al. (2019). Expert group meeting: aphasia – a report. [online] Available from https://aphasia.talkbank.org/publications/2019/Pauranik19.pdf. [Last accessed December, 2022].

5 CHAPTER

Testing the Cranial Nerves (I–VI)

Vinny Wilson, Vikram Asturkar, Arindam Mukherjee

CRANIAL NERVE I (OLFACTORY NERVE)

Introduction

The first cranial nerve is often ignored during cranial nerve examination partly because testing forms the least satisfactory part of the whole examination. And yet, examining the first cranial nerve can provide important clues to an underlying intracranial lesion.

Relevant Anatomy

First-order neurons: Bipolar sensory cells which lie in the olfactory epithelium, which occupies a small area on the superior nasal concha, upper nasal septum, and roof of the nose. Their peripheral ramifications are ciliated processes that penetrate the mucus membrane of the upper nasal cavity and cribriform plate of ethmoid bone and synapse with mitral and tuft cells. The second-order neurons, which reside mainly in the mitral cells, course posteriorly through olfactory tracts, which lie in olfactory grooves beneath the frontal lobes on the floor of the anterior cranial fossa.[1]

The olfactory tracts divide into medial and lateral olfactory striae that run on either side of the anterior perforated substance. Fibers of medial olfactory striae terminate in the medial surface of the cerebral hemisphere in the paraolfactory area, subcallosal gyrus, and inferior part of the cingulate gyrus. The lateral olfactory striae terminate in the uncus, anterior hippocampal gyrus, pyriform area, ethmoidal area, and amygdaloid nucleus. These structures are collectively referred to as the primary olfactory cortex. The parahippocampal gyrus sends impulses to the hippocampus, which further project to anterior hypothalamic nucleus mamillary bodies, which in turn project to the anterior nucleus of thalamus, cingulate gyrus, and mesencephalic reticular formation.[1]

Cranial Nerve Function

The olfactory nerve is a purely sensory nerve that subserves one function—smell.

The olfactory system works by way of chemosensory signal transduction. Specific odorants stimulate specific receptor cells. Only volatile substances soluble in lipid or water are perceived as odor. Olfactory information is processed in primitive areas of the brain and phylogenetically ancient system. Olfaction is the only sensation not directly processed in the thalamus.[2]

Objectives of Testing

- To detect any impairment of loss of smell sensation
- To detect whether the defect is unilateral or bilateral
- To detect whether the defect is a conductive deficit or sensorineural or neurogenic deficit

Method of Testing

Examine each nostril separately while occluding the other. Test substances used for smell can be clove, coffee, cinnamon, or oil of wintergreen present in mouthwash; soap can be used at the bedside. With the patient's eyes closed and one nostril occluded, bring the test substance near the open one. Ask the patient to sniff and indicate whether he smells and if so identify it.[2]

Repeat for the other nostril and compare the two sides.

Pearls and Pitfalls

- Always test the abnormal side first.
- Always occlude the other side while testing.
- Always ask the patient to sniff with eyes closed.
- Smell is always tested using a nonirritant stimulus, and avoid noxious substances such as ammonia, which may stimulate the trigeminal nerve instead of the olfactory nerve.
- Decreased smell function is not always pathological since it can occur with aging in an otherwise healthy individual (presbyosmia).
- Anosmia may be the first indicator of the presence of a neurodegenerative disease such as Parkinson's disease or Alzheimer's disease.[3]

- Perception of odor is more important than accurate identification. Perceiving the presence of an odor indicates continuity of the olfactory pathway, and identification indicates cortical function as well.[4]

CRANIAL NERVE II (OPTIC NERVE)

Introduction

The optic nerve is different from other cranial nerves. It is not a peripheral nerve in the true sense of the word but part of a central nervous system (CNS) fiber pathway that connects the retina to the brain. Myelin in the optic nerve is CNS myelin and formed by oligodendroglia. It is also a unique cranial nerve in that it represents a window to the brain that can be examined directly with an ophthalmoscope.[2]

Relevant Anatomy

There are nearly 1.2 million ganglion cells. Axons of retinal ganglion cells form the retinal nerve fiber layer (NFL) that further extends as the optic nerve. The photoreceptor layer, the deepest part of the retina, contains rods and cones. Rods respond to low-intensity stimulation and play a crucial role in detecting perception of movement, peripheral vision, and mediating night vision. Cones concentrated around the macula are important for color vision. The macula is responsible for the central 15 degrees of vision, for discrimination of colors, and in discerning fine visual details. Optic disc is the visible tip of the intraocular part of the optic nerve.[2] In addition to carrying visual impulses, they also transmit the impulses that mediate accommodation and reflex responses to light and other stimuli. The optic nerve fibers exit the globe and continue till optic chiasma where the nasal fibers decussate, which results in the grouping of all fibers of each hemifield in the opposite optic tract. In the process of decussation, fibers from the inferior nasal quadrant loop forward into the opposite optic nerve for a short distance before turning back to form Wilbrand's knee. The chiasma lies about 10 mm above the pituitary gland, separated by the suprasellar cistern. The majority of fibers in the optic tract carry visual afferents (~80%) while the remaining carry pupillary afferents. The optic tracts extend further to later geniculate body (LGB). Pupillary afferent fibers leave the optic tract just anterior to LGB and enter the pretectal area of the midbrain.[2]

Cranial Nerve Function

- To carry visual afferent impulses from the retina to optic chiasma and further via the optic tract to LGB
- To carry the afferent reflex responses to light and other stimuli via fibers traveling to the pretectal area of the midbrain

Objectives of Testing

- To directly inspect a part of the optic nerve, the fundus
- To measure the acuity of vision and assess color vision
- To chart visual fields

Fundus Examination

Method of Testing

A neurologist needs a good ophthalmoscope, large pupil, and still field to peek into a narrow sector of the retina. It is in many ways peering one-eyed into a dark cave with a torch light. The routine fundus examination in neurologic patients is undertaken via an undilated pupil. Mydriatic drops should be avoided in conditions where the assessment of pupillary size and function is crucial. When mydriatic drops are used, they should be mentioned in the examination notes. It requires practice and skill, especially in the technically difficult situations where fundus examination is the most critical. The patient should be instructed to look at a distant object or a point. It helps to tell the patient to use his free eye to focus on the distant point.[5] The patient must be instructed not to look at the light of the ophthalmoscope. The ambient illumination in the room should be diminished to overcome the light reflex. The direct ophthalmoscope had dials to adjust the light apertures. The large apertures should be used for examining a dilated pupil and small apertures for examining an undilated pupil. The red free filter is used to examine the NFL and blood vessels. Use the right eye to examine the patient's right eye while holding the ophthalmoscope in the right hand. To examine the left eye, shift sides to the left of the patient, change the ophthalmoscope to the left hand, and examine with your left eye. The disc is normally round or slightly oval. The nasal margins are slightly blurred compared to the temporal. The physiological cup is a slight depression in the center of the disc. The rim is elevated slightly above the cup. Sometimes when the patient has not followed correct instructions, and when the disc does not immediately come into view, it helps to find a retinal vessel and follow it to the disc. The color of the normal disc is yellowish white and paler temporally. Changes in the color of the disc, size of the cup, obliteration of the cup, clarity of disc margins, pulsation of blood vessels over the disc, and hemorrhage, if any, should be noted.[5]

Visual Acuity

Method of Testing

While examining a patient with a neurological disorder, only the patient's best corrected visual acuity is important. For distant vision measurement, a Snellen chart placed at 6 m (20 ft) is used. The patient should close one eye. The distance allows relaxation of accommodation and renders the light rays nearly parallel. The ability to resolve test characters (1 inch in height) at 6 m is normal visual acuity (6/6 or 20/20). Acuity is the line on Snellen chart where more than half of the characters are accurately read. By convention, the distance from the chart is the numerator. In infants and children, acuity may be estimated by following movements, blink to threat or bright light or pupillary reflex. Vision <20/800 (equivalent being 5/200) should be described as counting fingers (CFs), hand motion (HM), light perception (LP), or no LP. Improvement of vision while looking through a pinhole suggests impairment related to a refractive error. A pinhole permits only central light rays to enter the eyes, which are less likely to be disrupted by refractory errors. Other test types include Jaeger type card and others, but the general principles remain the same.[5]

Color Vision

Method of Testing

Color deficits may be partial or total. Color plates or pseudoisochromatic plates, e.g., Ishihara, are used to formally assess color vision. Ask the patient to identify the colors in a fabric such as a sari or T-shirt for a crude estimate. Red perception is usually lost first. The patient is asked to compare the redness of a cap or some other red-colored object in each hemifield. The flight of color phenomenon is a series of color perception that follows shining a bright light into the eye is reduced or absent with impaired color perception.[5]

Visual Fields

Method of Testing

When testing by confrontation method, the patient and examiner face each other at the same eye level with 18–24 inches between their eyeballs. If the examiner covers one eye, say the right eye, then the patient should cover his left eye. The patient must fix carefully on the examiner's pupil as the examiner moves test objects of varying size inward in each of the four quadrants from a point that is just outside the limits of his field. The patient should say the moment he sees the object. The examiner should move the test object from blind areas to areas of vision. The normal visual field extends 90–100° temporally, about 60° nasally, 50–60° superiorly, and 60–75° inferiorly. When testing children, keys, candy, or other interesting objects may be used, who will glance at or reach for the object.[5]

Pearls and Pitfalls

- Obliquity of optic nerves can give the impression of disc swelling. The examiner may be similarly misled in the presence of Drusen bodies, juxtapapillary choroiditis, and haziness of the vitreous.
- Small disc where edges appear blurred may be due to hypermetropia.
- Large eyebrows or an overgrown nose may produce curious bilateral defects in visual fields.
- Be suspicious of the accuracy of the small and concentrically constricted field if visual acuity is adequate.
- It is worthwhile to compare the degree of visual deficit claimed with what the patient can do when not under scrutiny.

CRANIAL NERVES III, IV, AND VI (OCULOMOTOR NERVES)

Introduction

Oculomotor nerve (III), trochlear nerve (IV), and abducens nerve (VI) are conventionally examined together. These cranial nerves supply the extraocular muscles and mediate conjugate eye movements. The IIIrd cranial nerve also carries fibers for eyelid elevators and the parasympathetic fibers.

Relevant Anatomy

The four rectus muscles (medial, lateral, superior, and inferior) arise from the annulus of Zinn, in the orbital apex. Superior and inferior recti insert into the globe, along its anatomic axis, and act maximally when the eye is slightly abducted. Superior and inferior obliques insert into the globe posteriorly and at an angle of about 30° and exert maximal pull with the eye slightly adducted. Because of the posterior insertion, the superior oblique pulls the back of the eye up, producing a downgaze, and the inferior oblique pulls the back of the eye down, producing an upgaze.[2] For optimum visual fixation, the extraocular muscles work in pairs that are yoked together, as shown in **Figure 1**.

Oculomotor Nerve

The oculomotor nuclear complex is situated in the midbrain, the uppermost part of which is the Edinger Westphal nucleus, that supplies parasympathetic innervation to ciliary muscle and iris via ciliary ganglion. *Another single midline subnucleus, placed caudally, caters to the levator palpebrae muscles bilaterally.* Only the superior rectus is innervated by the contralateral medial subnucleus.[2]

The nerve exits the brain stem at the interpeduncular fossa of the midbrain anteriorly, runs forward and parallel to the posterior communicating artery, passes through the lateral wall of the cavernous sinus, and divides in two branches to enter orbit.

Trochlear Nerve

The trochlear nucleus, located just anterior to the aqueduct at the level of the inferior colliculus, sends fibers that decussate within the substance of the brain stem and exit from the dorsal surface. It has the longest intracranial course of any of the cranial nerves and lies near IIIrd nerve in the cavernous sinus. *Cranial nerve IV terminates on the superior oblique muscle on the side opposite the nucleus of origin.*[2]

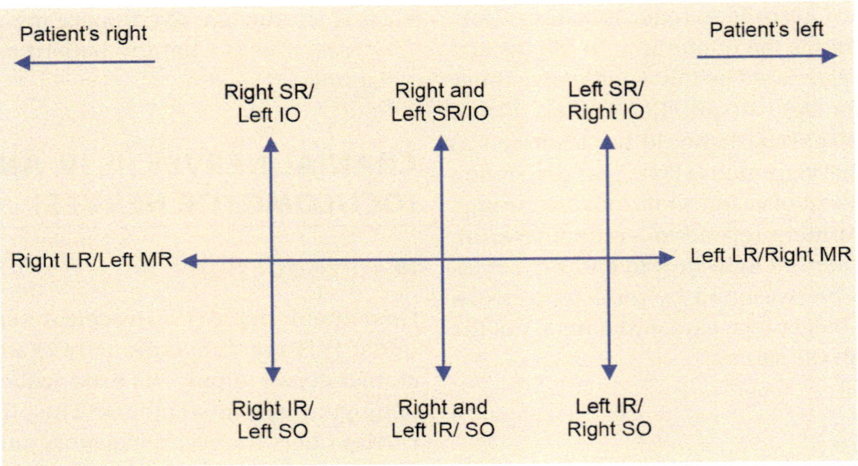

FIG. 1: Cardinal positions and yoke muscles.
(IO: inferior oblique; IR: inferior rectus; LR: lateral rectus; MR: medial rectus; SO: superior oblique; SR: superior rectus)

Abducens Nerve

The abducens nerve nucleus is situated in the pons within the floor of the fourth ventricle. The nucleus is encircled by the looping fibers of the facial nerve. The nerve exits anteriorly at the pontomedullary junction and crosses the internal auditory artery. It then passes over the surface of the clivus to enter the inferior petrosal sinus and then the cavernous sinus. It enters the orbit through the superior orbital fissure to supply the lateral rectus muscle.[2]

Understanding the Terminologies

Uniocular Movements (Ductions)

- *Abduction*: Outward horizontal movement of the eye along the vertical axis
- *Adduction*: Inward horizontal movement of the eye along the vertical axis
- *Supraduction (elevation)*: Upward movement of the eye along the horizontal axis
- *Infraduction (depression)*: Downward movement of the eye along the horizontal axis
- *Intorsion and extorsion*: Inward and outward rotation of the eyeball

Binocular Movements

- *Versions*: They are the conjugate movements of both eyes in the same direction.
- *Vergence*: They are the disconjugate movements of eyes, in which eyes move in the opposite direction to each other.
- *Strabismus (squint)*: It is the misalignment of the axis of both eyes.
- *Tropia*: It is the misalignment of both eyes while looking with both eyes uncovered.
- *Phoria (latent deviation)*: It is a misalignment of the eyes when binocular vision is broken, as can be detected by the cover–uncover test.

Objectives of Testing

- To perform a preliminary inspection of the eyes, examine ocular movements, and assess diplopia to determine the possible physiological and anatomical localizations of the lesion
- To detect and analyze nystagmus and other abnormal movements of the eyes
- To examine pupils for any abnormalities and determine whether the abnormality is because of local disease or autonomic involvement.

Methods of Testing

Inspection and Observation

The patient should be examined in a sitting position, and the examiner should be at eye level with the patient. Observe the position of the head during history taking. If the patient's head is turned to one side, it indicates horizontal diplopia. If head tilt is observed, it indicates vertical diplopia. The patient adopts these positions to minimize double vision.[6]

Note the position of both eyelids and their relation to the iris or cornea. Normally, the upper eyelid covers 1–2 mm of the cornea from the limbus, and the lower eyelid touches or just crosses the limbus. The palpebral fissure width is usually similar on both sides (normal is 9–12 mm). Note asymmetry in the position of eyelids. If asymmetry is noted, it indicates ptosis or lid retraction. When the cornea is covered partly or fully by the upper eyelid, it is ptosis, and when the upper eyelid is buried in the eyebrow revealing the sclera, it is called lid retraction. Ask the patient to open his eyes widely and notice the movements of eyelids as well as look for the frontalis muscle over action while elevating the upper eyelids. Frontalis contraction while looking straight ahead indicates the patient trying to compensate for ptosis. Determine whether the ptosis is partial or complete. Complete unilateral ptosis indicates IIIrd nerve palsy.[6]

Look for the protrusion of the eye or eyes. To assess exophthalmos, stand behind the patient, ask him/her to extend the neck slightly, and look down from above. Note the protrusion of the eyeballs on either side. Protrusion of eyes can also be assessed by standing by the side of the patient who is looking straight ahead and observing the bulge of eyes from both sides.

Examine the conjunctiva for congestion, hemorrhages, discoloration, or ulcers. Examine cornea for opacities, as it may further interfere in the assessment of vision and pupillary reaction. Examine the limbus of the cornea carefully for a color change. A golden-brown ring (Kayser–Fleischer ring), just inside the limbus, is diagnostic of hepatolenticular degeneration.[7]

Extraocular Movements

Ask the patient to look straight ahead at a distant object and observe the primary position of the eyes. Note any misalignment or abnormal movements in the primary position. Hold a finger or pen 50–100 cm in front of the patient's eyes and ask him/her to trace it as it moves. Move it slowly, in all nine cardinal directions, horizontally to right and left, vertically upward and downward in the midline, and when the eyes deviate to one side. Make sure that the finger or pen is held perpendicular to the axis of movement. The normal range of eye movements is about 45° to either side of the primary position. Normally at the terminal horizontal movements, the limbus gets buried in the corner of the eyes. Note down the observations as follows: (1) primary position of eyes, (2) lagging of one or both the eyes, (3) restriction of eye movements, (4) assess diplopia, and (5) abnormal movements.[7]

Diplopia Assessment

During the assessment of extraocular movements, look for the misalignment of the eyes and ask the patient whether he is perceiving a single image or two images. In the case of diplopia, one of the two images is false, and it appears less distinct. As the eyes move in the direction of action of the paretic muscle, the distance between the true and false images increases, and the false image becomes more peripheral and fainter. The false image comes from the paretic eye. There are different methods to detect false image. In the cover test, ask the patient to look in the direction where diplopia is maximum and cover one eye. If the more peripheral image disappears, the covered eye is the abnormal eye. Other tests are the red glass test and Maddox rod test. Prepare a diplopia chart and observe the following things: (1) Whether the diplopia is monocular or binocular, (2) Displacement of images, whether horizontal or vertical or a combination of both, (3) Whether the diplopia is present in the primary position or a particular gaze, (4) Whether the diplopia is more for near objects or distant objects, and (5) Notice the direction in which the distance between two images is maximum.[5]

For assessing pursuit movements move the finger, held at a 1-m distance in front of the patient's eyes, in a + pattern from the primary position. Notice whether the movements are smooth or jerky. To assess voluntary saccadic movements, sit in front of the patient at about a 1-m distance and hold up two fingers, one to the left of the center and the other to the right. Ask the patient to shift focus from one finger to another rapidly. Similarly, hold the fingers in vertical directions and ask the patient to look up and down. Observe undershooting, overshooting, or correction movements.[5]

Nystagmus

Method of Testing

Start observing the patient's eyes for any abnormal movements while taking history itself. Ask the patient to fix eyes on a specific object such as the examiner's finger or the tip of a pen held in front in the midline. Slowly move the object horizontally to right and then to left. Avoid moving objects to the extremes of gaze. Move the object not more than 30° from the midline. Similarly, assess for nystagmus in vertical directions from the midline. Hold the object in deviated position for at least 5 seconds. If not visibly obvious, low-amplitude nystagmus can be detected during fundus examination using an ophthalmoscope. Note down the following observations: (1) nystagmus or other abnormal movements in primary position, (2) assess the effect of gaze on nystagmus, (3) whether it is horizontal, vertical, torsional, or mixed nystagmus, (4) whether it is jerky or pendular nystagmus, (5) direction of fast component, (6) compare nystagmus in each eye, (7) degree of nystagmus, (8) is it associated with any ocular or gaze palsy, and (9) central or peripheral origin.[5]

Grades of Nystagmus

- *Grade 1*: Only when looking in the direction of the quick component
- *Grade 2*: If it is also present when looking straight ahead
- *Grade 3*: It is present when looking in the direction of the quick component, when looking straight ahead and when looking in the direction of the slow component

Optokinetic Nystagmus

At the bedside it is tested using optokinetic nystagmus (OKN) rotating drum or OKN tape. OKN drum, marked with the alternate black and white stripes, is rotated in front of the patient's eyes. Observe the smooth pursuit movements in the direction of rotation and the contralateral correcting saccades, occurring in succession till the time drum is rotating. Rotate the drum in opposite direction and observe similar movements. OKN is tested primarily to differentiate between the lesion in the occipital lobe or parietal lobe. It can also be used to make a crude assessment of vision in infants or patients with altered sensorium. It can be useful in assessing psychogenic blindness.[2]

Pupil Examination

The pupils should be checked for size, shape, regularity, and equality on both sides. The size of the pupils depends on the illumination of the examination room. The normal pupil size varies from 2 to 6 mm, and can be measured with a millimeter ruler.

Check for equality of pupils on both sides. The difference in the size of the pupils of two eyes is called anisocoria. The anisocoria can be physiological. More than a 2-mm difference in the size of pupils is considered significant. In physiological anisocoria, the inequality in the size of pupils is not affected by the ambient light, and the difference remains the same in dark and bright lights. In Horner's syndrome, the pupil becomes miotic, and the difference in the size of pupils becomes more marked in the dark, as the abnormal pupil fails to dilate. In the case of IIIrd nerve palsy, the abnormal pupil is dilated, and the difference in the size of pupils is more in bright light, as it fails to constrict.[5]

Pupillary reflex: It is tested preferably in a dimly lit room, and each eye is checked individually. Ask the patient to look straight ahead at a distant object and bring a bright pen torch from the side. Normal response is the brisk constriction of pupils. Repeat the same procedure for the other eye and notice the direct response to light. Following this, repeat the same steps and observe the response of the pupil in the opposite eye (consensual reflex) on which the light source is not shone. Normal response is equally brisk constriction of the opposite pupil. Swing light from one pupil to another to look for relative afferent pupillary defect (RAPD).[5]

Accommodation reflex: Ask the patient to fix the gaze on a distant object. Suddenly place an object such as a pencil or examiner's finger, about 22 cm in front of the patient's bridge of the nose, while asking him to shift focus toward it. A triple response is normal, which includes constriction of pupils, convergence of the eyes, and thickening of the lens by ciliary muscle contraction.[5]

Ciliospinal reflex: It consists of dilatation of the pupil on painful stimulation of the neck on the ipsilateral side. It indicates the integrity of the brain stem in comatose patients.[7]

Pearls and Pitfalls

Start observations while taking history:

- In case of doubt, please check the patient's old photograph to assess the symmetry of the eyelids.
- During the assessment of ptosis, if neuromuscular (NM) junction disorder is suspected, please look for ptosis time and perform an ice pack test.
- Before starting the examination of eye movements, ensure that the patient's visual acuity is not impaired. Ask the patient to wear glasses, if he is using one.
- Remember that nystagmus observed at extremes of gaze may be physiological.

CRANIAL NERVE V (TRIGEMINAL)

Introduction

The trigeminal nerve is the largest cranial nerve and subserves sensory, motor, and proprioceptive sensations.

Relevant Anatomy

Trigeminal nerve has a large sensory part and a smaller motor part. The sensory component has three divisions:

1. Ophthalmic division V1
2. Maxillary division V2
3. Mandibular division V3

The sensory portion of the first order neuron resides in the trigeminal/Gasserian ganglion, and contains unipolar sensory neurons whose central processes enter lateral pons through a large sensory root, while the peripheral processes subserve sensation to the face and head. There are two types of sensory neurons in the Gasserian ganglion; one mediates fine discriminate touch and pressure while the other carries pain and temperature. However, the two different sets of fiber take different roots to reach thalamus. The former synapses on the chief sensory nucleus and the latter take a circuitous note, first descending through lower pons and medulla into the spinal cord as far as C3/C4 and becoming continuous with Lissauer's tract and substantia gelatinosa of the posterior horn. The third sensory component, mesencephalic root of the V nerve, moves with the motor root and then extends posteriorly and cephalad from the level of the motor nucleus into the midbrain. It carries proprioceptive impulses from muscle supplied by the V nerve. The motor portion of the upper motor neuron (UMN) portion of the V nerve arises primarily from the lower third of the contralateral motor cortex fiber and descends into the corticobulbar tract to the pons where they desiccate. Motor root exits the lateral pons, passes beneath Gasserian ganglion, leaves the skull through foramen ovale, and supplies muscles of mastication and associated muscles—masseter, temporalis, and medial and lateral pterygoids.[8]

Objectives of Testing

- To detect whether there is a weakness of muscles of mastication, jaw movement, and tongue and if it is so then whether it is unilateral or bilateral

- To decide whether the sensory loss in the region innervated by the V nerve is organic or nonorganic
- To determine which modalities are involved
- To define the distribution of sensation loss
- To determine whether the lesion is supranuclear or infranuclear

Methods of Testing

Motor Function

1. Check for bulk and power of the masseter and pterygoids by palpating the nucleus as the patient clenches the jaw.
2. Place the finger anterior, not lateral, to the borders of masseter bilaterally; when the jaw is clenched, the finger will move forward symmetrically on both sides.
3. Careful observation of jaw opening should be made since it may provide the earliest clue to the presence of an abnormality.
4. Ask the patient to move the jaw from side to side and look for any deviation of the jaw.
5. Ask the patient to protrude and retract the jaw and bite on a tongue depressor and compare impression on two sides.
6. Elicit jaw reflex by placing the thumb over the middle of the patient chin, holding the mouth open about midway with jaw relaxed, and then tap the finger with a reflex hammer. Look for an upward jerk of the mandible.

Sensory Function

1. Check for touch, pain, and temperature over either side of the face—frontal, maxillary, and mandible regions—and look for any difference between the two sides and also between the perioral region to the posterior part of the face to exclude onion skin pattern.
2. Pain and temperature impairment should be compared to touch and exclude dissociated sensory loss.
3. Check for corneal reflex by lightly touching the cornea with a wisp of cotton or tissue and look for the blinking of the ipsilateral (direct reflex) and contralateral (consensual reflex) eyes.
4. Check for nasal and sneeze reflexes by stimulating nasal mucous membrane with cotton and look for wrinkling of the nose, closing of eyes often due to forceful exhalation, resembling forced sneeze.

Pearls and Pitfalls

- In testing for facial sensation, touch pain and temperature are examined and should be compared in each trigeminal division on both sides as well as in the perioral region.
- Compare the temperature with touch sensation in each V nerve division and perioral region to exclude dissociated sensory loss.
- During elicitation of corneal reflex stimulus must be delivered to the cornea, not the sclera.

REFERENCES

1. Zatorre RJ, Jones-Goytman M, Evans AC, Meyer E. Functional localization and lateralization of human olfactory cortex. Nature. 1992;360(6402):339-40.
2. Brazis PW, Masdeu JC, Biller J. Localization in Clinical Neurology, 7th edition. Philadelphia: Lippincott Williams & Wilkins; 2016.
3. Demarquay G, Ryvlin P, Royet JP. Olfaction et pathologies neurologiques: revue de la littérature [Olfaction and neurological diseases: a review of the literature]. Rev Neurol (Paris). 2007;163(2):155-67.
4. Dory RL. The olfactory system and its disorders. Semin Neurol. 2009;29(1):74-81.
5. Campbell WW, Barohn RI. Dejong's The Neurological Examination. Gurugram: Wolters Kluwer India Pvt. Ltd.; 2019.
6. Campbell WW. Clinical Signs in Neurology: A Compendium. Gurugram: Wolters Kluwer (India) Pvt. Ltd.; 2016.
7. Wilson-Pauwels L, Stewart PA, Akesson EJ, Spacey SD. Cranial Nerves: Function and Dysfunction, 3rd edition. New York: B.C. Decker Publications; 2010.
8. Kiernan JA, Rajakumar N. Barr's The Human Nervous System: An Anatomical Viewpoint, 10th edition. Philadelphia: Lippincott Williams & Wilkins; 2013.

6 CHAPTER

Testing the Cranial Nerves (VII–XII)

PC Gilvaz, Harisuthan T, Neena Baby

INTRODUCTION

There are 12 pairs of cranial nerves, of which the first two belong to the central nervous system (CNS) and the rest to the peripheral nervous system. A knowledge of the anatomy of the cranial nerve and its course is very important in the localization of a lesion affecting the nerves. This chapter gives an overview of the anatomy and basic examination, which helps in the clinical localization of the last six cranial nerves.

VII CRANIAL NERVE (FACIAL NERVE)

The motor component supplies the muscles of facial expression, stapedius, posterior belly of digastric, and stylohyoid. The sensory division carries taste from the anterior two-third of the tongue, and sensation from the eardrum and external auditory canal. The parasympathetic secretory fibers supply the submandibular, sublingual, and lacrimal glands.

Anatomy

Supranuclear motor fibers start from the lower precentral gyrus, emotional fibers from the frontal lobe anterior to the precentral gyrus, the supplementary motor area, medial temporal lobe, insula, and thalamus. The upper part of the face has bilateral supranuclear control.

Nucleus of the facial nerve is in the pons; it winds around VI nerve and forms the facial colliculus. The nervus intermedius carries the preganglionic parasympathetic fibers to submaxillary, pterygopalatine, and sphenopalatine ganglia. As the facial nerve leaves the brainstem, it contains the branchiomotor fibers to the muscles of the second branchial arch, parasympathetic fibers for lacrimation and salivation, and sensory fibers for touch, pain, temperature, and taste. All of these fibers begin and end in totally different nuclei.

The course of the facial nerve is divided into seven segments:

1. Brainstem segment from the facial nucleus to the exit point from the brainstem
2. Cisternal segment up to the internal acoustic meatus
3. Canalicular segment through the internal auditory canal to the entrance to the facial canal
4. Labyrinthine segment up to the geniculate ganglion
5. Horizontal segment up to the pyramidal eminence on the posterior wall of the tympanic cavity
6. Mastoid segment up to the exit through the stylomastoid foramen
7. Extratemporal segment

Examination

Facial nerve has to be examined by testing its different functions—motor, sensory, secretory, and reflexes.

Inspection

From above downward:

- Look for symmetry of the forehead furrows, palpebral fissures, nasolabial fold, and any asymmetry of the angle of the mouth.
- Observe for any facial asymmetry during spontaneous emotions, smiling, and normal conversation.
- Facial expression
- *Blink rate*: The normal blink rate is around 15/min and reduced in weakness of VII nerve.
- Atrophy of facial muscles
- Fasciculations
- Synkinetic movements and other involuntary movements

For upper face assessment, ask the patient to raise the eyebrows, frown, and close the eyes tightly.

For lower face assessment, ask the patient to smile or grin, blow out the cheeks, and whistle. Platysma can be examined by everting lower lip expressing the lower teeth.

Sensory function: Assess taste over anterior two-third of tongue on each side of the protruded tongue using sweet, salt, sour, and bitter tastes.

Reflexes

Bell's phenomenon: Ask the patient to close his eyes tightly. Normally, there is a symmetrical up and out rolling of eyes, which is not obvious due to the tight eyelid closure. However, this can be witnessed during lower motor neuron (LMN) facial palsy as there is incomplete closure of the eyelids on the ipsilateral side.

Orbicularis oculi reflex: Tap the forehead over the supraorbital ridge or glabella and look for bilateral blinking. Due to the phenomenon of habituation, this normally gets suppressed with repeated tapping.

Orbicularis oris reflex: Tap over the upper lip or side of the nose and observe for the angle of mouth elevation, lower lip protrusion, and puckering over the chin.

Frontal release reflexes: Palmomental, snout, and suck reflexes

Corneal reflex: The facial nerve forms the efferent arc of the reflex.

Secretory Function

- History of dry eyes, dry mouth, excessive tearing, or sialorrhea
- *Parasympathetic function*: Lacrimation is tested by inserting a filter paper of 0.5 mm width on each eye and quantifying the tear column in both eyes after 5 minutes. Usually, it can be up to 15 mm. A reading < 5 mm indicates dry eyes.

Table 1 points the clinical findings that help in differentiating between upper motor neuron (UMN) and LMN facial weakness.

How to differentiate bilateral UMN and LMN palsy?
Sparing of the upper face and Bell's phenomena will not be useful.

- In UMN palsy, there will be dissociation between emotional and motor fibers.
  Taste, hearing, and tearing will be preserved.

  Corneal and conjunctival reflexes will be well elicitable along with a brisk jaw jerk reflex in UMN palsy.
- In LMN facial palsy, both motor and emotional fibers are paralyzed.
  Facial reflexes will be depressed along with accompanying hyperacusis, taste, and parasympathetic involvement depending on the level of the lesion.

How to localize LMN facial palsy? (Box 1)

Other Points

- Melkersson–Rosenthal syndrome is characterized by recurrent orofacial swelling, relapsing facial paralysis, and a fissured tongue. It can be associated with autoimmune diseases.
- *Bilateral facial palsy*: Guillain–Barré syndrome, leprosy, polio, vasculitis, Lyme disease
- *Brain stem lesion*: Vascular causes are the most common, followed by demyelination.
- *Millard–Gubler syndrome*: Ipsilateral VI, VII, and contralateral hemiplegia
- *Eight-and-a-half syndrome*: VII nerve palsy with one-and-a-half syndrome due to paramedian pontine reticular formation (PPRF) and medial longitudinal fasciculus (MLF) involvement.

BOX 1 Localizing LMN facial palsy.

- Weakness of muscle supplied by only certain peripheral branches
- Impairment of taste in the anterior two-thirds of the tongue
- Impairment of taste, hyperacusis
- Impairment of taste, hyperacusis, and lacrimation
- Tinnitus, deafness, ataxia, facial sensory disturbances
- Ipsilateral VI nerve palsy and contralateral hemiparesis
- Lesion distal to stylomastoid foramen
- Lesion between the origin of nerve to stapedius and stylomastoid foramen
- Lesion between geniculate ganglion and nerve to stapedius
- Lesion at or between geniculate ganglion and internal auditory canal
- CP angle
- Pontine lesion

(CP: cerebellopontine; LMN: lower motor neuron)

TABLE 1: Clinical findings that help in differentiating between UMN and LMN facial weakness.

Clinical finding	UMN facial paralysis	LMN facial paralysis
Upper face	Spared	Affected
Dissociation between emotional and motor weakness	Can be present	No dissociation
Bell's phenomenon	Absent	Present
Hyperacusis	Absent	Can be present
Loss of taste over anterior two-third of tongue and tears	Not lost	Affected based on the level of the nerve involved
Facial reflexes	Brisk	Depressed
Hemiparesis	Present	Absent

(LMN: lower motor neuron; UMN: upper motor neuron)

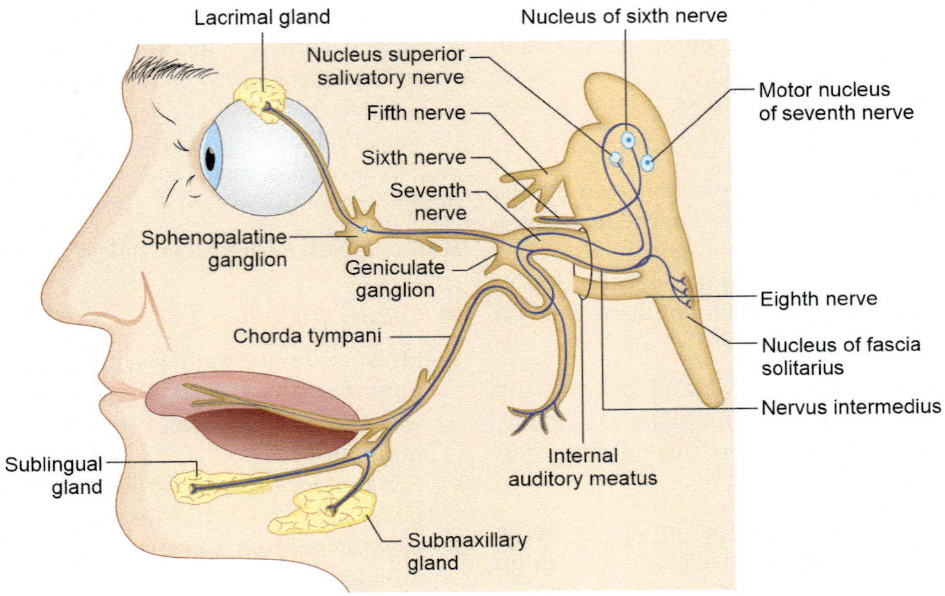

FIG. 1: Functional anatomy of the facial nerve.[1] Facial nucleus is in the caudal pons.

- Myasthenia gravis can produce markedly asymmetric facial weakness and can mimic Bell's palsy. Variability of weakness during the examination and fatigable ptosis gives a clue to the diagnosis.
- Aberrant regeneration of the nerves is common after Bell's palsy with the nerve intended for a particular muscle regrowing into another, leading to synkinesis, which may range from subtle manifestations to profound abnormalities. The inverted Gunn phenomenon, or the Marin-Amat sign, is suggestive of trigeminofacial regeneration, leading to the closure of eyes on opening the mouth.
- Gustatory lacrimal reflex, or the phenomenon of crocodile tears, occurs following the misdirected regeneration of salivary axons to the lacrimal gland, leading to lacrimation while consuming food.

Figure 1 shows the functional anatomy of the facial nerve.

The facial nerve courses dorsomedially and encircles the nucleus of the abducens (VI) cranial nerve.

Sensory cells located in the geniculate ganglion continue distally as the chorda tympani nerve, which carries taste fibers. Peripheral fibers of the nervus intermedius portion of the facial nerve initiate salivary, lacrimal, and mucous secretions.

VIII CRANIAL NERVE (VESTIBULOCOCHLEAR NERVE)

Anatomy

This special sensory afferent nerve consists of two components, the cochlear nerve and vestibular nerve, which unite to form a single trunk. Both the nerves originate in separate peripheral receptors and have distinct central connections.

The *cochlear nerve* receives its input from the auditory receptor, the organ of Corti.

The *vestibular nerve* derives its input from the saccule and utricle, which sense the linear acceleration, and the cristae of the semicircular canals, which detect angular acceleration of the head.

Clinical Assessment of the Cochlear Nerve

History

Sensorineural Deafness

- *Onset*: Acute or progressive
- *Pitch*: Sensorineural hearing loss (SNHL) is characterized by difficulty to hear high-pitched sounds.
- *Tinnitus*: Pulsatile or nonpulsatile
- *Pitch*:
  - *Low-roaring tinnitus*: Ménière's disease
  - *High-pitched tinnitus*: Presbycusis, vestibular schwannoma

Clinical Examination

- *Otoscopic examination*: External auditory meatus and tympanic membranes
- *Whispered voice*: Detects clinically significant hearing loss and has been recommended as a screening test. While using whispered voice, certain tones are heard better and at a greater distance than others. For example, short vowels such as a, e, and i are heard at a greater distance than o, u, or broad consonants such as l, m, n, and r.[2]

- *Finger rub test*: The noise made by rubbing the thumb and index finger together beside the external auditory canal1[3]
- It may be done binaurally, where the patient is asked to compare the sound intensity between the two ears.
- *Tuning fork tests*: A tuning fork of preferably 512 Hz is used to give more specific information and assess air conduction (AC) and bone conduction (BC).[4]
  - *Weber test*: A vibrating tuning fork is placed in the midline—vertex of the skull, nasal bridge, or forehead. Normally, the sound is heard equally in both ears.
    - *Conductive hearing loss (CHL)*: The sound is lateralized to the affected ear.
    - *SNHL*: The sound is better heard in the normal ear.
  - *Rinne's test*: Compares the patient's AC and BC. The vibrating tuning fork is initially placed over the mastoid bone and when no longer heard there, it is kept beside the ear. The fork should be heard twice as long by AC as by BC.
    - *CHL*: BC is better than AC—Rinne negative.
    - *SNHL*: Both AC and BC are reduced, but AC is better than BC—Rinne positive.
  - *Schwabach test*: The vibrating fork is held against the patient's mastoid process until he is unable to perceive any sounds. The examiner then places the tuning fork over his mastoid bone and compares the examiner's BC with that of the patient.
    - *SNHL*: The examiner perceives the vibrations after the patient no longer does.
    - *CHL*: The patient may hear the tuning fork longer than the examiner does.

Vestibular Nerve

Table 2 gives a clinical assessment of vestibular nerve.

- History for etiologic diagnosis should include: History of recent viral infections, head or neck trauma, toxin or drug exposure, alcohol abuse, and cardiovascular disease

Examination

The examination should include a complete otologic, audiologic evaluation and detailed neurologic examination.

- *Examination of ocular movements including*:
  - Observe the eye in primary gaze for 5–10 seconds
  - Smooth pursuit
  - Saccades
  - Fixation suppression
  - Spontaneous/gaze-evoked nystagmus/positional nystagmus
  - Skew deviation
- Bedside hearing assessment
- *Stance and gait*:
  - Gait speed, gait base, ability to walk in tandem
  - Observe for balance during and after quick turns
  - Cadence, stride length, arm swing
- *Romberg test*:
  - Observe the patient while he stands with eyes closed and feet together for 6–30 seconds. The patient tends to fall to the side of vestibular hypofunction.
  - Ask the patient to take three steps forward and three steps backward; there is a tendency to veer to one side, resulting in progressive deviation to the affected side, the steps resembling a star—"star gait."[6]

TABLE 2: Clinical assessment of vestibular nerve.[5]

Description	Onset	Duration	Triggers	Associated features	Syndrome
Spinning/rotating	Abrupt	5–60 seconds	Tilting head back, rolling in bed	Nausea	BPPV
Spinning/rotating	Abrupt	Days to weeks	No trigger, recent URTI	Worse with any head motion, nausea	Vestibular neuritis
Spinning/rotating	Abrupt	Days to weeks	No trigger	Unilateral hearing loss, nausea	Labyrinthitis
Severe spinning/ rotating	Abrupt	30 minutes to 12 hours	No trigger	Tinnitus, fluctuating hearing loss	Meniere disease
Unsteadiness is worse during movements	Insidious	Continuous	No trigger	Worse during head movements or in darkness	Bilateral vestibulopathy
Spinning, tilting	Insidious	Seconds to minutes recurrently	Loud sounds worsen the symptoms	Autophony, ear fullness, tinnitus	Superior canal dehiscence
Spinning, tilting	Abrupt or more gradual	Minutes to days	Motion-sensitive/visual stimuli	Migraine headache, photo- or phonophobia	Vestibular migraine
Swaying, floating	Insidious	Constant, with varying intensity	No trigger	Less severe when distracted	Persistent postural perceptual dizziness
Vertigo, ataxia	Abrupt	Resolves in 5–20 minutes	No trigger	Transient ataxia	Transient ischemic attack

(BPPV: benign paroxysmal positional vertigo; URTI: upper respiratory tract infection)

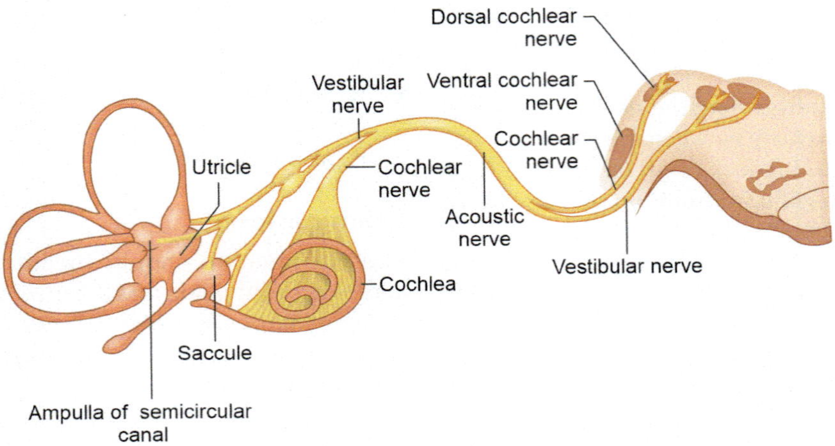

FIG. 2: Functional anatomy of the vestibulocochlear nerve.[8]

- *Provocative tests*:
  - *Head impulse test (HIT)*:
    - Bedside tests, mainly to document vestibular neuritis
    - Standing directly in front of the patient, the examiner holds the head firmly and instructs the patient to look at a fixed point. The examiner then abruptly rotates the patient's head but only to a small distance to the left and right. The rotation should be unpredictable in the timing and direction of the turn.
    - In a patient with unilateral vestibular deficit, the eyes move with the head, which is then followed by a rapid corrective saccade to bring the eyes back to the target.
  - *Hyperventilation test*: The patient takes 30 deep, forceful breaths and then his eyes are observed for nystagmus using Frenzel goggles. Hyperventilation-induced nystagmus suggests a partially conducting eighth nerve or central vestibular pathway.
  - *Provocative position maneuvers*:
    - *Dix-Hallpike test*:[7] It is done primarily to assess the particles in the posterior canal. To perform the test on the left side, the patient's head is turned 45° to the left; then the patient is quickly moved from sitting to a supine head-hanging position. The head should be tilted back approximately 20°, and then the eyes are observed for 10–15 seconds for nystagmus. The test is said to be positive when the nystagmus is triggered by it and is transient in duration, accompanied by symptoms of vertigo or nausea.
    - *Supine positional testing*:[7] It is to specifically move particles in the horizontal canal. Here, the patient starts in the supine position. Then the head is turned to one side and held there for 10–15 seconds, then brought back to the midline and turned to the opposite side and held for 10–15 seconds, and observed for nystagmus.
    - *Head shake test*: The patient's head is rotated for 30–45° to either side by the examiner in the horizontal plane for 20 cycles. Nystagmus that lasts 5 seconds or longer indicates an organic disease of the inner ear or CNS.
    - *Valsalva test*: This test is mainly performed if pressure or sound sensitivity symptom is elicited from history. The patient inhales a deep breath and strains for 10 seconds, while the examiner observes for nystagmus. Nystagmus at onset and release of pressure indicate a positive test. This test is mainly done to assess for superior canal dehiscence.

Figure 2 shows the functional anatomy of the vestibulocochlear nerve.

IX AND X CRANIAL NERVES (GLOSSOPHARYNGEAL AND VAGUS NERVES)[9]

Anatomy

The IX cranial nerve emerges from the medulla, takes its origin from the nucleus tractus solitarius, nucleus ambiguus, spinal nucleus of trigeminal nerve, and inferior salivary nucleus. It emerges from the posterolateral sulcus of the medulla, dorsal to the inferior olivary nucleus, and travels in close relation with the vagus and spinal accessory nerve in the jugular foramen. It emerges and forms the superior and inferior (also called petrosal) ganglia, followed by coursing down the neck between the internal jugular vein and internal carotid artery to finally wind around the stylopharyngeus muscle, supplying it, and forming the pharyngeal plexus along with the pharyngeal branch of the vagus supplying the pharyngeal constrictor muscles. The carotid sinus nerve carries the baroreceptive and chemoreceptive afferents from the carotid body and carotid sinus. Jacobson's nerve carries exteroceptive sensations from the mastoid, Eustachian tube, and tympanic membrane. Parasympathetic supply to the parotid gland originates in the inferior salivary nucleus and is carried by the Jacobson's nerve to the otic ganglion.

Supranuclear fibers arise from the primary motor cortex and synapse in the medulla in the rostral nucleus ambiguus. Bilateral innervation is present.

The vagus or pneumogastric nerve arises from nucleus tractus solitarius (NTS), nucleus ambiguus, dorsal motor nucleus of the vagus, and spinal nucleus of the trigeminal nerve, and emerges out of the medulla as multiple rootlets passing dorsal to the inferior olive, in close relation with glossopharyngeal nerve. It passes through the jugular foramen and forms the jugular and nodose ganglia, which gives off the meningeal branch to the posterior fossa dura mater, auricular ramus (Arnold's nerve) giving rise to the exteroceptive sensation in the concha. The pharyngeal ramus joins with the glossopharyngeal nerve to form the plexus supplying the constrictors of the pharynx. The superior laryngeal nerve is given off next, which divides into the external ramus supplying the cricothyroid muscle and the internal ramus carrying the sensory functions of the larynx. In the neck it also gives off the cardiac rami, which contribute to forming the cardiac plexus. At the root of the neck recurrent laryngeal nerve is given off, which winds around the aorta on the left side and the subclavian artery on the right side and supplies the laryngeal muscles except the cricothyroid. The pulmonary and esophageal branches enter the abdomen and supply the abdominal viscera **(Fig. 3)**.

Supranuclear innervation is bilateral and is present in the lower portion of the precentral gyrus.

Clinical Assessment

History

- *Is there difficulty in swallowing food?*
  Difficulty in consumption of liquids more than solids has been observed in IX and X nerve palsy. There is also associated history of nasal regurgitation of fluids.

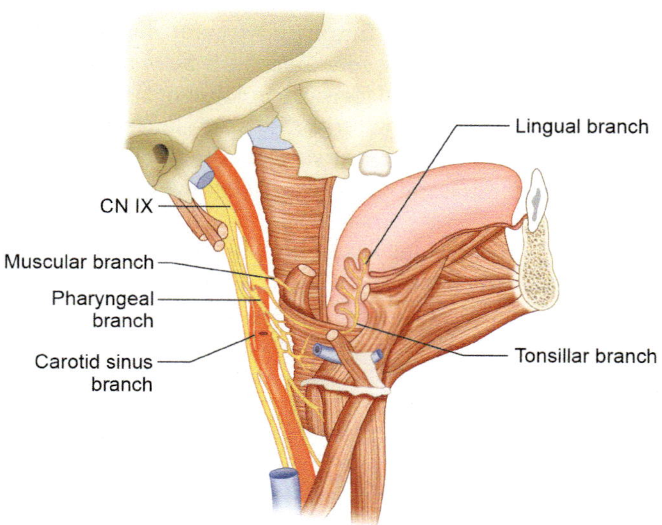

FIG. 3: Functional anatomy of the glossopharyngeal nerve.[10]
(CN IX: 9th cranial nerve)

- *Is there difficulty in speech?*
  The voice may acquire a nasal tone while talking, especially while bending the neck forward, which may normalize when lying back.[11] This indicates palatal weakness.
  If the patient chokes on his saliva while he is talking, it is an indication of both palatal and pharyngeal weakness.
  Unilateral LMN lesions of the vagus nerve may lead to the hoarseness of voice along with a nasal quality.
- *Is the patient dyspneic?*
  Bilateral vagal paralysis causes respiratory compromise associated with increased work of breathing and inspiratory stridor and can be life-threatening.

Examination

Inspection

- Mouth can be opened and examined for any asymmetry of the palatal arch. A few moments of waiting can avoid the use of the tongue blade, which may be used for better visualization.
- Patient is asked to repeat "ah" while breathing out and "ugh" while breathing in. This maneuver should be repeated multiple times to observe weakness with subsequent efforts.
- Soft palate musculature except the tensor veli palatini is supplied by the vagal nerve.
- Normally, the palate should move backward and upward symmetrically with a central uvula when two sides of the pharynx contract symmetrically.
- Unilateral UMN lesion does not produce any clinical symptoms as the innervation is bilateral.
- During phonation, no uvular deviation is noted, and symmetrical palatal elevation is noted.
- In unilateral LMN lesion there is a slight lowering of the ipsilateral palatal arch, which is noted. The median raphe of the uvula drifts toward the normal side on phonation. During laryngoscopy, ipsilateral vocal cord may have a cadaveric position.
- Bilateral lesions may cause an inability of the palate to elevate on phonation. Palatal droop is an inconsistent finding and is based on the function of the tensor veli palatini.
- On phonation, nasal quality is present in the speech as air escapes from the oral to the nasal cavity. Cough is impaired, and respiration may be severely affected.
- Abnormal movements may be noted such as the vertical oscillation of the palate also involving the pharynx, called palatal nystagmus/myoclonus, due to a lesion of the central tegmental tract.

Sensory

- Taste function on the posterior third of the tongue may be tested by using an applicator stick.
- LMN lesion of the glossopharyngeal nerve leads to ipsilateral loss of taste.[4]
- Pain and soft touch sensations are reduced in the soft palate, posterior third of the tongue, and tonsils.

Reflex

- Gag reflex: Afferent limb of gag reflex is the glossopharyngeal nerve, and the efferent is both the glossopharyngeal and vagal nerves.
- Stimulation of the anterior faucial pillar of the oropharynx, posterior pharyngeal wall, base of the tongue, and tonsils pharyngeal wall with an applicator stick or a tongue blade leads to the elevation and retraction of the muscles of the pharynx.[12]
- Palatal reflex: Stimulation when applied to the soft palate leads to elevation of the soft palate and uvular deviation to the ipsilateral side.
- Gag reflex and palatal reflex are considered for all practical purposes as same and are referred to as the gag reflex. It is a protective reflex and is composed of three components—elevation of the soft palate, pharyngeal constriction, and closure of the glottis to protect the airway.
- In unilateral LMN palsy, the gag reflex is absent on one side.[6]
- If this is due to the glossopharyngeal nerve weakness, the stimulation of the opposite side produces symmetrical movement on both sides.
- In the presence of pharyngeal weakness, the uvular raphe moves toward the normal side.
- When there is vagal palsy, even on stimulation of the normal side, there will not be palatal elevation and uvular deviation to the affected side.
- Hyperactive gag reflex is present in some individuals.
- It may also be the feature of pseudobulbar palsy and amyotrophic lateral sclerosis (ALS).

Pearls and Pitfalls

Hoarseness of voice and a nasal tone that increases toward the end of sentences may indicate myasthenia gravis.

In patients with sensitive faucial pillars and patients with complete insensitivity, observation of spontaneous movements on phonation and inspiration and swallowing with mouth open may give a lot of information without touching the palate.[11]

Figure 4 shows the functional anatomy of the vagus nerve.

XI CRANIAL NERVE (ACCESSORY NERVE)

Anatomy

Traditionally, the accessory nerve based on its origin is divided into spinal and cranial parts.[13]

The cranial root or internal ramus arises in the medulla from the caudal part of the nucleus ambiguus and dorsal motor nucleus of the vagus and exits via the lateral medulla below the roots of the vagus.

Spinal root or external ramus arises from the ventral horn cells in the upper six segments of the cervical cord, which are in continuity with the nucleus ambiguus. Roots arising from C1 and C2 innervate predominantly the ipsilateral

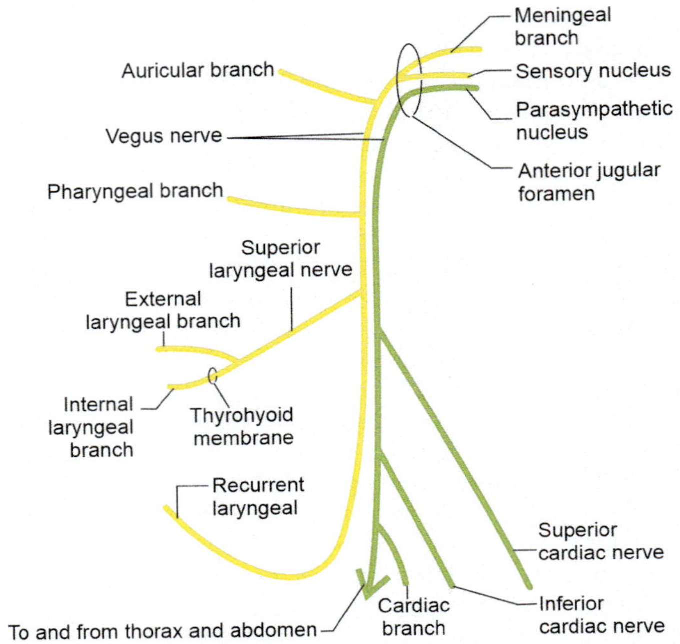

FIG. 4: Functional anatomy of the vagus nerve.

sternocleidomastoid (SCM) and those arising from C3 and C4 cord innervate ipsilateral trapezius.[14]

These fibers then unite to form the spinal part, ascend in the subarachnoid space, enter the skull through the foramen magnum, join its cranial counterpart, and exit together via the jugular foramen along with the ninth and tenth cranial nerves. Cranial root unites with the vagus, supplying the muscles of the pharynx and larynx. The spinal portion descends close to the internal jugular vein to enter the posterior aspect of the SCM. After innervating the SCM, it emerges from the middle of the muscle, passes through the posterior triangle of the neck to enter the trapezius and supply it.

Figure 5 shows the functional anatomy of the accessory nerve.

The SCM is the neck flexor and rotator of the head to the opposite side. Acting together, both SCMs cause neck flexion, bringing the head forward and downward.

Trapezius is a neck extensor. It also elevates, retracts, and rotates the shoulder, causing overhead abduction. Its lower fibers depress the scapula and stabilize it.

- *SCM*:
  - *Symptoms*: Usually presents with neck pain/difficulty to turn the neck

Clinical Examination

Inspection

- Volume and contour of the SCM muscles as the patient looks ahead
  - *Nuclear/infranuclear lesions*: Atrophy or fasciculations may be noted.
  - Head may fall backward in case of bilateral muscle weakness.

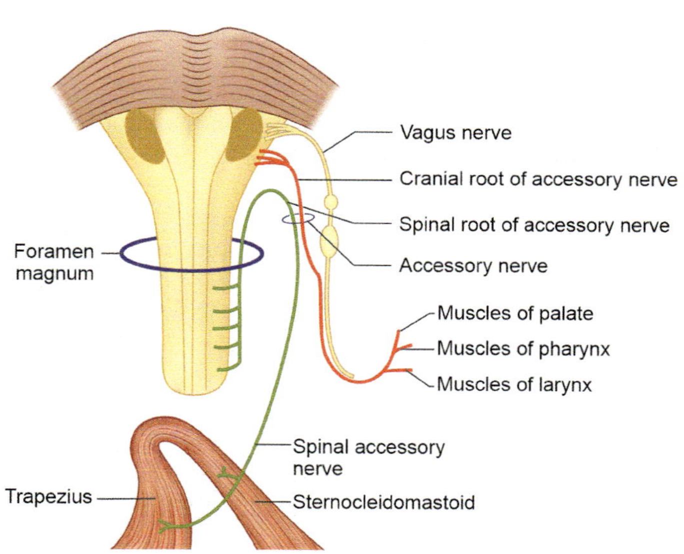

FIG. 5: Functional anatomy of the accessory nerve. The supranuclear innervation to trapezius and sternocleidomastoid (SCM) arises from the lower precentral gyrus. The corticobulbar fibers to trapezius are crossed, thereby innervating the contralateral muscle. However, the course of fibers to SCM is unknown, but is thought to terminate mainly in the ipsilateral nuclei. Two pathways have been proposed.[15]

- *Abnormal involuntary movements*:
  - *Head turning to one side*: An initial manifestation of seizure, where the head turns away from the side of the epileptogenic lesion (adverse seizure)
  - *Rigidity, akinesia, hyperkinesia*: Extrapyramidal lesions
  - *Torticollis, retrocollis*: As a part of cervical dystonia

Assessment of the Power

Test the right SCM muscle by facing the patient and placing the right palm on the patient's left cheek. Ask the patient to turn the head to the left, resisting the pressure that is being exerted in the opposite direction. At the same time, observe and palpate the right SCM. Then reverse the procedure to test the left SCM. The muscle usually stands out well, and its contraction can be palpated.

Both the SCM muscles can be simultaneously examined by placing the hand on the patient's forehead and pushing backward as the patient pushes forward.

- *Unilateral weakness*:
  - No significant change in the resting position of the head
  - Weakness in turning head to the opposite side on testing the muscle
- *Bilateral weakness*:
  - Weakness of neck flexion with the head tending to take an extended position

SCM Reflex

Tapping the muscle at its clavicular head results in prompt contraction.

Trapezius

- *Symptoms*:
  - *Pain*: Described as a dragging or pulling sensation in the neck. This may be due to traction on soft tissues of the neck, as the tip of the shoulder droops.[16]
  - *Weakness*: Mainly perceived as a decrease in strength of the affected arm with difficulty in such daily tasks as combing hair, putting on a shirt or blouse, and raising the arm above the horizontal plane.
- *Inspection*: Stand behind the patient and observe the shoulder contour for:
  - Hollowing, displacement, or winging of the scapula
  - Drooping of the shoulder
  - Flattening of the trapezius ridge
- *Assessment of power*:
  - The upper fibers are tested by placing the examiner's hands on the patient's shoulders and pressing down as the patient elevates or shrugs the shoulders.
  - Another method is by resisting the patient's attempt to approximate the occiput to the acromion.[4]
  - Middle and lower fibers are examined by placing the patient's abducted arm horizontally, palm up, and attempting to push the elbow forward.
  - Middle fibers are also tested by having the patient retract the scapula against resistance.
- *Unilateral trapezius weakness*:
  - Sagging of the shoulder, with the resting position of the scapula shifting downward
  - Loss of normal slant from the base of neck to the shoulder due to loss of the bulk of trapezius
  - Upper portion of scapula is displaced laterally with inferior angle moving inward, resulting in scapular winging. This winging is more prominent on lateral arm abduction.
  - Arm hangs lower on the affected side, and the fingertips touch the thigh at a lower level than on the normal side.
- *Bilateral trapezius weakness*:
  - Weakness of neck extension with head tending to fall forward, resulting in "dropped head syndrome"[17]

XII CRANIAL NERVE (HYPOGLOSSAL NERVE)

The XII nerve is a pure motor nerve, supplies the intrinsic and extrinsic muscles of the tongue. The nerve originates from the hypoglossal nucleus on the dorsal aspect of medulla, beneath the floor of fourth ventricle in the paramedian region. From rostral to caudal, the innervation is the intrinsic muscles, then genioglossus, hyoglossus, and styloglossus. The nuclei of both the sides lie in close proximity here; so a lesion in this area causes bilateral LMN palsy of hypoglossal nerve.

The nerve emerges through the hypoglossal canal[18] and descends vertically in neck, which joins with the C1 rami forming the ansa cervicalis/hypoglossi along with the other cervical plexus to the angle of mouth toward hyoid bone and tongue, innervating the extrinsic and intrinsic muscles of the tongue except the palatoglossus, which is supplied by the glossopharyngeal nerve.[19] The branches of the hypoglossal nerve are the meningeal, descending, thyrohyoid, and muscular.

Supranuclear control of the hypoglossal nerve is by corticobulbar fibers, originating from lower portion of precentral gyrus. These fibers pass through the internal capsule and descend to the pontomedullary junction, where they decussate. The genioglossus has only contralateral innervation; other tongue muscles have bilateral representation.[20] There are uncrossed fibers, which pass through the lateral aspect of the pons, which leads to ipsilateral lingual paresis.

The longitudinal intrinsic muscles on each side help to retract the tongue backward and ipsilaterally, while genioglossus protrudes and pushes the tongue to the other side. So, in a unilateral XII nerve palsy, the unprotruded tongue is deviated to the contralateral or healthy side; but on protrusion, it is deviated to the weaker or ipsilateral side.

Clinical Examination

History Taking

Hypoglossal paresis is associated more with signs than symptoms. In an analysis of 100 patients with hypoglossal nerve palsy, only 10 presented with symptoms pertaining to the tongue functions.[21]

- What was the onset of the deviation of the tongue?
    - *Acute*: Vascular insults, trauma, intraoperative procedures[22]
    - *Subacute/chronic*: Tumors, demyelination, syringobulbia, metastasis, occipital condyle syndrome[23,24]
- Is there any difficulty in protrusion of tongue?
    - Bilateral supranuclear palsy leads to difficulty in protrusion of tongue.
    - Ankyloglossia (tongue tie), seen in infants, can also lead to difficulty in protrusion and mobility of the tongue, causing difficulties in breastfeeding and maintenance of oral hygiene.[25]
- Is there a difficulty in speech?
    - Spastic dysarthria is seen associated with a strained quality, slow rate, and harsh speech seen predominantly in patients with bilateral UMN palsy.
    - Flaccid dysarthria associated with breathiness, hyper nasality of the voice may be seen in multiple cranial nerve palsy.
- What are the associated symptoms noted?
    - Involvement of other cranial nerves and structures such as medial lemniscus or of sympathetic chain in the nuclear and infranuclear pathway

Examination

Inspection

- Ask the patient to open his mouth, with tongue inside. Note the size, shape, position of tongue, tremors, chorea, dyskinesia, and fasciculations, if any.
- Look for any deviation of tongue on protrusion.
- Tongue dexterity can be tested by repeating the lingual sounds, la-la-la, or use words with the t or d phoneme.
- *Lateral movements*: Preserved in LMN lesions due to intrinsic muscles
- Facial palsy on one side causes lack of mobility of the corner of the mouth, leading to the appearance of tongue deviation on that side. This can be eliminated by assessing the relation of the tip of tongue with the upper incisors, tip of the nose, or by pulling up the corner of the mouth on the affected side.

Appearance

- *Macroglossia*: ALS, acromegaly, amyloidosis, Duchenne muscular dystrophy, Down syndrome, hypothyroidism, glycogen storage disorders, neurofibroma (NF), polymyositis, sarcoidosis
- *Fissured tongue*: Hypothyroidism, Down syndrome, vitamin B complex deficiency, Melkersson–Rosenthal syndrome
- *Strawberry tongue*: Kawasaki disease
- *Median rhomboid glossitis*: Human immunodeficiency virus (HIV) infection
- *Trident tongue, triple furrowed tongue, trissulcated tongue*: Myasthenia gravis[26]

Deviation

- On protrusion, tongue deviates to the ipsilateral side due to unopposed action of posterior fibers of genioglossus.
- In bilateral palsy, tongue may only be slightly protruded.
- *Bulk*: Atrophy is noted in LMN lesion on the involved side. In UMN lesion, the affected side may appear voluminous.
- On pressing the tongue to the lower lip, transient blanching is noted during the pressure release, which is seen in all ethnic groups and may be considered as a measure of the anterior and posterior fibers of the genioglossi **(Fig. 6)**.[27]

Abnormal Tongue Movement

- Fibrillations noted in LMN syndrome
- *Tremors*: Parkinson's disease, alcoholism, essential tremor
- *Chorea*: Bizarre lingual and irregular jerky movements along with an inability to maintain protrusion of tongue
- *Galloping tongue*: Episodic, rhythmic, involuntary movement of the tongue beginning in the midline and proceeding at 3 Hz/s[28]
- *Continuous lingual myoclonus*: Seen following head and neck trauma

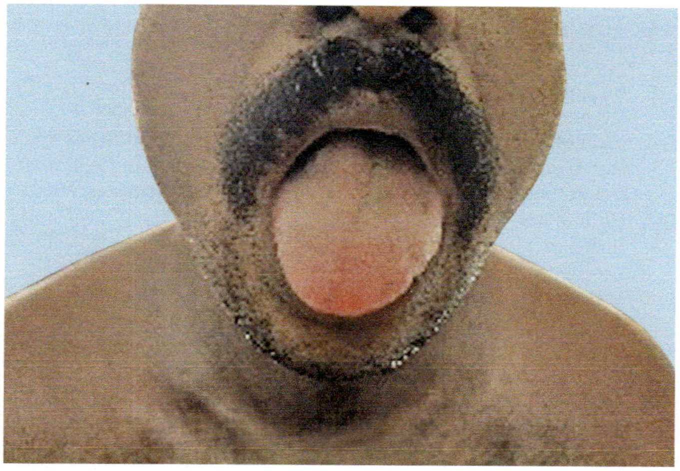

FIG. 6: Deviation of tongue to the right side on protrusion, suggestive of right hypoglossal nerve palsy.

Palpation

After wearing the gloves, feel the tone of tongue. Ask the patient to press one cheek with his tongue tip against examiners finger on the outer aspect of cheek and assess the power. Normally, tongue can push against the finger.

The patient may not be able to push the tongue against the cheek on the normal side but would be able to push it against the cheek on paretic side.[4]

With unilateral weakness, at rest, it may deviate or curl slightly toward the healthy side due to unopposed action of styloglossus, which draws tongue upward and backward. Lateral movements of the tip of nonprotruded tongue controlled by intrinsic muscles may be preserved.

Ipsilateral side weakness is noted with nuclear and infranuclear lesions.

Contralateral side weakness is noted with supranuclear palsy.

Bilateral supranuclear palsy leads to slow and irregular lateral tongue movements with no associated atrophy or fibrillation.

Tables 3 and 4 give the differences between unilateral and bilateral lesions and UMN and LMN lesions, respectively. **Figure 7** shows the functional anatomy of the hypoglossal nerve.

ACKNOWLEDGMENTS

We would like to acknowledge the assistance of my postgraduates, Dr Gayathri and Dr Nikhila, in the preparation of this article.

TABLE 3: Unilateral and bilateral lesions.

Unilateral lesion	Bilateral lesion
Atrophy, fasciculation on ipsilateral side	Atrophy, fasciculation on both sides
Deviation of tongue to the ipsilateral side	Inability to protrude the tongue
Minimal dysarthria and dysphagia	Marked dysphagia and dysarthria
Absence of dyspnea	Dyspnea present due to flaccid tongue falling backward

TABLE 4: UMN and LMN lesions.

UMN lesion	LMN lesion
Weakness present, no atrophy	Ipsilateral atrophy noted
Tongue protrusion to the opposite side of the supranuclear lesion	Tongue protrusion to the same side as the lesion
• Medial pontine lesions cause contralateral tongue deviation • Lateral pontine lesions cause ipsilateral tongue deviation	LMN lesion is ipsilateral with involvement of contiguous structures such as ascending or descending motor pathways and other cranial nerve nuclei
Spastic dysarthria	Flaccid dysarthria

(LMN: lower motor neuron; UMN: upper motor neuron)

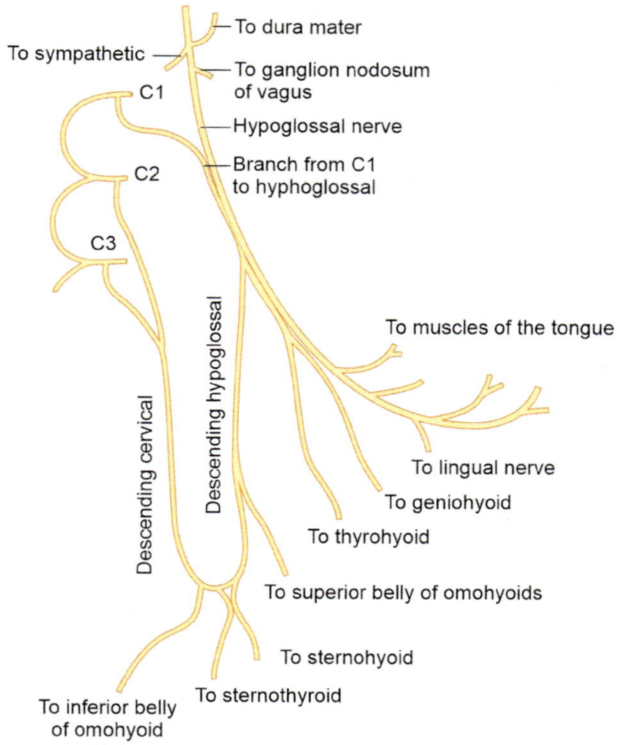

FIG. 7: Functional anatomy of the hypoglossal nerve.

REFERENCES

1. Khan A, Hussain N, Gosalakkal J. Bell's palsy in children—a review. J Pediatr Sci. 2011;3(2):e77.
2. Pirozzo S, Papinczak T, Glasziou P. Whispered voice test for screening for hearing impairment in adults and children: a systematic review. BMJ. 2003;327(7421):967.
3. Kugelberg E. Facial reflexes. Brain. 1952;75:385.
4. Campbell. Dejong's The Neurologic Examination, 7th edition. Philadelphia: Lippincott Williams and Wilkins; 2013.
5. Fife TD. Approach to the history and evaluation of vertigo and dizziness. Continuum (Minneap Minn). 2021;27(2):306-29.
6. Brazis P, Masdeu J. Localization of Clinical Neurology. In: Ranganathan LN (SA Ed). Gurugram: Wolters Kluwer India Pvt. Ltd.; 2020.
7. Hain TC, Cherchi M. Vestibular testing. Continuum (Minneap Minn). 2021;27(2):330-47.
8. Landau ME, Barner KC. Vestibulocochlear nerve. Semin Neurol. 2009;29(1):66-73.
9. Walker HK. Cranial nerves IX and X: The glossopharyngeal and vagus nerves. In: Walker HK, Hall WD, Hurst JW (Eds). Clinical Methods: The History, Physical, and Laboratory Examinations, 3rd edition. Boston: Butterworths; 1990.
10. Tubbs R, Shoja MM, Loukas M. (2015). Anatomy of the glossopharyngeal nerve. Nerves and Nerve Injuries. Amsterdam: Academic Press; 2015. pp. 317-83.
11. Kameshwar P, Spillane J, Yadav R (Eds). Bickerstaff's Neurological Examination in Clinical Practice, 7th edition. New Jersey: Wiley; 2013. pp. 109-13.
12. Bensard DD, Beauchamp KM, Hurt RT, McClave SA, Mills AM, Chen EH, et al. Gag Reflex. In: Encyclopedia of Intensive Care Medicine. Berlin, Heidelberg: Springer Berlin Heidelberg; 2012. pp. 961-3.
13. Brodal A. Neurological Anatomy in Relation to Clinical Medicine, 3rd edition. New York: Oxford University Press; 1981. pp. 457-9.
14. Manon-Espaillat R, Ruff RL. Dissociated weakness of sternocleidomastoid and trapezius muscles with lesions in the CNS. Neurology. 1988;38(5):796-7.
15. Geschwind N. Nature of the decussated innervation of the sternocleidomastoid muscle. Ann Neurol. 1981;10(5):495.
16. Kim DH, Midha R, Murovic JA, Spinner RJ, Teil R. Kline and Hudson's Nerve Injuries: Operative Results for Major Nerve Injuries, Entrapments, and Tumors. Philadelphia: Elsevier Health Sciences; 2007.
17. Hoffman D, Gutmann L, Griggs RC, Mendell JR, Miller RG. The dropped head syndrome with chronic inflammatory demyelinating polyneuropathy. Muscle Nerve. 1994;17(7):808-10.
18. Thompson EO, Smoker WR. Hypoglossal nerve palsy: a segmental approach. Radiographics. 1994;14(5):939-58.
19. Snell R. Clinical Neuroanatomy, 7th edition. Philadelphia: Wolters Kluwer; 2010. pp. 356-8.
20. Fisher CM. Ataxic hemiparesis: a pathologic study. Arch Neurol. 1978;35(3):126-8.
21. Keane JR. Twelfth-nerve palsy analysis of 100 cases. Arch Neurol. 1996;53(6):561-6.
22. Shah AC, Barnes C, Spiekerman CF, Bollag LA. Hypoglossal nerve palsy after airway management for general anesthesia: an analysis of 69 patients. Anesth Analg. 2015;120(1):105-20.
23. Rodríguez-Pardo J, Lara-Lara M, Sanz-Cuesta BE, Fuentes B, Díez-Tejedor E. Occipital condyle syndrome: a red flag for malignancy. Comprehensive literature review and new case report. Headache. 2017;57(5):699-708.
24. Capobianco DJ, Brazis PW, Rubino FA, Dalton JN. Occipital condyle syndrome. Headache. 2002;42(2):142-6.
25. Segal LM, Stephenson R, Dawes M, Feldman P. Clinical review prevalence, diagnosis, and treatment of ankyloglossia: methodologic review. Can Fam Physician. 2007;53(6):1027-33.
26. Matta APC, Andorinho AC, Ferreira F, Kirmse A, Damm AC, Gabriel J, et al. Antimusk positive myasthenia gravis and three semiological cardinal signs. Neurol Int. 2016;8:6361.
27. Bandyopadhyay S. Modified clinical examination of hypoglossal nerve (P4.170). Neurology. 2015;84(14 Suppl):P4.170.
28. Keane JR. Galloping tongue. Neurology. 1984;34(2):251.

7

CHAPTER

Testing the Motor System

Ayush Agarwal, Venugopalan Y Vishnu

INTRODUCTION

Motor system examination is one of the most important aspects of neurological assessment, which helps in the localization of the lesion. Motor deficits are broadly categorized into the upper motor neuron (UMN) and lower motor neuron (LMN) types. The major differences between the two are mentioned in **Table 1**. After identifying the lesion type (UMN vs. LMN), the next step requires identification of the distribution of weakness, i.e., hemiparesis, paraparesis, quadriparesis, monoparesis, proximal or distal predominant weakness, or weakness along a single nerve distribution only. This combination helps in arriving at a probable anatomical localization, following which relevant diagnostic tests can be conducted to arrive at the diagnosis.[1]

Upper motor neuron pathways extend from the cerebral cortex as corticobulbar and corticospinal tracts to the corresponding brainstem cranial nerve nuclei and anterior horn cells in the spinal cord, respectively. Lesions up to the brainstem result in contralateral UMN hemiplegia whereas spinal lesions result in ipsilateral UMN hemiplegia (cervical cord) or monoplegia (dorsal cord).

- *Cerebral cortex*: Nondense contralateral weakness with cortical signs such as seizures, aphasia, agnosia, apraxia, and hemineglect
- *Corona radiata*: Nondense contralateral weakness without cortical signs
- *Internal capsule*: Dense contralateral weakness
- *Thalamus*: Contralateral weakness with sensory loss (or hyperesthesia)
- *Brainstem*: Crossed hemiplegia (ipsilateral cranial nerve deficit with contralateral limb weakness)

Lower motor neuron lesions can occur from any pathology affecting the cranial nerve nuclei/anterior horn cell, radicle, plexus, peripheral nerve, neuromuscular junction, or muscle.

- *Anterior horn cell*: Radicular distribution of weakness with prominent wasting ± fasciculations
- *Root*: Radicular distribution of weakness with/without radicular pain
- *Plexus*: Nerve distribution of weakness with multiple nerves originating from the plexus afflicted. Usually, unilateral
- *Nerve*: Distribution depends on the nerve pathology: mononeuropathy, mononeuritis multiplex, polyneuropathy
- *Neuromuscular junction*: Fluctuating, proximal upper and lower limb weakness ± extraocular and bulbar involvement
- *Muscle*: Proximal upper and lower limb involvement with weakness more than wasting

TABLE 1: Differences between UMN and LMN lesions.

	UMN lesion	LMN lesion
Wasting	Mild or none	Moderate to severe
Tone	Spasticity	Hypotonia
Superficial reflexes	Absent	Absent/normal
Deep tendon reflexes	Exaggerated (unless acute)	Absent
Pathological reflexes	Present	Absent

(LMN: lower motor neuron; UMN: upper motor neuron)

EXAMINATION

Examination of the motor system involves the evaluation of bulk, muscle tone, and power.

Bulk

The patient should be inspected while seated or standing comfortably, with limbs in a symmetrical position and the area of interest exposed. The limbs should be evaluated for both muscle bulk and position. The bulk may be decreased in LMN disorders (muscle atrophy/wasting), which should be clearly documented for its position: Distal versus proximal, symmetrical versus asymmetrical, and unilateral versus bilateral. Any disorder affecting anterior horn cells, motor nerve root, plexus, and nerves can cause atrophy. Neuromuscular junction disorders usually do not cause atrophy, probably except for muscle-specific tyrosine kinase (MuSK) myasthenia gravis. In disuse atrophy, even though there is a marked reduction in volume, there may not be much reduction in muscle power. When wasting and weakness are comparable it is likely to be neurogenic, and when weakness is disproportionate to wasting it is likely myopathic. In an acute event, weakness precedes atrophy while in a chronic event atrophy precedes weakness. Patterns of atrophy may give some clue to etiology [e.g., split hand in amyotrophic lateral sclerosis (ALS), reverse split hand in Hirayama, inverted champagne bottle appearance in Charcot–Marie–Tooth disease (CMT), sternocleidomastoid atrophy in myotonic dystrophy, and fascioscapular muscle atrophy/Popeye arm in facioscapulohumeral muscular dystrophy (FSHD)]. Various endocrine diseases can cause muscle atrophy. Thyrotoxic myopathy can cause upper limb proximal atrophy; hyperparathyroidism can cause weakness, atrophy, hyperreflexia, and fasciculations mimicking ALS (Vical's syndrome); hypopituitarism can cause muscle weakness and atrophy; and asymmetric proximal weakness and atrophy are seen in diabetic amyotrophy.

Occasionally, an increase in bulk may also be seen, which could be true hypertrophy (myotonia congenita) or pseudohypertrophy (calf hypertrophy in Duchenne muscular dystrophy due to fat and connective tissue infiltration). Any persistent muscle contraction can cause muscle hypertrophy [e.g., sternocleidomastoid muscle (SCM) hypertrophy in cervical dystonia and enlarged masseter in bruxism]. Hypertrophic myopathy due to hypothyroidism in adults is known as the Hoffman syndrome. Other non-neurologic causes of muscle hypertrophy include myocysticercosis, trichinosis, sarcoidosis, and amyloidosis.

The contour and volume of muscle can be assessed by inspection, palpation, and measurement. Normal muscles are semielastic, hypertrophied muscles feel firm and hard, pseudohypertrophy has doughy and rubbery consistency, and atrophied muscles are soft and pulpy.

Some clinicians like to measure muscle bulk at fixed points above and below a joint: 7 cm above and 10 cm below the olecranon in the upper limbs and 15 cm above the superior patellar edge and 10 cm below the tibial tuberosity in the lower limbs. For uniformity, it is better to use two fixed points and measure at the maximally affected region and compare with the corresponding region on the other side.

Tone

Tone is defined as the resistance felt in the muscle (in a relaxed state) to passive stretch. The resting tone is maintained by the gamma loop (intrafusal fibers of muscle spindles are innervated by gamma afferents, which relay to the extrafusal fibers through the gamma efferents in the anterior horn cell).

The tone is assessed by passively moving the joint in various movements and at varying speeds and assessing the resistance to those movements. These can be either started proximally and moved distally or vice versa. Always compare with the corresponding part in the other side.

Upper limb tone is usually tested by holding the patient's hand or arm in the examiner's hand or arm (same side as the patient), and resistance is tested at the wrist and hand by rapid alternating flexion–extension movements conducted at the wrist, metacarpophalangeal joints, and interphalangeal (IP) joints. Supination and pronation at the forearm can also be done for the same.

Lower limb tone is assessed by rapid alternating flexion–extension movements at the hip and knee, with the patient lying supine in bed. It can also be tested by passive movement of the thigh while looking for adduction and abduction of the feet. Different disorders of tone are summarized in **Table 2**. A modified Ashworth scale is used to quantify spasticity **(Table 3)**.

Pronator catch and adductor catch: During testing the tone in the distal upper limb, after doing a few slow movements while shaking hands, the examiner should quickly flick the forearm from prone to supine position. If spasticity is present, a brief "catch" is felt at the midrange of rotation,

TABLE 2: Disorders of tone and their localization.

Abnormality	Description	Localization
Spasticity	• *Clasp knife pattern*: Velocity-dependent resistance (hypertonia) • Usually involves the antigravity muscles (flexors) in the upper limb and gravity muscles (extensors) in the lower limb	Corticospinal lesion
Rigidity	• *Hypertonia is present uniformly throughout the range of motion*: Lead pipe rigidity • Cogwheeling due to superimposed tremor	Extrapyramidal lesion
Gegenhalten (inhibitory paratonia)	Resistance is proportional to the force applied by the examiner	Frontal lobe
Mitgehen (facilitatory paratonia)	Patient actively assists examiner, and limb may continue to move even after the examiner releases it	Frontal lobe

Continued

Continued

Abnormality	Description	Localization
Myotonia	• Normal tone when muscle is relaxed but during muscle contraction there is tonic preservation with slow relaxation; usually improves with activity • *Paradoxical myotonia*: Worsens with activity	Muscle membrane
Hypotonia	Decreased resistance to stretch	• Anywhere from anterior horn cell to muscle • Upper motor neuron (UMN) lesions in shock • Chorea • Cerebellar lesions

TABLE 3: Modified Ashworth scale.

Score	Description
0	No increase in muscle tone
1	Slight increase in muscle tone (catch and release)
1+	Slight increase in muscle tone [catch and minimal resistance, less than half of range of motion (ROM)]
2	Marked increase in muscle tone throughout ROM but the examined part can be easily moved
3	Considerable increase in muscle tone and passive movements are difficult
4	Affected part is rigid in flexion and extension

TABLE 4: Medical Research Council (MRC) score.

Power	Movement present
0	No contraction
1	Flicker present
2	Movement with gravity eliminated only
3	Movement against gravity but not against resistance
4	Movement against partial resistance *4–*: Mild resistance *4*: Moderate resistance *4+*: Strong resistance
5	Normal power

following which it gets released and lets the movement proceed smoothly. This is known as the "pronator catch." A similar "catch" can be detected during adduction of hip as well.

Myotonia can be elicited while making a grip (grip myotonia), percussion of thenar muscles (percussion myotonia), forced eye closure (eyelid myotonia), and percussion of tongue (tongue myotonia: napkin ring sign).

Myoedema is a stationary muscle mounding (small swelling or ridge) at the point of muscle stimulation which may last for a few seconds, usually seen in hypothyroid myopathy. Close differential to myoedema is the idio-muscular contraction on direct muscle tapping, which causes depression in the muscle (and not swelling as in myoedema).

In tetanus, there is generalized rigidity and increased tone, starting from the face and jaw (trismus) and spreading to other parts leading to opisthotonos. The tone is increased in both agonists and antagonists. The curious half smile due to the retraction of the angle of the mouth is called risus sardonicus.

Painful muscle spasms and rigidity are seen in stiff person syndrome, especially involving paraspinal muscles. Tonic spasms are also seen in multiple sclerosis.

Power

Power is individually assessed for all movements in major joints of both upper and lower limbs (shoulder, elbow, wrist, hip, knee, and ankle). The power is graded on the Medical Research Council (MRC) score **(Table 4)**. The small muscles of the hand are tested separately and scored based on the percentage of weakness felt. The MRC scale is skewed toward the examination of very weak muscles. Even though MRC levels are clearly defined, they are not linear or evenly spaced. Any power less than Grade 5 is a significant weakness and less than Grade 4 is considered a severe weakness.[2]

This chapter will not discuss the examination of all muscles. Upper limb and lower limb muscles, their movements, nerve supply, and predominant root values are summarized in **Tables 5 and 6.** A summary of major joint movements and their examination in upper limbs, lower limbs, and small muscles of the hand are summarized in **Tables 7 to 10.**[3]

We enumerate here a few practice points to note during power testing:

- Proper strength/power testing requires good positioning and removing unnecessary movements.
- Always fix the proximal limb portion while testing the distal portion.
- Muscle power can be tested in two ways: placing a joint in a particular position and the examiner trying to break it or the patient trying to move against the examiner's resistance.
- Always rule out local causes of limitation of movement and also consider other factors which might affect power examination (e.g., pain).

TABLE 5: Upper limb major muscles, movements, predominant root value, and nerve supply.

Root value	Muscle/nerve supply	Movement
C5	Rhomboids/nerve to rhomboids	Retraction of scapula
	Supraspinatus/suprascapular nerve	First 15° arm abduction
	Infraspinatus/suprascapular nerve	External rotation
	Deltoid/circumflex nerve	Arm abduction between 15° and 90°
	Biceps/musculocutaneous nerve	Elbow flexion
C6	Brachioradialis/radial nerve	Pronation
	Serratus anterior/nerve to serratus anterior	• Overhead abduction • Protractor of scapula
C7	Triceps/radial nerve	Elbow extension
	Latissimus dorsi/nerve to latissimus dorsi	Adduction and internal rotation
	Extensor digitorum, extensor carpi ulnaris, extensor carpi radialis longus/radial nerve	Wrist and finger extension
C8	Flexor digitorum superficialis and profundus, flexor carpi radialis, and ulnaris/median and ulnar nerves	Wrist and finger flexion
C8–T1	Intrinsic muscles of hand/median, ulnar and radial nerves	All movements of the thumb and fingers

TABLE 6: Lower limb major muscles, movements, predominant root value, and nerve supply.

Root value	Muscle/nerve supply	Movement
L1, L2	Iliopsoas/lumbar plexus	Hip flexion
L2, L3	Adductor magnus/obturator nerve	Hip adduction
L3, L4	Quadriceps femoris/femoral nerve	Knee extension
L4, L5	Gluteus medius and minimus/superior gluteal nerve	Hip abduction
	Tibialis anterior/deep peroneal nerve	Foot dorsiflexion
	Tibialis anterior and posterior/posterior tibial nerve	Foot inversion
L5, S1	Gluteus maximus/inferior gluteal nerve	Hip extension
	Semitendinosus, semimembranosus/sciatic nerve	Knee flexion
	Peroneus longus and brevis/superficial peroneal nerve	Foot eversion
	Extensor digitorum brevis and extensor hallucis longus/deep peroneal nerve	Toe extension
S1	Gastrocnemius and soleus/posterior tibial nerve	Plantar flexion

TABLE 7: Testing of movements at major joints in the upper limb.

Area	Movement across	Fixation	Test	Pressure
Shoulder	Flexion	Shoulder joint	Ask the patient to flex the arm	The hand giving resistance is placed just above the elbow. Apply downward force at the contour of the patient's arm
	Extension	Shoulder joint	Ask the patient to extend the arm	The hand giving resistance is placed just above the elbow. Apply downward force at the contour of the patient's arm
	Adduction	Shoulder joint	Ask the patient to adduct the arm from an abducted position	Apply resistance on the arm against adduction
	Abduction	Shoulder joint or on the opposite shoulder to prevent any tendency to lean in the opposite direction	If patient can abduct the arm > 90°, ask the patient to position the shoulder to 90° with the elbow flexed and the forearm pronated	With shoulder in 90° of abduction, apply resistance just above the elbow

Continued

Continued

Area	Movement across	Fixation	Test	Pressure
	Internal rotation	Shoulder joint	With elbow flexed and by the side of body, ask the patient to move the forearm medially	Apply resistance outward on the forearm
	External rotation	Shoulder joint	With elbow flexed and by the side of body, ask the patient to move the forearm laterally	Apply resistance inward on the forearm
Elbow	Flection	Provide stabilization under elbow or anterior of the shoulder at proximal end the humerus	Ask patient to bend the elbow and touch the shoulder with the forearm supinated. Observe for substitution, specifically rotation of forearm to mid position—brachioradialis	Apply resistance on distal forearm
	Extension	Provide stabilization under elbow or anterior to the shoulder at proximal end of the humerus	Place the elbow in a midway between flexion and extension and ask the patient to extend the elbow	Apply resistance on distal forearm
		Shoulder joint	Ask the patient to pronate the forearm against resistance in forearm extension [pronator quadratus (PQ) > pronator teres] and forearm flexion (pronator teres and PQ)	Apply resistance against supination in distal forearm or wrist
	Pronation	Shoulder joint	Ask the patient to pronate the forearm against resistance in forearm extension (PQ and pronator teres) and forearm flexion (pronator teres and PQ)	Apply resistance against pronation in distal forearm or wrist
Wrist	Flexion	The examiner's other hand supports the patient's forearm, or rest the forearm on the table	Arm at the side, elbow flexed to 90° with the forearm supinated and the wrist fully flexed	The examiner's hand giving resistance is placed over the patient's hand first distal to the wrist
		The examiner's hand supports the patient's forearm, or rest the forearm on the table	Arm at the side, elbow flexed to 90° with the forearm pronated and the wrist fully extended	The examiner's hand giving resistance is placed over the back of the patient's hand just distal to the wrist

- Compare the power of muscles on both sides and also compare proximal and distal muscles.
- Always account for poor effort, and muscle power should be evaluated with a demonstration of maximal power.
- While assessing a weak muscle, it is a good practice to start with the movement against gravity. If the patient is not able to do it, proceed with movement with the elimination of gravity.
- When there is a disparity in the physical strengths of the examiner and the patient (e.g., a large powerful patient and a small weak examiner), the examiner can use a long lever (e.g., for deltoid, instead of applying force at lower one-third of the arm while testing deltoid, they can ask the patient to extend the elbow and apply force near the wrist). But the use of a long lever should be documented so that it is known to another examiner and findings are reproducible.
- MRC gradings 4+, 4, and 4– are subjective. A useful clinical tip depends on the examiner requiring the whole hand to break (4+), three fingers to break (4), or one finger to break (4–) a muscle.
- *Small muscles of hand*: Examiner should compare both sides and may compare with his own similar muscle.
- Look for endurance (ability to perform the repetitive motor activity) when there is a history of fatigability.
- Examining ankle plantar flexion in a sitting position or even a supine position may miss mild weakness. Making the patient lay on his abdomen and flexing the knee joint can allow plantar flexion examination against gravity. Asking the patient to walk on his toes may unravel subtle weakness.
- Pseudo-hand grip or finger abduction weakness noted in patients with wrist and finger drop is due to mechanical disadvantage. Always examine with wrist and fingers partially extended.
- Pseudo-radial nerve palsy due to stroke ("cortical hand") can be distinguished by the preserved synkinetic wrist extension after making a fist.

TABLE 8: Testing the small muscles of hand (except interossei).

Muscle	Fixation	Test	Pressure
Thenar muscles *Position: Sitting or supine*			
AP	The hand is stabilized by the examiner or rested on the table	Adduction of the thumb toward the palm	Against the medical surface of the thumb, toward thumb abduction
FPB	As above	Flexion of the interphalangeal joint of the thumb	Against the palmar surface of the distal phalanx, toward thumb extension
AbPB	As above	Abduction of the thumb initially from the palm	Against the proximal phalanx, toward adduction toward the palm
OP	As above	Flexion, abduction, and slight medical rotation of the metacarpal bone	Against the metacarpal bone, toward extension and adduction with lateral rotation
Hypothenar muscles			
ODM	As above	Opposition of the fifth metacarpal toward the first	Against the palmar surface, along the fifth metacarpal, toward the flattening palm of the hand
FDM	As above	Flexion of the metacarpophalangeal joint, with exclusion of interphalangeal joints	Against the palmar surface of the proximal phalanx, toward extension
AbDM	As above	Abduction of the little finger	Against the ulnar side of the little finger, in the direction of adduction toward the midline of the hand

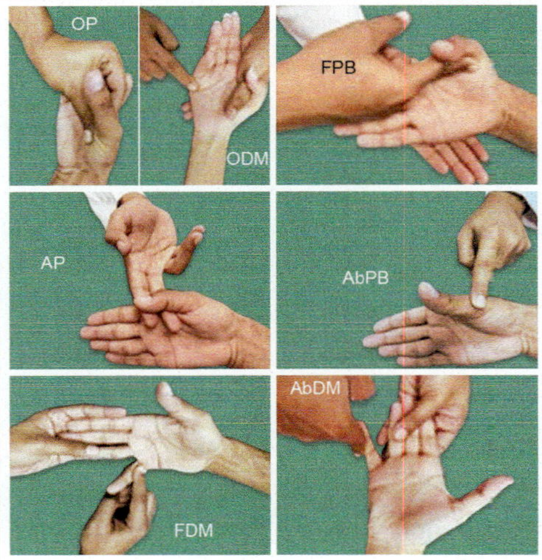

(AbDM: abductor digiti minimi; AbPB: abductor pollicis brevis; AP: adductor pollicis; FDM: flexor digiti minimi; FPB: flexor pollicis brevis; ODM: opponens digiti minimi; OP: opponens pollicis)

- Action of muscles may vary depending on:
  - *Part of muscle activated*: For example, the upper part of gluteus maximus (abduction) and lower part (hip adduction)
  - *Angle of joint during examination*: For example, when the hip is extended hip adductors act as flexors, and they act as extensors when the hip is flexed.
- In nonorganic weakness, contraction may be felt (palpated) in an apparently weak muscle, when the patient is asked to contract a synergistic muscle. Also, when asked to contract the weak muscle, the examiner may be able to feel the contraction in the antagonist in nonorganic weakness.
- Always look out for "trick movements" where the patient might use other muscles of similar function to compensate for the weak muscle.
- Neck flexion and extension are usually tested along with sternocleidomastoid and trapezius. For testing neck flexion, the examiner applies force to the forehead while the patient tries to place the chin on the chest and for neck extension, pressure is applied on the occiput while the patient tries to extend the neck.
- Examination of rhomboids is important to differentiate C5 radiculopathy from upper trunk plexopathy.
- Trapezius testing involves testing for upper, middle, and lower fibers. For upper fibers, ask the patient to shrug the shoulders against resistance. Middle fibers can be tested in a prone position with the shoulder abducted 90° and laterally rotated. The examiner applies pressure against the forearm in a downward direction. Lower fibers are tested in the prone position with the shoulder abducted diagonally overhead in line with lower fibers.
- Primary adductors of shoulder are pectoralis major (C5–T1) and latissimus dorsi (C6–C8). Pectoralis major is tested by asking the patient to adduct the horizontally abducted shoulder. Latissimus dorsi should be palpated while applying resistance to adduction of the horizontally and laterally abducted arm.

TABLE 9: Testing the palmar and dorsal interossei.

Muscle	Test	Pressure	
Interossei *Position*: Sitting or supine *Fixation*: Stabilization of the adjacent digits			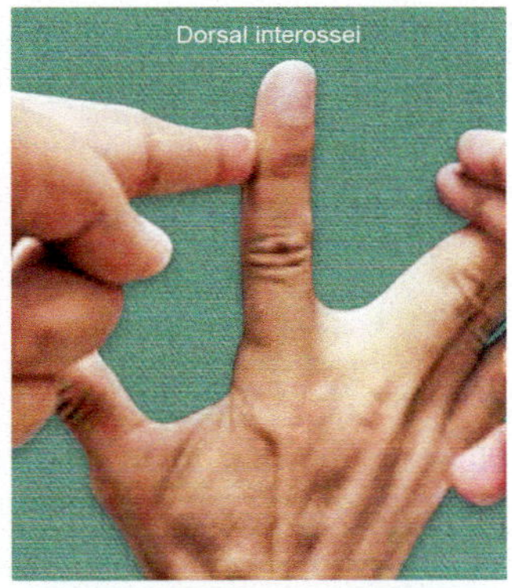
Dorsal interosseous 1	Abduction of the index finger toward the thumb	Apply pressure against the radial side of the index finger, toward the middle finger	
Dorsal interosseous 2	Abduction of the middle finger toward the index finger	Hold the middle finger, and pull toward the ring finger	
Dorsal interosseous 3	Abduction of the middle finger toward the ring finger	Hold the middle finger, and pull toward the index finger	
Dorsal interosseous 4	Abduction of the ring finger toward the little finger	Hold the ring finger, and pull toward the middle finger	
Palmar interosseous 1	Adduction of the thumb toward the index finger (acting with the adductor pollicis and first dorsal interosseous)	Hold the thumb, and pull in the radial direction	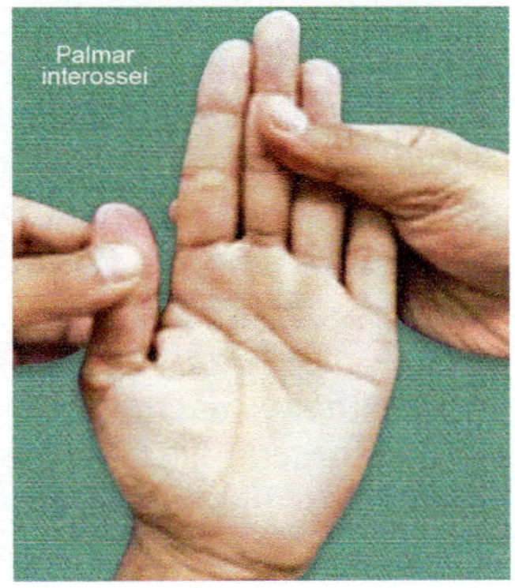
Palmar interosseous 2	Adduction of the index finger toward the middle finger	Hold the index finger, and pull toward the thumb	
Palmar interosseous 3	Adduction of the ring finger toward the middle finger	Hold the ring finger, and pull toward the little finger	
Palmar interosseous 4	Adduction of the little finger toward the ring finger	Hold the little finger, and pull in the ulnar direction	
Dorsal interosseous 1	Abduction of the index finger toward the thumb	Apply pressure against the radial side of the index finger, toward the middle finger	

TABLE 10: Testing of movements at major joints in the lower limb.

Area	Movement across joint	Fixation	Test	Pressure
Hip	Flexion	Stabilize hip joint or brace the anterior superior iliac spine on the opposite side	Ask the patient to raise the knee up as high as it will go. The patient attempts to flex the hip to 90° flexion or keep the hip at 90°. Knee is flexed and rests on the examiner's arm	The examiner's hand giving resistance is placed on distal anterior thigh just proximal to the knee, and pressure is applied in the direction of hip extension
	Extension	Hip joint with knee flexed and the patient prone	Ask the patient to extend the thigh against resistance	The hand giving resistance is placed on lower aspect of posterior thigh, and downward force is applied
	Adduction	Hip joint with knee extended	Ask the patient to adduct the extended leg against resistance	Apply resistance outward on the medial lower thigh or lower leg (if the examiner wants a longer lever)
	Abduction	Hip joint with knee extended	Ask the patient to abduct the extended leg against resistance	Apply resistance inward on the lateral lower thigh or lower leg (if the examiner wants a longer lever)
Knee	Flexion	Knee joint with the patient prone and knee in 90° flexion	Ask the patient to maintain the knee flexion at prone position	Examiner attempts to extend it by applying pressure on the posterior aspect of lower leg
	Extension	Place the arm under the tested knee, and rest the hand on the patient's distal thigh. This causes the tested knee to flex to approximately 15–30°	Ask the patient to straighten the knee against resistance	Apply downward force just proximal to ankle while the patient tries to extend the knee

Continued

Continued

Area	Movement across joint	Fixation	Test	Pressure
Ankle	Dorsiflexion	Hip and knee in flexion to keep foot on the bed to test Grade 3 power or hip and knee in mild flexion to test Grade 4 and above	Ask the patient to attempt dorsiflexion against resistance	Pressure is applied on dorsum of foot in the direction of plantarflexion
	Plantarflexion	Prone position with knee in 90° flexion	Ask the patient to attempt plantarflexion, in supine position and sitting position; it is difficult to identify subtle weakness	Pressure is applied on plantar aspect of the foot and on dorsiflexing it

- Teres major and latissimus dorsi form the posterior axillary fold.
- External rotators of the shoulder are infraspinatus and teres minor.
- Infraspinatus is the chief external rotator, and subscapularis is the chief internal rotator of the shoulder.
- *Shoulder flexors*: Anterior deltoid, pectoralis major, subscapularis, coracobrachialis, biceps brachii
- *Shoulder extensors*: Posterior deltoid, latissimus dorsi, triceps, subscapularis, and teres major
- *Rotator cuff muscles*: Subscapularis, supraspinatus, infraspinatus, and teres minor
- Biceps brachii is an elbow flexor and supinator of the forearm. It has maximum supination power when the elbow is flexed and pronated, and maximum flexion power when the forearm is supinated.
- Brachialis flexes elbow irrespective of forearm position.
- Brachioradialis acts as elbow flexor midway between pronation and supination; it supinates when the forearm is extended and pronated; it pronates when the forearm is flexed and supinated.
- *Bartender's sign*: It is a trick movement employed when the biceps is weak, and the patient employs brachioradialis by putting the arm in mid pronation or by pulling the elbow backward.
- *Chief elbow extensor*: Triceps brachii
- To detect mild weakness in the triceps, examine in full elbow flexion.
- Most powerful forearm supinator is the biceps brachii.
- *While testing for supination during elbow flexion*: Supinator and biceps are involved; during elbow extension, the supinator and brachioradialis are involved.
- Primary wrist flexors are flexor carpi radialis (FCR) and flexor carpi ulnaris (FCU), and primary wrist extensors are extensor carpi radialis longus (ECRL), extensor carpi radialis brevis (ECRB), and extensor carpi ulnaris (ECU).
- Most powerful wrist extensor is ECRL.
- In posterior interosseous neuropathy (PIN), there is a radial deviation of the wrist on extension due to an unbalanced pull of ECRL.
- Primary flexors of fingers are flexor digitorum superficialis (FDS) [proximal IP (PIP) joint] and flexor digitorum profundus (FDP) [distal IP (DIP) joint].
- Finger flexion at metacarpophalangeal (MCP) joint is by interossei and lumbricals.
- *Dorsal interossei*: Flex the MCP, extend PIP, and abduct the fingers.
- *Palmar interossei*: Flex the MCP, extend PIP, and adduct the fingers.
- *Lumbricals*: Extend the PIP and weak flexors of MCP.
- *Palmaris brevis sign*: On small finger abduction, there is wrinkling of skin over the hypothenar area, which indicates deep palmar branch of ulnar nerve involvement in case of weakness of ulnar intrinsic muscles.
- Ulnar claw hand is due to extension of MCP and flexion of PIP and DIP (due to weakness of interossei and lumbricals whose function is flexion of MCP and extension of IP joints).
- Ulnar claw hand predominantly affects little and ring fingers because both lumbricals and interossei are weak.
- Grip strength depends on the degree of flexion of MCP and IP joints, thumb position, and wrist extensors' action to stabilize the wrist. It predominantly gives a gross estimate of forearm muscles.
- Forearm muscles controlling the thumb are abductor pollicis longus (APL) (abducts thumb), extensor pollicis longus (EPL) (extends terminal phalanx), extensor pollicis brevis (EPB) (extends proximal phalanx), and flexor pollicis longus (FPL) (flexes distal phalanx).
- Abdominals, intercostals, and spine extensors are supplied by the thoracic nerves. Abdominal muscles are supplied by T5–T12 nerve roots and are examined in the upper and lower quadrants when the patient tries to lift their head or legs, respectively.
- Spine extensors arise from T1–T12 and are tested by making the patient lie prone and lift their upper chest and shoulder followed by both legs above the bed. Intercostal muscles are observed whilst the patient is doing quiet inspiration and expiration.
- *Beevor's sign and inverted Beevor's sign*:
  - In normal individuals, the rectus abdominis muscle contracts as a whole with no predominance between the upper or lower half and left part over the right. As a result, the umbilicus does not move on normal trunk flexion.
  - Beevor's sign is an abnormal upward movement of the umbilicus on truncal flexion in a supine position. It is elicited with the patient in the supine position who is asked to either flex the neck or sit up from this position without using the support of the arms. If the

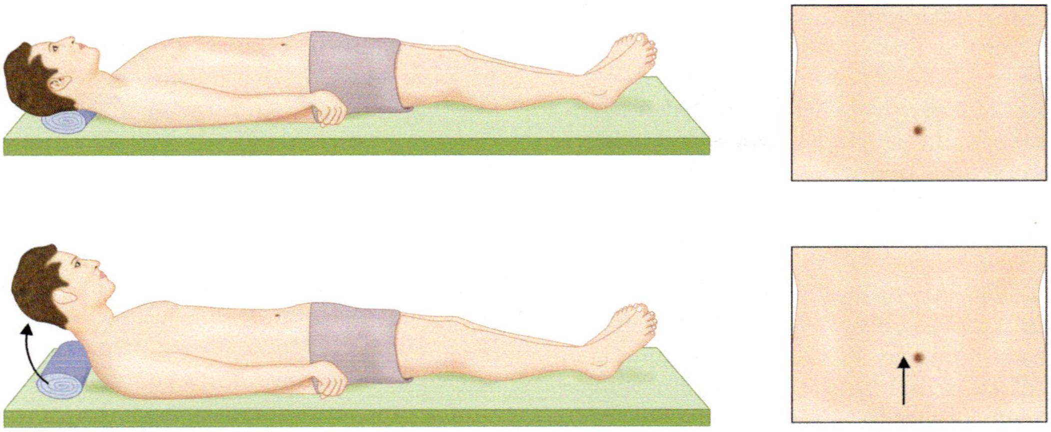

FIG. 1: Eliciting the Beevor's sign.

TABLE 11: Localization of foot drop.

	Tibialis anterior	Peroneus longus	Tibialis posterior	Hamstrings	Gluteus medius
	Ankle dorsiflexion	Ankle eversion	Ankle inversion	Knee flexion	Hip abduction
Deep peroneal nerve					
Common peroneal nerve					
Sciatic nerve					
Lumbosacral plexus					
L5 root					

umbilicus moves upward, it is a positive Beevor's sign. If it moves downward, it is an inverted Beevor's sign. It is normal if the umbilicus stays in its original position **(Fig. 1)**.

  - Beevor's sign is usually seen in a spinal cord lesion between T10 and T12 segments and in FSHD. It can rarely be seen in Pompe's disease, GNE myopathy, tubular aggregate myopathy, myotonic dystrophy, sporadic inclusion body myositis (IBM), and ALS. Inverted Beevor's sign can occasionally be seen in FSHD patients.

- Paraspinal weakness is commonly seen in FSHD and Pompe's disease.
- Chief hip flexor is iliopsoas, and the major hip extensor is the gluteus maximus. Primary hip abductors are gluteus medius, minimus, and tensor fascia lata.
- *Gower's sign*: It is characterized by the individual "climbing up" on their thighs with the aid of their hands. It is classically seen in Duchenne muscular dystrophy but can be seen in any condition associated with weakness of the pelvic girdle or proximal lower limb muscles.
- *Trendelenburg sign*: Gluteus medius and minimus muscles are essential in providing stability of the hip joint to maintain a midline center of gravity. Weakness of hip abductors leads to a contralateral pelvic drop with an ipsilateral rise during single-leg stance—positive Trendelenburg sign. This is because the pelvis cannot be maintained in a level plane by the lesioned abductors; the patient falls toward the good side and simultaneously the torso leans toward the lesioned side in order to maintain balance (Trendelenburg gait).
- Hip adductors are adductor longus, brevis, and magnus.
- Quadriceps are spared in GNE myopathy and affected predominantly in IBM.
- Ankle inversion weakness in the presence of foot drop points toward L5 radiculopathy. The localization of foot drop is summarized in **Table 11**.
- Extensor digitorum brevis (EDB) hypertrophy in the presence of weakness (proximal or distal) is seen in hereditary myopathies.
- *Identifying subtle weakness*: Pronator drift
  We ask the patient to extend both arms in front of them (nearly at shoulder height) with palms facing upward. They are observed in this position with eyes open for 20 seconds followed by eye closure for 20 seconds. A normal response consists of either no movement or slight pronation without downward drift of both upper limbs and the dominant hand (pseudodrift). In a *positive pronator drift with eyes open*, one side drops and pronates. This can occur when minimal amounts of corticospinal involvement are present in UMN pathologies. The selective weakness of shoulder abductors, external rotators, supinators, and elbow extensors is overcome by

their antagonists to cause pronation, elbow flexion, and downward drift. Other types of drifts seen are:

- *Sensory drift*:
  - *Positive with eyes closed*: The affected side rises upward without patient awareness due to loss of position sense ("updrift").
  - Lesion side is the parietal lobe contralateral to the drift.
- *Cerebellar drift*:
  - *Positive with eyes open or closed*: The affected side rises and moves outward or may drift aimlessly. Overcorrection may also be seen (on tapping the palm or the arm, it overcorrects and never goes back to the primary position).
  - Lesion is on the same side as the drift.
- *Conversion drift*:
  - *Positive with eyes open or closed*: The affected side drops without pronation.

- Hoover's sign is used to detect functional weakness in lower limbs. It is the absence of associated movement in the lower limb (absence of downward pressure of contralateral normal heel when "trying" to lift "paralyzed" limb and presence of downward movement of "paralyzed" limb while raising the unaffected lower limb).

CONCLUSION

Motor system examination is an integral part of neurological examination. The examiner should have a good understanding of neuroanatomy and the normal actions of muscles to examine them adequately. Always document the power charting including the position in which the patient was examined. Reproducibility is a major quality indicator of a good motor system examination.

REFERENCES

1. Brazis PW, Masdeu JC, Biller J. Localization in Clinical Neurology, 7th edition. Netherlands: Wolters Kluwer; 2016.
2. Campbell WW. Dejong's The Neurologic Examination, 7th edition. Netherlands: Wolters Kluwer; 2012.
3. Kendall FP, McCreary EK, Provance PG, Rodgers MM, Romani WA. Muscles: Testing and Function with Posture and Pain, 5th edition. Philadelphia: Lippincott Williams & Wilkins; 2005.

8 CHAPTER

Testing the Sensory System

Jayakumar Vaikundam, Harish Jayakumar, Rama Shankari Padmanabhan

INTRODUCTION

The evaluation of sensory system is highly dependent on the ability and desire of the patient to cooperate. Sensation is subjective and the examiner must, therefore, depend almost entirely on the patient's response.

One of the principal goals of the sensory examination is to identify meaningful patterns of sensory loss to localize the level of involvement.

Sensation can be categorized by various methods depending on anatomic or functional criteria.

An anatomic classification includes somatic and visceral sensations including general and special sensations. However, clinically only the somatic sensations can be assessed.

Functionally, the sensory nervous system was classified initially as protopathic (simple affective sensations) and epicritic (sensations that provide discriminative analysis) with respect to the environment.

However, Sherrington had devised a more practical scheme of classification and it remains the most useful for clinical analysis.

The major categories of sensory modalities that are quintessential for testing are:

- Exteroceptive sensations
- Proprioceptive sensations
- Cortical sensations

Exteroceptive sensations include pain (algesia) and temperature (thermesthesia).

Proprioceptive sensations include light touch, vibration sense (pallesthesia), joint position sense (arthresthesia), and joint movement sense (kinesthesia).

Cortical sensations include tactile localization (topagnosis), tactile discrimination, stereognosis, two-point discrimination (2PD), double simultaneous stimulation, graphesthesia, and barognosis.

General Principles in Sensory Testing

- Basic testing should sample the major functional subdivisions of the sensory systems.
- Since sensory testing is subjective and time-consuming, a good result is obtained when the patient is properly educated about the aims of testing and briefly describes how the testing is about to be performed.
- Explain to the patient what you are going to do and how they should respond.
- Properly expose the area to be examined and to be positioned in long sitting with legs, trunk, and thighs exposed.
- The patient's eyes should be closed throughout the sensory examination.
- For all modalities of testing, always test the affected side/area first and then the unaffected side. This prevents retained memory of the previously provided stimulus which might compromise assessment.
- Simultaneous assessment of certain modalities can be done; tactile localization and discrimination can be done immediately after confirming that touch is appreciable in the suspected area of impairment.
- Apply the stimulus to a normal area so that the patient is aware of what and how the normal sensation feels like.
- Stimuli should be applied at irregular intervals to avoid anticipation by the patient.
- When testing a sensation, compare two sides distal and proximal, and ask the patient whether the sensations are equal on both sides or not.
- To map the area of abnormal sensations, first examine the abnormal area and then move towards the normal area.
- Sensory tests are done from the distal to the proximal direction.
- If the superficial sensation is impaired then some impairment is also seen in deep and combined sensations, and the interpretation becomes difficult.

- Hence, it is important to examine in the following order:
  1. Superficial (exteroceptive) sensation
  2. Deep (proprioceptive) sensation
  3. Combined cortical sensations

SUPERFICIAL (EXTEROCEPTIVE) SENSATION

Pain (Pinprick) Sensation

It is tested by using a safety pin's sharp and blunt tip. The pointed end is used for the sense of sharpness and the rounded end for the sense of dullness. Whether using the dull or pointed end, light pressure is applied without moving the pin after the point of contact. The sensory level is determined accurately with this testing. Preservation of pinprick sensation is considered to have a good prognosis in spinal cord injury (SCI) patients.

Testing Method

- First the sharp and blunt sensations are clearly defined and referenced by touching the face—prior to testing the dermatomes. Individual dermatomes are then tested with the patient's eyes closed.
- Enquire if the given stimulus is sharp or blunt. Enquire by comparing the intensity with the pretest reference point at the face. Comparison with a similar site on the opposite side is then performed. Impairment is then mapped on the pictorial representation.
- If there are inconsistent responses, the same stimulus is given at the same pressure and 10 stimuli are given at each site. More than or equal to 8 out of 10 responses are considered normal.
- The sharp and dull ends are randomly applied perpendicular to the skin, and these should not be applied too close to each other or in a too rapid manner to avoid the summation of impulses.
- Make sure that the pinprick is not too strong (use constant pressure) and the tip is not too sharp to draw blood (hence avoid injection needles for testing pain), nevertheless it may still be possible to transmit communicable diseases by transferring small amounts of blood produced by pinprick, hence instruments should be cleaned or disposed off between patients **(Figs. 1A and B)**.
- A rolling pinwheel may also be utilized for testing for pain sensation, especially to delineate the affected large areas more precisely but should be sterilized before using it in the next patient **(Fig. 2)**.

Objective Scoring

- *0*: The patient is unable to differentiate the sensations of sharpness or bluntness.
- *1*: *Impaired*—The patient is able to differentiate different tips of the safety pin but states that there is a difference between the evaluated point and the face (more or less feeling).
- *2: Normal*—The patient is able to completely differentiate the sharp and blunt tips of the safety pin and states that there is no difference between the evaluated and reference points (the face).

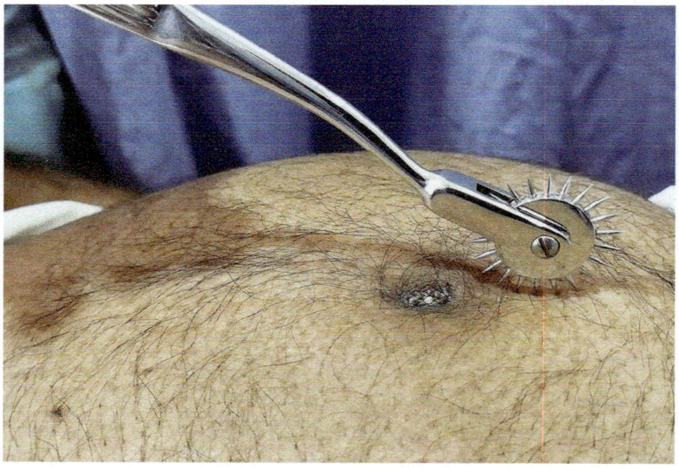

FIG. 2: Rolling pinwheel.

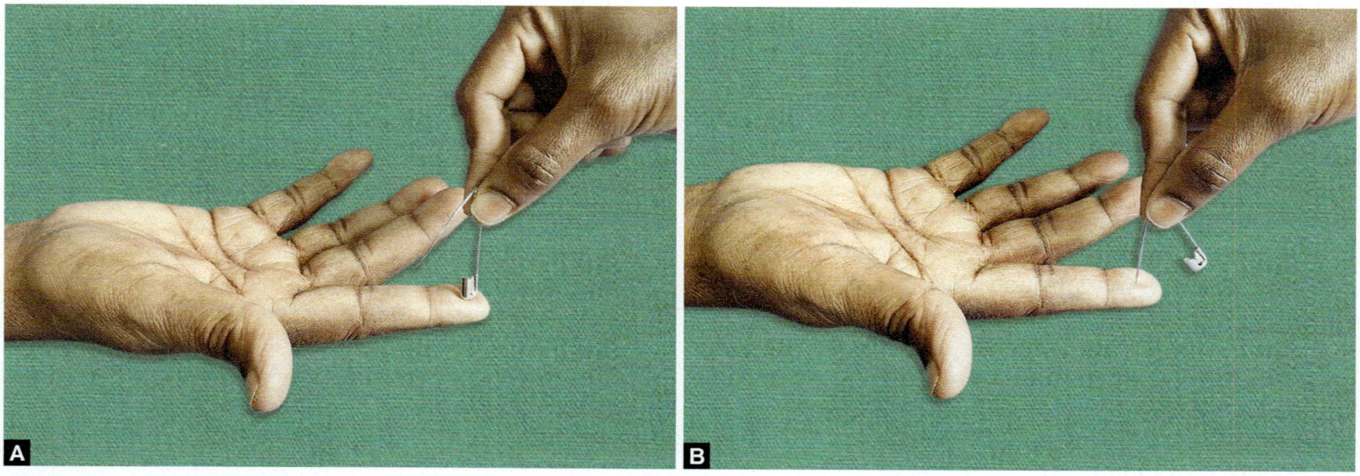

FIGS. 1A AND B: Testing pinprick: (A) Blunt end of the safety pin and (B) sharp end of the safety pin.

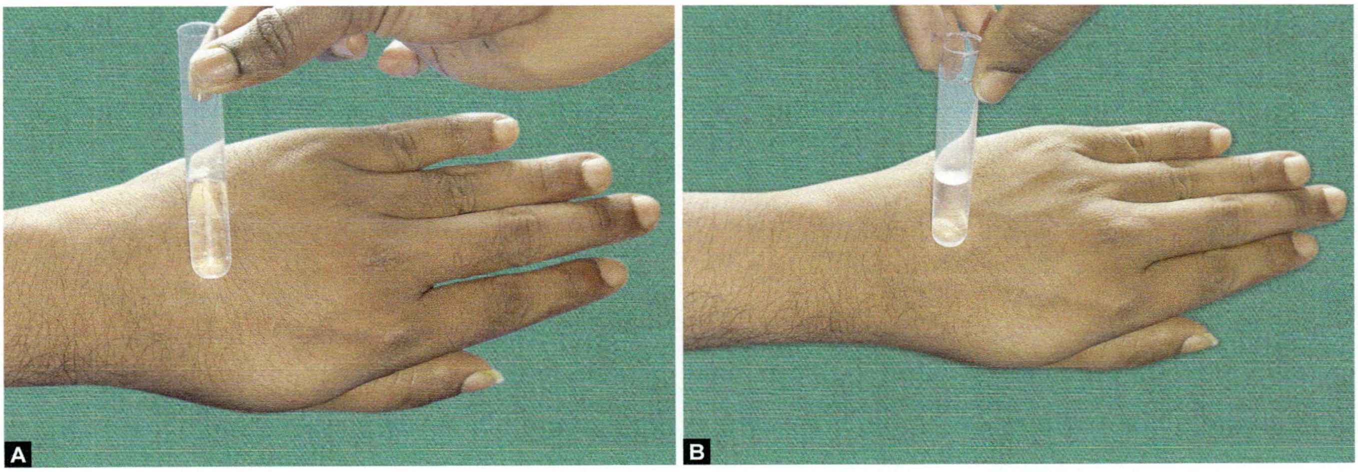

FIGS. 3A AND B: Testing temperature: (A) Use the sides of the test tube; (B) Avoid using the base of the test tube.

Temperature Sensation

- Two test tubes (metallic would be better because of better conductivity) with stoppers filled with warm water or cracked ice and water may be used for testing (sometimes cool ends of the tuning fork can also be used).
- One should be filled with cold water (between 5 and 10°C) and the other with warm water (40–45°C). Temperatures <5°C or >45°C elicits painful responses in addition to temperature and hence should be avoided.
- First demonstrate on an area of skin with intact sensation, the feeling of hot compared to cold.
- The test tubes are randomly placed over different areas of the skin area to be tested.
- Use the sides, not the bases of the test tubes **(Figs. 3A and B)**.
- Ask the patient to respond (with eyes closed) hot and cold after each stimulus application.
- Start distally in the arm/leg and in a random sequence, alternate between hot and cold test tubes with firm pressure for a short, equal period of time.
- Apply the stimulus for some time as the latency for detecting temperature is longer than for other sensory modalities.
- Pause after each stimulus awaiting response without prompting.
- Alternate between different surfaces in a random sequence. Note the number of correct responses and if there is any area with consistently wrong responses.
- The Lindblom roller (Rolltemp)[1] is designed for quick screening of temperature sensibility over large body areas. It uses two rollers on handles, one warm roller and the other cold **(Fig. 4)**.

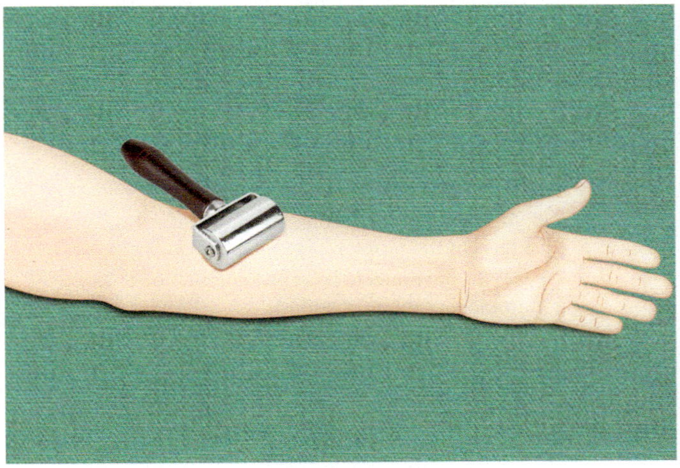

FIG. 4: Lindblom roller (Rolltemp).

Although both pain and temperature are carried through the lateral spinothalamic tract, one can occasionally encounter intact pain perception but lost or diminished temperature sensation in spinal cord lesions.[2] Hence, one cannot presume that if pain is felt normally there is no need to test for temperature.

According to American Spinal Injury Association (ASIA) international standard examination card, sensory testing (light touch and pinprick) should be done on 28 dermatomes at 56 key points (two for each dermatome) on each side which can be identified with anatomical bone indicators **(Table 1)**. The sensory levels are scored on a 0–2 scale for each dermatome.

- 0—the sensation is absent
- 1—the sensation is present but impaired
- 2—the sensation is normal

The maximum possible score is 112 points for each of them for a patient with normal sensation.

International Standards for Neurological Classification of SCI (ISNCSCI) Worksheet 2019 can be obtained from the site: *https://asia-spinalinjury.org/international-standards-neurological-classification-sci-isncsci-worksheet/*.

TABLE 1: Dermatomes—key sensory points to be examined.

Cervical	• *C2*: At least 1 cm lateral to the occipital protuberance (as alternative, 3 cm to the back of the ear) • *C3*: Supraclavicular fossa (behind clavicle) at midclavicular line • *C4*: On the acromioclavicular joint • *C5*: Side of antecubital fossa lateral (radial) (proximal to the elbow line) • *C6*: Thumb, dorsal aspect, and proximal phalanx • *C7*: Middle finger, dorsal aspect, and proximal phalanx • *C8*: Small finger, dorsal aspect, and proximal phalanx	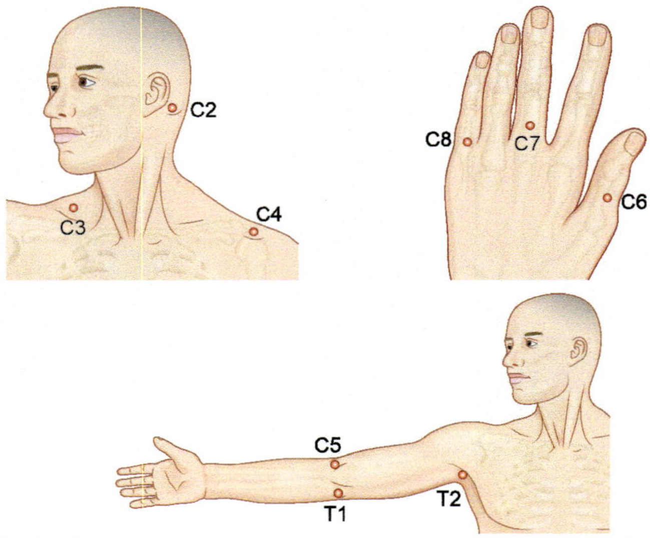
Thoracic	• *T1*: Antecubital fossa medial (ulnar) side and proximal to the humerus medial epicondyle • *T2*: Axilla apex • *T3*: On the midclavicular line and in the 3rd intercostal space (IS); determined by palpating the 3rd rib and the space just below that 3 IS • *T4*: On the midclavicular line and in the 4th IS (level of the nipple) • *T5*: On the midclavicular line and in the 5th IS (middle point of T4 and T6) • *T6*: On the midclavicular line and in the 6th IS (xiphisternum level) • *T7*: On the midclavicular line and in the 7th IS (middle point of T6 and T8) • *T8*: On the midclavicular line and in the 8th IS (middle point of T6 and T10) • *T9*: On the midclavicular line and in the 9th IS (middle point of T8 and T10) • *T10*: On the midclavicular line and in the 10th IS (umbilicus) • *T11*: On the midclavicular line and in the 11th IS (middle point of T10 and T12) • *T12*: On the midclavicular line and the middle point of the inguinal ligament	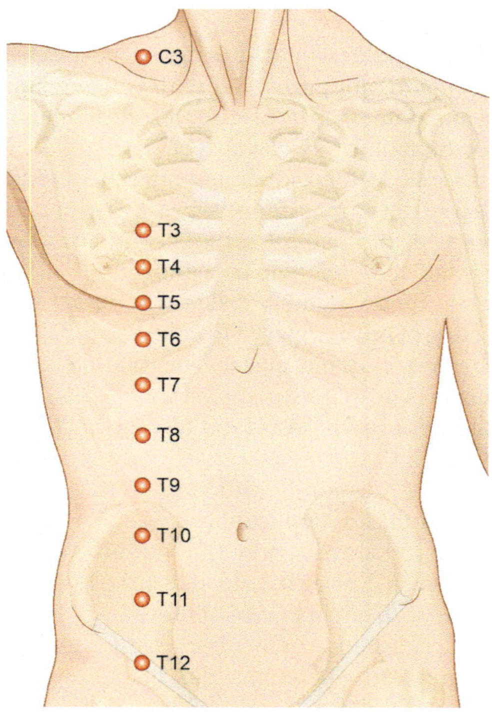
Lumbar	• *L1*: Middle of the distance between T12 and L2 sensory key points • *L2*: In the anterior–medial femur, the middle point of the line between the middle point of the inguinal ligament (T12) and the medial femoral condyle • *L3*: Above the medial condyle on the knee • *L4*: Medial malleolus • *L5*: 3rd metatarsophalangeal joint on the dorsum of the foot	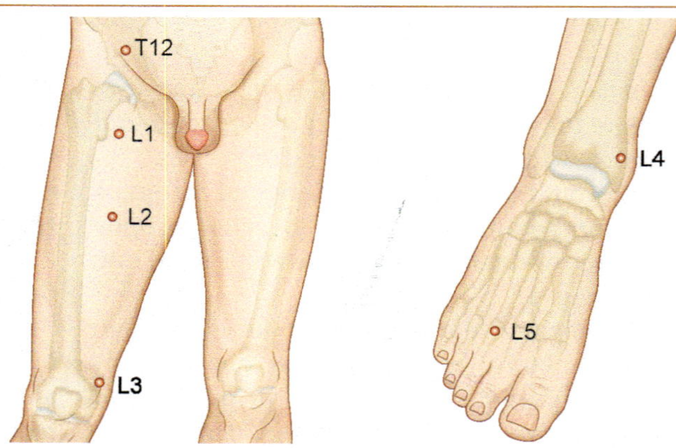

Continued

Continued

Sacral	• *S1*: Lateral heel (calcaneus) • *S2*: Middle point of the popliteal fossa • *S3*: Ischial tuberosity or infragluteal fold • *S4–5*: Perianal region, <1 cm lateral to the mucocutaneous junction (a single level is accepted)	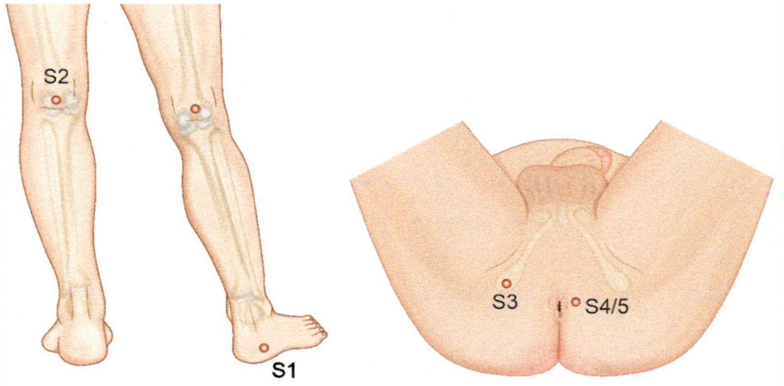

PROPRIOCEPTIVE SENSATIONS

Light Touch

- *Crude touch*—refers to a less discriminative form of touch, where the patient feels that something has touched and is unable to localize where he was touched and is modulated through spinothalamic tracts.
- *Fine touch*—refers to more discriminative light touch that allows a subject to sense and localize the sensation and is modulated through posterior columns.

Explain the procedure including the purpose of the assessment like—*"I am going to test the feeling in your arm/trunk/leg, let me know what you feel."*

1. Use a cotton swab, wisp of cotton, or finger to lightly touch or jab the patient's skin with his eyes closed. Do not drag the stimulus as it tends to cause a different form of stimulation, such as tickling. The area touched by the cotton should not be >1 cm **(Fig. 5)**.
2. Await a response from the patient without prompting them. Then ask the patient what it feels like (tactile discrimination) and where he felt it (tactile localization).
3. Commence testing in the suspected area of impairment. Start distally in arms or legs by gently touching but rapid stroke using equal pressure throughout. Compare the sides. Proceed testing in a caudocranial manner.
4. Ensure that you switch to the opposite side without manual handling so as to reduce sensation learning.
5. Evaluate whether the touch is appreciated and whether it is comparable in intensity to identical places on the other half of the body and from other body parts.
6. Every time, the patient appreciates a touch and after randomly touching different body regions, ask the patient to count while keeping their eyes closed.
7. To avoid the patient's anticipated prediction of the next stimulus, alter the rate of stimulus and also alternate by applying and withholding the stimulus to make sure he does not routinely answer "yes" even in the absence of any stimulus.

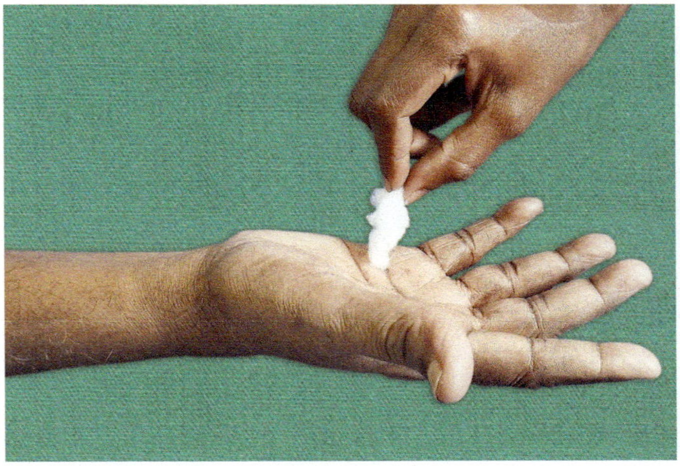

FIG. 5: Cotton wisp for touch perception.

8. Should there be an impairment, compare with the normal side (similar site on the opposite side) and elicit the percentage of impairment in the abnormal side.
9. Graphically or pictorially represent the area of impairment in a line diagram to assess the pattern of involvement.
10. Assess the pattern of impairment, if it is dermatomal, segmental, or in the distribution of the peripheral cutaneous nerve

Semmes–Weinstein Monofilament Examination

The 10-g monofilament is commonly used. It is an objective and simple instrument used to screen the diabetic foot for loss of protective sensation **(Fig. 6)**.[3,4]

- First apply the monofilament perpendicular to the skin surface on the patient's hands or forehead and apply sufficient force to cause the filament to bend or buckle for 1 cm. Make sure that the patient could feel the sensation with eyes closed **(Fig. 6)**.
- Then start examining three sites or more on both feet as indicated in **Figure 7**.

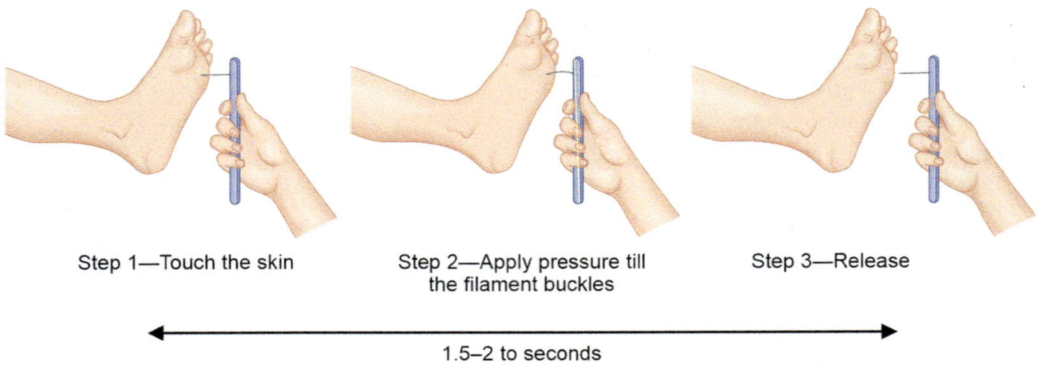

FIG. 6: Semmes–Weinstein monofilament test.

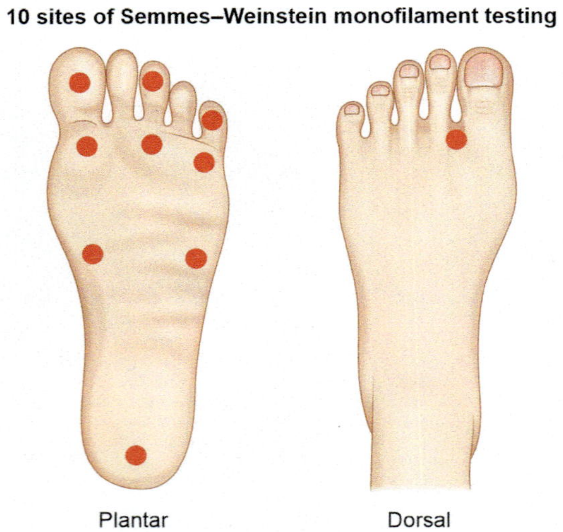

FIG. 7: Monofilament testing sites.

- It should be applied, held, and released over 1–2 seconds for each test.
- Repeat this test twice at the same site but alternate this with at least one "mock" test without applying the filament.
- The filament should be applied along the perimeter of (not on) an ulcer site, callus, scar, or necrotic tissue.
- Do not slide or wiggle the filament or make repetitive contact at the testing area.
- If the patient is unable to identify correctly two out of three times at each site, then he has a high risk of developing an ulcer.

Pressure Sensation

It is tested by applying pressure on deep structures (such as muscles, tendons, and nerves) or by firm touch on the skin using finger pressure or a blunt object.

Although pressure sensation is closely related to touch, but it involves the perception of pressure from the deeper subcutaneous structures rather than a light touch from the superficial skin.

It is also closely related to position sense and is mediated via the posterior columns.

- Deep pressure elicits deep pain which may be absent in disorders like Tabes dorsalis in relation to testicles (Pitres' sign), the ulnar nerve (Biernacki's sign), Achilles tendon (Abadie's sign).
- Retained testicular sensation (unpleasant feeling elicited by squeezing or pressure) in a diabetic with impotence indicates that the impotence is unlikely to be due to autonomic neuropathy.[5]

Vibration Sense

Testing Method

1. Use a tuning fork with a 128-Hz frequency, as this frequency provides a clearer separation of normal from abnormal than 64- or 256-Hz tuning forks.
2. Make sure that the patient can distinguish between the vibrating and nonvibrating tuning forks by demonstrating to them how the vibrating ("this is vibrating or buzzing") and nonvibrating ("this is just touching") forks feel.
3. Also demonstrate and confirm that he clearly understands the difference between pressure and vibration.
4. The examiner should hold the stem of the tuning fork with two fingers, similar to gripping a dart so as not to touch the vibrating tines **(Figs. 8A and B)**.
5. Ask the patient to close his eyes and start testing from distal to proximal parts, from lower limbs to upper limbs in a sequential manner (e.g., over the toes, the medial, lateral malleoli, tibial tuberosity, anterior iliac spine, over the spinous processes, fingertips, interphalangeal joint, metacarpophalangeal joint, wrist, elbow, and shoulder).
6. Ask the patient if he can feel the vibration and must be able to appropriately identify it as soon as it stops. One can also compare the patient's response to his own by checking if he can still feel the vibrations after the patient has stopped feeling it.

Timed Vibration Sense

- Use a 128-Hz tuning fork, strike it and apply it on the dorsum of distal phalanx of the thumb of the patient. Use a stopwatch to calculate the time from the start of perceiving the vibration till its cessation.

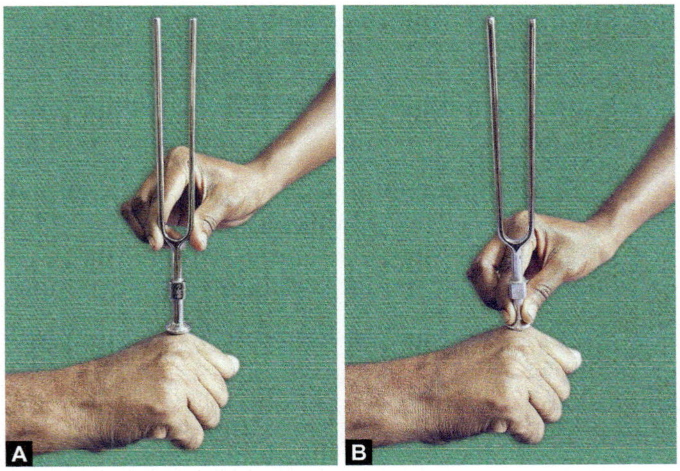

FIGS. 8A AND B: (A) Vibration sense—wrong way; (B) Vibration sense—right way.

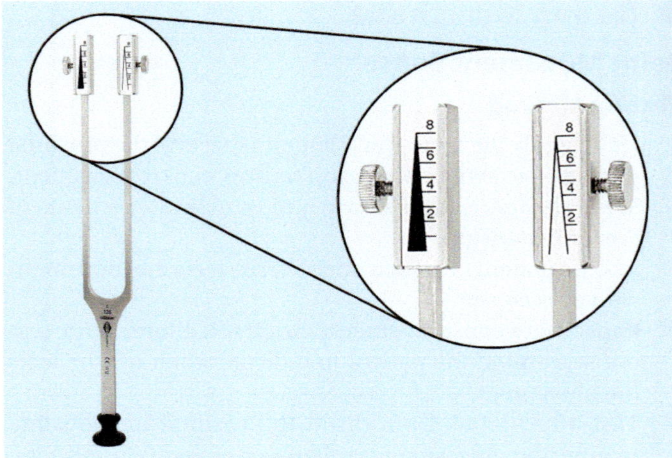

FIG. 9: Rydel–Seiffer tuning fork.

- Then apply the tuning fork on the dorsal aspect of the distal phalanx of the examiner's thumb. The time (in seconds) at which vibration sensation is no longer perceived by the examiner is also recorded.
- Test for timed vibration over the dorsum of the distal phalanx of the great toe, medial malleolus, tibial tuberosity, and dorsum of the distal phalanx of the index finger. Compare the timing between similar sites on the opposite side.[6]

Interpretation

- A difference of >8 seconds in the great toe indicates impairment (sensitivity—85%, specificity—42.8%)
- It is a reliable bedside examination when performed using a standardized protocol.[7]

Rydel–Seiffer Tuning Fork

The Rydel–Seiffer tuning fork (RSTF) is a 64-/128-Hz tuning fork which allows semiquantitative assessment of vibration perception. There is a black and white display of two arrows and two sets of numbers from 0 to 8 on the tines. During vibration, the numbers and arrows blur out. Once vibrations decrease, the triangles appear to intersect on the graduated scale of 0–8. Once the patient says that he is no longer able to feel the vibration, he can read the value at the apex of the single triangle formed from the initial two triangles. That value is called the "vibratory threshold" **(Fig. 9)**.[8]

A more detailed description can be accessed at: https://neurosigns.org/wiki/Vibration_testing_with_the_Rydel-Seiffer_tuning_fork.

A reference value chart is available for various ages and for both upper and lower extremities.[9]

Quantitative vibration testing with the RSTF correlated well with the amplitude of the sural sensory nerve action potential in a series of 184 subjects.[10]

It also appears to be an inexpensive device for screening diabetic patients with high-risk foot.[11]

Few Caveats

- A normal young adult should perceive vibration for at least 15 seconds at the great toe; this value decreases by about 1 second per decade. Perception for <10 seconds at the great toe is abnormal at any age.
- Loss of vibratory sensation is an early and sensitive indicator of demyelination of the peripheral nerves or the posterior columns.
- Testing vibration sense can be helpful in detecting psychogenic sensory disorders in addition to proprioception.

A vibrating tuning fork activates Pacinian corpuscles very rapidly and widely across the periosteum of the skull or the sternum.

Patients who can feel the vibration in the center of the forehead or sternum but not over the affected side which is only a few mm away are likely to have psychogenic symptoms. This finding is known as "splitting the sternum" or "splitting the forehead" for vibration sense.[12]

- It has been observed that the combination of intact vibratory sensation and impaired joint position sensation may predict ataxia of spinal origin even without other myelopathic findings.[13]
- It appears that the dorsolateral funiculus (not the posterior columns) is the main ascending spinal cord pathway for joint position sense, kinesthesia, and vibration sense in human beings.

Diseases that specifically affect the dorsal columns do not affect these senses. However, disorders that affect the dorsolateral portions of the spinal cord selectively affect position sense and vibration with preservation of tactile and nociceptive sensation.[14]

Testing Kinesthesia

Joint Movement Sense

Testing Method

- Hold lightly the medial and lateral aspects of the proximal phalanx—to avoid giving extra sensory cues to the patient.
- Move the toe/thumb slowly into random increments of flexion/extension.
- Ask the patient to inform once he/she feels the movement with eyes closed.
- Pause between movements briefly, if there is no response, remind the patient to indicate when he/she feels the movement.
- Test other joints from distal to proximal in the same manner by assessing one plane of movement for each joint.
- It is better to start the testing with finger or toe slightly flexed or extended as the sensitivity is less when the joint is in mid position.
- Once the responses are consistently correct, proceed to test joint position sense.

Joint Position Sense

Testing Method

- First ask the patient to watch the up- or downward movement of the great toe with eyes open to make sure that he can understand the procedure properly.
- Then with eyes closed by grasping the great toe at its sides, move the toe up or down, hold it steady for some time, and ask the patient to indicate whether the toe has been moved up or down.
- Slowly move the thumb/toe into flexion/extension with smaller degrees of movement.
- Briefly pause between movements and ask the patient "Is that moving up or down?" to make sure that he does not make automatic guesses.
- Test ankle/wrist, knee/elbow, and hip/shoulder in the same way, only one plane of movement needs to be assessed for each joint.
- For larger joints, move one joint and ask the patient to copy the position with their opposite limb (e.g., move right knee into 90° flexion, the patient keeps the left knee in a similar position).

Few Caveats

- Joint movement should be tested slowly, over 1–2 seconds, instead of rapidly (since the sensitivity of the test is inversely related to the velocity of the movement).
- To avoid stimulation of tactile, pressure receptors that may give clues to the direction of movement, it is important to hold the digit laterally, parallel to the plane of movement **(Figs. 10A and B)**.
- The great toe should be separated from adjoining toes to eliminate all contact which can possibly give a suggestion of the direction of movement of the great toe.
- The distal interphalangeal joint and phalanx of the middle finger are the joints of choice for the upper limbs to test.[15]
- One can demonstrate definite involvement of position sense in the 4th digit when it is preserved in the other digits in dorsal column involvement. The reason being when compared to 3rd and 4th digits, other digits of the hands and feet have the richest innervation and the largest cortical representation. Hence, a larger lesion is required to manifest the involvement of other digits **(Figs. 11 and 12)**.
- The patient should be instructed not to attempt any active and/or any anticipatory movement of the body part that is being tested.
- Normally, people can correctly identify movements to the tune of one degree or less over the finger joints and three degrees at the toes.
- Mild impairment of position sense usually occurs first in the digits, then followed by impairment of the sense of movement.
- These sensations are affected earlier in the small toes before the great toe in the foot, and in the hand, involvement of the little finger may precede involvement of the ring, middle, or index finger or thumb.

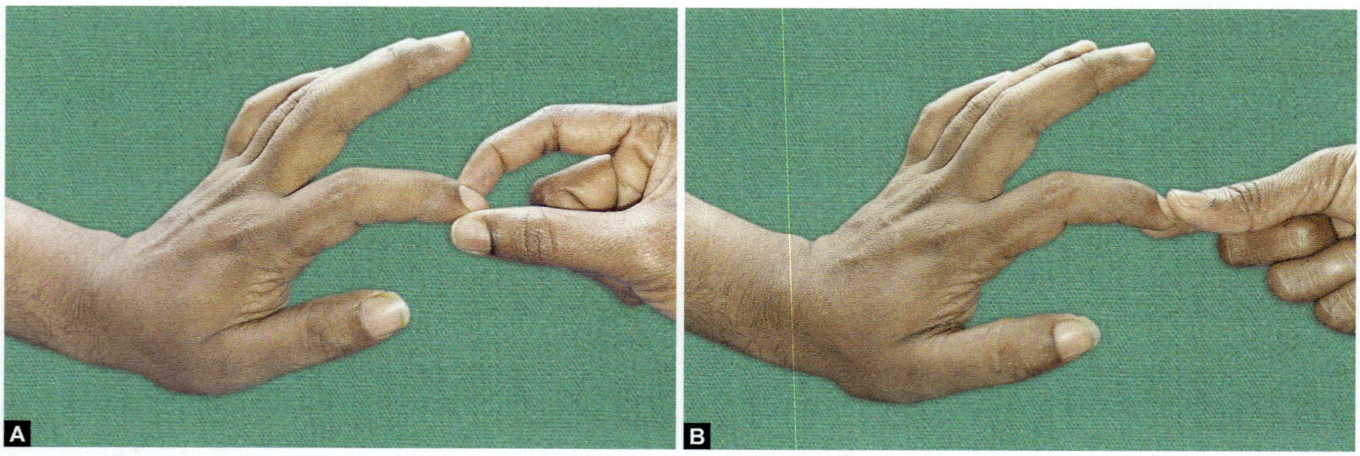

FIGS. 10A AND B: (A) Testing JP sense (right way); (B) Testing JP sense (wrong way).

- If there is an impairment at the great toe, proceed to test by advancing more proximally, e.g., at the ankle. If position sense is impaired there also, proceed with testing successively at the knee and at the hip. Then test the upper limb from fingers, wrist, elbow, and shoulder joints successively up to the level at which the subject could identify correctly.
- One should remember that Romberg's sign need not be positive in a patient who has impairment of joint sense distally especially confined to the great toe.
- Abnormality in Joint position sensory testing (JPST) correlates well with the severity of neuropathies and appears to be a good clinical marker for increased risk of ulceration in patients with known diabetic neuropathy.[16]

Dual Joint Position Test

Described by Yesim Yetimalar Beckmann et al. seem to have a better clinical utility to demonstrate lemniscal system dysfunction apart from demonstrating other digits are more sensitive to demonstrate the abnormal perception of the position sense than the great toes **(Figs. 13 and 14).**[17]

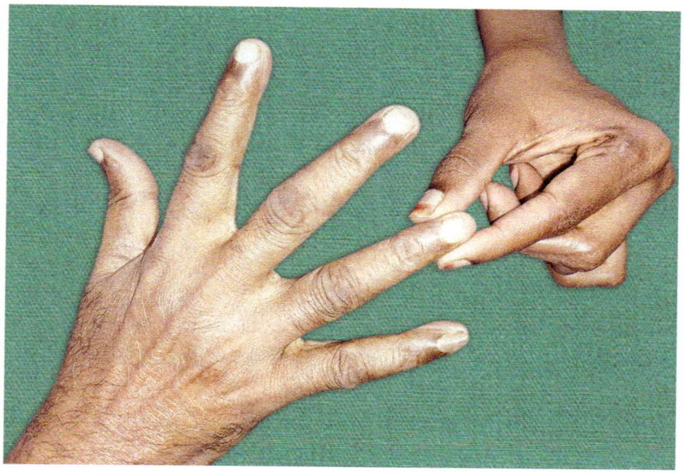

FIG. 11: Fourth digit is important.

Romberg Test[18]

Method of Testing

- Ask the patient to remove shoes and stand with both feet together.
- Then ask him to hold his arms next to the body or crossed in front of the body.
- Observe for any swaying or unsteadiness.
- Ask the patient to stand erect with his eyes closed for 1 minute.
- Observe for imbalance

The Romberg test is considered positive when the patient loses balance (evidenced by increased body swaying, foot movement in the direction of the fall, or falling) with his eyes closed.[19]

A positive Romberg test denotes sensory ataxia due to posterior column involvement (seen commonly in tabes dorsalis, vitamin B12 deficiency, and in myelopathies)

Measures to increase the sensitivity:

- *Sharpened Romberg test*: Perform the test with feet in a heel-to-toe tandem position thereby narrowing the patient's base.
- *The modified Romberg test using a foam pad ("MRuFP")*: Here, the test is done by asking the patient to stand on a foam rubber pad instead of a firm surface (to abolish the proprioceptive inputs from the feet). This is a test of the vestibular system rather than that of posterior column.[20]

Variations of the Romberg test include the following:

- Single-leg-stance test (SLST)[21]
- Sitting-rising test (SRT)[22]
- Get-up and Go test[23]

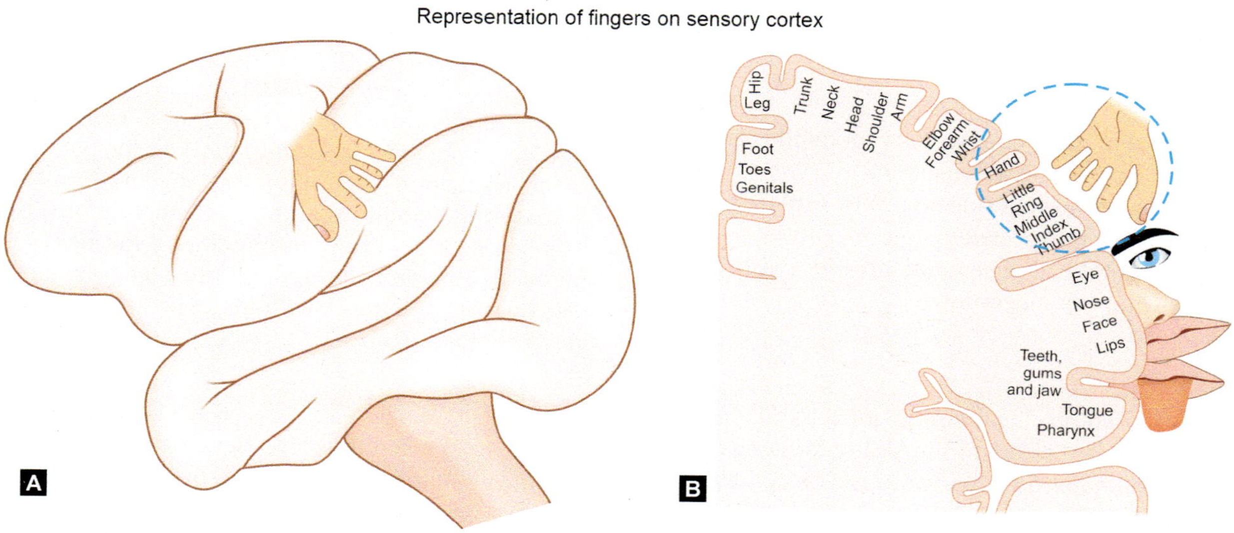

FIGS. 12A AND B: Cortical representation of digits.

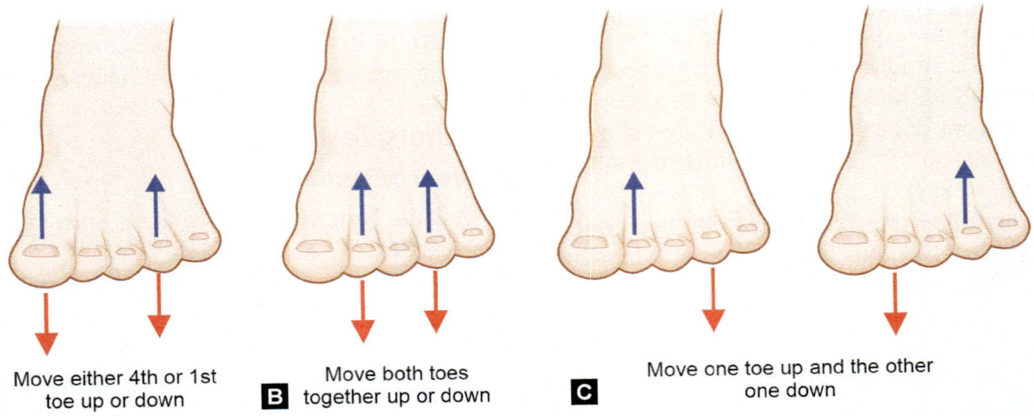

FIGS. 13A TO C: (A) Single joint position sense; (B and C) Dual joint position sense.

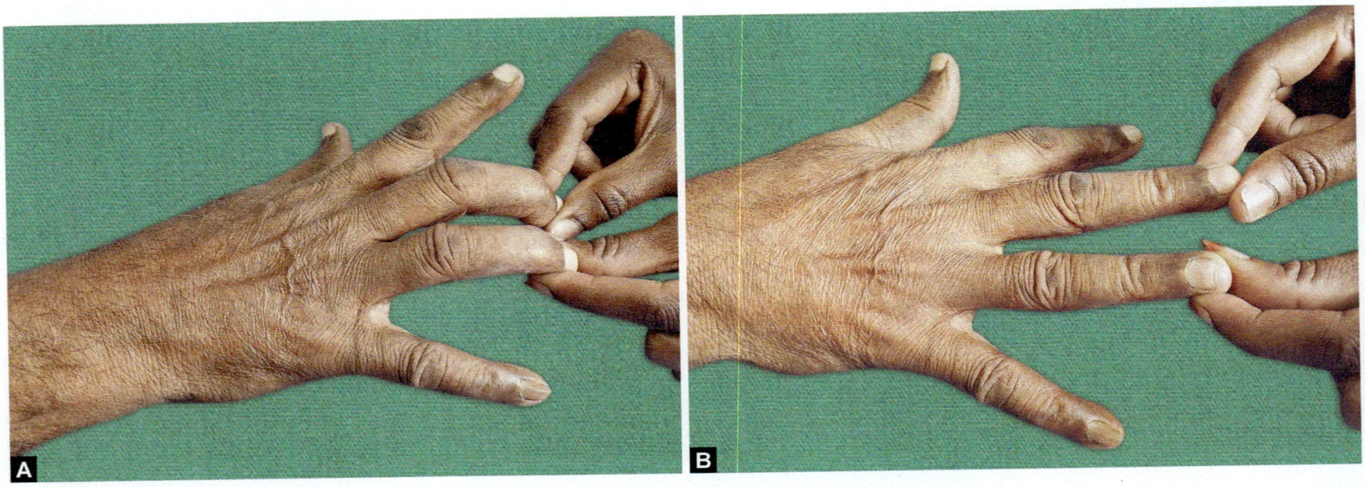

FIGS. 14A AND B: (A) Dual joint position sense flexion; (B) Dual joint position sense extension.

COMBINED CORTICAL SENSATIONS

Cortical sensations are interpretative sensory functions that require analysis of individual sensory modalities by the parietal lobes to provide discrimination.

Few caveats:

- Make sure that individual sensory modalities are intact before testing for cortical sensations.
- First test on the normal side after fully explaining to the patient what he is expected to do.
- Ask him to close his eyes and proceed with the test without giving any suggestions.

Stereognosis

Stereognosis ("stereo," meaning solid, and "gnosis," meaning knowledge) refers to the ability to recognize and identify the size, shape, form, and nature of objects by feeling them without visual, auditory, or other cues.[24]

- *Size identification*: It is tested by using objects of the same shape but different sizes (e.g., different-sized balls)
- *Shape identification*: It is tested with objects of simple shape (e.g., plastic or cardboard cut square, triangle, and circle objects)
- *Identification of form*: It is tested by using solid objects of different geometry (e.g., ball, cube, and pyramid)
- *Object recognition*: It is tested by placing commonly used three-dimensional objects (e.g., pen, comb, key, coin, safety pin, paper clip, and button) on the patient's hand and asking him to identify it by feeling it **(Figs. 15A to C)**.

Loss of this ability is known as astereognosis. Stereognosis can be tested only in hands and the deficit will be unilateral. However, the inability to recognize objects by feeling with either hand, with intact primary modalities, is known as tactile agnosia.

Graphesthesia

It refers to the ability to recognize letters, symbols, or numbers written on the skin purely by the sensation of touch with eyes closed **(Fig. 16)**.

Its name is derived from the Greek "grapha" (writing) and "aisthesis"" (perception).

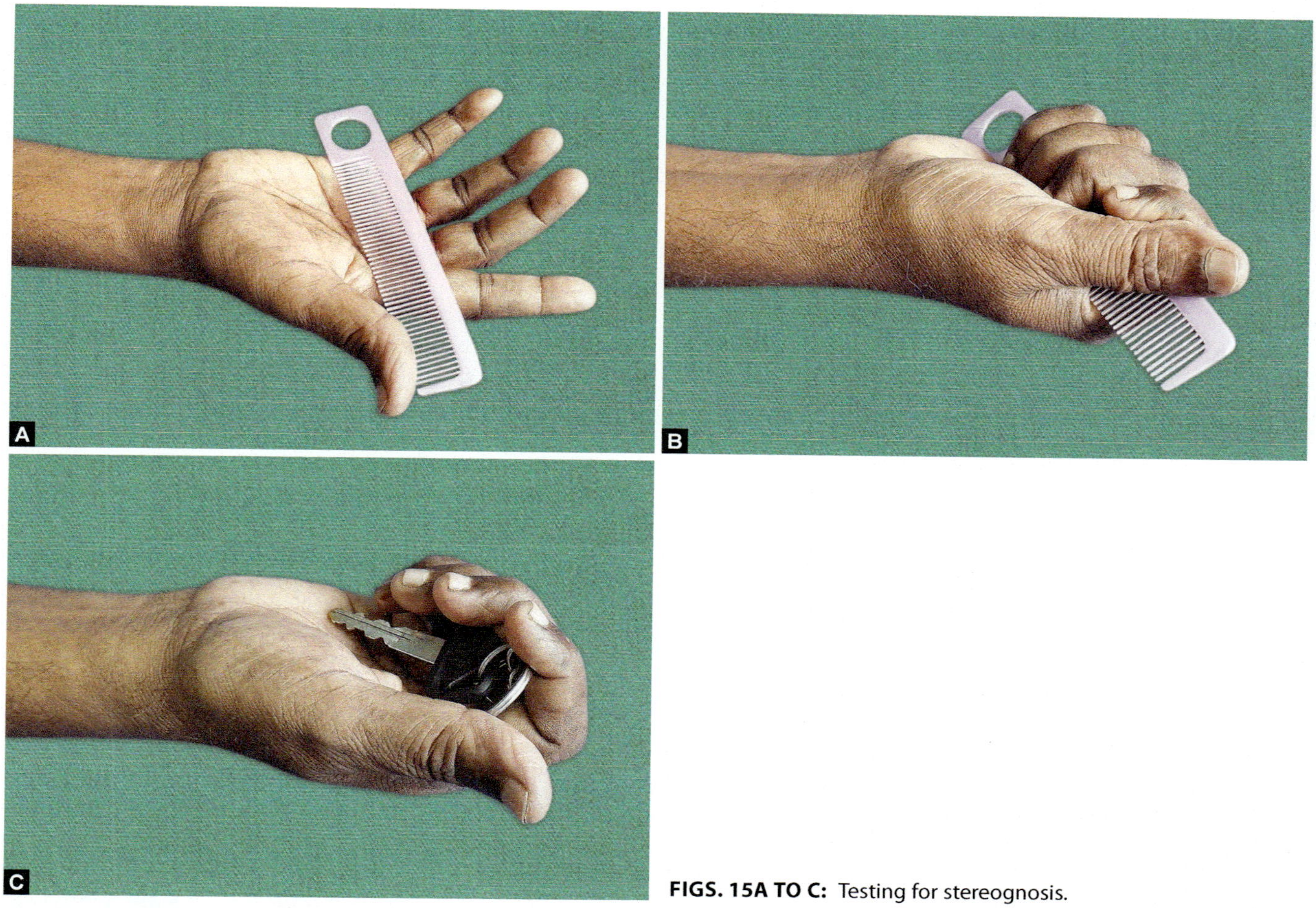

FIGS. 15A TO C: Testing for stereognosis.

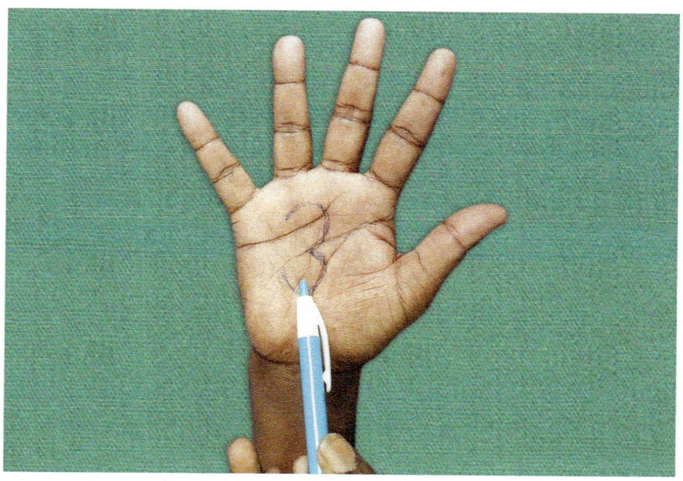

FIG. 16: Testing for graphesthesia.

Testing Method

Testing can be done over the finger pads, palms, or dorsum of the feet (some patients may be hypersensitive on the soles).

Let the patient see his palm or foot and make him understand which is the upper and which is the lower part. With the blunt end of a pen or pencil, write slowly a large number on the patient's palm. Then repeat it with eyes closed. Make sure he is able to understand and identify correctly.

Few Caveats

- Write letters or numbers of about 1 cm in height on the finger pads, larger in other places.
- Use easily identifiable, dissimilar numbers (e.g., 3 and 4 rather than 3 and 8).
- Initially start with numbers 8, 4, and 5 and later with numbers 6, 9, and 3.
- Write with a continuous stroke without taking the stimulus in-between.
- It does not generally matter whether the numbers are written as how the patient would "read" them or "upside down".
- Repeat testing for four or five times and use numbers/letters with an unpredictable sequence.
- Even a mild peripheral sensory impairment can give a negative response.
- This test can come in handy when stereognosis testing becomes difficult to perform, e.g., in the presence of motor weakness, arthritis, or other conditions that prevent the patient from manipulating an object well enough to identify it.

Loss of this ability is known as agraphesthesia or graphanesthesia.

Tactile Movement Sense (Directional Cutaneous Kinesthesia)

It refers to the ability to tell the direction of movement of a light scratch stimulus drawn for 2–3 cm across the skin.

- Ask the patient to inform whether the object moved up or down initially with eyes open.
- After two trials, test with eyes closed, make 10 trials in random up or down directions (normal person should be able to identify all).
- If he makes mistakes, increase the distance to 5 cm and then to 10 cm to get a quantitative assessment.

Hankey and Edis (1989) found this test superior to joint position and vibration sense and a sensitive sign of posterior column function.[25]

Tactile Localization (Topognosis)

It refers to the individual's ability to perceive where on the skin he was touched with a light touch.

- Touch briefly a point on the patient's skin with his eyes closed.
- Then ask the patient to open both eyes and point to the place where he was touched.
- He must be able to identify correctly.

Tactile localization is most accurate on the palmar surfaces of the fingers, especially the thumb and index finger. The term "topagnosia" refers to the absence of this ability (a person with intact touch perception fails to locate the site of stimulus).

Double Simultaneous Stimulation

Double simultaneous stimulation (DSS) (also known as sensory extinction) examines the ability to perceive a simultaneous touch stimulus on opposite sides of the body, proximally and distally on a single extremity, or proximally and distally on one side of the body **(Figs. 17A to C)**.

Method of Testing

- Inform the patient that you may touch one or both sides.
- With the patient's eyes closed, touch one area on one side and the corresponding area on the opposite side both randomly and simultaneously with your index finger or a wisp of cotton.

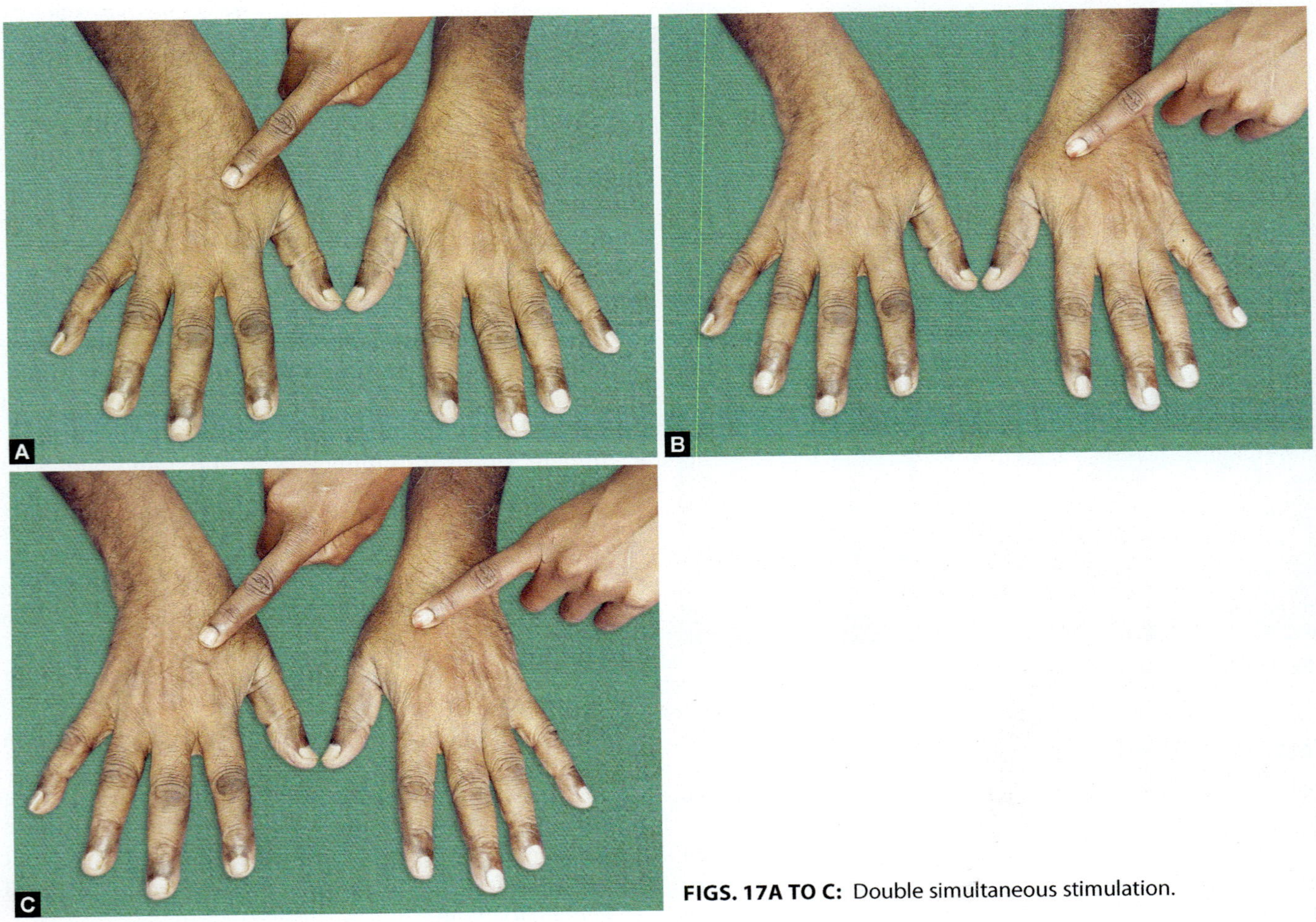

FIGS. 17A TO C: Double simultaneous stimulation.

- Ask him to identify where he was touched. Repeat the test randomly by touching one area and simultaneously both areas.
- Test can be done between two opposite sides or proximally and distally on a single extremity, or proximally and distally on one side of the body.
- Make sure that he could identify two different stimuli when two areas are simultaneously touched.
- Consistent failure to identify two separate points when two stimuli are applied simultaneously is termed sensory extinction or inattention.

Few Caveats

Inattention is most prominent after right parietal lobe lesions, where the patient fails to attend to the stimulus on the left.

Two-point Discrimination Test

It simply refers to the minimum distance between two points, which is necessary to feel two contacts when applied simultaneously **(Figs. 18A and B)**.

Testing Method

A bent paper clip or drawing compass with a blunt-pointed tip or a measured blunt caliper (unfolded paper clip or a discriminator) is generally used.

- First explain the patient clearly by touching the two points widely separated so that he can differentiate them as two points.
- Then with the patient's eyes closed, touch the testing area with one point or two points at random starting far apart and gradually approximating them until he fails to identify the two points.
- Apply two-point stimulus for 1 second, then repeat.
- Note the minimum distance at which the patient can reproducibly differentiate two points which is called the patient's "two-point threshold".
- Although the finger pads (especially the tip of the index finger) are tested generally, other areas also can be tested if required.
- The threshold of a normal person on different body parts are as follows (Dejong 1967):
    - *Tongue tip*: 1 mm
    - *Lips*: 2–4 mm
    - *Fingertip*: 2–4 mm
    - *Dorsum of fingers*: 4–6 mm
    - *Palm*: 8–12 mm
    - *Dorsum of hand*: 20–30 mm
    - *Forearm*: 12–35 mm
    - *Shins*: 30–40 mm
- *There are two types of 2 point descrimination—static and moving*:
    1. To test static 2PD (first reported by Weber[26]), the test instrument is held in place for a few seconds on the site to be tested.
    2. The moving test of 2PD (m2PD) was described by Dellon[27,28] where the two ends of the paper clip are pulled longitudinally from proximal to distal, along the fingertip and across the papillary ridges. Randomly alternate the testing stimulus from one to two points, and if the patient correctly identifies the changes, then proceed to the next lower value. Seven out of 10 correct responses are required before proceeding to the next lower value. Based on this Dellon developed a device (an easy to handle and a validated tool for neurosensory testing)—Pressure Specified Sensory Device (PSSD) to measure how hard the skin had to be pressed to decide if one or two rounded objects were moving or in constant contact on that skin's surface.

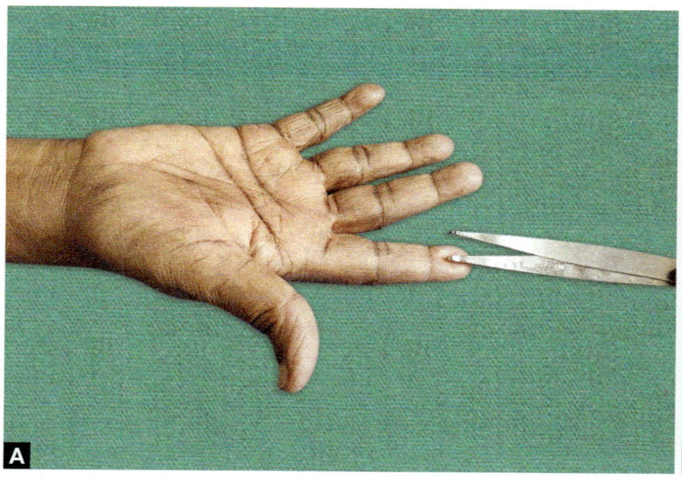

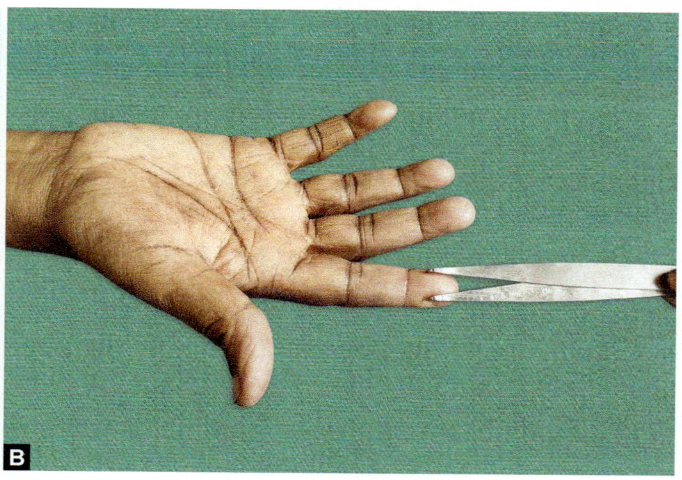

FIGS. 18A AND B: Two-point discrimination test.

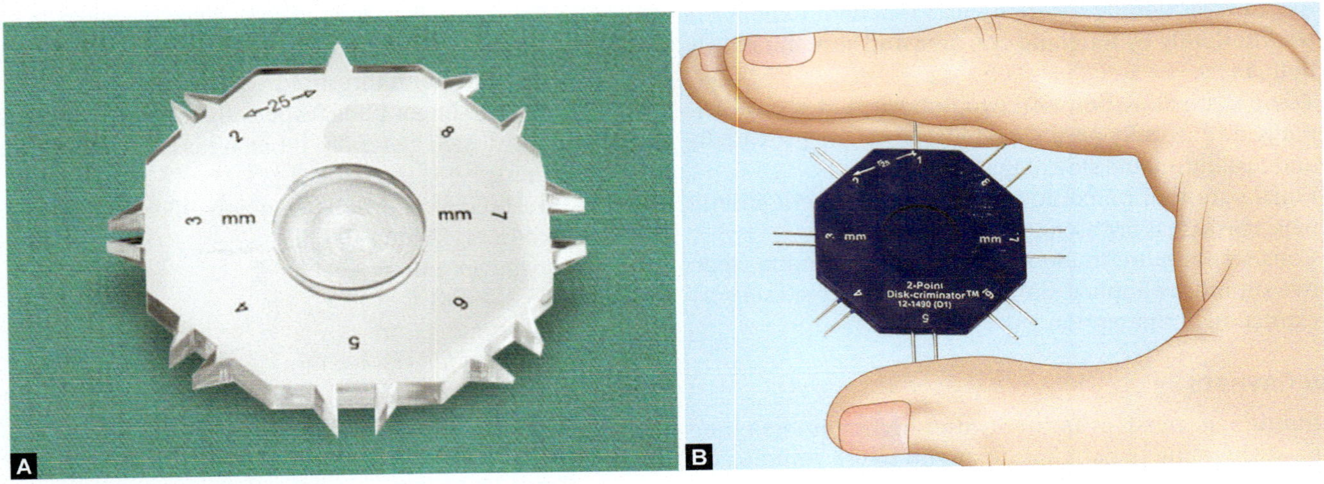

FIGS. 19A AND B: Two-point discrimination test "Greulich star".

Few Caveats

- Applying too much of pressure is a common mistake, which can change the result as more pressure will bring more receptors into the field of stimulation and cause more deformation on the skin.[29]
- "Wriggling" of the finger by the patient to induce sufficient pressure to provoke a result may invite the risk of including nondenervated receptors in the nearby skin territories.
- In patients with neuropathies or repaired nerve injuries, measurable 2PD can be obtained by performing "just blanching the skin technique".[30]
- It is important to remember that only blunted ends on the testing instrument should be used to ensure that touch and not pain is assessed.
- The test can also easily and rapidly be done by using the commercially available device, such as the "Greulich star"[31] or any other similar device which can be indigenously made **(Fig. 19)**.[32] A 2PD test with a greater value of 6 mm was defined as pathological.
- Gelberman et al. (1978) and Fess et al. (1978) have suggested a classification that has been adopted by the American Society for Surgery of the Hand (ASSH): 2PD test value <6 mm is normal, 6–10 mm is fair, and 11–15 mm is poor (ASSH, 1983).[30]

Two-point orientation discrimination: In this, patient attempts to discern the orientation (vertical or horizontal) of two points of contact.[33] Unlike 2PD, two-point orientation discrimination measures tactile spatial acuity in a better way.

Barognosis

- Barognosis ("baros" weight, "gnosis" knowledge) refers to the ability to estimate or perceive differences in the weight of an object.
- *Abarognosis*: It refers to loss of the ability to sense weight or difference in weight between two objects.

SENSORY TESTING FOR ALTERED SENSATIONS

Pain-oriented Sensory Testing

Allodynia

"Allo" means other and "dynia" means pain simply meaning pain due to a stimulus that does not normally provoke pain (nociceptive sensation elicited by a non-nociceptive stimulus). It can occur with mechanical, thermal, or chemical stimuli (e.g., tactile allodynia and heat allodynia).

Hyperpathia

It is an abnormally painful reaction to a repetitive (cutaneous) stimulus along with an increased threshold.

Hyperalgesia

It is an increased pain response to a (noxious) stimulus that normally provokes pain.[34]

A detailed account of various (quantitative) sensory testing methods in relation to the above-mentioned painful conditions which are important to assess the severity and to assess efficacy of various treatment modalities is available as Pain-Orientated Sensory Testing (POST) Guidelines (2018) at: *https://www.anzca.edu.au/getattachment/554e8dd9-a45d-4f6d-8cdc-1b0793dba926/POST-Guidelines.*

Quantitative Sensory Testing

Quantitative sensory testing (QST) is a psychophysical method for assessing somatosensory functions in a quantitative way, although originally evolved to measure the thermal and vibratory stimuli, it has now developed into a standardized tool where multiple parameters are measured.

The QST protocol developed by the German Research Network on Neuropathic Pain assesses nearly 13 parameters, including thermal, mechanical, pain thresholds, vibration thresholds, dynamic mechanical allodynia, wind-up ratio, pressure pain threshold, etc.[35,36] The detailed account of them is beyond the scope of this chapter.

CONCLUSION

Sensory examination forms an integral part of clinical localization. Being highly dependent on the cooperation of the patient and partly subjective, findings need to be interpreted carefully. Experience is required for carrying out a meaningful sensory examination and repeating the testing protocol may be necessary in some patients.

REFERENCES

1. Marchettini P, Marangoni C, Lacerenza M, Formaglio F. The Lindblom roller. Eur J Pain. 2003;7:359-64.
2. Rosner J, Hubli M, Hostettler P, Jutzeler CR, Kramer JLK, Curt A. Not Hot, but Sharp: Dissociation of Pinprick and Heat Perception in Snake Eye Appearance Myelopathy. Front Neurol. 2018;9:1144.
3. Schaper NC, Van Netten JJ, Apelqvist J, Lipsky BA, Bakker K; International Working Group on the Diabetic Foot. Prevention and management of foot problems in diabetes: A Summary Guidance of Daily Practice 2015, based on the IWGDF Guidance Documents. Diabetes Metab Res Rev. 2016;32(Suppl 1):7-15.
4. Suchitra D, Hulke SM, Wakode SL, Khadanga S, Thakare AE, Bharshankar RN, et al. Effectiveness of Semmes Weinstein 10 gm monofilament in diabetic peripheral neuropathy taking nerve conduction and autonomic function study as reference tests. J Family Med Prim Care. 2022;11(10):6204-8.
5. Campbell IW, Ewing DJ, Clarke BF, Duncan LJ. Testicular pain sensation in diabetic autonomic neuropathy. Br Med J. 1974;2(5920):638-9.
6. Prabhakar AT, Suresh T, Kurian DS, Mathew V, Shaik AIA, Aaron S, et al. Timed vibration sense and joint position sense testing in the diagnosis of distal sensory polyneuropathy. J Neurosci Rural Pract. 2019;10(2):273-7.
7. Botez SA, Liu G, Logigian E, Herrmann DN. Is the bedside timed vibration test reliable? Muscle Nerve. 2009;39(2):221-3.
8. Panosyan FB, Mountain JM, Reilly MM, Shy ME, Herrmann DN. Rydel-Seiffer fork revisited: Beyond a simple case of black and white. Neurology. 2016;87(7):738-40.
9. Martina IS, van Koningsveld R, Schmitz PI, van der Meche FG, van Doorn PA. For the European Inflammatory Neuropathy Cause and Treatment (INCAT) group. Measuring vibration threshold with a graduated tuning fork in normal aging and in patients with polyneuropathy. J Neurol Neurosurg Psychiatry. 1998;65:743-7.
10. Pestronk A, Florence J, Levine T, Al-Lozi MT, Lopate G, Miller T, et al. Sensory exam with a quantitative tuning fork: rapid, sensitive and predictive of SNAP amplitude. Neurology. 2004;62:461-4.
11. Vijay V, Snehalatha C, Seena R, Ramachandran A. The Rydel Seiffer tuning fork: an inexpensive device for screening diabetic patients with high-risk foot. Pract Diab Int. 2001;18(5):155-6.
12. Gilman S. Joint position sense and vibration sense: Anatomical organisation and assessment. J Neurol Neurosurg Psychiatry. 2002;73:473-7.
13. Kanazawa M, Katsumi K, Tokutake T, Endo N, Onodera O, Nishizawa M. Dissociation between intact vibratory sensation and impaired joint position sensation may predict ataxia of spinal origin. Interdiscipl Neurosurg. 2016;6:68-70.
14. Brazis PW. (2002). Anatomy of joint-position sense and vibration sense. [online] Available from https://www.jwatch.org/jn200212270000005/2002/12/27/anatomy-joint-position-sense-and-vibration-sense. [Last accessed April, 2023].
15. Crumbie L, Mytilinaios D. (2022). Neurological examination of the sensory system. [online] Available from https://www.kenhub.com/en/library/anatomy/neurological-examination-of-the-sensory-system. [Last accessed April, 2023].
16. Sebastianes FM, Zanoni PH, Feitosa ACR, Nery M, Parisi MC. Sensitivity of joint position sense test, tuning fork test, Semmes-Weinstein Monofilament Examination and Michigan Neuropathy Screening Instrument in the diagnosis of diabetic polyneuropathy. Rev Med (São Paulo). 2021;100(3):246-53.
17. Beckmann YY, Çiftçi Y, Ertekin C. The detection of sensitivity of proprioception by a new clinical test: The dual joint position test. Clin Neurol Neurosurg. 2013;115(7):1023-7.
18. Pearce JM. Romberg and his sign. Eur Neurol. 2005;53(4):210-3.
19. Lanska DJ, Goetz CG. Romberg's sign: development, adoption, and adaptation in the 19th century. Neurology. 2000;55(8):1201-6.
20. Halmágyi GM, Curthoys IS. Vestibular contributions to the Romberg test: Testing semicircular canal and otolith function. Eur J Neurol. 2021;28(9):3211-9.
21. Chomiak T, Pereira FV, Hu B. The single-leg-stance test in Parkinson's disease. J Clin Med Res. 2015;7(3):182-5.
22. Ng SS, Fong SS, Chan WL, Hung BK, Chung RK, Chim TH, et al. The sitting and rising test for assessing people with chronic stroke. J Phys Ther Sci. 2016;28(6):1701-8.
23. Podsiadlo D, Richardson S. The timed "Up & Go": a test of basic functional mobility for frail elderly persons. J Am Geriatr Soc. 1991;39(2):142-8.
24. Schermann T, Tadi P. (2022). Stereognosis. [online] Available from https://www.ncbi.nlm.nih.gov/books/NBK556003/. [Last accessed April, 2023].
25. Hankey GJ, Edis RH. The utility of testing tactile perception of direction of scratch as a sensitive clinical sign of posterior column dysfunction in spinal cord disorders. J Neurol Neurosurg Psychiatry. 1989;52:395-402.
26. Weber E. Ueber den tastsinn. Arch Anat Physiol Wissensch Med. 1835;52:152-60.
27. Dellon AL. The moving two-point discrimination test: clinical evaluation of the quickly adapting fiber/receptor system. J Hand Surg Am. 1978;3(5):474-81.
28. Dellon AL, Mackinnon SE, Crosby PM. Reliability of two-point discrimination measurements. J Hand Surg. 1987;12(5):693-6.
29. Moberg E. The unsolved problem – how to test the functional value of hand sensibility. J Hand Ther. 1991;4:105-10.
30. Lundborg G, Rosén B. The two-point discrimination test—time for a re-appraisal? J Hand Surg Br. 2004;29(5):418-22.
31. Boesch CE, Medved F, Held M, Bender D, Schaller HE, Fuchsberger T. Analysis of the two-point discrimination test in daily routine practice. Eur J Plast Surg. 2017;40:333-6.
32. Agarwal P, Mukati P, Kukrele R, Sharma D. Simple indigenous two-point discrimination testing device. Neurol India. 2021;69(1):147-8.

33. Tong J, Mao O, Goldreich D. Two-point orientation discrimination versus the traditional two-point test for tactile spatial acuity assessment. Front Hum Neurosci. 2013;7:579.
34. International Association for the Study of Pain. (2011). IASP Taxonomy. [online] Available from http://www.iasp-pain.org/Content/NavigationMenu/GeneralResourceLinks/PainDefinitions/default.htm. [Last accessed April, 2023].
35. Jensen TS, Karlsson P, Gylfadottir SS, Andersen ST, Bennett DL, Tankisi H, et al. Painful and non-painful diabetic neuropathy, diagnostic challenges and implications for future management. Brain. 2021;144(6):1632-45.
36. Rolke R, Baron R, Maier C, Tölle TR, Treede DR, Beyer A, et al. Quantitative sensory testing in the German Research Network on Neuropathic Pain (DFNS): standardized protocol and reference values. Pain. 2006;123(3):231-43.

9 CHAPTER

Testing the Coordination

Guruprasad Hosurkar, Mayank Kumar Shrivastava

INTRODUCTION

Action of the proximal and distal muscles at various joints of the limbs with different sensory inputs is required for precise, smooth, controlled voluntary motor movements to achieve specific tasks. Similarly, orolingual, and pharyngeal muscles coordinate to produce normal speech. The cerebellum along with basal ganglia through the brainstem and spinal cord has a major influence on speech and coordinated limb movements **(Fig. 1)**. Damage to the cerebellum and or sensory tracts which mediate coordination leads to disruption of smooth and efficient movements leading to ataxia associated with awkward, inaccurate movements **(Table 1)**. Coordination can be affected in isolation or can be involved along with motor weakness, and sensory loss. Clinician's responsibility is to take a detailed history and perform a neurological examination related to coordination along with other assessments to make an impression of the presence or absence of ataxia, extent or severity of involvement, localization of the lesion, and the possible etiologies.

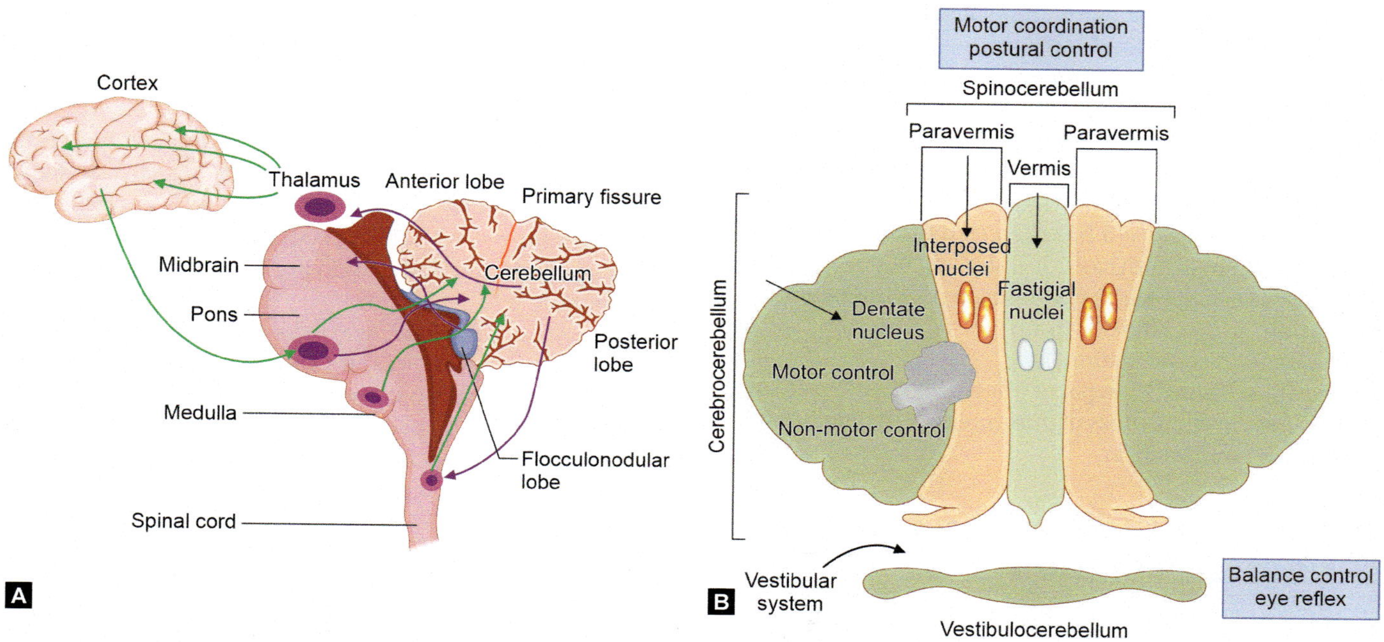

FIGS. 1A AND B: Cerebellar functional anatomy. (A) Scheme of the circuits connecting the cerebellum with other brain areas. Afferent connections are represented in green, efferent connections are represent in violet. (B) Schematic representation of the functional regions of cerebellum: the vestibulocerebellum, consisting of the flocculonodular lobe, the spinocerebellum which includes the vermis and the medial part of the hemispheres (paravermis) and the cerebrocerebellum corresponding to the remaining parts of the lateral hemispheres.
Source: Farini D, Marazziti D, Geloso MC, Sette C. Transcriptome programs involved in the development and structure of the cerebellum. Cell Mol Life Sci. 2021;78(19-20):6431-51.

TABLE 1: Various signs of incoordination—anatomic correlate (tracts/connections).

Signs of incoordination	Localization
Titubation	Cerebellar vermis
Truncal ataxia	Vermian/paravermian zone of cerebellum
Dysmetria	Lateral cerebellar hemisphere
Limb ataxia	• Lateral cerebellar hemisphere • Corticospinal tract • Proprioceptive pathway
Dysdiadochokinesia	Lateral cerebellar hemisphere
Intentional tremors	Lateral cerebellar hemisphere

HISTORY TAKING

History taking related to coordination needs to be focused on eliciting details on the onset, progression, extent, symmetry of involvement of the limbs, interference of the incoordination to day-to-day activities, and the present disability.

Some of the leading questions to elicit details on coordination:

1. Ability to perform smoothly day-to-day manual activities like brushing, drinking, eating, shaving, writing, wearing a dress, etc.
2. Is the person clumsy or overshoots the target while doing the above act, spills while eating, drinking, etc.?
3. Does the person have tremulousness throughout the act or only during the final act?
4. Does the person have a normal stance or a broad one while standing?
5. Does the person sway to one side or both sides while standing or walking, does it worsens in dark rooms or while closing eyes?

Above history should be taken into account symptoms of slurring of speech (dysarthria), shaking of objects in front of the eyes (oscillopsia), tremulousness of the head, trunk (titubation, truncal ataxia) to further localize the neuraxis involvement in coordination.

Previous historical aspects related to motor weakness, sensory loss, and slowness of movements will help to further analyze the coordination.

METHODS OF EXAMINATION AND THEIR INTERPRETATION

Examination of the coordination begins as the person walks into the OPD chamber by observing gait, stance, posture, balance, arm swing, ability to carry bag or file in the upper limbs smoothly, tremulousness, whether assisted for walking, ability to sit on the chair in the OPD, his or her speech and gestural response on greeting, etc. There will be occasions when coordination needs to be assessed in some patients seated in wheelchair at the OPDs, some completely bedbound in the wards or intensive care unit (ICU) with or without altered sensorium. Examination of coordination may not be adequate and satisfactory in such situations. Here the examiner has to innovate and modify the below described tests to elicit as much information as possible. For example, a patient on a wheelchair can be asked to do a knee heel test while sitting or if the proximal upper limb is immobilized due to a fracture, one can test for dysdiadochokinesia in the hands and get relevant information on coordination. In this age of advanced neuroimaging and its wide availability, there is a tendency to circumvent the neurological examination, and quickly go towards seeing the images. It is always better to thoroughly examine the patient, make a good clinical impression, and later interpret neuroimaging, and correlate it with clinical findings.

Consciousness

Ideally, patient needs to be fully conscious with motor and verbal components in the Glasgow Coma scale (GCS) being maximum (6 and 5 respectively) for a good assessment of coordination. However, if the patient's GCS is low, one needs to watch the motor movements in the limbs while localizing to pain, speech, etc. Patients under sedation in the ICU should undergo periodic neurological assessments including coordination after lightening the sedation.

Cranial Nerve Examination and Speech

Coordinated and smooth eye movements, articulation of the speech are intricately related with the coordination of the limbs and the whole body. Various types of nystagmus such as gaze-evoked nystagmus, downbeat nystagmus, and rebound nystagmus are specifically associated with defects in certain structures of the cerebellum and its connections. Examination of the saccades, pursuit eye movements, and vestibulo-ocular reflex (VOR) will assist in further localizing the lesion and classifying the disorder related to coordination.

Assessment of speech involves checking phonation, prosody, articulation, respiration, and resonance. The initial oromotor examination involves examining accuracy, range, strength, and speed of facial, lips, jaw, and lingual movements. One also has to look at the symmetry of the face, lips, and jaw during the resting state. A person is asked to count 1–10, read aloud (words, phrases, and sentences) and the examiner encourages the patient to have a brief conversation. A person is also asked to repeat lingual (tah, tah), labial (pah, pah), pharyngeal consonants (kah, kah), and some of the vowels (aa, ee, etc.).[1] Changes in pitch, tone, loudness, speech rate, accuracy, and intelligibility of speech production are closely observed for when the patient is speaking or articulating. Other aspects of language are covered in the chapter on language and aphasia.

The patient is diagnosed to have *dysarthria* if there is abnormal articulation of the speech or phonemes distorting its speed, strength, prosody, tone, pitch, loudness, and respiration. Dysarthria happens because of dysfunction of the CNS (mainly brainstem, basal ganglia, and corticobulbar tracts), cranial nerves (V, VII, IX, X, and XII), neuromuscular junction, or muscles involved in speech mechanism (facial, jaw, lingual, pharyngeal, and laryngeal muscles). Patients with dysarthria will have specific difficulty in repeating consonants. Total loss of articulation is called anarthria. Local structural abnormalities in the tongue, palate, and lips like cleft palate or lip causing a change in speech are not included in dysarthria. Detailed clinical approach to dysarthria, its different types, and differential features have been described in **Table 2.**

Testing coordination of the limbs usually follows an examination of motor strength, tone, and deep tendon reflexes. Analysis of the coordination tests should take into account the sensory examination findings since posterior column sensory loss can cause incoordination and *ataxia*.

Coordination in the limbs is evaluated by testing the patient's ability to perform rapid alternating movements, accuracy in moving to a target, smoothness, and efficiency of movements, position holding, steadiness of gait, and stance.

Rapid Alternating Movements

Ask the patient to sit and to keep the hands on the thighs, turn the hand repeatedly over and back rapidly (supination and pronation) with slightly lifting it off from the thigh. It is repeated similarly on the other side. Alternately, the patient can also be told to perform the rapid alternate movements of the hand placing it over the other hand and vice versa while sitting **(Fig. 2)** or standing. Inability or clumsiness in performing the act is called dysdiadochokinesia. One needs to take into account that rapid alternating movements will also be affected in Parkinson's disease or spastic weakness but the movements are slow and effortful rather than clumsy.

Finger Nose Test

Ask the patient while sitting to use the index finger to touch the tip of "his" nose and the outstretched examiner's finger back and forth a few times on both sides **(Fig. 3)**. Next, the examiner can move his hand to different positions with the patient trying to track, follow it quickly, and touch the tip of the examiner's finger using his index finger. Later, the patient can close his eyes and repeat the act of the finger nose test. Normally, a person should be able to perform the finger nose cleanly, with proper speed and control. A person with abnormal coordination will demonstrate *dysmetria* wherein the finger will overshoot the target, *intentional tremors* as he reaches the target, and clumsiness of the whole act with improper control of speed and accuracy **(Fig. 4)**. If the person can perform the finger nose test accurately with the eyes open but is clumsy in his act while closing his eyes, involvement of posterior columns, or its relay in the parietal cortical sensory area is a possibility.

Knee Heel Testing

Ask the patient while lying supine to lift his right or left leg, place the heel on the other knee, take it along the shin till the ankle, and repeat with the other leg **(Fig. 5A)**. Ask the patient to repeat the test couple of times on each side. A person should be able to perform the act smoothly without the heel falling off the shin, wavering while moving it, or overshooting the ankle every time. Inability to perform

TABLE 2: Types of dysarthria, its clinical manifestations, and localization—differential diagnosis.

Types of dysarthria	Localization	Clinical manifestations	Clinical conditions/ differential diagnosis
Spastic	Pyramidal tracts	Effortful, strained voice, strangled, and syllables run into one another	Strokes, primary lateral sclerosis
Flaccid	Brainstem nucleus, lower cranial nerve palsy, neuromuscular junction	Breathy quality with nasal intonation of voice, sometimes hoarseness	Myasthenia gravis, bulbar MND, medullary stroke
Ataxic	Cerebellum	Words broken into separate syllables separated by pauses and spoken with varying volume, leading to scanning speech	Stroke, degenerative disorder of cerebellum
Hypokinetic	Extrapyramidal tracts (basal ganglia circuits)	Low volume, monotonous, rapid rate, sometimes palilalia	Parkinson disease
Hyperkinetic	Extrapyramidal tracts (basal ganglia circuits)	Strained voice, inappropriate halts and variable rate	HD, dystonia

(HD: Huntington's disease; MND: motor neuron disease)

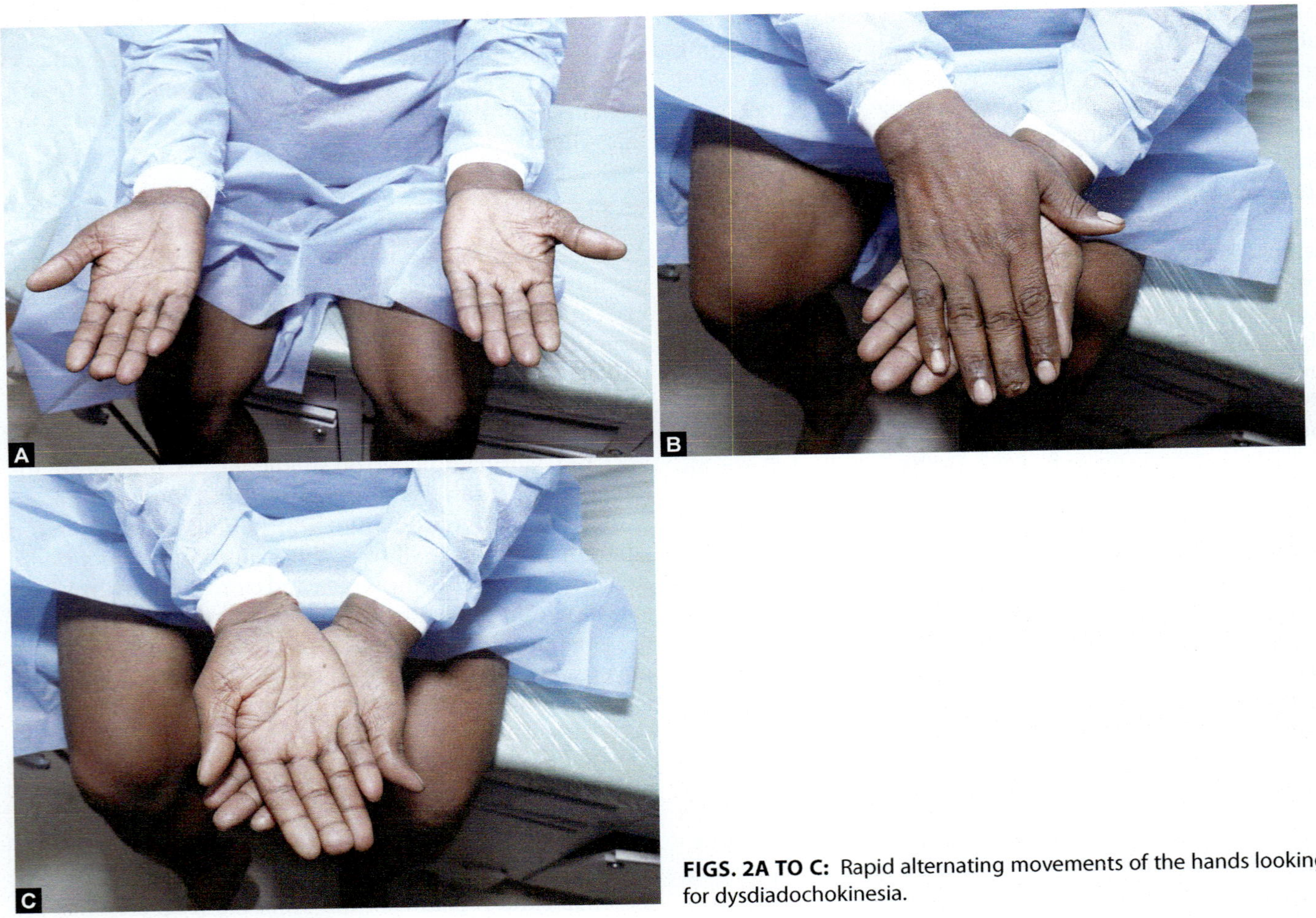

FIGS. 2A TO C: Rapid alternating movements of the hands looking for dysdiadochokinesia.

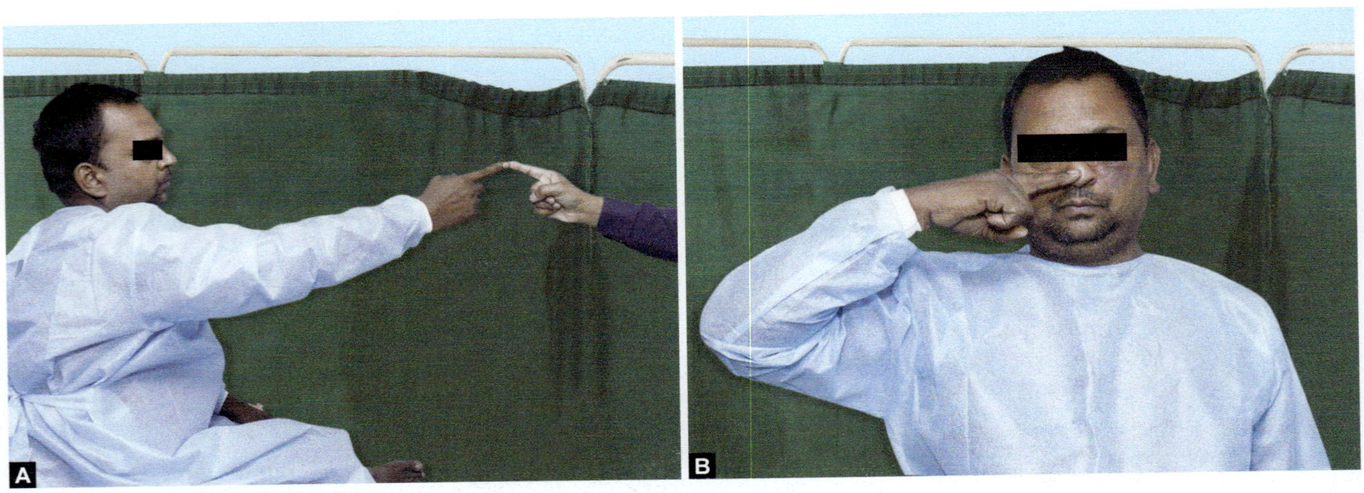

FIGS. 3A AND B: Finger nose testing.

the motion accurately, smoothly, and rapidly is abnormal coordination **(Fig. 5B)**.

Abnormal finger nose and knee heel test is suggestive of ipsilateral cerebellar involvement in the presence of preserved motor strength and sensory function in the limb.

The *rebound phenomenon* is a reflex that occurs when the patient attempts to resist and tries to maintain the outstretched or flexed upper limb that has been pulled and released. Normally, there is gradual recoil to the original position after some movements in the direction of the pull, whereas if there is an exaggerated response in the spastic limb, it overshoots the original position. A complete absence of rebound phenomenon is seen with cerebellar disease because of failure of the contraction of the antagonist muscles.

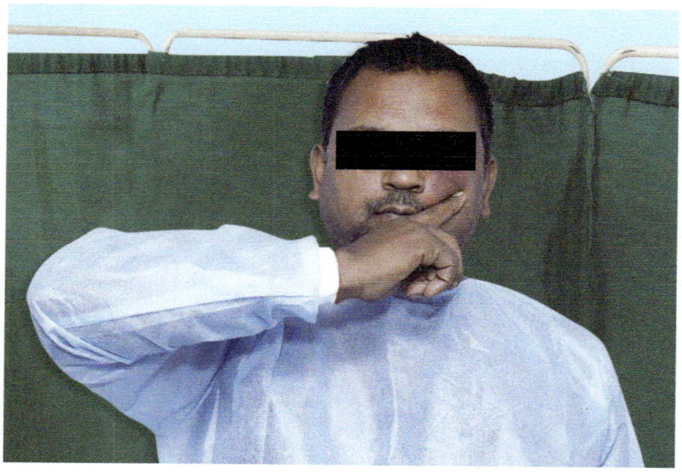

FIG. 4: Finger nose testing depicting dysmetria (testing with eyes closed).

Stance, Posture, and Gait

Patient is asked to stand erect with the upper limbs on the sides and then made to walk inside the OPD room for few minutes which includes turning around the corner of the room. Once this task is completed comfortably, the patient is asked to walk with heel-to-toe in a straight line across the room **(Fig. 6)**. The patient is observed closely for his ability to maintain posture while standing, maintain balance while walking normally, and heel-to-toe. Examiner needs to comment on stance, posture while standing, arm swing, length of steps, strides, speed, balance while walking, and smoothness in turning. Wide-based stance, irregular steps, unsteadiness, and swaying on either side with worsening while turning is seen in ataxia due to various etiologies **(Table 3)**.

Romberg's Sign

Ask the patient to stand with their feet together, arms by the sides, and close eyes. Stay close to the patient to prevent any falls. If the patient sways even before the eyes are closed or feet together, there is the possibility of cerebellar dysfunction or severe sensory ataxia, or vestibular defect. If the patient starts swaying and has the tendency to fall after closing his eyes, it is more likely suggestive of sensory ataxia or vestibular dysfunction.

Scale for the Measurement of Ataxia

The International Cooperative Ataxia Rating Scale (ICARS) and scale for the assessment and rating of ataxia (SARA) are the commonly used rating tools for assessing coordination in clinical trials. SARA scale has eight items which include: (1) gait, (2) stance, (3) sitting, (4) speech, (5) finger-chase test, (6) nose-finger test, (7) fast alternating

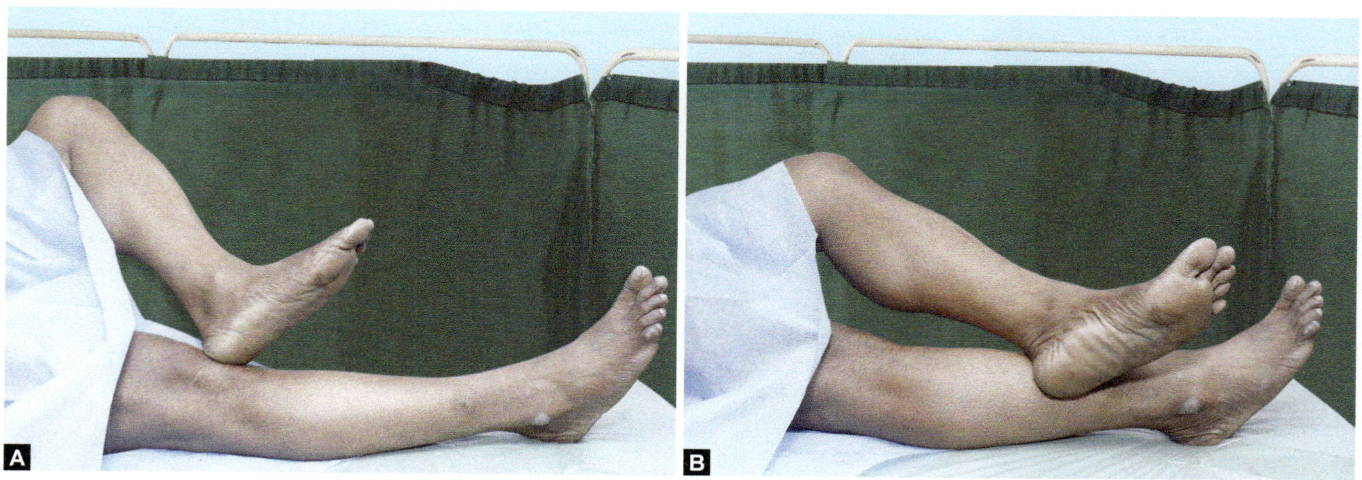

FIGS. 5A AND B: Knee heel test. (A) Initiation of the knee heel test; and (B) Abnormal test—heel falling off the shin.

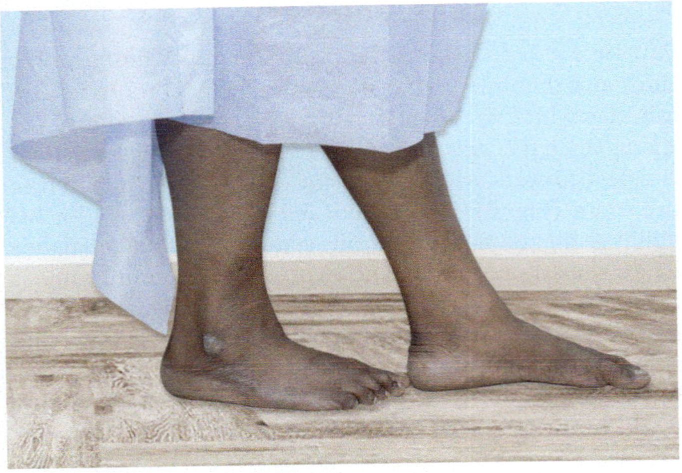

FIG. 6: Heel-to-toe or tandem walking test.

movements, and (8) heel-to-shin test with scores ranging from 0 (no ataxia) to 40 (severe ataxia). It can be used in acute or chronic conditions, is simpler, well-validated, and has good inter-rater reliability, and reproducibility.[2,3] These tools can also be used in the clinical practice setting for monitoring the progress of ataxia on treatment.

CONCLUSION

Accurate and complete testing of the coordination of the limbs, speech, and gait is an important aspect of the neurological examination. It adds immense value to the localization and extent of neurological involvement. The establishment of clinical diagnosis of the neurological condition after detailed history taking and examination of various components of coordination will help in further decisions on diagnostics and therapeutics.

TABLE 3: Components of gait, types of gait, clinical implications, and localization value, differential diagnosis.

	Cerebellar ataxia	Sensory ataxia	Parkinsonism	Frontal lobe	Spastic	Proximal muscle weakness	Psychogenic
Stance	Broad based	Broad based	Narrow base (except in MSA-C)	Broad based	Narrow based	Broad based	Variable
Posture	Leans forward	Stooped	Stooped sometimes camptocormia	Erect	Upright, asymmetric posture with more weight on unaffected side	Exaggerated lumbar lordosis	Normal or abrupt change in the posture
Steps	Staggering, lurching	High steppage, ataxic with swinging on both sides, cautious	Short steps, decreased arm swing, shuffling	Initiation difficulty, short steps, shuffling	Circumduction on the affected side, scissoring	Bilateral waddling, effortful	Bizarre gait, irregular steps, may mimic one of the other patterns or mixed
Speed	Normal, slow	Normal, slow	Slow, festinant, impaired acceleration and deceleration	Slow	Slow	Slow	Changes speed quickly, unpredictable
Turning corners	Sways, needs support	Minimal effect	Slow with occasional gait freezing	Slow	Impaired, needs support	Minimal effect	Minimal effect
Romberg's test	Sways even with eyes open	Positive	Negative	Negative	Negative	Negative	Negative or falsely positive even with eyes open
Heel-to-shin test	Abnormal, clumsy, heel drops from the shin multiple times, overshoots the ankle	Abnormal, clumsy, more after closing eyes	Slow, heel drops from the shin if there is associated tremors in the legs	Normal	Difficulty in initiating and performing the act, inaccurate, slow, and clumsy	Normal, initial difficulty in lifting the leg	Normal
Falls	Rare	Common	Common	Common	Uncommon	Buckling at the knees with falls	Rare

(MSA: multiple system atrophy)

REFERENCES

1. Fabus R, Gironda F. Assessment of articulation and phonological disorders. In: Stein-Rubin C, Fabus R (Eds). A Guide to Clinical Assessment and Professional Report Writing in Speech-Language Pathology. Clifton Park, NY: Delmar Publications; 2011.
2. Schmitz Hübsch et al. Scale for the assessment and rating of ataxia: development of a new clinical scale. Neurology. 2006;66(11):1717-20.
3. Kim BR, Lim JH, Lee SA, Park S, Koh SE, Lee IS, et al. Usefulness of the scale for the Assessment and Rating of Ataxia (SARA) in Ataxia Stroke patients. Ann Rehabil Med. 2011;35:772-80.

10

CHAPTER

Testing the Reflexes

Vaibhav Wadwekar, Rajeswari Aghoram

INTRODUCTION

A sensory stimulus may lead to an involuntary response in the form of muscle contraction, pupillary reaction, secretions, etc. This involuntary response is known as reflex. Any reflex thus elicited has an afferent loop, which takes the sensations and delivers its "efferent" loop via which the signal reaches the response organ, and a reflex is elicited. In this chapter, we will be concerned with motor reflexes. A reflex is called motor if the response is seen in the form of visible or palpable muscle contraction often associated with the movement at the concerned joint. Depending on the location of the sensory organ which perceives the sensory stimulus, the reflex may be further classified as "superficial and deep reflexes."

Reflex elicitation is one of the most important aspects of neurological examination for many reasons. First of all, being involuntary, it is one of the most objective tests in neurology. Additionally, it is a part of the bedside examination, easy to observe, does not require sophisticated equipment, and is nonpainful to the patient. However, the onus of correct elicitation of reflex and interpretation of the observed results in the context of history and other findings lie with the examiner.[1]

HISTORY TAKING

A detailed history is the first and possibly the most important prerequisite for "testing the reflexes." A proper and detailed history arms the examiner with the knowledge of what to expect in the reflexes. A discrepancy between the history and examination is an important warning sign that the diagnosis we are about to make may be wrong. As far as motor reflexes are concerned, the following points in history should be asked diligently.

- *History suggesting hyperreflexia*:
  - History of persistent tightness in the limbs, which the patient usually complains as walking with some weight tied, walking underwater, or just tightness-indicated spasticity
  - History of sudden flexion of libs at night, indicating flexor spasms
  - History of involuntary rhythmic movement when the sole is being put in a particular position indicates clonus. Some people move their legs due to habit or when being anxious in a similar manner but those are voluntary and can be immediately stopped when noticed.
- *History suggesting hyporeflexia*:
  - Patients do give a history of flailness or flaccidity of the joints. The patient may give a history of tripping or falling, especially while climbing the stairs, in cases of foot drop. When a patient gives such a history, it usually means severe hypotonia.
  - Milder/subtle hypotonia is more difficult to differentiate from normal tone just on a historical basis. Hence, if one does not get a history of flailness/flaccidity from the patient, milder and more subtle hypotonia may still be found during examination.

PHYSIOLOGY

Muscle fibers resist any sort of passive stretching. They do so by contracting, which again reduces their length. This property is utilized to elicit the deep tendon reflexes (DTRs) where a sudden stretch of muscle is caused by hitting its tendon with a percussion hammer. The tendons have spindles that when stretched send impulses via afferents to the spinal cord. These afferents synapse directly with motor neurons in the spinal cord without any intervening interneuron. The alpha motor neuron in turn supplies the muscle fibers of the same muscle, leading to their contraction. This whole circuit is called a "monosynaptic reflex" as the afferent and efferent loops form the synapse directly without an intervening interneuron.

METHODS OF EXAMINATION AND THEIR INTERPRETATION

Deep Tendon Reflexes

Equipment: Percussion Hammer

Note: A good-quality percussion hammer is imperative for the elicitation of correct DTRs. This usually means a hammer with a heavy, soft rubber head and a long, flexible handle. A lighter head may lead to nonelicitation of reflexes, and a nonsoft head is painful to the patient. Similarly, a rigid handle may not generate the appropriate force needed to elicit the reflex due to inadequate swing action.

Prerequisites

- DTRs are tested only after one has tested bulk, tone, power, abnormal movements, and sensory system evaluation.
- While testing the above, it should be noted that there is no pain, contracture, spasm, or dystonia and that the joint has full passive movement. The presence of any of the above and restricted passive joint movement limits the elicitation of proper reflexes.
- Environment where reflexes are being tested should be comfortable and silent. Excessive cold/hot or crowded room and sounds may make it difficult for the patients to relax.
- Patients should be explained the procedure and assured that elicitation of reflex is nonpainful. They may be specifically anxious about being hit by the hammer. A simple demonstration of hitting the percussion hammer about to be used on your tendon/arm easily allays this anxiety.
- Concerned muscle should be uncovered fully.
- Muscle to be tested should be in a relaxed state (this should be confirmed with gentle palpation of the muscle). In this regard, it is important to note that an anxious patient is rarely able to relax the muscle fully. Some patients are very anxious, in which case it is better to make them lie down and rest for about 5–10 minutes.

Procedure

1. Positioning of the limb is an important aspect of the proper elicitation of reflex. A limb is positioned in such a manner that the muscle to be tested is fully relaxed. This aspect has been described in more detail in the forthcoming text under individual reflex description.
2. Procedure of eliciting itself is simple. The hammer is held in the hand and then its head end is "swung" in such a manner that it hits the tendon of the muscle being tested. The word "swing" here means that the action should come from the free movement of the wrist joint.
3. In most cases, the tendon of the muscle to be tested is hit directly but in a few like "biceps reflex or finger flexion reflex," thumb/finger of the other hand (one not holding the hammer) may be kept above the tendons.
4. Examiner should start with a light swing at the wrist hitting the tendon with lesser force and then increase the force in the next one or two hits till the reflex is elicited.
   Note: One should not try to elicit a reflex more than three times at a single go. This is important because of the "habituation" property of reflex. It is normal for a reflex to wean off after three-to-four hits, and it may be erroneously reported absent.

Precautions/Pearls

- While eliciting the reflex, the examiner should make sure to percuss the tendon and *not* the muscle itself. A muscle may contract if percussed directly even though the DTR is absent.
- Complementary reflexes of either limb should be tested together and compared, e.g., right and left knee reflexes should be tested together (consecutively). Examiner should not give in to the tendency of testing all the reflexes of the right limb followed by the left limb.
- In case of hemiparesis or monoparesis, the normal side should be tested first.
- Instruction to the patient to "relax the muscle" may lead to an exactly opposite result. Instead, it is better to instruct the patient to close his eyes and relax his whole body. Distracting the patient and gently massaging the muscle of which reflex is about to be elicited also helps in achieving the relaxation of the muscle.

Grading of Reflexes

Most neurologists grade reflexes as follows:

- *Grade 0*: Absent
- *Grade 1+ (or +)*: Present but diminished, present only on Jendrassik maneuver (JM)
- *Grade 2+ (or ++)*: Normal
- *Grade 3+ (or +++)*: Exaggerated
- *Grade 4+ (or ++++)*: Markedly hyperactive with clonus

Certain Phenomenons

- *Habituation of reflex*: Repetitive elicitation of DTR renders the reflex diminished or nonelicitable for a short duration of time. Hence, the examiner should try to elicit reflexes within the first two-to-three percussions of tendons. If there is any doubt or another examiner is eliciting the same reflex, it should be done after waiting for a brief period (a minute or 2 should suffice) and allowing habituation to wane off.
- *Spread or irradiation of reflex*: It is normal to note reflex being elicited in the muscles adjacent, neighboring to the muscle where the examiner is trying to elicit the reflex. For example, it is normal to note slight contraction of the fingers while eliciting brachioradialis reflex, or contraction of hip adductors while eliciting knee

extensor response. Spreading is more pronounced when reflexes are hyperactive or exaggerated but it can occur during normal reflexes also.

- *Jendrassik maneuver (JM)*: In cases where reflexes are markedly diminished it is difficult to comment whether they are absent or not. In such a scenario reflexes can be reinforced. Reinforcement can be done by various techniques, the simplest being contraction of muscles where reflex is not being elicited. While eliciting the lower limbs, it is achieved by interlocking and then pulling both hands and at the same time clenching the teeth. In the case of the upper limb, it is done by clenching teeth and making a fist with the contralateral limb. This procedure is known as JM. Any DTR should be noted as absent only after JM has been performed. The effect of JM lasts for a few seconds only after the contraction. Hence, the DTR should be elicited as soon as the reinforcement is done by the patient and compared with the prereinforcement reflex. Moreover, the patient should be clearly instructed not to contract the limb which is being tested and keep it relaxed.
- *Inverted reflex*: A reflex is called inverted if the reflex being elicited is absent but instead opposite reflex (that is reflex controlled by the antagonist muscle) is elicited, e.g., elicitation of biceps reflex while eliciting triceps reflex. This indicates that the reflex loop of the triceps is affected, and biceps are being elicited because of preserved reflex arc and spread.

Jaw Jerk[2]

Jaw jerk is the highest elicitable DTR.

Root value: Both the afferent and the efferent are carried by the trigeminal nerve.

Elicited by: The mouth should be partially open and relaxed. This can be done by asking the patient to breathe quietly through his mouth. A finger is placed over the chin of the patient and struck with a percussion hammer in a downward direction.

Response: Normal response is a small amplitude, often an imperceptible upward movement of the jaw caused by contraction of the temporalis, masseter, and medial pterygoid muscles. Exaggerated responses are abnormal and seen in conditions with corticobulbar involvement. Occasionally, clonus may also occur.

Upper Limb Reflexes

The biceps, triceps, brachioradialis, and finger flexor are the routinely elicited important reflexes and we will discuss these.

Position of the Upper Limb

When the patient is lying in bed:

- Examiner stands on the right side of the patient.
- Patient is made to lie supine.
- Elbow should rest on the bed.
- Palm of the patient should be placed over the patient's abdomen in a semipronated position.

When the patient is sitting or standing:

- Examiner faces the patient.
- Patient's elbow rests on the examiner's palm while being flexed at 90°.
- Patient's hand rests on the examiner's elbow.

Bicep Reflex

Root value: C5, C6

Nerve: Musculocutaneous nerve

Technique:

a. If the patient is lying on the bed (position I), the examiner places his index finger over the bicep tendon and elicits the reflex.
b. If the patient is sitting or standing (position II), the examiner places his thumb on the bicep tendon and elicits the reflex.
c. If needed, reinforcement may be done by making a fist of the contralateral upper limb and clenching the jaw.

Normal response: Visible contraction of the biceps muscle and slight flexion + supination at the elbow.

Brachioradialis (Supinator) Reflex

Root value: C6

Nerve: Radial nerve

Technique: Either in position I or in position II, the reflex is elicited by percussing just above the styloid reflex.

Normal response: Visible contraction of brachioradialis muscle and slight flexion and supination at the elbow.

Triceps Reflex

Root value: C7

Nerve: Radial nerve

Technique: Either in position I or in position II, the reflex is elicited by tapping the triceps tendon just above the insertion on the olecranon fossa.

Normal response: Visible contraction of triceps muscle and slight extension at the elbow.

Finger Flexor Reflex

It is also called Wartenberg's reflex.

Root value: C8, T1

Nerve: Median and ulnar

Position and technique: Patient's hand is placed on a hard surface such as a table in the supine position. The patient is asked to keep his fingers relaxed. The examiner then places his finger against the patient's fingers (palmar aspect) and taps on the back of his fingers.

Normal response: Absent or slight flexion of fingers.

Lower Limb Reflexes

Knee and ankle reflexes are the routinely elicited important reflexes, and we will discuss these.

Position of Lower Limb

When the patient is lying in bed:
- Examiner stands on the right side of the patient.
- Patient is made to lie supine.
- Limb being tested is semiflexed at the knee with heels resting on the bed.
- After this, the position depends on the reflex being tested.

When the patient is sitting (lower limb reflex cannot and should not be tested in a standing position):
- Patient sits with feet placed slightly apart.
- Patient's knee should be semiflexed at about 90°.
- Patient's soles should fully rest on the ground. Alternative legs may be kept dangling from the examination table (for knee reflex only).

Knee Reflex

Root value: L2, 3, 4

Nerve: Femoral

While done in a patient lying in bed (position I, after point d):
a. Abduct the knee slightly, while the whole limb is still supported by the heel on the bed.
b. While palpating the tendons of hamstrings in the popliteal fossa, wait for a few seconds.
c. You should elicit a knee reflex only when you feel these tendons are fully relaxed. This is a surrogate marker that his quadriceps are also relaxed.
d. Now elicit the knee reflex with a hammer by percussion of the patellar tendon.

While done in a patient in a sitting position (position II, after point c):
a. Ensure that the quadriceps muscle is relaxed by palpation.
b. Now elicit the knee reflex with a hammer by percussion of the patellar tendon.

Normal response: Contraction of quadriceps muscles (should also be palpated, especially if diminished) with a slight extension of knee joint.

Precaution: As the reflex elicitation leads to the extension of the knee, there are chances that the great toe and other toes may be injured if they hit an obstacle, especially if the knee reflex is brisk. Hence, there should be no obstacle before the limb while eliciting this reflex, thus allowing a full range of movement.

Ankle Reflex (Ankle Jerk)

Root value: S1

Nerve: Sciatic nerve

While done in a patient lying in bed (position I, after point d):
a. Abduct the knee fully, so that the whole limb lies on the bed in a semiflexed (at knee and hip) position.
b. Place one hand under the foot and dorsiflex the foot to achieve an "appropriate" stretch of the Achilles tendon.
c. *Note*: The knowledge of this appropriate stretch comes with experience and is difficult to objectify.
d. Now elicit the ankle reflex with a hammer by percussion of the Achille's tendon.

While done in a patient in a sitting position (position II, after point c):
a. Ensure that the soleus muscle is relaxed by palpation.
b. Now elicit the knee reflex with a hammer by percussion of the Achille's tendon.

Normal response: Contraction of calf muscle and slight plantar flexion of ankle.

Superficial Reflexes

Abdominal Reflex

Root value:
- *Upper quadrants*: T7, 8, 9, 10 via intercostal nerves.
- *Lower quadrants*: T10 to upper lumbar via intercostal, iliohypogastric, and ilioinguinal nerves.

Elicited by: Gently stroking the abdominal wall with a *blunt* pin or cotton wisp segment-wise in particular directions (shown in **Fig. 1**).

Response: Umbilicus is pulled toward the direction of response.

Note: Some patients may be extremely sensitive to stroking (tickling) and may need a much gentler approach. It may lead to injury or abrasion over the skin if a sharp object is used or forceful stroking is done.

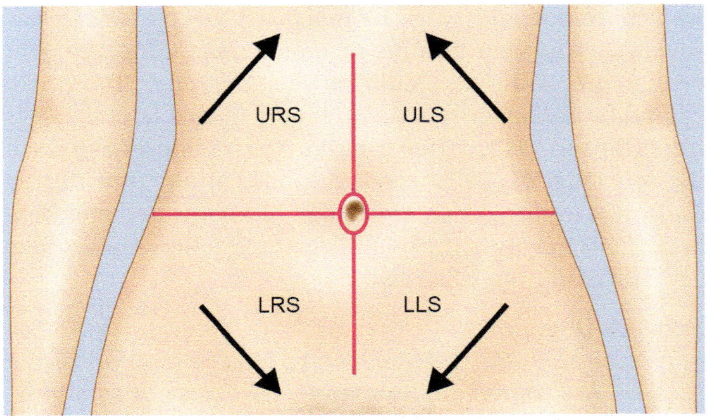

FIG. 1: Elicitation of abdominal reflex.
(LLS: lower left side quadrant; LRS: lower right side quadrant; ULS: upper left side quadrant; URS: upper right side quadrant)

Cremasteric Reflex

Root value: L1, 2

Nerve: Genitofemoral nerve

Elicited by: Gently stroking the inner aspect of the upper thigh. This can be done by using a blunt pin or cotton wisp. This part is extremely sensitive and delicate, and utmost precaution must be taken not to cause injury or pain.

Response: Contraction of the ipsilateral cremasteric muscle and elevation of the ipsilateral testis.

Note: May be absent normally in elderly males.

Anal Reflex

Root value: S2–5

Nerve: Inferior hemorrhoidal nerve, usually a branch of the pudendal nerve.

Elicited by: Gently stroking the perianal region. This can be done by using a blunt pin or cotton wisp. This part is extremely sensitive and delicate, and utmost precaution must be taken not to cause injury or pain.

Response: Contraction of external anal sphincter.

Plantar Reflex[3,4]

Root value: L4–S2

Elicited by: With the patient supine, flex the knee and externally rotate the hip, and hold the foot by the ankle. A mild nociceptive stimulus is then applied over the lateral aspect of the heel toward the ball of the great toe slowly. Blunt objects such as a key should be used, and the firmness of the stroke can be progressively increased depending upon the response elicited. The force required to elicit the response varies from patient to patient. Some patients have extremely sensitive/ticklish skin where a lighter force is adequate. However, patients, especially those who work/walk barefoot and work in fields, may have thick, less sensitive skin with fissures or cracks. In such cases, you need to give a firmer stimulus to elicit the reflex. The stroke should be in the form of an arch and started laterally. It is important to restrict the stimulus to the lateral aspect of the sole **(Fig. 2)**. An extensor response at any time during the stroke is considered abnormal. In infants and children, fingernails may be sufficient to elicit the reflex. Always take care not to injure the patient.

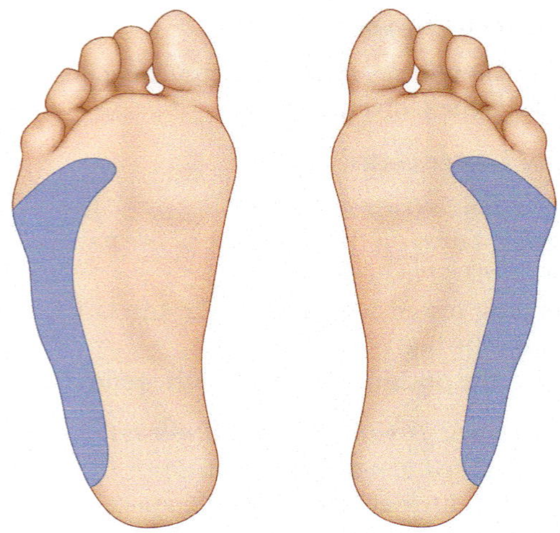

FIG. 2: The area where Babinski reflex should be elicited.

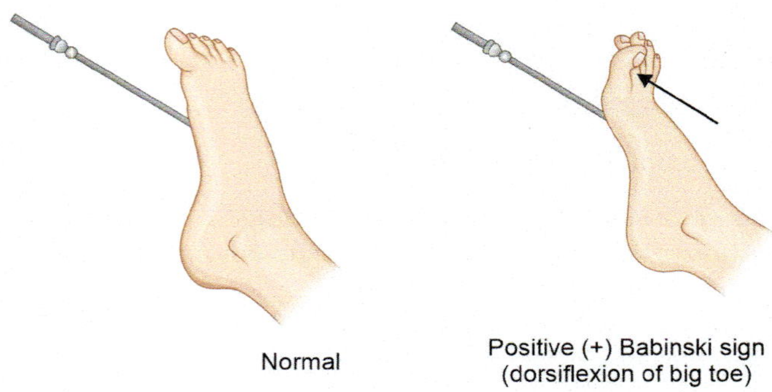

FIG. 3: Babinski reflex.

Source: Earl Lawrence House and Ben Pansky. Wikimedia Commons. (1960) (Public Domain).

Response **(Fig. 3)**:

- *Flexor response*: Plantar flexion and adduction of the toes. Associated mild hip and knee flexion may also be there. This is the normal response after infancy.
- *Extensor response*: There is dorsiflexion of the great toe with fanning and extension of other toes. Such an extensor response is often normal in infancy. In addition, dorsiflexion of the ankle and flexion of the hip and knee may be seen. This contraction of the tibialis anterior, hamstrings, and tensor fascia lata is called the triple response or Babinski sign. A true Babinski sign is not inhibited by pressure over the base of the great toe. When highly exaggerated, it may culminate in an extensor or flexor spasm.

In certain conditions such as neuropathy, this reflex may be nonelicitable.

Variants of Babinski response:

- *Minimal Babinski*: Only contraction of hamstring and tensor fascia lata is seen.
- *Tonic Babinski reflex*: In a lesion of the frontal lobe with extrapyramidal involvement, a slow contraction of the toe extensors may be seen.
- *Crossed extensor response*: Unilateral stimulation produces a bilateral response.
- *Spontaneous Babinski*: Passive extension of the knee or passive flexion of the hip and knee may result in a spontaneous Babinski response in extensive upper motor neuron (UMN) lesions.

Other named methods to elicit extensor plantar response are given in **Table 1**.

TABLE 1: Other named methods to elicit extensor plantar response.

Name	Method of eliciting
Oppenheim sign (shin-toe reflex)	Pressure is applied by knuckles or the thumb and index finger on the shin above downward. The response occurs toward the end of the stimulus
Strumpell sign	Forceful pressure over the anterior tibia
Gordon sign (Calf-toe sign)	Squeezing or pinching of the calf muscles or tendo Achilles
Schaefer sign (Achilles-toe reflex)	Squeezing the tendo Achilles
Gonda sign/Allen sign (toe-pull reflex)	Snapping of the distal phalanx of the second or fourth toe
Stansky sign	Abduction and sudden release of the fourth toe
Cornell sign	Scratching the dorsum of the foot along the inner side of the great toe extensor tendon
Throckmorton sign	Percussion of the dorsum of the metatarsophalangeal joint of the great toe
Bing sign	Pinprick on the dorsum of the foot
Chaddock sign	Stroking the skin around the lateral malleolus in a circular motion
Moniz sign	Forceful passive plantar flexion of the ankle

CONCLUSION

Reflexes play a very important role in the anatomical localization of the lesion in the nervous system. A sound method of elicitation needs to be practiced and perfected by clinicians to develop confidence in their findings and extrapolations thereof.

REFERENCES

1. Campbell WW, DeJong RN, Ranganathan LN. DeJong's The Neurologic Examination, South Asian edition. Philadelphia: Lippincott Williams & Wilkins; 2020. pp. 655-74.
2. Pearce JMS. The jaw jerk: an instance of misattribution. J Neurol Neurosurg Psychiatry. 2011;82(3):351-2.
3. Taksande A, Saqqaf SY, Panwar ASR. Planter reflex: an important superficial reflex. Int J Pediatr Neonatol. 2020;2(1):1-3.
4. van Gijn J. (1977). The plantar reflex: a historical, clinical, and electromyographic study. [online] Available from http://hdl.handle.net/1765/26189. [Last accessed December, 2022].

11

CHAPTER

Testing the Gait and Stance

Abhishek Srivastava, Nirmal Surya, Guhan Ramamurthy

INTRODUCTION

In the process of evolution, humans have assumed a bipedal stance, making the gait a highly efficient process requiring balance and coordination compared to the predecessors in the evolutionary tree. The gait provides freedom of locomotion and in humans provides an additional degree of freedom to the hands that can be used for dexterous activities. The intricacies of the gait as the person negates through the pathways of daily life normally go unnoticed, and one becomes aware of it in the presence of dysfunction. The visual story narrated by the gait of the patient, as he steps into the clinician's room, to the trained eye of the examiner provides clues to the diagnosis of the clinical condition of the patient. The gait of a patient may be affected by both neurological and non-neurological conditions. The addition of sensors and instrumental gait analysis in the current era of technological evolution has further expanded the armamentarium of gait analysis.

HISTORY OF GAIT ANALYSIS

The first history of gait analysis in the precomputer era dates to the comments recorded on walking in humans by Aristotle. In the 17th century, the progress in gait analysis was made further by Giovanni Borelli through his experiments. In the 19th century, Willhelm and Eduard Weber made simple measurements of gait. Jules Etienne Marey and Eadweard Muybridge made advancements in the technology that is used to measure gait. In the 20th century, the advancements in the use of force plate was used that helped in the understanding of the kinetics and kinematics of movement. Further advancements were made in the clinical applications of gait. The computerization of gait analysis has opened several avenues in gait assessment. Nevertheless, the systemic examination of gait holds the ground and forms the basis of neurological examination.[1]

NEUROPHYSIOLOGY OF GAIT CONTROL

The complex and extraordinary process of gait comprises locomotion or movement, balance and coordination, and adapting to environmental challenges. A normal gait requires coordinated interaction between (1) the sensory system, which includes proprioception, visual, and vestibular systems; (2) the motor system, which includes muscles, bones, and joints; and (3) suprasegmental control of the afferent and efferent systems by the brain and spinal cord of the central nervous system.[2]

The central pattern generators (CPGs) in the spinal cord generate the sequence of events in the activation of muscle in a coordinated pattern to produce gait. The mesencephalic locomotor region located anterior to the superior colliculus, which contains the pedunculopontine nucleus, cuneiform and sub cuneiform nucleus, and the locus coeruleus, median raphe and dopaminergic neurons of the lateral hypothalamus send facilitatory input to the CPG in the spinal cord through the reticulospinal tract. The mesencephalic locomotor region receives inhibitory input from basal ganglia, the output of which is modulated by cortical structures, premotor cortex, and supplementary motor cortex.[3]

The sensory input from peripheral structures is integrated at multiple levels in the spinal cord, midbrain, and basal ganglia. The sensory input from the primary somatosensory cortex, visual cortex, and vestibular cortex is integrated with the posterior parietal cortex. This information about the body schema in space is transferred to the supplementary motor areas (SMAs). The SMA in association with basal ganglia and cerebellum generates the necessary motor sequence, which is transferred to the motor cortex to produce the goal-oriented gait.[4]

The three perspectives on the evaluation of gait include:

1. Gait cycle
2. Temporal and spatial parameters of gait
3. Functionality of gait

Gait Cycle

The gait cycle is the sequence of events in gait that occurs from the first heel strike of one limb to the subsequent heel strike of the same limb **(Fig. 1)**. Each limb has a stance phase and a swing phase. The stance phase is when the limb is in contact with the ground which constitutes 60–70% of the gait cycle. The swing phase is from the point of toe-off to the heel strike, which constitutes the remaining time of the gait cycle. The time when both feet are in contact with the ground is the double support phase, which constitutes 25% of the gait cycle. The double support phase decreases during running and increases during cautious or senile gait.

Temporal and Spatial Parameters of Gait

The temporal and spatial parameters of gait that measure the metrics of gait are summarized in **Table 1**.[2,5]

Functionality of Gait

In functionality of gait, the initial point of heel contact or toe-off and other functionalities are assessed. The kinematics of gait measures the dynamic motion range. Kinetics refers to various forces that act on the body while moving. The kinematics of the range of motion can be analyzed based on clinical observation or in a gait laboratory. The kinetics involved in gait is assessed in a laboratory setting.[6]

CAUSES OF GAIT DISORDERS

Physiological Causes

The physiological causes of gait dysfunction are cautious gaits in the elderly whose neurological examination is normal.

Gait Disorders due to Neurological Causes

The categories of gait disorders are summarized in **Table 2**.

Lower-level Gait Disorders

- *Myopathic gait*: In myopathic gait, there is an increased rotation of the hip, waddling of the trunk, and flexion of the hip arising from weakness of hip extension, resulting

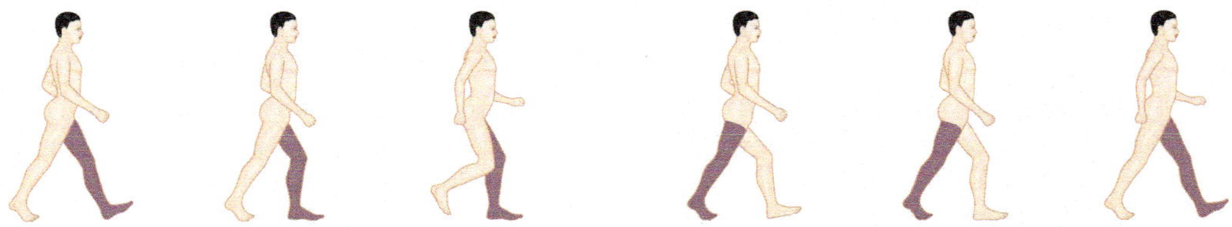
Left heel strike
Right toe off
Left mid-stance
Right swing
Right heel strike
Left toe off
Left heel strike

FIG. 1: Gait cycle, which consists of the sequence of events in gait that occurs from the first heel strike of one limb to the subsequent heel strike of the same limb.

TABLE 1: Spatial and temporal parameters of gait.

Gait parameter	Definition
Gait velocity	• The distance walked is measured as a function of time • Distance walked/time
Cadence	The step count that the patient walks every minute is measured as steps/min
Step length	The distance covered by the leg from "toe-off" to "heel strike," which is the swing phase of the leg
Stride length	The distance covered by the leg from one heel strike to the subsequent heel strike of the same leg
Step width	The distance between the two feet for a given step
Step height	The highest distance between the ground and the foot during the swing phase of the feet
Coordination	The timing and uniformity in the sequence of events in comparison between the two feet in a gait cycle
Variability	The variability in the indices of the spatial and temporal parameters of gait

TABLE 2: Levels of gait disorders.

Level	Gait disorder
Lower-level gait disorders	Gait disorders due to lesions of the peripheral structures such as muscle or nerve
Middle-level gait disorders	Gait disorder due to lesions of the corticospinal tracts, cerebellum, hypokinetic gait, and gait in hyperkinetic movement disorders
High-level gait disorders	Gait disorders that cannot be explained by peripheral nerve, muscle, spinal tracts, and basal ganglia lesions

in exaggerated lumbar lordosis. Though this pattern of weakness is classically seen in myopathy, neuropathic causes of bilateral proximal weakness can result in a similar pattern.[7]

- *Neuropathic gait*: Neuropathic causes of dorsiflexion weakness include peroneal nerve palsy, L5 radiculopathy, and sciatic nerve palsy. The patient walks with a high steppage gait in which he walks with high steps to clear the ground. In patients with weakness of plantar flexion, they walk with a shallow gait, as they are unable to propel the toe off the ground.
- *Sensory ataxic gait*: The absence of proprioceptive input from the lower limbs results in a slow cautious gait guided by visual input with the slapping of the foot on the ground. The gait worsens in dark or poor light situations. Romberg test is positive, and large fiber and posterior column sensations are decreased in the lower limbs.

Middle-level Gait Disorders

- *Spastic gait*: In patients with unilateral spasticity of the upper and lower limbs, the shoulder is adducted and internally rotated, the elbow is flexed, the forearm is pronated, wrist and fingers are flexed. The lower limb is slightly flexed at the hip, with the knee in extension, ankle in plantar flexion, and inverted. As the patient walks, the trunk lurches to the opposite side, and the lower limb circumducts to clear the ground. In patients with spasticity of both lower limbs, such as in spastic paraparesis, the patient presents with circumduction of both lower limbs, resulting in a scissoring gait.
- *Cerebellar ataxic gait*: In lesions of the anterior lobe of the cerebellum, vermis, or other midline structure, the patient adopts a wide-based stance with short steps, stiffens the legs, and lurches forward to improve stability. There may be a superimposed titubation. In lesions of the flocculonodular lobe, the truncal sway is multidirectional with stance and truncal ataxia. The truncal stability is affected in ataxic gait, resulting in frequent falls.
- *Parkinsonian gait*: In Parkinsonism, the patient has a narrow base, stooped forward posture, hesitation at the start of the gait, freezing of gait, and festination with a progressive decrease in step length. There may be a tendency to fall forward. In progressive supranuclear palsy, the patient may have backward falls. There is a reduction in arm swing and associated movements of the limb.
- *Gait in patients with hyperkinetic movement disorder*: In patients with chorea, the choreiform movement is superimposed on the limb and trunk, resulting in a dancing gait. The chorea may be accentuated as the patient walks, compared to the resting state. In dystonia, the patient presents with action dystonia of the lower limbs. In primary dystonia, the dystonia of the foot may be evident in walking forward and disappearing as the patient walks backward. The striatal toe may be present. In dopa-responsive dystonia, the difficulty in walking may develop toward the evening, and disappear with a nap and administration of levodopa. Paroxysmal kinesigenic dyskinesia is brief jerks that occur when the patient begins to walk, assuming a standing position from a seated position.

High-level Gait Disorders

A high-level gait disorder is characterized by a wide base, short steps, freezing, and postural disequilibrium. The various terms used to describe the gait are frontal gait, apraxia of gait, and lower body parkinsonism. These patients can cycle while lying in the bed but have difficulty in walking. The patient may exhibit gait initiation failure and hesitation at the initiation.

ASSESSMENT OF GAIT AND BALANCE

Assessment of Gait

Indications for gait analysis are summarized in **Box 1**.

Assessment of gait includes clinical observational assessment, functional and performance-based assessment, and instrumental or computer-based gait analysis.

Clinical Observational Assessment

Clinical assessment by the physician is to observe any deviation from normalcy and approach using pattern recognition in detecting the underlying disorder. It depends on the proficiency, competency, and experience of the clinician. The clinical assessment of gait begins with a history and detailed assessment of stance and gait. It is imperative to assess the risk of falls. The presence of falls or near falls in the preceding 6 months to 1 year is a predictor of falls, and advice on the suitable preventive measure should be adopted. The clinical observation of the gait focuses on the sagittal plane observations of pressing hip extension, midswing hip flexion, position of the knee at initial contact and midstance, and peak flexion of the knee, and the position of the ankle at initial contact, mid stance, plantar flexion at preswing and midswing **(Fig. 2)**. This can be done with any video camera mounted on a tripod or handheld phone camera. The recording can then be analyzed later to mark these key events on the gait cycle at the hip, knee, and ankle.[8]

The clinical assessment of gait involves the analysis of deficits. It is also very important to consider the compensation that arises due to the deficit in gait. A patient with poor balance may have a cautious gait with a widening of gait width and increase in the double support phase if

BOX 1 Indications for gait analysis.

- Identify the cause of gait impairment
- Assess the extent and severity of functional impairment
- Monitor the progressive course of the disease
- Assess the response to therapeutic intervention and outcomes

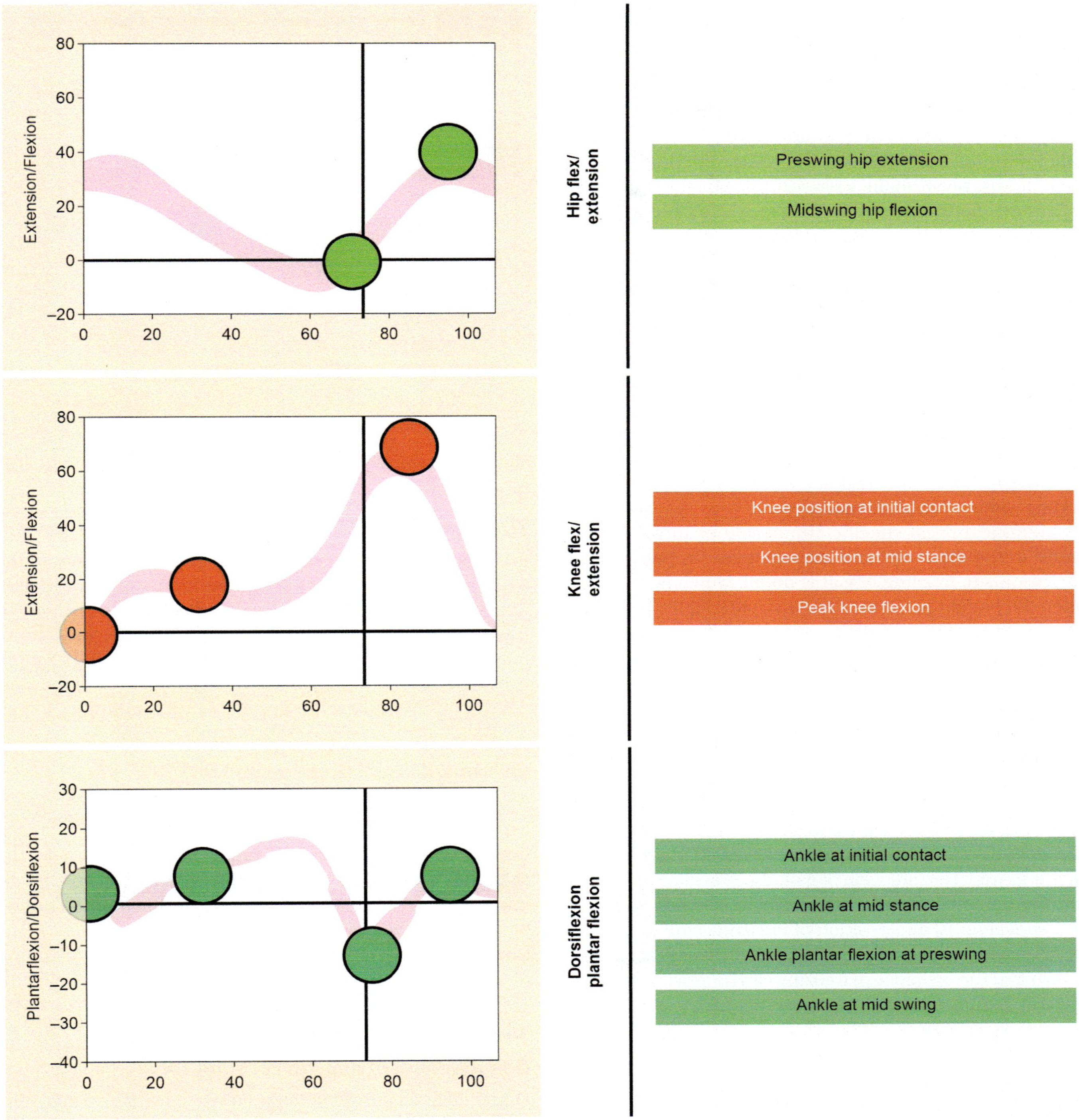

FIG. 2: Key events in the clinical observation of the hip, knee, and ankle in the gait analysis.

the patient is aware of the imbalance or a reckless gait with frequent falls if the patient is unaware of the imbalance. A patient with an ataxic gait will have a broad-based gait with locking of the knee to compensate for medial-to-lateral instability and reduce hypermetria.[2,9]

The assessment of limb and trunk features such as proximal weakness and distal weakness of the lower limbs can aid in the localization and identification of possible structure involved. In proximal weakness (myopathy, neuromuscular junction disorder) the trunk alternately sways to either side laterally with augmented hip elevation. In the distal weakness of the legs due to weakness of dorsiflexion, which results in foot drop either unilaterally or bilaterally, the patient has a high steppage gait as he attempts to lift and flex the affected lower limb to clear the ground. In the distal weakness of the legs due to weakness of plantar flexion, the patient finds it difficult to push the feet off the ground and hence drags the feet on the ground. In a patient with quadriceps weakness, the patient hyperextends the knee and flexes the trunk forward. In patients with an increased tone of the lower limb, the leg is extended with plantar flexion with a circumduction gait. When the tone of both lower limbs is increased, the patient circumducts both lower limbs, resulting in a scissoring gait, which increases with the increasing velocity of the gait as the spasticity is velocity dependent. Hyperkinetic movement such as dyskinesia and factors that destabilize the gait such as myoclonic jerks and hyperekplexia may be visualized in the limbs.[2]

The clinical observation to look for spatial and temporal features of gait gives clue to the diagnosis. A decrease in step length is noted in Parkinsonism and spastic gait. Increased and irregular step length is noted in patients with hypermetria due to cerebellar disease. Wide step width is seen in cerebellar disorders, atypical Parkinsonism, and normal pressure hydrocephalus. It may be a nonspecific finding when an imbalance is present.[10]

Identification of specific abnormalities in gait may be useful in the diagnosis and management. In patients with Parkinsonism, freezing of gait is noted, which is prominent when the patient performs dual-task paradigms. In an older adult with walking difficulty, the physician must bear in mind non-neurological causes such as cardiopulmonary causes, and vascular insufficiency in both lower limbs.[1,7]

A systemic and comprehensive clinical assessment of gait should be performed. As the patient rises from sitting to standing position, the proximal strength, coordination of movements between trunk and limbs, stance width, and stability can be assessed. In a standing position, the posture of the patient, stance width and stability of the base, Romberg test, and pull test can be assessed. As the patient begins to walk the initiation of gait, the presence of freezing, step length, stride length, cadence, gait velocity, associated limb movements, and position of the trunk can be assessed. As the patient turns while walking, the number of steps taken to turn and the presence of freezing can be assessed. The use of other maneuvers such as tandem walking and walking backward can provide further clues.[7]

Functional and Performance-based Measurement

The various performance-based measures of gait discussed below include:[11]

- Timed up and go (TUG) test
- Rivermead visual gait assessment
- Gait assessment and intervention tool
- Wisconsin gait scale
- Tinetti performance-oriented mobility assessment (POMA)

Other various functional and performance-based tests are summarized in **Box 2**.[5,9]

BOX 2 Performance-based assessment of gait analysis.

Gait scales

- 6-minute walk test
- 10-meter walk test
- Dynamic gait index
- Functional gait assessment
- Visual assessment of hemiplegic gait
- Gait abnormality rating scale
- 12-item multiple sclerosis scale
- Emory functional ambulation
- Salford gait tool
- Observational gait scale
- Gait and a balance scale
- Edinburgh visual gait score
- Bath assessment of walking inventory
- Hemiplegic gait assessment form

"Further details are available in the following web link https://ifnr.org/public/core/kar.php"

TUG Test

It is a performance-based measure of gait that assesses the patient as he gets up from a seated position, walks in a straight line for 3 m, turns around, and walks back to the seated position. A time duration of >14.9 seconds is a predictor of fall risk. The TUG test is also an estimate of cognition and executive function. It is a measure of completion of the task, and it does not assess the deviations from normalcy in gait analysis.[5]

Rivermead Visual Gait Assessment

It is a 20-item gait assessment scale with components assessing the upper limb, trunk, and lower limb, and each limb is assessed separately, rated on a scale of 0–3. The scale has good inter-rater reliability. This can further be augmented by training the examiner in the administration of the scale. The use of scale can also be used to assess the improvement in gait metrics following the administration of intervention. However, the gait is scored subjectively. This scale is useful in the assessment of gait in patients with multiple sclerosis and traumatic brain injury.[8]

Gait Assessment and Intervention Tool

Designed by a neurorehabilitation specialist, it uses a 31-item scale to assess the gait metrics. It uses 4 items to assess the upper limbs and trunk and 27 items to assess the lower limbs and trunk (14 items for the stance phase and 13 items for the swing phase). The items are graded on a scale of 0–3 with 0 denoting normalcy and 3 denoting maximum deviation. The scale has excellent inter-rater reliability. It is more sensitive in demonstrating improvement following gait rehabilitation and can be used as a monitoring tool in assessing treatment response to various interventions. It is most useful in the assessment of gait in stroke as it has been studied in this patient population.[8,12]

Wisconsin Gait Scale

It was designed to assess and analyze the gait of patients with stroke. The scale uses 14 items. 13 items are used to analyze the lower limbs, and 1 item is used to analyze the gait while the patient is using a gait aid held in the hand. The items are graded on a scale of 1–3. The first item assessing the handheld gait assist device is graded on a scale of 1–5, and the 11th item in the scale, which assesses the knee flexion during the swing phase, is graded on a scale of 1–4. The scale has good inter-rater reliability. The scale is useful in the monitoring of gait improvement following a gait training program. It shows a good correlation with functional outcomes such as the Barthel index and Brunnstrom stages of recovery.[8,13]

Tinetti POMA

The Tinetti gait scale, which was initially designed to study gait in the elderly, has also been extrapolated to study the gait in patients with neurological disorders such as Parkinson's disease. It is commonly used in the assessment of gait in clinics as it is easy to administer. The scale contains two subscales: the gait subscale and the balance subscale. The balance subscale has a maximal score of 16 and the gait subscale 12, summing to a total of 28. The gait subscale was sensitive to identifying fall risk in patients with Parkinson's disease. The Tinetti POMA scale was also a good predictor of mortality after 7 years in patients with Parkinson's disease. The scale was also useful in the assessment of gait in stroke patients. The scale has good inter-rater reliability.[8,14,15]

Instrumented and Computerized Gait Analysis

The technological evolution in the current era aids in the objective measure of gait, which is useful in modern-day clinical examination and research analysis.

The instrumented and computerized gait analysis is categorized as nonwearable and wearable sensors. The nonwearable sensors utilize external sensors to analyze the gait parameters and are limited to gait research labs. The gait analysis has shifted from sampling a few steps in the lab to continuous assessment and monitoring of gait in the community.

The wearable sensors can be extended for out-of-lab monitoring of gait at home. Nonwearable sensors are based on floor sensors or image-processing devices. The use of a force platform in the gait lab is useful in the assessment of power and forces of gait. Multiple trials are used to average the gait parameters of the patient **(Fig. 3)**.[14]

The motion capture system utilizes a camera, infrared sensors, and laser scanners. The use of the motion capture system provides a three-dimensional analysis of the gait in space. The analysis of the kinetics and kinematics of the movement in the space and the pattern of muscle activation aid in the identification of the deficit in gait and compensatory strategies used **(Figs. 4A to C)**.

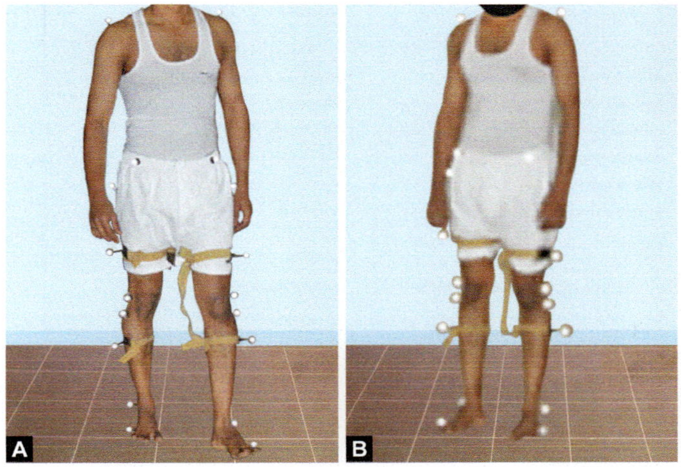

FIGS. 3A AND B: Three-dimensional instrumented gait analysis laboratory.

Three-dimensional instrumented gait analysis has been widely used in cerebral palsy, and specific gait patterns have been identified in spastic diplegia and spastic hemiplegia. The patterns can be identified, and treatment of these difficult problems can thus be standardized accordingly.[16]

However, its use is limited by the limited availability of technical expertise, space required, and high cost **(Box 3)**.[17,18]

The use of insole sensors analyses the gait at the community and household levels. It analyses the gait impairments and risk of falls in the elderly by applying pattern recognition approaches in the data obtained from the insoles.[19] The body-fixed sensors such as the inertial measurement unit are unobtrusive devices, which are light-weighted portable devices that are attached to the ankle, knees, wrists, trunks, and other joints. The various gait parameters can be assessed from devices containing a magnetometer and accelerometer that are recorded over long periods and provide temporal variations in gait over the day. Gait variability and regularity can be calculated from the data. Now, it is feasible to record gait parameters over 3–7 days using body-fixed sensors. It helps to capture and identify episodic events such as freezing of gait in Parkinson's disease.[19,20]

Assessment of Balance

The importance of the assessment of balance lies in the identification of imbalance and cause of the balance disorder.

Functional and Performance-based Measurement

The balance can be assessed using the TUG test and balance subcomponent of the Tinetti balance and gait test. The other scales that are useful in the analysis of balance are

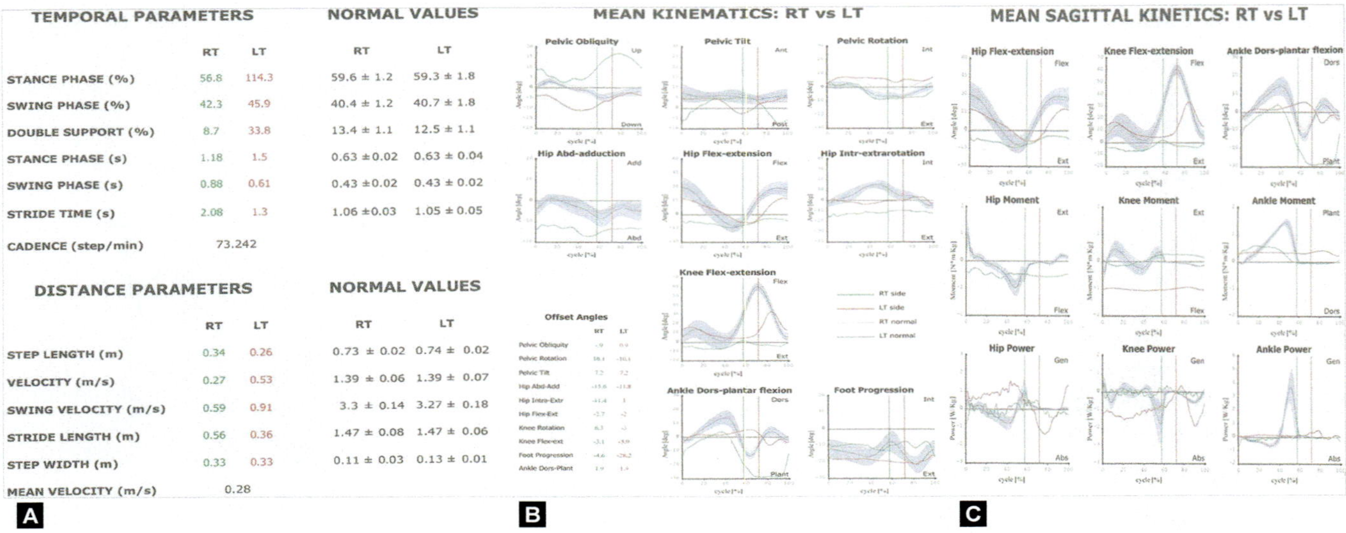

TEMPORAL PARAMETERS	RT	LT	NORMAL VALUES RT	NORMAL VALUES LT
STANCE PHASE (%)	56.8	114.3	59.6 ± 1.2	59.3 ± 1.8
SWING PHASE (%)	42.3	45.9	40.4 ± 1.2	40.7 ± 1.8
DOUBLE SUPPORT (%)	8.7	33.8	13.4 ± 1.1	12.5 ± 1.1
STANCE PHASE (s)	1.18	1.5	0.63 ±0.02	0.63 ± 0.04
SWING PHASE (s)	0.88	0.61	0.43 ±0.02	0.43 ± 0.02
STRIDE TIME (s)	2.08	1.3	1.06 ±0.03	1.05 ± 0.05
CADENCE (step/min)	73.242			

DISTANCE PARAMETERS	RT	LT	NORMAL VALUES RT	NORMAL VALUES LT
STEP LENGTH (m)	0.34	0.26	0.73 ± 0.02	0.74 ± 0.02
VELOCITY (m/s)	0.27	0.53	1.39 ± 0.06	1.39 ± 0.07
SWING VELOCITY (m/s)	0.59	0.91	3.3 ± 0.14	3.27 ± 0.18
STRIDE LENGTH (m)	0.56	0.36	1.47 ± 0.08	1.47 ± 0.06
STEP WIDTH (m)	0.33	0.33	0.11 ± 0.03	0.13 ± 0.01
MEAN VELOCITY (m/s)	0.28			

FIGS. 4A TO C: Report of three-dimensional instrumented gait analysis showing (A) temporal and spatial parameters of gait, (B) kinematics, and (C) kinetics.

(LT: left; RT: right)

BOX 3 Limitations in the use of instrumented gait analysis.

- Paucity of evidence that instrumented gait analysis augments clinical improvement in specific diseases
- Limited guidelines in the application of various gait analysis technique in clinical evaluation and treatment
- Limited therapeutic options in the management of adult gait disorders
- Limited understanding of instrumented gait analysis data by the clinicians

discussed further. Timed single-leg stance is an old test in the identification of imbalance. The Berg balance scale is easy to administer with high inter-rater reliability, and low sensitivity. A score which is >45 is used to identify patients with a low risk of falls. Activities of balance confidence is a self-reported questionnaire based on 16 activities performed during daily living and is a very useful test is assessing imbalance.[21] In the functional reach test, the patient is asked to reach forward as much as possible without falling. It is used to identify patients with an increased risk of falls.[22]

The systems assessment for the evaluation of balance includes balance evaluation system test and physiological profile approach. The former focuses on six components of the balance system. This clinical test includes external disturbances to balance and postural vertical perception. The balance test helps to identify the type of deficit in balance and provides targeted treatment to patients. It includes components from the Berg balance scale, get up and go test, functional reach test, and clinical test of sensory integration for balance. The test requires 30 minutes to administer.[23] The later test includes a brief and comprehensive version. The brief version includes an assessment of vision, cutaneous sensation, power in the legs, time to react, and swaying while standing and requires 15 minutes for assessment. The comprehensive assessment includes an expanded version. A score of >2 indicates an increased risk of falls.[24]

Instrumented Assessment

The objective assessment of balance is done using posturography and wearable sensors. These tests provide objective quantification of the imbalance with a reduction in variability and improved sensitivity. The posturography is static or dynamic. Static posturography assesses the truncal sway while the patient attempts to stand still. This can be assessed by measuring the displacement from the foot sensor on a force plate, accelerometers attached to the low back, and wearable inertial sensors.

Dynamic posturography is useful to assess the balance in response to external perturbations, surface changes, and changes in visual conditions **(Figs. 5A and B)**. Adaptations to rapid perturbations are used to assess the latency, and adaptations to slow perturbations are used to assess the adaptation, anticipation, and motor learning. It also helps to identify the impairment that contributes to imbalance.[25]

Though dynamic posturography is a gold standard in assessing the motor and sensory components of balance, its widespread use is limited by high cost, and requirement for technical expertise.[26]

The development of wearable inertial sensors with the advent of technological advancement overcomes the limitations of high cost, space, and time required. The sensors contain accelerometers and a gyroscope that are used to measure the movements of limbs, and the trunk. These sensors can measure the dynamic balance while the patient walks in a real-world scenario. More evidence is required for its clinical use. And further, it can help provide increasing clinical information regarding balance in various neurological disorders.[27]

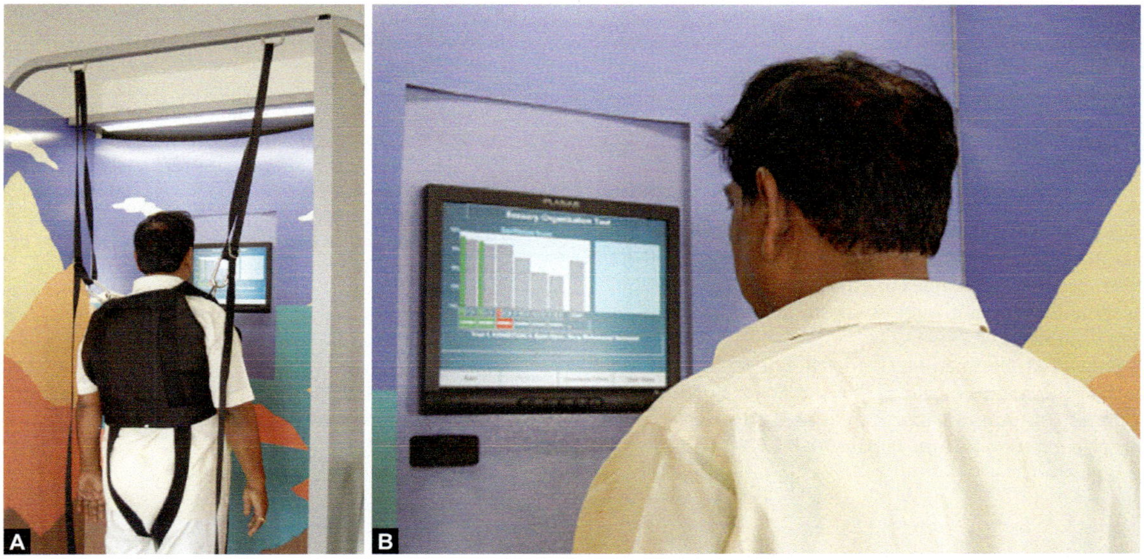

FIGS. 5A AND B: Dynamic posturography used to assess the balance in response to external perturbations, surface changes, and changes in visual conditions.

CONCLUSION

The systematic and comprehensive clinical assessment of the gait as the patient walks into the clinician's examination couch provides diagnostic clues to the trained eye **(Box 4)**. Further, the use of technologies in the analysis of gait increases the sensitivity to identify the gait deficits and compensatory strategies and helps in monitoring the gait parameters and their response to therapeutic interventions. The use of various rehabilitative strategies to provide task-oriented and deficit-oriented gait training is useful in the functional restoration of the patient.

BOX 4 Importance of gait assessment in clinical practice.

Why assess gait in clinical practice?

- Biomechanical basis of pathological gait
- Severity of gait impairment
- Plan treatment strategy
- Prescription of orthotic devices
- Target muscles for intervention
- Plan surgical treatment
- Evidence of the efficacy of intervention

REFERENCES

1. Baker R. The history of gait analysis before the advent of modern computers. Gait Posture. 2007;26(3):331-42.
2. Fasano A, Bloem BR. Gait disorders. Contin Lifelong Learn Neurol. 2013;19(5):1344-82.
3. Pahapill PA, Lozano AM. The pedunculopontine nucleus and Parkinson's disease. Brain. 2000;123(9):1767-83.
4. Mirelman A, Shema S, Maidan I, Hausdorff JM. Gait. Handb Clin Neurol. 2018;159:119-34.
5. Kharb A, Saini V, Jain YK, Dhiman S. A review of gait cycle and its parameters. Int J Comput Eng Manag. 2011;13:78-83.
6. Chambers HG, Sutherland DH. A practical guide to gait analysis. J Am Acad Orthop Surg. 2002;10(3):222-31.
7. Thompson PD, Nutt JG. Gait disorders. Bradleys Neurol Clin Pract E-Book. 2021;334.
8. Gor-García-Fogeda MD, de la Cuerda RC, Tejada MC, Alguacil-Diego IM, Molina-Rueda F. Observational gait assessments in people with neurological disorders: a systematic review. Arch Phys Med Rehabil. 2016;97(1):131-40.
9. Bakker M, Allum JH, Visser JE, Grüneberg C, van de Warrenburg BP, Kremer BH, et al. Postural responses to multidirectional stance perturbations in cerebellar ataxia. Exp Neurol. 2006;202(1):21-35.
10. Lundin-Olsson L, Nyberg L, Gustafson Y. Stops walking when talking as a predictor of falls in elderly people. Lancet. 1997;349(9052):617.
11. Ridao-Fernández C, Pinero-Pinto E, Chamorro-Moriana G. Observational gait assessment scales in patients with walking disorders: systematic review. Biomed Res Int. 2019;2019:2085039.
12. Zimbelman J, Daly JJ, Roenigk KL, Butler K, Burdsall R, Holcomb JP. Capability of 2 gait measures for detecting response to gait training in stroke survivors: gait assessment and intervention tool and the Tinetti gait scale. Arch Phys Med Rehabil. 2012;93(1):129-36.
13. Rodriquez AA, Black PO, Kile KA, Sherman J, Stellberg B, McCormick J, et al. Gait training efficacy using a home-based practice model in chronic hemiplegia. Arch Phys Med Rehabil. 1996;77(8):801-5.
14. Morita Y, Osaki Y, Doi Y. Factors associated with falling in patients with Parkinson's disease and atypical Parkinsonism: an assessment using the Tinetti gait and balance scale. Geriatr Gerontol Int. 2006;6(4):234-43.
15. Gray WK, Hildreth A, Bilclough JA, Wood BH, Baker K, Walker RW. Physical assessment as a predictor of mortality in people with Parkinson's disease: a study over 7 years. Mov Disord. 2009;24(13):1934-40.

16. Rodda J, Graham HK. Classification of gait patterns in spastic hemiplegia and spastic diplegia: a basis for a management algorithm. Eur J Neurol. 2001;8:98-108.
17. Muro-De-La-Herran A, Garcia-Zapirain B, Mendez-Zorrilla A. Gait analysis methods: an overview of wearable and nonwearable systems, highlighting clinical applications. Sensors. 2014;14(2): 3362-94.
18. Wren TA, Gorton III GE, Ounpuu S, Tucker CA. Efficacy of clinical gait analysis: a systematic review. Gait Posture. 2011;34(2):149-53.
19. Di Rosa M, Hausdorff JM, Stara V, Rossi L, Glynn L, Casey M, et al. Concurrent validation of an index to estimate fall risk in community dwelling seniors through a wireless sensor insole system: a pilot study. Gait Posture. 2017;55:6-11.
20. Weiss A, Brozgol M, Dorfman M, Herman T, Shema S, Giladi N, et al. Does the evaluation of gait quality during daily life provide insight into fall risk? A novel approach using 3-day accelerometer recordings. Neurorehabil Neural Repair. 2013;27(8):742-52.
21. Myers AM, Fletcher PC, Myers AH, Sherk W. Discriminative and evaluative properties of the activities-specific balance confidence (ABC) scale. J Gerontol A Biol Sci Med Sci. 1998;53(4):M287-94.
22. Duncan PW, Weiner DK, Chandler J, Studenski S. Functional reach: a new clinical measure of balance. J Gerontol. 1990;45(6):M192-7.
23. Horak FB, Wrisley DM, Frank J. The balance evaluation systems test (BESTest) to differentiate balance deficits. Phys Ther. 2009;89(5):484-98.
24. Lord SR, Menz HB, Tiedemann A. A physiological profile approach to falls risk assessment and prevention. Phys Ther. 2003;83(3):237-52.
25. Srivastava A, Taly AB, Gupta A, Kumar S, Murali T. Poststroke balance training: role of force platform with visual feedback technique. J Neurol Sci. 2009;287(1-2):89-93.
26. Visser JE, Carpenter MG, van der Kooij H, Bloem BR. The clinical utility of posturography. Clin Neurophysiol. 2008;119(11):2424-36.
27. Mancini M, Horak FB. The relevance of clinical balance assessment tools to differentiate balance deficits. Eur J Phys Rehabil Med. 2010;46(2):239.

12

CHAPTER

Systemic Examination in Neurological Disorders

Steven L Lewis

INTRODUCTION

The purpose of the neurologic history and neurologic examination is to look for clues to the cause of a patient's neurologic symptoms. This means that the history and neurologic examination are performed to try to determine the localization of the disease process (i.e., where in the nervous system the problem is), as well as the mechanism of the disease process (i.e., how that neurologic problem is occurring), paving the way for the most appropriate diagnostic studies, when indicated.[1] The neurologic diagnostic process typically refers to the historical assessment of neurologic symptoms and the neurologic examination for neurologic signs; however, systemic assessment by attainment of a systemic history and, when appropriate, focused systemic examination can also be critical in neurologic diagnosis as determined for each unique clinical circumstance.

In the context of systemic assessment in neurologic diagnosis, neurologic disorders with systemic symptoms and/or signs can be divided into two main categories:

1. Neurologic disorders with systemic historical features or examination findings as a clue to a primary neurologic disease process (e.g., abdominal symptoms in a patient with migraine)
2. Neurologic disorders with systemic historical features or examination findings as a clue to a primary underlying systemic disease process (e.g., hepatic signs and symptoms in a patient with Wilsonian or non-Wilsonian hepatolenticular degeneration)[2]

In addition to neurologic diagnosis, however, systemic assessment/examination can be important in the investigation of systemic complications of neurological disease (e.g., deep vein thrombosis in a hospitalized patient with stroke) or a complication of neurological disease therapy (e.g., skin rash from an antiseizure medication).

This chapter addresses the role of, and performance of, the systemic history and examination in the diagnostic assessment of neurologic disorders. It should be noted that in this chapter, the term *systemic* refers to any historical or examination features not directly related to the nervous system, i.e., not related to the primary senses, strength, coordination, reflexes, or gait.

HISTORY TAKING FOR SYSTEMIC ASSESSMENT IN NEUROLOGIC DISORDERS

In neurologic diagnosis, the patient's history should invariably be obtained prior to performing the examination. This includes features including the history of the present illness, past medical history, past surgical history, medications, social history, and review of systems. Although the term *past* is included in "past medical history," the past medical history typically refers to illnesses within any of the following categories:

- Previously diagnosed and presumably resolved medical illnesses (e.g., viral exanthems as a child)
- Ongoing chronic medical illnesses (e.g., hypertension or diabetes)
- Current and recently diagnosed medical illnesses (e.g., recently diagnosed systemic cancer) for which treatment might still be ongoing

Obtaining the past medical history should be agnostic to the history of the present illness; that is, a patient's past medical history should be the same at any moment in time regardless of the history of the present illness; the relevance (or lack thereof) of any element of the patient's past medical history can only be determined during the diagnostic synthesis of the current problem. Selectively prodding the patient only for specific medical issues—or conversely, prematurely excluding any items from the past medical history that are offered by the patient—may lead to inaccurate neurologic diagnoses via both biased and insufficient information.

Unlike the patient's past medical history, which should be obtained in an agnostic fashion independent of the

BOX 1	Fourteen major category elements in a review of systems.[3]

1. Constitutional symptoms (e.g., fever and weight loss)
2. Eyes
3. Ears, nose, mouth, throat
4. Cardiovascular
5. Respiratory
6. Gastrointestinal
7. Genitourinary
8. Musculoskeletal
9. Integumentary (skin and/or breast)
10. Neurological
11. Psychiatric
12. Endocrine
13. Hematologic/lymphatic
14. Allergic/immunologic

Source: With permission from Center for Medicare and Medicaid Services. (2022).[3]

current clinical context, the review of systems—sometimes alternatively referred to as *review of symptoms*—represents a set of symptoms, mostly systemic in nature, where the specific symptoms inquired about might vary depending on the clinical context. Although it would be optimal to inquire about all elements of a review of systems in every individual diagnostic encounter (and this option is indeed available in certain previsit assessments via the electronic health record or printed forms), in many cases the decision as to which systemic elements to inquire about is dependent on the clinician's reasoning process that is informed by the history of present illness.

The typical elements of a review of (primarily systemic) systems are outlined in **Box 1**. As mentioned above, although the specific sets of elements inquired about in the review of systems might vary depending on the clinician's developing suspicions during the historical process, in this author's opinion, the presence or absence of constitutional symptoms (e.g., fevers, chills, weight loss, or weight gain) should be assessed in every new diagnostic patient encounter, as the presence of these symptoms is particularly sensitive, albeit nonspecific, in raising the suspicion of an ongoing or recent systemic process.

METHODS OF SYSTEMIC EXAMINATION AND THEIR INTERPRETATION

The complete neurologic examination (described elsewhere in this textbook) has required elements—as well as optional elements—that are typically performed in a standard order, although variations in the order of performance of each element are dependent on the neurologist's preference and style. Unlike the purely neurologic components of the neurologic examination, however, the need for the performance of many components of the systemic

BOX 2	Major elements of a non-neurologic (systemic) examination.*

- Vital signs†
- Eyes
- Mouth
- Ears
- Neck (including assessment for meningismus)
- Lungs
- Cardiac/cardiovascular
- Abdomen
- Extremities
- Skin

*Not all of these examination elements need to be performed by the neurologist as part of routine neurologic assessments.
†Should be assessed in all patient encounters, especially during the initial encounter.

examination in neurologic assessment is less consistent and might vary depending on any of the following:

- Clinical milieu (e.g., inpatient vs. outpatient)
- Disease acuity (e.g., emergent vs. chronic)
- The need to search for systemic clues as suggested by the history (e.g., a historical detail pointing directly to the need to look for a specific systemic finding, such as the patient's complaint of a skin rash)
- The need to search for systemic origins to an underlying neurologic diagnosis as suggested by the history (e.g., assessment for Kayser–Fleischer rings in a patient with possible Wilson disease)

This section highlights the systemic examination in neurologic diagnosis and provides details including when the examination elements may be most likely to be reasonably performed by the neurologist, while also pointing out when such assessment might be more optimally provided by a primary care physician or medical subspecialist. The main elements of the systemic (non-neurologic) examination are listed in **Box 2**.

Vital Signs

Assessment and recording of vital signs is an integral and invariable part of all new patient encounters and can also be extremely valuable in routine follow-up encounters. Assessment of respiratory rate, blood pressure, and resting pulse rate provides basic details of a patient's airway, breathing, and circulation (the so-called *ABC*s), while providing a clue to patient stability. Palpating the radial or brachial pulse by the clinician can also suggest clues as to the underlying heart rhythm, with an irregularly irregular pulse highly suggestive of atrial fibrillation, an important risk factor for cardioembolic stroke.

Routine assessment of a patient's temperature provides a clue to systemic infectious or inflammatory illnesses, particularly when fever is present, while the presence of hypothermia also provides clues to a similar systemic disorder and might also suggest an underlying endocrine or hypothalamic process.

Assessment of orthostatic blood pressure and pulse by the neurologic clinician can be extremely valuable and should be performed in all patients who present with symptoms suggestive of orthostatic hypotension, including patients with lightheadedness, dizziness, or imbalance on standing, or patients with unexplained syncope. Assessment for orthostatic hypotension entails checking the patient's blood pressure and pulse in the supine position, and then rechecking the patient's blood pressure and pulse after approximately 3 minutes of quiet standing (if the patient is unable to stand, assessment in the sitting position may substitute for the standing assessment but is less sensitive for orthostasis). An orthostatic drop of systolic blood pressure of at least 20 mm Hg or a reduction of diastolic blood pressure of at least 10 mm Hg is consistent with orthostatic hypotension.[4] A lack of compensatory increase in pulse rate despite the blood pressure drop is most consistent with autonomic dysfunction (i.e., autonomic/sympathetic failure), whereas the presence of a compensatory increase suggests hypovolemia (e.g., dehydration) with an intact sympathetic nervous system.[1]

Head, Eye, Ear, and Neck Examination

Some assessment and observation of the head, eyes, oropharynx, and neck are unavoidable during the routine neurologic examination of cranial nerves, and special additional assessments of these regions beyond what is encountered during the neurologic examination may not always be needed.

Routine fundoscopic assessment, by the neurologist allows for the detection of additional systemic clues for chronic medical illnesses or infectious disorders that include retinitis (though in the current era best recognized on formal ophthalmological examination by an ophthalmologist); the neurologist, however, should be able to recognize optic disc edema suggesting increased intracranial pressure or an inflammatory/infiltrative optic disc process.

Assessment of pupillary function showing small pupils with light-near dissociation (constriction to light without constriction to near vision) can suggest the Argyll Robertson pupil of tabes dorsalis (neurosyphilis), though can also be seen in other disorders including pseudotabes from diabetes mellitus.[5]

A multitude of neurologic disorders can be suggested, or even diagnosed, on examination of the retina, optic disc, pupil, and iris (including on fundoscopic and slit lamp examinations, the latter including assessment for Kayser–Fleischer rings or Lisch nodules for neurofibromatosis type 1[6] in the appropriate clinical scenarios), but these usually require formal ophthalmological expertise and equipment.

Regarding the assessment of the ears, otoscopic assessment of the ear canals is not typically performed routinely on neurologic examination but can be extremely valuable in the setting of possible meningeal infection from an otitic source, or the assessment for a cerebrospinal fluid (CSF) leak.

On examination of the neck, specific maneuvers to assess for meningismus should be performed by the neurologist when meningeal inflammation, and particularly infection or subarachnoid hemorrhage, is suspected. Nuchal rigidity is assessed by passively flexing the patient's neck forward and assessing for rigidity, resistance, or pain with this maneuver.[1] The presence of nuchal rigidity can be a helpful sign of meningismus but is insensitive particularly in patients who are obtunded or comatose. The Kernig sign is assessed by passively flexing the patient's hip so that the thigh is held up at about 90 degrees; the examiner then attempts to passively extend (i.e., straighten) the patient's leg at the knee, looking for resistance and pain with this maneuver. The Brudzinski sign is assessed by passively flexing the patient's neck forward, with a positive sign consisting of flexion of the hips and legs with this maneuver.[1] An analysis by Mehndiratta and colleagues showed that Kernig and Brudzinski signs are not very sensitive for detecting meningitis, and that their absence should therefore not be interpreted as evidence to exclude it; however, due to their high specificity, the presence of either of these signs suggests a high likelihood for meningitis.[7]

Cardiac and Cardiovascular Examination

Assessment of cardiac function is inherent in the routine assessment of vital signs discussed above, particularly the measurement of blood pressure and the bedside assessment of cardiac rhythm by palpation of an extremity pulse. In addition, in certain clinical situations, and particularly in the assessment of patients with a possible cerebrovascular disorder, auscultation of the heart and neck vessels can provide additional potentially useful diagnostic information; auscultation for carotid bruits continues to be utilized routinely in bedside neurologic assessment, although the findings are insensitive (particularly for complete occlusion) and nonspecific,[8] and their absence or presence should not alter the clinician's decision to perform noninvasive vascular assessment when clinically indicated.

Lungs and Abdominal Examination

Bedside physical examination of the lungs and abdomen may be appropriate in the routine medical care of a neurologic patient (e.g., a critically ill or other hospitalized inpatient), and are standard in primary care (medical) evaluations but will rarely provide the neurologist with additional specific neurologic diagnostic information that was not otherwise inferred from the neurologic history.

It is worth mentioning in this regard that certain examination elements, including assessment of the abdomen (or genitals), particularly when deemed outside of the realm of routine neurologic examination techniques, may require consideration that a chaperone be present for patient comfort and possible medicolegal implications.[9]

Extremities

Like the head and neck examination, some assessment and observation of the extremities is unavoidable during the routine neurologic examination of motor strength and distal sensation. During this routine neurologic assessment, for example, observation for edema or cyanosis can be helpful, with edema and Homan sign being helpful in the assessment for deep vein thrombosis in a hospitalized neurologic patient, and cyanosis being relevant to the strong consideration of a peripheral vascular cause of symptoms in a patient in whom vascular, rather than neurogenic, claudication remains in the differential diagnosis for exertion-related extremity pain. Similarly, assessment of pedal pulses by palpation can easily be incorporated, when appropriate, into the examination concomitant to when distal sensation is being assessed.

Assessment for joint deformities by simple observation can also yield clues to a systemic disease, such as the findings inherent in the hand and finger joints that may be suggestive of the various inflammatory arthritides that may be associated with neurologic disease.[10]

Skin

Finally, examination of the skin may in many cases be the most relevant and highly accessible systemic assessment available to the neurologist,[11] providing clues to the wide variety of neurologic disorders discussed in this textbook, even in the absence of a specific patient complaint or symptom referable to the skin. By definition, cutaneous manifestations may be highly suggestive, and even diagnostic, of any of the wide variety of neurocutaneous (hereditary) syndromes[6] seen in neurologic practice. In addition, cutaneous manifestations are inherent in a multitude of toxic disorders of the nervous system, with skin and nail manifestations particularly associated with peripheral nervous system toxins (e.g., Mees' lines in arsenic and thallium toxicities).[12] Neurovascular and neurorheumatologic disorders can be suggested by cutaneous signs such as livedo reticularis.[11]

The skin may also provide critically important and sometimes highly specific clues to the diagnosis of neuroinfectious diseases discussed throughout this volume, ranging from the classic vesicular rash of herpes zoster (a viral infection of the dorsal root ganglia) to the petechial rash of meningococcemia and meningococcal meningitis.[11]

CONCLUSION

The systemic history and systemic examination can play important roles in neurologic diagnosis, including the diagnosis of primary neurologic disease with systemic manifestations, the diagnosis of a neurologic disease that is secondary to a primary systemic disease, and an assessment of systemic complications of neurologic disease or its treatment.

The systemic history should always include a detailed history of the past medical (and surgical) history independent of any considerations suggested by the history of present neurologic illness, so that the clinician can have as much information as possible for neurologic reasoning of underlying disease mechanism. The review of systems/symptoms, however, can often be honed somewhat depending on the clinical suspicion, but should always include a review of constitutional symptoms.

Unlike the neurologic examination, where many examination elements are invariably performed regardless of the pretest probability, the elements of the systemic examination that are performed by the neurologist may vary depending on the clinical suspicion and even on provider expertise.

In summary, this chapter reviewed the role of systemic history and examination in neurologic diagnosis. The potential systemic historical and examination findings relevant to neurologic diagnosis are myriad, and always expanding, especially as new disorders (including pandemics) arise. Neurologists should incorporate the systemic history, and appropriately, thoughtfully, and judiciously assess for potentially clinically relevant systemic examination clues during neurologic assessment for optimal patient diagnosis and management.

REFERENCES

1. Lewis SL. Field Guide to the Neurologic Examination. Philadelphia: Lippincott Williams and Wilkins; 2005.
2. Lewis SL (Ed). Neurological Disorders due to Systemic Disease. Oxford: Wiley-Blackwell; 2012.
3. Center for Medicare and Medicaid Services. (2022). Evaluation and management services guide. [online] Available from https://www.cms.gov/outreach-and-education/medicare-learning-network-mln/mlnproducts/downloads/eval-mgmt-serv-guide-icn006764.pdf. [Last accessed December, 2022].
4. Palma J-A, Kaufmann H. Management of orthostatic hypotension. Continuum (Minneap Minn). 2020;26:154-77.
5. Aziz TA, Holman RP. The Argyll Robertson pupil. Am J Med. 2010;123(2):120-1.
6. Rosser T. Neurocutaneous disorders. Continuum (Minneap Minn). 2018;24:96-129.
7. Mehndiratta M, Nayak R, Garg H, Kumar M, Pandey S. Appraisal of Kernig's and Brudzinski's sign in meningitis. Ann Indian Acad Neurol. 2012;15:287-8.
8. Johannson EP, Wester P. Carotid bruits as predictor for carotid stenoses detected by ultrasonography: an observational study. BMC Neurol. 2008;8:23.
9. Pimienta AL, Giblon R. The case for medical chaperones. Fam Pract Manag. 2018;25(5):6-8.
10. Miloslavsky E, Cho TA. Clinical approach to neurorheumatology. Semin Neurol. 2014;34:371-7.
11. Warburton KL, Wakerley B. Dermatological clues to neurological diagnoses. Pract Neurol. 2011;11:289-95.
12. Chauhan S, D'Cruz S, Singh R, Sachdev A. Mees' lines. Lancet. 2008;372:1410.

2

SECTION

Applied Neuroanatomy and Neurophysiology

13

CHAPTER

Applied Neuroanatomy and Neurophysiology of the Basal Ganglia

Ruchika Tandon, Ajay Chavan, Saurabh Nigam, Sanjeev Jha

INTRODUCTION

The brain's subcortical nuclei, which regulate movements, executive functions, control behavior and emotions, and facilitate in learning motor skills, constitute basal ganglia.[1] Generally, the basal ganglia comprise nuclei buried deep inside the cerebral hemispheres [striatum or caudate-putamen combined and the globus pallidus (GP)], as well as the related nuclei situated in the areas of the brain other than the cerebral hemispheres such as in the diencephalon [subthalamic nucleus (STN)], in the mesencephalon (substantia nigra), and in the pons [pedunculopontine nucleus (PPN)] **(Fig. 1)**.[1-3] In this chapter, we strive to discuss the present and emerging understanding of the neuroanatomy and neurophysiology of the basal ganglia and related structures with a view to further apply this knowledge to the clinical aspects of the functioning of extrapyramidal system/basal ganglia.

NEUROANATOMICAL POINTS AND THEIR RELEVANCE

Human striatum composed of caudate nucleus and putamen regulates movement and helps in reinforcement, learning, reward, cognitive functioning, and addiction. Age

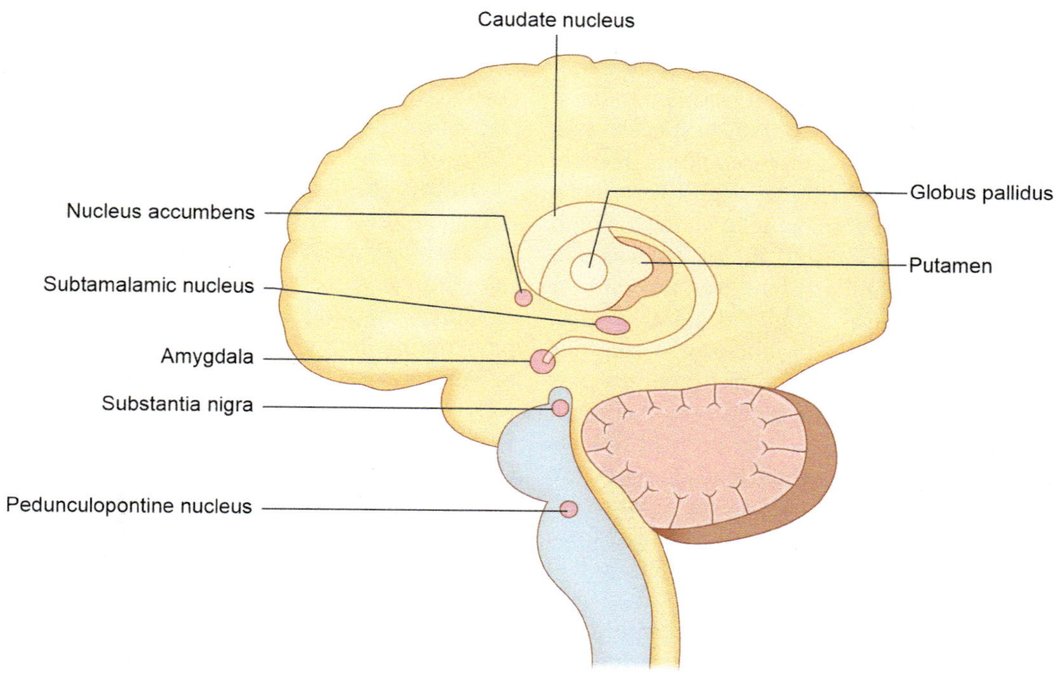

FIG. 1: Basal ganglia and related structures.

reduces the volume of this structure.[4] There may be right–left asymmetry in the affinity of dopamine binding to dopamine D1 receptors and in dyskinetic rats, the affinity is significantly higher in left than in the right striatum.[5,6] Striatum may also regulate appetite perception and eating behavior, which changes in schizophrenic individuals.[7] According to some researchers, dopaminergic changes in the frontostriatal circuits may lead to depressive symptoms.[8]

Increasing the speed of decision-making process and regulating human emotions are the functions of STN of the brain.[9] People traditionally believed that this nucleus has three parts, which are the medial tip-regulating limbic functions, a ventromedial cognitive area, and a dorsolateral area for movements. However, the immunocytochemical studies reveal that these boundaries may not be absolute, although the anatomy of the STN may not be homogeneous either.[9] The brain imaging studies show groups of corticostriatal projections in narrow, elongated, or spherical subspaces extending across the entire striatum in mammals.[10]

Amygdala and its basal ganglia–cortical networks may help in processing gustatory/visceral and visual information,[11] and amygdala and its connections with the prefrontal cortex, anterior cingulate cortex, and insula play a part in depression and insomnia.[12] Basal ganglia may compensate for cortical deficits in the visual processing areas in adults with strabismus.[13]

Magnetic resonance imaging (MRI) studies of attention-deficit/hyperactivity disorder (ADHD) show volume differences in the basal ganglia and cerebellar region of these children.[14] Volume of the ventral portion of basal ganglia may be less in autistic adult males with late language acquisition, probably giving an insight into the role of basal ganglia in the acquisition of language.[15] A functional MRI (fMRI) study on patients suffering from schizophrenia demonstrated that in these people, processing of the second noun only starts after the processing of first noun and that these speech tasks activate bilateral caudate nuclei and cerebellum. Hence, basal ganglia may play a role in these cognitive/speech tasks.[16] Due to its effect on the basal ganglia activity, a high altitude increases vowel duration and increases errors in speech motor sequencing.[17] Similarly, children who stutter have dysfunctional corticobasal ganglia–thalamocortical loops.[18] The volume of the nucleus accumbens, which carries out cognitive, emotional, and psychomotor functions, may increase in schizophrenics.[19] Increase in tissue iron content of the striatum region of the basal ganglia in fMRI reflects maturation of the adolescent brain, which leads to sensation seeking in adolescents.[20] Basal ganglia may have links with the perception of time.[21] We should also not shy away from acknowledging the contributions of Dr Thomas PS Powell in the circuitry of basal ganglia.[22]

Damage to basal ganglia may cause micrographia but not always Parkinsonism.[23] Furthermore, the scientists have observed functional reorganization in Parkinson's disease (PD) patients in both the motor basal ganglia-thalamocortical circuitry and cortical areas for vocal speech. This could be due to dopaminergic therapy or due to compensatory mechanism in PD.[24] Emerging vistas of regenerative medicine and tissue engineering may replace the lost neuronal tissues of the nigrostriatal region, thereby treating PD in the future.[25]

With regard to the role of STN stimulation in the management of drug refractory obsessive–compulsive disorder (OCD), STN affects decision-making and the action-selection mechanisms of humans, which, when dysfunctional, may cause OCD and the nonmotor STN affects the checking behavior of these individuals. STN neurons in OCD patients fire at a lower rate, have less frequent but longer bursts, have greater burst activity in the anterior ventromedial area, an asymmetrical left-sided burst distribution, and oscillations in the δ-band. Therefore, STN–DBS (deep brain stimulation) may interrupt the dysfunctional information processing, causing normalization of connectivity within the corticobasal ganglia-thalamocortical circuits.[26] Advances in TSE T2 sequence using 3 T-MRI demonstrate only 0.2- to 0.3-mm right–left asymmetry in the anteroposterior and superoinferior length of the STN but greater variations in the sagittal plane angulation, transverse dimension, and most inferior border of STN in different individuals. These observations have an implication in STN–DBS surgery.[27]

Employing high-resolution fMRI studies, investigators found activation in the thalamus, head of caudate nucleus, rostral or caudal cingulate cortex, and anterior insula, demonstrating thalamo-striato-cortical loops during sexual arousal. Along with hypothalamus and ventral striatum, paraventricular thalamus may integrate cognitive and emotional aspects of human behavior like sexual processing.[28] In cases of OCD, we know that the symptoms' severity correlates with higher connectivity pattern within cortico-striatal-thalamo-cortical circuits and repetitive transcranial magnetic stimulation (rTMS) may target this circuit, thereby improving OCD.[29]

Huntington's disease patients may have a greater damage to the striatal neurons than cortical neurons due to greater number of mitochondria in the striatum, as seen by a mitochondrial toxin study.[30]

Since, the basal ganglia regions, especially the anterior part of the head of caudate nucleus, have numerous opioidergic receptors, these relate to pain function as well.[31,32] This pain could be a nonmotor manifestation of PD. Using single-photon emission computed tomography (SPECT), a study's investigators found out that the nigrocaudate function affects executive capabilities in PD but not in healthy individuals and that motor severity in PD patients relates to nigroputaminal impairment and visuospatial dysfunction.[33] Furthermore, we know that the GP connects with nucleus ventralis lateralis of the thalamus, which may degenerate following stereotactic pallidotomy.[34]

NEUROPHYSIOLOGICAL POINTS AND THEIR RELEVANCE

Recently, the researchers have described regulatory interactions between the dopaminergic and renin-angiotensin systems in the substantia nigra and striatal regions of the brain. In animal models, once the brain depletes dopamine, it hyperactivates the local renin–angiotensin system, which then activates NADPH-oxidase, causing activation of the microglia, leading to oxidative stress. This makes the dopaminergic neurons more prone to destruction. Hence, angiotensin-converting enzyme inhibitors and angiotensin receptor blockers may be neuroprotective to the dopaminergic neurons, thereby, slowing the progression of PD.[35] Mutations in the *GBA1* gene coding for glucocerebrosidase and others such as *LRRK2*, *PINK1*, and *DJ-1* gene pose a risk of development of synucleinopathies like PD and dementia with Lewy bodies (DLB). Decreased glucocerebrosidase may increase aggregation of misfolded alpha-synuclein in the substantia nigra in PD and DLB due to changes in lipid metabolism, autophagy, mitochondrial dysfunction, endoplasmic reticulum stress, and cytotoxicity.[36] Moreover, an injection of adeno-associated viral vectors coding for *GBA1* and mutated forms of alpha-synuclein in rats prevented nigral dopaminergic neurons from neurodegeneration in a study.[36] A novel treatment promoting α-synuclein clearance utilizing genes to increase the activity of glucocerebrosidase may come up soon.[37] LRRK2 (leucine-rich repeat kinase 2) regulates the levels of dopamine and presynaptic glutamate release using D2-dependent synaptic plasticity and dopamine-receptor signal transduction.[38] In synucleinopathies, Lewy bodies appear in the locus coeruleus before the appearance of α-synuclein aggregates in the substantia nigra and neurons in the locus coeruleus and substantia nigra pars compacta show both α-synuclein and Tau proteins in progressive supranuclear palsy (PSP) patients. In Alzheimer's disease, there is an abnormally phosphorylated Tau protein in the subcortical nuclei such as the nucleus basalis of Meynert and the locus ceruleus.[36]

Of late, people have been using viral vectors in nonhuman primates to deliver genes to modify basal ganglia circuits. Viral vectors may cause the controlled release of neurotrophic factors, may silence either temporarily or permanently any basal ganglia circuit, may convert existing cells into dopaminergic-like neurons, and may improve levodopa efficacy by targeting aromatic L-amino acid decarboxylase.

The rat striatum expresses angiotensin II type 1 (AT1) receptors, which form heteromers with dopamine D2 receptors. Therefore, AT1 receptor-selective drugs may change the functional response of D2 receptors.[39] In PD-affected rat's striatum, modulating the AMPA receptors, the NMDA receptors along with dopamine, alters neurotransmission and synaptic plasticity, and this throws light on the role of amantadine, which inhibits the NMDA receptors in the treatment of PD.[40-42] Following reward-related learning, scientists have identified long-term depression of glutamatergic synaptic transmission in the dorsal striatum and in the nucleus accumbens.[43] The reward may also induce burst firing of dopaminergic neurons in the caudate nucleus of monkeys.[44]

Exogenous glial cell line-derived neurotrophic factor (GDNF) may require striatal transforming growth factor-β (TGF-β) for neuroprotection against PD.[45] We now know that the striatal microglial activation in a PD model may relate to levodopa-induced dyskinesia and that the activated microglial cells are sensitive to cannabinoids, hence, one may target cannabinoid receptors for treating levodopa-induced dyskinesias.[46] In PD, we see the burst firing of STN neurons and the dopamine D5 receptors may contribute to this firing and may serve as targets of treatment for these patients.[47] One sees the tyrosine hydroxylase enzyme, which converts tyrosine to dopamine, in the amygdala as well as in the striatum and this may explain the behavioral alterations in PD.[48] According to published literature, the neurotransmitter dopamine induces fibroblast growth factor 2 (FGF-2) in the striatal astroglial cells, which also increases the growth of dopaminergic midbrain neurons.[49]

Earlier, traditional wisdom conceptualized a direct pathway and an indirect pathway, depicting connections within the brain starting from the cerebral cortex, involving the basal ganglia and the thalamus, and culminating at the cerebral cortex once again. The direct pathway may on the whole be excitatory to the cerebral cortex and the indirect pathway inhibitory in nature **(Figs. 2 and 3)**.[50] Also, we know that the direct pathway (cortical-putaminal-GP pars interna) transmits information for starting movements and this decreases in PD causing akinesia/bradykinesia.[51] Dopamine depletion may also increase the GP pars externa-STN-GP pars interna (indirect pathway) network. As the drug treatment does not restore this physiology, so motor complications may arise.[52] However, earlier people used to think that these corticostriatal circuits act in parallel, but now we know that there are cross-connections between them. The dorsal and ventral striata do not have opposing actions, but they interact in a way that the body needs for its normal motor functioning. The striatum coordinates learning and memory and it does not merely convert cortical cognitive, motor, or emotional information into actions. Interestingly, glucose-sensitive neurons of the pallidum contain task-related and taste- and smell-responsive units for regulating feeding behavior and the ventral pallidum helps in memory consolidation.[53,54] According to a study, the hippocampal–ventral striatal connections suggest the role of basal ganglia in sleep, the dorsolateral striatum's neural activity changes during habit formation, and the striatum has its own activity of fast-spiking interneurons, which coordinates with that of the cortex.[55] With regard to motor learning, basal ganglia and thalamus may fire almost simultaneously, probably via a common external source and the striatopallidal fibers rather than striatonigral fibers of the

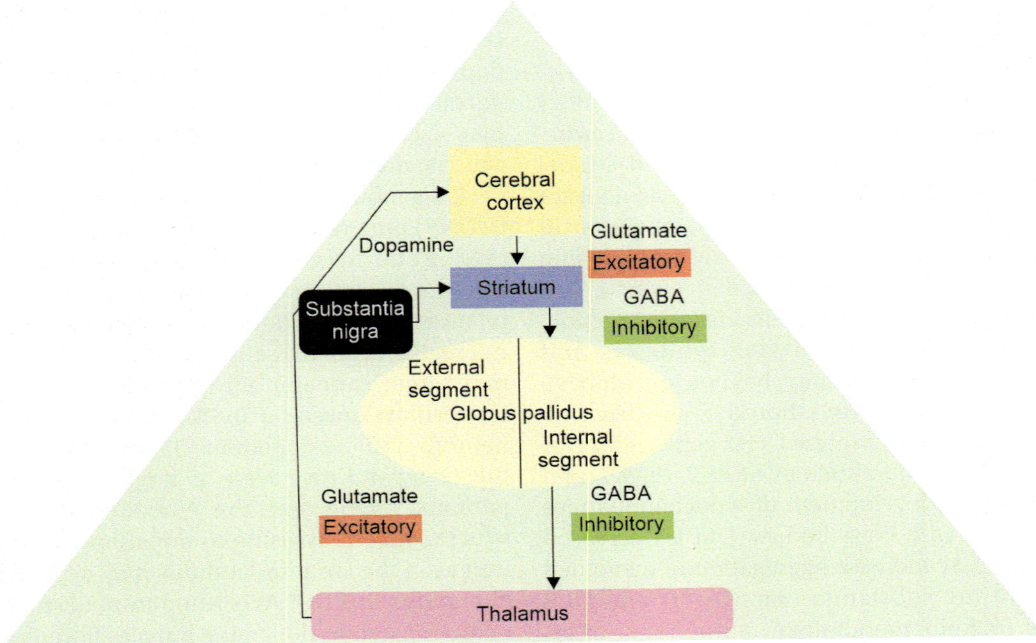

FIG. 2: Direct pathway which is excitatory to the cortex.
(GABA: γ-aminobutyric acid)

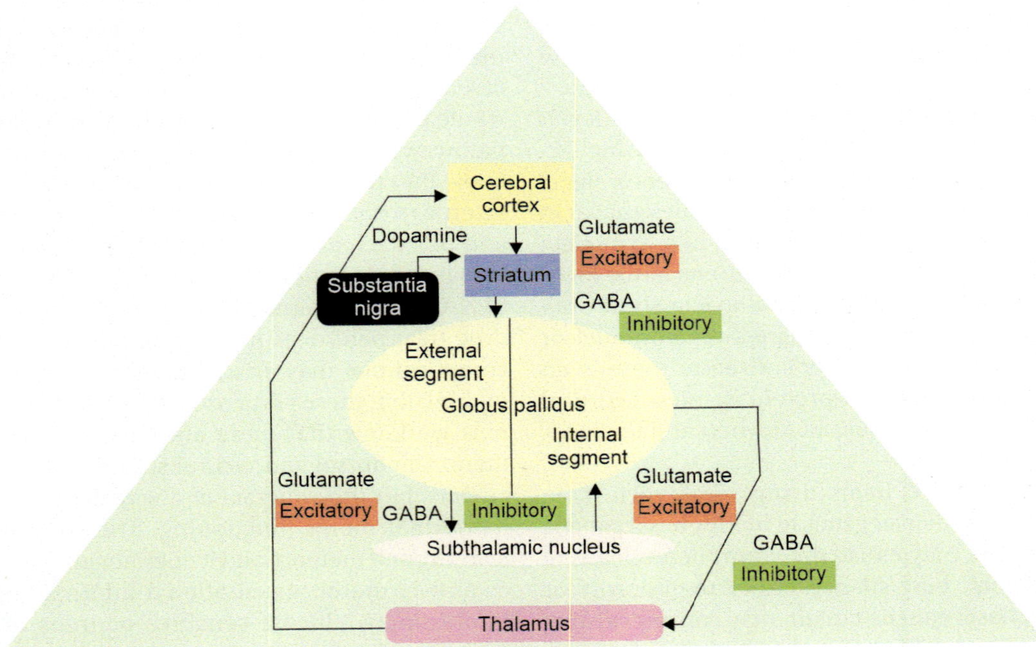

FIG. 3: Indirect pathway which is inhibitory to the cortex.
(GABA: γ-aminobutyric acid)

basal ganglia help in motor learning.[56,57] Also, researchers believe that dopaminergic and cholinergic mechanisms together with taurine transporter and glycine receptors enhance corticostriatal synaptic transmission.[58] β4 subunits of voltage-gated sodium channels in the striatum regulate cell adhesion, migration, and neurite outgrowth in this region.[59]

The success of DBS requires the neurophysiological properties of basal ganglia and other nuclei. Novel DBS pulse generators, using adaptive DBS technology, can record local field potentials (LFPs) generated by the STN. One may observe a decrease in β-band (8–35 Hz) activity by dopaminergic drugs or DBS and this relates to an improvement in akinesia, bradykinesia, and rigidity, but not in tremor. STN-LFP recordings may offer clues about tremors, freezing of gait, and differentiate between speech and movement activities. Surface electromyography (EMG) and wearable sensors can detect tremors, freezing of gait, bradykinesia, and dyskinesias. On/off amplitude modulation systems in akinetic-rigid PD patients stimulate when STN β-LFP exceeds a certain threshold while on/off systems in tremor-dominant PD patients start stimulating several seconds before tremor reoccurs using machine-learning algorithms to predict tremors.[60] While undergoing surgery for DBS, these LFPs may decrease following propofol but not dexmedetomidine (0.2 μg/kg/h). Consequently, dexmedetomidine may be a better choice as an anesthetic agent for DBS procedures.[61] In the past, investigators have observed that parkinsonian rest tremor, arising from the STN, and ventrolateral thalamus may respond to low-frequency stimulation without amplitude modulation but low-frequency thalamic stimulation in essential tremor, with origins in the ventrolateral thalamus, has a narrower frequency–amplitude tolerance and hence needs amplitude modulation.[62] This knowledge facilitates DBS programming in these two disease states. The cortico-subthalamic synchronization in 14–35-Hz oscillations positively correlates with accuracy in lexical decisions in PD patients. Hence, these oscillations affect the nonmotor manifestation of this disease as well.[63] Knowing about and measuring the oscillatory activity of the motor cortex and basal ganglia for motor control and in the diseased state may also help in noninvasive brain stimulation using rTMS and transcranial direct current stimulation (tDCS). Neurostimulation pulses may resemble normal firing patterns or oscillatory activity.[64] The β-band hypersynchronization in the basal ganglia associates with lesser brain flexibility, which in turn may give rise to cognitive impairment in persons suffering from PD.[65] Surprisingly, STN–DBS may even modulate the genes like the major histocompatibility complex (MHC)-related genes, probably reducing the disease progression.[66]

The pedunculopontine tegmental nucleus (PPTg) connects with the main basal ganglia nuclei and transmits basal ganglia activity to thalamic and brainstem nuclei and to the spinal effectors. Cerebellar nuclei also transmit signals from PPTg to thalamic and brainstem nuclei. PPTg, therefore, plays a role in arousal, attention, reward, action selection, and other motor functions. It may transfer glutamatergic monosynaptic input to the dopaminergic neurons of the substantia nigra and in turn mediate excitotoxic degeneration of these neurons. Knowing these actions may lead us to neuroprotective strategies in the management of PD.[67] According to a recent trial, suppression of low β power in the globus pallidus internus (GPi) and a 1–8-Hz modulation in the PPN correlates with gait, with the PPN feature governing the walking speed in human beings. GPi β desynchronization and PPN low-frequency synchronization occur when these people started walking from a resting state.[68] Furthermore, the cortical inputs to the GP and entopeduncular nucleus (EPN) are locally inhibitory and globally excitatory in nature.[69] Employing transcranial magnetic stimulation, researchers demonstrated that cortical disinhibition is an early, may be prodromal feature of PD.[70] Along with cortical disinhibition, the regional functional connectivity of striato-frontal, temporal, occipital, and limbic connections also decreases in PD and affects cognitive pathology progression in these patients.[71]

In adults with ADHD, the bottom-up circuit causes increased emotions in the amygdala and the orbitofrontal cortex also plays a part in regulating these emotions. The vagal nerve also mediates high-frequency heart rate variability with the uncontrolled emotional state in these individuals.[72] Even, Tourette syndrome (TS) may have basal ganglia links, as the abnormalities in the motor and limbic corticobasal ganglia pathways highlight.[73] The presence of micrographia in OCD and irregular handwriting speed in depression also throws light on the role of basal ganglia in the pathophysiology of these disorders.[74,75] Microstimulation and electroconvulsive stimulation of the striatum may help people with psychotic symptoms, proving thereby that their symptoms relate to the striatum.[76]

A study on rodents showed that oxytocin receptors are frequent in the central nucleus of the amygdala, which relates to learning, memory, anxiety, and reinforcing mechanisms and that dopamine reinforces these effects of oxytocin.[77] According to neurophysiology research, serotonin ($5\text{-}HT_{1A}$) receptors in the amygdala control the antiepileptic effects and improve memory following low-frequency stimulation.[78,79] The basal ganglia also relate to the control and propagation of ictal activity.[80] RFRP-1 (RFamide-related peptide-1) and NPFF-1 (neuropeptide FF receptor-1) receptors positively reinforce the reward-based learning mechanisms of the amygdala.[81] As we all are aware, the disorders of basal ganglia may manifest in motor and nonmotor ways and the motor ones may be either hyperkinetic (movement disorders) or hypokinetic (PD). The movement disorders include tremors, chorea, athetosis, ballism, and dystonia (sometimes tics and dyskinesias). Brain circuitry for rhythmic activity involving the primary motor cortex presents as tremors in the nigrostriatal pathway in PD.[82] In EMG, in ballism, one sees regular movements of around 1 Hz with torsion of the proximal part of the limbs, while in chorea, successive involuntary contractions occur at irregular intervals; however, in both chorea and ballism, the single motor contractions are brief, there is an underlying muscular hypotonia and sudden, brief involuntary stoppage of tonic voluntary contraction in the affected muscles.[82] In athetosis and dystonia, as well as in some cases of Huntington's disease, tonic and phasic involuntary contractions take place in both the flexors and extensors simultaneously with normal to hyperactive muscle tone. Experimental damage to the GP results in a correctable flexed posture but damage to both the GP and substantia nigra results in a fixed flexed posture and rigidity results from substantia nigra pathology. On the other hand, dystonia involves the GP more than the substantia nigra. In cerebral palsy, dystonic posture may be due to the striatum pathology and stereotaxic surgery of the GP or thalamus slightly lessens rigidity, without improving voluntary movement. Moreover, in idiopathic torsion dystonia, there is no histopathological change in the neurons or interconnecting fibers in the basal ganglia but functional brain imaging techniques show an increase in metabolic activities in the posterior putamen, GP, cerebellum, and supplementary motor cortex in this variety of dystonia. As such, GPi DBS surgery shows benefits in these persons. Ordinarily, clinicians did not achieve much success in the treatment of freezing of gait and postural abnormalities in PD patients. Nonetheless, utilizing gait analysis proves that freezing of gait in PD may improve by external cues due to a shift in the acting motion center from a center for automatic stepping to that for voluntary stepping and basal ganglia coordinate elementary motor patterns with sensory feedback to produce a purposeful action. The cerebral cortex saves this information for purposeful action beforehand.[82]

CONCLUSION

In this chapter, what we are mentioning is just a glance at the ongoing research on the neurophysiology and anatomy of the basal ganglia and related structures and as the knowledge base on this subject is ever-expanding, we are gaining new insights into the possible applications of this subject on human beings suffering from the dysfunction related to the basal ganglia. Consequently, knowing the neurophysiology and neuroanatomy of a particular individual, for instance, about different brain waves using the approaches described above may soon usher in an era of personalized medicine.

REFERENCES

1. Lanciego JL, Luquin N, Obeso JA. Functional neuroanatomy of the basal ganglia. Cold Spring Harb Perspect Med. 2012;2(12):a009621.
2. Wikimedia Commons. (2020). File:Basal ganglia and related structures (2).svg. [online] Available from https://commons.wikimedia.org/wiki/File:Basal_ganglia_and_related_structures_(2).svg. [Last accessed February, 2023].
3. Pal GK, Pal P, Nanda N. (2017). Limbic System. Comprehensive Textbook of Medical Physiology (Volume 2), 1st edition. [online] Available from https://www.jaypeedigital.com/book/9789386107688/chapter/ch137 [Last accessed February, 2023].
4. Koikkalainen J, Hirvonen J, Nyman M, Lötjönen J, Hietala J, Ruotsalainen U. Shape variability of the human striatum--Effects of age and gender. Neuroimage. 2007;34(1):85-93.
5. Franco R, Casado-Anguera V, Munoz A, Petrovic M, Navarro G, Moreno E, et al. Hints on the Lateralization of Dopamine Binding to D1 Receptors in Rat Striatum. Mol Neurobiol. 2016;53(8):5436-45.
6. Farre D, Munoz A, Moreno E, Reyes-Resina I, Canet-Pons J, Dopeso-Reyes IG, et al. Stronger Dopamine D1 Receptor-Mediated Neurotransmission in Dyskinesia. Mol Neurobiol. 2015;52(3):1408-20.
7. Grimm O, Vollstadt-Klein S, Krebs L, Zink M, Smolka MN. Reduced striatal activation during reward anticipation due to appetite-provoking cues in chronic schizophrenia: a fMRI study. Schizophr Res. 2012;134(2-3):151-7.
8. Hickie I, Lloyd A, Dixon G, Halliday G, McRitchie D, Scott E, et al. Utilising molecular biological and histopathological techniques to study the dopaminergic system in patients with melancholia. Aust N Z J Psychiatry. 1997;31(1):27-35.
9. Alkemade A, de Hollander G, Miletic S, Keuken MC, Balesar R, de Boer O, et al. The functional microscopic neuroanatomy of the human subthalamic nucleus. Brain Struct Funct. 2019;224(9):3213-27.
10. Zakiewicz IM, Majka P, Wojcik DK, Bjaalie JG, Leergaard TB. Three-Dimensional Histology Volume Reconstruction of Axonal Tract Tracing Data: Exploring Topographical Organization in Subcortical Projections from Rat Barrel Cortex. PLoS One. 2015;10(9):e0137571.
11. Hintiryan H, Dong HW. Brain networks of connectionally unique basolateral amygdala cell types. Neurosci Insights. 2022;17:26331055221080175.
12. Bagherzadeh-Azbari S, Khazaie H, Zarei M, Dimigen O, Sommer W. Neuroimaging insights into the link between depression and Insomnia: A systematic review. J Affect Disord. 2019;258:133-43.
13. Chan ST, Tang KW, Lam KC, Chan LK, Mendola JD, Kwong KK. Neuroanatomy of adult strabismus: a voxel-based morphometric analysis of magnetic resonance structural scans. Neuroimage. 2004;22(2):986-94.
14. Castellanos FX, Acosta MT. Neuroanatomia del trastorno por deficit de atencion con hiperactividad [The neuroanatomy of attention deficit/hyperactivity disorder]. Rev Neurol. 2004;38 (Suppl 1):S131-6.
15. Lai MC, Lombardo MV, Ecker C, Chakrabarti B, Suckling J, Bullmore ET, et al. Neuroanatomy of Individual Differences in Language in Adult Males with Autism. Cereb Cortex. 2015;25(10):3613-28.
16. Creyaufmüller M, Heim S, Habel U, Mühlhaus J. The influence of semantic associations on sentence production in schizophrenia: an fMRI study. Eur Arch Psychiatry Clin Neurosci. 2020;270(3):359-72.
17. Lieberman P, Morey A, Hochstadt J, Larson M, Mather S. Mount Everest: a space analogue for speech monitoring of cognitive deficits and stress. Aviat Space Environ Med. 2005;76(6 Suppl):B198-207.
18. Neef NE, Korzeczek A, Primabin A, Wolff von Gudenberg A, Dechent P, Riedel CH, et al. White matter tract strength correlates with therapy outcome in persistent developmental stuttering. Hum Brain Mapp. 2022;43(11):3357-74.
19. Lauer M, Senitz D, Beckmann H. Increased volume of the nucleus accumbens in schizophrenia. J Neural Transm (Vienna). 2001;108(6):645-60.
20. Larsen B, Luna B. In vivo evidence of neurophysiological maturation of the human adolescent striatum. Dev Cogn Neurosci. 2015;12:74-85.
21. Fontes R, Ribeiro J, Gupta DS, Machado D, Lopes-Júnior F, Magalhães F, et al. Time Perception Mechanisms at Central Nervous System. Neurol Int. 2016;8(1):5939.
22. Jones EG. Making brain connections: neuroanatomy and the work of TPS Powell, 1923-1996. Annu Rev Neurosci. 1999;22:49-103.
23. Inzelberg R, Plotnik M, Harpaz NK, Flash T. Micrographia, much beyond the writer's hand. Parkinsonism Relat Disord. 2016;26:1-9.
24. Rektorova I, Mikl M, Barrett J, Marecek R, Rektor I, Paus T. Functional neuroanatomy of vocalization in patients with Parkinson's disease. J Neurol Sci. 2012;313(1-2):7-12.
25. Harris JP, Burrell JC, Struzyna LA, Chen HI, Serruya MD, Wolf JA, et al. Emerging regenerative medicine and tissue engineering strategies for Parkinson's disease. NPJ Parkinsons Dis. 2020;6:4.

26. Mulders AEP, Plantinga BR, Schruers K, Duits A, Janssen MLF, Ackermans L, et al. Deep brain stimulation of the subthalamic nucleus in obsessive-compulsive disorder: Neuroanatomical and pathophysiological considerations. Eur Neuropsychopharmacol. 2016;26(12):1909-19.
27. Hoch MJ, Bruno MT, Faustin A, Cruz N, Mogilner AY, Crandall L, et al. 3T MRI Whole-Brain Microscopy Discrimination of Subcortical Anatomy, Part 2: Basal Forebrain. AJNR Am J Neuroradiol. 2019;40(7):1095-105.
28. Metzger CD, Eckert U, Steiner J, Sartorius A, Buchmann JE, Stadler J, et al. High field FMRI reveals thalamocortical integration of segregated cognitive and emotional processing in mediodorsal and intralaminar thalamic nuclei. Front Neuroanat. 2010;4:138.
29. Mantovani A, Neri F, D'Urso G, Mencarelli L, Tatti E, Momi D, et al. Functional connectivity changes and symptoms improvement after personalized, double-daily dosing, repetitive transcranial magnetic stimulation in obsessive-compulsive disorder: A pilot study. J Psychiatr Res. 2021;136:560-70.
30. Singh S, Misiak M, Beyer C, Arnold S. Brain region specificity of 3-nitropropionic acid-induced vulnerability of neurons involves cytochrome c oxidase. Neurochem Int. 2010;57(3):297-305.
31. Sprenger T, Berthele A, Platzer S, Boecker H, Tölle TR. What to learn from in vivo opioidergic brain imaging? Eur J Pain. 2005;9(2): 117-21.
32. Lianfang H, Ruiliang L, Shouyuan Z, Xuegui Z, Xiaoping P. Possible involvement of opioid peptides of caudate nucleus in acupuncture analgesia. Pain. 1985;23(1):83-93.
33. Nobili F, Campus C, Arnaldi D, De Carli F, Cabassi G, Brugnolo A, et al. Cognitive-nigrostriatal relationships in de novo, drug-naïve Parkinson's disease patients: a [I-123] FP-CIT SPECT study. Mov Disord. 2010;25(1):35-43.
34. Larson SJ, Sances A Jr, Wetzel N. Cerebello-pallido-thalamic connections in man. Appl Neurophysiol. 1982;45(6):549-62.
35. Labandeira-Garcia JL, Rodriguez-Pallares J, Dominguez-Meijide A, Valenzuela R, Villar-Cheda B, Rodríguez-Perez AI. Dopamine-angiotensin interactions in the basal ganglia and their relevance for Parkinson's disease. Mov Disord. 2013;28(10):1337-42.
36. Dopeso-Reyes IG, Sucunza D, Rico AJ, Pignataro D, Marín-Ramos D, Roda E, et al. Glucocerebrosidase expression patterns in the non-human primate brain. Brain Struct Funct. 2018;223(1):343-55.
37. Pignataro D, Sucunza D, Rico AJ, Dopeso-Reyes IG, Roda E, Rodríguez-Perez AI, et al. Gene therapy approaches in the non-human primate model of Parkinson's disease. J Neural Transm (Vienna). 2018;125(3):575-89.
38. Beccano-Kelly DA, Volta M, Munsie LN, Paschall SA, Tatarnikov I, Co K, et al. LRRK2 overexpression alters glutamatergic presynaptic plasticity, striatal dopamine tone, postsynaptic signal transduction, motor activity and memory. Hum Mol Genet. 2015;24(5):1336-49.
39. Martinez-Pinilla E, Rodriguez-Perez AI, Navarro G, Aguinaga D, Moreno E, Lanciego JL, et al. Dopamine D2 and angiotensin II type 1 receptors form functional heteromers in rat striatum. Biochem Pharmacol. 2015;96(2):131-42.
40. Blanpied TA, Clarke RJ, Johnson JW. Amantadine inhibits NMDA receptors by accelerating channel closure during channel block. J Neurosci. 2005;25(13):3312-22.
41. Skiteva O, Yao N, Nouhi M, Chergui K. High frequency stimulation induces LTD of AMPA receptor-mediated postsynaptic responses and LTP of synaptically-evoked firing in the dorsolateral striatum. Neurosci Lett. 2018;666:11-6.
42. Nouhi M, Zhang X, Yao N, Chergui K. CIQ, a positive allosteric modulator of GluN2C/D-containing N-methyl-d-aspartate receptors, rescues striatal synaptic plasticity deficit in a mouse model of Parkinson's disease. CNS Neurosci Ther. 2018;24(2):144-53.
43. Zhang X, Yao N, Chergui K. The GABAA receptor agonist muscimol induces an age- and region-dependent form of long-term depression in the mouse striatum. Learn Mem. 2016;23(9):479-85.
44. Yoshimi K, Naya Y, Mitani N, Kato T, Inoue M, Natori S, et al. Phasic reward responses in the monkey striatum as detected by voltammetry with diamond microelectrodes. Neurosci Res. 2011;71(1):49-62.
45. Schober A, Peterziel H, von Bartheld CS, Simon H, Krieglstein K, Unsicker K. GDNF applied to the MPTP-lesioned nigrostriatal system requires TGF-beta for its neuroprotective action. Neurobiol Dis. 2007;25(2):378-91.
46. Navarro G, Borroto-Escuela D, Angelats E, Etayo Í, Reyes-Resina I, Pulido-Salgado M, et al. Receptor-heteromer mediated regulation of endocannabinoid signaling in activated microglia. Role of CB1 and CB2 receptors and relevance for Alzheimer's disease and levodopa-induced dyskinesia. Brain Behav Immun. 2018;67: 139-51.
47. Chetrit J, Taupignon A, Froux L, Morin S, Bouali-Benazzouz R, Naudet F, et al. Inhibiting subthalamic D5 receptor constitutive activity alleviates abnormal electrical activity and reverses motor impairment in a rat model of Parkinson's disease. J Neurosci. 2013;33(37):14840-9.
48. von Bohlen und Halbach O, Schober A, Hertel R, Unsicker K. MPTP treatment impairs tyrosine hydroxylase immunopositive fibers not only in the striatum, but also in the amygdala. Neurodegener Dis. 2005;2(1):44-8.
49. Reuss B, Unsicker K. Survival and differentiation of dopaminergic mesencephalic neurons are promoted by dopamine-mediated induction of FGF-2 in striatal astroglial cells. Mol Cell Neurosci. 2000;16(6):781-92.
50. Henley C. Basal Ganglia. Foundations of Neuroscience. [online] Available from https://openbooks.lib.msu.edu/neuroscience/chapter/basal-ganglia/. [Last accessed February, 2023].
51. Chiken S, Takada M, Nambu A. Altered dynamic information flow through the cortico-basal ganglia pathways mediates Parkinson's disease symptoms. Cereb Cortex. 2021;31(12):5363-80.
52. Obeso JA, Marin C, Rodriguez-Oroz C, Blesa J, Benitez-Temiño B, Mena-Segovia J, et al. The basal ganglia in Parkinson's disease: current concepts and unexplained observations. Ann Neurol. 2008;64(Suppl 2):S30-46.
53. Peczely L, Ollmann T, Laszlo K, Kovács A, Gálosi R, Szabó A, et al. Effects of ventral pallidal D1 dopamine receptor activation on memory consolidation in morris water maze test. Behav Brain Res. 2014;274:211-8.
54. Karadi Z, Faludi B, Lenard L, Czurkó A, Niedetzky C, Vida I, et al. Glucose-sensitive neurons of the globus pallidus: II. Complex functional attributes. Brain Res Bull. 1995;37(2):157-62.
55. Pennartz CM, Berke JD, Graybiel AM, Ito R, Lansink CS, van der Meer M, et al. Corticostriatal interactions during learning, memory processing, and decision making. J Neurosci. 2009;29(41):12831-8.
56. Schwab BC, Kase D, Zimnik A, Rosenbaum R, Codianni MG, Rubin JE, et al. Neural activity during a simple reaching task in macaques is counter to gating and rebound in basal ganglia-thalamic communication. PLoS Biol. 2020;18(10):e3000829.
57. Ena SL, De Backer JF, Schiffmann SN, de Kerchove d'Exaerde A. FACS array profiling identifies Ecto-5' nucleotidase as a striatopallidal neuron-specific gene involved in striatal-dependent learning. J Neurosci. 2013;33(20):8794-809.
58. Chepkova AN, Sergeeva OA, Haas HL. Long-lasting enhancement of corticostriatal transmission by taurine: role of dopamine and acetylcholine. Cell Mol Neurobiol. 2005;25(3-4):767-76.
59. Miyazaki H, Oyama F, Inoue R, Aosaki T, Abe T, Kiyonari H, et al. Singular localization of sodium channel β4 subunit in unmyelinated fibres and its role in the striatum. Nat Commun. 2014;5:5525.
60. Habets JGV, Heijmans M, Kuijf ML, Janssen MLF, Temel Y, Kubben PL. An update on adaptive deep brain stimulation in Parkinson's disease. Mov Disord. 2018;33(12):1834-43.
61. Martinez-Simon A, Alegre M, Honorato-Cia C, Nuñez-Cordoba JM, Cacho-Asenjo E, Trocóniz IF, et al. Effect of Dexmedetomidine

and Propofol on Basal Ganglia Activity in Parkinson Disease: A Controlled Clinical Trial. Anesthesiology. 2017;126(6):1033-42.
62. Cagnan H, Little S, Foltynie T, Limousin P, Zrinzo L, Hariz M, et al. The nature of tremor circuits in parkinsonian and essential tremor. Brain. 2014;137(Pt 12):3223-34.
63. Hohlefeld FU, Ewald A, Ehlen F, Tiedt HO, Horn A, Kühn AA, et al. Neural correlates of lexical decisions in Parkinson's disease revealed with multivariate extraction of cortico-subthalamic interactions. Clin Neurophysiol. 2017;128(4):538-48.
64. Benninger DH. Parkinson's disease. Handb Clin Neurol. 2013;116: 469-83.
65. Sorrentino P, Rucco R, Baselice F, De Micco R, Tessitore A, Hillebrand A, et al. Flexible brain dynamics underpins complex behaviours as observed in Parkinson's disease. Sci Rep. 2021;11(1):4051.
66. Grieb B, Engler G, Sharott A, von Nicolai C, Streichert T, Papageorgiou I, et al. High-frequency stimulation of the subthalamic nucleus counteracts cortical expression of major histocompatibility complex genes in a rat model of Parkinson's disease. PLoS One. 2014;9(3):e91663.
67. Vitale F, Capozzo A, Mazzone P, Scarnati E. Neurophysiology of the pedunculopontine tegmental nucleus. Neurobiol Dis. 2019;128: 19-30.
68. Molina R, Hass CJ, Sowalsky K, Schmitt AC, Opri E, Roper JA, et al. Neurophysiological correlates of gait in the human basal ganglia and the PPN region in Parkinson's disease. Front Hum Neurosci. 2020;14:194.
69. Ozaki M, Sano H, Sato S, Ogura M, Mushiake H, Chiken S, et al. Optogenetic activation of the sensorimotor cortex reveals "local inhibitory and global excitatory" inputs to the basal ganglia. Cereb Cortex. 2017;27(12):5716-26.
70. Ammann C, Dileone M, Pagge C, Catanzaro V, Mata-Marín D, Hernández-Fernández F, et al. Cortical disinhibition in Parkinson's disease. Brain. 2020;143(11):3408-21.
71. De Micco R, Agosta F, Basaia S, Siciliano M, Cividini C, Tedeschi G, et al. Functional connectomics and disease progression in drug-naïve Parkinson's disease patients. Mov Disord. 2021;36(7): 1603-16.
72. Christiansen H, Hirsch O, Albrecht B, Chavanon ML. Attention-deficit/hyperactivity disorder (ADHD) and emotion regulation over the life span. Curr Psychiatry Rep. 2019;21(3):17.
73. Israelashvili M, Loewenstern Y, Bar-Gad I. Abnormal neuronal activity in Tourette syndrome and its modulation using deep brain stimulation. J Neurophysiol. 2015;114(1):6-20.
74. Mavrogiorgou P, Mergl R, Tigges P, El Husseini J, Schröter A, Juckel G, et al. Kinematic analysis of handwriting movements in patients with obsessive-compulsive disorder. J Neurol Neurosurg Psychiatry. 2001;70(5):605-12.
75. Mergl R, Juckel G, Rihl J, Henkel V, Karner M, Tigges P, et al. Kinematical analysis of handwriting movements in depressed patients. Acta Psychiatr Scand. 2004;109(5):383-91.
76. Pavlasek J, Masanova C, Haburcak M, Murgas K. Catecholamine overflow within rat striatum: the influence of microstimulation and electroconvulsive stimulation as observed with voltammetry. Exp Physiol. 1994;79(3):327-35.
77. Laszlo K, Peczely L, Geczi F, Kovács A, Zagoracz O, Ollmann T, et al. The role of D2 dopamine receptors in oxytocin induced place preference and anxiolytic effect. Horm Behav. 2020;124:104777.
78. Gharib A, Sayyahi Z, Komaki A, Barkley V, Sarihi A, Mirnajafi-Zadeh J. The role of 5-HT1A receptors of hippocampal CA1 region in anticonvulsant effects of low-frequency stimulation in amygdala kindled rats. Physiol Behav. 2018;196:119-25.
79. Gharib A, Komaki A, Manoochehri Khoshinani H, Saidijam M, Barkley V, Sarihi A, et al. Intrahippocampal 5-HT1A receptor antagonist inhibits the improving effect of low-frequency stimulation on memory impairment in kindled rats. Brain Res Bull. 2019;148:109-17.
80. Vuong J, Devergnas A. The role of the basal ganglia in the control of seizure. J Neural Transm (Vienna). 2018;125(3):531-45.
81. Lenard L, Kovács A, Ollmann T, Péczely L, Zagoracz O, Gálosi R, et al. Positive reinforcing effects of RFamide-related peptide-1 in the rat central nucleus of amygdala. Behav Brain Res. 2014;275: 101-6.
82. Yanagisawa N. Functions and dysfunctions of the basal ganglia in humans. Proc Jpn Acad Ser B Phys Biol Sci. 2018;94(7):275-304.

14

CHAPTER

Applied Neuroanatomy and Neurophysiology of the Eye Movements

Sujit Kumar, Aastha Takkar, Padma Youron

INTRODUCTION

In order to maintain a single binocular vision, the image of objects must fall on both foveae simultaneously. This requires, apart from a properly functioning afferent visual apparatus, extraocular muscles and their corresponding nerve supply (IIIrd, IVth, and VIth), an intact supranuclear apparatus. Abnormalities in this axis, which range from higher cortical centers to gaze centers in the brainstem, result in gaze disturbances with intact vestibulo-ocular reflex (VOR). In contrast, lesions in the nuclear and infranuclear pathways result in gaze palsies that are not overcome by VOR. This chapter focuses on the basic anatomy and physiology of ocular motility, along with a brief description of gaze disturbances.

SUPRANUCLEAR PATHWAYS AND EYE MOVEMENTS

There are several types of supranuclear ocular movements such as:

- Saccades
- Pursuits
- Vestibulo-ocular reflex
- Optokinetic nystagmus (OKN)
- Vergence
- Fixation

Saccades

They are fast eye refixation movements, which serve to change fixation from one target to another. They are fast movements and, once initiated, cannot be aborted. If the visual target moves during a saccade, then the eyes must complete the saccade and then refixate on the new location. Saccadic eye movements can reach velocities of as much as 700° per second. There are four major types of saccadic eye movements:[1,2]

1. *Reflexive*: They are visual or auditory stimulus guided (externally triggered). The rapid conjugate eye movement that occurs in response to a loud sound or a visual target is an example.
2. *Volitional*: These are visual and memory-guided (internally triggered); such as when searching for an object.
3. *Spontaneous*: These occur throughout the day such as scanning of an individual's surroundings. They are present even during sleep.
4. *Anti-saccades*: This is a type of volitional saccade in which gaze is voluntarily directed away from an object.

Saccades can be assessed by asking the subject to make eye movements from the primary position to an eccentric target and back again. While assessing saccades, the following points are to be noted:[3]

- *The primary position*: It is important to note any saccadic intrusions.
- Whether the initiation of the saccade is prompt or delayed.
- *Conjugacy and range*: If any limitation is noted in range of motion, it is important to do VOR.
- Whether the speed of the saccade is slow or rapid.
- Whether the saccade is hypo- or hypermetric.

Important higher cortical centers for both horizontal and vertical saccades include:[4,5] Frontal eye field (FEF), which initiates command for volitional saccades along with controlling amplitude of all types of saccades; parietal eye field (PEF), which initiates command for reflexive saccades; prefrontal cortex including dorsolateral prefrontal cortex (DLPFC) that is involved in planning of volitional saccades along with inhibition of unwanted saccades.

The higher cortical centers are connected to each other and ultimately the FEF sends impulses to either the horizontal gaze center in pons—the pontine paramedian reticular formation (PPRF) or the vertical gaze center in midbrain—the midbrain paramedian reticular formation (MPRF). These impulses are sent both directly from the cortex and indirectly via the basal ganglia, cerebellum, and superior colliculus.

The eyes move together as a unit. It is the brainstem integrator which sends impulses to the extraocular nerve nuclei to move the corresponding muscles of both eyes, to function as a "yoked pair." For instance, equal impulses are sent to the lateral rectus of one eye and the medial rectus (MR) of the other eye, so as to make the eyes move in a coordinated pattern, in one direction. The vertical eye movements are a little more complex, as the direction of the eye along the horizontal axis determines which muscles are stimulated.

The PPRF is located ventral to the VIth nerve nucleus in the pons, and is responsible for horizontal conjugate eye movements, through its projections within the medial longitudinal fasciculus (MLF), to the contralateral IIIrd nerve nucleus.

The MPRF, which is the corresponding center for vertical eye movements, is located in the tectum of the midbrain and the pretectum, just rostral to the beginning of the midbrain. It includes the nucleus of Darkshevich, the rostral interstitial nucleus of the medial longitudinal fasciculus (riMLF), interstitial nucleus of Cajal (INC), and the nucleus raphe interpositus.

The medullary paramedian reticular formation (MRF) and the nucleus prepositus hypoglossi (PPH), adjacent to the vestibular nuclei and caudal to the abducens nucleus, may integrate visual and vestibular inputs and project the information to PPRF/MPRF centers for initiation and maintenance of saccades.

The Role of Basal Ganglia in Saccades

The substantia nigra usually tonically inhibits the superior colliculus, thereby preventing unwanted saccades. On receiving commands from FEF, the caudate nucleus causes inhibition of the substantia nigra, thereby releasing the superior colliculus from tonic inhibition, so that saccades can be generated.[6]

The Role of Cerebellum in Saccades

The flocculonodular lobe and the vermis are the main integrators in the cerebellum for eye movements. These phylogenetically old and midline centers receive retinal input and respond to visual tracking. They project to the brainstem integrator and help stability of fixation and coordination of VOR. It also plays a role in saccadic movement accuracy.[2]

The Center for Horizontal Saccades

The PPRF has two population of cells: Excitatory burst neurons (EBNs) and inhibitory burst neurons (IBNs). EBNs generate the final command—the burst of tonic discharge (also known as pulse command) for gaze initiation that is transmitted to the ipsilateral VIth nerve nucleus, resulting in an ipsilateral saccade. IBNs lie caudally and send axons inhibiting the contralateral VIth nerve nucleus, during the ipsilateral saccades.

Omnipause neurons (OPNs) tonically inhibit the burst neurons till a saccade command is generated. Generation of a saccade command by FEF results in inhibition of OPNs both directly and indirectly via the superior colliculus, thereby releasing the burst neurons. In order to maintain gaze in this new position, once a saccade is generated, tonic discharge (also known as step command) is required so that eyes do not deviate back to the primary position. This mathematical integration to convert the velocity-coded information to position-coded information is carried on by the neural integrators (NIs). NIs for horizontal saccades are the MRF and PPH **(Figs. 1 to 3)**.[2,5]

The Center for Vertical Saccades

The MPRF in the midbrain includes burst neurons, OPNs, and the NI. The riMLF contains the burst neurons for vertical gaze. EBNs for upward gaze project to bilateral elevators, superior rectus (SR), and inferior oblique (IO). EBNs for downward gaze project to ipsilateral depressors, inferior rectus (IR), and superior oblique (SO). OPNs are constituted by the nucleus raphe interpositus. The NI is formed by the

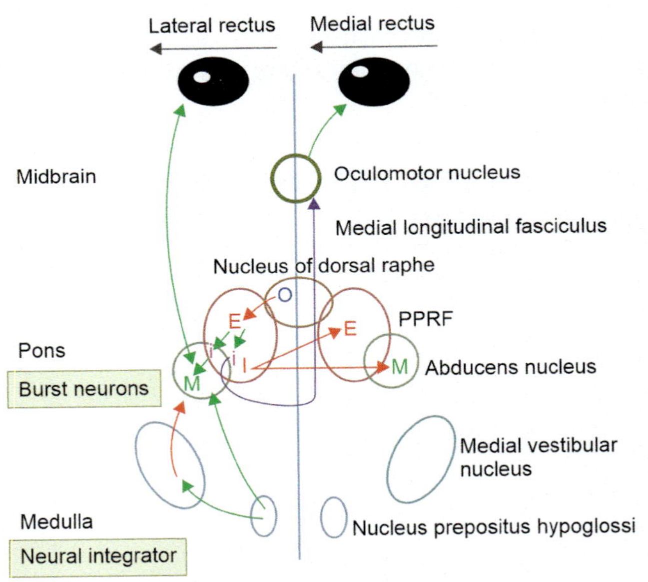

FIG. 1: Horizontal saccade pathway: Excitatory burst neurons (EBN: E) generates the final command which stimulates the motor neurons of the abducens nuclei ipsilaterally and oculomotor neurons contralaterally (through) the medial longitudinal fasciculus. The activity and discharge of the EBN and the motor neurons are also controlled by the omnipause neurons, nucleus prepositus hypoglossi and the medial vestibular nucleus.

(E: excitatory burst neurons; I: inhibitory burst neurons; O: omnipause neurons; M: motor neurons; i: interneurons; PPRF: pontine paramedian reticular formation)

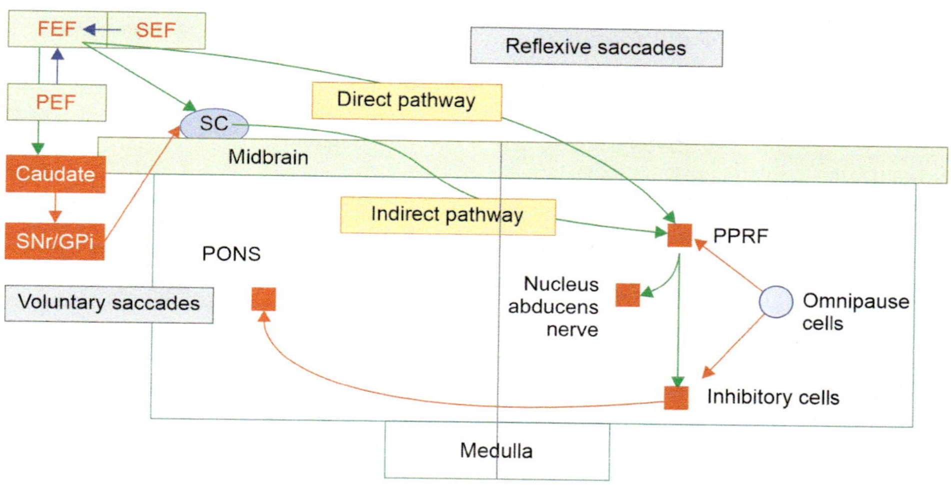

FIG. 2: Direct and indirect pathway of reflexive and voluntary saccades.
(FEF: frontal eye fields; PEF: parietal eye field; PPRF: pontine paramedian reticular formation; SEF: supplementary eye field)

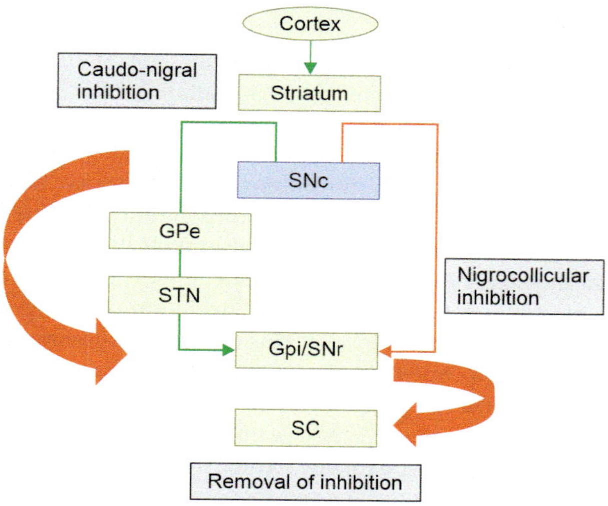

FIG. 3: The removal of the tonic inhibition of superior colliculus allows the generation of saccades.

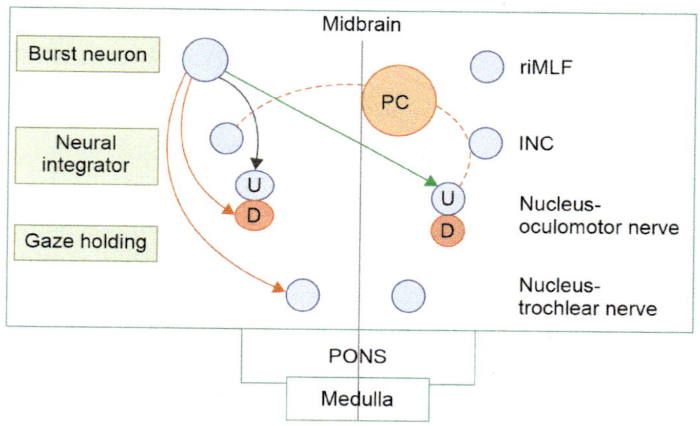

FIG. 4: Vertical saccades.
(PC: posterior commissure; U: elevators; D depressors; INC: interstitial nucleus of Cajal; riMLF: rostral interstitial nucleus of medial longitudinal fasciculus)

INC. Fibers from the INC travel posteriorly and cross the midline in the posterior commissure, to ultimately control contralateral elevators and depressors. However, fibers for upward gaze are located more posteriorly in the posterior commissure. Thus, any dorsal midbrain lesion will first result in upward gaze restriction **(Fig. 4)**.

Overview of Pathology of Saccades[7]

Impairment of saccades can be seen in disorders involving different structures **(Table 1)**.

TABLE 1: Pathology of saccades.

Structure	Saccadic abnormality
FEF/PEF/superior colliculus	Impaired saccadic latency and amplitude
Flocculonodular nucleus and dorsal vermis	Impaired accuracy (hypo- and hypermetric saccades)
Basal ganglia	Impaired volitional saccades
Omnipause neurons	Ocular flutter and opsoclonus
PPRF	Slow horizontal saccades
MPRF	Slow vertical saccades

(FEF: frontal eye field; MPRF: midbrain paramedian reticular formation; PEF: parietal eye field; PPRF: pontine paramedian reticular formation)

Saccadic intrusions: Spontaneous eye movements. with initial rapid movement (as against the initial slow drift in nystagmus) disrupting the fixation, characterize a saccadic intrusion. Square wave jerks and macrosaccadic oscillations are saccadic intrusions with intersaccadic interval, whereas ocular flutter and opsoclonus are saccadic intrusions without an intersaccadic interval. Ocular flutter constitutes involuntary back-to-back saccades, in the horizontal plane, as against opsoclonus which has been described as multidirectional, irregular, conjugate, chaotic, and partially continuous rapid eye movements.

Apart from these, there are other periodic ocular deviations that are usually seen in non-/semiresponsive

TABLE 2: Periodic ocular deviations in semi-/unresponsive patients.

Type of movement	Direction of movement	Site of lesion/etiology
Ocular bobbing	Downward fast/ slow upward	Pons, posterior fossa lesions
Reverse bobbing	Upward fast/slow downward	Pons, metabolic encephalopathy
Ocular dipping	Downward slow/ fast upward	Pons, hypoxic encephalopathy
Reverse ocular dipping	Upward slow/ downward rapid	Metabolic encephalopathy/ viral encephalitis
V pretectal pseudo bobbing	V pattern down-ward movement	Obstructive hydrocephalus

patients, where the initial movement can be either slow or fast. Ocular bobbing is a distinctive eye movement disorder, characterized by abnormal spontaneous vertical eye movements, which have an abrupt, spontaneous rapid downward jerky component, followed by a slow upward return. **Table 2** shows various other periodic ocular deviations.

Pursuits

These are smooth, slow, tracking conjugate eye movements to maintain fixation of a target on the fovea. Vestibular input helps to maintain the slow movement, fixing on the target, when the target is moving. Compared to saccades, the pathways of pursuit movements are less well known.[5]

Higher cortical centers include:
- *FEF*: Which generates volitional pursuit
- *Parieto-temporo-occipital cortex (PTO)*: Which generates reflexive pursuit

From the FEF and PTO, impulses are sent directly to the ipsilateral dorsolateral pontine nucleus (DLPN), the center for the pursuit eye movements. From the DLPN, impulses are sent to the contralateral vestibular nucleus (VN) and cerebellum (vermis and flocculus), which in turn sends impulses to the contralateral VIth nerve nucleus. Due to this double decussation, cortical centers control ipsilateral pursuit movements **(Fig. 5)**.

Vertical pursuits are similar to horizontal pursuit pathways. Upward pursuit pathways decussate in the posterior commissure, while downward pursuit pathways decussate anterior to the aqueduct of Sylvius. Therefore, in dorsal midbrain lesions downward pursuit movements may be spared, with restricted upward pursuit, along with impaired upward and downward saccades, as previously mentioned.[1,8]

Vestibulo-ocular Reflex

Three semicircular canals (anterior, posterior, and horizontal) send impulses to the ipsilateral VN, to ensure foveation during accelerating and decelerating head movements.

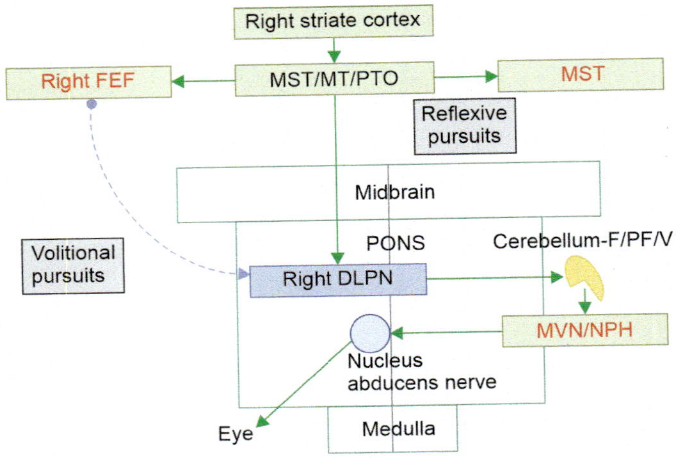

FIG. 5: The horizontal pursuit pathway.

(FEF: frontal eye field; MST: medial superior temporal lobe; MT: middle temporal lobe; PTO: parieto-temporo-occipital cortex; DLPN: dorsolateral pontine nuclei; F: flocculus, PF: paraflocculus; V: vermis; MVN: medial vestibular nucleus; NPH: nucleus prepositus hypoglossi)

During a horizontal head movement, for instance, a horizontal semicircular canal is stimulated, which sends impulses to the ipsilateral VN and then to the contralateral VIth nerve nucleus, resulting in a horizontal gaze opposite to the direction of head movement.[5,9] This pathway passes through the MLF. There is also a multisynaptic pathway via the reticular formation to the pontine and midbrain centers.

In the cold caloric test, when cold water is injected into the external ear, it results in a slow deviation of the eyes to the same side as the injection. This is, however, followed by a corrective saccade (fast component) that brings the eyes back to the primary position, indicating intact VOR on that side. If no corrective saccade occurs, it indicates a lesion anywhere in the VOR pathway.[7] Thus, in comatose patients, the fast corrective saccade is not seen and if the brainstem is intact, a slow deviation is seen.

Optokinetic Nystagmus

When a series of moving targets are presented to an individual in one direction, there is a slow pursuit movement following the target to the point where the eyes are deviated to their maximum degree, followed by a corrective saccadic movement. Unlike pursuit movements, it requires full visual field stimulation by the moving object. Although higher cortical centers are not delineated, OKN is defective in parieto-occipital lesions. In any patient with suspected functional visual loss, the presence of OKN implies intact afferent visual function.[10]

During an optokinetic stimulation, if the lights are turned off, the nystagmus persists for a short time. This is called optokinetic after nystagmus (OKAN).

Vergence

These are disconjugate eye movements to maintain the foveation of objects moving along the depth axis of the visual field. They include convergence and divergence. They are believed to arise from the occipital cortex, which sends projections to the dorsal midbrain and from there to the ipsilateral ocular motor neurons.

Fixation

It is a mechanism to prevent fading of the fixed image. Higher cortical centers include FEF, supplementary eye field (SEF), DLPFC, and parietal cortex which send impulses to the substantia nigra. This, in turn, tonically inhibits the rostral superior colliculus, till a saccade command is generated by FEF. Also, OPNs tonically inhibit PPRF and MPRF, so that during fixation, no eye movements occur.

INTERNUCLEAR PATHWAYS

The VIth nerve nucleus in the pons contains two groups of neurons: Motor neurons that supply the ipsilateral lateral rectus and interneurons that cross the midline as the MLF, which ascends to the IIIrd nerve MR subnucleus, to supply the contralateral MR **(Fig. 6)**.

Lesion of the MLF results in ipsilateral internuclear ophthalmoplegia (INO). A lesion of the right MLF results in impaired adduction of the right MR during left horizontal gaze, resulting in left adducting nystagmus. However during convergence, the right MR adducts normally, indicating an intact right MR nucleus and nerve.[11]

Lesions of bilateral MLF result in wall-eyed bilateral INO (WEBINO); impaired adduction in both directions of horizontal gaze with adducting nystagmus. VOR is, however, intact.[12]

Lesions of the ipsilateral MLF extending to the VIth nerve nucleus result in one-and-a-half syndrome. In lesions of the right VIth nerve nucleus (damage to both motor and interneurons) with right MLF, apart from the impaired

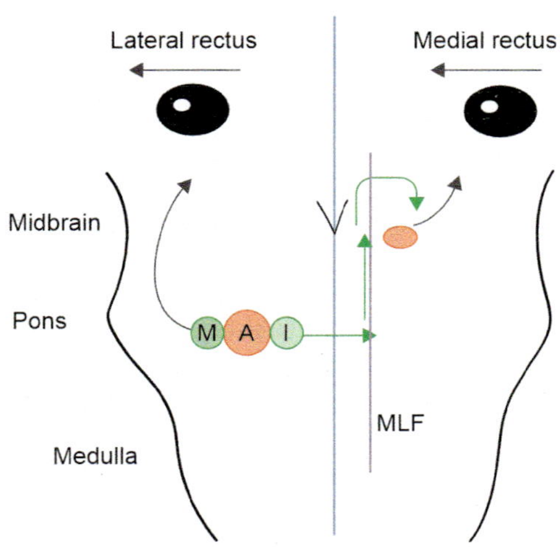

FIG. 6: The final common pathway of gaze.
(A: abducens nucleus; M: motor neurons; I: interneurons; MLF: medial longitudinal fasciculus)

TABLE 3: Internuclear syndromes of ocular motility.

Internuclear syndromes of ocular motility	Structures involved
One-and-a-half syndrome	Ipsilateral MLF, VIth nerve nucleus
Eight-and-a-half syndrome	Ipsilateral VIIth nerve nucleus + one-and-a-half syndrome
Nine syndrome	Eight-and-a-half syndrome + ipsilateral medial lemniscus and corticospinal tract
Thirteen syndrome	Eight-and-a-half syndrome + ipsilateral Vth nerve paresis
Fifteen-and-a-half syndrome	One-and-a-half syndrome + bilateral facial nerve paresis
Sixteen-and-a-half syndrome	Eight-and-a-half syndrome + ipsilateral facial and corticospinal tract

adduction of right MR with left eye adducting nystagmus on left horizontal gaze, the patient is unable to look to the right. Therefore, the only horizontal eye movement the patient can do is left eye abduction.[11]

In the eight-and-a-half syndrome, apart from the structures involved in one-and-a-half syndrome, the VIIth nerve is also affected as it winds around the VIth nerve nucleus, resulting in ipsilateral VIIth nerve lower motor neuron palsy **(Table 3)**.[13]

NUCLEAR AND INFRANUCLEAR PATHWAYS

IIIrd Nerve

The IIIrd nerve nucleus is a pear-shaped structure, present in the periaqueductal gray matter of the rostral midbrain. It is further divided into following subnuclei—the SR subnucleus supplies the contralateral SR muscle, the decussation occurring at the nuclear level. The IR, MR, and IO subnuclei supply the ipsilateral muscles. A single midline subnucleus supplies the bilateral levator palpebrae superioris (LPS). A large midline Edinger–Westphal nucleus provides parasympathetic innervation to bilateral iris sphincter and ciliary muscles.

The IIIrd nerve fascicle emerges and travels ventrally in the midbrain close to the crus cerebri, from where it enters the interpeduncular fossa, between the midbrain and pons. It then passes beneath the posterior cerebral artery and then lateral to the posterior communicating artery (PCOM). It passes between the tentorial edge and lateral aspect of the posterior clinoid process, to pierce the dura and enter the cavernous sinus. It then passes through the superior orbital fissure to divide into a superior division which supplies the SR and LPS muscles and an inferior division which supplies the MR, IR, and IO muscles. The parasympathetic fibers travel with the inferior division and supply the ciliary ganglion, ciliary body, and pupillary sphincter muscle. Third nerve fibers are arranged such that—the parasympathetic fibers are dorsomedially wrapped—around the fibers supplying the EOMs.[5,14]

Nuclear lesions result in bilateral SR palsy along with bilateral ptosis, due to bilateral LPS involvement and ipsilateral palsy of other muscles supplied by IIIrd nerve. Involvement of IIIrd nerve fascicle, before its exit from the midbrain, results in ipsilateral IIIrd nerve palsy along with the involvement of other midbrain structures resulting in many named syndromes:

- *Claude syndrome (IIIrd and superior cerebellar peduncle)*: Ipsilateral IIIrd nerve palsy with contralateral ataxia
- *Benedikt syndrome (IIIrd and red nucleus)*: Ipsilateral IIIrd nerve palsy with contralateral chorea.
- *Weber syndrome (IIIrd and cerebral peduncle)*: Ipsilateral IIIrd with contralateral hemiparesis.

In the subarachnoid space, due to arrangement of the nerve fibers, the superficially located parasympathetic fibers are more likely to be affected by compressive etiologies: PCOM aneurysm with clinical presentation, as headache and anisocoria with spared extraocular movements (EOMs). However, EOMs may be affected along with pupillary involvement, in aneurysmal compression as well. Conversely, in microangiopathies like diabetes mellitus, pupils may be spared due to the involvement of vasa nervorum and more tenuous blood supply of the deeper fibers.

Due to proximity to the medial temporal lobe, uncal herniation due to raised intracranial pressure (ICP) results in ipsilateral IIIrd nerve compression manifested in early stages by poorly reactive ipsilateral pupillary constriction, due to nerve fiber irritation. As compression increases, ipsilateral pupillary dilatation sets in (Hutchison's pupil). Further compression then involves the contralateral IIIrd nerve in the same manner.

In the cavernous sinus, the IIIrd nerve is affected along with other contents of the cavernous sinus: IVth nerve, VIth nerve, and V1, V2 distribution of Vth nerve, internal carotid artery (ICA) and sympathetic plexus. The cavernous sinus is further divided into anterior, middle, and posterior segments (Jefferson or Ishikawa classification). Malignancies including metastasis involve predominantly the posterior segment, while vascular etiologies, like ICA aneurysm, involve the middle segment, and infections, especially fungal ones, involve the anterior segment. Depending upon the structures involved, neurological deficits that can be seen involve contralateral hemiparesis due to ICA involvement, anisocoria due to the involvement of sympathetic plexus, parasympathetic fibers present in IIIrd nerve, ptosis, ophthalmoplegia (due to the involvement of III, IV, and VI), and impaired sensation in ipsilateral V1/V2 distribution.[15] An important point to note is that—vision loss is not usually seen in cavernous sinus pathologies, as the IInd nerve is not a content. However, ICA involvement can lead to sudden onset ipsilateral vision loss, owing to a vascular event, secondary to impaired blood supply via the ophthalmic artery.

In the orbital apex, divisional palsy may be seen. Apart from the IIIrd to VIth nerves along with IInd nerve involvement are seen. Due to the involvement of draining ophthalmic veins, chemosis, lid edema, and proptosis are common associated features.[15]

After an injury to the IIIrd nerve (usually compressive), frequently, aberrant innervation occurs, resulting in a variable combination of signs: Upper eyelid elevation on attempted downgaze (pseudo-Von Graefe phenomenon), pupillary constriction with adduction, and others.

IVth Nerve

The IVth nerve nucleus lies in the periaqueductal gray matter of the midbrain, at the level of the inferior colliculi, caudal to and continuous with the oculomotor nucleus. The fascicles emerge from the nucleus, curve around the Sylvian aqueduct, decussate within the anterior medullary velum, and then travel dorsally. This is the only cranial nerve to leave the midbrain from its dorsal aspect. It then turns around to travel ventrally in the subarachnoid space, between the posterior cerebral and superior cerebellar arteries to reach the cavernous sinus. It then enters the superior orbital fissure to supply the SO, which is contralateral to the nucleus of origin.[14]

Superior oblique causes intorsion and depression in the adducted position. Therefore, palsy results in hypertropia in the affected eye, with vertical or oblique diplopia, when the eye is depressed and adducted—such as during reading and descending stairs. To compensate for this, a person with SO palsy tilts the head in the opposite direction, as it results in extorsion of the affected eye and resolution of diplopia.

Nuclear lesions in isolation are rare and usually are associated with other long-tract signs. They result in contralateral SO palsy. They usually occur in tumors, multiple sclerosis, and vascular malformations. Fascicular lesions also occur in tumors, vascular malformations, and demyelinating lesions.

In the subarachnoid space, cavernous sinus, and orbital apex, it is usually affected in combination with other cranial nerves such as the third and fifth.[14]

VIth Nerve

The VIth nerve nucleus lies in the caudal paramedian pontine tegmentum, on the floor of the fourth ventricle, medial to the vestibular nuclei. It passes ventrally and exits from the lower pons. It then rises over the ventral pons, being crossed by the anterior inferior cerebellar artery. It then passes through the clival dura, beneath the petroclinoid ligament (Gruber's ligament), and then over the petrous tip of the temporal bone, underneath the petrosphenoid ligament (Dorello's canal). It then passes through the cavernous sinus and supplies the lateral rectus muscle.

Lesions involving the VIth nerve nucleus produce ipsilateral conjugate gaze paresis, owing to its connection through the MLF to the contralateral IIIrd nerve nucleus. Bilateral lesions of the VIth nerve nucleus produce complete bilateral conjugate gaze palsy. Owing to the proximity of the VIIth nerve looping fibers, very often the VIIth nerve is also involved.

Fascicular lesions are caused by ischemia, tumors, infection, and demyelination. The following syndromes have been described:

- *Foville syndrome*: Horizontal conjugate gaze palsy, ipsilateral deafness, ipsilateral Horner's syndrome, ipsilateral Vth and VIIth nerve palsies
- *Millard-Gubler syndrome*: Ipsilateral VIth and VIIth nerve palsies and contralateral hemiparesis
- *Raymond's syndrome*: Ipsilateral VIth and contralateral hemiparesis

The subarachnoid space syndrome can occur due to stretching of the VIth nerve, secondary to raised ICP.

Gradenigo syndrome with ipsilateral VIth and VIIth nerve paresis with ipsilateral deafness can occur with mastoiditis and inflammation of the adjacent meninges of the petrous bone.

Further, the VIth nerve can be involved with the Vth, IVth, and IIIrd nerves in the cavernous sinus and superior orbital fissure syndromes.

CONCLUSION

Every area of the brain is related to some aspects of ocular motility control. Understanding the pathways helps in localization and diagnosis at the early stages of the disease process. In general, supranuclear pathway lesions result in conjugate eye movement abnormalities, while intranuclear pathway lesions result in ipsilesional eye movement abnormalities. As a general rule, VOR is intact in supranuclear disorders, while it is impaired in infranuclear lesions.

REFERENCES

1. Bender MB. Brain control of conjugate horizontal and vertical eye movements. Brain. 1980;103(1):23-69.
2. Sparks DL. The brainstem control of saccadic eye movements. Nat Rev Neurosci. 2002;3(12):952-64.
3. Kennard C. Disorders of higher gaze control. In: Kennard C, Leigh RJ (Eds). Handbook of Clinical Neurology, 1st edition, Volume 102. Amsterdam: Elsevier B.V.; 2011. pp. 379-402.
4. Pierrot-Deseilligny C, Müri RM, Ploner CJ, Gaymard B, Rivaud-Péchoux S. Cortical control of ocular saccades in humans: A model for motricity. Prog Brain Res. 2003;142:3-17.
5. Vinny PW, Lal V. Gaze disorders: A clinical approach. Neurol India. 2016;64(1):121-8.
6. Lal V, Truong D. Eye movement abnormalities in movement disorders. Clin Park Relat Disord. 2019;1:54-63.
7. Strupp M, Kremmyda O, Adamczyk C, Böttcher N, Muth C, Yip CW, et al. Central ocular motor disorders, including gaze palsy and nystagmus. J Neurol. 2014;261:S542-58.
8. Mehta S, Takkar A, Ray S, Lal V. Ophthalmological findings in movement disorders. Ann Mov Disord. 2021;4(1):10-20.
9. Termsarasab P, Thammongkolchai T, Rucker JC, Frucht SJ. The diagnostic value of saccades in movement disorder patients: a practical guide and review. J Clin Mov Disord. 2015;2(1): 1-10.
10. Papanagnu E, Brodsky MC. Is there a role for optokinetic nystagmus testing in contemporary orthoptic practice? Old tricks and new perspectives. Am Orthopt J. 2014;64(1):1-10.
11. Menon V, Gogoi M, Saxena R, Singh S, Kumar A. Isolated "One and a half syndrome" with brainstem tuberculoma. Indian J Pediatr. 2004;71(5):469-71.
12. Chakravarthi S, Kesav P, Khurana D. Wall-eyed bilateral inter nuclear ophthalmoplegia with vertical gaze palsy. QJM. 2014;107(2): 165.
13. Nandhagopal R, Krishnamoorthy SG. Eight-and-a-half syndrome. J Neurol Neurosurg Psychiatry. 2006;77(4):463.
14. Brazis PW, Masdeu JC, Biller J. Localisation in Clinical Neurology, 8th edition. Riverwoods, IL: Wolters Kluwer Health/Lippincott Williams & Wilkins; 2020. pp. 261.
15. Bhatkar S, Goyal MK, Takkar A, Modi M, Mukherjee KK, Singh P, et al. Which classification of cavernous sinus syndrome is better - Ishikawa or Jefferson? A prospective study of 73 patients. J Neurosci Rural Pract. 2016;7(5):S68-71.

15
CHAPTER

Applied Neuroanatomy and Neurophysiology of the Brainstem

Birinder Singh Paul, Dhananjay Gupta, Gagandeep Singh

INTRODUCTION

The brainstem is a small stalk-like structure that connects the cerebrum with the spinal cord. It is composed of three distinct parts: (1) midbrain (mesencephalon), (2) pons (metencephalon), and (3) medulla oblongata (myelencephalon) **(Fig. 1)**, and it has a critical role in controlling vital functions of the body, such as swallowing, breathing, and vasomotor tone. All cranial nerve nuclei, except those associated with olfaction and vision, are located in the brainstem, providing motor and sensory supply to structures of the cranium, including the facial muscles, tongue, pharynx, larynx, as well as supplying the senses of taste, equilibrium, and hearing. The brainstem also has nuclei important for autonomic functions. All efferent and afferent pathways between the cerebrum and cerebellum course through the brainstem, and many of them decussate, or cross, within.[1]

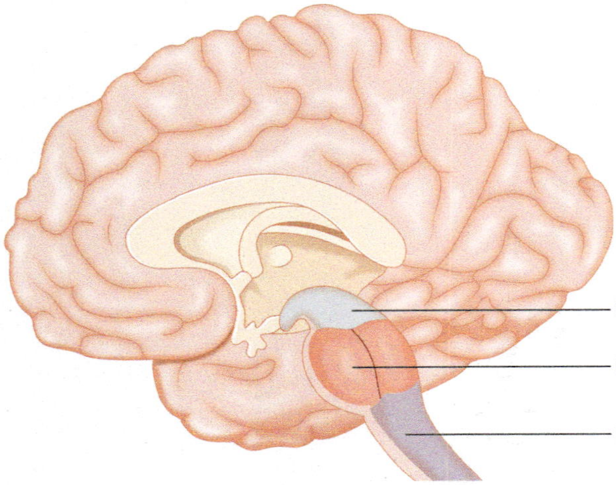

FIG. 1: The three parts of brainstem are depicted in this sagittal view.

MIDBRAIN

The midbrain (mesencephalon) is the most superior and the smallest. The rostral boundary of the midbrain is formed by the superior colliculi and the caudal boundary is marked by a plane caudal to inferior colliculi. Midbrain may be divided into dorsal tectum (containing colliculi), central tegmentum, and ventral cerebral peduncles. The corpora quadrigemina are made up of four rounded eminences arranged in pairs, the superior and the inferior colliculi. The superior quadrigeminal brachium forms a pathway between the superior colliculus and the retina and the inferior quadrigeminal brachium conveys fibers from the lateral lemniscus and inferior colliculus to the medial geniculate body. The tegmentum contains ascending and descending tracts along with reticular nuclei. The paired cerebral peduncles are white matter structures separated anteriorly in the midline by the interpeduncular fossa. The peduncles contain white matter tracts including frontopontine fibers in their medial fifth, corticospinal tract in the middle three fifth and temporopontine fibers in their lateral fifth. There is a somatotopic arrangement of corticospinal fibers within the peduncles as arm fibers are placed medially, leg fibers laterally with trunk fibers in-between. The decussation of the superior cerebellar peduncles can be seen centrally at the level of the inferior colliculus.[1,2]

The substantia nigra—a pigmented nucleus that separates the two regions of the cerebral peduncles—is posteriorly placed. It is divided into—the pars reticulata (anterior) and pars compacta (posterior).

There are two main cranial nerve nuclei present in the midbrain **(Figs. 2A and B)**. The oculomotor nerve nucleus lies rostral to the trochlear nucleus beneath the superior colliculus (CN III) and the nerve exits between the peduncles. The trochlear nucleus is located in the ventral part of the central gray matter at the level of the inferior colliculus. Inferiorly, the trochlear nerve (CN IV) emerges

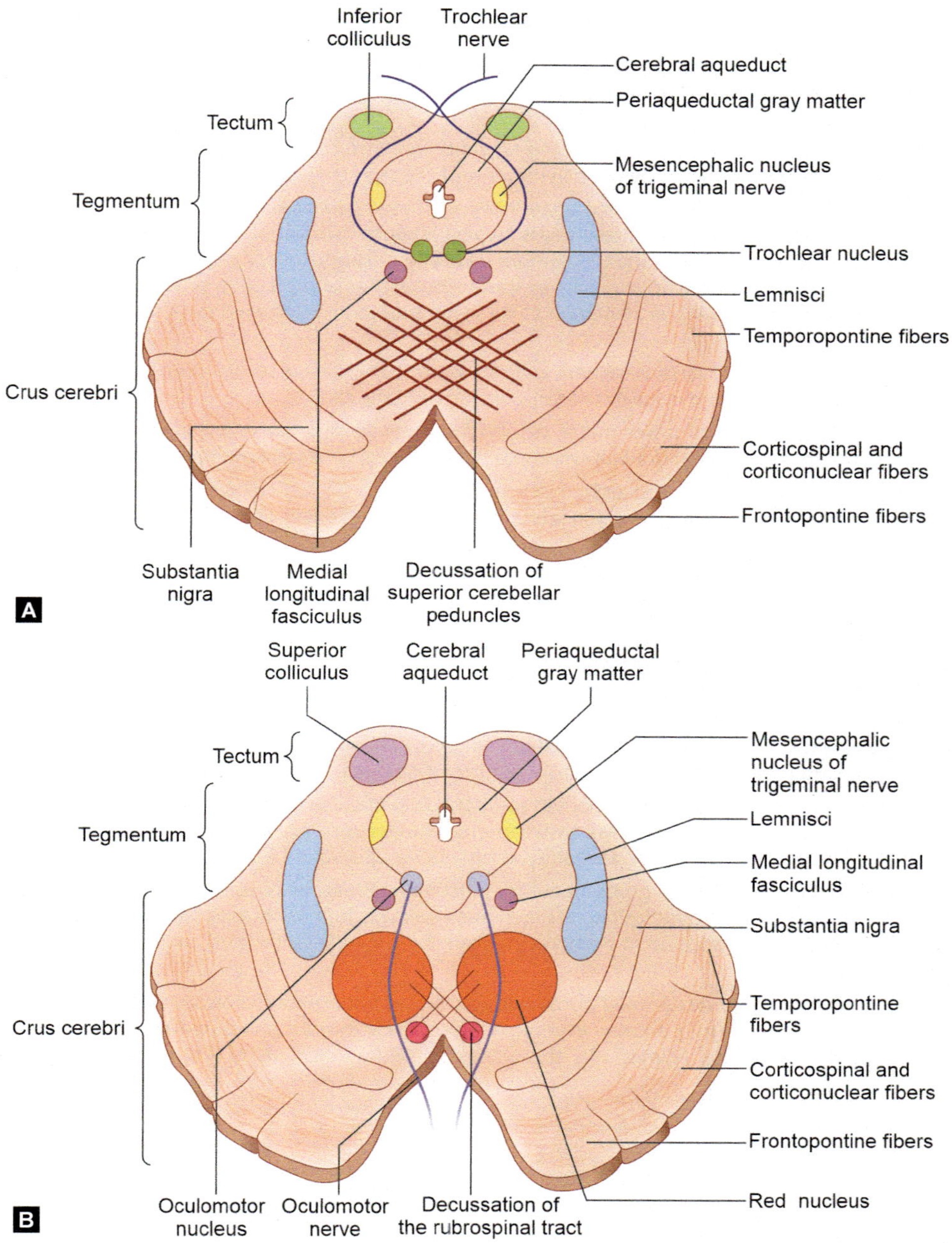

FIGS. 2A AND B: (A) Cross-section of midbrain at level of the inferior colliculi. (B) Cross-section of midbrain at level of the superior colliculus.

from the dorsal surface at this level before sweeping across to the anterior surface.

The cerebral aqueduct is a midline structure surrounded by central gray matter and the periaqueductal gray matter. Within this gray matter lies the mesencephalic nucleus of the trigeminal nerve, as well as the trochlear nucleus with its fibers continuing around the gray matter to exit from the midbrain. The medial longitudinal fasciculus (MLF) is also located in the midline anteriorly. Other mesencephalic tracts present include—the medial, spinal and trigeminal lemniscus, MLF, medial tegmental tract, and the dentatorubrothalamic tract descending and ascending in the midbrain **(Box 1)**.[2,3]

Vascular Supply

The midbrain receives vascular supply from the basilar artery and its branches, i.e., circumferential and paramedian arteries. The circumferential arteries include the posterior cerebral artery (PCA), superior cerebellar artery (SCA), and posterior choroidal artery. These predominantly supply cerebral peduncles and the two colliculi in the mesencephalon.

Thalamoperforating and peduncular arteries are paramedian arteries that originate from the PCA itself and supply the thalamus and other midline structures located in the midbrain, respectively **(Fig. 3)**.[3]

BOX 1 "Halves" and other numerical neuro-ophthalmic brainstem syndromes.[14,15]

- *Internuclear ophthalmoplegia (INO)*: This unique and characteristic syndrome occurs due to involvement of the medial longitudinal fasciculus (MLF) secondary to a small dorsal brainstem infarction. Isolated INO presents as impaired adduction of the ipsilateral eye with nystagmus in the contralateral abducting eye
- *WEBINO*: Wall-eyed bilateral INO is a rare neuro-ophthalmological condition characterized by bilateral adduction impairment, abduction nystagmus, and primary exotropia and has been described in mesencephalic tegmental strokes and multiple sclerosis
- *One-and-a-half syndrome*: Combination of ipsilateral conjugate horizontal gaze paresis and ipsilateral INO leads to this horizontal ocular movement disorder. The only horizontal movement preserved is the abduction in the contralateral eye, which is associated with nystagmus The usual cause is a lesion in the paramedian pontine tegmentum involving the abducens nucleus, the MLF, and the parapontine reticular formation (PPRF). One-and-a-half syndrome was originally proposed by Fischer and recently many additions have been made to the spectrum of "one-and-a-half syndrome". Careful examination of these mathematical numbered syndromes helps in precise localization of these lesions
- *Seven-and-a-half syndrome*: Combination of facial weakness and INO leads to the clinical seven-and-a-half syndrome (VII + INO = 7.5). The lesion is localized to the paramedian pons and involves the facial nucleus and the MLF
- *Eight-and-a-half syndrome*: A combination of lower motor neuron fascicular facial palsy (VII) and one-and-a-half syndrome leads to a constellation of symptoms described as eight-and-a-half syndrome (VII + 1.5 = 8.5). It is localized to the dorsal tegmentum of the lower pons
- *Nine syndrome*: Additional contralateral hemiparesis or hemisensory loss (0.5) to the ipsilateral facial palsy, horizontal gaze palsy, and INO leads to the recently described "nine" syndrome. The lesion is localized to the paramedian and dorsal pontine tegmentum
- *Thirteen-and-a-half syndrome*: Dorsal pontine tegmental lesions involving the fifth and seventh cranial nerve nuclei can lead to a combination of ipsilateral trigeminal palsy and eight-and-a-half syndrome (5 + VII + INO = 13.5). The patient can complain of hemifacial pain, numbness, or can have objective sensory loss over the face along with corneal erosions and ulcers. Very few case reports exist in literature and have been attributed to pontine mass lesions like cavernomas and lymphomas
- *Fifteen-and-a-half syndrome*: Bilateral pontine tegmental lesions can damage the bilateral abducens nuclei, bilateral facial nuclei, and the MLF. This leads to bilateral horizontal gaze restriction, INO, and bilateral facial weakness and has been described as fifteen-and-a-half syndrome (VII + 1.5 + VII = 15.5). The limited case reports of this rare entity have been described with bilateral tegmental infarctions
- *Sixteen syndrome*: The most recent addition to the list is the sixteen syndrome characterized by one-and-a-half syndrome, bilateral peripheral facial palsy, and contralateral hemiparesis (1.5 + VII + VII + 0.5 = 16), occurring due to bilateral paramedian pontine infarction
- *Sixteen-and-a-half syndrome*: Involvement of the lateral pons in addition to paramedian tegmentum can lead to additional hearing loss in the ipsilateral ear due to damage to the auditory nerve. This constellation of one-ana-a-half syndrome with ipsilateral peripheral facial weakness and auditory involvement is referred to as sixteen-and-a-half syndrome (1.5 + VII + VIII = 16.5)
- *Twenty-and-a-half syndrome*: Involvement of the pontomedullary junction, medulla, or cerebellar peduncles along with paramedian and lateral pons can lead to one-and-a-half syndrome, ipsilateral trigeminal weakness, hemifacial anesthesia, and bifacial weakness with bilateral absent corneal reflexes. This combination adds up to twenty-and-a-half (1.5 + V + VII + VII = 20.5) and has been described with small-vessel ischemic disease of the brainstem
- *Twenty-four-and-a-half syndrome*: Sometimes a small pontine lesion causes widespread clinical deficits due to the perilesional edema and mass effect. This was described in right pontine cavernoma which leads to right one-and-a-half syndrome, right facial weakness, bilateral hearing loss, and left hemiataxia. Numerically this was described as the twenty-four-and-a-half syndrome (1.5 + VII + VIII + VIII = 24.5)

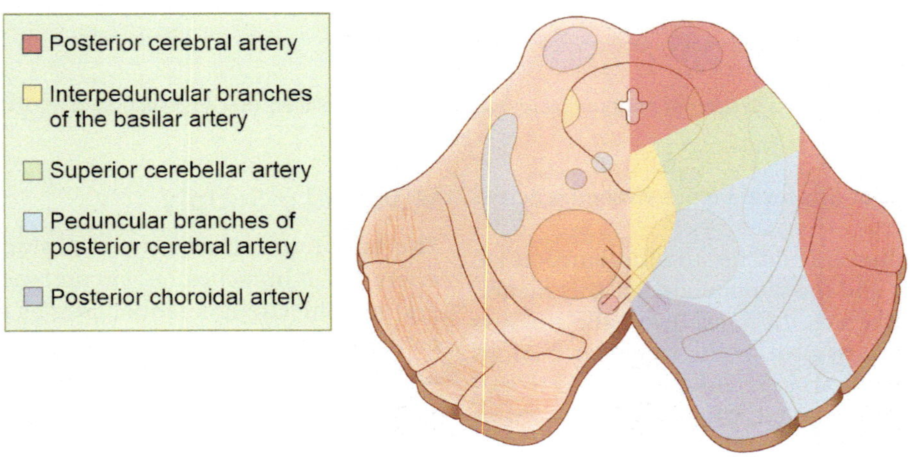

FIG. 3: Vascular supply of the midbrain.

Midbrain Syndromes

Depending on the blood supply, the midbrain is divided into the following regions: the anteromedian region supplied by the PCA, the anterolateral midbrain region supplied by the PCA and the anterior choroidal artery, the lateral midbrain region along with superior cerebellar peduncles supplied by the cerebellar arteries, choroidal artery and the collicular artery, and the posterior midbrain supplied by the SCA along with posterior choroidal artery **(Box 1)**.[4,5]

Anteromedian (Paramedian) Midbrain Syndromes

This is the most common pattern of midbrain ischemia, commonly seen in up to 50% of midbrain strokes. The lesion involves the midbrain tegmentum, comprising the third (or fourth) cranial nerves along with corticospinal tracts, MLF, red nucleus, and substantia nigra. As sensory tracts are located in the dorsolateral midbrain, sensory affection is uncommon with paramedian syndromes. Eponymous paramedian midbrains syndromes include:

- *Weber syndrome*: Weber syndrome clinically presents with an incomplete ipsilateral oculomotor nerve palsy (ptosis with ophthalmoplegia) and contralateral hemiparesis or -plegia due to involvement of the corticospinal tracts. The usual cause is occlusion of paramedian perforators of the basilar artery or the PCAs.
- *Claude syndrome*: This is characterized by dorsomedian midbrain infarction and presents with ipsilateral oculomotor palsy with contralateral hemiataxia due to the involvement of the superior cerebellar peduncle and cerebello-rubrthalamic tracts at or near the red nucleus. As there is sparing of the crus cerebri, there is minimal weakness, but predominant ataxia.
- *Benedikt syndrome*: This is another paramedian syndrome that involves the midbrain tegmentum and occurs due to the involvement of branches of the PCAs. It clinically presents with fascicular oculomotor involvement with contralateral hemiparesis, hemiataxia with or without Holmes tremor and choreoathetosis. The hemichorea (or ballismus) occurs due to the involvement of the subthalamic nucleus.
- *Holmes (Rubral tremor)*: Holmes tremor is classically seen in Benedikt syndrome and is attributed to the affection of the rubrothalamic tracts and the red nucleus. It is characterized by intentional, postural, as well as action tremors. It is usually a subacute to chronic presentation, developing weeks to months after a midbrain stroke.
- *Lilliputian peduncular hallucinations*: Lesions of the thalamus or midbrain may cause very vivid, colorful visual hallucinations of objects and people, often of "lilliputian" sizes. They occur more during evening and night and are thought to be due to the involvement of the pars reticulata of the substantia nigra.

Anterolateral Midbrain Syndromes

Anterolateral syndromes are less common (20–30%) and present with predominant crus cerebri involvement. They can present with ataxic hemiparesis, clumsy hand syndrome, or dysarthria-clumsy hand syndrome and spare the cranial nerves.

Dorsal Midbrain Syndrome (Parinaud or Sylvian Aqueduct or Pretectal Syndrome)

Compression of the tectum of the midbrain at the level of superior colliculus presents with a triad of upward gaze palsy, light-near dissociation, and convergence-retraction nystagmus. The usual cause of this presentation is a structural lesion causing a mass effect on the dorsal midbrain, near the posterior commissure or the pineal region. The anatomical substrate of upward gaze restriction is the vertical gaze center [rostral interstitial nucleus of medial longitudinal fasciculus (riMLF) and the interstitial nucleus of Cajal (INC) and its connections]. riMLF is responsible for vertical saccades and INC controls vertical eye movements and skew deviations. Unilateral involvement causes upward gaze restriction and bilateral involvement leads to downgaze restriction; hence, downgaze is preserved till the late stages. Light-near pupillary dissociation is caused by damage to the pretectal and the Edinger-Westphal nuclei. Damage to midbrain supranuclear fibers causes convergence-retraction nystagmus and Collier's sign (bilateral lid retraction).

Nothnagel Syndrome

Nothnagel syndrome is a very rare entity, characterized by oculomotor palsy along with cerebellar ataxia, and results from the involvement of the midbrain tectum (quadrigeminal plate) with extension into the superior cerebellar peduncles. It should be emphasized that the involvement of the superior cerebellar peduncle causes ataxia ipsilateral to the oculomotor weakness and differentiates this from Claude syndrome, which causes contralateral hemiataxia.

Top of Basilar Syndrome (Tip of Basilar Syndrome or Rostral Brainstem Infarction)

Thromboembolic occlusion of the distal basilar artery leads to infarction of the bilateral thalami and midbrain. This clinically presents as alternating disorientation, drowsiness, unresponsive, hallucinations, behavioral abnormalities, and alternating disorientation.

Artery of Percheron Syndrome

This is a rare anatomical variant in which a single perforator supplied the bilateral thalami. Occlusion of artery of Percheron (AOP) leads to bilateral paramedian thalamic infarctions with or without midbrain involvement.

PONS

Surface Anatomy

Pons is the largest part of the brainstem. "Pons" in Latin means *bridge* and here it functions as a connecting link between the cerebrum and cerebellum. It is a horseshoe-shaped structure located in the anterior part of the posterior cranial fossa. Anatomically, it is related to the cerebellum posteriorly separated by the fourth ventricle, medulla oblongata lying inferiorly, and the midbrain superiorly. The basilar artery is present in the midline on the ventral surface in the basilar groove in the pons **(Figs. 4A and B)**. The pontomedullary junction is an important anatomical landmark defined by the angle between the lower border of the pons and the superior border of the medulla. Another important anatomical landmark, relevant for intracranial growth, is the cerebellopontine angle formed at the junction of the pons, medulla, and cerebellum. At this angle, the cerebellar flocculus, the ventricular choroid plexus, and the emerging cranial nerves—VII and VIII surround the lateral apertures of the fourth ventricle (the foramen of Luschka).

Internal Anatomy

The pons is comprised of two major components—the ventral *basis pontis* and the dorsal portion, referred as the *tegmentum*. The *basis pontis* mainly contains the pontine nuclei and multidirectional nerve fiber bundles, which are responsible for coordinating movement. Transverse pontocerebellar fibers from the pontine nuclei cross the midline on the ventral surface and form the middle cerebellar peduncles on their way to the cerebellum. The other tracts passing through the pons include descending corticospinal tracts (motor control of the body), descending corticobulbar tracts (subserving motor control of face, head, and neck), and ascending spinothalamic tracts (subserving pain and temperature sensation). MLF, the white matter tract connecting the third nerve nucleus with the opposite sixth nerve nucleus, is situated dorsomedially. The ascending medial lemniscus tract that transmits fine touch, vibration, and proprioception lies dorsal to the corticospinal tract at the level of pons. The pons also has the lateral lemniscus conveying auditory impulses along with the nucleus of the lateral lemniscus, trapezoid body, and superior olivary complex, completing the auditory pathway.[5]

The tegmentum is the older part of the pons that is composed of the reticular formation, a set of nuclei found throughout the brainstem rostrally, continuing with the medullary reticular formation. This reticular core is divided into a medial large group of neurons called the magnocellular region and lateral parvocellular region that are responsible for arousal and attentiveness.

The pons comprises several important cranial nerve nuclei originating from the ventral surface. The main sensory and the motor nuclei of the trigeminal nerve are located at the level of mid-pons, and the fibers originate from the lateral aspect of the pons. The main sensory nucleus receives somatosensory information from the face. The other important nuclei located in the pons include the cochlear nucleus and the lateral and superior vestibular nuclei.

The sixth cranial nerve, abducens, originates from the pontomedullary junction, close to the midline. Ventromedian to the abducens nucleus is the paramedian pontine reticular formation (PPRF) that plays an important role in the control of horizontal saccadic eye movements. The motor nucleus of the facial nerve (CN VII) is situated ventrolaterally. Fibers from this nucleus transverse dorsomedially toward the floor of the fourth ventricle, make a sharp bend around the

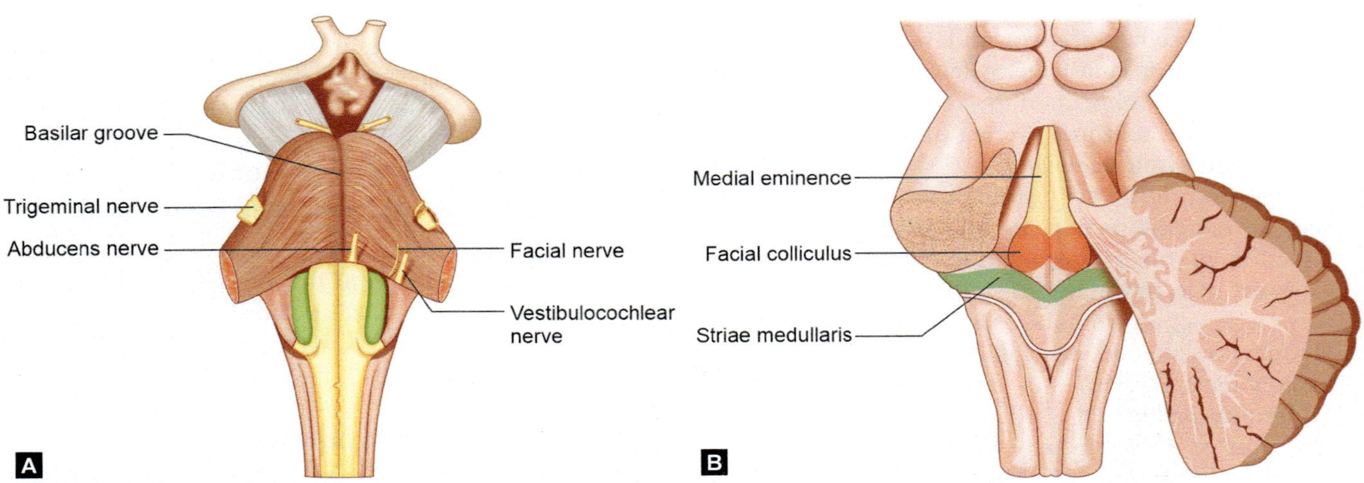

FIGS. 4A AND B: (A) Ventral (anterior) surface anatomy of the pons. (B) Dorsal (posterior) surface anatomy of the pons.

abducens nucleus (facial colliculus), and then turn laterally through the pons to exit lateral to fibers of the abducens nerve. Lastly, vestibulocochlear nerve (CN VIII) originates lateral to the facial nerve. The cochlear and vestibular nuclei are located dorsolaterally in the inferior pons.

Vascular Supply

The blood supply of the pons is mainly from the branches of the vertebrobasilar system. These branches can be broadly classified into three groups—(1) long circumferential arteries, (2) paramedian, and (3) short circumferential arteries. The long circumferential arteries arise from the basilar artery or its branches and are responsible for the vascularity of most of the pons.

- The superior cerebellar artery supplies dorsolateral pons, basis pontis, dorsal reticular formation, and periaqueductal area in the pons.
- The anterior inferior cerebellar artery (AICA) supplies the lateral tegmentum of the lower two-thirds of the pons and ventrolateral cerebellum.
- The internal auditory artery branch of the anterior inferior artery or occasionally from the basilar artery supplies the auditory, vestibular, and facial cranial nerves.

There are four to six paramedian vessels that also arise from the basilar artery and supply medial basal pons, pontine nuclei, pyramidal tracts, and medial lemniscus.

The short circumferential arteries also arise from the basilar artery and supply the ventrolateral part of basis pontis.

Venous drainage of the pons mainly consists of the anterior pontomesencephalic vein, which drains superiorly into the basal vein, which in turn drains into the cerebral veins. Inferiorly, the pons drains into the inferior petrosal sinus, which drains into the internal jugular vein.

Pontine Syndromes

The pons is supplied by the perforators from the basilar artery along with medial branches of the SCA and the AICAs. Depending on the arteries, it is divided into anteromedian pons (supplied by basilar artery perforators), anterolateral pons (supplied by the AICA), and the lateral pons (supplied by the lateral pontine perforators, SCA, and the AICA).[4,5]

Unilateral Anteromedian and Paramedian Pontine Syndromes

The pontine affection may involve only the basal region, only the tegmental region or a combined basal-tegmental region. The basal region (basis pontis) contains the corticospinal and corticobulbar motor fibers. Conversely, the tegmental region contains the medial lemniscus resulting in hemisensory syndromes and the cranial nerve nuclei **(Box 1)**.

- *Basal pons infarctions*: Can cause pure motor weakness or ataxic hemiparesis.
- *Raymond syndrome (crossed abducens hemiplegia)*: This anteromedian pontine syndrome presents with ipsilateral abducens palsy (lateral gaze weakness) along with a contralateral facial weakness and hemiparesis (or hemiplegia). The difference with Foville syndrome is that there is no ipsilateral facial weakness.
- *Millard-Gubler syndrome (ventral pontine syndrome)*: This is one of the classical and common brainstem crossed syndromes causing ipsilateral facial weakness with a contralateral hemiparesis (or plegia). Although the original descriptions of Auguste Millard and Adolphe Gubler did not include abducens palsy, subsequent reports have reported ipsilateral abducens palsy also in Millard-Gubler syndrome.
- *Foville syndrome (inferior medial pontine syndrome)*: Foville syndrome presents with ipsilateral abducens and facial palsy, conjugate gaze palsy (VI and VII nerve nuclei) along with contralateral hemiparesis (corticospinal involvement), and hemisensory loss (medial lemniscus involvement). The common etiology is occlusion of the pontine perforators causing infarction of the pontine tegmentum.
- *Facial colliculus syndrome*: Lesions of the pontine tegmentum near the facial colliculus may lead to a constellation of abducens nerve palsy, nuclear or lower motor neuron type facial weakness, diplopia, conjugate gaze paresis, and internuclear ophthalmoplegia (due to impairment of the MLF). There is a loss of taste sensation and hyperacusis as the facial nerve involvement occurs proximal to the geniculate ganglion.

Bilateral Pontine Syndromes

Locked-in syndrome: Bilateral ventral pontine affection causes a characteristic and devastating neurological condition mimicking a coma. It leads to bilateral abducens palsy, loss of horizontal eye movements, bifacial weakness, bulbar palsy, dysphagia, dysarthria, quadriplegia, and whole-body sensory loss. Pathological crying or laughter may be seen in less severe cases. Cognition, hearing, and vertical eye movements along with blinking are classically preserved. Hence, the patient can only communicate via blinking or vertical ocular movements. Ocular bobbing with sudden downward and slow upward movements is an ominous sign of extensive pontine infarction.

Central Pontine Myelinolysis (Osmotic Demyelination Syndrome)

This is a rare syndrome that occurs due to too rapid correction of hyponatremia and causes symmetrical involvement of the basis pontis. An acute stage of encephalopathy and seizures is followed by bulbar weakness and spastic quadriparesis in the second week. Most severe cases can lead to catatonia, locked-in state, and coma.

MEDULLA OBLONGATA

Surface Anatomy

The medulla oblongata (medulla) is the most caudal portion among the three regions that make up the brainstem. It is continuous above with the pons and below with the spinal cord at the level of foramen magnum. The medulla is conical in shape, decreasing in width as it extends inferiorly. It is approximately 3 cm long and 2 cm wide at its largest point. On the anterior surface of the medulla is the anterior median fissure, which is continuous along the length of the spinal cord. There are two sulci on its surface—the ventrolateral and the posterolateral sulcus **(Fig. 5)**.[6,7]

Internal Anatomy

Cross-sectionally, the medulla contains the ascending and descending nerve tracts, cranial nuclei, and the roots. Within the medulla are situated multiple cranial nerves and their roots. Arising from the junction between the pons and medulla is the abducens nerve (CN VI). Emerging out of the ventrolateral sulcus is the hypoglossal nerve (CN XII), which arises from the centrally located hypoglossal nucleus under the eminence called the hypoglossal trigone. Laterally, in the medullary reticular formation, the nucleus ambiguous is located and in the posterolateral sulcus, three cranial nerves jointly exit the medulla (CN IX, X, and bulbar XI). Dorsal nucleus of the vagus lies dorsolateral to the hypoglossal while the nucleus and tractus solitaries (CN VII, IX, and X) are situated dorsally in the medullary reticulum **(Fig. 5)**.

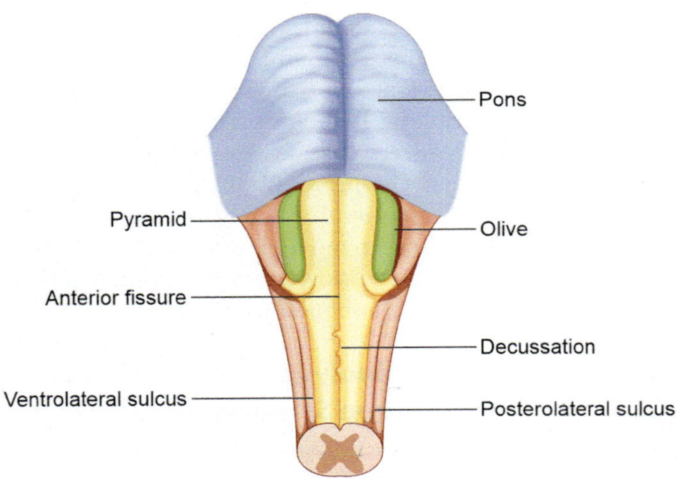

FIG. 5: Anterior surface anatomy of the medulla.

The two vestibular nuclei (medial and inferior) are both located near the midline while the two cochlear nuclei are found above and below the inferior peduncle (restiform body). The spinal tract of the trigeminal nerve and nucleus is seen adjacent to the peduncle. The large inferior olivary nucleus is located within the olive.[7,8]

Lateral from the midline, the fasciculus gracilis and fasciculus cuneatus are located, separated by the posterior intermediate sulcus located in the dorsal medulla. Internal arcuate fibers run from the nucleus gracilis and nucleus cuneatus around and anterior to the central gray matter to form the medial lemniscus, which is dorsomedial to the pyramids. Lateral to the medial lemniscus, the trigeminal nucleus and spinal tract can once again be seen descending caudally to the level of C3.

The pyramids are paired swellings found between the anterior median fissure and the ventrolateral sulcus. The pyramids are the major decussation point of the descending motor fibers. Nearly 75–90% of motor fibers cross diagonally and posteriorly and continue down the spinal column as the lateral corticospinal tracts. The rest of the corticospinal tract descends homolaterally to form the anterior corticospinal tract. In addition, there is the somatotopic organization of the corticospinal fibers within the pyramid with fibers of the lower extremities placed more laterally than the fibers of the upper extremities **(Figs. 6A and B)**.[7-9]

The other structures present in the medulla include the spinocerebellar tracts (ventral and dorsal) located laterally, with the lateral spinothalamic tract situated between them. Medial and lateral reticulospinal tracts, rubrospinal and descending sympathetic pathway descend laterally. In addition, there is continuation of the substantia gelatinosa of the spinal cord.[4,6,7]

Vascular Supply

The vasculature of the medulla is complex and the vessels that supply the medulla include the anterior spinal, the posterior spinal, the posterior inferior cerebellar, the anterior inferior cerebellar, and vertebral arteries. The blood supply of the medulla is subdivided as the paramedian branches, bulbar branches, and lateral bulbar branches **(Fig. 7)**.

Throughout the medulla, the anterior spinal artery, a branch of the vertebral artery, supplies a region beginning at the central canal (or anterior border of the fourth ventricle), and fans out to encompass the pyramids. Below the level of the olives, the posterior spinal artery supplies the posterior half of the medulla. In cross-section through the olives, both the posterior inferior cerebellar and vertebral arteries supply the posterolateral and anterolateral areas, respectively. At the highest point in the medulla, the AICA supplies the outermost portions of the posterior region.[1,3,5]

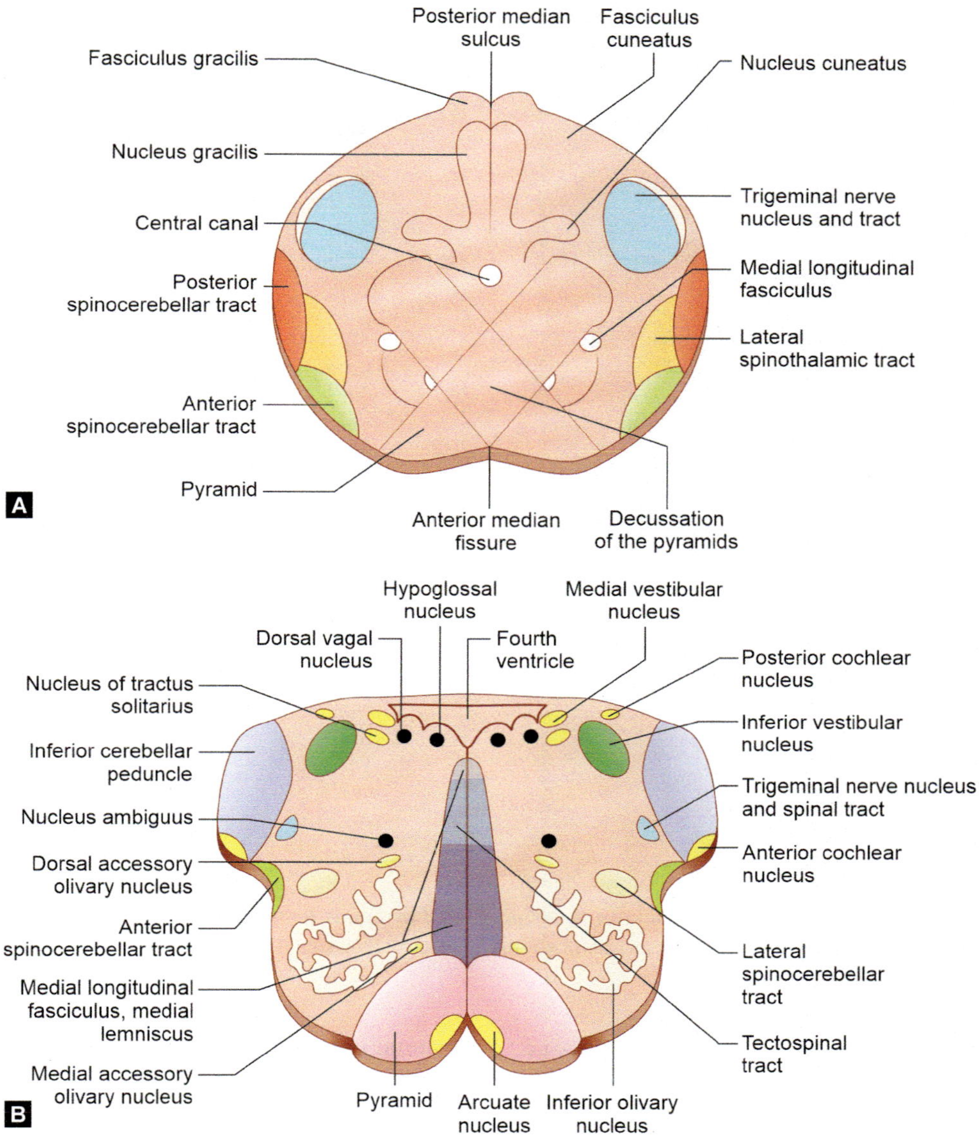

FIGS. 6A AND B: (A) Cross-section of the medulla at the level of the decussation of the pyramids. (B) Cross-section of the medulla at the level of the olives.

Vascular Lesions of the Medulla Oblongata

There are two main vascular lesions of the medulla—namely the medial medullary and lateral medullary syndromes. The former is uncommon in comparison to the latter, which is also better characterized.[3,4,6]

Paramedial Medullary Infarction (Medial Medullary Syndrome)

This was perhaps first described by Dejerine as the "anterior bulbar syndrome". It involves the vascular territory of the anterior spinal artery, which is formed from the union of one branch each from both vertebral arteries. Hence, the medial medullary syndrome can occur as a result of occlusion of either the anterior spinal artery, the vertebral artery, or rarely the proximal basilar artery. The vascular territory of the anterior spinal artery includes mainly the paramedian region of the medulla and, hence, the pyramids, the medial lemnisci, and the hypoglossal nerves and nuclei. When unilaterally affected, the clinical features include—(1) ipsilateral paresis and atrophy of the tongue, hence away from the side of hemiplegia (see below) and toward the side of the lesion on MRI, (2) contralateral hemiplegia, sparing of course, and the face, and (3) contralateral loss of vibration and joint position sensation.

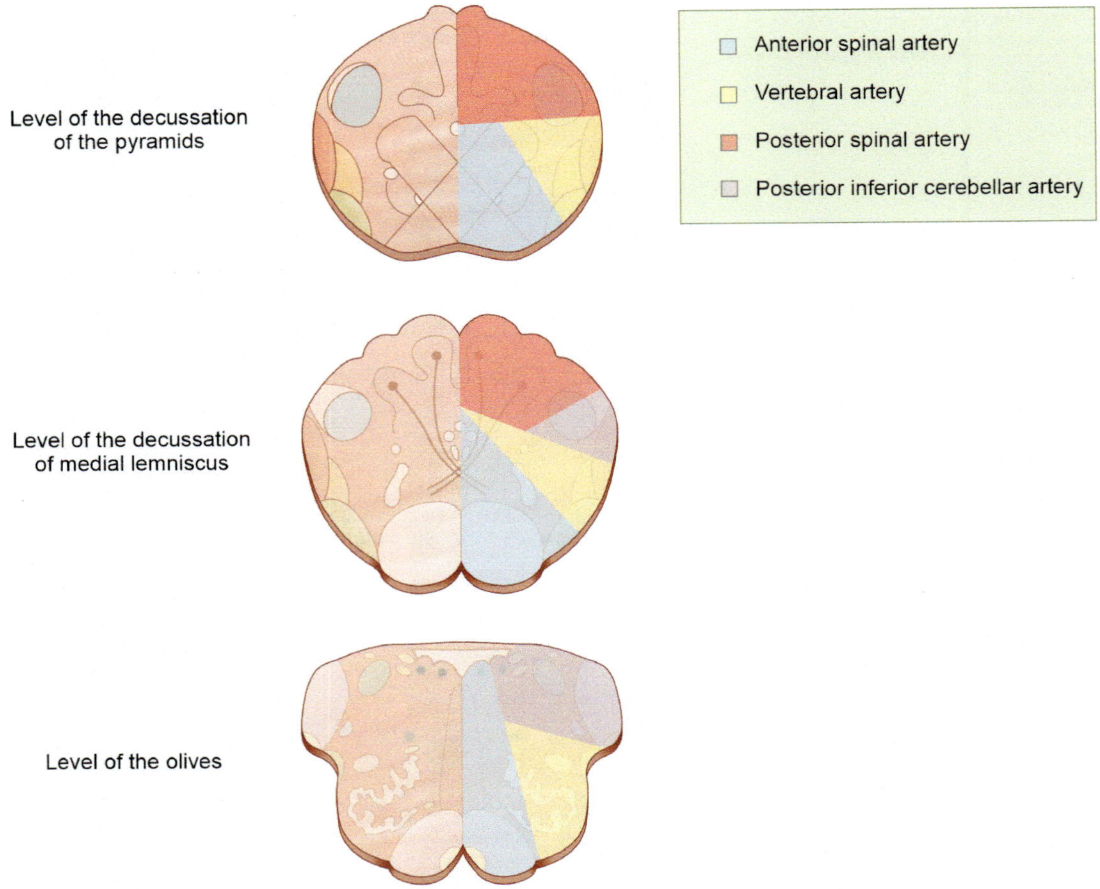

FIG. 7: Blood supply to the medulla at level of decussation of pyramids, lemnisci, and at the olives level.
Source: https://teachmeanatomy.info/neuroanatomy/brainstem/medulla-oblongata/

The occlusion frequently involves the large vessels, i.e., most often the vertebral artery and hence, dissection is an important cause. In addition, it can frequently lead to bilateral infarction and symptoms and signs. The clinical presentation is one of quadriplegia and respiratory paralysis. In such cases, MRI (including diffusion-weighted scans) frequently discloses a heart-shaped lesion.

Nystagmus can occur and is frequently under-recognized in paramedian medullary infarction. Most typical is a primary position upbeat nystagmus, in which the eye beats upward, more so in upgaze. This nystagmus occurs as a result of a lesion in the nucleus prepositus hypoglossi, located in the floor of the fourth ventricle in the vicinity of the hypoglossal nuclei in the lower pons and upper medulla. This nucleus is reciprocally connected with the flocculus of the cerebellum, the medial vestibular nuclei, and the pontine paramedian reticular formation. By virtue of its connections with the medial vestibular nuclei, it maintains a vertical balance, which, if disturbed, leads to a slow downward movement of the eyes and rapid upward correction. Besides a primary position upbeat nystagmus, torsional upbeat nystagmus can also occur in paramedian medullary infarction due to the involvement of the pathways originating from the anterior semicircular canal.

Lateral Medullary (Wallenberg's) Syndrome

Infarction of the posterior and lateral part of the medulla with or without the inferior portion of the cerebellum characterizes the lateral medullary syndrome. This is typically supplied by branches of the vertebral artery and the posterior inferior cerebellar artery (PICA). Common and uncommon features of the lateral medullary syndrome are listed in **Tables 1 and 2**. These features are the result of lesions involving the descending spinal nucleus of the trigeminal nerve and the trigeminothalamic tract (leading to ipsilateral thermoanesthesia and analgesia or hypoalgesia of the face), descending spinothalamic tracts (leading to contralateral hemithermoanesthesia and hemianalgesia or hemi-hypoalgesia of the body), inferior cerebellar peduncle (leading to ipsilateral cerebellar signs), dorsal motor nucleus of the vagus (dysphagia), and area postrema (vomiting and hiccups).[8-13]

TABLE 1: Common manifestations of lateral medullary syndrome.[8-13]

Ipsilateral manifestation	Contralateral manifestation	Other manifestation	Basis
Ipsilateral facial hypoalgesia and thermoanesthesia. Ipsilateral facial pain is common			Trigeminal spinal nucleus and tract involvement
	Contralateral trunk and extremity hypoalgesia and thermoanesthesia		Due to damage to the spinothalamic tract
Ipsilateral palatal, pharyngeal, and vocal cord paralysis with dysphagia and dysarthria			Due to involvement of the nucleus ambiguous
• Ipsilateral Horner syndrome • Ipsilateral hypohidrosis of the body may occur, probably due to interruption of the mostly uncrossed excitatory sweating pathway, which descends from the hypothalamus through the tegmental area of the mesencephalon and pons and, more caudally, through the posterolateral area of the medulla to synapse with the sympathetic sudomotor neurons of the intermediolateral cell column of the spinal cord			Due to affection of the descending sympathetic fibers
		Vertigo, nausea, and vomiting	Due to involvement of the vestibular nuclei
Ipsilateral cerebellar signs and symptoms			Due to involvement of the inferior cerebellar peduncle and cerebellum
Occasionally, hiccups (singultus) attributed to lesions of the dorsolateral region of the middle medulla and diplopia			Perhaps secondary to involvement of the lower pons

TABLE 2: Uncommon manifestations of lateral medullary syndrome.[8-13]

Manifestations	Basis
Wild arm ataxia	Lateral cuneate nucleus
Clumsiness of the ipsilateral upper limb	Subolivary area
Central	Interruption of the sympathetic pathways
Contralateral hyperhidrosis with ipsilateral anhidrosis	Interruption of the sympathetic pathway
An inability to sneeze	Sneezing center located at the ventromedial margin of the descending tract and nucleus of the trigeminal nerve
Loss of taste	Rostral and the lateral zone of the nucleus tractus solitaries
Autonomic dysfunction	Caudal and medical zone of the nucleus tractus formation
Failure of automatic breathing	Nucleus ambiguous and the adjacent reticular formation
Body lateropulsion	Descending lateral vestibulospinal tract
Axial lateral pulsion	Vestibulospinal and spinocerebellar tracts
Pure sensory stroke	
Ipsilateral hemiparesis	Lower most caudal end of the medulla
Central hypoventilation	
Poststroke facial	

REFERENCES

1. Singh V. Textbook of Anatomy Head, Neck, and Brain; Volume III, 2nd edition. 2014. p. 363.
2. Haines D, Mihailoff G. Fundamental Neuroscience for Basic and Clinical Applications, 5th edition. 2018.
3. Brainstem | Definition, Structure, & Function. Encyclopedia Britannica. 2020-05-13.
4. Cranial Nerve Nuclei and Brain Stem Circulation. Neuroanatomy Online. 2020-05-13.
5. Gowda SN, Jesus O. Brainstem infarction. [Updated 2022 Aug 15]. In: StatPearls [Internet]. Treasure Island (FL): StatPearls Publishing; 2023 Jan. Available from: https://www.ncbi.nlm.nih.gov/books/NBK560896/Kolb B, Whishaw IQ (2009). Fundamentals of human neuropsychology: Sixth edition. New York, NY: Worth Publishers.
6. Snell R. Clinical neuroanatomy, 10th edition. Philadelphia: Wolter Kulwer/Lippincott Williams & Wilkins; 2010.
7. Carpenter, Malcolm. Core text of neuroanatomy (3rd ed.). Williams & Wilkins, 1985. pp. 42-43.
8. Paul W Brazis, Joseph C Masdeu, Joese Biller. Localization in Clinical neurology. 6th edition. Lippincott Williams & Wilkins; 2011.
9. Guyton A, Hall J. Textbook of medical physiology, 11th edition. India: Elsevier Saunders; 2007.
10. Netter F. Atlas of human anatomy, 6th edition. Philadelphia: Elsevier Saunders; 2014.
11. Standring S, Gary H. Gray's anatomy, 42nd edition. Edinburgh: Churchill Livingstone/ Elesevier; 2008.
12. Basinger H, Hogg JP. Neuroanatomy, Brainstem. StartPearls (Internet); 2020. Available from: https//www.ncbi.nlm.nih.gov/books/NBK544297/
13. Nolte J. The Human Brain: An Introduction to its functional Anatomy. St Louis: Mosby; 1993.
14. Xue F, Zhang L, Zhang L, Ying Z, Sha O, Ding Y. One-and-a-half syndrome with its spectrum disorders. Quant Imaging Med Surg. 2017;7(6):691-7.
15. Bridge F, Bennett T, Buzzard K. Sixteen syndrome: a rare presentation of central demyelination. BMJ Case Rep. 2023;16(1):e250440.

16

CHAPTER

Applied Neuroanatomy and Neurophysiology of the Pyramidal System

Hiral Halani, Satish V Khadilkar

INTRODUCTION

The initial references to motor weakness resulting from contralateral head trauma appeared from the writings of Hippocrates (the fourth century before the Christian era). Mistichelli, Professor of medicine at Pisa, explained the phenomenon of crossed hemiplegia by the crossing of fibers in the bulbs, i.e., pyramidal decussation, hence also named "Mistichelli decussation". It may seem surprising that the anatomical fact of pyramidal crossing was debated in past for some time before universal acceptance. Moritz Heinrich Romberg once stated, "The most established fact, and rarely threatened by a single exception, is the law of crossing conduction." The course of the pyramidal tract was first elaborated by Ludwig Turck and Charcot in the 19th century.[1]

A succinct account of the nervous system can be taken from the statement of John Hughlings Jackson (1883): "A whole nervous system is a sensorimotor machine, a coordinating system from top to bottom."[2] Complying with this statement, the motor system in higher vertebrates can be construed in various hierarchical levels both anatomically as well as functionally **(Fig. 1)**. These levels are the spinal cord lower motor neurons (LMNs), subcortical level, and cortical level.

The pyramidal level functioning governed by the cerebral cortex is phylogenetically recent. There has been a transition in motor control from the subcortical centers in lower vertebrates to the cerebral cortex in higher mammals. The evolutionary development of the motor system in primates coincides with the emergence of highly skilled fine motor abilities.[3] Bernstein termed this higher-level flexible

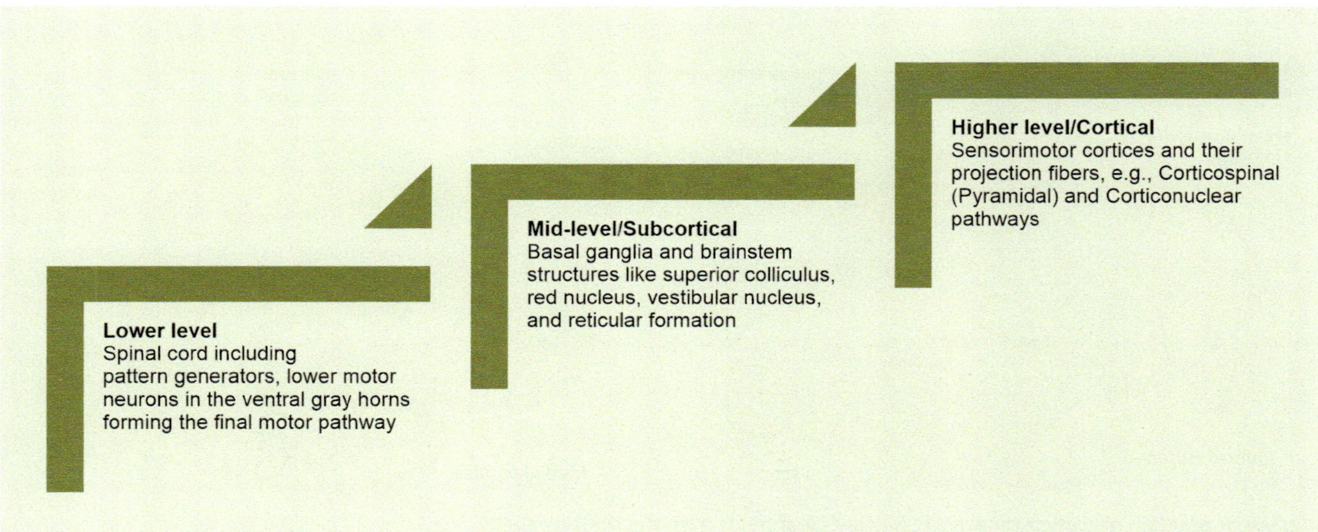

FIG. 1: Hierarchical control of the motor system.

functionality or motor wit as "Dexterity".[4] This is primarily the function of the "pyramidal system," or corticospinal pathways. Recently, the multifunctional aspects of the pyramidal system are being explored including modulation of sensory inputs at the spinal cord level. This chapter focuses on the development, neuroanatomical, and physiological aspects of the pyramidal system and its clinical relevance.

NEUROANATOMY

Embryology

The development of the corticospinal tract (CST) begins in a very immature cortical plate. The outgrowing axons from the sensorimotor cortex descend to the caudal medulla by day 23, then follow a long waiting period. The pyramidal decussation is completed by the 17th gestational week and thereafter a significant increase in the number of axons occurs in the cervical cord region. The lower thoracic and lumbosacral cord levels are reached subsequently by the 19th and 29th week, respectively. The target-derived chemotropic factors guide the growing axons to predestined connections. Early in development, the pattern of corticospinal terminations is more extensive including ipsilaterally. Therefore, neonates can have ipsilateral corticospinal responses that recede by about 18 months of age. A set of molecules "ephrins" expressed in the midline spinal cord, identified from animal studies, are shown to play role in constraining corticospinal terminal axons. The postnatal refinement corticospinal terminations are driven by cortical activity in motor areas and motor experience. The myelination of the pyramidal tract begins by the end of the second trimester and is not complete until the age of 2–3 years. The central conduction times reach adult values approximately by 2–4 years.[5]

Structural Anatomy

The CST is the principal motor efferent pathway for control of voluntary movements. These are the major corticofugal pathways involved in the execution of the fine dexterous and precise movement of limbs; for example, pincer grip. The term "pyramidal" is derived from the pyramid-shaped prominences formed by their axons on the ventral surface of the medulla.[6] This was identified before the discovery of pyramidal cells in the motor cortex as their cells of origin. The corticonuclear (older term corticobulbar) pathways are organized in parallel with the corticospinal pathway. It projects to cranial nerve nuclei and reticular formation in the brainstem, hence not per se part of the "pyramidal" system.[7]

Origin, Course, and Termination

Origin ***(Fig. 2)***: The cortical neurons giving rise to corticospinal and corticonuclear tracts are distributed largely in the frontal and parietal lobes.

- The primary motor cortex [Brodmann area 4/(M1)] occupying the precentral gyrus contributes approximately 30% of corticospinal neurons. The characteristic feature is the presence of giant pyramidal cells in the lamina V of this agranular cortex. These are large (60–100 μ diameter) projection neurons known as Betz cells. Their distribution is heterogeneous in terms of size, shape, and clustering. The largest ones are located medially in the leg and foot area, probably for the farther distance traveled by their axons. It has now been demonstrated that only 2–3% of CST fibers are formed by these cells, which were once thought to be the sole source of CST.[8] There are about 30,000 Betz cells in total whereas each medullar pyramid harbors about 1 million axons. Therefore, it appears that most fibers in CST originate from neurons other than Betz cells.[9]

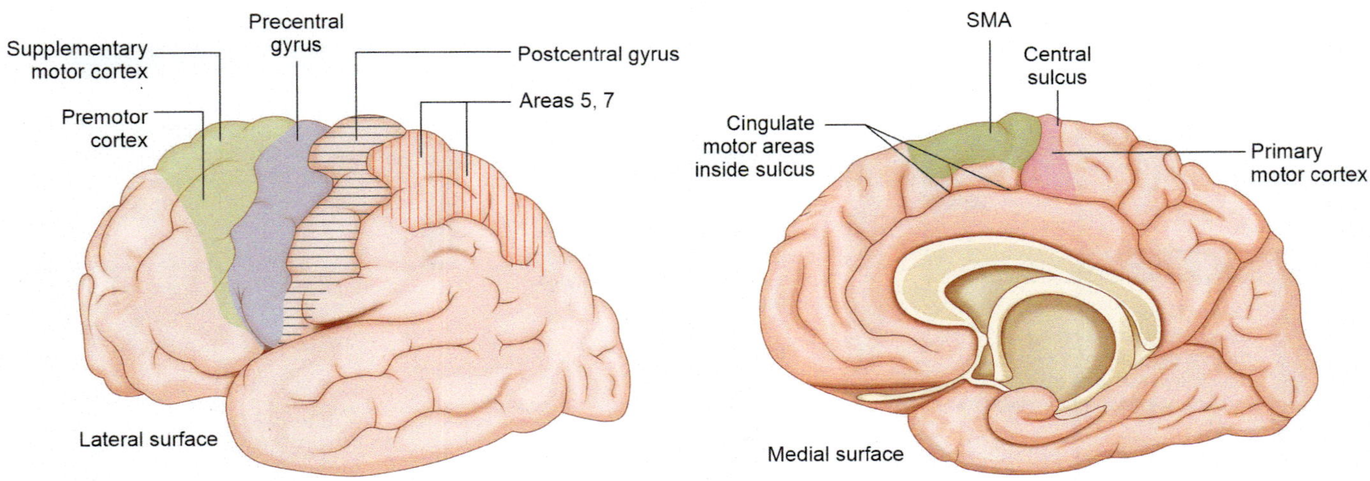

FIG. 2: Areas of origin of corticospinal and corticonuclear tracts from the cerebral cortex.

- Premotor (area 6) and supplementary motor cortices contribute about a similar proportion (~30%) to CST fibers. They are involved in the preparation and planning of the movement. The two differing points to note here are: (1) premotor cortex despite being histologically similar to the primary motor cortex/M1 lacks giant pyramidal cells. (2) Secondly, a proportion of fibers originating from the premotor cortex pass ipsilaterally. They communicate with the extrapyramidal system, (i.e., basal ganglia and its connections) and are involved in axial and proximal limb movement as well as postural responses.[8] Their connection with brainstem nuclei including superior colliculus, red nucleus, and vestibular nucleus account for the movement of head and trunk in response to visual, auditory, and somatosensory stimuli. This is in opposition to fine distal extremity movements governed by CST. The supplementary motor cortex (M2) is probably involved in the integration of bilateral body movements.
- The next contribution (~40%) comes from the somatosensory cortex (area 3,1,2) in the postcentral gyrus, superior parietal lobule, and parts of the cingulate gyrus.

Somatotopic organization: The corticospinal neurons are somatotopically organized within the motor cortex. The neurons projecting to lumbosacral segmental levels arise from the most medial part of the precentral gyrus. The control of lower extremities and perineal musculature is placed in the paracentral lobule in medial frontal cortex. The neurons from the medial two-thirds of the cortex project to the thoracic and cervical cord innervating the trunk and upper limb muscles. The corticonuclear tract originates from the lateral third of the motor cortex. This part of motor homunculus represents the areas of the tongue, face, and neck. From here axons travel to the cranial nerve nuclei innervating the pertinent muscles. The proportion of the cortex allocated to a particular body part is in accordance with its degree of innervation and functional specialization **(Fig. 3)**.[10] The topographical organization of the premotor cortex is nearly the same as that of the primary motor cortex.

Course ***(Figs. 4 and 5)****:* The corticospinal and corticonuclear tracts follow a descending course from the sensorimotor cortex. The fibers first course through centrum semiovale subjacent to the cortex. The centrum semiovale is a semioval-shaped paired mass of white matter above the lateral ventricles and corpus callosum. Inferolaterally, these fibers are continuous with the corona radiata. It is so named because of its appearance of a broad fan-shaped array

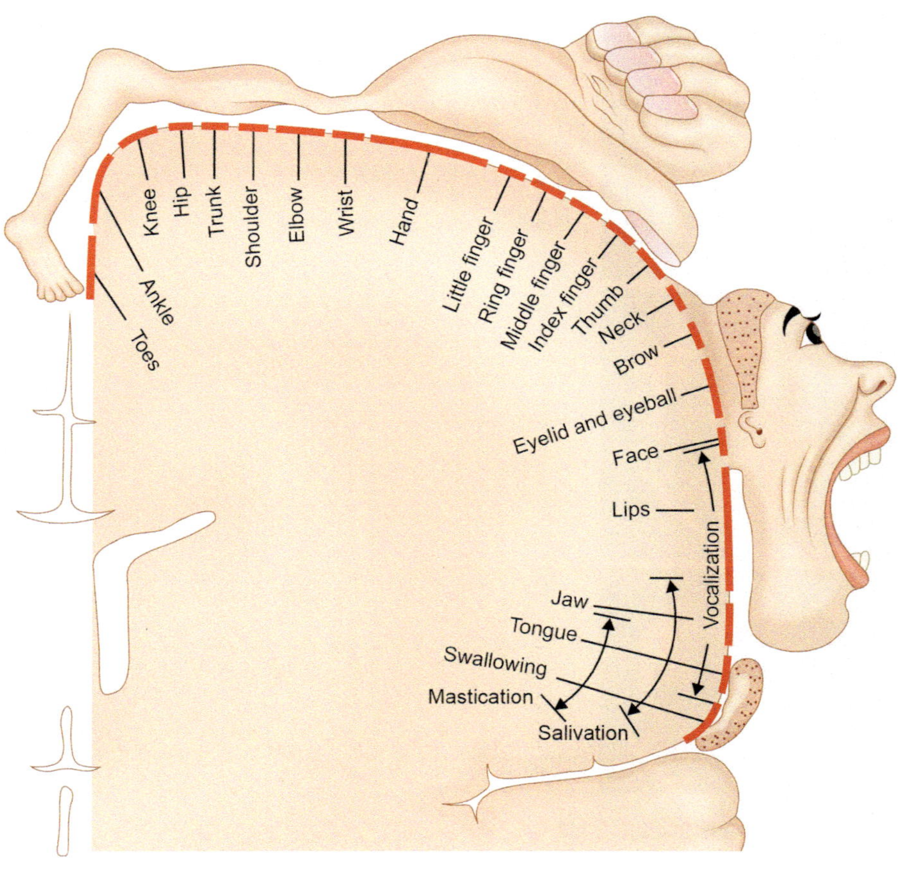

FIG. 3: Homunculus in the motor cortex.

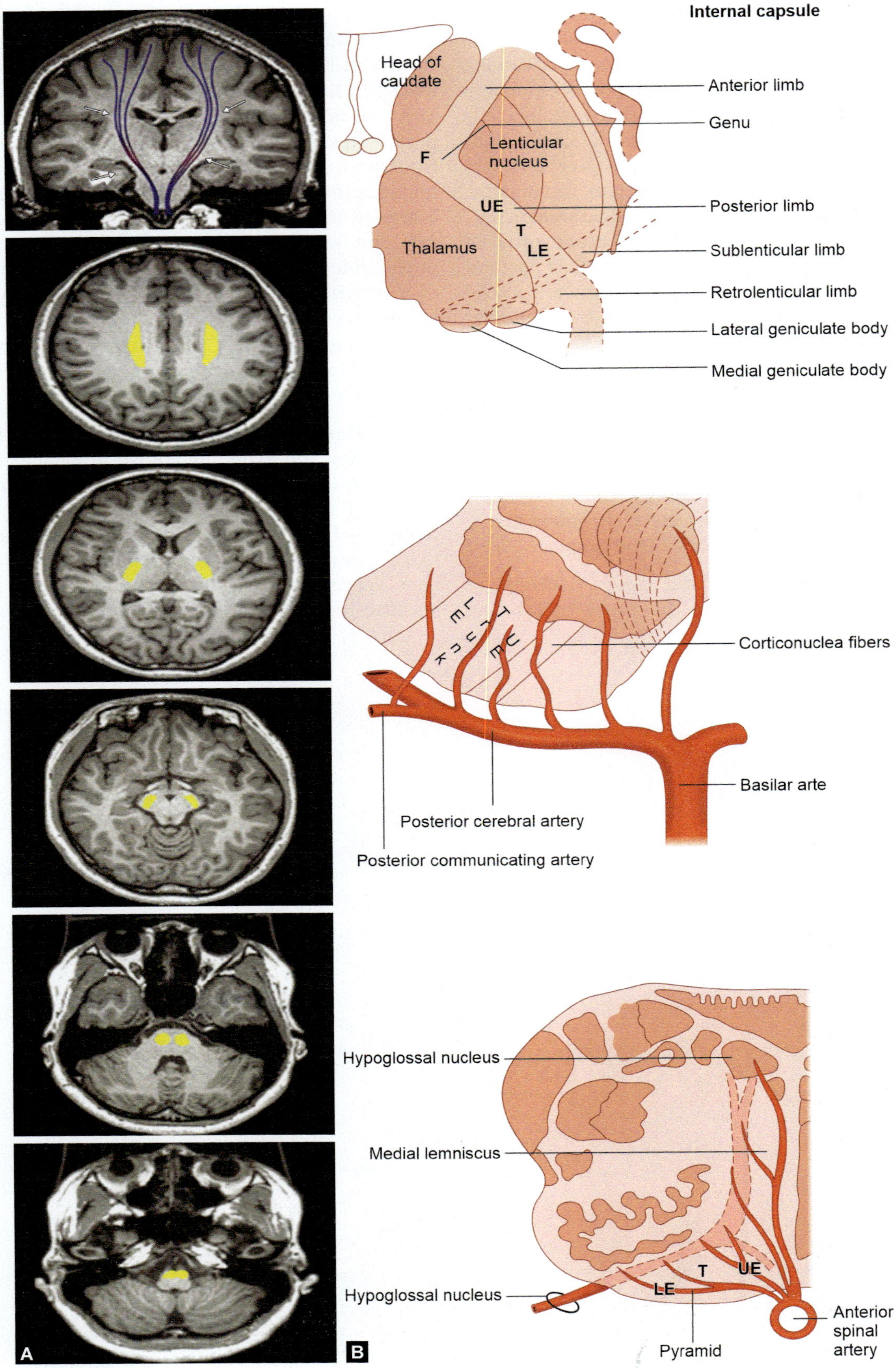

FIGS. 4A TO C: *Continued*

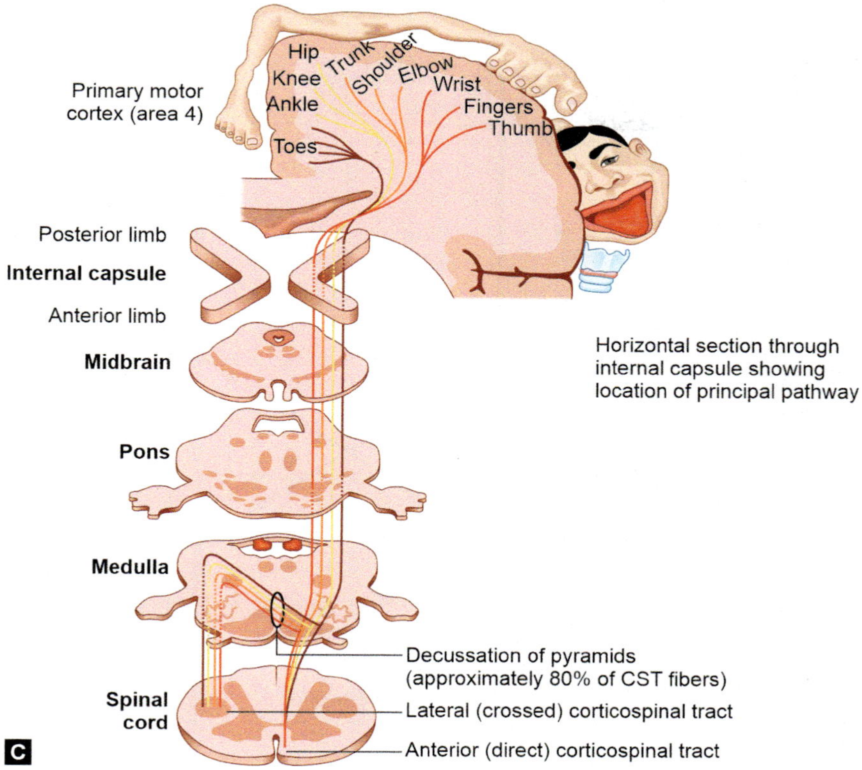

FIGS. 4A TO C: Corticospinal pathway: Course and somatotopy.

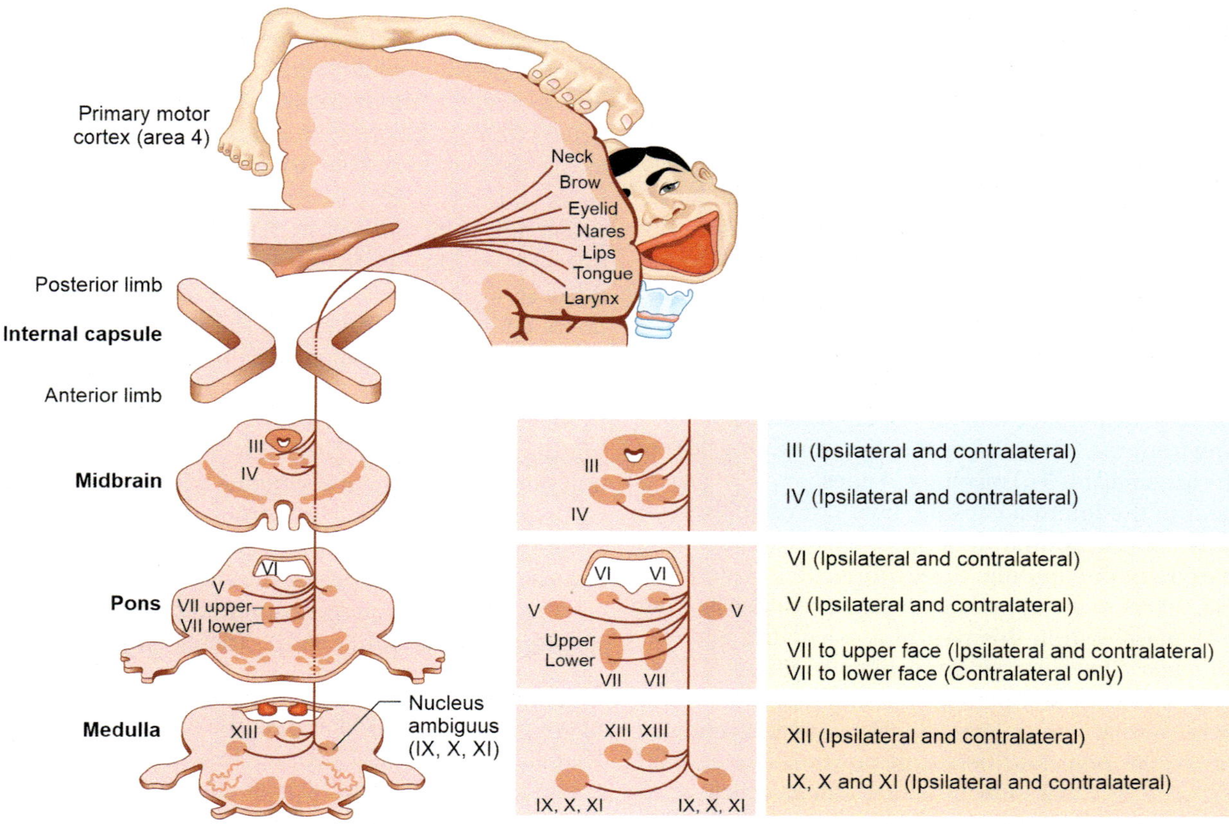

FIG. 5: Corticonuclear pathway.

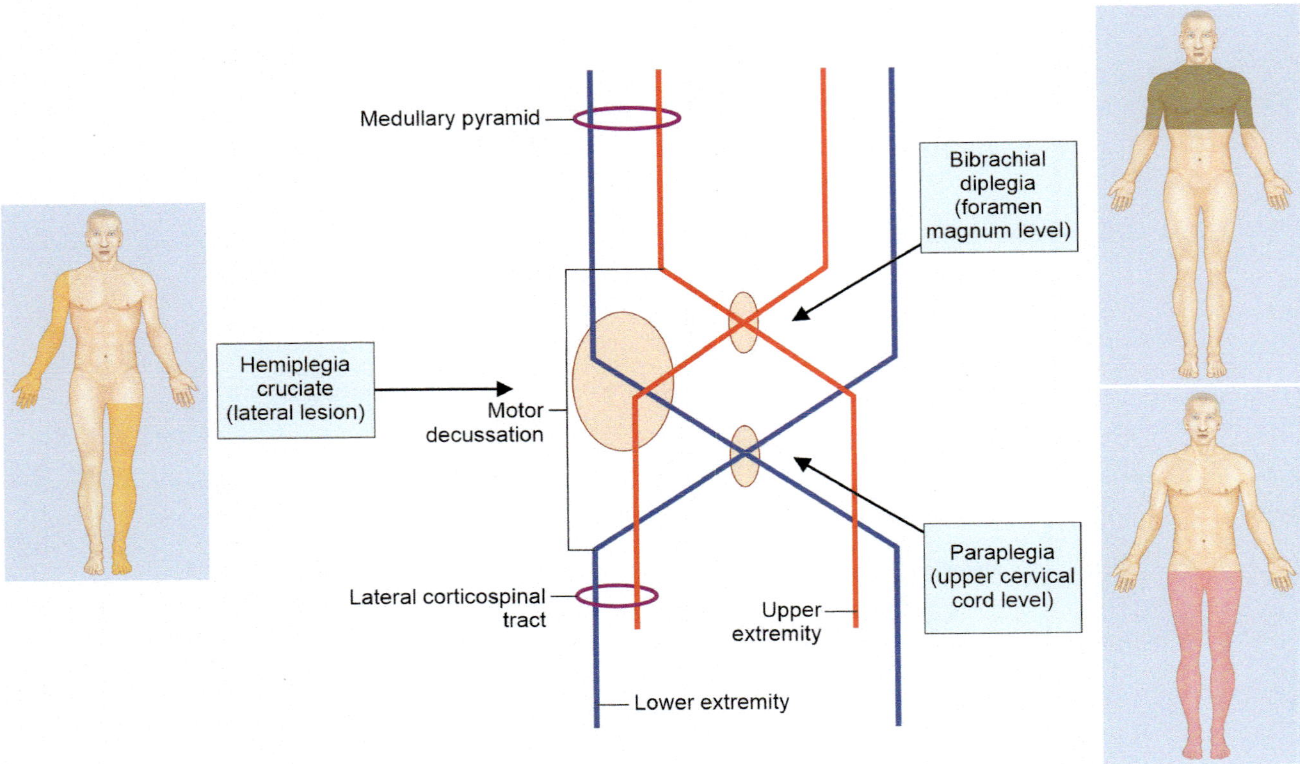

FIG. 6: Pyramidal decussation and its lesions.

of fibers converging down into the internal capsule. The internal capsule is a compact lamina of afferent and efferent fibers located between the caudate and thalamus medially and the lentiform nucleus laterally. Corticobulbar fibers occupy the genu of the internal capsule. In the posterior limb of the internal capsule, the fibers are somatotopically organized. From the anteromedial to dorsolateral direction are the fibers to upper limbs, trunk, and lower limbs. The corticospinal fibers move further posteriorly to reside in the posterior third of the posterior limb as the capsule descends. This often is seen as a subtle T2 hyperintensity on axial magnetic resonance imaging (MRI), which probably points to the heavily myelinated fibers of the pyramidal tract. These large (10–20 μ) myelinated and rapidly conducting fibers are stemming from the Betz cells in M1. The remaining 90% of the fibers are small (4–5 μ) myelinated ones.

Caudal to the internal capsule, fibers traverse through the brainstem. At the midbrain level, corticospinal fibers are located in the middle three-fifths of the cerebral peduncle. Fibers to the upper and lower extremities lie from medial to lateral within this part of crus cerebri, whereas corticonuclear fibers are situated most medially.[11] Next at the pontine level, the pyramidal tract passes ventrally through the basilar pontis. Here, the fibers get intermingled with transverse pontine fibers and pontine nuclei. MRI mapping analyses have shown that the topographical arm/leg distribution somewhat breaks down at this level.[12] Though the fibers controlling proximal muscles are placed dorsally compared to those innervating distal muscles. In the medullary pyramids, corticospinal fibers to hands and legs are arranged in a mediolateral direction.[11] At the caudal end of the medulla, approximately 85–90% of pyramidal fibers decussate ventrally (pyramidal or mistichelli decussation) to the opposite side **(Fig. 6)**. The decussation is shown to be asymmetrical with the more extensive crossing of fibers projecting from the left hemisphere than the right. The fibers to the upper extremities decussate more rostrally than those to the lower extremities. Thereafter the decussating fibers continue to descend in the lateral funiculus of the spinal cord as the lateral CST. The remaining 10–15% of the CST fibers do not decussate and descend ipsilaterally in the anterior funiculus, known as the anterior CST (Turck bundle). Eventually, these fibers also decussate in the anterior commissure of segmental cord levels. The anterior CST along with the small proportion of truly uncrossed fibers (about 2%, named as "bundle of Barnes") are involved in the control of axial and proximal muscles.[13]

The somatotopic organization of corticospinal fibers at different levels is mentioned in **Tables 1 and 2**.

Termination: Corticonuclear fibers terminate on the cranial nerve nuclei **(Fig. 5)** including the trigeminal nucleus (CN V), facial nucleus (CN VII), nucleus ambiguous (CN IX,X), accessory (CN X1), and hypoglossal nucleus (CN X11). The distribution is bilateral except: (1) the facial nucleus for the lower face receives exclusively contralateral innervation,

TABLE 1: Somatotopic organization of corticospinal tract and its clinical relevance.

Structure	Somatotopic arrangement	Clinical relevance
Motor cortex	• As per the motor homunculus **(Fig. 3)** • Muscles of legs, thigh, and perineum: medial part of MC and anterior paracentral gyrus • *Trunk and upper limbs*: Medial two-thirds of the precentral gyrus • Craniofacial-oral musculature: Ventrolateral part of precentral gyrus	• Disproportionate hemiparesis occurs in corticosubcortical stroke • For example, faciobrachial predominant weakness in laterally placed lesions and crural predominance in medial paracentral region of contralateral hemisphere[15] • Paraparetic weakness can result from parasagittal cerebral lesions, e.g., parasagittal meningioma • *CSO*: Dilated perivascular spaces and signal abnormalities in CSO are closely related to small vessel disease, amyloid aggregation, and aging[16]
Subcortical—CSO, CR	• CSO: Hand fibers are located laterally • Leg fibers are located medioposterior to hand fibers. • CR: Hand fibers are placed more anteriorly to foot fibers	
Internal capsule	Upper extremity fibers are positioned lateral and anterior to lower extremity fibers	• Lesions of posterior limb of IC leads to pure motor hemiplegia, which is usually proportionate, (i.e., a similar degree of weakness of the face, upper, and lower limbs) • Lesions of genu leads to involvement of corticobulbar fibers
Cerebral peduncles at midbrain level	Hand fibers are medial to leg fibers	"Crossed" signs (e.g., ipsilateral cranial nerve palsy and contralateral hemiparesis) and involvement of cranial nerves point to brainstem localization (individual brainstem vascular syndromes are discussed in detail in Chapter 15 Brainstem)
Pons	• *Fibers to proximal muscles*: Dorsally • *Fibers to distal muscles*: Ventrally • The somatotopy is much less defined in caudal pons	
Medullary pyramids	• *Fibers to the upper extremity*: Medial and decussate rostrally • *Fibers to the lower extremity*: Lateral and decussate caudally as compared to those to upper limbs	
Pyramidal decussation **(Fig. 6)**	Fibers to upper extremities decussate rostral and medial to lower extremities	• A lesion at caudal medulla or cervical-medullary junction can lead to bibrachial weakness and a lesion at a lower level (C1 cord) can lead to bicrural paresis • Hemiplegia cruciata (ipsilateral arm and contralateral leg weakness) in a laterally placed lesion[17] • Aberrancy in decussation could account for the development of mirror movements, though they are generally thought to result from deficient contralateral cortical inhibition[18]
Spinal cord lateral funiculus	• *Fibers of distal muscle groups*: Lateral • *Fibers of proximal and axial muscle groups*: Medial	Ipsilateral UMN type of weakness below the level of lesion, may be accompanied by LMN signs at the segmental level

(CSO: centrum semiovale; CR: corona radiata; IC: internal capsule; LMN: lower motor neuron; UMN: upper motor neuron)

TABLE 2: Vascular supply.[15,19]

The level of CST pathway	Blood supply
Motor cortex	Terminal branches of MCA and ACA
Corona radiata and posterior limb of Internal capsule	Small perforators including lenticulostriate branches of MCA, anterior choroidal artery
Genu of Internal capsule	Anterior choroidal artery
Crus cerebri	Paramedical branches from PCA (P1) and branches from PCom
Basis pontis	Paramedical branches from basilar artery
Medullary pyramids and pyramidal decussation	Vertebral artery and anterior spinal artery
Lateral and anterior funiculus of spinal cord	Anterior spinal artery from vertebral artery

(ACA: anterior cerebral artery; MCA: middle cerebral artery; PCA: posterior cerebral artery, PCom: posterior communicating artery)

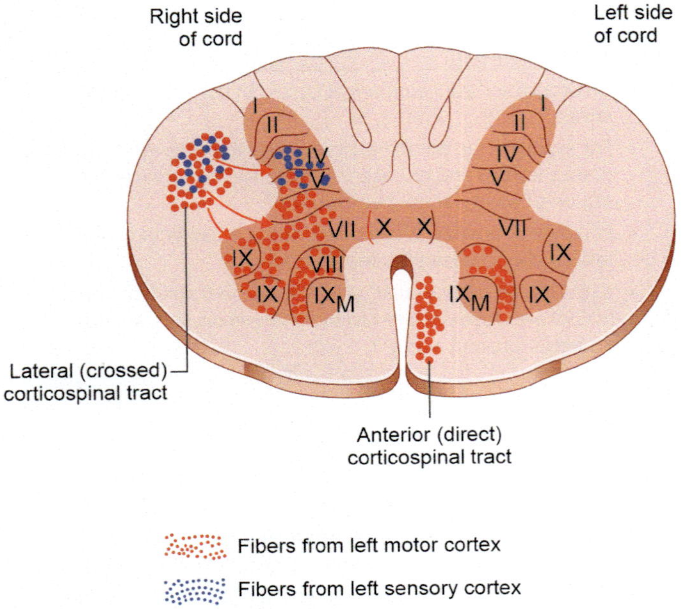

FIG. 7: Termination of corticospinal tract on the ventral gray horn.

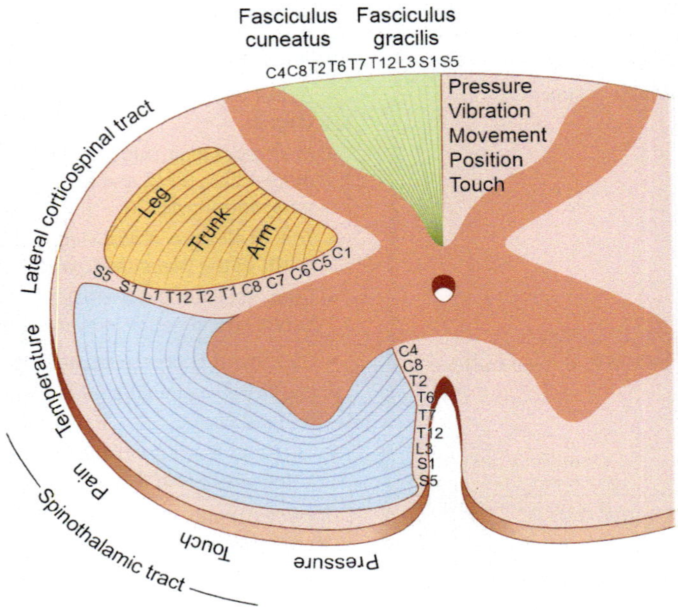

(2) corticobulbar tract (CBT) axons to hypoglossal nucleus are largely contralateral, and (3) those to spinal accessory nucleus are largely ipsilateral. The nuclei of the 3rd, 4th, and 6th CN receive inputs from frontal and parietal eye fields involved in the control of eye movements.[7]

The lateral CST terminates at various levels in the spinal cord. The axons terminating to the cervical cord are situated most medially in the tract whereas those extending to lumbosacral levels are lateral. Approximately, half of the fibers end at the cervical level. Out of the remaining half, about 20% of fibers end at the thoracic level and 30% continue till the lumbosacral levels and the tract ends at the S4 level. The anterior CST terminates at mid-thoracic segments.

The corticospinal fibers projecting from the frontal cortex terminate in lamina VII-IX in the intermediolateral gray column and anterior horn **(Fig. 7)**. The fibers synapse on the alpha and gamma motor neurons both directly as well as indirectly through the interneurons.[14] There is topographic organization of motor neurons in ventral horns. The spinal neurons supplying axial muscles are collected most medially in a column extending the length of the spinal cord. The neurons supplying limb muscles are largely collected in cervical and lumbosacral enlargement. Laterally are the neurons supplying distal muscles and those to proximal muscles are found medially. A portion of CST fibers originating from the parietal lobe terminate in dorsal horns (lamina IV-VI).

NEUROPHYSIOLOGY[20]

The voluntary movements are initiated by the motor cortex. The cells in motor cortex are arranged in vertical columns, each column functioning as a unit that stimulates a group of synergistic muscles. The cortical neurons encode the speed, force as well as direction of a movement. Evarts and colleagues have shown using the single cell recording techniques that a pyramidal cell fires about 60 ms before the onset of a movement. Two populations of pyramidal neurons are excited—dynamic neurons firing at a high rate cause the initial rapid development of the force, whereas the much slower firing by static neurons continues to maintain the force of contraction for longer periods. These motor signals are transmitted to the spinal cord effector segment directly through corticospinal pathways and indirectly through various accessory pathways involving basal ganglia, cerebellum, and brainstem nuclei. The somatosensory feedback signals provided by the muscle spindles and tactile receptors help with the precision of movement. Studies on rehabilitation after a stroke have shown that cortico-subcortical lesions are associated with the functional reorganization and increased task related activity in contralateral sensorimotor cortices. This indicates that contralesional (ipsilateral) CST accounts for the poststroke recovery of limb movements.

The phenomenon of midline crossing of tracts is obscure and poorly understood. According to Cajal's hypothesis, motor decussation follows the crossing of visual and tactile pathways, for fine motor skills necessarily depend on the sensory inputs. This allows the gathering of sensory and motor information in the brain.[21]

Lawrence and Kuypers elucidated the functional organization of descending motor fibers in three groups:[22]

1. Corticobulbar and corticospinal fibers projecting to the brainstem and spinal cord, the "lateral motor system". The corticospinal neurons influence spinal motor neurons through direct and indirect connections. The

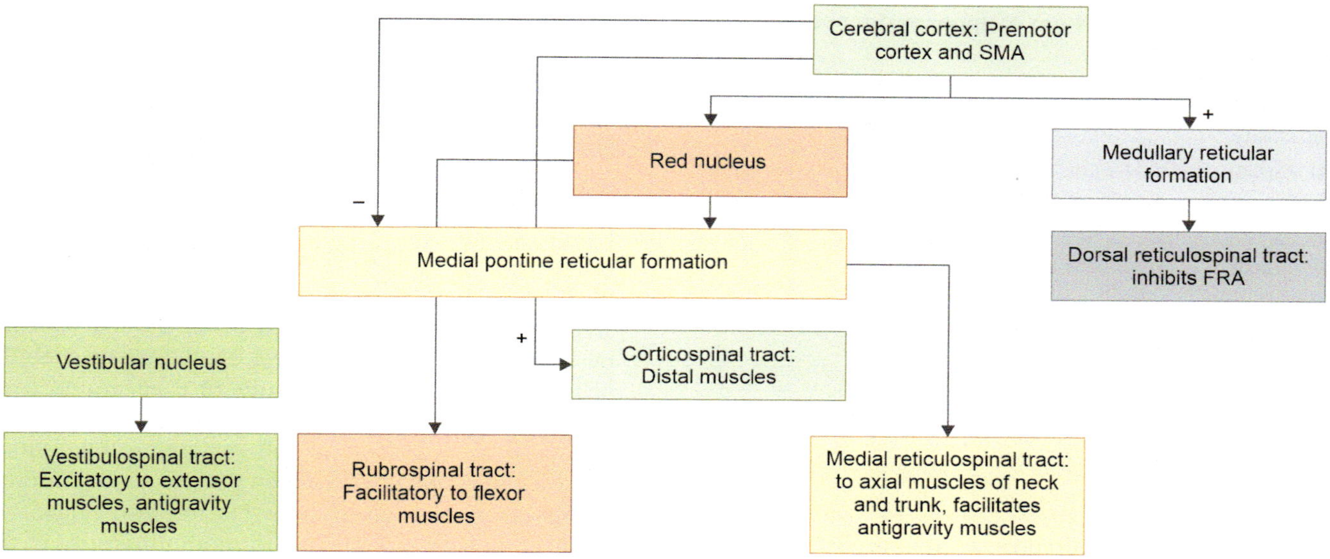

FLOWCHART 1: Descending pathways.

excitatory neurotransmitter in the CST is glutamic acid, whereas the interneurons function through inhibitory neurotransmitters γ-aminobutyric acid (GABA) and glycine. The direct excitatory synapses on alpha motor neurons (direct corticomotoneuronal connection) are found in about 10% of fibers and characteristically present only in primates. These are particularly important in fine discrete movements of hands and fingers such as grasping. The unique feature of the corticospinal synapse is a progressively larger excitatory postsynaptic potential generation with successive cortical stimuli. The indirect connection made through interneurons regulates a larger number of muscles and hence the multijointed movements such as reaching. The fraction of CST fibers projecting from the sensory cortex to dorsal horns appears to be involved in the control of sensory inflow to the cortex. They also function in the modulation of movement by sensory afferents.

2. The dorsolateral pathway mainly includes the cortico-rubrospinal system which deserves some attention here. The red nucleus situated in the midbrain tegmentum plays a critical role in motor control in humans. It receives inputs from the prefrontal and sensorimotor cortices as well as the dentate nucleus of the contralateral cerebellum. The magnocellular portion of RN contains the somatographic representation of limb muscles which is much less detailed than the motor cortex. From here, the rubrospinal tract descends to the contralateral cervical cord in the dorsolateral funiculus. The pathway is excitatory and the main neurotransmitter is glutamate. It primarily facilitates flexor activity and has a greater influence on distal musculature. It has been proposed that this could serve as an accessory pathway to CST and adds to the capacity of distal hand movements. The parvocellular portion of RN projects to the ipsilateral olivary nucleus in the central tegmental tract. This pathway is thought to be involved in movement learning and antinociception, though its function is not entirely clear. But these rubro-olivary projection fibers are more numerous and actively participate in motor control than rubrospinal fibers in humans.
3. The ventromedial pathway, which includes the reticulospinal, vestibulospinal, and tectospinal tracts terminating on the internuncial cells in the ventromedial gray matter of the spinal cord. This system primarily functions in the control of posture and axial movements.

Other Corticofugal Pathways (Flowchart 1)

In most vertebrates, the extrapyramidal system (the popular term used for basal ganglia and its connection) is considered the dominant motor system. This conforms with the perpendicular orientation of their body axes to gravity. Coextending with the adoption of erect bipedalism in humans, functional reorganization of the motor system led to the pyramidal system becoming the dominant one. This was associated with the unprecedented increase in the bulk of pyramidal tracts and decreased overall bulk of other descending pathways including rubrospinal, reticulospinal, vestibulospinal, and tectospinal tracts.[23] These pathways are described in detail in Chapter 21 (Applied Neuroanatomy and Neurophysiology of the Spinal Cord), the table on the descending pathways in the spinal cord.

CLINICALLY RELEVANT ASPECTS OF THE PYRAMIDAL SYSTEM

Upper motor neuron (UMN) lesions can result from injury to corticospinal/nuclear pathways anywhere from the cerebral cortex, subcortical structures, brainstem, or

TABLE 3: Signs and symptoms of upper motor neuron lesions.

Positive components	Negative components
• Spasticity	• Weakness
• Hyperreflexia of deep tendon jerks	• Hyporeflexia of superficial reflexes
• Clonus (involuntary rhythmic contractions in response to a passive sudden stretch)	• Easy fatigability
• Babinski sign, other pathological reflexes	• Loss of dexterity and slowed movements
• Spastic contraction during movement	
• Flexor and extensor spasms	

spinal cord before termination. Animal experiments have shown that a pure pyramidal tract lesion does not result in spasticity. Therefore, the term "pyramidal syndrome" appears to be a misnomer as there are other nonpyramidal (or parapyramidal) fibers that are usually involved in the production of spasticity and other pyramidal signs. The clinical features of UMN syndromes are mentioned in **Table 3**.

Some of the important UMN signs are discussed below:

- *Weakness*: Pyramidal tract lesions mainly lead to slowness and weakness of the distal hand and finger movement, causing loss of dexterity and precision.
  Concept of "pyramidal weakness"[24-26]: This suggests a lesion of corticofugal pathways in the cortex or subcortical white matter, but not in the caudal neuraxis. The term "pyramidal weakness" is defined manifoldly and the literature regarding its use is confusing. By and large, weakness sparing the antigravity muscles is said to be in pyramidal distribution. It preferentially involves the extensors of the elbow, wrist, and fingers (which are physiologic flexors) and shoulder abductors and external rotators and forearm supinators in the upper limb. In the lower limbs, foot dorsiflexors, knee flexors and hip flexors, and internal rotators are weak, with sparing of hip and knee extensors and foot plantar flexors.

  The controversy around the term stems from the conjecture that pyramidal weakness cannot result from the lesioning of CST alone. The mechanisms postulated include affection of other corticofugal pathways mainly reticulospinal, vestibulospinal, and rubrospinal tracts. The dorsal reticulospinal tract receives facilitatory cortical inputs and in turn inhibits the flexor reflex afferent (FRA). Conversely, medial RST appears to be under the inhibitory cortical influence and has an excitatory effect on stretch reflex circuitry. The medial RST along with the vestibulospinal tract facilitates antigravity muscles, i.e., flexors in the upper limb and extensors in the lower limbs. Similarly, the rubrospinal tract has a flexor tone facilitatory effect. Therefore, the CST lesion after a cerebral insult leads to uninhibited increases in medial RST, vestibulospinal, and rubrospinal influences on flexors of the upper limb and extensors of the lower limb, resulting in their preservation of strength. Additionally, the inherent strength of antigravity muscles could also account for this. Together this sums up what is traditionally called a pyramidal pattern of weakness.
- *Hyperreflexia*: Abnormal processing of proprioceptive information within the spinal cord probably underlies the hyperexcitability of phasic and tonic stretch reflexes. Hyperexcitable tonic stretch reflexes are thought to be the basis for spasticity. On the other hand, hyperexcitability of phasic stretch reflexes results in exaggerated deep tendon reflexes, irradiation of reflexes, and clonus. Clonus is a rhythmic and self-sustaining involuntary contraction evoked by a sudden passive stretch. Clonus results from the alternative contraction-relaxation cycles of muscle spindles set in motion because of the hyperexcitability of alpha and gamma motor neurons.
- *Spasticity*[27]
  - Tone, as we know, is the resistance offered by a resting muscle to passive stretching. The normal tone is contributed by mainly two factors: firstly the viscoelastic properties of a muscle itself and secondly, the gamma motor neuron activity in the spinal cord segment, which in turn is modulated by supraspinal pathways. Disorders of tone can result from the affection of the nervous system at various levels, i.e., UMN/LMN/cerebellar level. UMN lesions classically result in spasticity along with one or more features mentioned in **Table 3**.
  - *Definition of spasticity*: "A disordered sensorimotor control resulting from an UMN lesion, presenting as intermittent or sustained involuntary activation of muscles" (ref). The characteristic is velocity dependency which results from hyperexcitability of the tonic stretch reflexes.
  - *"Clasp-knife phenomenon"*: While passively stretching the muscle, more resistance is felt in the initial part and with continued stretching, there occurs a sudden release of resistance. The presumed mechanisms are: (1) velocity sensitivity of stretch reflex, i.e., the initial resistance slows down the movement and reduces the threshold of the stimulus for the reflex contraction to occur and the resistance declines. (2) The length dependency of a tonic stretch reflex implicates its decline with increasing length and the resistance goes away once the muscle reaches a critical length.
  - *Pathophysiology of spasticity*: The factors responsible for the development of spasticity are both spinal and supraspinal, described in **Figure 8**.

Clinically measurement of spasticity can be done using various methods **(Box 1)**.

- *The extensor plantar response or Babinski sign*: This is the most important sign of UMN syndrome linked to pyramidal tracts. Extension/dorsiflexion of the toe is

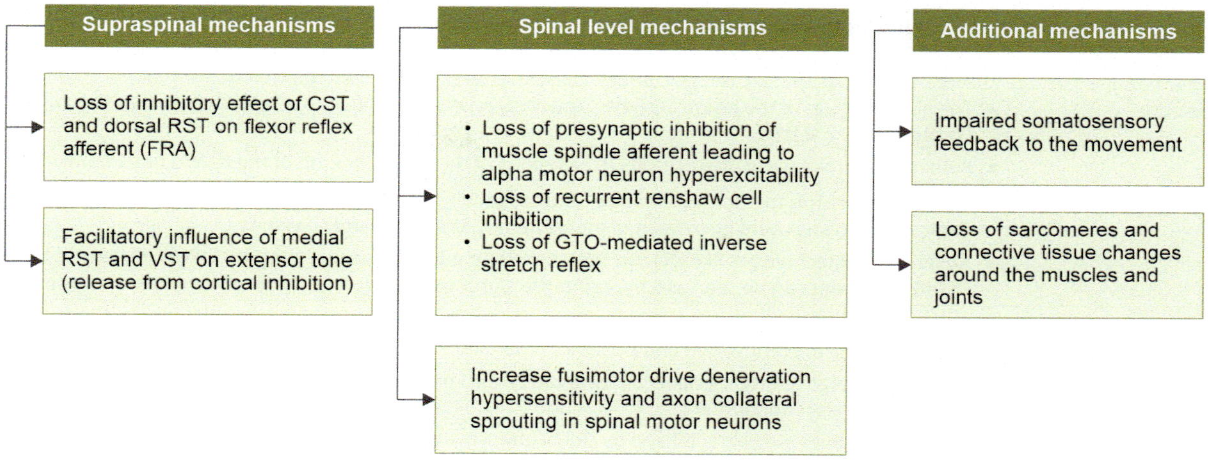

FIG. 8: Pathomechanisms of spasticity.
(CST: corticospinal tract; GTO: Golgi tendon organ; RST: reticulospinal tract; VST: vestibulospinal tract)

BOX 1 Clinical measurement of spasticity.

- *Measurement of spasticity*:
  - Modified Ashworth scale
  - Tardieu scale
  - Pendulum test
  - Spasm frequency score
  - Neurophysiological parameters: H reflex, T reflex, and F waves
- *Modified Ashworth scale*:
  - 0 = No increase in muscle tone
  - 1 = Slight increase in muscle tone
  - 1+ = Slight increase in muscle resistance throughout the range
  - 2 = Moderate increase in muscle tone throughout the range of motion; passive movement is easy
  - 3 = Marked increase in muscle tone throughout the range of motion; passive movement is difficult
  - 4 = Marked increase in muscle tone; affected part is rigid

physiologically considered as flexion and is a part of the triple flexion synergy/withdrawal response. Such a response is normally present in infants. With the maturation of the nervous system and pyramidal tracts this reflex is modified to adapt to an upright walking posture. In lesions of pyramidal tracts, this flexion withdrawal returns and response includes dorsiflexion of toes and ankle along with flexion of hip and knee. The site and the intensity of stimulation on the sole are important.[28] The plantar reflex is evoked by a non-nociceptive stimulus over the lateral border of the sole and ball of the foot. The stimulation over the medial aspect of the sole normally would result in flexion of the toes and can be misleading. Similarly, a painful stimulus can produce a withdrawal response which should be differentiated from a pathological response. Voluntary withdrawal does lead to hip and knee flexion, but the distinguishing point is the movement at the ankle. The ankle movement is usually more prominent than the toes in a withdrawal response and it rarely causes dorsiflexion at the ankle.

- *Flexor and extensor spasms*: These are essentially disinhibited and distorted manifestations of spinal reflexes.
- *Pseudobulbar palsy*: Bilateral lesions of corticonuclear pathways cause bulbar dysfunction, spastic speech, exaggerated jaw jerk, and frontal release reflexes. Pseudobulbar affect or emotional incontinence, (i.e., spontaneous and unprovoked laughter and crying) is common.

CLINICOPATHOLOGICAL CORRELATION[27]

The clinical picture of UMN syndrome to a great extent depends upon the location of the lesion in the neuraxis. UMN syndrome resulting from cerebral lesions is somewhat different from that of spinal cord lesions. From cerebral lesions, spasticity tends to be less severe, more in extensors with a posture of the lower limb in extension. The other features of the clasp-knife phenomenon, clonus and spasms are rarely seen. On the contrary, spinal cord lesions cause severe spasticity, particularly involving flexors with a posture of the lower limb in flexion (paraplegia in flexion) along with flexor spasms, prominent clasp-knife phenomenon, and clonus. The pathophysiological substrate for this could be the intact corticoreticular inhibitory influence on the brainstem centers and release of FRA (responsible for flexor spasms) from CST and dorsal RST in spinal cord lesions.

Corticospinal tract abnormalities result from various pathologies including vascular lesions, degenerative diseases, immune/inflammatory processes, demyelinating or dysmyelinating processes, toxic/metabolic disorders, malignancies, etc. **(Table 4)**.

TABLE 4: Common pathologies involving the pyramidal system.

Etiologies	Remarks
Vascular lesions	• The anatomic site of the lesion and the somatotopic organization at that level determine the clinical deficits **(Table 1)** • Pure motor stroke particularly results from lesions of the posterior limb of the IC and basis pontis
Demyelinating (MS, ADEM, PML, etc.)	• Multiple sclerosis is the demyelinating CNS disease, white matter T2 hyperintense lesions are the hallmark. Clinical symptoms could be in form of mono/hemi/paraparesis and spasticity • Advanced MR techniques like DTI can detect the altered corticospinal integrity in NAWM early in the disease. CST involvement can be seen as a hyperintense signal in the IC (early phase) and periventricular region (late)
• Neurodegenerative disorders • Neurogenetic disorders	• Degeneration of corticospinal neurons is typical of ALS and PLS. This can be visualized as altered signal intensity in the precentral gyri and posterior limb of IC[29] • Other degenerative diseases like Parkinsonian syndromes, e.g., MSA, PSP, FA, SCA, etc., are associated with corticospinal tract impairment • Leukodystrophies are characterized by signal abnormalities along the corticospinal pathways. For example, adrenoleukodystrophy, Krabbe disease, adult-onset polyglucosan body disease, etc.
Tumors	Result in progressive deficits like hemiparesis, cortical signs are usually present
Migraine	• Migraine with aura is particularly linked with white matter abnormalities on MRI and a higher risk of stroke[30] • Certain uncommon types of migraine like hemiplegic migraine and basilar migraine manifest with short-lasting stroke-like symptoms along with headache • Sustained deficits can result from a rare sequel of migrainous infarction
Developmental malformation	• Aplasia or hypoplasia of pyramids can be seen in induction defects like holoprosencephaly, and microcephaly; neuronal migration disorders like lissencephaly, abnormal axonal guidance mechanisms due to L1CAM mutation • Anomalies of pyramidal decussation can be found in posterior fossa malformation like Dandy walker malformation and Joubert syndrome[5]

(ADEM: acute disseminated encephalomyelitis; ALS: amyotrophic lateral sclerosis; CST: corticospinal tract; CNS: central nervous system; DTI: diffusion tensor imaging; FA: fatty acid; MRI: magnetic resonance imaging; MS: multiple sclerosis; MSA: multiple system atrophy; NAWM: normal appearing white matter; PLS: primary lateral sclerosis; PML: progressive multifocal leukoencephalopathy; PSP: progressive supranuclear palsy; SCA: spinocerebellar ataxia)

CONCLUSION

The pyramidal system is the major cortical efferent system for the control of voluntary movements, especially fine and skilled movements. The knowledge of their course and topographic distribution is important for the localization of the lesion. In addition, there are other corticofugal pathways responsible for axial and postural control. Together, these descending motor pathways contribute to the syndrome of UMN lesions. CST dysfunction can arise from heterogeneous etiologies. Advanced MRI of white matter as with DTI can help detect the early involvement of these fibers in many diseases.

REFERENCES

1. Rezende-Cunha F, Oliveira-Souza R de. The pyramidal syndrome and the pyramidal tract: a brief historical note. Arq Neuropsiquiatr. 2011;69(5):836-7.
2. An Introduction to the Life and Work of John Hughlings Jackson. Med Hist. 2006;50(S26):1-34.
3. Welniarz Q, Dusart I, Roze E. The corticospinal tract: Evolution, development, and human disorders: Corticospinal Tract Human Disorders. Dev Neurobiol. 2017;77(7):810-29.
4. Merel J, Botvinick M, Wayne G. Hierarchical motor control in mammals and machines. Nat Commun. 2019;10(1):5489.
5. ten Donkelaar HJ, Lammens M, Wesseling P, Hori A, Keyser A, Rotteveel J. Development and malformations of the human pyramidal tract. J Neurol. 2004;251(12):1429-42.
6. Drake R, Vogl AW, Mitchell AWM. Gray's Anatomy for Students E-Book. Amsterdam: Elsevier Health Sciences; 2009.pp. 1139 .
7. Felten DL, O'Banion MK, Maida MS. Motor Systems. Netter's Atlas of Neuroscience. Amsterdam: Elsevier; 2016. pp. 391-420.
8. Campbell WW, DeJong RN. DeJong's the Neurologic Examination. Philadelphia: Lippincott Williams & Wilkins; 2005. pp. 732.
9. Lassek AM. The human pyramidal tract. II. A numerical investigation of the Betz cells of the motor area. Arch Neurol Psychiat. 1940;1940(42):872-6.
10. Catani M. A little man of some importance. Brain. 2017;140(11): 3055-61.
11. Jang SH. Somatotopic arrangement and location of the corticospinal tract in the brainstem of the human brain. Yonsei Med J. 2011;52(4):553.
12. Marx JJ, Iannetti GD, Thömke F, Fitzek S, Urban PP, Stoeter P, et al. Somatotopic organization of the corticospinal tract in the human brainstem: A MRI-based mapping analysis. Ann Neurol. 2005;57(6):824-31.
13. Afifi AK, Bergman RA, Bergman R. Functional Neuroanatomy: Text and Atlas, 2nd Edition. Philadelphia: McGraw Hill Professional; 2005. pp. 518.

14. Porter R. The corticomotoneuronal component of the pyramidal tract: corticomotoneuronal connections and functions in primates. Brain Res. 1985;357(1):1-26.
15. Ranganathan LN. Localization of Clinical Neurology. Gurugram: Wolters Kluwer India Pvt. Ltd.; 2020. pp. 964.
16. Munoz DG, Hastak SM, Harper B, Lee D, Hachinski VC. Pathologic Correlates of Increased Signals of the Centrum Ovale on Magnetic Resonance Imaging. Arch Neurol. 1993;50(5):492-7.
17. Maramattom B, Joseph S. Cruciate bibrachial diplegia due to an acutely trapped fourth ventricle. J R Coll Physicians Edinb. 2018;48(4):328-31.
18. Schott GD, Wyke MA. Congenital mirror movements. J Neurol Neurosurg Psychiatry. 1981;44(7):586-99.
19. Nuñez M, Guillotte A, Faraji AH, Deng H, Goldschmidt E. Blood supply to the corticospinal tract: A pictorial review with application to cranial surgery and stroke. Clin Anat. 2021;34(8):1224-32.
20. Hall JE, Hall ME. Cortical and Brain Stem Control of Motor Function. Guyton and Hall Textbook of Medical Physiology, 14th Ed. Amsterdam: Elsevier; 2020.
21. Vulliemoz S, Raineteau O, Jabaudon D. Reaching beyond the midline: Why are human brains cross wired? Lancet Neurol. 2005;4(2):87-99.
22. Lemon RN. Descending pathways in motor control. Annu Rev Neurosci. 2008;31(1):195-218.
23. Oliveira-Souza R. The clinicoanatomic uniqueness of the human pyramidal tract and syndrome. J Neurol Neuromedicine. 2017;2(2):1-5.
24. Castle-Kirszbaum M, Goldschlager T. Pyramidal weakness: Is it time to retire the term? Clin Anat. 2021;34(3):478-82.
25. Thijs RD, Notermans NC, Wokke JHJ, van der Graaf Y, van Gijn J. Distribution of muscle weakness of central and peripheral origin. J Neurol Neurosurg Psychiatry. 1998;65(5):794-6.
26. Wiles CM. Pyramidal weakness. Pract Neurol. 2017;17(3):241-2.
27. Esquenazi A. Upper motor neurone syndrome and spasticity. Lancet Neurol. 2009;8(6):517.
28. Khadilkar SV, Chheda AH. A systematic and quantitative evaluation of plantar stimulation: The effect of type, pattern, force of stimulation in eliciting an accurate plantar response. Clin Neurol Neurosurg. 2018;168:83-90.
29. Toosy AT. Diffusion tensor imaging detects corticospinal tract involvement at multiple levels in amyotrophic lateral sclerosis. J Neurol Neurosurg Psychiatry. 2003;74(9):1250-7.
30. Planchuelo-Gómez Á, García-Azorín D, Guerrero ÁL, Aja-Fernández S, Rodríguez M, de Luis-García R. White matter changes in chronic and episodic migraine: a diffusion tensor imaging study. J Headache Pain. 2020;21(1):1.

17 CHAPTER

Applied Neuroanatomy and Neurophysiology of the Cerebellar System

Priyanka Sehrawat, Divya M Radhakrishnan, Roopa Rajan

INTRODUCTION

The cerebellum (Latin for "little brain") is a vital part of the hindbrain and lies in the posterior fossa. It is connected to both the brainstem and the cerebrum via cerebral peduncles. Cerebellum was earlier called the "silent" area of the brain, as electrical stimulation of this area did not lead to either conscious sensation or any muscle contraction. The cerebellum and its circuitry play a crucial role in motor processing and motor planning. The role of the cerebellum in cognitive and affective functions has been increasingly recognized in recent studies.[1] Understanding the anatomy and physiology of the cerebellum helps to understand its functions in the human body. This chapter summarizes the neuroanatomy and neurophysiology of the cerebellum and its clinical relevance.

NEUROANATOMY

The cerebellum is a small structure of the hindbrain, weighing approximately 120 g. It represents approximately 10% of brain volume in adults and 5% in neonates.[2] Despite its small size, it contains almost 80% of all brain neurons that play an important role in motor, cognitive, and affective functions.[3]

Embryology

The cerebellum originates from the dorsal portion of the hindbrain and its development can be summarized in four steps: (1) organization of cerebellar territory, (2) establishment of cerebellar progenitors (GABAergic and glutamatergic ones), (3) migration of granule cells, and (4) formation of cerebellar nuclei. Cerebellar development starts at 4–5 weeks of gestation and continues for approximately 20 weeks postnatally.[4]

The development and maturation of the cerebellum revolve around a morphogenic factor known as the sonic hedgehog (*Shh*) gene. The Shh signaling pathways are active in the ventricular germinal zone. They play an important role in the propagation of progenitor cells derived from the ventricular germinal zone. The Purkinje cells secreted Shh then upkeeps the amplification of two postnatal neurogenic niches, the external granular layer and the prospective white matter that produce excitatory granule cells and inhibitory interneurons, respectively. The Shh signaling also affects Bergmann glial cell differentiation, leading to the characteristic foliation during the development of the cerebellum.[5] With this basic foundation, we move forward to discuss the structural as well as the vascular anatomy of the cerebellum.

Structural Anatomy

The cerebellum is located dorsal to pons and medulla oblongata in the posterior fossa, separated from the cerebrum by a layer of dura mater called tentorium cerebelli. It comprises two hemispheres and a midline structure vermis. Falx cerebelli, a layer of dura mater, separates the two-cerebellar hemispheres **(Fig. 1)**. The cerebellar surface is globally composed of many leaf-like subdivisions, called folia,[6] giving it an onion-like appearance. Two main transverse fissures: (1) the primary fissure, and (2) the posterolateral fissure define the three lobes: [(i) anterior lobe, (ii) posterior lobe, and (iii) flocculonodular lobe] of the cerebellum. The primary fissure divides the cerebellum into the small anterior and large posterior lobe. The posterolateral fissure separates the flocculonodular lobe from the rest of the cerebellar hemispheres and vermis. Each lobe is divided into lobules; the vermis has 10 lobules **(Fig. 2)**. Functionally cerebellum is divided into three parts, (a) the archicerebellum, (b) paleocerebellum, and (c) neocerebellum in the order of development **(Fig. 3)**.

Archicerebellum

The archicerebellum *(also called vestibulocerebellum)* is the oldest lobe phylogenetically. It comprises the flocculonodular lobe that receives inputs (position of head and neck) from the vestibular nerve, and nuclei. A unique feature of this lobe is that it sends outputs directly to the vestibular nuclei, bypassing the deep nuclei. The medial vestibulocerebellum primarily controls axial musculature by modulating the activity of the vestibular nuclei, whereas the lateral vestibulocerebellum is involved in the coordination of head and eye movements and pursuit movement of the eyes.[3]

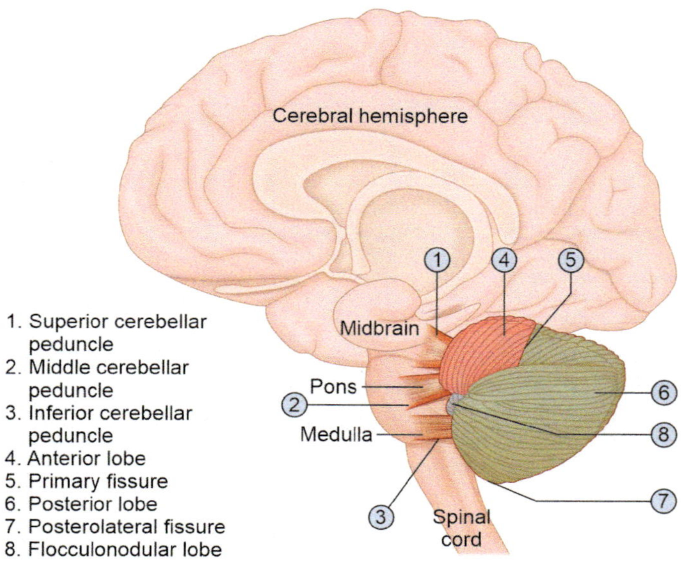

FIG. 1: Relation of cerebellum with rest of the central nervous system (lateral surface).

Paleocerebellum

The paleocerebellum *(also called spinocerebellum)* comprises vermis and paravermian areas on both sides. The vermis receives visual, auditory, vestibular, and sensorimotor inputs from the head, trunk, and proximal portions of limbs.

> *Tip to remember:*
> *The midline structure of the cerebellum handles the midline structures of the body.*

It sends outputs through the fastigial nucleus to the cortex and the brainstem, thus leading to control of proximal muscles of limbs, trunk, and head and neck movements. The paravermian areas send output to the corticospinal and rubrospinal systems, thus leading to control of the distal muscles of limbs. Overall, the outputs of these pathways are involved in postural control, balance, and locomotion.[7]

Neocerebellum

The neocerebellum *(also called cerebrocerebellum)* is the newest addition to the cerebellum phylogenetically. Neocerebellum encompasses the largest part of the cerebellum and is connected with the cerebral cortex. Lateral cerebellar hemispheres project to the contralateral ventrolateral thalamic nucleus and red nuclei via output fibers passing through the dentate nucleus. Axons of these thalamic nuclei project to the premotor cortex and primary motor area of the frontal lobe. Lesions in the cerebellar hemispheres could lead to deficits in motor planning, delays

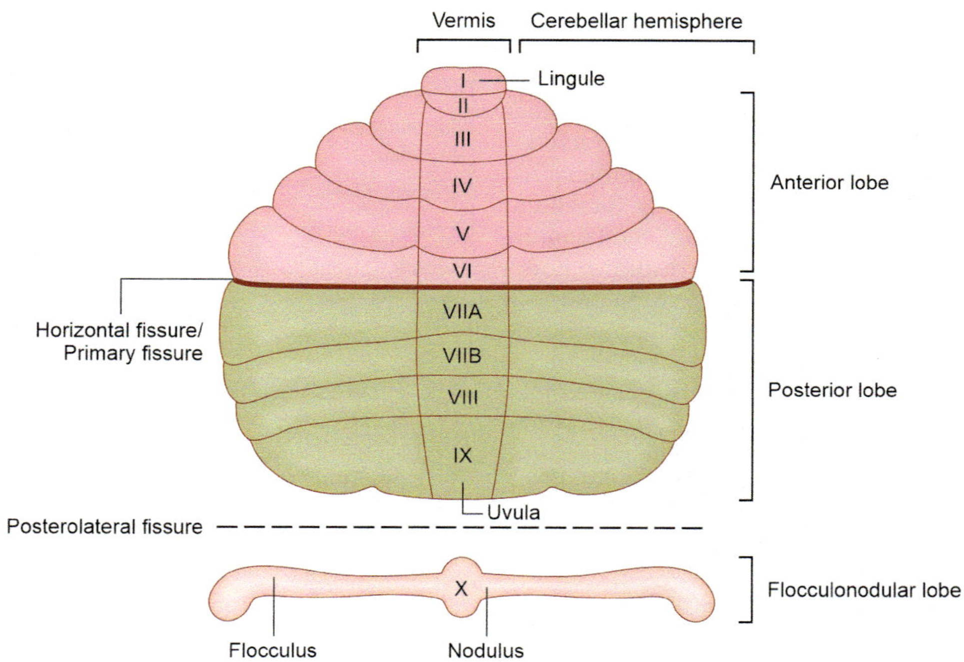

FIG. 2: Unfolded view of cerebellar structures.

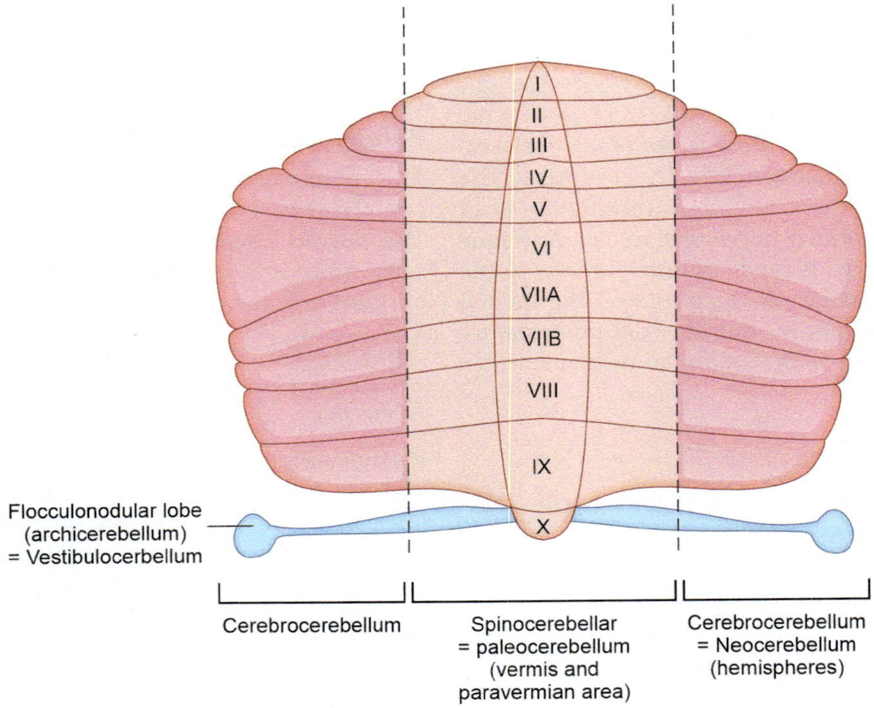

FIG. 3: Phylogenetic/functional segregation of cerebellum.

in the onset of movements, and irregularities in the timings of movement components.[8]

Tips to remember/Mnemonics:
- *Archicerebellum = Vestibulocerebellum = Flocculonodular lobe (AVF)*
- *Paleocerebellum = Paravermian area and vermis*
- *Neocerebellum = Cerebrocerebellum = Cerebellar hemispheres (NCC)*

Cerebellar Peduncles

The cerebellum is connected to the cerebral hemispheres via cerebral peduncles: Superior, middle, and inferior cerebellar peduncles. The superior cerebellar peduncle (brachium conjunctivum) carries information to and from the spinal cord (ventral). The middle cerebellar peduncle (brachium pontis) contains information from the contralateral pontine nuclei. The inferior cerebellar peduncle (restiform body) receives information from the spinal cord through dorsal tracts, the pontine nuclei, and also the reticular nuclei. The major afferent and efferent fibers of the cerebellum are enumerated in **Table 1**.[9] The afferent fibers include fibers passing through vestibular nuclei, reticular nuclei, spinal cord, inferior olivary nucleus, and the trigeminal tract. The efferent fibers include fibers through cerebellar nuclei to the red nucleus, thalamus, and vestibular nucleus.

Pearl of wisdom:
Cerebellum is not responsible for the initiation of movements, and hence does not cause paralysis. Cerebellar dysfunction leads to difficulty in maintaining balance, posture, and tone.

TABLE 1: Afferent and efferent fibers of cerebellum.

Afferent fibers	
Inferior cerebellar peduncle	• Vestibulocerebellar tract (ipsilateral) • Dorsal spinocerebellar tract (ipsilateral) • Cuneocerebellar tract (ipsilateral) • Reticulocerebellar tract (bilateral) • Trigeminocerebellar tract (ipsilateral) • Olivocerebellar tract (contralateral)
Middle cerebellar peduncle	Pontocerebellar tract (contralateral)
Superior cerebellar peduncle	Anterior spinocerebellar tract (ipsilateral)
Efferent fibers	
Inferior cerebellar peduncle	Cerebellovestibular tract (ipsilateral)
Superior cerebellar peduncle	• Cerebellothalamic tract (contralateral) • Cerebellorubral tract (contralateral)

Vascular Supply

Arterial Supply

The three main arteries originating from the vertebrobasilar system, the superior cerebellar artery (SCA), anterior inferior cerebellar artery (AICA), and the posterior inferior cerebellar artery (PICA) supply the cerebellum.

The superior cerebellar artery, a branch of the basilar artery, is given off just before the basilar artery divides into two posterior cerebral arteries. SCA then passes below

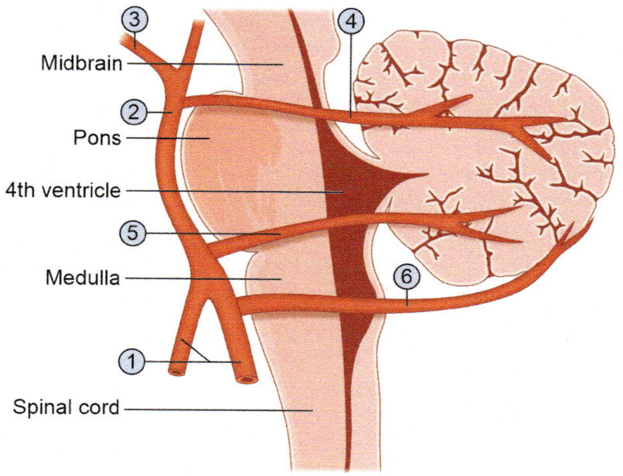

Blood vessel	→ Branch of
1. Vertebral arteries	→ Subclavian artery
2. Basilar artery	→ Confluence of vertebral arteries
3. Posterior cerebellar artery	→ Basilar artery
4. Superior cerebellar artery (SCA)	→ Basilar artery
5. Anterior inferior cerebellar artery (AICA)	→ Basilar artery
6. Posterior inferior cerebellar artery (PICA)	→ Vertebral artery

FIG. 4: Vascular supply of cerebellum.

the oculomotor nerve, encircles the brainstem below the oculomotor nerve and above the trigeminal nerve, and splits into two branches: (1) medial and (2) lateral. The medial branch supplies the mesencephalon, inferior and superior colliculi, superior portion of the vermis, and the superomedial cerebellar cortex. The lateral branch of SCA supplies the superolateral cerebellar cortex.[10,11]

The AICA, after its origin from the basilar artery, divides into two branches: one supplies the anterior inferior cerebellum while the other supplies the flocculus, choroid plexus, and the middle cerebellar peduncle **(Fig. 4)**. PICA takes origin from the V4 segment of the vertebral artery. It passes between the cerebellum and the medulla and supplies the cerebellar nuclei, the inferior surface of the vermis, and the inferior surface of the cerebellar hemisphere. Medulla oblongata and the choroid plexus of the fourth ventricle are also supplied by PICA.[10,11]

Venous Drainage

The superior and inferior cerebellar veins drain the superior and inferior surfaces of the cerebellum, respectively. The superior cerebellar veins end in the straight sinus and the inferior cerebellar veins drain into the superior petrosal sinus, transverse sinus, and occipital sinus.[10,11]

CLINICAL RELEVANCE OF NEUROANATOMY

The peculiarly layered structure of the cerebellum leads to differentiated topography and localization of various symptoms. Before discussing the topodiagnosis of cerebellar dysfunction, one should know the definitions of a few terms, which are given in **Box 1**.[12] Cerebellar dysfunction leads to dysmetria, dysdiadochokinesia, dyssynergia, stance ataxia, gait ataxia, etc. The signs and symptoms of cerebellar dysfunction (head-to-toe) are enumerated in **Box 2**.[13,14]

BOX 1 Definitions.

- *Dysmetria*: Inaccurate judgment of rate, range, force and direction of movement
- *Dysdiadochokinesia*: Inability to perform rapid alternating muscle movements
- *Ataxia*: Derived from Greek word "a-taxis" meaning "without order": lack of coordination in movements
- *Tremor*: Involuntary, rhythmic, and oscillatory muscle movement
- *Tone*: Resistance to passive movement
- *Titubation*: Oscillatory movements of head over a central axis which may be horizontal or vertical
- *Saccades*: Rapid fixating movements of the eye. Derived from the word "saccar" meaning horse's reins
- *Nystagmus*: Involuntary, rhythmic, and oscillatory movements of eyeballs

BOX 2 Signs and symptoms of cerebellar dysfunction.

- Memory problems, personality changes, and impaired communication skills [cerebellar cognitive affective syndrome (CCAS)]
- Head tremor/titubation
- *Oculomotor dysfunction*: Dysmetric saccades, gaze-evoked nystagmus/downbeat nystagmus/rebound nystagmus/oscillopsia/broken pursuits
- Scanning/staccato speech, cerebellar mutism
- Dysmetria, dysdiadochokinesia, dyssynergia, rebound phenomenon
- Appendicular ataxia, intention tremor (coarse, <5 Hz)
- Hypotonia, postural sway/axial ataxia
- Gait ataxia (wide stance, uncoordinated gait, swaying on the ipsilateral side, impaired tandem gait)

Pearl of wisdom:
Cerebellar dysfunction causes ipsilateral symptoms and signs.

Topodiagnosis

Topodiagnosis refers to the localization of various symptoms to different parts of the cerebellum. Because of its extensive connections with the brainstem and cerebellar cortex, pathological involvement of the cerebellum results in a wide spectrum of clinical manifestations. Gait ataxia and wide base stance occur due to the involvement of the rostral vermis, a part of the anterior lobe. Dysfunction of the caudal vermis (posterior lobe) and adjacent paravermian area leads to gait and truncal ataxia, and truncal titubation. The floccular lobe connects the cerebellum to the vestibular system and pathology involving this circuitry results in oculomotor dysfunction. Involvement of the dentate nucleus and its connections can

TABLE 2: Localization of cerebellar symptoms.

Clinical features	Localization
Wide base stance, gait ataxia	Rostral vermis
Gait ataxia, truncal titubation, truncal ataxia	Caudal vermis and adjacent paravermian area
Ipsilateral appendicular ataxia	Cerebellar hemispheres
Dysarthria, intention tremors	Dentate nucleus and its connections
Oculomotor dysfunction	Flocculonodular lobe and its connections

TABLE 3: Topographical organization and cerebellar syndromes.

Topographic organization	Area involved	Syndrome	Features
Sensorimotor cerebellum	Anterior lobe and parts of lobule VI	Cerebellar motor syndrome	Dysmetria, dysarthria, ataxia, oculomotor disorders
Cognitive cerebellum	Posterior lobe, lobule VI, VII	Cerebellar cognitive affective syndrome	Executive, visuospatial, and linguistic impairments (agrammatism), and affective dysregulation
Limbic cerebellum	Vermis and paravermian area	Neuropsychiatric disorders	Anger, depression

cause cerebellar dysarthria. The cerebellar hemispheres control the posture and coordination of the limbs and hence, when affected, lead to appendicular ataxia, dysmetria, dysdiadochokinesia, rebound phenomenon, and intention tremors.[15] The clinical features and localization are summarized in **Table 2**.

The topographic distribution of cerebellar syndromes, including cerebellar motor syndrome, cerebellar cognitive affective syndrome (CCAS; Schmahmann's syndrome), and neuropsychiatric disorders are given in **Table 3**.[16] Stroke syndromes of the cerebellum occur due to the occlusion of PICA (40%), AICA (5%), SCA (35%), and watershed zone (20%).[10] The symptoms and signs vary according to the vascular territory involved.

NEUROPHYSIOLOGY

The cerebellum comprises a tightly folded layer of cortex with white matter beneath, in which the deep cerebellar nuclei (lateral to medial: dentate nucleus, emboliform nucleus, globose, and fastigial nucleus) are embedded.

Cerebellar Cortex

The cerebellar cortex has three layers: (1) the granular layer (the deepest layer), (2) the Purkinje layer (the middle layer), and (3) the molecular layer (the most superficial layer).

BOX 3 Cerebellar cortex.

- *Layers of cerebellar cortex:*
  - Granular layer
  - Purkinje layer
  - Molecular layer
- *Excitatory cells in cerebellar cortex:*
  - Unipolar brush cells
  - Glial cells
  - Granule cells
- *Inhibitory cells in cerebellar cortex:*
  - Golgi cells
  - Stellate cells
  - Basket cells
  - Purkinje cells

The cells of the cerebellar cortex are broadly divided into inhibitory cells and excitatory cells. Inhibitory cells of the cerebellar cortex are stellate cells, basket cells, Purkinje cells, and Golgi cells. Three excitatory cells of the cerebellar cortex are: (i) unipolar brush cells, (ii) glial cells, and (iii) granule cells **(Box 3)**.

The granular layer contains many granular cells (excitatory) that present a single ascending axon projecting to the molecular layer, where it splits in a T-shaped pattern, thus forming the parallel fibers.[17] Each granule cell dendrites has synaptic contact with inputs from the mossy fibers. The mossy fibers (a major afferent cerebellar pathway) coalesce to form the synaptic structure known as "glomerulus" which is nothing but a bundle of fibers.[18] The Purkinje cell layer contains flask-shaped Purkinje cells arranged in a single layer and the axons of the Purkinje cells (cell bodies in the Purkinje layer) cross the granular layer to reach the deep cerebellar nuclei, thus leading to the formation of the cerebellar efferent fibers **(Fig. 5)**. A few of the Purkinje cell axons pass directly to the end in the vestibular nuclei in the brainstem. The dendrites of the Purkinje cells undergo profuse branching in the molecular layer, making synapses both with the parallel fibers and with the axons of the stellate cells. The molecular layer contains outer stellate cells and inner basket cells, which are scattered among dendritic arborizations and many thin axons that run parallel to the long axis of the folia. Neuroglial cells are present between these structures. The cerebellar afferent fibers (mossy fibers and climbing fibers) are the excitatory pathways and activate the cerebellar cortex, which then inhibits the deep cerebellar nuclei. The cortical circuitry, therefore, operates as a feedback loop regulating the activity of the four deep cerebellar nuclei, which are the only output pathway from the cerebellum **(Fig. 6)**.

Deep Cerebellar Nuclei

The deep cerebellar nuclei are present in the white matter of the cerebellum. The cerebellar white matter has a treelike

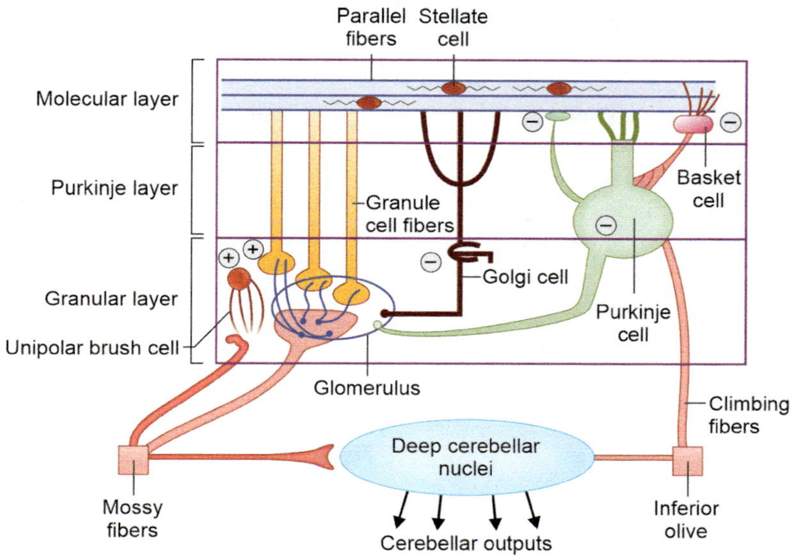

FIG. 5: Schematic representation of the cerebellar cortex.

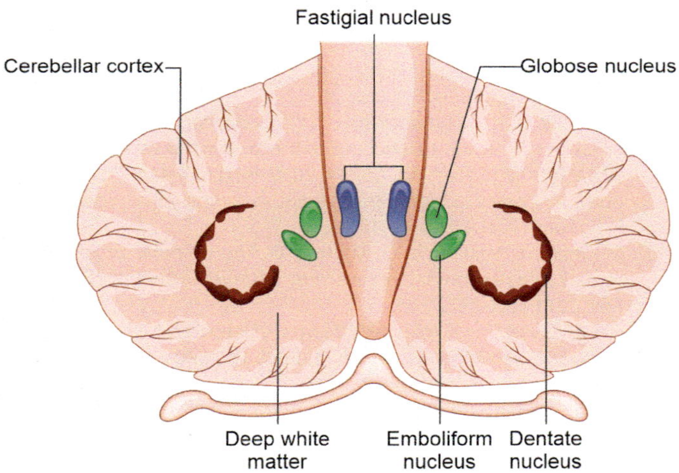

FIG. 6: Arrangement of deep cerebellar nuclei.

branching appearance known as "arbor vitae". It contains both the afferent and efferent fibers conveying sensorimotor information to and from the cerebellum. Four pairs of nuclei are present in the deep cerebellar white matter. From the medial to lateral direction, they are fastigial nuclei, globose nuclei, emboliform nuclei, and dentate nuclei **(Fig. 6)**. These deep cerebellar nuclei receive inhibitory (GABAergic) inputs from Purkinje cells in the cerebellar cortex and excitatory (glutamatergic) inputs from both the mossy fibers and climbing fiber pathways. Most output fibers of the cerebellum originate from these deep nuclei. The fibers from the flocculonodular lobe synapse directly on vestibular nuclei and have no connections to the deep cerebellar nuclei.[19]

CLINICAL RELEVANCE OF NEUROPHYSIOLOGY

The cerebellum operates as a feed-forward controller by increasing the excitatory input to the cortex. Studies of cerebellar neuronal activities in vitro and in vivo, under natural and artificial conditions, have contributed to the current knowledge and understanding of the physiologic basis underlying the motor, cognitive, and affective functions of the cerebellum. These studies explain that, along with the firing rate, the spatiotemporal firing pattern of the Purkinje cells also plays an important role in cerebellar functioning. The firing of Purkinje cells occurs as simple and complex spikes; simple spikes are single action potentials, while the complex spikes represent multiple short action potentials. Climbing fibers convey error signals to the cerebellum, which helps in adapting to the motor functions based on errors from prior movements. These fibers activate the Purkinje cells in the cerebellar cortex that control (inhibitory) the deep cerebellar nuclei. The deep cerebellar nuclei then send output signals from the cerebellum to the spinal cord, vestibular nucleus, red nucleus, and olivary nucleus.[20]

The cerebellar plasticity and learning depend on the activation timings of the climbing (afferent) fibers and parallel fibers. The differences between the two result in synergic plasticity at various synapses in the cerebellar circuitry. Defective channels in the cerebellar synapses lead to the excitability of the cells, and can also alter their firing pattern, thus leading to the varied symptoms and signs of cerebellar dysfunction/diseases.[3] Cerebellum regulates the neuronal activity in different brainstem nuclei, including the red nucleus, vestibular nuclei, and the reticular nucleus.

Along with the descending pyramidal tracts, the cerebellum modifies and modulates the firing of these nuclei. The cerebellum plays a crucial role in gait by modulating the swing and stance phases. This modification and modulation disappear when the cerebellum is inactivated or lesioned. The vestibular nucleus stimulates the alpha motor neurons, whereas the reticular nuclei and red nucleus stimulate the gamma motor neurons. Cerebellum, by controlling these nuclei, also regulates the muscle tone, myotatic reflex, and muscle contraction. The connections of the cerebellum to the premotor areas and prefrontal cortex regulate motor planning.

CONCLUSION

The cerebellum is aptly called the "little brain" because of its extensive connections to the rest of the central nervous system, including the cortex, brainstem, and spinal cord. Cerebellum plays a crucial role in motor and nonmotor control. From knowing about the role in motor function to exploring the role in cognitive functions, the cerebellum still remains a fascinating and unexplored area of research. It is imperative to know the topography, anatomy, and physiology to understand the disease process involving the cerebellum.

REFERENCES

1. Amore G, Spoto G, Ieni A, Vetri L, Quatrosi G, Di Rosa G, et al. A focus on the cerebellum: from embryogenesis to an age-related clinical perspective. Front Syst Neurosci. 2021;15:646052.
2. Solov'ev SV. The weight and linear dimensions of the human cerebellum. Neurosci Behav Physiol. 2006;36(5):479-81.
3. Roostaei T, Nazeri A, Sahraian MA, Minagar A. The human cerebellum: a review of physiologic neuroanatomy. Neurol Clin. 2014;32(4):859-69.
4. Ten Donkelaar HJ, Lammens M, Wesseling P, Thijssen HO, Renier WO. Development and developmental disorders of the human cerebellum. J Neurol. 2003;250(9):1025-36.
5. De Luca A, Cerrato V, Fucà E, Parmigiani E, Buffo A, Leto K. Sonic hedgehog patterning during cerebellar development. Cellular and molecular life sciences. 2016;73(2):291-303.
6. Voogd J, Glickstein M. The anatomy of the cerebellum. Trends Neurosci. 1998;2(9):307-13.
7. Manni E, Petrosini L. A century of cerebellar somatotopy: a debated representation. Nat Rev Neurosci. 2004;5(3):241-9.
8. Kandel ER, Schwartz JH, Jessell TM, Siegelbaum SA, Hudspeth AJ. Principles of Neural Science, 5th edition. New York: McGraw-Hill Education; 2013.
9. Standring S. The Anatomical Basis of Clinical Practice, 40th edition. Philadelphia: Elsevier Churchill Livingstone; 2008. pp. 978-80.
10. Delion M, Dinomais M, Mercier P. Arteries and veins of the cerebellum. Cerebellum (London, England). 2017;16(5):880-912.
11. Matsushima K, Yagmurlu K, Kohno M, Rhoton AL. Anatomy and approaches along the cerebellar-brainstem fissures. J Neurosurg. 2016;124(1):248-63.
12. Javalkar V, Khan M, Davis DE. Clinical manifestations of cerebellar disease. Neurol Clin. 2014;32(4):871-9.
13. Marsden JF. Cerebellar ataxia. Handb Clin Neurol. 2018;159:261-81.
14. Sokolov AA, Miall RC, Ivry RB. The cerebellum: adaptive prediction for movement and cognition. Trends Cogn Sci. 2017;21(5): 313-32.
15. Ranganathan LN. Localization of Clinical Neurology. Gurugram: Wolters Kluwer India Pvt. Ltd.; 2020.
16. Stoodley CJ, Schmahmann JD. Evidence for topographic organization in the cerebellum of motor control versus cognitive and affective processing. Cortex. 2010;46(7):831-44.
17. Buffo A, Rossi F. Origin, lineage and function of cerebellar glia. Prog Neurobiol. 2013;109:42-63.
18. Mugnaini E, Sekerková G, Martina M. The unipolar brush cell: a remarkable neuron finally receiving deserved attention. Brain Res Rev. 2011;66(1-2):220-45.
19. Habas C, van Dun K, Manto M, Marien P. Deep Cerebellar Nuclei and language, In: Mariën P, Manto M (Eds). The linguistic cerebellum. London, UK: Academic Press; 2016.
20. Habas C, Manto M. Probing the neuroanatomy of the cerebellum using tractography. Handb Clin Neurol. 2018;154:235-49.

18 CHAPTER

Applied Neuroanatomy and Neurophysiology of the Sensory System

Birinder Singh Paul, Nahush Roop Bansal, Gunchan Paul

INTRODUCTION

The sensory system is part of the nervous system that allows us to perceive sensory information both from inside the body and the outside environment. This complex system, distributed peripherally and centrally, integrates with the motor system for the normal functioning of the nervous system in the body. A sensory impulse, perceived foremost by receptors, travels through the peripheral nerves, sensory dermatomes (roots), and somatosensory pathways in the spinal cord and brainstem to eventually reach the thalamus and parietal cortex. A clear understanding of the structure and function of each of these components plays a pivotal role in delineating the site and etiology of sensory loss.

FUNDAMENTAL NEUROANATOMY AND NEUROPHYSIOLOGY

Receptors: Cutaneous Senses

Receptors can be structurally classified into encapsulated and nonencapsulated receptors.[1] Functionally, sensory receptors are of five types: (1) mechanoreceptors—which respond to mechanical deformation, (2) thermo-receptors—respond to temperature changes, (3) nociceptors—detect pain by responding to tissue damage, (4) electromagnetic—respond to light intensity and wavelengths, (5) chemoreceptors—respond to chemical changes.[2] Primary modalities of sensations subserved by distinct end organs include: Meissner corpuscles—touch; Merkel disk—pressure; Ruffini—warmth; Krause end bulbs—cold; Pacinian corpuscles—vibration; and free nerve ending—pain. The role of neural plasticity in the nociceptors is now recognized as the basis and possible interventional target for chronic pain. Hyperalgesia caused by tissue injury, nerve injury, and opioids is characterized by increased pain sensation due to the increased sensitivity of the nociceptors. Meissner's corpuscles, by virtue of their extreme sensitivity to touch, assist in close two-point tactile discrimination testing.

Peripheral Nerves

Fibers mediating superficial sensations are located in sensory or mixed sensorimotor nerves. **Table 1** depicts the fibers involved in carrying various sensations and their characteristic features. The conduction velocity is directly proportional to the fiber diameter and extent of myelination. All sensory neurons have their cell bodies in the dorsal root ganglia. The peripheral extension of these cells constitutes the sensory nerve, which is connected to several receptors in the skin, to a higher center on the other end.

Dorsal Roots and Ganglion

The central projection of the cell bodies in the dorsal root ganglia forms the posterior (dorsal) roots and enters the spinal cord. Each dorsal root receives sensation from the skin, muscles, connective tissue, tendons, joints, bones, and viscera that lie within a single body segment (somite). The nerve roots may lie in the intervertebral foramen above or below the corresponding vertebral bodies depending on their spinal level. The skin area supplied by a single spinal cord segment is called a dermatome, illustrated in **Figure 1**.

Spinal Tracts

Sensory impulses within the spinal cord travel via different tracts, each responsible for carrying a different sensation.[3] **Figure 2** illustrates the major sensory tracts of the body. They are as follows.

Posterior Column

The large myelinated fibers form the posterior column that enter the spinal cord medial to the dorsal horn and ascend upward.[4] The posterior column demonstrates somato-trophic lamination which means that the longest fibers from

TABLE 1: Neuroanatomy of different receptors and nerve fibers.

Receptor	Sensations	Fiber				Tracts involved
		Type	Myelination status	Diameter (μm)	Conduction velocity (m/s)	
Free nerve endings	Pain	A delta (fast)	Small myelinated axon	2–5	12–30	Lateral spinothalamic, spinal lemniscus
		C (slow)	Unmyelinated axon	0.4–20	0.5–2.0	
• Free nerve endings • Krause's end bulbs	Temperature	A delta	Small myelinated axon	2–5	12–30	Lateral spinothalamic, spinal lemniscus
• Free nerve endings • Merkel's disks	Light touch and pressure	A beta	Myelinated axons	5–12	30–70	Anterior spinothalamic, spinal lemniscus
Muscle spindles, Golgi tendon organs, deep tissue mechanoreceptors	Proprioception	A alpha	Myelinated axons	12–20	70–120	Posterior column, medial lemniscus
Meissner's corpuscles, Pacinian corpuscles	Vibration	A alpha	Myelinated axons	12–20	70–120	Posterior column, medial lemniscus

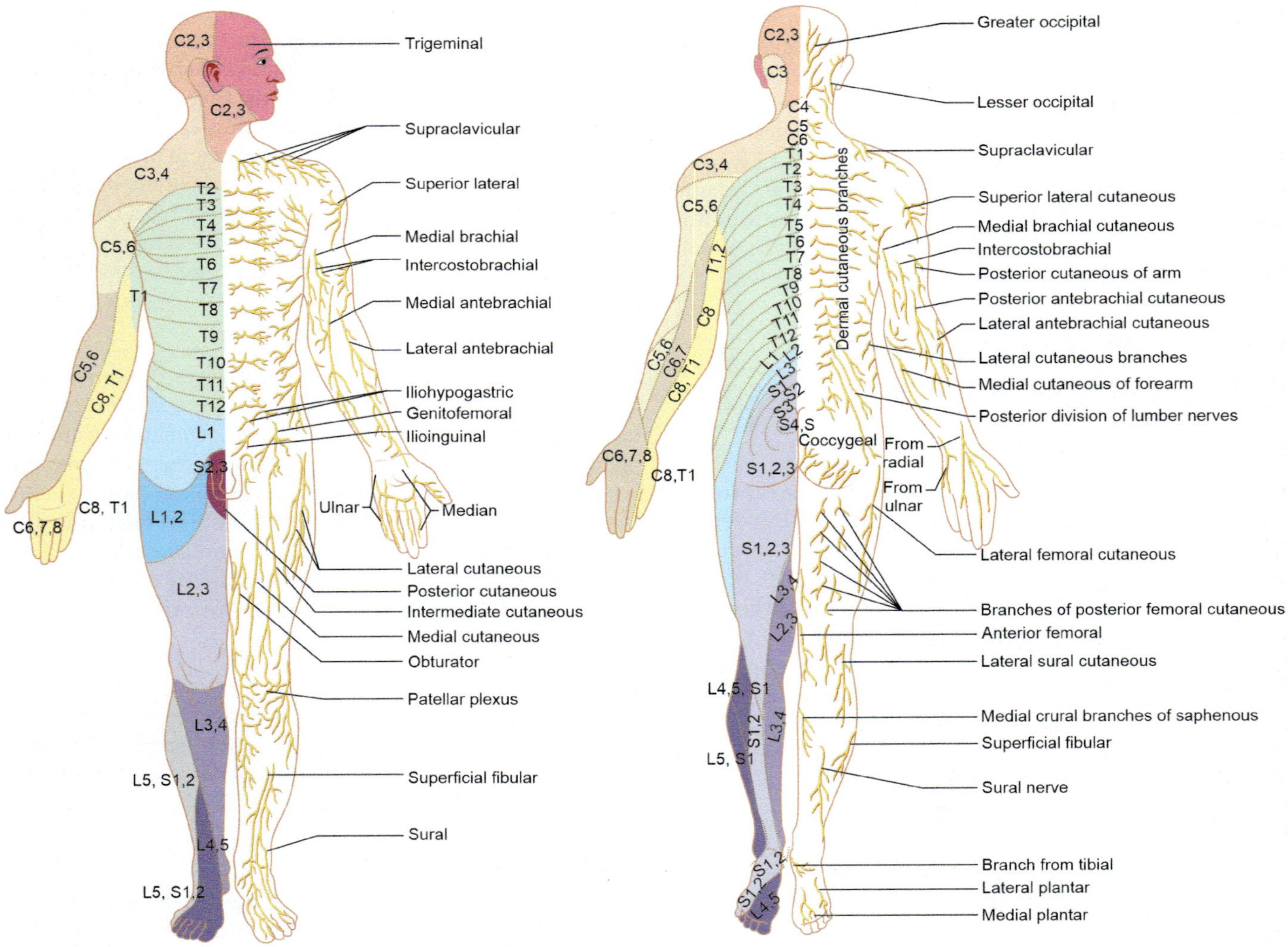

FIG. 1: Dermatomal and the individual nerve distribution in the body.

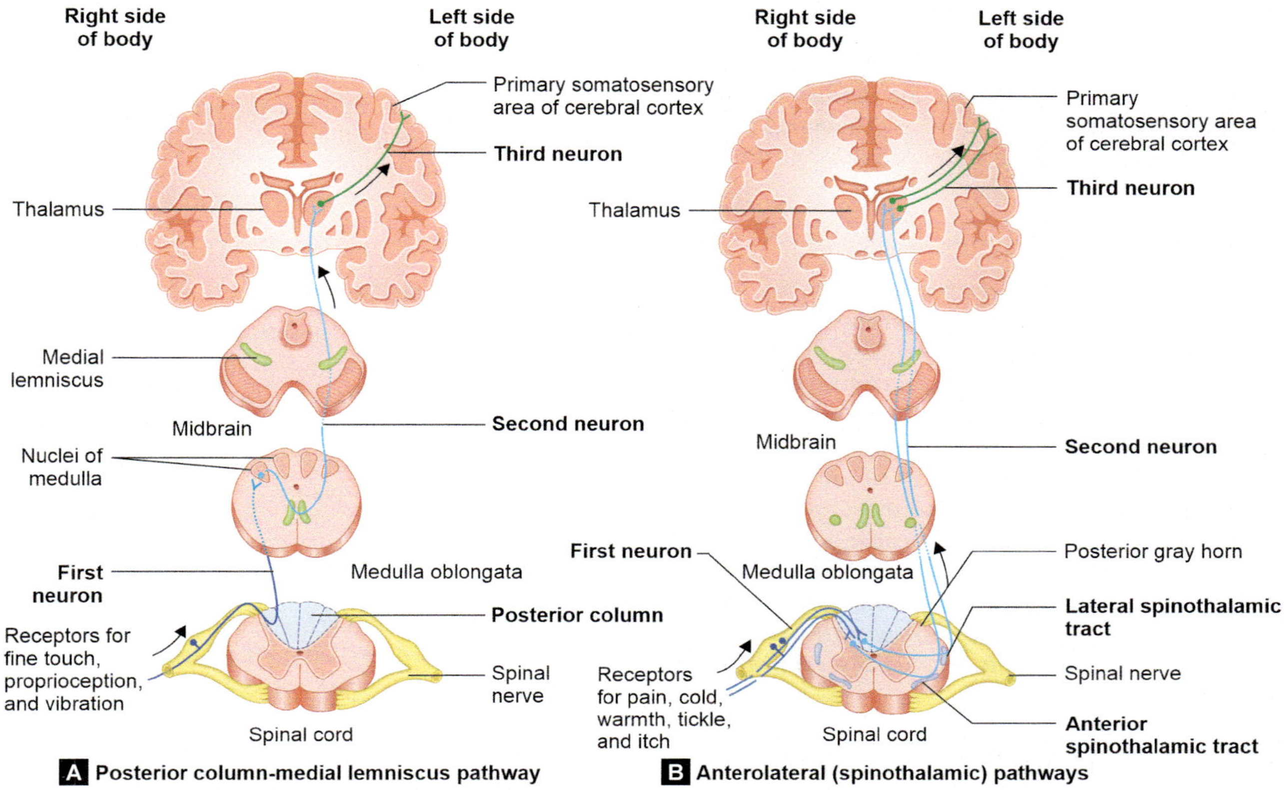

FIGS. 2A AND B: Major sensory pathways.

the sacral segments lie in the medial and deeper part, and subsequent fibers from the lumbar, thoracic, and cervical segments occupy a more lateral and superficial position. These fibers stay in the ipsilateral portion of the spinal cord to eventually synapse in the gracile and cuneate nuclei located in the upper cervical cord and medulla. The nerve cells of these nuclei give rise to a second-order neuron that crosses the midline in the medulla and ascends as medial lemniscus to the posterior thalamus. The posterior pathway is responsible for the sense of touch, vibration, direction, and position of joints.

Spinothalamic Tracts

Thin myelinated and unmyelinated fibers subserving pain, touch, temperature, and pressure enter the cord lateral to the dorsal horn. These first-order neurons ascend briefly for 1–2 segments, forming the posterolateral tract of Lissauer and synapse at a level within one to two segments of their entry point. The axons of the second-order neurons now decussate to the opposite side and ascend further as the lateral and anterior spinothalamic tracts. As these fibers ascend, the novel fibers from the consequent upper segments are added to the anteromedial aspect of the tract. Thus, in the upper cervical cord segments, the sacral and the cervical fibers occupy the most lateral and medial positions, respectively. The spinothalamic tract forms the spinal lemniscus, which travels through the brainstem to terminate at the posterior thalamic nuclei. Lateral spinothalamic tracts carry pain and temperature, whereas the anterior spinothalamic tracts are responsible for light touch and pressure sensations.

Trigeminal Tracts

For the face and head region, pathways mediating various sensations convey signals to the brainstem by the trigeminal system. The pain and temperature fibers run caudally in the medulla to terminate in the spinal trigeminal nucleus in the pons. The spinal trigeminal nucleus extends to the second and the third cervical segment of the cord. Axons of the second-order neurons arising from this nucleus cross the midline and ascend further as the trigeminal lemniscus.

Brainstem

The white matter conveying sensory signals from the various tracts passes through the brainstem before reaching the thalamus. As discussed before, unlike the spinothalamic tracts, the first-order neurons of the posterior column relay in the nuclei of the medulla oblongata. The second-order neurons from the various pathways carried in the spinal, medial, and trigeminal lemniscus also have to transcend through the brainstem and can thus be involved in lesions at this site.

Thalamus

The ventral posterior lateral (VPL) and median (VPM) thalamic nuclei are relay centers for medial lemniscal, spinal lemniscal, and trigeminal tracts. Thalamus projects the third-order neurons to the somatosensory cortex in the brain.

Cortex

The third-order neurons eventually reach the higher somatosensory regions of the brain after ascending through the internal capsule and corona radiata. The primary somatosensory area occupies the postcentral gyrus in the parietal lobe and comprises four distinct regions known as Brodmann's areas 3a, 3b, 1, and 2. In the contralateral sensory cortex, fibers have a somatotropic distribution, with the leg represented in the uppermost and the face in the lowermost portion. Accurate localization of sensory modalities (tactile location and discrimination) and the ability to recognize shapes (stereognosis) depend on the integration of information by the sensory cortex. A feedback loop from the higher centers is possibly seen at every sensory level.

CLINICAL APPLICABILITY: SENSORY EXAMINATION

Examining the sensory system is the most challenging aspect of a neurological examination as there is no measure to objectively determine or quantify the sensory loss. Given the high reliability of subjective interpretations and responsiveness, sensory examination in different subjects can demonstrate considerable variations. The sensory examination may be normal in people having symptoms and vice versa.

Sensory symptoms may be positive or negative.[5] Negative symptoms may be reported as feeling numb, lack of pain on contact, and inability to feel clothing or water while bathing. On the contrary, various descriptors may be used for abnormal positive sensations like feeling a band of tightness, an ant crawling, a needle pricking, or being wrapped in a bandage.

Testing Sensory Functions

Testing for various sensory modalities and noting the regions involved play a huge role in delineating the site and the extent of the sensory lesion. The following considerations are essential to note whenever examining the sensory system.

- Always test and compare both sides simultaneously to check for symmetry in sensory involvement.
- It is always easier for the patient to appreciate the sensory level when the physician proceeds from the abnormal area toward the normal area.
- Rather than asking leading questions like "Do you feel this?" when examining, it is a good practice to engage the patients actively. This can be done by asking patients to close their eyes and count every time they feel the sensation.[6]
- Finally, the sensory findings should be accurately noted on a chart by highlighting or shading the affected regions on the sketch of the body.

Various bedside tests to detect sensory functions are discussed here.

Testing for Tactile Sensation

This is done with a wisp of cotton. First, familiarize the patient with the stimulus applied to the normal part of the body (like the face). With eyes closed, the patient is asked to count serial numbers if he/she feels a sensation when the body parts are touched. Moving stimulus is more sensitive for detecting tactile sensory loss.

Testing for Pain Perception

It is important to underscore to the patients that they need to report the feeling of sharpness rather than just a feeling of contact of a pinpoint. Testing is done by a pinprick at an adequate speed of one per second. To compare any two areas, ask the patients to report the pin sensation on a scale of 0–100. Clear demarcation of the involved area should be done to note whether the sensory impairment corresponds to the distribution of the peripheral nerve, dermatome, or sensory tract.

Testing for Temperature Sense

This examination requires a careful assessment, considering extreme temperatures can evoke a pain sensation. Testing is done using two test tubes containing hot (45°C) and cold (20°C) tap water, with temperatures verified using a thermometer. The side of each test tube is applied successively to the skin for a few seconds, and the patient is then asked to report whether he feels hot, less hot, cold, or less cold compared to the normal part.

Testing for the Proprioceptive Sense

Proprioception testing incorporates testing for the sense of position and movement. Sense of movement is first tested in the toes and fingers by grasping the digit at the sides (not on the nail) perpendicular to the plane of movement. The digit is then gently moved 10–30° up and down. Patients are instructed to report movement as being up or down from the original position, given that they can perceive it. The test should be repeated several times to eliminate chance and compared with the opposite side.

More proximally, the knee joint proprioception can be tested by displacing the limb from its original position and asking the patients with their eyes closed to place the other leg in the same position and angle. Romberg's sign demonstrates proprioception in the axial structures. The patient is asked to stand with feet together while the examiner stands in front with arms encircling the patient.

Romberg's sign is positive when the patient sways or steps sideways or backward on closing the eyes. A positive sign indicates possible abnormalities in peripheral nerves, the posterior column, or the vestibular apparatus. Loss of proprioception can occur at higher levels and can also be demonstrated by asking the patients to stand and outstretch their arms with their eyes closed. The affected arm will wander from its original position and is accompanied by the undulating movements of fingers (pseudoathetosis).

Testing for Vibration Sense

Vibration and position senses are typically impaired in similar conditions and pathologies. Loss of vibration can also occur in the distal parts of the body like toes and ankles and can be seen in normal aging. Testing is carried out using a 128-Hz tuning fork (due to its low rate of decay and longer duration vibration) over the bony prominences. Patients should be instructed to report the feeling of buzzing and not the touch or pressure of a fork. The handle of the vibrating fork is placed over the dorsal aspect of the great toe and allowed to run down until the vibration is no longer perceived. The fork is then transferred to the corresponding part of the examiner to detect any vibration after it ceases for the patient. The perception of vibration is tested at the ankle, patella, and anterior superior iliac spine to ascertain length-dependent neuropathy or establish a level in spinal cord disorders (by testing over the spinous process of the dorsal vertebra).

Testing for Cortical Sensations

It is crucial to establish the integrity and the normalcy of the primary sensory modalities before testing discriminative sensory functions.

Two-point discrimination: It is tested by applying the blunt ends of a compass simultaneously. The minimum distance at which such stimuli can be recognized (as two separate points) varies with the body region tested; it is roughly 1 mm at the tip of the tongue, 2–3 mm on lips, 3–5 mm at the fingertips, 8–15 mm on palm, 20–30 mm on dorsal hands and feet, and 4–7 cm on the trunk. Abnormalities in two-point discrimination are characteristically seen in the lesion of the sensory cortex.

Graphesthesia: Testing graphesthesia for tactile or painful stimuli is done by touching various points on the patient's body and asking him to place the finger on the point stimulated. Recognition of the letters or numbers traced on the skin (letters or numbers should be more than 4 cm in size) is another method of testing this cortical sensation. Identifying the direction of a line drawn across the skin can also be done for patients with low literacy.

Appreciation of texture, shape, and size (stereognosis): Testing for stereognosis is performed by asking the patients to recognize and identify the objects by palpating them with closed eyes. Inability to do so (astereognosis) is seen in the right or left hemisphere lesions leading to the abnormality on the opposite side.

CLINICAL RELEVANCE: LOCALIZATION OF SENSORY ABNORMALITIES

Sensory abnormalities can present in variable patterns in the terms of type of modalities affected and the area involved. Recognition of the pattern of sensory involvement forms the foundation for accurate localization **(Table 2)**.

Peripheral Nerve

A lesion solely in the peripheral nerve is known as neuropathy, which can be mono or poly depending on the number of nerves involved. Compression of the nerve is the most common cause of mononeuropathy, which manifests initially with paresthesias followed by progressive loss of various sensations. Loss of tactile and vibration sense occurs first, followed by the loss of cold and heat sensations in the anatomical distribution of the affected nerve. Certain provocative maneuvers that can provide essential clues in diagnosing mononeuropathies include the Tinel sign, which is characterized by a tingling sensation felt upon repetitive tapping of the regenerating peripheral nerve. Some tests are more specific to detect nerve involvement; for instance, the Phalen sign, characterized by paresthesias in the median nerve territory on wrist flexion, helps to diagnose carpal tunnel syndrome.

Polyneuropathy is typically characterized by sensory anomalies accompanied by varying degrees of motor and reflex loss.[7] The characteristic stocking and glove distribution of sensory loss in the lower and upper limbs is due to the involvement of long and large sensory fibers.[8] Neuropathies can occur due to demyelination, axonal damage, or both. Demyelinating neuropathies cause a disproportionate loss of the position and vibration sensations with a relative sparing of the pain and temperature, whereas the opposite pattern is seen in axonal neuropathies. This can be attributed to large-fiber involvement in the demyelinating neuropathies and small myelinated/unmyelinated fiber involvement in the axonal types. Nerve conduction velocity (NCV) studies also aid in differentiating as demyelinating disorders are primarily associated with slowed conduction velocities, whereas reduced amplitudes are predominant in axonal damage. Guillain–Barré syndrome is a typical example of demyelinating neuropathy whereas length-dependent axonal neuronopathies are seen in many clinical conditions such as diabetes, excessive alcohol consumption, vitamin B12 deficiency, and amyloidosis.

Dorsal Ganglion (Sensory Neuronopathy)

Lesions of the dorsal root ganglion lead to a dermatomal sensory loss pattern. Widespread involvement of sensory

TABLE 2: Common patterns of sensory abnormalities.

Pattern of sensory loss	Description	Site of lesion	Etiology
Distal sensory loss	Loss in the distal portion of limbs, typically legs > arms	Peripheral nerve (length-dependent neuropathy)	Peripheral neuropathy due to metabolic (diabetes, uremia), toxic (alcoholism, chemotherapy), infective (leprosy, HIV)
Proximal sensory loss	Loss in the trunk region with sparing of the limbs	Peripheral nerve with predominantly proximal involvement	Neuropathy due to—diabetes, porphyria, inflammatory demyelinating neuropathy
Dermatomal sensory loss	Pain and/or loss in the dermatome of a single nerve root	Nerve root involvement	Radiculopathy due to disk herniation, tumor, osteophytes
Whole-limb sensory loss	Loss of sensations in the entire limb completely	Plexus or involvement of multiple nerves simultaneously	Autoimmune plexitis, mechanical compression (hematoma, tumor, or infiltration)
Crossed sensory loss	Involvement of ipsilateral face and contralateral body	Brainstem lesions	Lateral medullary syndrome
Loss of different sensory modalities on different sides of body	Pain and temperature loss on right side and vibration and proprioception loss on the left side (or vice versa)	Spinal cord lesions	Hemisection of the spinal cord (Brown–Sequard syndrome)
Dissociated or suspended sensory loss	Selective loss of one sensory modality like pain and temperature and sparing of other sensory modality	Spinal cord lesions affecting only a single type of tract	• Syringomyelia • Posterior cord syndrome
Sacral sparing	Sensory loss in the legs and trunks with preserved perianal sensations	Spinal cord lesions predominantly affecting the central portion of the cord	Trauma, intrinsic tumors of cord

ganglia can cause a sensory loss in the body's proximal areas, including the face, oral mucosa, trunk, and genitalia.[9] Additionally, loss of proprioception and deep tendon reflexes is evident in the distal and proximal body parts. A positive Romberg sign depicting sensory ataxia and pseudo athetoid movements of fingers on clinical examination are classical features of sensory neuronopathy. The recognition of this pattern is vital for diagnosing sensory neuronopathies, commonly seen in paraneoplastic syndrome (anti-Hu),[10] Sjögren syndrome, toxic/drug exposure, or inflammatory disorders.

Pain originating from the nerve roots is described as radicular pain. Radicular pain is characterized by its sharp and shooting nature (lancinating) typically going along the course of nerve roots. Features such as numbness, tingling, muscle weakness, and loss of reflexes may also be present. Given the vulnerable location of the nerve roots, they can be easily compressed by various spinal pathologies, including disk herniation, degenerative disk disease, osteoarthritis of the spine, epidural abscess, and spinal tumors. The surface anatomy of the dermatomes of the sensory nerve roots is the most helpful guide for the localization of the lesion. However, it is crucial to note that there is considerable overlap in the dermatomal supply of nerve roots, and a sound clinical judgment is necessary to delineate the affected roots. The extent of overlapping is more at certain locations (more in the trunk than extremities) and is more for certain sensations (more for pain and thermal sensations as opposed to tactile sensations).

Spinal Cord

Sensory Spinal Cord Syndromes

Based upon the level and the portion of the spinal cord affected, patients may have sensory loss ranging across various modalities and involving different body parts. **Table 3** depicts an overview of various spinal cord syndromes.

Complete cord syndrome: Complete transverse disruption of the spinal cord characteristically causes loss of motor functions and loss of all forms of sensation below the level corresponding to the lesion site. Given the spinothalamic tract's pathway, the loss of pain, temperature, and crude touch begins one to two segments below the lesion. A narrow zone of hyperesthesia may be noticed above the anesthetic zone. Impairment in the bowel, bladder, sexual, and motor function is also noticed in the complete cord syndrome.

Central cord syndrome: The central portion of the spinal cord is constituted primarily by the decussating spinothalamic fibers in the anterior commissure. Hence, any lesion here will lead to loss of pain and temperature but will preserve the tactile sensations carried by the posterior column. This

TABLE 3: Spinal cord syndromes.

Syndrome	Area affected (representative diagram)	Sensory tracts affected	Ipsilateral sensory findings	Contralateral sensory findings	Accompanying symptoms	Etiology
Complete cord syndrome	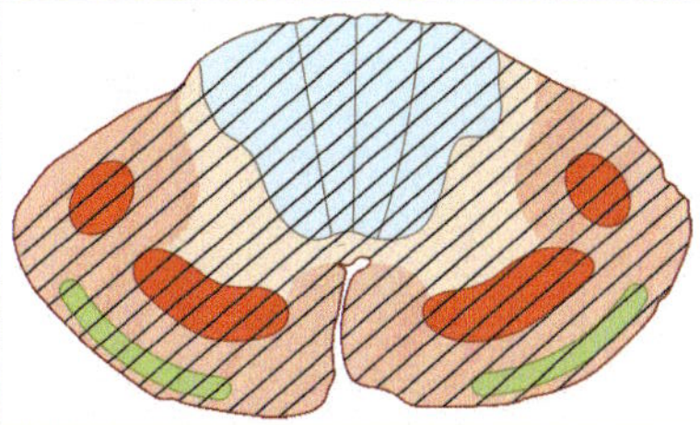	All the sensory tracts are affected bilaterally	Loss of all sensory modalities below the level of lesion		• Bowel, bladder, and sexual dysfunction • Motor and autonomic impairment	Transverse myelitis (infective, inflammatory)
Central cord syndrome	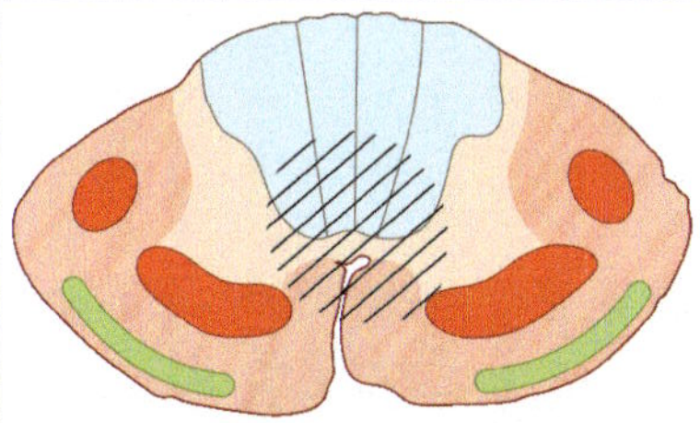	Lateral and anterior spinothalamic tracts (anterior commissure decussation)	None	Loss of pain and temperature 1–2 segments below the lesion	In the advanced stages, it can cause flaccid paralysis and reflex loss at lesion level, and spastic paralysis below lesion	• Syringomyelia • Intramedullary tumor • Spondylosis
Brown–Sequard syndrome	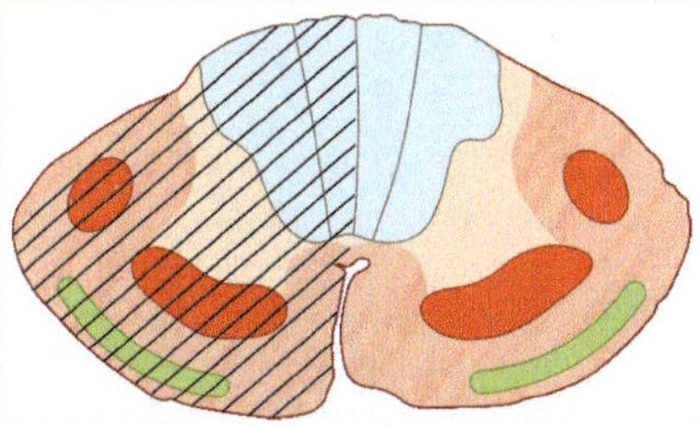	• Lateral and anterior spinothalamic tracts • Dorsal column	Loss of proprioception, vibration, and fine touch below the lesion	Loss of pain and temperature 1–2 segments below the lesion	• Ipsilateral flaccid paralysis at the lesion level and spastic paralysis below the level • Ipsilateral Horner syndrome for lesions above T1	• Multiple sclerosis • Trauma (sharp edge injury or bullet injury) • Compression
Posterior cord syndrome	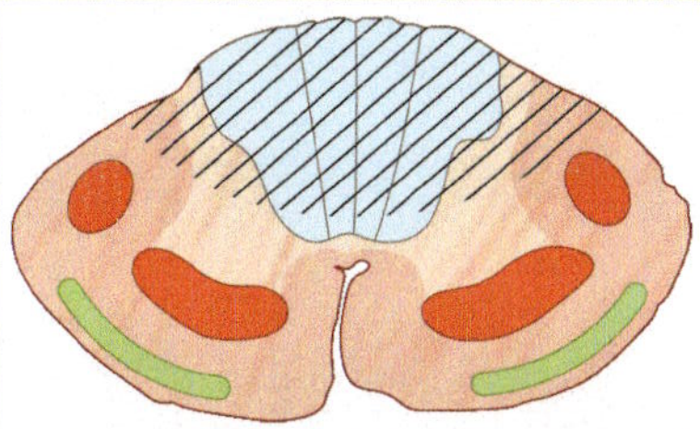	Dorsal column	Loss of proprioception, vibration, and fine touch below the lesion	None	"Lhermitte sign"—transient electric shock like sensation extending down the spine and extremities upon neck flexion	• Posterior spinal artery occlusion • Cervical spondylosis (posterior) • Multiple sclerosis
Anterior cord syndrome	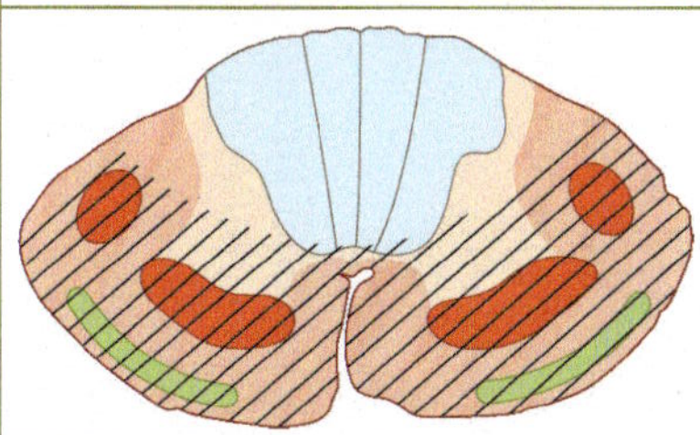	Bilateral lateral and anterior spinothalamic tracts	Cause loss of pain and temperature over the whole body 1–2 segments below the level of lesion		• Flaccid paralysis and reflex loss at lesion level • Bladder typically involved • Spastic paralysis below the lesion	• Anterior spinal artery occlusion • Trauma

selective loss of sensory modalities, known as dissociative sensory loss, is a hallmark feature of central cord syndrome. Typically, the upper limbs are involved more than the lower limbs. Associated segmental amyotrophy and reflex loss are also seen at the same segmental level. As the lesion expands further, the involvement of other tracts like the corticospinal tracts occurs. Common causes of central cord syndrome are centrally located developmental or acquired syringomyelia, intramedullary tumor, and trauma. The closest differential diagnosis is pseudosyringomyelia syndrome, which is related to small-fiber neuropathies.

Hemisection cord syndrome (Brown-Sequard syndrome): A lesion confined to one side of the cord causes contralateral loss of pain and temperature sensations beginning from one or two segments below the lesion and ipsilateral loss of proprioception from just below the lesion. Fracture dislocation of the vertebral column by a bullet or a stab wound, or an expanding tumor, can lead to hemisection of the cord.

Posterior column syndrome: Complete and selective lesion of the posterior column leads to ipsilateral loss of vibration and position sense below the level of lesion with a relative sparing of temperature and pain sensation. Clinically, the patients may report a characteristic girdle or band-like sensation or diffuse burning pain. Etiologies leading to posterior cord syndrome include multiple sclerosis, vitamin B12 deficiency, copper deficiency, HIV infection, and tabes dorsalis. A key feature that distinguishes between large-fiber neuropathy and posterior column lesions where both present with disproportionate loss of vibration and position is the examination of reflexes. Deep tendon reflexes will be intact in the posterior column lesions but lost in the neuropathies.

Anterior cord syndrome: The most typical cause of anterior cord syndrome is spinal cord infarction in the anterior spinal artery territory, affecting the ventral portion of the cord. The hallmark feature is loss of pain and temperature sensation below the level of the lesion with the sparing of position and vibration sense (posterior column). Accompanying paraparesis is seen due to corticospinal tract involvement.

Brainstem

Based on the fiber arrangement, various sensory modalities are affected in different lesions affecting the brainstem. A classical syndrome is the Wallenberg syndrome (lateral medullary infarction), presenting with crossed sensory abnormalities. It is characterized by ipsilateral loss of pain and temperature on the face and a contralateral loss of the same sensations in the body. This pattern occurs due to the involvement of the ipsilateral trigeminal tract and crossed spinothalamic tract on the side of the infarcted brainstem region.

In the upper medulla and lower pons, the crossed spinothalamic and the uncrossed trigeminothalamic tracts run together to cause characteristic loss of pain and temperature on the opposite half of the face and the body. Additional features may include cranial nerve palsies, cerebellar ataxia, and motor paralysis. Isolated sensory loss in the brainstem lesions is rare.

In the upper pons and the midbrain, the spinal and medial lemniscus become confluent and are thus involved together in lesions. This leads to contralateral loss of all the sensory modalities in the body.

Thalamus

The thalamic lesions can be attributed most commonly to hemorrhage or thrombosis in the arterial supply system or damage occurring due to neoplastic invasion. Involvement of the ventral posterolateral and ventral posteromedial nucleus will lead to the loss of all sensory modalities on the opposite side of the body. When a patient recovers from a thalamic infarct, the severe debilitating pain occurring in the body opposite to the side of the lesion is known as *thalamic pain*. This type of pain is characterized by spontaneous onset, hyperarousal to light stimuli, and a failure to respond to potent analgesics.

Cortex

Cortical sensory loss can be noticed when the parietal area is affected by stroke. If the somatosensory cortex is impaired, the thalamus can provide awareness of primary sensory modalities. However, corresponding to the cortex functions, the patients lose the ability to localize, discriminate, and quantify the intensity of sensations. The characteristic loss of discriminative sensations like stereognosis and graphesthesia is seen in the cortical sensory loss.

Key phenomena recognized only in the cortical sensory losses are sensory extinction, neglect, or inattention. Sensory extinction is illustrated by the simultaneous application of stimuli on both sides of the body and the patient's ability to perceive only one stimulus on the affected side of the body. Hemi-neglect is seen when the nondominant parietal lobe is affected. This is characterized by complete ignorance of the contralateral half of the body and extra personal space.

Functional Sensory Loss

Distinguishing the subjective functional sensory complaints from an actual organic pathology can be challenging. It can be done by eliciting the presence of any accompanying nonorganic symptoms and by noting variations in the sensory loss distribution displayed by the patient from the known anatomically consistent patterns. For instance, a person complaining of sensory loss in the lower half of the face (trigeminal distribution) can be rendered functional if there is a concomitant loss of sensations behind the angle of the mandible (C2 distribution) due to anatomical discrepancy. Other common complaints which can direct a physician toward functional over organic etiology include complete hemisensory loss with a sharp midline demarcation, reduced hearing and vision on one side, and impaired vibration sense just over one-half of the sternum or skull.

ELECTROPHYSIOLOGICAL EVALUATION

History and neurological examination provide information but sometimes may not be enough to define the nature of pathologic changes in nerve involvement. Electrophysiological studies play an essential role in the detailed characterization of pathology, especially when imaging can be equivocal as in functional sensory symptoms such as nonorganic neuropathies. Electrodiagnostic tests include nerve conduction studies (motor and sensory) and needle electromyography (EMG) studies. Sensory nerve conduction testing demonstrates abnormalities in sensory transmission, thus providing objective evidence of sensory system disease, which may be crucial for the diagnosis.[11] This testing significantly enhances diagnostic accuracy by assessing the functional integrity of sensory nerve fibers.

The standard sensory electrophysiological examination typically consists of nerve conduction studies and somatosensory evoked potentials (SEPs) to non-noxious stimuli. These techniques, widely available, explore the non-nociceptive pathways, namely large myelinated (Aβ) fibers in the periphery and the dorsal column-medial lemniscus at the central level. Additionally, evaluating thermonociceptive pathways (peripheral nerve fibers, dorsal roots, or spinothalamic–cortical systems) is crucial for the objective evaluation of common sensory complaints like neuropathic pain. These specific pathways are activated by heat stimuli or laser pulses.

The sensory response is recorded as the sensory nerve action potential (SNAP), representing the sum of a single nerve fiber action potential either orthodromically in the direction of normal nerve conduction or antidromically when measured in the distal part of the major peripheral nerves. The primary goal of sensory nerve conduction studies is the assessment of: (1) the number of functioning axons (amplitude of SNAP) and (2) the degree of myelination in the nerves (conduction velocity of SNAP).

In axonal neuropathies (common prototype-diabetic), the primary feature is a marked reduction in SNAP as there is a linear relationship between the number of axons lost and the amplitude of SNAP while conduction velocity is slightly reduced or preserved. In contrast, demyelinating neuropathies [common prototype—acute/chronic inflammatory demyelinating polyneuropathy (AIDP/CIDP)] lead to a profound slowing in conduction velocity with or without minor alterations in the action potential.

Sensory nerve conduction testing, in some instances, may become abnormal earlier in the course of a disease relative to motor nerve conduction parameters. Additionally, abnormalities in sensory nerves localize the anatomic basis of lesions, especially in carpal tunnel syndrome or entrapment neuropathies in which motor fibers are spared. A normal SNAP and velocity in the presence of active sensory complaints like numbness indicate a pathologic process proximal to the dorsal root ganglion or may suggest a functional sensory deficit. These facts emphasize the need to clinically correlate the sensory abnormalities in electrophysiology with the sensory examination.

Quantitative sensory testing (QST) is the preferred method in addition to NCV studies in patients with small-fiber neuropathies or painful sensory neuropathies. QST uses graded and reproducible stimuli for estimating sensory and nociceptive thresholds for assessing small-fiber neuropathies. However, QST is not an objective test as it relies on the patient's subjective response. The electrophysiological recording of neural responses, on the bright side, can assess and quantify somatosensory deficits to a variety of calibrated peripheral sensory stimuli. Electrical, thermal, vibration, or tactile stimuli are chosen to assess distinct neuroanatomic pathways with discrete fiber populations. Abnormal QST suggests that the lesion can lie anywhere along the sensory pathway between the receptor apparatus and the primary sensory cortex. The quantitation of an individual patient's sensory perceptions, when compared with normative values, gives a clearer distinction between normal and abnormal responses.

CONCLUSION

Lesions in the entire sensory pathways from the receptors to the cortex can present with some unique and overlapping features. **Table 4** summarizes the localizing features of the sensory lesions at different sites. A sound sensory examination, supplemented with electrophysiological testing, is vital to localize and determine the extent of the lesion. When examining, noting the type of sensory modalities impaired is as important as marking the area affected. Loss of certain modalities, in isolation or combination, can assist in establishing the site of the lesion. For instance, isolated impairment of touch and pinprick sensations indicate a likely peripheral nerve lesion. Similarly, isolated loss of pain and temperature indicate a spinothalamic lesion whereas isolated loss of vibration and proprioception point toward posterior column lesion. The involvement of higher centers in the thalamus and the internal capsule is indicated by the loss of all sensory modalities on one side of the body. For establishing the definitive etiology of sensory abnormality, it is necessary to correlate the sensory findings to the accompanying symptoms of motor and autonomic involvement.

TABLE 4: Sensory localization of different lesion sites.

Sensory lesion site	Sensory loss pattern	Distribution	Characteristics	Accompanying symptoms	Other features	EMG studies
Peripheral nerves	Pan sensory loss involving all modalities	• Individual nerve distribution (mononeuropathy) • Symmetrical glove and stocking distribution (polyneuropathy)	Tingling may be described as pins or needles sensation	Loss of reflexes and weakness of the muscle supplied by the nerve	Distal areas of limb are usually affected first	Drop SNAP
Nerve root	• Sensory loss can be seen in various extents • May be absent in some cases	Dermatomal distribution	Radicular pain—sharp and shooting pain	• Loss of reflexes pertaining to the involved dermatome • Involvement of two or more adjacent roots leads to sensory symptoms corresponding to the plexus division	• Pain is worsened by maneuvers that increased intraspinal pressure like cough, sneeze or straining • Moving the limb to stretch the nerve root (like SLR) may worsen pain	Preserved SNAP
Spinal cord	Affected sensory modalities depend on the extent and site of lesion in spinal cord	A definitive sensory level is present with a band of hyperesthesia at upper level	• Sensations described in dorsal column lesions • Band or girdle like diffuse burning sensation	• Depending on extent and site of lesion, may have paralysis • Bowel and bladder involvement • Ipsilateral Horner syndrome above the T1	• Depending on the syndrome, patients may have a dissociative or a suspended sensory loss • Sacral sparing	Normal
Thalamus	Complete loss of all sensory modalities	Contralateral body, including the face is involved	Thalamic pain is characterized by spontaneous onset, extreme sensitivity to touch and failure to respond to analgesics	• Sensory loss may split the midline • Sensory loss without weakness is highly suggestive of pure thalamic lesion	Sensory ataxia involving contralateral body	Normal
Cerebral cortex	Loss of cortical sensations like stereognosis, graphesthesia, and tactile discrimination	Contralateral body is involved corresponding to the homunculus affected by lesion	None	Nondominant parietal lobe lesion leads to complete inattention and sensory extinction on the contralateral side	In pure cortical loss, all the primary sensory modalities like pain, temperature, and proprioception are intact	Normal

(EMG: electromyography; SLR: straight leg raising; SNAP: sensory nerve action potential)

REFERENCES

1. Splittgerber R. Snell's Clinical Neuroanatomy, 8th edition. Philadelphia: Wolters Kluwer; 2019.
2. Johnson KO. The roles and functions of cutaneous mechanoreceptors. Curr Opin Neurobiol. 2001;11(4):455-61.
3. DeMyer W. Chapter 31. Anatomy and clinical neurology of the spinal cord. In: Baker AB, Baker LH (Eds). Clinical Neurology. Philadelphia: Harper and Row; 1984.
4. Ropper A, Samuels M, Klein J, Prasad S. Adams and Victor's Principles of Neurology, 11th edition. New York: Mc Graw Hill Education; 2019.
5. Brazis PW, Masdeu JC, Biller J. Localization in Clinical Neurology, 8th edition. Philadelphia: Wolters Kluwer; 2022.
6. Campbell WW. DeJong's The Neurologic Examination, 7th edition. Philadelphia: Wolters Kluwer; 2013.
7. Watson JC, Dyck PJ. Peripheral neuropathy: a practical approach to diagnosis and symptom management. Mayo Clin Proc. 2015; 90(7):940-51.
8. Gwathmey KG, Pearson KT. Diagnosis and management of sensory polyneuropathy. BMJ. 2019;365:l1108.
9. Sheikh SI, Amato AA. The dorsal root ganglion under attack: the acquired sensory ganglionopathies. Pract Neurol. 2010;10(6): 326-34.
10. Camdessanché JP, Antoine JC, Honnorat J, Vial C, Petiot P, Convers P, et al. Paraneoplastic peripheral neuropathy associated with anti–Hu antibodies: A clinical and electrophysiological study of 20 patients. Brain. 2002;125(1):166-75.
11. Daroff RB, Jankovic J, Mazziotta JC, Pomeroy S. Bradley's Neurology in Clinical Practice, 7th edition. New York: Elsevier; 2016.

19

CHAPTER

Applied Neuroanatomy and Neurophysiology of the Urinary Bladder

Lakshmi Narasimhan Ranganathan, Srividhya S, Durgam Sathya Tejaswini, Guhan Ramamurthy

INTRODUCTION

The kidneys filter around 180 L of blood per day excreting nearly 1 L as urine, which is transported through the ureters to the bladder. The ureters pass obliquely through the bladder wall and form a one-way valve at the uretero-vesicular junction to prevent the retrograde reflux of urine from the bladder to the kidneys. It is the oblique course of the ureter that maintains this one-way valve mechanism.[1]

The bladder is divided into dome or the body, consisting of smooth muscle called detrusor, and the base which includes the trigone and the bladder neck. The bladder outlet has two sphincters—(1) internal (smooth muscle) and (2) external (striated muscle) urethral sphincters.

The lower urinary tract (LUT) function is controlled by neural pathways which are organized in the form of a simple switching-on-off mechanism to maintain a reciprocal relationship between urinary bladder and urethral outlet. The two important phases of LUT activity are storage and voiding.

The neural control of the urinary tract can be viewed as:

- Afferent connections
- Efferent connections
- Central control

The central control can further be classified as:

- Cortical
- Subcortical
- Brainstem
- Spinal

AFFERENT CONNECTIONS OF THE BLADDER

Afferent connections of bladder start from the urothelium, carried by pelvic nerves to spinal cord and from there to periaqueductal gray (PAG) matter.

Urothelium

- It prevents the passage of toxins in the urine into the bladder interstitial tissue, thereby acting as a passive barrier.
- A few sensory nerve fibers also extend through the urothelium into the bladder cavity to transduce both physical and chemical stimuli.
- Chemical mediators such as acetylcholine (ACh), adenosine triphosphate (ATP), and nitric oxide (NO) are released by urothelium, which either excite or inhibit bladder afferents. The urothelium may also express muscarinic, adrenergic, or purinergic receptors.
- It also communicates with the afferent nerves, because of its sensory and signaling properties.

Afferent Axons

- Afferent information on bladder filling is transmitted by sensory fibers in the dense suburothelial and muscular plexuses.
- The pelvic, hypogastric, and pudendal nerves carry afferent axons which transmit information from the LUT to the second order neurons in the lumbo-sacral spinal cord.
- Pelvic nerve afferents are divided into small myelinated A delta fibers and unmyelinated C fibers. Both synapse in the caudal lumbosacral dorsal root ganglia and the main neurotransmitter involved is glutamate.
- The A delta fibers transmit sensory information related to bladder wall distention and trigger micturition, whereas C fibers respond to painful stimuli. Most of the C fibers are inactive during normal micturition but can get activated in pathological conditions such as suprasacral spinal cord injury. Moreover, the C fibers have a high activation threshold and mediate a spinal micturition reflex (apparent after spinal transection).[2]

Spinal Cord

- Sacral afferent pathways from the pelvic nerve project into Lissauer's tract at the apex of the dorsal horn and send collaterals both laterally and medially around the dorsal horn into laminae 5–7 and 10. Central terminations of pudendal nerve afferent pathways are similar to those of other bladder afferents in laminae 1, 5–7, and lamina 10. Many bladder afferent nerve fibers project to the sacral parasympathetic nucleus and synapse with both preganglionic neurons and local interneurons mediating the segmental spinal reflexes.[3]
- The sensation of bladder filling is carried by the posterior column whereas pain is carried through the spinothalamic tracts.

Higher Centers

- The sensory information from dorsal horn is transmitted rostrally to the PAG region.
- Some ascending projections terminate in the gracile nucleus and parabrachial nucleus, both of which convey the afferent input from the bladder to the thalamus and insular cortex (IC).

EFFERENT CONNECTIONS TO THE BLADDER

The LUT is innervated by three sets of peripheral nerves involving the parasympathetic, sympathetic, and the somatic nervous systems **(Fig. 1)**.

Parasympathetic

Parasympathetic excitatory transmission to the bladder is mediated by ACh acting on postjunctional muscarinic receptors. Both M2 and M3 receptor subtypes are expressed in the bladder smooth muscle, with M3 subtype being the principal receptor.[3] Activation of M3 receptors triggers intracellular calcium release whereas activation of M2 receptors inhibits adenyl cyclase. Activation of the muscarinic receptors produces detrusor contractions while parasympathetic activation in the proximal urethra causes release of NO leading to urethral smooth muscle relaxation. Stimulation of parasympathetic nerves also produces noncholinergic contraction mediated by ATP. ATP excites the smooth muscle by acting on the P2X receptors which are ligand gated ion channels, called as purinergic transmission.[3] Purinergic transmission appears to play an important role in pathological conditions such as detrusor overactivity or chronic urethral outlet obstruction.

Sympathetic

Sympathetic preganglionic pathways that arise from T11-L2 spinal segments can synapse either in the sympathetic chain ganglia, or the prevertebral ganglia (such as the inferior mesenteric plexus), or in the paravertebral ganglia (superior hypogastric and pelvic plexuses) or also to the short adrenergic neurons in the bladder and urethra.[4] Sympathetic postganglionic nerves that release norepinephrine provide an excitatory input to the smooth muscle of the urethra and bladder base and an inhibitory input to the detrusor muscle, and an inhibitory input to the vesical parasympathetic ganglia.

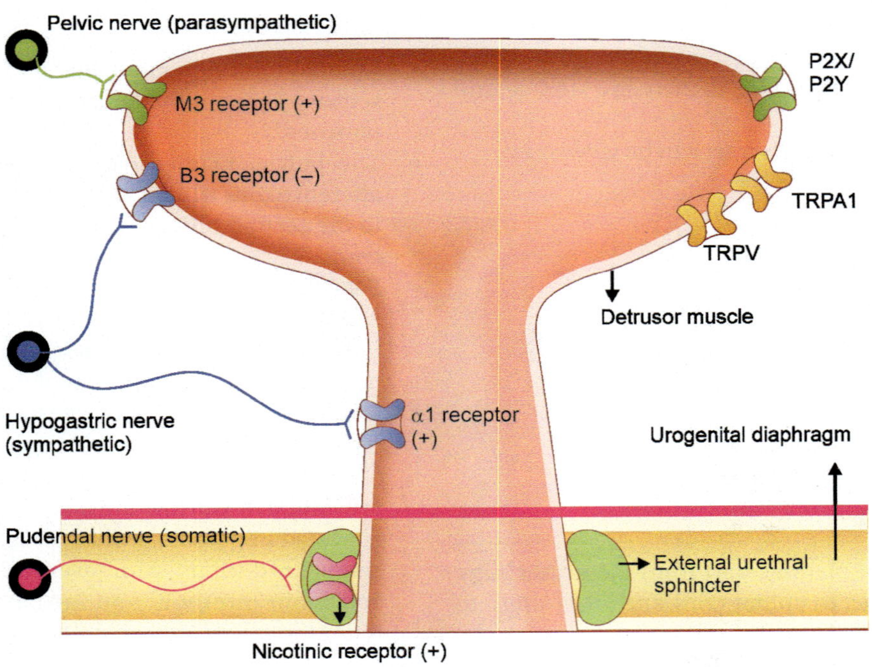

FIG. 1: Receptors in the neural control of bladder.

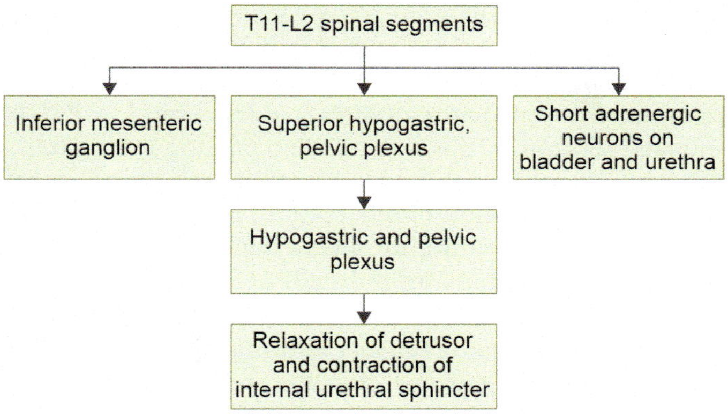

FLOWCHART 1: Sympathetic supply to bladder.

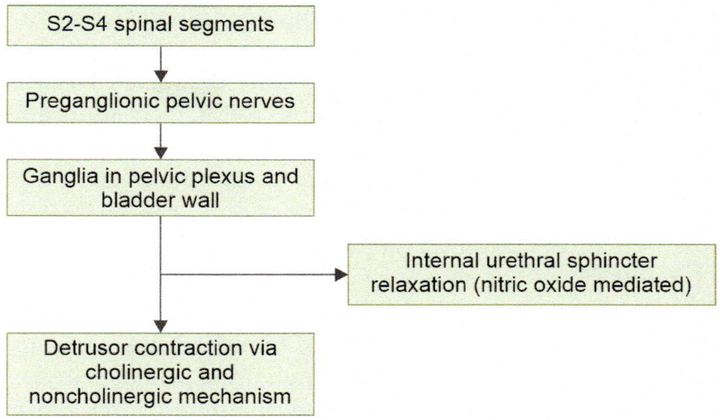

FLOWCHART 2: Parasympathetic supply to bladder.

Alpha adrenergic receptors (alpha-1a, alpha-1d, and alpha-2) are concentrated in the bladder base and proximal urethra whereas beta adrenergic receptors (beta-3) are more prominent in the bladder body.[3] The neurotransmitter involved in sympathetic postganglionic nerves is norepinephrine, which causes relaxation of detrusor muscle via the beta-3 receptors and contraction of bladder neck through alpha-1 receptors. They also inhibit synaptic transmission in the parasympathetic ganglia through alpha-2 receptors. The alpha-1A adrenergic receptor subtype is most prominent in a normal bladder the alpha-1B subtype receptor is upregulated in bladder outlet obstruction.[5]

Somatic

External urethral sphincter (EUS) motor neurons are located in the Onuf's nucleus in the ventral horn of the sacral spinal cord (S2–S4). Efferent connections from the cortical and subcortical micturition centers descend through the pyramidal tracts to the pudendal nuclei (Onuf's nucleus), whose motor neurons, carried via the pudendal nerve innervate the striated EUS.[6] Muscle supplied by the pudendal nerve include ischiocavernosus, erector clitoritis (males), bulbospongiosus (females), EUS, external anal sphincter, and levator ani. Hence, it plays a major role in erection, ejaculation, urinary, and fecal continence. Onuf's nucleus does not have recurrent inhibition system mediated by Renshaw cells (inhibitory interneurons). This allows tonic contraction of EUS.[3]

Sympathetic, parasympathetic, and somatic controls are summarized in **Flowcharts 1 to 3**, respectively.

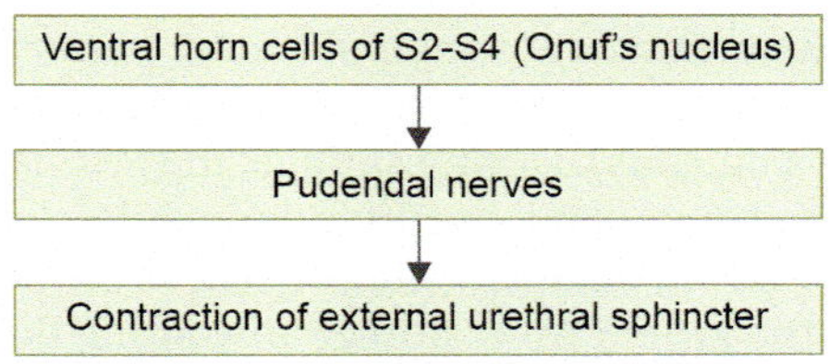

FLOWCHART 3: Somatic supply to bladder.

CENTRAL CONTROL

Cortical and Subcortical Control

There are three forebrain circuits involved in storage and voiding:

1. *Circuit 1—prefrontal cortex*: The medial prefrontal cortex (MPFC), which is a part of default mode network (DMN) is activated during voiding and has a role in the voluntary control of micturition. In case of involuntary voiding or leakage, the excitatory input from the insula reduces the output to the MPFC via inhibitory connections, resulting in MPFC deactivation and thus leads to reduced input to the PAG. This helps in maintaining continence.[3,6,7]
2. *Circuit 2—anterior cingulate cortex (ACC), insula and supplementary motor area (SMA)*: Salience network, involving ACC, IC, and supplemental motor area (SMA), is associated with generation of sensation of filling, desire to void, however, it promotes continence, when emotionally inappropriate. The insula receives afferent input from the spinal cord, after a relay in the thalamus. Afferent information regarding the degree of bladder filling is the most critical part of this input. This has been evidenced by the presence of insular activation during the storage phase of micturition. The activation of the ACC suppresses voiding via sympathetic activity that inhibits bladder contraction and contracts urethral smooth muscle. Coactivation of dorsal ACC and the adjacent SMA occurs in association with the contraction of the pelvic floor and the striated sphincter muscles.[3,7]
3. *Circuit 3—subcortical circuit involving parahippocampal complex*: This circuit is probably involved in subconscious monitoring of bladder. During bladder filling, when the bladder volume is small, a subcortical network involving the PAG and parts of the inferior or middle parahippocampal cortex is activated. In this situation, the cortical regions are uninvolved, as

consistent with the absence of bladder filling sensation. Hypothalamus, which is considered a part of subcortical circuit, is involved in providing "safe" or "unsafe" signal to the pontine micturition center (PMC). In addition, dopaminergic modulation of the micturition reflex also occurs. D1 receptors mediate a tonic inhibition of the micturition reflex via gamma-aminobutyric acid (GABA) in the PAG while D2 receptors facilitate the micturition reflex.[6-8]

In addition, the ascending limb of voiding reflex provides information regarding the state of bladder filling. It is to mainly assess whether there is enough urine available in the bladder for micturition. This is called *circuit zero*. Circuits are depicted in **Figure 2**.

Brainstem Control

The brainstem has two principal nuclei concerned with voiding—the PAG and the PMC (also called as M-region or Barrington's nucleus). During storage, the PAG is activated by afferent input from the bladder while the PMC is inactive. When the bladder volume exceeds the micturition threshold, the switch from storage to voiding occurs. This is associated with PMC activation and enhanced PAG activity. The PAG projects to many parts of the forebrain, receives ascending afferent activity from the bladder, and sends efferent signals back to the bladder and urethra. PAG has three paired and one unpaired column. The paired columns are ventrolateral (vlPAG), dorsolateral (dlPAG), and lateral column. The dorsomedian column is unpaired. Afferent information about bladder filling is relayed to the vlPAG and stimulation of this column results in detrusor contraction and voiding through excitation of the PMC. GABAergic projections from the dlPAG inhibit the vlPAG resulting in inhibition of PMC, and thereby, suppressing micturition.[9] Ascending sensory information on the degree of the bladder filling reaches the PAG and then is relayed to the hypothalamus and thalamus, ACC, insula, and MPFC. These regions inhibit the PAG which itself has excitatory input to the PMC. The hypothalamus also has excitatory influences on the PAG. When the conscious decision to void occurs, the MPFC inhibition of PAG is interrupted. Simultaneously, the hypothalamus stimulates the PAG, leading to net effect of excitation of the PMC, producing voiding.[6]

Periaqueductal gray—leaky bucket: The PAG can be viewed as a leaky bucket, which is partly filled with water, wherein it receives inputs from bladder afferents and MPFC. When bladder is filling, excitatory inputs to PAG

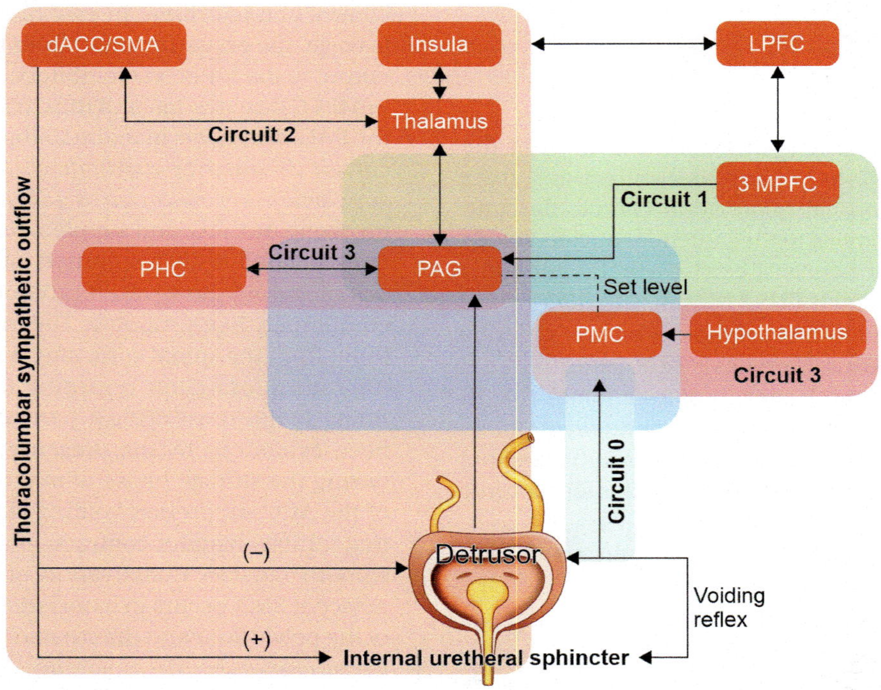

FIG. 2: Cortical circuits involved in storage and voiding; circuit 0 (light blue color)—sensory afferents, circuit 1 (green color), circuit 2 (red color), and circuit 3 (pink color).

(DACC: dorsal anterior cingulate cortex; IUS: internal urethral sphincter; MPFC: medial prefrontal cortex; LPFC: lateral prefrontal cortex; PMC: pontine micturition center; PAG: periaqueductal gray; PHC: parahippocampal cortex; SMA: supplemental motor area)

Source: Modified from Griffiths D, (2015).[7]

increase, suggesting a rise in water level. When the water level reaches set point, switch to voiding occurs, starting the voiding reflex. After voiding, afferent signals reduce and water level falls below set point. By increasing inflow from MPFC to PAG (rise in water level), one can voluntarily initiate voiding.[7]

There is a third brainstem nucleus, lateral and ventral to the PMC, called as the L-region or the pontine urine storage center (PUSC). Excitation of this region is results in contraction of the urinary sphincter.[6]

To summarize, the brain bladder control network maintains inhibition of the voiding reflex during urine storage. At small bladder volumes, the subcortical network is activated. Further bladder filling generates a desire to void, reflected as insular activation. Despite the increasing sensation, in normal individuals, voiding reflex does not occur unless it would not only be mechanically appropriate but also emotionally safe and socially appropriate.

Spinal Control

From the Barrington's nucleus, efferents to the spinal cord descend by reticulospinal tracts (located medially and anteriorly in the anterior funiculus) to the detrusor motor neurons in the intermediolateral cell columns of the sacral gray matter. Also, efferent connections from the cortical and subcortical micturition centers descend by the pyramidal tracts to the pudendal nuclei (Onuf's nucleus). Parasympathetic preganglionic neurons are located in the intermediolateral gray matter in the sacral segments of the cord (laminae 5–7) whereas sympathetic preganglionic neurons are located in the medial (lamina 10) and lateral (laminae 5–7) sites.[3]

Involuntary or reflex voiding is mediated through the spinobulbospinal reflex, when the volume of urine exceeds the micturition threshold. Increased afferent firing from tension receptors in the bladder produces firing of the sacral parasympathetic pathways and inhibition of the sympathetic and somatic pathways, which produces voiding. This type of voiding is normally seen in infants.

The PMC-PAG Switching Circuits

Griffith et al. proposed a computer model of PMC-PAG switching circuits.[7]

Storage Switch

Storage switch is shown in **Flowchart 4**.

Voiding Switch

Voiding switch is shown in **Flowchart 5**.

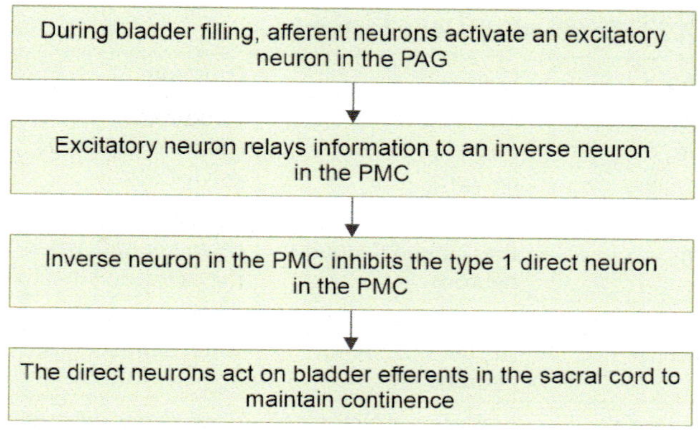

FLOWCHART 4: Storage switch.
(PAG: periaqueductal gray; PMC: pontine micturition center)

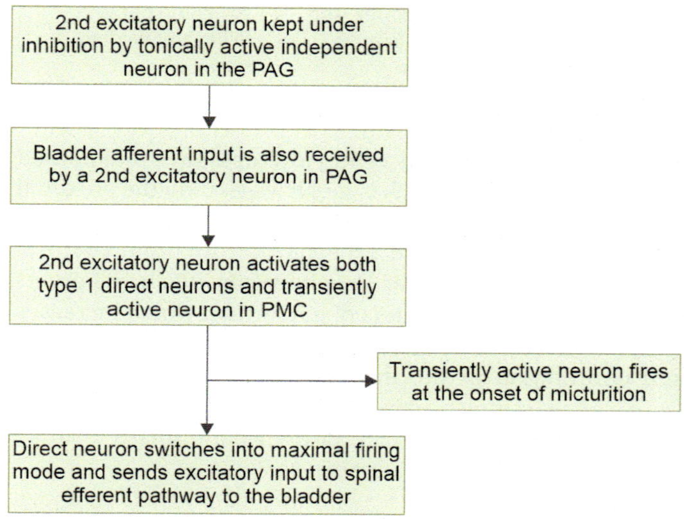

FLOWCHART 5: Voiding switch.
(PAG: periaqueductal gray; PMC: pontine micturition center)

STORAGE AND VOIDING

As mentioned before, the two important phases of LUT activity are storage and voiding. Normal storage capacity of bladder is 400–600 mL. While the first desire to micturition occurs at 300–400 mL, the urge to void urine occurs when the volume crosses 400 mL. Bladder filling occurs at a low pressure.[1] Continence is promoted by both passive and reflex activities. During the passive filling phase, there is minimal increase in the intravesical pressure initially due to the elastic property of the smooth muscle and connective tissues of the bladder wall. Reorientation of the detrusor muscle, thinning of the lamina propria and flattening of the urothelium, maintains the normal compliance throughout

TABLE 1: The Bradley's loop system.

Loop	Connections	Function
Corticospinal loop	Motor cortex to pudendal motor neurons	Voluntary control of sphincters and the pelvic floor
Urethral reflex loop	Urethral afferents to the pudendal motor neurons	Maintains the sphincter tone when the detrusor is inactive
Detrusor reflex loop	Detrusor afferents to pudendal motor neurons	Sphincter relaxation when detrusor is active
Cord loop	Brainstem structures to the conus medullaris	Coordinates detrusor and sphincter contraction and relaxation
Cerebral loop	Includes the brainstem, cerebral cortex, and the basal ganglia structures	Initiates and inhibits switching between filling and voiding states

the filling phase. As a result of this, low pressure is maintained in the bladder cavity, which is much lesser than the proximal urethral pressure, thus maintaining continence.[2,10] When the intravesical pressure exceeds the proximal urethral pressure, then the reflex mechanisms occur. There is stimulation of frontal centers of micturition which increases sympathetic activity resulting in inhibition of the detrusor and contraction of the internal urethral sphincter. The Onuf's nucleus is also activated which causes contraction of EUS and pelvic floor muscles. Both mechanisms contribute to the maintenance of continence.[5]

Voiding is normally a voluntary act, which happens as a result of the coordinated relaxation of the urethral sphincter and contraction of the detrusor. When appropriate circumstances are present, the cortical inhibition of the PAG is removed, activating the PMC via PAG, which in turn activates the detrusor reflex and inhibits the sphincter.

The Bradley's Loop System of Classification

The central pathways concerned with micturition and sphincter control are summarized in **Table 1**.[11]

PATHOPHYSIOLOGY AND TYPES OF NEUROGENIC BLADDER

Neurogenic bladder is classified based on the location of the neurological lesion:[1]

- *Uninhibited bladder*: Lesions above PMC
- *Upper motor neuron (UMN) bladder*: Lesions between the pons and the sacral spinal cord
- *Mixed type A bladder*: Sacral cord lesions that damage the detrusor nucleus but spare the pudendal nucleus
- *Mixed type B bladder*: Sacral cord lesions that spare the detrusor nucleus but affect the pudendal nucleus
- *Lower motor neuron (LMN) bladder*: Sacral cord or sacral nerve root injuries

In uninhibited neurogenic bladder, there is reduced awareness of bladder fullness and a low-capacity bladder due to reduced inhibition of the PMC by cortical and subcortical lesions, usually bilateral. As the PMC is intact, the normal opposition of the detrusor and internal/external sphincter tonus is maintained and hence there are no high bladder pressures leading to renal damage. It is seen in conditions such as cerebrovascular disease and cerebral atrophy with dementia.

Upper motor neuron bladder dysfunction is characterized by detrusor sphincter dyssynergia (DSD). There is simultaneous contraction of detrusor and urinary sphincter generating pressures up to 80–90 cm H_2O, leading to vesicoureteral reflux (VUR) resulting in renal damage. The spinal cord lesions, especially above T10, render the bladder and sphincters spastic. The bladder capacity is reduced secondary to high detrusor tone (detrusor hyperreflexia) which occurs due to excessive ACh release facilitated by the activation of prejunctional M1 receptors. Hypertrophy of the detrusor muscle secondary to bladder hypertonicity, alters the normal oblique course of the ureter leading to VUR. When the detrusor pressure exceeds sphincter pressure, incontinence may occur. It is seen in conditions such as transverse myelitis, spondylosis, trauma, and tumors of the cord.

In the mixed type A bladder, detrusor nucleus damage renders the detrusor flaccid (detrusor areflexia), while the intact pudendal nucleus produces spastic EUS. The large, low-pressure bladder along with spastic EUS produces urinary retention. However, both incontinence and VUR are uncommon as the detrusor pressure is low.

The mixed type B neurogenic bladder is characterized by a flaccid EUS (pudendal nucleus lesion) and spastic bladder (disinhibited detrusor nucleus). Thus, the bladder capacity is low but vesicular pressures are not elevated since there is little outflow resistance, and incontinence usually occurs.

An autonomous neurogenic bladder is seen with complete lesions below the T12 segment that involve the conus medullaris and cauda equine (examples, sacral myelomeningocele and tumors of the conus-cauda region). This also occurs during the initial phase of spinal shock. As the tone of the detrusor muscle is abolished, urinary retention occurs with distension of bladder, however, there is impaired awareness of the state of fullness. Inability to initiate micturition, overflow incontinence and increased residual urine volume develop. Associated features include saddle anesthesia, absence of bulbocavernosus, and anal reflexes. Anal sphincter control is often similarly affected.

A sensory paralytic bladder is caused by the impairment of afferent pathways innervating the bladder or the posterior columns or lateral spinothalamic tract at the level of the spinal cord. Voluntary initiation of micturition is maintained; however, urinary retention, overflow incontinence, or urinary tract infection occurs. The bulbocavernosus and superficial anal reflexes may be absent, decreased, or present. It is seen in tabes dorsalis, syringomyelia, or diabetes mellitus (DM).

URODYNAMIC STUDIES

The urodynamic test involves noninvasive assessment of bladder emptying and the invasive assessment of bladder storage and emptying. Usually, a multichannel urodynamic test consists of following components:

- *Uroflowmetry*:
    - Urinary flow, time taken to reach maximum flow, maximum and average flow rates, and the voided volume are calculated.
    - The volume of urine expelled per unit time is called the flow rate (Q). The total volume expelled via urethra (in mL) is called voided volume (V_{void}). The maximum measured value of the flow rate is called the maximum flow rate (Q_{max}). A flow time is the time over which measurable flow occurs. The average flow rate (Q) is obtained when voided volume is divided by flow time.
    - A normal uroflowmetry test is characterized by a bell-shaped curve with Q_{max} reached in initial one-third of voiding time.
    - A significant neurogenic bladder is unlikely if the patient has a normal bladder capacity and urinary flow rate.
- *Cystometry*:
    - Measures the pressure-volume relationship in the bladder. The difference between the intravesical and intra-abdominal pressures is the detrusor pressure.
    - In cystometry, the following five parameters are assessed—(1) detrusor function, (2) bladder sensation, (3) bladder compliance, (4) bladder capacity, and (5) urethral function.
    - Detrusor overactivity can either be phasic or terminal. In phasic detrusor overactivity, there is urgency and incomplete emptying, whereas in terminal detrusor overactivity, there is urgency and complete bladder emptying.
    - Detrusor hyperreflexia is characterized by unstable contractions of the bladder (rise in detrusor pressure > 15 cm of water), reduced bladder capacity, and loss of compliance.
    - Detrusor hyporeflexia, on the other hand, is characterized by an increased bladder capacity during filling phase, considerable abdominal pressure generated during voiding correlating with the interrupted urinary flow.
    - Reduced or absent bladder sensation is indicative of autonomic dysreflexia.
    - Bladder compliance (C) is defined as change in bladder volume (V) divided by change in pressure (C = V/Pdet; Pdet - detrusor pressure). A value > 30–40 cm H_2O, indicates reduced bladder compliance.
    - Detrusor leak point pressure (DLPP) is the detrusor pressure at which urine leak occurs in the absence of detrusor overactivity or abdominal straining. Safe bladder capacity is defined as the volume of fluid at pressures below 40 cm of water.
    - Abdominal leak point pressure is the vesical pressure at which leak occurs during voluntary increase of abdominal pressure in the absence of detrusor overactivity.
- *Urethral pressure profile*: Urethral length and competence is measured and is typically done in women to identify the cause of stress incontinence.
- Electromyography of pelvic floor muscles.

CLINICAL IMPLICATIONS

Frontal Lobe Lesions

Conditions such as stroke, hydrocephalus, subdural hematoma, frontotemporal dementia neoplasms, affecting frontal lobe especially medial, and anterior frontal lobe results in urinary disturbances in form of urgency, nocturnal urge incontinence, and frequency. Prefrontal cortex, along with other cortical centers mentioned earlier, has a role in voluntary control of bladder, and lesions lead to impaired awareness of need to void. In urodynamic studies, frontal lobe lesions are characterized by detrusor hyperreflexia, uninhibited sphincter relaxation.[12]

Parkinson's Disease

Urinary disturbance in Parkinson's disease (PD) is multifactorial, and occurs in 38–71% of patients with PD. The most common symptom is nocturia, followed by urgency and frequency. Urodynamic studies show detrusor hyperreflexia with low postvoidal residual volume (PVR). Studies showed chronic levodopa treatment, subthalamic nucleus deep brain stimulation (DBS) reduced these symptoms, by increasing bladder capacity and delaying first desire to void in PD patients.[13]

Multisystem Atrophy

Urinary disturbances in MSA patients are significantly higher than in PD patients. It can be initial manifestation of MSA.[14] Common symptoms include urgency, frequency, urge incontinence, and incomplete bladder emptying. Involvement of sacral preganglionic nuclei, Onuf nucleus, and PMC leads to these kind of urinary symptoms in MSA. Urodynamic studies show large postvoidal residual urine.[6]

TABLE 2: Therapeutic strategies for neurogenic bladder.

Condition	Therapeutic strategy	Effects
Detrusor overactivity	*Pharmacological*: Antimuscarinic drugs: • Oxybutynin • Tolterodine • Solifenacin • Darifenacin Beta-3 agonist: • Mirabegron	• Competitively inhibit muscarinic receptors • Detrusor relaxation • Intravesicular pressure reduction • Detrusor relaxation • Not a first line agent
	Surgical: Bladder augmentation—enterocystoplasty	• Portion of small intestine or stomach is used • Increases bladder capacity and compliance

	Others:
	• Botulinum toxin type A injection
	• *Sacral neuromodulation*:
	  ○ Direct sacral root stimulation by implanted simulator
	  ○ Dorsal rhizotomy
	• Intravesical administration of Vanilloids
		• Under cystoscopy guidance, 200–300 units injected into 20–30 equidistant sites on detrusor
		• Restores detrusor stability
		• For patients with detrusor overactivity despite behavioral, pharmacological therapies
		• Not recommended in routine use
		• Reserved for patients with severe detrusor overactivity, complete urinary retention
		• Desensitizes C fiber sensory afferents
		• Reduces detrusor hyperreflexia due to spinal cord lesions

Detrusor under activity	*Nonpharmacological*: • Behavioral therapy bladder retraining, fluid schedules, techniques to perform timed voids—Credé technique and Valsalva maneuver Intermittent self-catheterization Long term indwelling catheters/suprapubic catheter	• Triggers detrusor contraction • Periodic bladder emptying method using catheter • Frequency of catheterization depends on bladder functional capacity, fluid intake, urodynamic parameters—bladder compliance, filling pressure, and involuntary contractions • Suprapubic catheters are preferred over indwelling catheters
Mixed type A bladder	*Pharmacological*: Cholinergic agonists: Urecholine Benzodiazepines: Diazepam GABAB agonists	• Promotes detrusor contraction • Acts on gamma-aminobutyric acid type A (GABAA) receptor • Reduces skeletal muscle tone, including external urethral sphincter • Allows more complete emptying of bladder • Reduces skeletal muscle tone including external urethral sphincter

Spinal Cord Lesions

Traumatic spinal cord injuries, demyelinating lesions are most common spinal causes of neurogenic bladder.[6] Urinary disturbances after acute spinal cord lesion include initial areflexic bladder due to loss of supraspinal control, followed by development of detrusor over activity along with DSD, mediated by spinal reflex.[5]

Systemic Causes

Diabetes mellitus is one of the most frequent causes of bladder dysfunction. Urinary disturbances in patients with DM vary from bladder overactivity causing storage symptoms to bladder underactivity leading to voiding symptoms. Hyperglycemia-associated osmotic diuresis leading to increased intravascular pressure and detrusor muscle hypertrophy initially contributes to storage symptoms. As hyperglycemia persists, in due course in time, due to toxin accumulation and associated neuropathy, decompensation of detrusor with detrusor areflexia occurs, leading to voiding symptoms. This is called as temporal theory of diabetic bladder dysfunction.[15,16] Treatment depends on the symptomatology.

THERAPEUTICS—NEUROGENIC BLADDER

Therapeutic strategies for neurogenic bladder are given in **Table 2**.[1,17,18]

CONCLUSION

The neural control of the urinary bladder is a highly complicated yet interesting subject. The underlying concepts may be used to simplify many areas in neurourology.

REFERENCES

1. Dorsher PT, McIntosh PM. Neurogenic bladder. Adv Urol. 2012;2012:816274.
2. Clemens JQ. Basic bladder neurophysiology. Urol Clin North Am. 2010;37(4):487-94.
3. de Groat WC, Griffiths D, Yoshimura N. Neural control of the lower urinary tract. Compr Physiol. 2015;5(1):327-96.
4. Continuum (Mineapp Minn) 1998;4(4, Neuroanatomy, neurophysiology and neuropharmacology of the urinary bladder):7-20.
5. Fowler CJ, Griffiths D, de Groat WC. The neural control of micturition. Nat Rev Neurosci. 2008;9(6):453-66.
6. Benarroch EE. Neural control of the bladder: Recent advances and neurologic implications. Neurology. 2010;75(20):1839-46.
7. Griffiths D. Neural control of micturition in humans: A working model. Nat Rev Urol. 2015;12(12):695-705.
8. Seki S, Igawa Y, Kaidoh K, Ishizuka O, Nishizawa O, Andersson KE. Role of dopamine D1 and D2 receptors in the micturition reflex in conscious rats. Neurourol Urodyn. 2001;20(1):105-13.
9. Zare A, Jahanshahi A, Rahnama'i MS, Schipper S, van Koeveringe GA. The role of the periaqueductal gray matter in lower urinary tract function. Mol Neurobiol. 2019;56(2):920-34.
10. Yeates WK. Neurophysiology of the bladder. Spinal Cord. 1974;12(2):73-82.
11. Continuum (Mineapp Minn). 1998;4(4, Classification of neurogenic bladder disease):29-41.
12. Pettersen R, Stien R, Wyller TB. Post-stroke urinary incontinence with impaired awareness of the need to void: clinical and urodynamic features. BJU Int. 2007;99(5):1073-7.
13. Herzog J, Weiss PH, Assmus A, Wefer B, Seif C, Braun PM, et al. Subthalamic stimulation modulates cortical control of urinary bladder in Parkinson's disease. Brain J Neurol. 2006;129(Pt12):3366-75.
14. Sakakibara R, Panicker J, Simeoni S, Uchiyama T, Yamamoto T, Tateno F, et al. Bladder dysfunction as the initial presentation of multiple system atrophy: a prospective cohort study. Clin Auton Res Off J Clin Auton Res Soc. 2019;29(6):627-31.
15. Daneshgari F, Moy ML. Current indications for neuromodulation. Urol Clin North Am. 2005;32(1):37-40,vi.
16. Liu G, Daneshgari F. Diabetic Bladder Dysfunction. Chin Med J (Engl). 2014;127(7):1357-64.
17. Fowler CJ, O'Malley KJ. Investigation and management of neurogenic bladder dysfunction. J Neurol Neurosurg Psychiatry. 2003;74(suppl 4):iv27-31.
18. Truzzi JC, de Almeida FG, Sacomani CA, Reis J, Rocha FET. Neurogenic bladder—concepts and treatment recommendations. Int Braz J Urol. 2022;48(2):220-43.

20 CHAPTER

Applied Neuroanatomy and Neurophysiology of Balance

Anirban Biswas, Gargi Kar

INTRODUCTION

The maintenance of balance is possibly the most complicated mechanism in the human body. It has deep ramification in different parts of the body from head to foot which involves the central, the peripheral, the psychic, the cognitive system, the musculoskeletal, the vestibular system, and organs like the brain, ears, and eyes.

Each of these systems and organs vie with each other in respect to the complexities of the structure and function that is packed into them.

BASIC MECHANISM OF MAINTENANCE OF BALANCE

The central nervous system (CNS) collects information about the static and dynamic position of the body about the ground and the surroundings from certain sensors in different parts of the body.

From these sensors, the brain gets aware of the external environment, i.e., the stability of the ground where we are positioned, the stability of the surroundings and the stability and position of the internal environment, i.e., the position of the body in the surrounding three-dimensional space and the position of the body parts how the head is positioned on the shoulder.

Information from different sensors integrated into the brain and compared with previously stored experiences.

So, when the brain is retrieving information about the stability of the ground and the surroundings, it is simultaneously also retrieving information from the. Vestibular memory about the similar condition of the stability of the ground and the surroundings from the past vestibular memory about the experiences and later combines and compares them and formulates a motor output by which the body's balance is best maintained in that particular situation and hence it is imperative to mention to achieve that we need to have an efficient vestibular memory and equally efficient system for retrieving the requisite information in obtaining a similar balance situation from the vestibular memory as when required.

Hence it is imperative to state that a cognitive system plays a very important role in maintaining the balance system, the more efficacious the cognitive system the better the storage capacity of the brain to store information.

- Vestibular labyrinths-which is in the ear of the human body which is again one of the most complex organs of the body, sense different types of body movement in different planes and hence inform the brain about the individual's position in respect to the ground and the surroundings and the contiguous orientation. The vestibular labyrinths are the internal sensors of the balance system which sense the static and dynamic position of the individual.

  Hence, all this information is collected by the vestibular labyrinths and sent to the brain through the vestibular nerve.
- *The eyes*: The information about the stability of the surrounding is informed to the brain by the eyes, regarding its visual environment, whether stable or moving.
- *The proprioceptors*: The sensors which are present in the soles of the feet, in the buttocks, and the back inform the brain about the stability of the ground and the surroundings, i.e., walking/standing/sitting or even inclined in a plane, the brain senses this with the help of the proprioceptors.
- Cerebellum fine-tunes the motor output, the cognitive system determines the nature of the response, and higher centers in the brain modulate the motor response.

The motor output evolved by the brain is directed to two groups of muscles:

1. *The limbs and trunk, i.e., the skeletal muscles*: This correction of the body posture is always a very precise and almost accurate 100% correct. The motor output is fine-tuned by the cerebellum. The cerebellum calculates the contraction of muscle, the contraction to perform,

and the time of contraction. Nevertheless, the cerebellum also considers what would be the best response based on stored memory and acts on the response accordingly. The cognitive system is simultaneously relevant in retrieving past experiences in that specific situation from vestibular memory.

2. *The external muscles of the eyes, i.e., the extraocular muscles*: The image of the object falls in the retina, on the most sensitive area called as the fovea, which is effected by the contraction of the six extraocular muscles, namely, the lateral, medial, inferior, and superior rectus muscles, and the inferior and superior oblique muscles.

These extraocular muscles will contract in a very precise way and the image will remain fixed in the fovea and there will be no retinal slip whatsoever. If there is any retinal slip, the subject will feel vertiginous. Here, too, the cerebellum will take control of each extraocular muscle and will contract depending upon the extent, and duration so that the image remains fixed and stable in the fovea despite being in motion.

In normal individual have a very effective and efficient vestibular system that senses the head movement and brings about a movement of the eyes in the opposite direction at the same speed as that of the head movement, ensuring thereby that the image of the car remains fixed in the fovea and there is no retinal slip whatsoever.

But for the individual whose sensitivity to the vestibular system is compromised, the vestibular inputs and the visual inputs sends contradictory information to the brain. So, the brain gets confused which results in a balance disorder.

Any retinal slippage of the visual images from the fovea will not only cause a vertiginous sensation but also cause a sharp drop in visual acuity.

MOTOR MECHANISMS OF THE VESTIBULAR SYSTEM

The *vestibulospinal reflex (VSR) system* and the *vestibulo-ocular reflex (VOR) system* are the two reflex systems that maintain our balance system.

The cerebellum fine-tunes the motor output, the cognitive system determines the nature of the response. The cognitive system retrieves from the vestibular memory a similar situation and determines that under a particular situation what will be the best response (motor output) to maintain stability. If the cognitive system is intact, the correct direction is given to the motor system hence the best possible results are achieved.

Later, the higher centers in the brain will modulate the motor response because the neural signals to the muscles of the limbs and the trunk as well as that to the eyes will traverse from the motor cortex of the brain passing through different stations of the brain, as the internal capsule, the thalamus, basal ganglia, reticular formation, etc.

These stations of the brain are the relay sections of the neural signals which carry the motor cortex to the relevant muscles and each of these relay stations has some function in modulating the motor response.

Parts of the CNS Involved in the Motor Output for Maintenance of Balance

- Cerebral cortex
- Pyramidal and extrapyramidal tracts
- Basal ganglia
- Reticular formation
- Thalamus
- Cerebellum
- Ascending/descending tract in the spinal cord

Defects in any of these structures will affect the body's balance.

The connections between the motor cortex in the forebrain and motor neurons within the brainstem that houses the motor nuclei of the nerves for eye movement are made up of two tracts or systems, viz., (1) the pyramidal system, and (2) the extrapyramidal system.

These tracts are concerned with the different motor activities of the body and any defect in these tracts leads to abnormalities in the execution of any motor activity. Since maintenance of balance involves movement of body parts executed by contraction of muscles, any disorder in the pyramidal or extrapyramidal system especially, the extrapyramidal remarkably jeopardizes the balance function as well as a movement disorder. Hence, the clinician who is practicing, neurology needs to evaluate the functionality of these two systems thoroughly in all patients presenting with vertigo/dizziness/unsteadiness.

The pyramidal system: Pyramidal system is the pathway for direct activation of the skeletal muscles in the limbs and the trunk. All of the motor impulses emanating from the cerebral cortex of the brain travel through this tract. This pathway supplies the voluntary muscles of the head, neck, and limbs. Neurons of this tract originate in the postcentral gyrus or primary motor cortex. This neural network from the motor area of the cerebral cortex down to the motor nucleus of the cranial nerves as well as to the anterior horn cells in the spinal cord is called the pyramidal pathway.

The pyramidal system has two tracts—(1) *corticobulbar tract,* and (2) *corticospinal tract.* The corticobulbar tract originates in the motor cortex in the precentral gyrus of the cerebral cortex in the brain and descends to the genu of the internal capsule and then enters the basilar part of the pons, and finally terminates in the motor nuclei of the cranial nerves of the opposite side. These fibers are responsible for the motor activity of the head and neck muscles, which include the extraocular muscles of the eyes that execute eye movement and are hence in the control of gaze stabilization which is the primary function of the vestibular system. Any defect in the corticobulbar tracts or the genu of the internal capsule will lead to abnormalities in gaze stabilization and hence cause vertigo.

The nerve fibers of the corticospinal tract originate in the motor area of the cerebral cortex which travels down through the corona radiata, radiate, the posterior half of the lateral ventricle, the posterior limb of the internal capsule and then enter the midbrain through the cerebral peduncle, and after that the medulla where they form medullary pyramids on either side of the midline. After this most fibers of the corticospinal tract decussate, i.e., cross over to the other side and descend in the contralateral side of the spinal cord as the lateral corticospinal tract and synapse (i.e., terminate) at the anterior horn cells. From the anterior horn cells, the next neurons start and through the peripheral motor nerves, and reach the muscles of the limbs and trunk, mainly the limbs. Some fibers do not decussate at the level of the medulla and travel downward through the spinal cord as the anterior corticospinal tract and decussate lower down in the spinal cord and mostly supply the trunkal muscles.

In its passage from the motor cortex to the final destination, which is the skeletal muscles, the corticospinal tracts pass through some relay stations in the brain like the thalamus. The final activity of motor neurons is therefore a result of activity within the cerebral cortex and/ or the thalamus. The thalamus effectively acts as a relay station from the cerebrum and cerebellum before neurons enter the motor pathways of the spinal cord. Disorders of the thalamus will hence lead to faulty muscular contraction, as malfunctioning thalamus will abnormally change the motor output that has originated in the cerebral motor cortex.

Any defect in the entire pathway right from the cerebral motor cortex to the skeletal muscles as well as that in the relay stations, will cause defective contraction of the muscles of the limbs/trunk and lead to postural instability. Hence to maintain an erect posture and to prevent a fall, this corticospinal tract has to function perfectly and hence any defect in the pathway or the relay stations will lead to imbalance. Therefore, imperative to mention, that the functional integrity of the relay systems like the thalamus needs to be evaluated in patients presenting with imbalance.

Signs of Disorder in the Pyramidal Tract—Areflexia, Hyperreflexia, Abnormal Babinski Reflex, Hypotonia, and Hypertonia

Extrapyramidal system: The descending fibers from the cerebrum, cerebellum and brainstem that enter the spinal cord after relaying in subcortical nuclei, mainly the basal ganglia, are known as the extrapyramidal tracts.

Extrapyramidal tracts are responsible for maintenance of postural balance as well as control of the movement of the eyes. They modify neural impulses that originate in the cerebral cortex, and then fine-tune the involuntary movements. The impulses generated at the primary motor cortex areas are sent via the extrapyramidal fibers to the basal ganglia. The neural impulse passing through these tracts are in turn modulated by various parts of the CNS, including the nigrostriatal pathway, the basal ganglia, the cerebellum, the vestibular nuclei, and different sensory areas of the cerebral cortex.

Maintenance of balance, especially postural balance, involves the coordinated movement of groups of muscles in a very precise and controlled fashion; defects in the extrapyramidal tracts jeopardize this coordination of groups of muscles and result in imbalance. Hence, evaluation of the extrapyramidal tract should be keenly done by a Neurologist in examining a patient with a balance disorder.

Extrapyramidal tract disorder includes resting tremors, posture (hunched over), slow monotonal speech, expressionless facial expression, sialorrhea (drooling) due to bradykinesia of swallowing, fine eyelid tremor when closing eyes, muscular bradykinesia, rigidity, hypotonia, and low-frequency tremor, gait-difficulty in initiating and stopping movements" shuffling "gait with small steps, leaning forward to initiate movements, festinate gait (starting slow and speeding up as they continue to walk), etc.

There are two types of vestibulospinal tracts—*(1) the lateral and (2) the anterior*. The lateral vestibulospinal tract maintains the VSR and also exerts an excitatory effect on the extensor antigravity muscles. It plays a major role in the maintenance of muscle tone and body posture. Tonic contraction of body muscles, which is a vital function of the vestibular system, is controlled by this tract. The vestibular-bulbar tract has a similar effect on the extraocular muscles. The anterior or medial vestibulospinal tract originates in the medial vestibular nucleus and descends up to the upper cervical part of the spinal cord. It receives afferents from the vestibular labyrinth, mainly the three semicircular canals. Its primary function is the adjustment of the head and body during angular and linear acceleration and is also concerned with manipulating conjugate horizontal eye movement and the integration of eye and head movement. In conjunction with the tectospinal and tectobulbar tracts, it influences head movement in response to auditory and visual stimuli.

Tectospinal and Tectobulbar Tracts

The tectospinal tract neurons synapse with motor neurons of the cervical muscles and facilitate reflex postural movements. Its function is the control of head movement in response to auditory and visual stimuli. The neurons of the tectobulbar tracts terminate in the nuclei of the cranial nerves and mediate eye movements in response to auditory/ visual stimuli.

Olivospinal Tract

The olivospinal tract function is to control the reflex of head movements in response to proprioceptive inputs.

Rubrospinal Tract

The rubrospinal is also involved in the maintenance of muscle tone and has a facilitatory influence on flexor muscles and an inhibitory effect on the extensor muscles, i.e., the opposite of the lateral vestibulospinal tract.

Reticulospinal Tract[1]

The reticulospinal tract comprises the medial and lateral tracts that connect the reticular formation with the spinal cord. The tracts integrate information from the motor systems to coordinate automatic, i.e., nonvoluntary movements that are required for locomotion and the maintenance of posture. The reticulospinal tract also influences the maintenance of muscle tone and mediates some autonomic functions.

Disorders of the extrapyramidal system disorders such as Parkinsonism, chorea, athetosis, dystonia, tardive dyskinesia, etc., all these disorders patients present with imbalance and unsteadiness in the initial stages when all the typical features may not have been overtly manifested.

Most of the commonly used antivertigo drugs, especially prochlorperazine and cinnarizine, and the commonly used antiemetic drugs as well as most psychotropic drugs induce extrapyramidal disorders. Hence, whenever a patient presents with unsteadiness or the clinician suspects an extrapyramidal disorder, the clinician should essentially ask whether such drugs have been used. Cinnarizine and flunarizine used for a prolonged period can induce Parkinsonism which is the commonest extrapyramidal disorder. Cinnarizine is the most common cause of drug-induced Parkinsonism.

Medial Longitudinal Fasciculus[2]

It has a major role in the maintenance of oculomotor function and the maintenance of gaze stabilization.

Whenever the head moves in any particular plane, the movement is accurately sensed by the vestibular labyrinths and all details of the speed, nature, intensity, plane, and direction of the head movement sensed by the vestibular labyrinths is then fed to the oculomotor system.

The balance system is the only system in the body where so many different and diverse systems are involved. This is what makes the anatomy and physiology of the balance system so very complex.

THE REFLEX PATHWAY FOR MAINTENANCE OF BALANCE

A reflex arc is the neural pathway traversed by the nerve impulses from the part, which is stimulated to generate the reflex, to the part where the involuntary response is generated. All reflexes have a reflex arc that consists of:

- *An afferent sensory organ* that needs to be stimulated to generate the reflex.
- *An afferent neural pathway* that carries the neural impulse generated at the afferent sensory organ to the center of the reflex arc.
- *The center of the reflex* where the motor neural signal is generated.
- *An efferent neural pathway* that carries the neural signal generated in the center of the reflex to the effector motor organ.
- *An effector motor organ* where the final response takes place.

The vestibular labyrinth in the ear, which is the afferent sensory organ for the reflex arc of the vestibular system, collects the information about the stability of the head/body and passes this information in the form of neural codes or action potentials (AP) through the vestibular nerve (8th cranial nerve), which in this case is the afferent neural pathway, and reaches the center of the reflex, which is the vestibular nucleus; from the vestibular nucleus the neural impulse passes through the efferent neural pathway (also termed as the efferent motor pathway), which is the medial longitudinal fasciculus (MLF), and the descending tracts of the spinal cord to the motor nuclei of the eye muscles (nuclei of the 3rd, 4th, and 6th cranial nerves) and from there to the extraocular muscles of the eyes to move the eyes and to the anterior horn cells of the spinal cord, and from there to the muscles of the limbs and trunk to move the body muscles **(Fig. 1)**.

This is how the entire system works.

If any one part of this reflex arc is defective or is performing subnormally, the entire body's balance system gets jeopardized and the subject feels vertiginous and/or has a feeling of unsteadiness.

The Reflex Pathway

The optic nerve is the afferent sensory pathway from the eyes. The efferent pathway of the reflex arc for the proprioceptors and of the eyes is the same as that described for the vestibular labyrinths, i.e., the descending column in the spinal cord anterior horn cells, peripheral nerves for the body (skeletal) muscles that carry out the contraction of muscles of the limbs and the trunk and the 3rd/4th and 6th cranial nerves, which are the efferent motor pathways for the eye movement.

Vestibular Labyrinth and Its Different Functions and Connections

The vestibular labyrinth senses head and body movement. It has five different sensors for this purpose: the three semicircular canals and the two otolith organs, viz., the utricle and the saccule. Each part of the vestibular labyrinth monitors one particular type of movement. Linear and/or translational movement is sensed by the otolith organs, i.e., the saccule and the utricle, and angular movement in different planes is sensed by the semicircular canals.

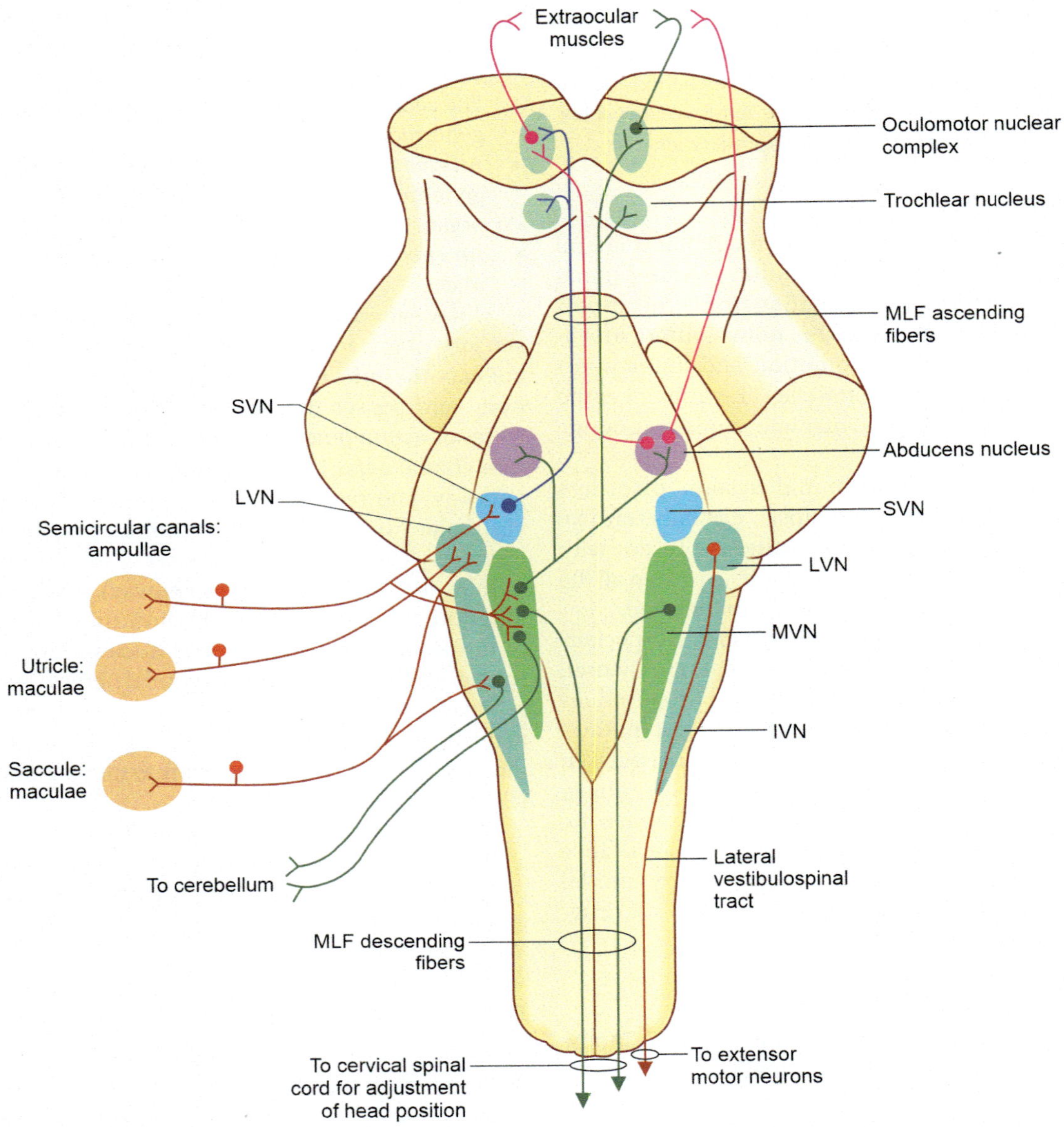

FIG. 1: The connections of the vestibular system.

(IVN: inferior vestibular nucleus; LVN: lateral vestibular nucleus; MLF: medial longitudinal fasciculus; MVN: medial vestibular nucleus; SVN: superior vestibular nucleus)

Up-down movement is monitored by the *saccule*, and *forward-backward and side-to-side movements* are monitored by the *utricle*. The three *semicircular canals* monitor *angular movement* in different directions.

Functions and Connections of Vestibular Labyrinth in Maintenance of Balance

Within each semicircular canal, there is a special sensory epithelium, *the ampulla,* which gets stimulated whenever the head suddenly moves and remains stimulated till the head movement attains a fixed speed. This happens as the semicircular canals are sensitive to acceleration only, which is the measurement of the change of speed (either increase or decrease of speed). The semicircular canals open at both ends into the utricle. The semicircular canal contains *endolymph,* which is displaced during rotational movements of the head because of its inertia. The ampulla is an enlargement or swelling at one end of each semicircular canal *the cupula* is a pliable structure that seals the inner diameter of the semicircular canal at the ampulla. In the cupula, there are hair cells that function more or less in the same way as hair cells of the cochlea. The hair cells in the cupula are arranged in a set pattern from large to small (tallest to shortest). The longest/tallest hair cell at one end is called the kinocilium and the others are called stereocilia. The movement of the endolymph in the semicircular canals bends the hair jutting out from the hair cells. Even when there is no movement, the hair cells are not moving but constantly discharging AP (spikes) with a firing rate of about 80–100 spikes per second, which is called the resting potential of the hair cells.

But when the head moves in any direction there is bending of the hair of the hair cells as the endolymph is displaced within the semicircular canal. Bending of the hair in a particular direction opens the filament between the hair of each hair cell. When the filament opens, the endolymph (which is high in K^+ and low in Na^+) that surrounds the hair of the hair cells can enter the hair cells. The endolymph has a +80 mv charge concerning the hair cell that is negatively charged. The endolymph's positive voltage pushes K^+ into the negatively-charged hair cell. When this happens, the hair cell depolarizes, releasing a neurotransmitter. This neurotransmitter excites the neuron attached to the hair cells which starts firing and causes an increase in the frequency of generation of AP in the vestibular nerve afferent fibers. These afferent fibers are the neurons of the vestibular nerve that originate from the hair cells.

This increase of AP caused by the bending of the hair cells toward the kinocilium is called depolarization or excitation of the cells. The opposite of depolarization/excitation is called hyperpolarization or inhibition. Hyperpolarization or inhibition occurs when the projecting hair of the hair cells is moved away from the kinocilium. Depending on the direction of movement of the endolymph in the semicircular canal, either toward the ampulla or away from the ampulla, there will be either depolarization or hyperpolarization in the particular semicircular canal.

Any movement or displacement of the endolymph within a semicircular canal deflects the cupula. The movement of endolymph toward the ampulla is called ampullopetal movement and the movement of endolymph away from the ampulla is called ampullofugal movement.

VESTIBULO-OCULAR REFLEX

The information on head-turning generated in the semicircular canals traverses in the form of neural impulses (or stimuli) from the vestibular nuclei through the MLF to the oculomotor centers and finally generates a precise contraction of the extraocular muscles. This contraction brings about the corrective eye movement for gaze stabilization. While traversing the neural pathway, it undergoes some neural processing influenced by the inputs from the cerebellum and other parts of the brain in such a way that the eye movement generated based on the information about head movement obtained from the semicircular canals is very precise and perfectly tuned as per the head movement.

Otolith organs (i.e., the utricle and the saccule) have a huge role to play in the maintenance of balance and are probably more important than the semicircular canals. The semicircular canals can only sense angular movements. But in our day-to-day life, we are always executing front-back, up-down, and side-to-side movements, which can only be sensed by the otolith organs. So, in a patient with vertigo we need to evaluate the otolith organs perfectly.

One of the primary functions of the balance system is also maintaining our correct *sense of verticality*.

All five sensors of each vestibular labyrinth sense completely different types of head/body movements. Hence defect in any of the semicircular canals can lead to incorrect posture for which the brain can perceive the correct information and hence instability or balancing defect will be present. This will result in deranged gaze stabilization and deranged postural stabilization due to which the subject will feel giddy and unsteady. Hence, a combination of angular and linear movements involves stimulation of the semicircular canals as well as the otolith organs maintain the posture or balance of the body.

FUNCTIONS OF BALANCE SYSTEM—GAZE STABILIZATION (VOR), POSTURAL STABILIZATION (VSR), CORRECT PERCEPTION OF VERTICALITY (OTOLITH ORGANS)

The eye movements on stimulation of the different semicircular canals.

Stimulation of individual semicircular canals induces different types of eye movements. The eyes always move in the direction of movement of the endolymph in the semicircular canals. Stimulation of the semicircular canals generates a slow movement of the eyes away from the central/neutral position. But after the eyes have moved away from the central/neutral position of the orbit to the sides, the CNS brings the eyes back to the center of the orbit by a fast movement in the opposite direction. The alternate slow and fast eye movement is nystagmus. Nystagmus has a slow phase generated by the semicircular canals which is immediately followed by a corrective fast phase in the opposite direction generated by the CNS. Since nystagmus is designated by the fast phase, the nystagmus generated by the stimulation of the different canals will always be opposite to the eye movement.

- *The posterior canals*: Stimulation of the posterior semicircular canals makes the eyes of both sides move vertically downward and torsionally inward (intorsion).
- *The anterior canals*: Stimulation of the anterior semicircular canals makes the eyes of both sides move vertically upward and torsionally inward (intorsion), i.e., the torsion is toward the other eye.

Hence, the nystagmus (i.e., the fast phase of nystagmus) on stimulation of the different semicircular canals will be as follows:

- *Right lateral canal*: Left beating pure horizontal nystagmus
- *Left lateral canal*: Right beating pure horizontal nystagmus

- *Right posterior canal*: Up-beating torsional nystagmus upper pole beating to the right
- *Left posterior canal*: Up-beating torsional nystagmus upper pole beating to left
- *Right anterior canal*: Down-beating torsional nystagmus upper beating to the right
- *Left anterior canal*: Down-beating torsional nystagmus beating to left

Gaze Stabilization; the part played by the higher Centers—gaze stabilization is primarily carried out by the VOR but other mechanisms like the oculomotor system and the cerebellar systems that work in conjunction and modulate the VOR are also involved in the execution of the VOR.

Supranuclear Oculomotor System

The supranuclear oculomotor centers are neural centers/nuclei which are higher in the hierarchy of the oculomotor system than the nuclei of the oculomotor nerves (i.e., the 3rd,4th, and 6th cranial nerves) and hence control and mediate the functioning of the three oculomotor nuclei.

Supranuclear Oculomotor Centers in the Brain

The important supranuclear oculomotor centers in the brain are:

- *riMLF*: Rostral interstitial nucleus of medial longitudinal fasciculus (upper midbrain)
- *INC*: Interstitial nucleus of Cajal (upper midbrain)
- *PPRF*: Paramedian pontine reticular formation (in pons)
- *NPH*: Nucleus prepositus hypoglossi
- *PC*: Posterior commissure (connects the riMLF of two sides)

Supranuclear Oculomotor Mechanisms

- *Smooth pursuit system*
- *Saccadic system*
- *Convergence system*
- *Visual fixation with a gaze-holding system*
- *VOR and suppression of VOR by visual fixation*
- *Optokinetic system*

Smooth Pursuit

The smooth pursuit/tracking system (SPS) allows the eyes to closely follow a moving object very often against a fixed visual backdrop and even when there is no backdrop.

The smooth tracking system functions only when the eyes track a moving object that is traversing a predictable trajectory and is moving at a speed of <1.2 Hz. The smooth pursuit system works best under this condition only and fails if the speed is >1.2 Hz or the trajectory is uneven, i.e., if the moving object abruptly changes speed or follows an unpredictable and changing trajectory.

Pursuit system: Control of smooth pursuit eye movements is a complex process. The stimulus for pursuit movement is the movement of an image across the fovea at velocities >3–5 deg/sec but <50–70 deg/sec. Visual (striate and peristriate) cortex projects to the parietal temporo-occipital region (PTO) as well as to the frontal eye field (FEF). The PTO projects via the internal sagittal striatum and the posterior limb of internal capsule to ipsilateral dorsolateral and lateral pontine nuclei (DLPN). Pursuit pathways control ipsilateral tracking, hence, undergo double decussation.

CNS involvement: The vestibulo-cerebellum (flocculus, nodulus, and posterior vermis) plays a dominant role in smooth pursuit; the remainder of the cerebellum, portions of the brain stem, and cortical areas also partic. Defects in smooth tracking may be due to disorders in the visual cortex, extrapyramidal system, the dorsolateral pontine nuclei, the cerebellum, and also in the oculomotor nuclei.

Saccade System

It is for stabilizing the image of a visual target at the end of the visual field in the fovea by a rapid single eye movement. It facilitates visual tracking when SPS fails and when speeds of movement of the visual target are >1.2 Hz as SPS fails beyond this speed.

Functions: The saccadic system's function is to suddenly move the eyes and fix them over the visual object of interest not only at the end of the visual field, but at any point of the visual field. However, the function of the saccadic system is not to keep the eyes fixed over there and its function finishes immediately after taking the eyes to the new object of interest.

The videonystagmography (VNG) test allows very accurate documentation of all these parameters of the saccadic system. Tests for saccades are done both in the horizontal and the vertical axes.

Gaze-holding System

The function of the gaze-holding system is to maintain the static position of the gaze that the saccadic system has placed the image of the visual target stationed at the periphery of the visual field on the fovea. Fixating images of objects at the upper and lower ends of the visual field in the fovea is the function of the vertical gaze-holding system. The faculty of gaze-holding both in the horizontal as well as in the vertical axis is tested clinically by the clinical gaze test and precisely documented by the VNG gaze test.

Optokinetic System

The optokinetic system allows us to keep images in the fovea when the entire visual field is moving.

The optokinetic test can be perfectly recorded on VNG. VNG accurately records the speed of the slow phase of the induced nystagmus. The optokinetic response is a combination of a saccade and smooth pursuit eye movements.

TABLE 1: Manifestations of cerebellar lesions.[3]

Vermis lesions cause	Flocculus lesions cause	Nodulus lesions cause
Dysmetric saccade-like hypermetria	Defect in smooth pursuit	Periodic alternating nystagmus
Downbeat nystagmus	Impaired VOR suppression and/or positional nystagmus	Central positioning nystagmus
Gaze-evoked nystagmus	Rebound nystagmus	

BOX 1 Cerebellar control of ocular movements.[4]

The cerebellum coordinates the ocular motor system to drive the eyes smoothly and accurately and is richly supplied by afferent fibers conveying ocular information from the vestibular system, afferent visual system, and the premotor centers, e.g., PPRF, INC, etc.

- Dorsal vermis and fastigial nuclei determine the accuracy of saccades by modulating saccadic amplitude also; they adjust innervations to each eye selectively to ensure precise conjugate movements. Lesions of these structures result in saccadic dysmetria (often overshoot dysmetria that is greater centripetally), macrosaccadic oscillations, and disorders of vergence
- Flocculus—it is a part of the vestibulo-cerebellum which is responsible for matching saccadic pulse and step appropriately and for stabilizing images on the fovea. Lesions of the flocculus result in gaze holding deficits, such as gaze-evoked, rebound, and downbeat nystagmus. Floccular lesions impair smooth pursuit and cancellation of VOR by pursuit system during combined head and eye tracking
- Nodulus—lesions of cerebellar nodulus cause loss of GABA-mediated inhibition from the Purkinje cells to vestibular nuclei leading to instability in the velocity storage mechanism. Postrotational response is excessively prolonged leading to periodic alternating nystagmus. Some authorities believe that lesions in the nodulus may also cause central positioning nystagmus
- Deep cerebellar fastigial nuclei dysfunction leads to pendular nystagmus

(GABA: gamma-aminobutyric acid; INC: interstitial nucleus of Cajal; PPRF: paramedian pontine reticular formation; VOR: vestibulo-ocular reflex)

Convergence Divergence System

In order to look at an object closer by, the eyes rotate toward each other (convergence), while for an object further away, they rotate away from each other (divergence).

Vestibulo-ocular Reflex

This suppression of the VOR and consequently the cessation of the generation of nystagmus when the head is moved with the eyes open helps in fixating the gaze and is one of the oculomotor mechanisms of gaze stabilization during head movement with eyes open.

But if the subject is without visual fixation, then the examiner will be able to perceive the nystagmus in the subject's eyes as the subject moves the head. A jerky eye movement will be felt in the fingers which is the generated nystagmus. But when eyes are open, then no nystagmus is generated because of the VOR system.

Testing: In central oculomotor disorders, the VOR system is jeopardized and visual fixation does not suppress the nystagmus generated by head movement, and hence head movement with eyes open causes vertigo which is abnormal.

This mechanism can be tested by VNG, as well as by VHIT.

It is estimated that around 5% or more cases of the acute vestibular syndrome (AVS) occur due to stroke (CVA).

Acute vestibular syndrome is defined as a sudden onset of vertigo that lasts over seconds/minutes/hours and is accompanied by symptoms like nausea and vomiting, gait instability, nystagmus, and intolerance of change in posture which lasts for more than a day. It can happen due to vestibular neuritis, labyrinthitis, or other causes of acute peripheral vestibulopathy, but Identification of stroke from other AVS is crucial and requires prompt intervention.

MECHANISM OF MAINTENANCE OF POSTURAL STABILITY

The narrow base of support and multisegmental body architecture results in a potential instability of the erect posture. Postural stability involves the synchronization of strategies to stabilize the center of the body's mass during disturbances of stability induced by external destabilizing forces as well as by those initiated by the subject himself. The exact response strategy chosen by the body's balance mechanism to counter the destabilization depends not only on the characteristics of the postural displacement induced by the external destabilizing force (or self-induced, like while ballet-dancing), but also on the particular person's objectives, and expectations of the outcome, and on prior experience which is retrieved from the vestibular memory at that particular time. Anticipatory adjustments of posture and stance before initiation of movement of the trunk or the limbs help to sustain postural stability by counteracting and responding to the destabilization associated with moving the trunk or the limbs.

All this requires a huge amount of cognitive processing, as determining the best anticipatory postural adjustment and the selection of the best strategy that is most suited for a particular form of destabilization depends on the cognitive skills of the person. The extent of cognitive processing required for postural control depends both on the complexity and nature of the destabilizing force and on the proficiency of the subject's posture control system. Cognitive deficiencies that occur in old age hence lead to postural imbalance and falls. Multiple mechanisms are involved in postural control/stabilization which are more complex but less studied than gaze stabilization. Too many biological mechanisms and processes are involved in the control of posture and even a subclinical constraint, not necessarily a full-fledged pathology, can jeopardize the mechanism of maintenance of postural stability.

PERCEPTION OF VISUAL VERTICAL AND GRAVICEPTION

The third function of the balance system is the perception of verticality or graviception. It is the sense of verticality and the correct feeling of the line of the force of gravity acting on the body. To keep ourselves erect and to feel that we are not tilted or unsteady, the correct perception of the line of gravity is essential. This is a vestibular function carried out by the otolith organs but some contribution from the semicircular canals and may be from the cerebral cortex is also probably there. For proper orientation of the visual surroundings and for getting a sense of self-localization in three-dimensional space, the brain perceives the coordinates of verticality and horizontality and based on this perception, we get the feeling of how we are oriented or placed in the surroundings. To get the correct orientation our perception of verticality, i.e., what we consider as vertical, has to perfectly tally with the gravitational vertical. The sense of horizontality is at right angles to our perception of verticality. If the sense of verticality is deranged, the sense of horizontality is also correspondingly deranged and what we perceive around us will appear as tilted. This will contradict the inputs from the other sense organs (eyes and the proprioceptive system) giving rise to sensory conflicts and the feeling will be that we are not standing straight and that our body is tilted.

Otolithic Function

The otolithic function is to perceive verticality. The otolithic organs in the vestibular system sense gravity, both the utricle and saccule are responsible for the sense of verticality. So, in cases where otoliths or the neural pathway that transmits impulses from the otoliths or any aural part to the brain is damaged, the sense of perception of verticality will be altered.

Otolithic Dysfunction

In otolithic dysfunction, the otoliths provide erroneous information for control of posture and gaze stabilization in the horizontal and vertical planes. This leads to the incorrect sensation of upright posture, of a sense of self-motion and an incorrect spatial orientation of the body.

Subjective Visual Vertical Test

The subjective visual vertical test (SVV) is the test to ascertain the sense of verticality of a subject.

Central and Peripheral Disorders—What is the Difference?

From the clinical perspective, vertigo and imbalance can be due to any disorders in the brain (cerebral cortex, brainstem, cerebellum, and subcortical structures) or the spinal cord or because of the vestibular labyrinths, the eyes, proprioceptors in different parts of the body, or by disorders in the neural connections between all these organs. If occurs because of disorders in the vestibular labyrinths it is called peripheral disorders and if caused by disorders in the brain (and the other organs) are called central disorders.

Though most peripheral disorders will induce some functional central changes and vice versa. Any acute lesion of the vestibular labyrinth will induce some changes in the brainstem for the development of vestibular compensation and the final result will be a combination of the peripheral lesion including functional change in the brain.

CONCLUSION

Over the last two decades, our understanding of vestibular physiology has much evolved and today the pathophysiology of most vestibular disorders can be fathomed with much more clarity due to advancements in demystifying many of the hitherto unravelled complexities of vestibular physiology.

REFERENCES

1. Cheney PD, Fets EE, Mewes K. Neural mechanisms underlying corticospinal and rubrospinal control of limb movements. Prog Brain Res. 1991;87:213-52.
2. Fiester P, Baig SA, Patel J, Rao D. An anatomic, imaging, and clinical review of the medial longitudinal fasciculus. J Clin Imaging Sci. 2020;10:83.
3. Banerjee S. An introduction to Neurotology: Anirban. Indian J Otolaryngol Head Neck Surg. 1998;50(4):401.
4. Zee DS, Walker MF, Ramant S. The cerebellar contribution to eye movements based upon lesions: binocular three-axis control and the translational vestibulo-ocular reflex. Ann NY Acad Sci 2002;956:178-89.

21

CHAPTER

Applied Neuroanatomy and Neurophysiology of the Spinal Cord

Tejaswini Shanubhogue, Devangi Desai, Soaham Desai

INTRODUCTION

The spinal cord is a tubular structure connecting the brain and the peripheral nervous system. Information is relayed to and from peripheral organs such as skin, muscle, and viscera to the brain via the various ascending and descending tracts traversing the spinal cord. In addition, autonomic outputs to viscera also travel through the spinal cord. The spinal cord has intrinsic functions in addition to serving as a conduit to the functional tracts.

NEUROANATOMY OF SPINAL CORD AND ITS SIGNIFICANCE

Brief Anatomy of Vertebral Column

The vertebral column is composed of 33 vertebrae—7 cervical, 12 thoracic, 5 lumbar, 5 sacral (fused to form the sacrum), and 4 coccygeal (the lower 3 are commonly fused). It measures 65 cm in length. It is a segmented flexible structure made up of vertebrae, joints, and intervertebral discs.[1]

In a typical vertebra, the spinal cord with its covering lies in the vertebral foramen, encircled by the body of the vertebra anteriorly and vertebral arch posteriorly **(Fig. 1)**. The sides of the vertebral arch are formed by a pair of cylindrical pedicles and comprise a pair of flattened laminae posteriorly. Posteriorly, it gives rise to the spinous process from the junction of two laminae, and from the junction of pedicles and the laminae, it gives rise to transverse processes on either side and four articular processes (two superior and two inferior). Muscles and ligaments are attached to the spinous and transverse processes, and synovial joints are formed between the two superior articular processes of one vertebral arch with the two inferior articular processes of the arch above. The segmental spinal nerves with their dural sheath and vascular structures exit through the intervertebral foramina, which is formed by the notches on the superior and inferior borders of the pedicles of the adjacent vertebrae. The adjacent vertebral bodies have intervertebral discs of fibrocartilage between them, which are thickest in the cervical and lumbar regions, and they serve as buffers to shocks/movements. The discs contain a central, gelatinous, fluid structure called nucleus pulposus, which makes the forward/backward movements of vertebral bodies possible. It is surrounded by fibrocartilaginous annulus fibrosus.[1,2]

The anterior longitudinal ligament (ALL) and posterior longitudinal ligament (PLL) lie anterior and posterior to the vertebral body, respectively. PLL is weak and narrow compared to the ALL. Other ligaments include the supraspinous ligament between the connecting tips of the adjacent spine, an interspinous ligament between adjacent spinous processes, and an intertransverse ligament between the adjacent transverse process and ligamentum flava between laminae of adjacent vertebrae. In the cervical region, the nuchal ligament is formed by the thickening of supraspinous and interspinous ligaments.

Clinical significance:

- In sudden compressive load, the flattening of the nucleus pulposus is initially accommodated by the surrounding annulus fibrosus but occasionally may cause the annulus to rupture, leading to bulging of the nucleus pulposus causing impingement of nerve roots/spinal cord.
- With age, the nucleus pulposus is replaced by fibrocartilage, and collagen of the annulus also generates, decreasing its resilience and predisposing it to disc herniation and myeloradiculopathy.[1]

Anatomy of the Spinal Cord

Surface Anatomy

The spinal cord is an oval-shaped tubular structure measuring 42–45 cm, flattened anteroposteriorly with cervical (C3–T1, measuring 38 mm) and lumbar (L1–S3, measuring

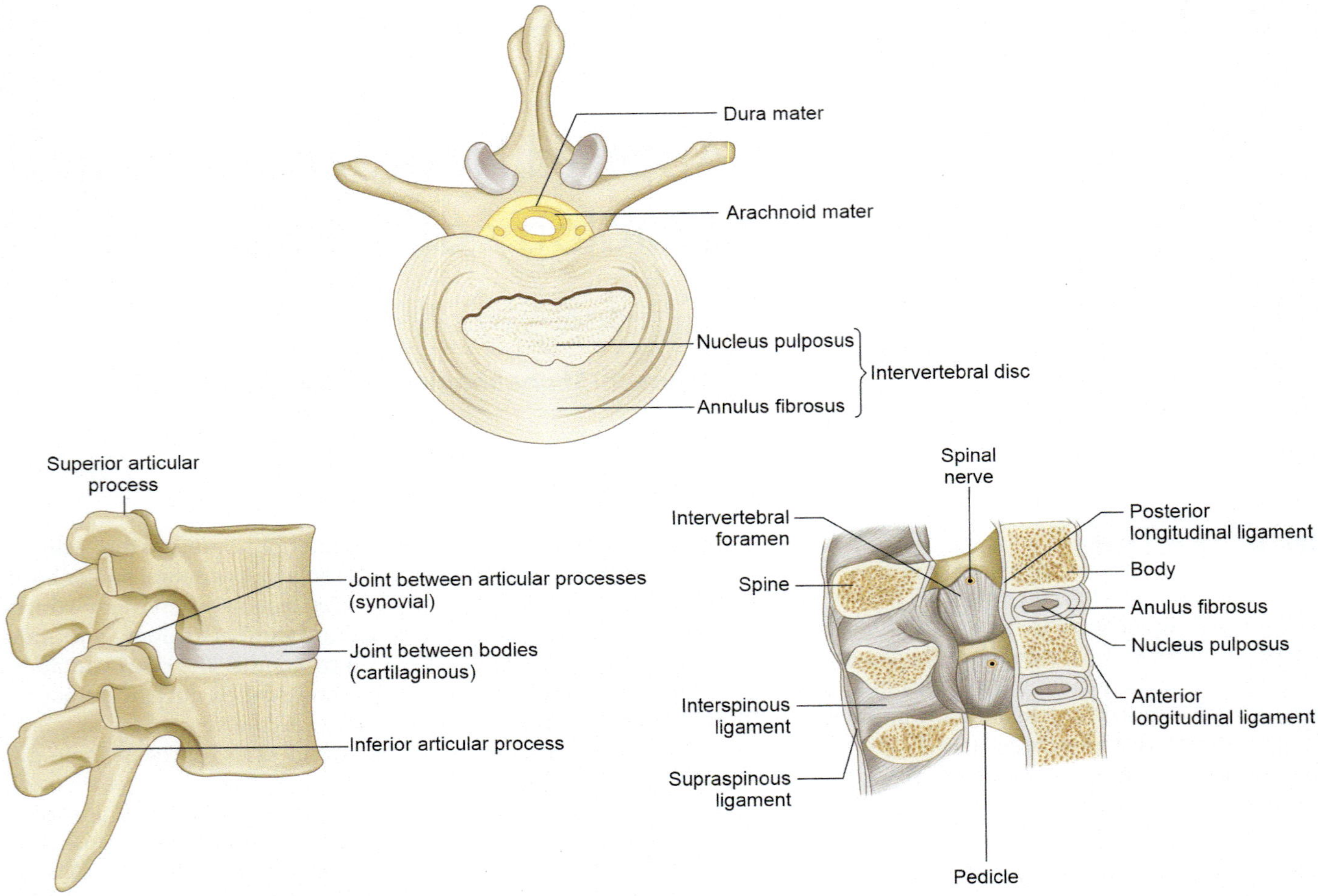

FIG. 1: Vertebral column: Intervertebral joints and ligaments.

35 mm) bulges, corresponding to the nerves of the limbs. It extends from the foramen magnum and terminates in the conus medullaris.

The spinal cord ends at the third vertebral level at birth (L3) and L1–L2 in adults due to differential growth of the vertebral canal and the body as compared to the spinal cord. As the spinal cord segments do not correspond to the vertebral segments, the nerve roots must travel in a downward direction to reach their proper entry and exit levels between the vertebrae, especially for the lower spinal cord roots **(Table 1)**. These nerve roots traveling through the cerebrospinal fluid (CSF)-filled lumbar cistern from the end of the spinal cord at the L1–L2 level are collectively called the cauda equina.

The spinal cord is marked by a deep anterior median fissure, shallower posterior median sulcus, and the anterolateral and posterolateral sulci are the longitudinal grooves along the spinal cord **(Fig. 2)**. Filaments from anterolateral and posterolateral sulci form the anterior and posterior roots, respectively. The spinal nerve is formed by joining together one anterior root and the corresponding posterior root on each side just distal to the dorsal root ganglion. Each mixed nerve gives a ventral ramus which supplies the anterolateral body wall, muscles, and skin of

TABLE 1: Relation between vertebral level and spinal segment.

Vertebral level	Spinal segment
C1–C4	Same segment
C5–C7	Add one to the number of vertebrae
T1–T6	Add two to the number of vertebrae
T7–T9	Add three to the number of vertebrae
T10	L1–L3 segments
T11	L3–L4 segments
T12	L5–S1 segments
L1	S2-coccyx segments

the limbs, and a dorsal ramus which supplies the muscles and skin of the back **(Fig. 3)**. Corresponding to each pair of spinal nerves, the spinal cord is organized into segments, namely 8 cervical, 12 dorsal or thoracic, 5 lumbar, 5 sacral segments, and 1 coccygeal.

The spinal cord is covered by three meningeal layers akin to the brain. The pia mater, the innermost cover, tightly adheres to the surface of the cord and continues above as the cranial pia mater. Pial modifications include 21/22 pairs of ligament denticulata (tooth-like attachments) from the spinal cord to the inner aspects of the dura mater, filum terminale attaching the lower end of the spinal cord to the posterior aspect of the coccyx, and linea splendens, which is a shiny band at the anteromedian fissure. The arachnoid is a transparent middle layer that extends up to the second sacral vertebra and is separated from the inner pia mater by the CSF-containing subarachnoid space **(Fig. 4)**. It continues rostrally with the cranial arachnoid mater and the subarachnoid space. The outermost layer, the dura mater, is continuous with the cranial dura where it is fused with the endosteum at the foramen magnum and hence the absence of true epidural space in the skull physiologically. Caudally, it extends up to the second/third sacral vertebra and is separated from the bony vertebral periosteum by the epidural space in the vertebral canal, containing fat and a thin-walled vertebral venous plexus (Batson's plexus). Dura extends over the dorsal and ventral roots of the spinal nerve up to the intervertebral foramina and is attached to its margins. The three meningeal layers then continue and attach to the coccyx as the coccygeal ligament.[1-3]

Clinical significance:

- Epidural anesthesia is given in the epidural space and spinal anesthesia in the subarachnoid space. Less anesthetic is required in spinal anesthesia. Epidural anesthesia is especially preferred in labor. Caution needs to be exercised as inadvertent injury to the venous plexus may cause an epidural hematoma. In caudal epidural anesthesia, a needle is passed through the sacral hiatus to anesthetize the perineal area supplied by S4/S5 nerve roots.
- Lumbar puncture for diagnostic/therapeutic purposes can be done in the lumbar cistern without risk of injury to the spinal cord as it terminates at L1. The lumbar cistern is the subarachnoid space that extends from L1–S2 as the dura and the arachnoid mater extends up to S2 **(Fig. 5)**.

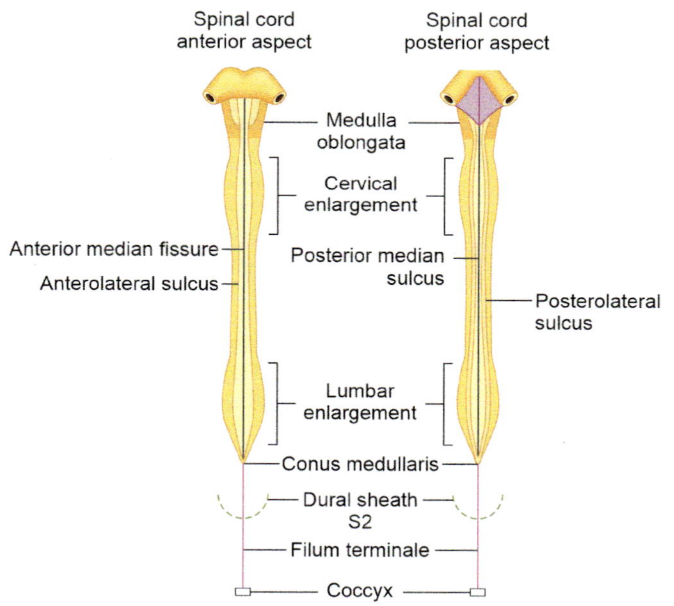

FIG. 2: Surface anatomy of spinal cord.

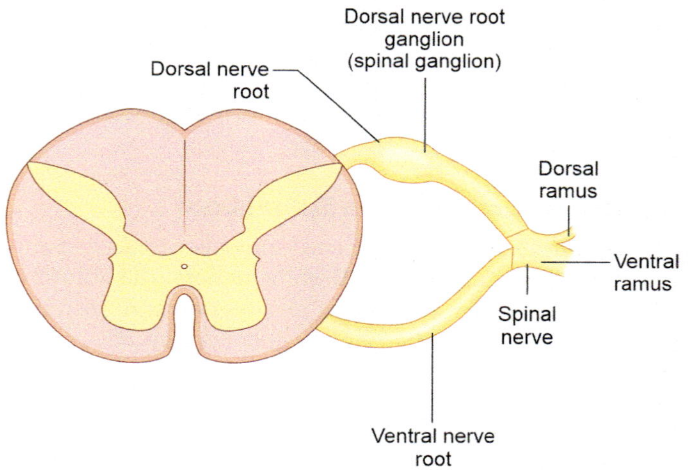

FIG. 3: Spinal nerve: Relation of a spinal nerve to the spinal cord.

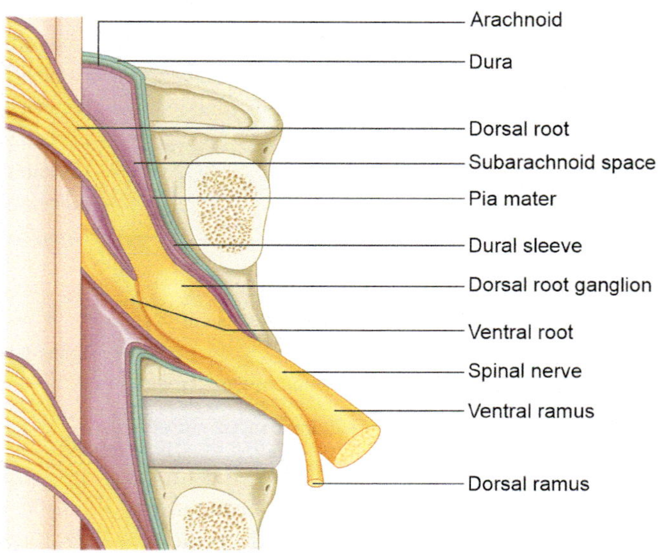

FIG. 4: Spinal cord meninges and spaces.

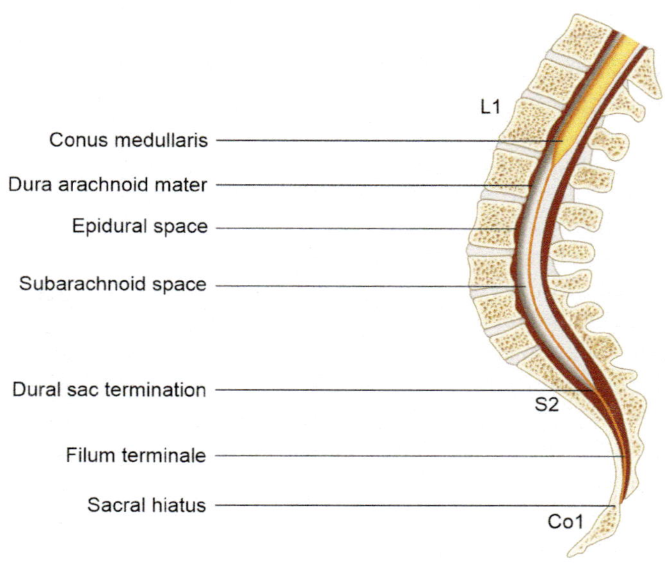

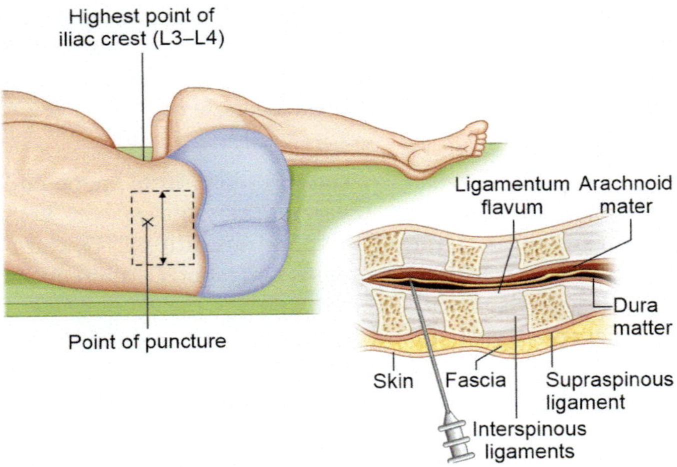

FIG. 5: Lumbar puncture.

- In pediatric patients, filum terminale may pull on the spinal cord known as tethered cord syndrome. It can cause numbness of feet, asymmetrical muscle atrophy of calf/thigh, upper motor neuron (UMN) signs, bladder/bowel dysfunction, foot deformities or scoliosis, etc. Once, it is confirmed by imaging studies; management includes surgically resecting it to relieve spinal cord tension.[1,4]

Internal Structure of the Spinal Cord

On the transverse section, the cord substance is divided into the central gray and peripheral white matters. The butterfly-shaped gray matter consists of an anterior and posterior horn on each side, united by the gray commissure, in the middle of which lies the central canal.

Gray Matter of Spinal Cord

Gray matter is divided into I–X Rexed laminae. I–VI constitute the posterior horn, VII–IX refer to the anterior horn, and X surrounds the central canal **(Table 2 and Fig. 6)**. Gray matter is divided into anterior, posterior, and lateral horns. The gray matter of both sides is connected by a gray commissure that is traversed by the central canal. Rostrally, it continues as the central canal of the medulla oblongata, and caudally it expands to form a terminal ventricle in conus medullaris and continues for a while in filum terminale.[2] The amount of gray matter is maximum at cervical and lumbar enlargements supplying the limb muscles. In the cervical spinal cord, the arrangement from medial to lateral of the motor neurons destined for specific spinal segments are cervical, thoracic, lumbar, and sacral, which is similar to the ascending fibers in the spinothalamic tracts. But, contrary to this, the fibers from the lower limbs lie medial to those from the upper limbs in the posterior columns **(Tables 3 and 4)**.[2,5]

TABLE 2: Rexed laminae of spinal cord gray matter.

Laminae	Localization	Important structures and functions
I	Posterior horn, below tract of Lissauer	Dorsal root mediating pain, touch, temperature, posteromarginal nucleus
II	Posterior horn	Substantia gelatinosa neurons mediating pain transmission
III and IV	Posterior horn	Proper sensory nucleus receiving inputs from substantia gelatinosa and contributing to anterolateral system carrying pain, temperature, and touch
V	Posterior horn	Afferents from skin, muscle, and viscera
VI	Present in cervical and lumbar segments	Clarke's nucleus (C8–T2), muscle/tendon afferents from spinocerebellar tract
VII	Most anterior part of posterior horn	Intermediolateral column carrying sympathetic and parasympathetic preganglionic from T1–L2, S2–S4, and Renshaw cells
VIII and IX	Anterior horn	Alpha and gamma motor neurons innervating skeletal muscles. Medial aspect carries vestibulospinal and reticulospinal tracts innervating axial muscle and maintain balance and posture. Lateral aspect contains corticospinal tract, rubrospinal tract, and innervates distal musculature
X	Gray matter surrounding spinal cord	

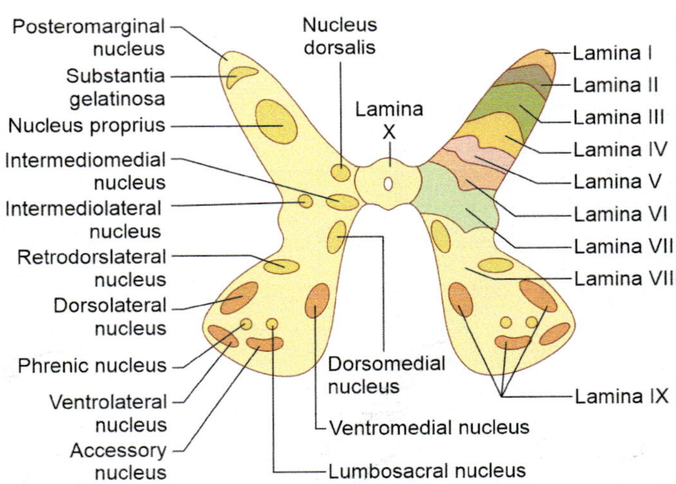

FIG. 6: Rexed laminae of spinal cord.

TABLE 3: Nerve cell groups (gray matter of spinal cord).

Anterior gray column	Posterior gray column	Lateral gray column	Gray commissure and central canal
• *Medial group of nerves*: Supply the axial muscles • *Central group*: ○ *One phrenic nucleus*: C3–C5, to diaphragm ○ *Two accessory nuclei*: C1–C5 accessory branch of XI nerve to sternocleidomastoid and trapezius ○ *Three lumbosacral nuclei*: L2–S3 to unknown distribution • Lateral group in cervical and lumbosacral segments innervates the skeletal muscles of limbs	• Posteromarginal nucleus • Substantia gelatinosa of Rolando (sensory neurons cell body, small-sized neurons, interneurons), and above continuous with spinal tract of V nerve, traversed by fiber of dorsal nerve roots carrying pain, temperature, touch from posterior root, and receive descending fibers from supraspinal levels, which modulate the pain pathways • Nucleus proprius anterior to substantia gelatinosa and carries proprioception, two-point discrimination, and vibration • Nucleus dorsalis extends from C8–L3/L4 and consists of large cells with proprioceptive endings to neuromuscular and tendon spindles • Visceral afferent nucleus is lateral to nucleus dorsalis (extends from T1–L3) and receives afferent information	• Intermediolateral group of cells form small lateral gray column from T1–L2 carrying preganglionic sympathetic fibers along anterior nerve root and reaches sympathetic chain via white rami communicans • In S2–S4, group of cells forms lateral column carrying preganglionic parasympathetic fibers, forms pelvic splanchnic nerves	Gray commissure resembles "H" with central canal, which divides it into anterior gray commissure and posterior gray commissure

TABLE 4: Types of neurons in spinal gray column.

Anterior gray horn	Posterior gray horn	Lateral gray horn
• *Alpha motor neurons*: Innervate skeletal muscles (lamina IX) • *Gamma motor neurons*: Sensory information from intrafusal fibers and muscle spindles reach alpha motor neurons (lamina IX) • Modulatory interneurons (lamina VIII) • *Renshaw cells*: Regulate alpha motor neuron activity *Note*: The somatotropic representation of flexor muscles is posterior to extensor muscles, and distal muscles are represented lateral to proximal muscles. It is larger in C5–T1 and L2–S4	• Internuncial neurons • *Intersegmental/ascending tracts*: Carrying afferent information from central processes of dorsal root ganglion (DRG)	• Preganglionic neurons sympathetic in T1–L2 • Preganglionic neurons parasympathetic in S2–S4

Clinical significance:

- Spinal cord can be affected by tumors, either within the cord (intramedullary) or outside the cord (extramedullary). These tumors cause cord compression, and the evolution of symptoms is according to the involvement of different tracts of the spinal cord.[1]

White Matter of Spinal Cord

The white matter is divided into three columns, namely the anterior column between the anterior fissure and the anterior horn of gray matter, the lateral column between the ventral and dorsal roots, i.e., the anterolateral and posterolateral sulci, and the posterior column, between the posterior median septum and the posterior horn of gray matter and its dorsal root **(Fig. 7)**. The sympathetic autonomic fibers descend in the intermediolateral columns of the gray matter on each side in the thoracic cord and upper lumbar segments, and parasympathetic in the anterior horns of the gray matter of sacral segments. There are ventral and dorsal gray commissures connecting the white matter of both halves of the spinal cord. The amount of white matter at upper levels is more than at lower levels due to the addition of ascending fibers at higher cord segments and the termination of descending levels before the lower cord segments.[2,5]

Blood Supply of the Spinal Cord

Arteries

Two posterior spinal arteries, derived from the corresponding vertebral or posterior inferior cerebellar artery, lie either in front of or behind the dorsal nerve roots of the spinal nerve in the posterolateral sulci and give off coronal

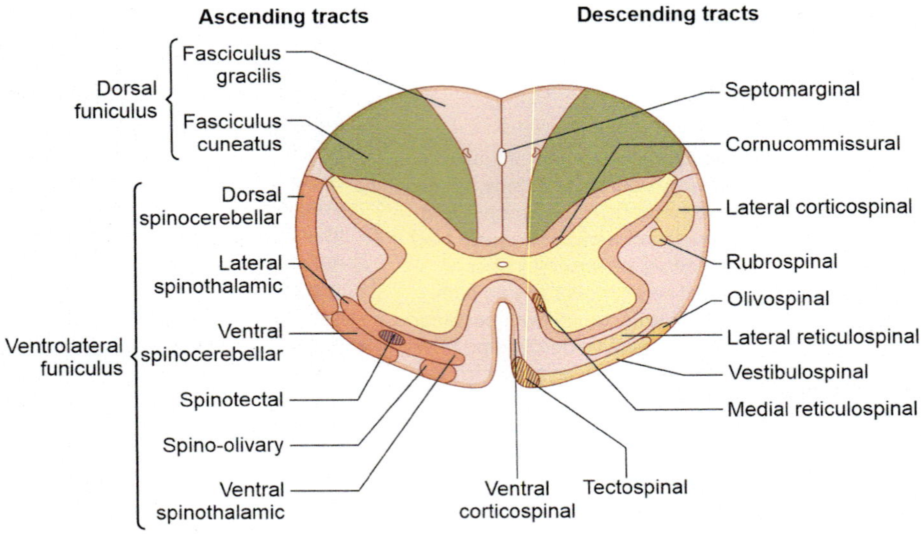

FIG. 7: White matter tracts of spinal cord.

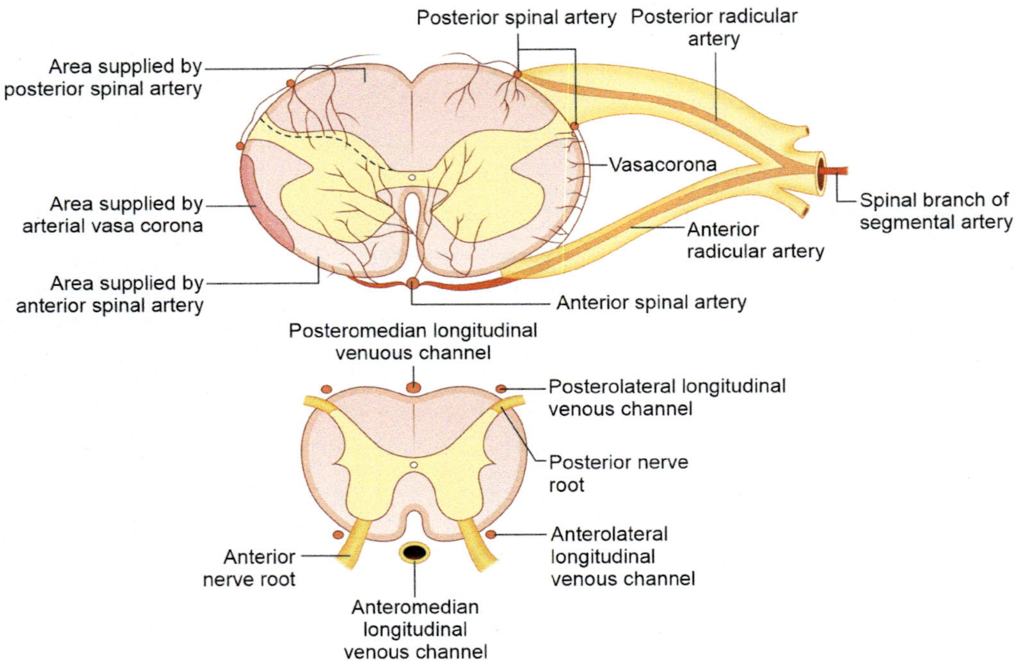

FIG. 8: Blood supply of spinal cord.

branches, which anastomose with the segmental branches of the aorta. The posterior spinal arteries supply the posterior one-third of the spinal cord including the posterior columns, the posterior root entry zone, the Lissauer tract, and substantia gelatinosa along with some portions of the corticospinal tract **(Fig. 8)**.

A single anterior spinal artery lies in the anterior median fissure along the whole length of the cord, and it is formed by the union of branches of vertebral artery on either side. It supplies the anterior two-thirds of the spinal cord to the base of the posterior horn. Additionally, vertebral costocervical trunk, intercostal and lumbar arteries contribute to the spinal cord blood supply by giving off segmental arteries, which enter through the intervertebral foramina. The one in the lower cervical region at C6 and the great anterior radicular artery of Adamkiewicz, commonly between the T5 and T8 segments (may enter at any level from T5 to L4), are the segmental arteries that need special mention.

Few circumferential vessels run over the cord surface at each segment and form anastomoses between the anterior and posterior spinal vessels, sending some horizontal branches to the white matter and the posterior horns of the gray matter.

Conus medullaris and cauda equina are supplied by the iliolumbar and lateral sacral branches of the internal iliac arteries in addition to the descending branches of the spinal arteries. At the conus, anterior spinal artery and posterior spinal artery are joined by the ansa of the conus.[2]

Clinical significance:
- Artery of Adamkiewicz may be injured in spinal cord surgeries, injuries, or during aortic aneurysm repair and may be an important cause of lumbosacral cord ischemia.
- Spinal cord perfusion is initially maintained by autoregulatory mechanisms. Damage occurs when there is prolonged ischemia with failure of autoregulation usually in 20–30 minutes. Anterior horn cell is affected first due to high metabolic demand.
- Anterior spinal cord syndrome presents with neck pain, areflexic paraplegia, loss of pain, and temperature sensations below the level of involvement with preserved joint position sense and vibration. In posterior cord syndrome, joint position and vibration, i.e., posterior column, is affected by sparing of motor functions.
- Spinal cord vascular malformations can present with acute as well as chronic myelopathy **(*See* Table 12)**.[1,6]

Veins

The six longitudinal spinal veins run in the pia mater and drain via the veins of the medulla oblongata into the intracranial venous sinuses. The posterior medullary veins drain the posterior half of the spinal cord. One lateral and two medial groups of the anterior medullary veins drain the anterior part of the cord **(Fig. 8)**.[2]

Clinical significance:
- Anatomical pattern of venous drainage explains the clinical features of venous infarction of the cord. Thrombophlebitis may reach the spinal veins through the venous drainage through the intervertebral foramina. The epidural venous plexus of the spinal cord is a possible site for metastases from pelvic (including prostate) tumors.[1,5]

Spinal Cord Segments and Nerve Roots

The spinal cord is divided into parts according to the region innervated: Cervical (8 spinal roots), thoracic (12 spinal roots), lumbar (5 spinal roots), sacral (5 spinal roots), and coccygeal (1 root). Areas of skin are supplied by a spinal segment by its nerve root called its dermatome. There is a significant overlap between the adjacent dermatomes. The muscles supplied by a spinal segment by its motor root are called its myotome. A single muscle may be innervated by multiple nerve roots, and a single root may innervate multiple muscles. The spinal cord is enlarged in the cervical region and the lumbosacral segments, the roots of which form the brachial and lumbosacral plexus, respectively. The spinal cord tapers and its lowermost portion is called the conus medullaris, and it corresponds approximately to the sacral segments **(Table 5 and Fig. 9)**.

TABLE 5: Spinal level localization.

Level involved	Motor system	Sensory system	Others
C1–C4	Quadriparesis or quadriplegia	Sensory involvement of trunk and all four limbs	Lesions above C4 may involve diaphragm. Downbeating nystagmus and ataxia may be seen if lesion at foramen magnum
C5/C6	Rhomboids, deltoids, Brachialis, biceps, and brachioradialis weakness and atrophy and spastic paralysis below the level. Biceps, radial jerks absent/diminished/inverted	Sensory involvement of lower limbs, trunk, and medial arm	
C8/T1	Wrist and finger flexors and small hand muscles weakness + atrophy; preserved upper limb DTRs. UMN signs below the lesion	Sensory involvement of lower limbs, trunk, medial arm, and forearm, and occasionally little finger is seen	Rarely, Horner's syndrome may also be seen
T2–T8	Atrophic paralysis confined to the intercostals at the segment involved with spastic paralysis of the muscles of abdomen and lower limbs below it	A sensory level is found on the trunk	Diaphragm is normal
T9–T10	Lower halves of abdominal recti paralyzed with normal upper halves. Umbilicus is drawn upward when the patient raises his head against resistance. There is spastic paralysis of the lower limbs. Upper abdominal reflexes are lost with preserved lower abdominal reflexes	Sensory signs are found below the level of the umbilicus	
T12–L1	The abdominal recti are normal, but the lower fibers of obliquus internus and transversus abdominis are paralyzed. The abdominal reflexes are preserved, but the cremasteric reflexes are diminished or lost. There is spastic paralysis of the lower limbs	Sensation is impaired throughout the lower limbs	

Continued

Continued

Level involved	Motor system	Sensory system	Others
L3/L4	Flexion of the hip is preserved. There is weakness and wasting of the quadriceps and of the hip adductors, with diminution and loss of knee jerks, and spastic paralysis of the remaining muscles of the lower limbs, with exaggeration of the ankle jerks and extensor plantar responses	Sensory loss is found below the knees, on the posterior aspect of the thighs, the buttocks, and perineum	
S1/S2	Flexion of the hip, adduction of the thigh, extension of the knee, and dorsiflexion of the foot are preserved. There is atrophic paralysis of the intrinsic muscles of the foot and those of the calf, with weakness of knee flexion and hip abduction and extension. The knee jerks are preserved; the ankle jerks and plantar reflexes are lost. The anal and bulbocavernosus reflexes are retained	Sensory impairments involve the buttocks, perineum, and posterior aspects of the lower limbs, including the soles of the feet	
S3/S4	The large bowel and bladder are paralyzed with retention of urine and feces, due to the uninhibited action of the sympathetic nerve supply. The external sphincters are paralyzed, and the anal and bulbocavernosus reflexes are lost. The motility and reflexes of the lower limb are normal	There is usually sensory loss in the perineum and buttocks in a "saddle" distribution	

(DTR: deep tendon reflex; UMN: upper motor neuron)

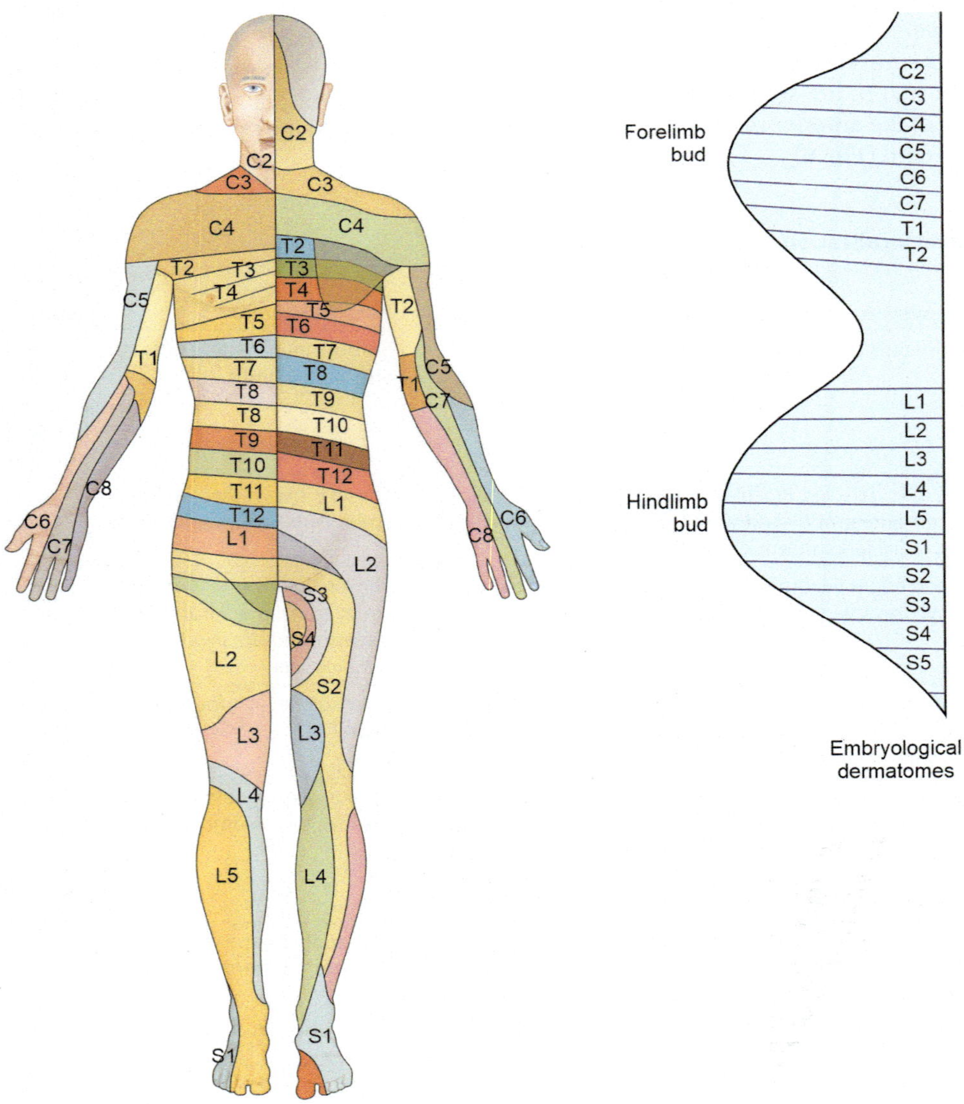

FIG. 9: Dermatomes.

Clinical significance:
- Knowledge of spinal cord segments and the dermatomes and myotomes helps in interpreting the neurological examination findings to localize the injury or disease (called the lesion) at the spinal cord (segmental) level. Nerve roots may be compressed by intervertebral disc herniation or protrusion/degenerative changes at the joints connecting the discs. The most commonly involved nerve roots in back injuries are L4/L5 or L5/S1. Nerve roots can be anesthetized by local anesthetic injection in the epidural region. This technique is used to anesthetize the sensory nerve roots in the perineal region during childbirth.
- Pain from viscera is felt in the skin or body wall supplied by the same nerve root. For example, pain from the diaphragm is referred to as C4, heart to lower cervical/upper thoracic, stomach to T7–T9, intestine to T7–T10, appendix to T10, gallbladder to the inferior angle of the scapula (T7), cervix/pelvis to low back and S2–S4.
- Herpes zoster affects the dorsal root ganglion and may cause painful rash and eruptions along with the dermatomal distribution of the nerve root as well as neuralgia.[5]

NEUROPHYSIOLOGY OF THE SPINAL CORD AND ITS RELEVANCE

Ascending and Descending Tracts of the Spinal Cord

The uncrossed anterior corticospinal tracts run in the anterior column. The lateral column consists of the lateral corticospinal tracts, the spinocerebellar tracts laterally, and the spinothalamic tracts anteriorly. The other tracts in the lateral column include the ascending spino-olivary tract and the descending rubrospinal tract. The posterior column contains the fasciculus gracilis medially and fasciculus cuneatus laterally. The fibers to/from cervical segments lie medial most; then thoracic, lumbar, and sacral fibers are the most lateral in the case of the lateral corticospinal tract and spinothalamic tract. However, the reverse is true for the posterior column where the sacral fibers lie medially.

Other ascending pathways include spinoreticular pathways, which are partially crossed, lying in the ventrolateral spinal cord, and terminate in the reticular formation of the medulla and pons and function in pain modulation.

Spino-olivary and spinotectal are other ascending pathways **(Tables 6 and 7)**. See **Figures 10 to 15** for various ascending tracts of the spinal cord and **Figures 16 to 19** for various descending tracts of the spinal cord.[2,5]

Clinical significance:
- Spinal cord disorders may present with sensory, motor, and sphincter deficits in varying combinations. Symptoms may include difficulties in walking with stiff/dragging/unsteady gait or upper limb function with weakness below the level of the lesion. There may be painful muscle spasms in the lower limbs. Sensory symptoms may include numbness, tingling, pins and needles, hyperalgesia, allodynia, burning sensations, altered temperature sensation, and tight-band-like feelings below the level of the lesions.
- Except for acute transverse lesions, where bladder involvement in the form of acute urinary retention is the rule, spinal cord disease usually presents with urgency, frequency, and urge incontinence rather than hesitancy or retention. Constipation is common, though fecal incontinence may also happen.

TABLE 6: Different sensations and their ascending pathways of the spinal cord.

Sensation	Receptor	First-order neuron	Second-order neuron	Third-order neuron	Pathways	Crossing	Destination
Pain and temperature	Free nerve endings	Posterior root ganglia	Substantia gelatinosa	Ventral postero-lateral nucleus of thalamus	Lateral spinothalamic, spinal lemniscus	Ventral white commissure	Posterior central gyrus
Light touch and pressure	Free nerve endings	Posterior root ganglion	Substantia gelatinosa	Ventral postero-lateral nucleus of thalamus	Anterior spinothalamic, spinal lemniscus	Ventral white commissure	Posterior central gyrus
Discriminative touch, vibratory sense, conscious muscle joint sense	Meissner's corpuscles, Pacinian corpuscles, muscle spindles, tendon organs	Posterior root ganglion	Nuclei gracilis and cuneatus	Ventral posterolateral nucleus of thalamus	Fasciculi gracilis and cuneatus, medial lemniscus	Crossing in sensory decussation in medulla	Posterior central gyrus
Unconscious muscle joint sense	Muscle spindles, tendon organs, joint receptors	Posterior root ganglion	Nucleus dorsalis		Anterior and posterior spinocerebellar		Cerebellar cortex

TABLE 7: Descending pathways in spinal cord.

Tract	Origin	Crossing	At spinal cord	Function
Corticospinal tract (CST)	Cerebral cortex motor, premotor, and somatosensory areas	Lower end of medulla. 80% cross and form lateral CST. Uncrossed descend as anterior CST and cross at the level	Gray matter at various levels	Voluntary movement
Rubrospinal tract	Red nucleus in upper midbrain	Lower part of tegmentum	Lateral funiculi anterior to lateral CST	Facilitatory to flexors, inhibitory to extensors
Tectospinal tract	Superior colliculus of midbrain	Upper part of tegmentum of midbrain	Anterior funiculi of spinal cord	
Medial reticulospinal	Medial part of reticular formation of pons	Cross in pons	Anterior funiculus	Facilitation to extensor of trunk and limbs. Some inhibition to neck
Lateral reticulospinal	Medulla reticular formation	Cross in medulla	Lateral funiculus	Facilitation to flexors of trunk and limbs Automatic breathing Pain modulation
Medial vestibulospinal	Medial vestibular nucleus in medulla	Uncrossed	Anterior funiculus	Inhibits muscles of neck and back, maintains equilibrium
Lateral vestibulospinal	Lateral vestibular nucleus in medulla	Uncrossed	Anterior funiculus	Inhibits flexors, supplies extensors of neck, back, limb, maintains equilibrium
Descending autonomic	Paraventricular hypothalamus	Uncrossed	Dorsolateral funiculus	Autonomic functions

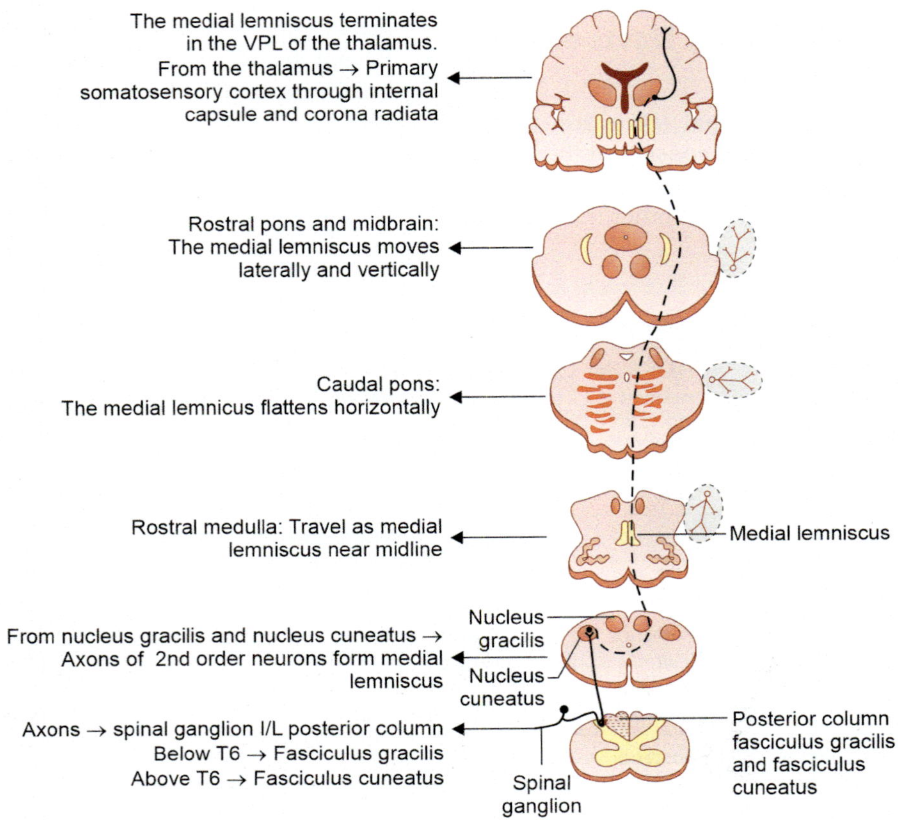

FIG. 10: Posterior column medial lemniscus pathway.
(VPL: ventroposterolateral nucleus)

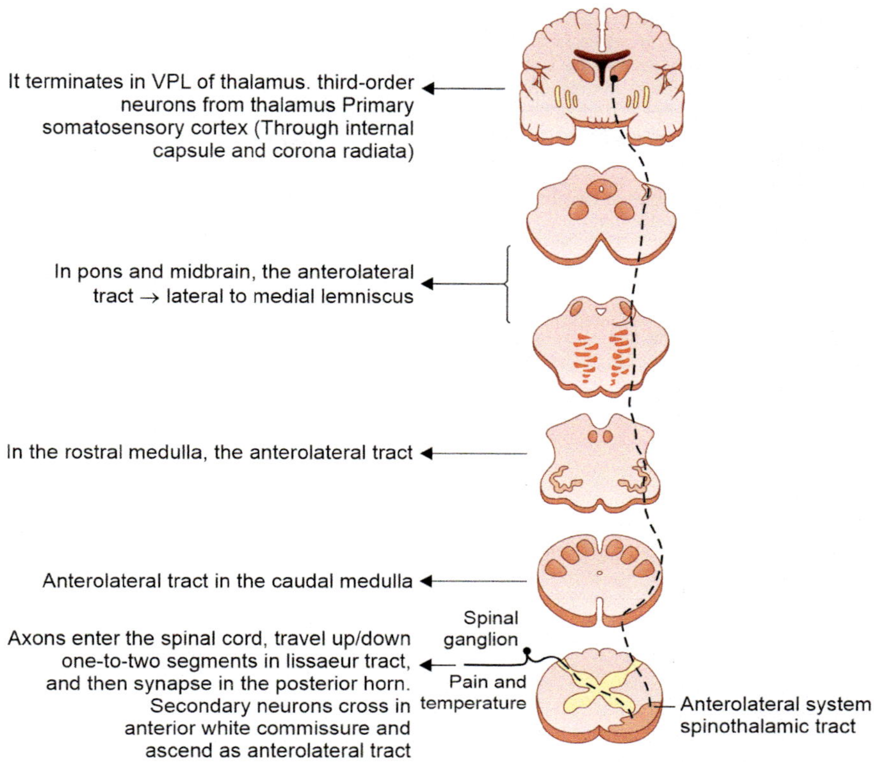

FIG. 11: Spinothalamic tract.
(VPL: ventroposterolateral nucleus)

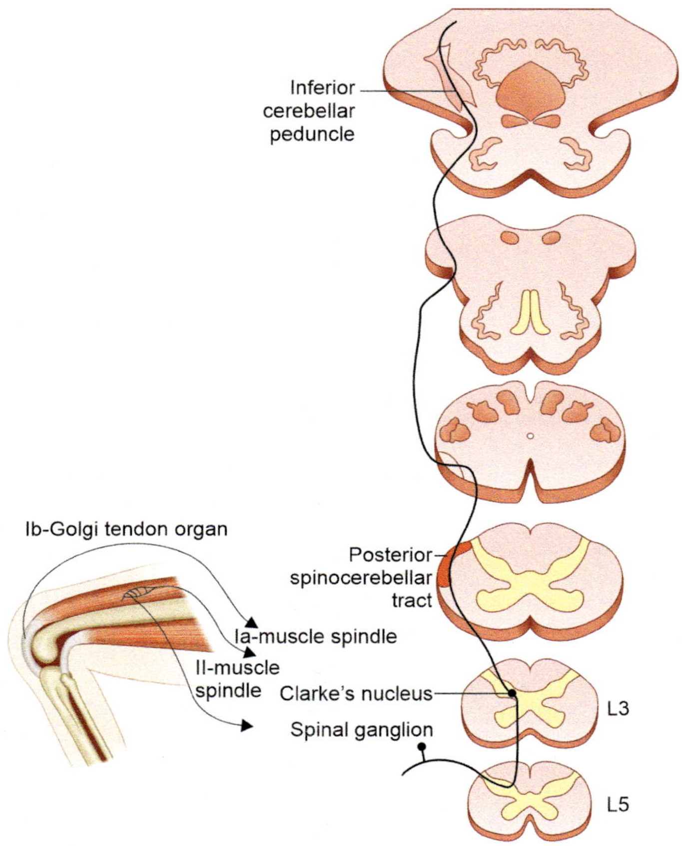

FIG. 12: Posterior spinocerebellar tract.

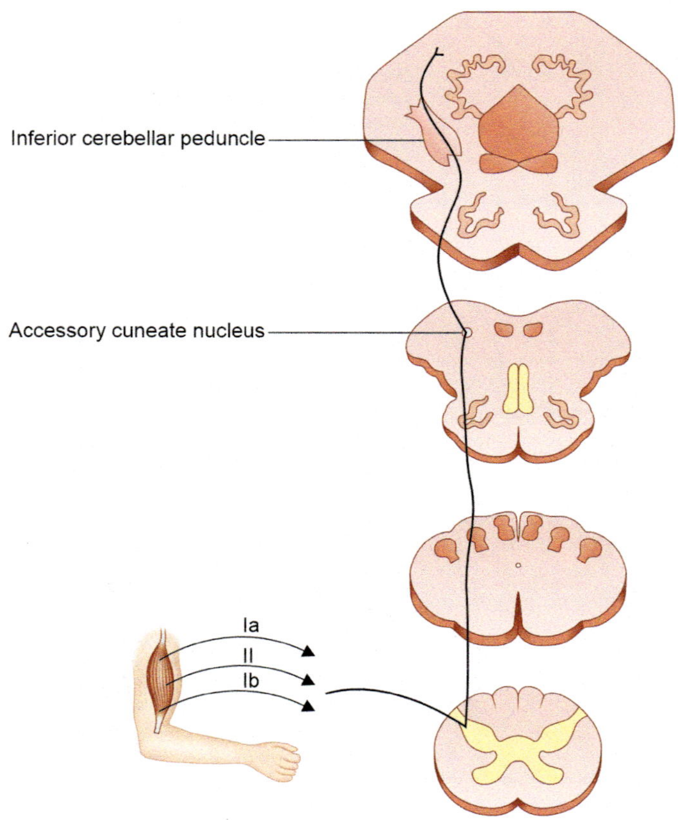

FIG. 13: Cuneocerebellar tract.

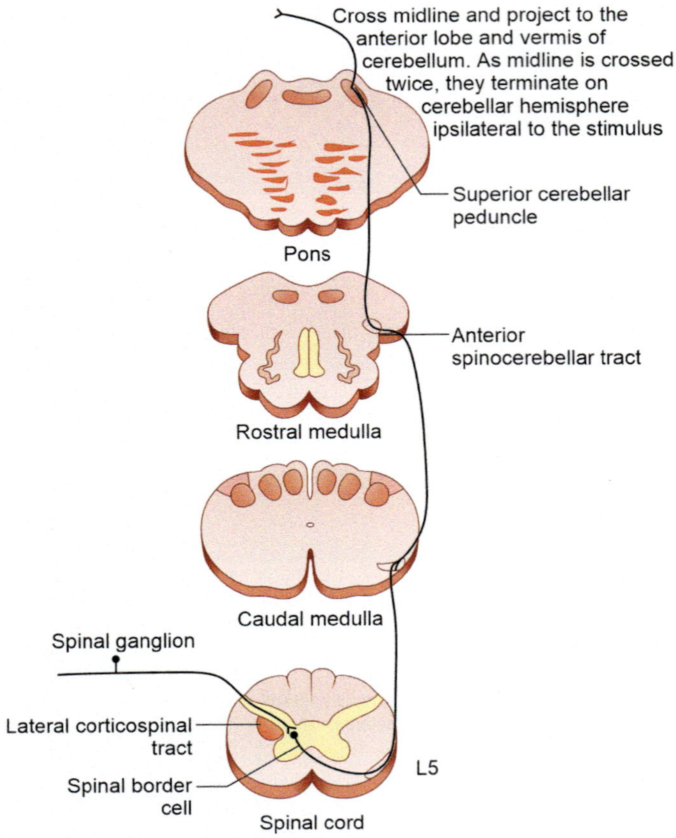

FIG. 14: Anterior spinocerebellar tract.

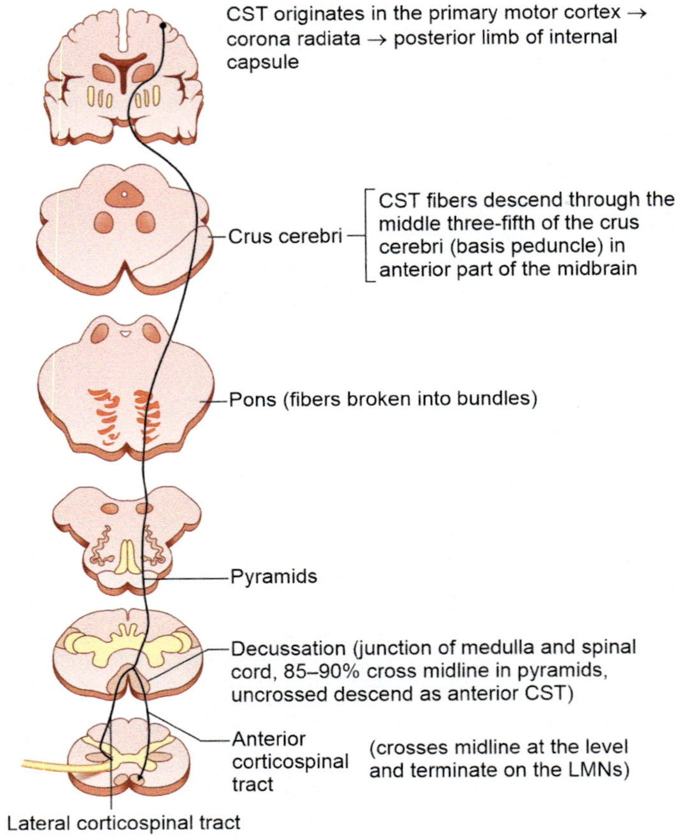

FIG. 16: Corticospinal tracts.

(CST: corticospinal tract; LMN: lower motor neuron)

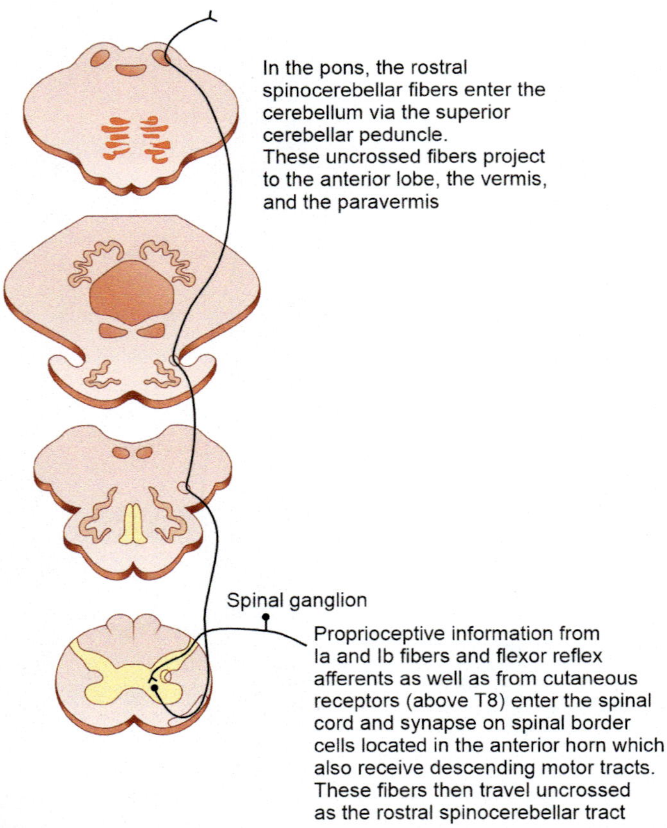

FIG. 15: Rostral spinocerebellar tract.

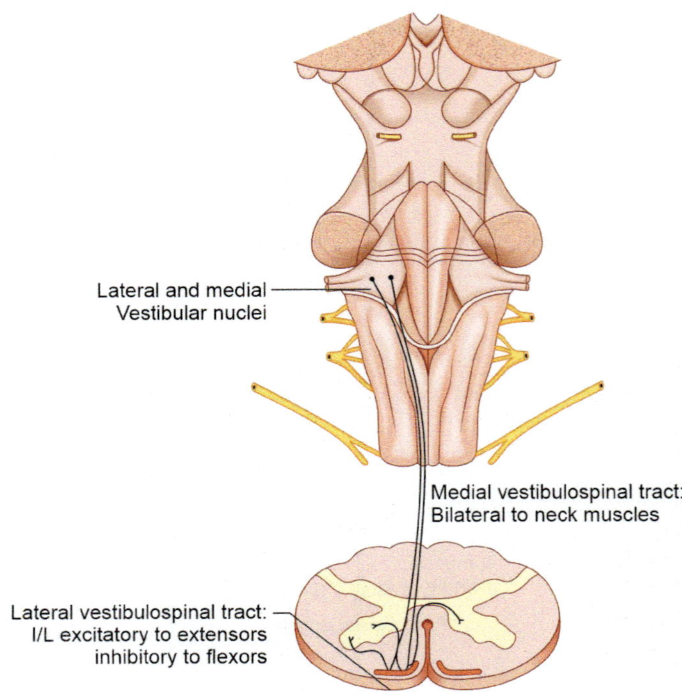

FIG. 17: Vestibulospinal tract.

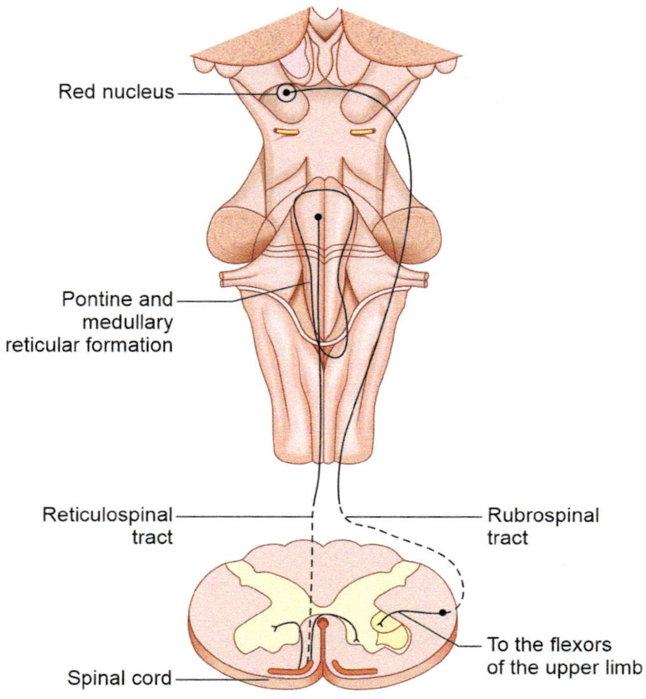

FIG. 18: Reticulospinal tract and rubrospinal tract.

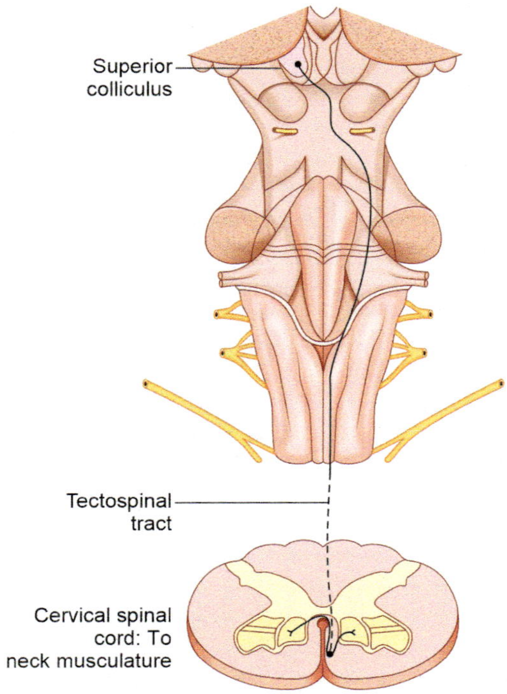

FIG. 19: Tectospinal tract.

- In males, erectile dysfunction is a common symptom.
- Autonomic symptoms, such as excessive sweating or vasomotor disturbances below the site of the lesion and Horner's syndrome in cervical cord lesions, may also be seen.

TABLE 8: UMN versus LMN lesion.

Feature	UMN	LMN
Paralysis	Groups of muscles paralyzed	Individual muscles paralyzed
Muscle tone	Increased	Decreased
Deep tendon reflexes	Exaggerated	Absent
Superficial reflexes	Extensor	Absent
Plantar response	Extensor	Mute
Muscle atrophy	May be absent/mild	Early and severe
Fasciculations and fibrillations	Absent	Commonly present

(LMN: lower motor neuron; UMN: upper motor neuron)

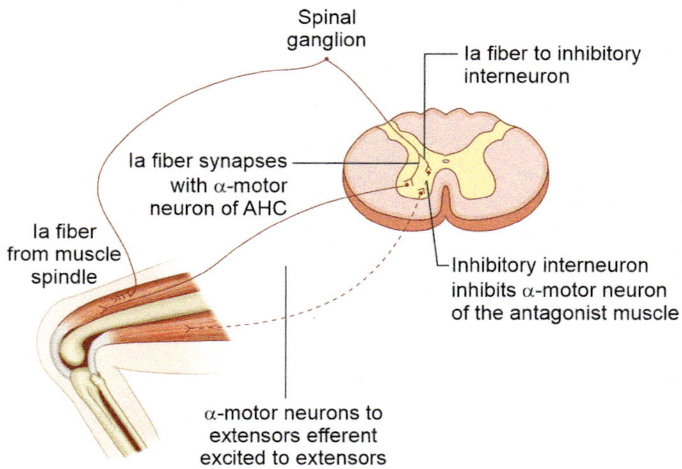

FIG. 20: Stretch reflex.
(AHC: anterior horn cell)

- If the corticospinal tract is involved, UMN type of weakness results and if the anterior horn cell or distal pathway is involved, lower motor neuron (LMN) type of paralysis results. See **Table 8** for UMN versus LMN lesions.[1,4,7]

Spinal Reflexes

Myotactic/Stretch Reflex

Sudden tapping on muscle tendon causes contraction of muscles. Proprioceptive signals are carried from the muscle spindle to the spinal cord, where they synapse with motor neurons, and fibers from motor neurons supply muscles resulting in muscle contraction. It is exaggerated in UMN lesions **(Fig. 20)**.

Flexor Reflex

In response to a painful stimulus, there is a withdrawal of the limb due to the activation of limb flexors. Normally, the response is inhibited by descending pathways, which prevents reflex withdrawal to harmless stimuli. This is a superficial polysynaptic reflex **(Fig. 21)**.

Clinical significance:

- Superficial polysynaptic spinal reflexes are abolished in lesions of the spinal cord, and deep reflexes like stretch reflexes are exaggerated. The Babinski sign is a part of the flexion withdrawal reflex of the lower limb, where there is dorsiflexion of the great toe and fanning of other toes in injury to the corticospinal tract or in intoxicated patients.[2]

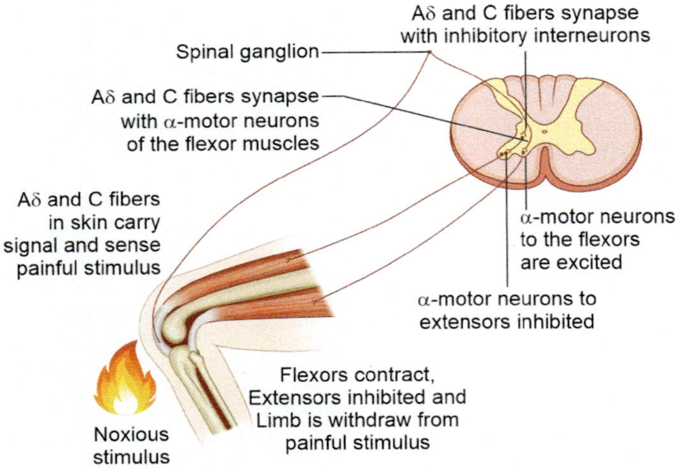

FIG. 21: Withdrawal reflex.

Bladder, Bowel, and Sexual Functions in the Spinal Cord

Bladder Innervation

There is a total of five loops in the innervation of the bladder **(Figs. 22 and 23)**:

1. Corticospinal tract is involved in voluntary control of the sphincter and pelvic floor. It descends from cortical and subcortical regions to pudendal nuclei (Onuf) in S2–S4. Motor neurons in S2–S4 via pudendal nerves supply the striated muscle around the urethra.
2. *Urethral reflex loop*: Urethral afferents to pudendal motor neurons are involved in maintaining sphincter tone when the detrusor is inactive.
3. *Detrusor reflex loop*: Detrusor afferents to pudendal motor neurons, sphincter relaxation when detrusor is active

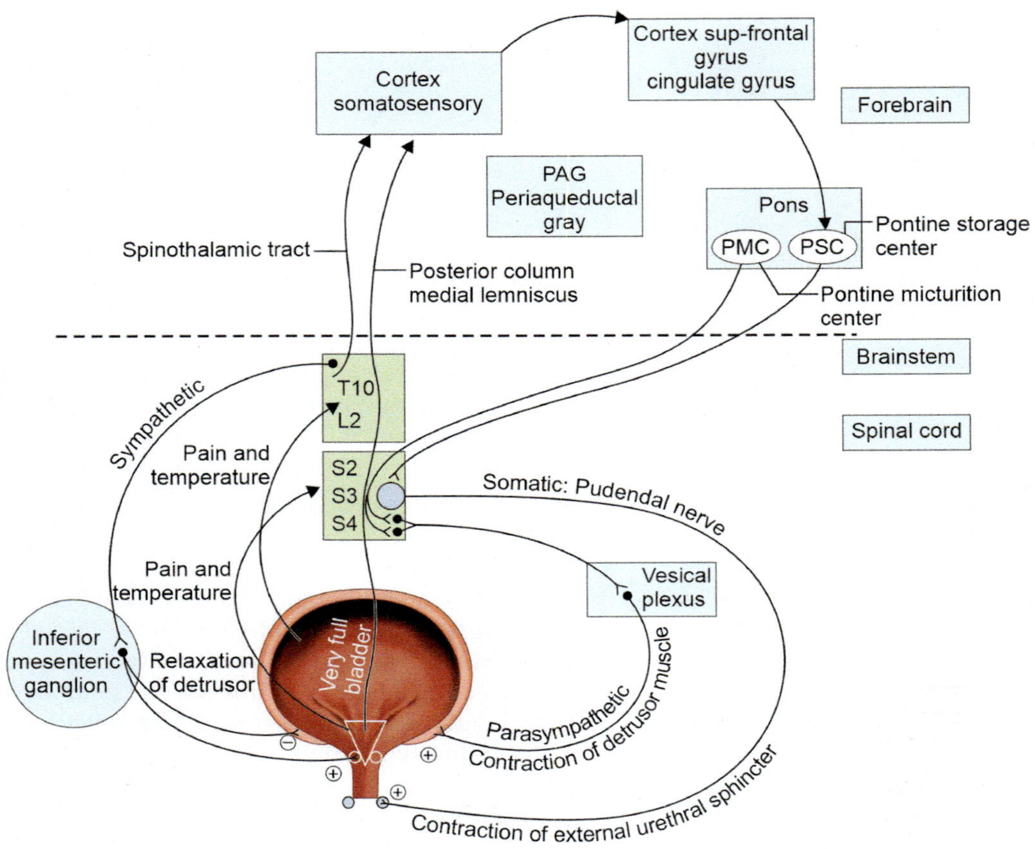

FIG. 22: Innervation of bladder.

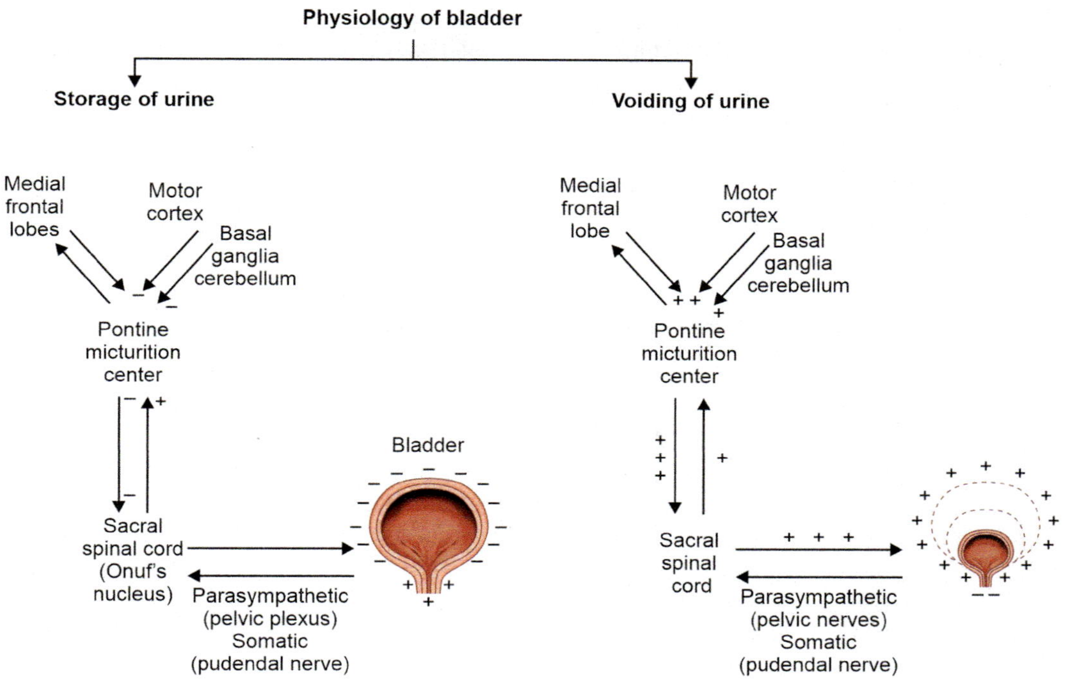

FIG. 23: Physiology of bladder.

TABLE 9: Various types of neurogenic bladder.

Type of bladder	Lesion	Symptoms	Ability to initiate micturition	Residual volume	Anal/bulbo-cavernosus reflex	Bladder sensation	Comments
Hyperreflexic spastic bladder	Between pontine micturition center and sacral cord	Urgency, frequency, urge incontinence	Not preserved	Increased	Preserved	Preserved	Mass reflex with fullness of bladder with bradycardia, hypertension, and headache
Autonomous Neurogenic bladder	Complete lesion below T12 level	Paralyzed bladder, retention, overflow incontinence	Not preserved	Increased	Lost with saddle anesthesia	Absent	Seen in conus–cauda lesion/spinal shock
Motor paralytic bladder	Efferent motor fibers to detrusor	Painful retention	Not preserved	Increased	Absent	Present	Seen in lumbar stenosis, hysterectomy
Sensory paralytic	Afferent pathways, posterior column, lateral spinothalamic tract	Urinary retention, overflow incontinence	Preserved	Increased	Absent/ decreased/ present	Absent	Diabetes mellitus

4. *Cord loop*: From brainstem to conus, coordination of sphincter and detrusor contraction and relaxation
5. *Cerebral loop*: Cortex (frontal cingulate region, genu of corpus callosum), basal ganglia, and pontine micturition center. Functions in initiation and inhibition of switching between voiding and filling states of the bladder[8]

Clinical significance: Different types of neurogenic bladder result from different types of lesions **(Table 9)**.[8]

Bowel Innervation

The internal anal sphincter, which is responsible for 80% of resting sphincter tone, is made of smooth muscle and is under autonomic control. External anal sphincter and puborectalis form the voluntary sphincter, formed of slow-twitch striated muscle supplied by the pudendal nerve.

Clinical significance:

- Diabetes, pudendal neuropathy, and cauda equina cause decreased rectal sensation and incontinence. Sensory roots of S3–S4 involvement or conus lesions also decrease anal sphincter tone, decreased perianal sensations, and loss of anal wink.

- *Double incontinence*: As the segments and tracts involved in bladder/bowel innervation are the same, sacral spinal cord lesions cause double incontinence, i.e., both urinary and fecal incontinence.[8]

Sexual Function

Male Function

Erection: It has both psychogenic and reflex components. Conus medullaris is the reflex center. Sympathetic outflow at T12, via hypogastric, pelvic, and pudendal nerves, supplies the genitals. Parasympathetic outflow in S2–S3 segments via the pelvic plexus, supplies corpus cavernosa by the cavernous nerve. The somatic pathway is by the pudendal nerve. Descending pathways from cerebrum travel in the lateral column of the spinal cord and also play a role in erection pathways. Limbic and hypothalamic regions travel in the medial forebrain bundle, midbrain tegmentum, ventrolateral pons, lateral fasciculus, and lumbosacral center and play an important role in penile erection.[8]

Clinical application:

- If the lesion is above the T12 level, psychogenic erection is impaired. In conus-cauda lesions, reflex erection is abolished. If a complete lesion occurs below T12–L2, psychogenic erection through sympathetic outflow is still possible.

Ejaculation: Hypothetical center is presumed at the T12–L1 level, which receives sensory information from the glans and frenum and consolidates information from ascending and descending pathways in the lateral column. Afferents are via S2–S3 and efferents via T10–L2.

Clinical significance:

- If the spinal cord lesion is above T10, ejaculation may be impaired, but reflex ejaculation can still be induced as afferents (S2–S3) and efferents (T10–L2) are intact. If T12–L2 is destroyed, reflex ejaculation cannot be obtained.[8]

Female Function

The female sexual function consists of four phases namely arousal, plateau, orgasm, and resolution. *Arousal* consists of two pathways: *The reflex pathway* and the *psychogenic pathway*. In the reflex pathway, dorsal clitoral nerve synapses in sacral segments S2–S4 with parasympathetic preganglionic pelvic nerves, which synapse with postganglionic cavernous nerve through the uterine-vaginal plexus. This leads to vaginal lubrication, clitoral erection, functional elongation of the vagina by anterior elevation of the uterus, and congestion of labia majora and minora. *Plateau* phase results after maximal congestion of vestibular bulbs, clitoral structures, and suspensory ligament contraction, which leads to vaginal orgasm characterized by the rhythmic contraction of perineal muscles and autonomic response in the form of hypertension, tachycardia, hyperventilation, flushing, shivering, etc., resulting from activation of hypogastric nerves and sympathetic chain. Vasocongestion is cleared and autonomic functions return to normal in the resolution phase. The psychogenic pathway of arousal consists of psychogenic stimuli from the brain entering either the sacral pathway or the thoracolumbar pathway through the paravertebral sympathetic chain and entering the uterovaginal plexus.

Clinical significance:

- If spinal cord injury lies above T10, reflex arousal in response to stimulation of the clitoris, vulva, and cervix in the form of clitoral erection, vaginal lubrication, and labial congestion is preserved.
- In lower lesions, psychogenic stimulation allows better vaginal lubrication.
- With a higher level of complete lesion, orgasm is achieved with local stimulation of the clitoris, vagina, or cervix through the retrograde transmission of sympathetic activity to the hypothalamus and brainstem nuclei as well as sympathetic plasticity in females.
- In complete lesions, orgasm is hardly ever achieved with psychogenic stimulation.
- Women with LMN lesions have greater difficulty in achieving orgasm than women with UMN lesions.[8]

ABNORMALITIES OF SPINAL CORD FUNCTION

Disorders related to spinal cord dysfunction are referred to as myelopathy.

Detailed history taking, physical examination, and logical reasoning are required to differentiate amongst causes of spinal cord dysfunction. The pointers to a possible localization of pathology to be in the spinal cord are: (1) weakness of bilateral lower limbs (paraparesis) or all four limbs (quadriparesis), (2) bilateral sensory deficit with sensory level, (3) bladder and bowel dysfunction, and (4) flexor or extensor spasms with spasticity **(Table 10)**.

When a patient presents with classic spastic quadriplegia with sensory level and bladder involvement, a diagnosis of myelopathy is easy. However, it is not uncommon for myelopathy to present as a chameleon, leading to pitfalls in investigations and management.

Progressive evolving spinal cord pathologies may have asymmetric involvement or intermittent symptoms, and so have a diagnostic delay, leading to delayed initiation of treatment as well. Associated neuropathy may hide features of myelopathy in patients presenting with myeloneuropathy **(Table 11)**. A systematic approach to diagnostic reasoning,

TABLE 10: Clinical features and their association with myelopathy.

Strongly suggestive of myelopathy	Signs suspicious of but not diagnostic of myelopathy	Signs suggestive of alternative diagnosis
Sensory level on the torso	Sensory loss in glove and stocking distribution in the presence of brisk reflexes (suggest myeloneuropathy rather than only myelopathy)	Spasms without spasticity (suggest stiff-person syndrome)
Crossed spinal tract findings (unilateral pyramidal with contralateral spinothalamic features)	Hypotonia/hyporeflexia (can be in state of spinal shock and also in neuropathy)	Paratonic rigidity (suggests frontal subcortical involvement)
Spinal tract specific features (suspended band of spinothalamic sensory loss, selective spinothalamic loss with preserved dorsal column sensation)	Unilateral or bilateral upper motor neuron signs (can also be seen with bilateral cerebral or brainstem or anterior horn cell disorders)	Cognitive impairment (suggests cerebral involvement)
Urinary retention with/without bowel dysfunction	Ataxia/nystagmus/oculomotor abnormality (suggestive of associated brainstem/cerebellar involvement)	Dysarthria, dysphagia, fasciculations of tongue and/or brisk jaw jerk (suggest brainstem or anterior horn cell disease)
Spasticity with flexor or extensor spasms	Weakness of all four limbs (can also be seen with cerebral or brainstem or nerve lesions)	Rigidity (lead pipe/cogwheel), dystonia/myoclonus or other involuntary movement suggestive of a movement disorder

TABLE 11: Certain presentations of myelopathy when pitfalls in diagnosis may occur.

Incorrect diagnosis thought of instead of myelopathy	Examples	Reasons for pitfalls in diagnosis
Motor neuron disease	Atlantoaxial dislocation, infiltrative myeloradiculopathy/myeloarachnoiditis	Combined UMN + LMN features
Stroke	Brown–Séquard syndrome/asymmetric myelitis	Unilateral motor weakness
Brachial plexopathy	Monomelic presentation of high cervical cord lesion	Unilateral upper limb weakness and pain
Lumbar canal stenosis	Conus medullaris + cauda equina lesions	Asymmetric lower limb weakness and exercise-dependent radicular pain
Guillain–Barré syndrome	Acute myelopathy in stage of spinal shock	Quadriplegia with generalized areflexia
Chronic neuropathy	Myeloneuropathy incomplete cord involvement	Incomplete evolution of lesion or combined involvement
Peripheral vascular disorder or metabolic myopathy	Cauda–conus lesions	Exercise-dependent symptoms
Hip, knee disorders	Chronic myelopathies	Spastic gait misinterpreted

(LMN: lower motor neuron; UMN: upper motor neuron)

detailed history, and examination and thorough knowledge of varied presentations of myelopathies are important to avoid pitfalls in evaluation and management.[9]

There are various ways to approach myelopathies:
- *Based on the time course of symptom onset*: Acute, subacute, intermittent or chronic **(Table 12)**
- According to different cord syndromes based on the horizontal degree of involvement of various tracts of the cord **(Table 13 and Fig. 24)**
- According to the vertical level of involvement as cervical myelopathy (again further as high cervical or low cervical), dorsal myelopathy, or lumbosacral myelopathy
- Etiologies of compressive or noncompressive myelopathies **(Table 14)**. Although there are certain features to clinically differentiate between compressive or noncompressive myelopathies **(Table 15)**, appropriate imaging is mandatory to rule out compressive etiology in all cases of spinal cord dysfunction.

Although classic textbooks describe myelopathies as either compressive or noncompressive myelopathies, all etiologies of myelopathies cannot be classified as either compressive or noncompressive as some etiologies may have indeterminate or mixed features.

Hence, newer ways to classify spinal cord disorder have used the terms extrinsic lesions, intrinsic lesions, or mixed/

TABLE 12: Differential diagnosis of myelopathies on the basis of time course of evolution.

Hyperacute *Deficit occurs suddenly*: Seconds, minutes, hours	• *Vascular causes*: Infarction, hematomyelia • Trauma
Acute: Spinal cord dysfunction which lasts for at least 48 hours and reaches to maximum deficit within 3–4 weeks	• *Compressive*: Abscess, tumor, prolapsed disc • Demyelination (MS/NMOSD/ADEM) • Infectious/parainfectious • Post vaccination (influenza, rabies, measles) • Systemic disease (SLE, Sjögren's syndrome, neurosarcoidosis, MCTD)
Subacute: Spinal cord dysfunction occurs over weeks to a month	• Metabolic (e.g., vitamin B12 deficiency) • Compressive (tumor, tuberculosis, metastasis) • Inflammatory (systemic disorders)
Chronic: Spinal cord dysfunction which is insidious in onset and gradually progressive over months to years	• Compressive (spondylosis, tumor) • Heredodegenerative (hereditary spastic paraplegia, Friedreich's ataxia, adrenomyeloneuropathy) • Toxin (fluorosis, lathyrism) • Infections (HIV, HTLV, tabes dorsalis) • Vascular (dural AV fistula) • CNS demyelinating disease (primary progressive MS) • Craniovertebral junction anomaly/syringomyelia
Intermittent episodic symptoms	• Demyelination (MS, NMOSD, systemic inflammatory disorders) • Spinal AVM/dural AV fistula

(ADEM: acute disseminated encephalomyelitis; AV: arteriovenous; AVM: arteriovenous malformation; CNS: central nervous system; HIV: human immunodeficiency virus; HTLV: human T-lymphotropic virus; MCTD: mixed connective tissue disease; MS: multiple sclerosis; NMOSD: neuromyelitis optica spectrum disorder; SLE: systemic lupus erythematosus)

TABLE 13: Features of various spinal cord syndromes.

Syndrome	Common features	Certain examples

Complete transection of spinal cord	• *Motor*: Weakness below the level of lesion
	• *Sensory*: All modalities of sensations are lost below the level of lesion
	  ○ Bowel and bladder dysfunction
	  ○ Initially there is stage of spinal shock with flaccidity, areflexia, and urine retention
		Traumatic
		Postinfectious acute transverse myelitis

Brown–Séquard hemicord syndrome	I/L weakness with I/L loss of proprioception below the level of lesion, C/L loss of pain and temperature few segments below the level of lesion	Traumatic/demyelination/bullet injury
Central cord syndrome	• Motor weakness (upper limbs > lower limbs); sensory impairment: dissociated sensory loss for pain and temperature with preserved position and vibration sense, cape-like sensory deficit may be present • Bladder dysfunction (usually urinary retention)	Syringomyelia Ependymoma
Posterior–lateral cord syndrome	Spastic paraparesis and sensory ataxia	*SACD*: Vitamin B12 or folic acid deficiency, zinc toxicity leading to copper deficiency, HIV myelopathy, neurosyphilis
Anterior spinal cord syndrome	*Deficits below the level of lesion*: • *Motor*: Weakness • *Sensory*: Pain and temperature loss with preserved position and vibration • *Autonomic*: Bladder, bowel, and sexual dysfunction • Initially there will be spinal shock with hypotonia and areflexia, which is followed by gradual increase in reflexes to hyperreflexia and spasticity	Anterior spinal artery occlusion
Posterior column syndrome	• Impaired position, vibration, and light touch sensation • Sensory ataxia	Tabes dorsalis Posterior spinal artery syndrome
Anterior horn cells and pyramidal tract syndrome	• Asymmetric involvement of different limbs • LMN signs such as atrophy and fasciculations are seen along with UMN signs such as spasticity and hyperreflexia • Sparing of sensory and autonomic functions	Amyotrophic lateral sclerosis (*not a myelopathy*)

(C/L: contralateral; HIV: human immunodeficiency virus; I/L: ipsilateral; LMN: lower motor neuron; SACD: subacute combined degeneration of cord; UMN: upper motor neuron)

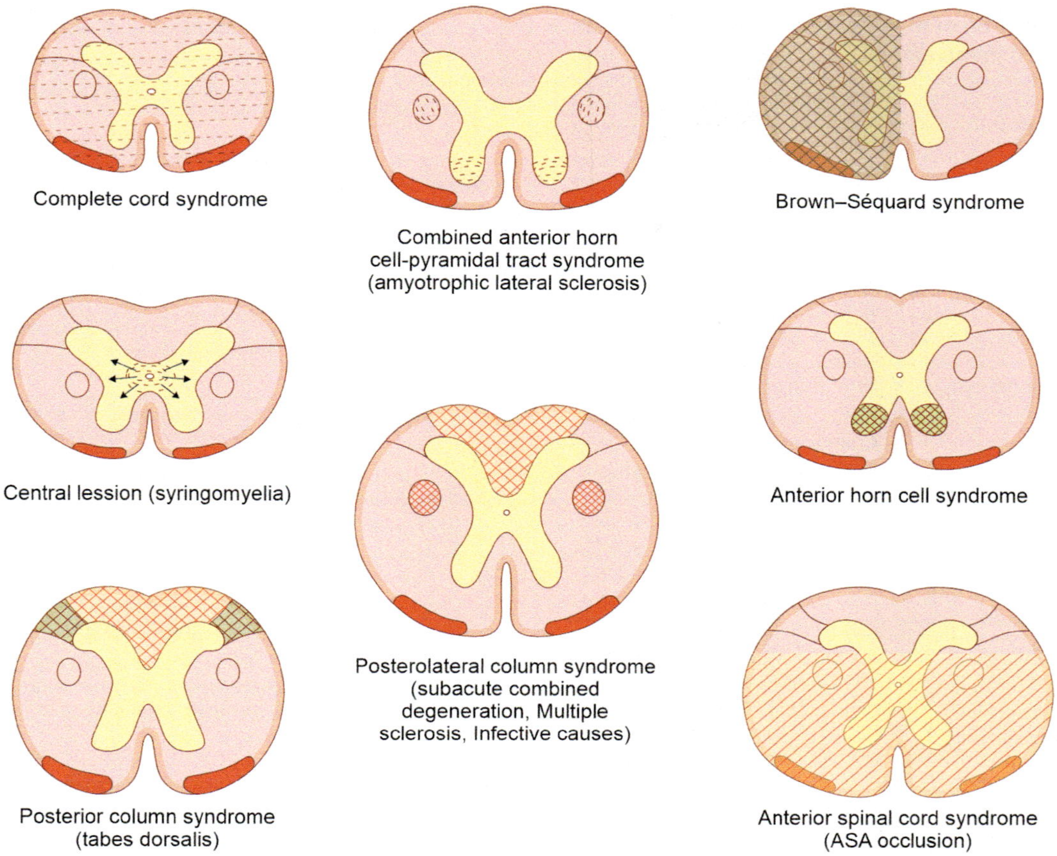

FIG. 24: Various cord syndromes.
(ASA: anterior spinal artery)

TABLE 14: Etiologies of compressive and noncompressive myelopathies.

Compressive	Noncompressive
• Degenerative disease (e.g., compression by osteophytes) • Traumatic (e.g., disc herniation and bone lesion) • Neoplastic (extra- or intradural tumors) • Infection (abscess) • Vascular (e.g., AV malformation, AV fistula, and aneurysm) • Syringomyelia	• Infection (transverse myelitis due to viral/bacterial/fungal) • CNS demyelinating disorders (MS/NMO/ADEM) • Systemic inflammatory disease (e.g., SLE and sarcoidosis) • Spinal cord infarction • Toxic (e.g., lathyrism, nitrous oxide, and radiation) • Metabolic (e.g., vitamin B12 or E deficiencies and hepatic disease) • Paraneoplastic • Degenerative (e.g., hereditary spastic paraplegia, SCA, Friedreich's ataxia)

(ADEM: acute disseminated encephalomyelitis; AV: arteriovenous; CNS: central nervous system; MS: multiple sclerosis; NMO: neuromyelitis optica; SCA: spinocerebellar ataxia; SLE: systemic lupus erythematosus)

TABLE 15: Some features differentiating compressive and noncompressive myelopathy.

Features	Compressive myelopathy	Noncompressive myelopathy
Radicular pain	Present	Absent
Local tenderness	Present	Absent
Onset	Gradual	Acute
Symmetry	Usually asymmetrical	Usually symmetrical

indeterminate lesions concerning spinal cord involvement. And the etiology may also be classified as congenital, genetic, traumatic, inflammatory, infective, and vascular. Such a combined approach to classifying myelopathy can give a further idea about the etiology of the myelopathy **(Table 16)**.

Also, a detailed approach to acute-subacute causes of myelopathies as well as chronic myelopathies is important for neurologists. **Flowchart 1 and Tables 17 to 20** give a gist of the approach to evaluation and clinical clues to different types of myelopathies.

TABLE 16: Classification of myelopathies based on etiology and manner of cord involvement.

Type of lesion	Extrinsic	Indeterminate/ mixed	Intrinsic
Etiology			
Genetic	Mucopolysaccharidosis		• HSP • Adrenomyeloneuropathy • SCA • Friedreich's ataxia
Congenital	Arachnoid cyst	• Syringomyelia • Craniovertebral junction anomaly • Spinal dysraphism	
Traumatic	Vertebra fracture dislocation		
Infective	• Epidural abscess • Tuberculous osteomyelitis		• Acute viral/ bacterial myelitis • Tuberculosis • Neurocysticercosis • HIV, HTLV • Syphilis
Inflammatory	• Rheumatoid arthritis • Ankylosing spondylitis		• MS • NMOSD • Post vaccinal • Idiopathic • Connective tissue disease
Vascular	Epidural hematoma	Dural AV fistula	• Infarct • Hematomyelia
Neoplastic	Metastasis		• Ependymoma • Lymphoma
Toxic	• Intrathecal methotrexate • Myodil arachnoiditis • Fluorosis	• Radiation • Electric injury • Acute myelopathy in asthma	• Lathyrism • Konzo • Nitrous oxide
Metabolic	Paget's disease		• B12 deficiency • Folic acid deficiency • Vitamin E deficiency • Copper deficiency
Degenerative	• Spondylosis • Disc prolapse		Motor neuro disease

(AV: arteriovenous; HIV: human immunodeficiency virus; HSP: hereditary spastic paraplegia; HTLV: human T-lymphotropic virus; MS: multiple sclerosis; NMOSD: neuromyelitis optica spectrum disorder; SCA: spinocerebellar ataxia)

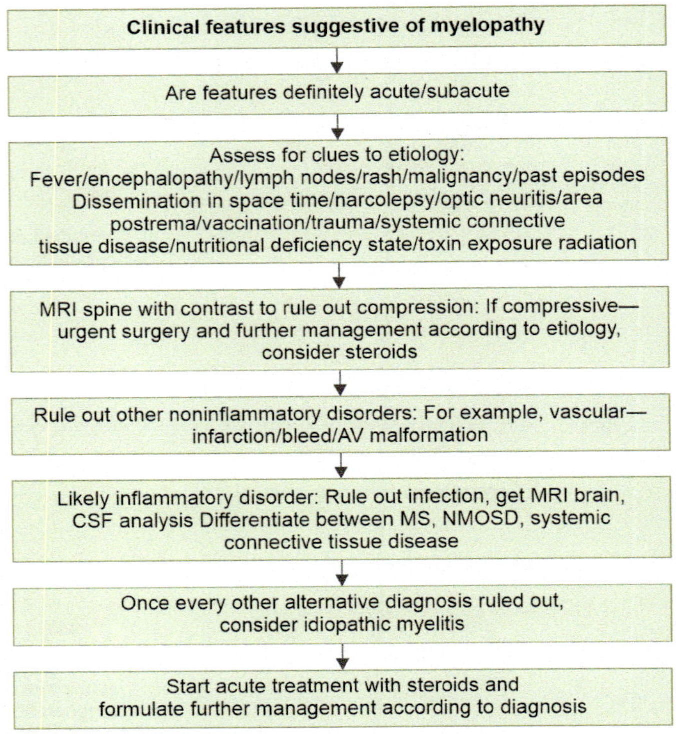

FLOWCHART 1: Approach to acute/subacute myelopathy.

(AV: arteriovenous; CSF: cerebrospinal fluid; MRI: magnetic resonance imaging; MS: multiple sclerosis; NMOSD: neuromyelitis optica spectrum disorder)

TABLE 17: Neoplastic compressive myelopathies according to localization.

Extradural	Intradural extramedullary	Intradural intramedullary
• Lymphoma • Primary bone tumor of spine (e.g., osteoblastoma, giant cell tumor, and Ewing's sarcoma) • Metastasis from other source (e.g., carcinoma of breast, lung, and prostate)	• Meningioma • Schwannoma • Malignant nerve sheath tumor • Neurofibroma • Leptomeningeal spread from other source (e.g., leukemia, lymphoma, and melanoma)	• Ependymoma • Astrocytoma • Hemangioblastoma • Cavernous angioma • Intramedullary spread from other source (e.g., carcinoma of lung, breast, and renal cell)

TABLE 18: Features differentiating intramedullary and extramedullary pathologies.

Features	Intramedullary	Extramedullary
Radicular pain	Unusual	Common
Funicular pain	Common	Unusual
UMN signs	Late	Early
LMN signs	Predominant	Unusual, may occur at the segmental level
Bladder involvement	Early	Late
Trophic changes	Common	Unusual

(LMN: lower motor neuron; UMN: upper motor neuron)

TABLE 19: Types of spinal AVMs.

Type 1	Spinal dural AV fistula
Type 2	Intramedullary glomus AVM
Type 3	Juvenile
Type 4	Intradural perimedullary AV fistula
Subtype 1	• Single arterial supply • Single small fistula • Slow-ascending perimedullary venous drainage • Multiple arterial supply
Subtype 2	• Multiple medium fistula • Slow-ascending perimedullary venous drainage • Multiple arterial supply
Subtype 3	• Single giant fistula • Large ectatic venous drainage

(AV: arteriovenous; AVM: arteriovenous malformation)

Appropriate imaging and investigations are important to evaluate different types of myelopathies. **Table 21** delineates a summary of different investigations required for the diagnosis of different spinal cord disorders. **Figures 25 and 26** give examples of different spinal cord disorders, which can be diagnosed by appropriate imaging of the spinal cord and brain. It is not uncommon to find situations when clinically the diagnostic reasoning would suggest spinal cord dysfunction but the imaging of the spinal cord may be normal. These situations further require a unique approach to further evaluation of such patients as listed in **Table 22**. Such spinal cord disorders further reemphasize the importance of a strong knowledge of spinal cord anatomy and physiology in approaching evaluation and treatment of spinal cord disorders.[9]

TABLE 20: Causes of chronic myelopathies and salient features.

Etiology/Disorder	Salient features
Nutritional	• *Vitamin B12/folic acid deficiency*: SACD with associated polyneuropathy, macrocytic anemia, low serum levels, raised homocysteine, methylmalonic acid • *Copper deficiency*: SACD, normal B12, folic acid, no anemia, low serum copper, high serum zinc • *Vitamin E deficiency*: Spinocerebellar ataxia, retinal dysfunction, low serum alpha-tocopherol
PPMS	Abnormal MRI brain, short-segment spine lesions, raised CSF OCB/IgG index, excluded other causes of demyelination/inflammation/infection
Spinal AV dural fistula	Elderly male with slow progressive myelopathy with T2 hyperintensity in cord with peripheral hypointensity, with perimedullary flow voids, with diagnostic spinal angiogram
Toxic myelopathy	• *History of exposure*: Intravenous/intrathecal methotrexate, cytarabine, cisplatin, cladribine, for chemotherapy of cancers with posterolateral cord syndrome • *Konzo/lathyrism*: Chronic dietary exposure to specific toxin, endemicity in the local region
Infections	• *HIV vacuolar myelopathy*: SACD—with normal B12, copper with positive HIV, and low CD4 • *Neurosyphilis*: Tabes dorsalis (dorsal cord syndrome with neuropathy) with Argyll Robertson pupil and positive VDRL/TPHA/RPR • *HTLV*: Progressive predominant motor myelopathy with normal imaging, with abnormal HTLV Ab
Neoplastic	• Compressive extradural lesions would present subacutely with pain (metastasis) • *Extramedullary intradural*: Meningioma, astrocytoma, metastasis • *Intramedullary*: Ependymoma • *Lumbosacral filum terminale*: Myxopapillary ependymoma • *Recurrent progressive cord-enhancing lesions with initial response to steroids followed by no response, with negative workup for NMOSD and systemic connective tissue diseases*: Primary spinal lymphoma
Delayed postradiation myelopathy	• History of >45 Gy radiation to cord, usually with combined chemotherapy, before months to years • Progressive myelopathy with sensory symptoms, T2 hyperintensity with cord swelling, variable enhancement
Genetic	• *Hereditary spastic paraplegia*: Positive family history, posterolateral syndrome, multiple subtypes according to features, and genetic abnormality • *Friedreich's ataxia/spinocerebellar ataxia*: Predominant associated cerebellar dysfunction, extraocular movement abnormality, cerebellar atrophy • *Adrenomyeloneuropathy*: In males, predominantly motor involvement, adrenal dysfunction, typical MRI brain and spine, low VLCFA, and ABCD1 mutation
Motor neuron disease	• *Various different syndromes*: Sporadic and genetic forms • *Isolated UMN syndrome*: Primary lateral sclerosis • *Combined UMN + LMN syndromes*: Amyotrophic lateral sclerosis, focal segmental amyotrophy • *Isolated LMN syndromes*: SMA (proximal/distal syndromes), Kennedy's disease (X-linked bulbospinal atrophy)

(AV: arteriovenous; CSF: cerebrospinal fluid; HIV: human immunodeficiency virus; HTLV: human T-lymphotropic virus; IgG: immunoglobulin G; LMN: lower motor neuron; MRI: magnetic resonance imaging; NMOSD: neuromyelitis optica spectrum disorder; OCB: oligoclonal band; RPR: rapid plasma regain; SACD: subacute combined degeneration of cord; SMA: spinal muscular atrophy; TPHA: treponema pallidum hemagglutination assay; UMN: upper motor neuron; VDRL: venereal disease research laboratory; VLCFA: very-long-chain fatty acid)

TABLE 21: Important investigations useful for diagnosis of myelopathies.

Investigation	Relevance
Spine MRI	• Diagnosis of compression and vascular abnormalities • Confirm parenchymal (intrinsic) cord pathologies
Brain MRI	To diagnose demyelination/leukodystrophy
Chest X-ray/CT thorax	Diagnose tuberculosis, occult neoplasm, sarcoidosis
CSF study (cell, TC, DC, protein, glucose, OCB, IgG index)	Evidence of inflammation/infection
CSF cytology	Spinal neoplasm
Hematology, peripheral smear, B12 estimation	SACD
Panels for autoimmune disorders	For specific connective tissue disorders
Panels for infections	For diagnosing specific infection based on associated clinical features
Visual evoked potentials	To diagnose associated optic nerve involvement
Spinal angiogram	Vascular malformations of cord
EMG NCV	For associated neuropathy/consideration of anterior horn cell disease
NMO Ab and MOG Ab	For considering NMOSD and MOG syndromes
Paraneoplastic Ab Whole body PET CT scan	Paraneoplastic myelopathies
Serum copper/zinc	Copper deficiency myelopathy
VLCFA	Adrenomyeloneuropathy
Genetic testing: NGS/WES panels	Hereditary spastic paraplegia

(CSF: cerebrospinal fluid; CT: computed tomography; DC: differential cell count; EMG: electromyography; IgG: immunoglobulin G; MOG: myelin oligodendrocyte glycoprotein; MRI: magnetic resonance imaging; NCV: nerve conduction velocity; NGS: next-generation sequencing; NMO: neuromyelitis optica; NMOSD: neuromyelitis optica spectrum disorder; OCB: oligoclonal band; PET: positron emission tomography; SACD: subacute combined degeneration of cord; TC: total cell count, Differential count; WES: whole exome sequencing)

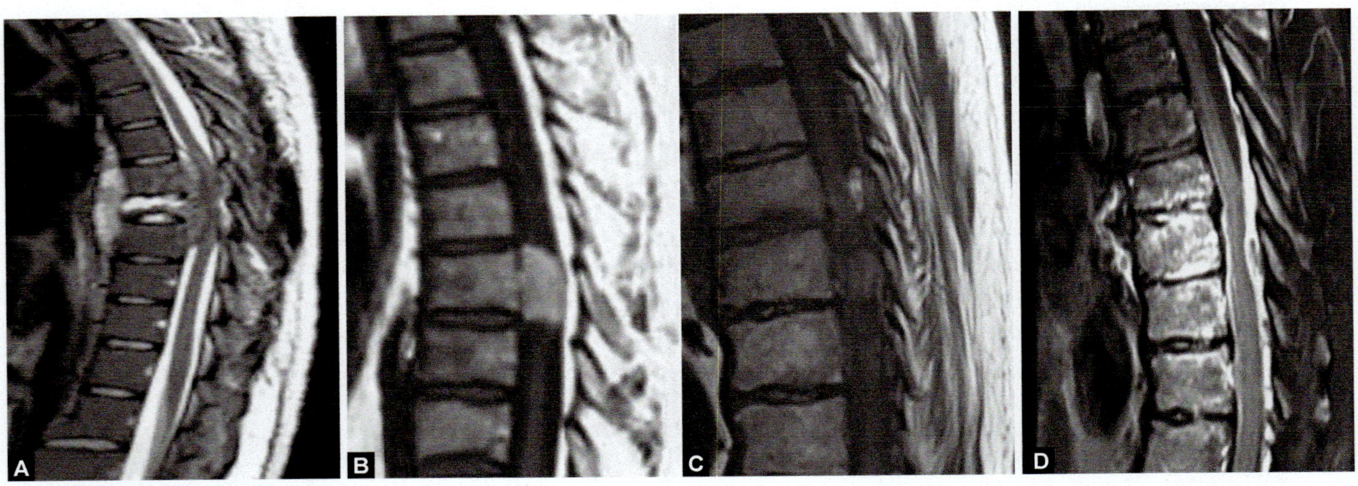

FIGS. 25A TO H: *Continued*

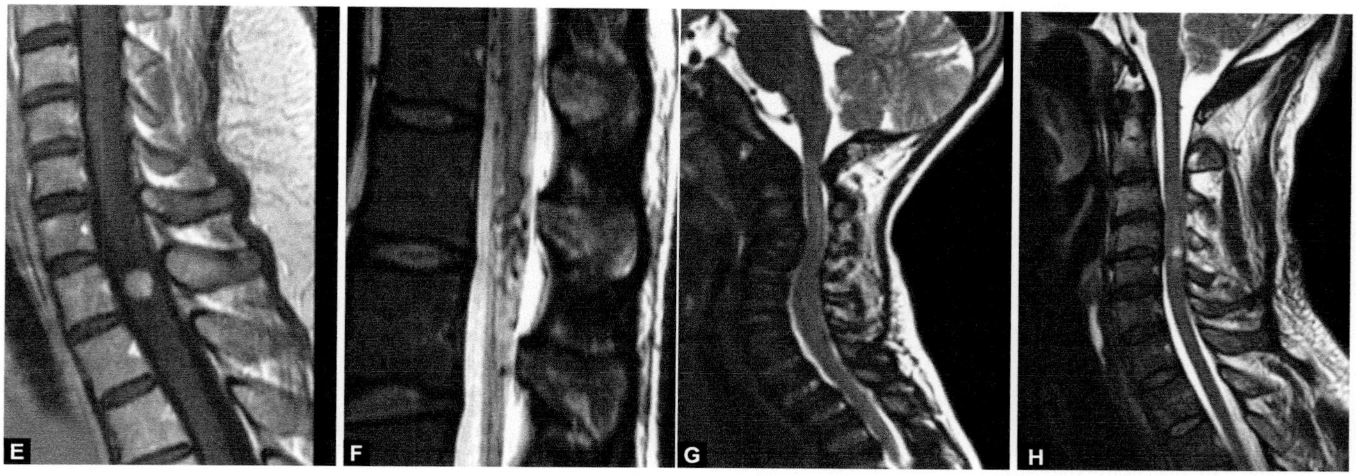

FIGS. 25A TO H: MRI patterns in different compressive myelopathy. (A) T2-enhanced spine showing osteomyelitis with discitis with cord compression secondary to TB spine; (B) T1 post contrast enhancing intraparenchymal lesion: meningioma; (C and D) T1 intensity change at endplate and post contrast enhancement in epidural region suggestive of epidural abscess; (E) T1 contrast enhancing intramedullary lesion: ependymoma; (F) T2 images showing flow voids in dorsal cord suggestive of spinal AV malformation; (G) Chronic myelopathy with CV junction anomaly with T2 hyperintensity with thickening of cord; (H) Acute post-traumatic myelopathy with T2 hyperintense signal at C4–C5 level.

(AV: arteriovenous; CV: craniovertebral; MRI: magnetic resonance imaging)

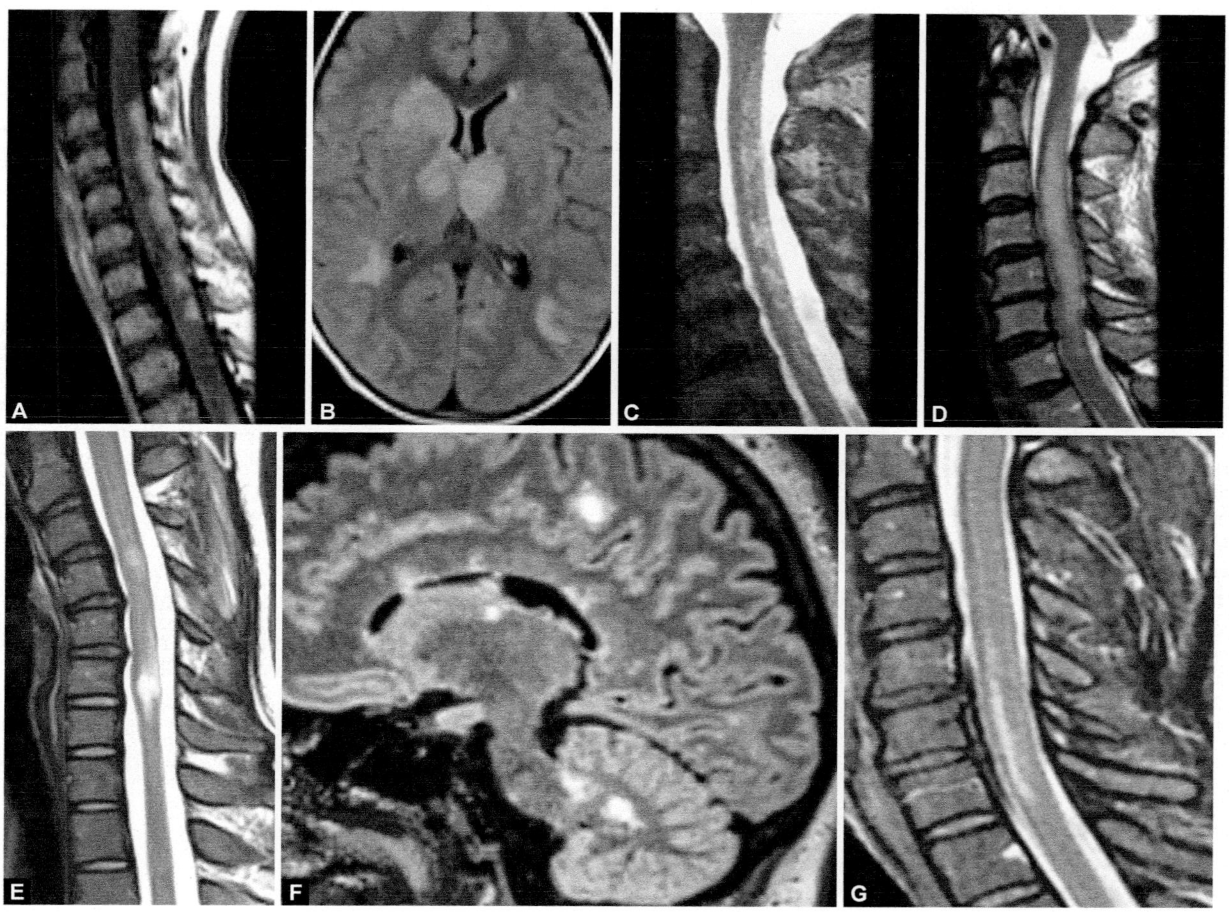

FIGS. 26A TO G: MRI patterns in different noncompressive myelopathy. (A and B) Patchy spinal lesions with asymmetric basal ganglia and subcortical lesion in ADEM; (C) Patchy posterolateral T2 hyperintense signal in SACD; (D) Long-segment myelitis: in a patient with NMOSD; (E) Short-segment myelitis in a patient with MS; (F) MRI brain in a patient with MS showing multiple juxtacortical, periventricular, and infratentorial lesions; (G) Anterior spinal hyperintense signal in anterior spinal artery thrombosis with infarct.

(ADEM: acute disseminated encephalomyelitis; MRI: magnetic resonance imaging; MS: multiple sclerosis; NMOSD: neuromyelitis optica spectrum disorder; SACD: subacute combined degeneration)

TABLE 22: Approach to "myelopathy" with normal imaging spine: Important considerations for review.

What else could this be?	Examples
Is the MRI quality good?	• Low Tesla scan (0.3/0.5 T) • Motion artefact • Gadolinium contrast not done in situations where contrast study is important • *CISS sequence not taken*: Posterior flow voids missed in reporting
Compressive etiology possibly missed?	• Epidural lipomatosis • Dynamic compression of cord in flexion/extension of neck
Is it a myelopathy mimic?	• *Sensory ganglionopathy*: Sjögren's, autoimmune, toxic, paraneoplastic • *Polyneuropathy*: GBS/CIDP • *Plexopathy*: Brachial/lumbosacral • Anterior horn cell disease • *Brain disorder*: Parasagittal pathology, ACA disease, hydrocephalus, vascular parkinsonism
Acute presentation is on the background of subacute to chronic progressive myelopathy	• HIV, HTLV, syphilis • B12, folic acid deficiency • Nitrous oxide toxicity, lathyrism, konzo • Hereditary spastic paraplegia
Scan done too early in the disease	To repeat scan
Does the patient have functional neurologic disorder?	Look for specific clinical features of functional symptoms

(ACA: anterior cerebral artery; CIDP: chronic inflammatory demyelinating polyneuropathy; CISS: constructive interference in steady state; GBS: Guillain–Barré syndrome; HIV: human immunodeficiency virus; HTLV: human T-lymphotropic virus; MRI: magnetic resonance imaging)

CONCLUSION

Knowledge of the cord anatomy and physiology and the different clinical cord syndromes can help make early diagnosis and initiate early management in treatable conditions. Early anticipation of possible deficits, prompt evaluation and treatment, proper care, pharmacotherapy, physiotherapy, rehabilitation, management of autonomic disturbances, occupational therapy, and management of spasticity have improved outcomes in spinal cord injury.

REFERENCES

1. Splittgerber R, Snell RS. Snell's Clinical Neuroanatomy. Philadelphia: Wolters Kluwer; 2019.
2. Krebs C, Weinberg J, Akesson EJ. Neuroscience. Philadelphia: Lippincott Williams & Wilkins; 2012.
3. Mancall EL, Brock DG, Gray H. Gray's Clinical Neuroanatomy: The Anatomic Basis for Clinical Neuroscience. Philadelphia: WB Saunders Co Ltd; 2011.
4. Ropper AH, Samuels MA, Klein J, Sashank Prasad. Adams and Victor's Principles of Neurology. New York: McGraw Hill Education; 2019.
5. Brain R, Donaghy M. Brain's Diseases of the Nervous System. Oxford: Oxford University Press; 2009.
6. Doppman JL, Di Chiro G, Oldfield EH. Origin of spinal arteriovenous malformation and normal cord vasculature from a common segmental artery: angiographic and therapeutic considerations. Radiology. 1985;154(3):687-9.
7. Kasper DL, Fauci AS, Hauser SL, Longo DL, Jameson L, Loscalzo J. Harrison's Principles of Internal Medicine, 19th edition. New York: McGraw Hill Professional; 2015.
8. Brazis PW, Masdeu JC, Biller J. Localization in Clinical Neurology. Lippincott Williams & Wilkins; 2021.
9. Jacob A, Weinshenker B. An approach to the diagnosis of acute transverse myelitis. Semin Neurol. 2008;28(1):105-20.

22

CHAPTER

Applied Neuroanatomy and Neurophysiology of the Plexuses and Peripheral Nerves

Madhu Nagappa

INTRODUCTION

The peripheral nervous system (PNS) is composed of a network of nerve fibers and is organized into roots, plexuses, and peripheral nerves. Disorders affecting the PNS have varied etiologies, though they share many clinical features in common. The PNS may be the primary site of pathology, or it may be affected as a part of a multiaxial neurological disease, in which case the clinical deficits related to the PNS may range from overt to subclinical, and may be overshadowed by other system involvement. Importantly, dysfunction of the PNS may be a manifestation of an underlying systemic condition such as connective tissue disorder or cancer.

There is limited data on the overall burden of these disorders in the community.[1] About 2–8% of the general population suffers from peripheral neuropathy. Studies from India suggest that the prevalence of peripheral neuropathies ranges from 5 to 2,400 per 100,000 population. In the hospital setting, neuropathies constitute 7.7–14% of neurological diagnoses. These epidemiological findings are greatly influenced by the geographical location and population studied. Thus, the incidence of neuropathy is higher in the elderly, diabetics, chemotherapy recipients and those residing in the arsenic belt, etc., while there is no data on the community prevalence of plexopathy, their occurrence, such as in the setting of road traffic accidents, perinatal trauma, and neoplasms have been reported.

The changes in the trend of various PNS disorders with time have not been studied. However, it may be expected that these disorders are on the rise because of the aging population, and an increase in disorders that predispose to neuropathy such as diabetes mellitus. Therefore, it is of paramount importance to be thoroughly familiar with the anatomy of various components of the PNS, particularly the cutaneous innervation and muscles supplied, as well as the physiology of impulse conduction through the nerve fibers. Application of this knowledge and understanding will enable accurate interpretation of the symptoms and signs, which is useful for anatomical localization, planning electrophysiological testing, deciphering the pathology, and listing the possible etiologies. This chapter will focus on the approach to disorders of the plexuses and peripheral nerves, including applied neuroanatomy and neurophysiology.

ORGANIZATION OF THE PERIPHERAL NERVOUS SYSTEM

The PNS conducts information to and from the central nervous system (CNS). Each nerve fiber with its myelin sheath is surrounded by a connective tissue called as the endoneurium. Bundles of nerve fibers, or fascicles, are surrounded by the perineurium, and the nerve itself, comprising of multiple fascicles, is bounded by the epineurium. The sensory fibers are the afferent fibers that transmit various modalities of sensation from the peripheral receptors to the spinal cord and brain, while the motor fibers are the efferent fibers that carry impulses to the skeletal muscles to initiate voluntary movements. The cell bodies of the sensory nerve fibers are in the dorsal root ganglia, while the cell bodies of the motor nerve fibers reside in the gray matter of the spinal cord (anterior horns). Apart from these, the autonomic fibers innervate the blood vessels and viscera, etc.

The axons are surrounded by myelin sheaths which are derived from the Schwann cells. These are discontinuous segments, the lengths of which range from 250 to 1,000 μm. The gaps in the myelin sheath where the axolemma is in direct contact with the extracellular fluid are the nodes of Ranvier. The thickness of the myelin sheaths also varies. The myelin sheath enhances the speed of propagation of the action potentials, since depolarization occurs only at the nodes of Ranvier (saltatory conduction). The speed of conduction is proportionate to the thickness of the myelin sheath. Erlanger and Gasser's classification of nerve fibers takes into account the diameter and conduction velocities **(Table 1)**. Ultrastructurally, a nerve fiber can be divided

TABLE 1: Erlanger and Gasser's classification of nerve fibers and their functions.

Fiber type	Fiber diameter (μm)	Conduction velocity (m/s)	Functions
A			
Alpha (α)	12–20	70–120	Proprioception, somatic motor
Beta (β)	5–12	30–70	Touch, pressure
Gamma (γ)	3–6	15–30	Motor to muscle spindles
Delta (δ)	2–5	12–30	Pain, cold, touch
B	< 3	3–15	Preganglionic autonomic
C	0.4 to 1.2	0.5–2.0	Pain, temperature
C (sympathetic)	0.3–1.3	0.5–2.3	Postganglionic sympathetic

into distinct zones, which are the nodes, paranodes, juxtaparanodes, and internodes. The node of Ranvier has a high concentration of voltage-gated sodium channels. The paranode is covered by uncompacted myelin and has a high concentration of voltage-gated potassium channels. The internode is bound by compact myelin. Along with these ion channels, various proteins such as the gangliosides, neurofascins, contactin, and contactin-associated proteins are differentially distributed along the node-paranode complex. This molecular organization is central to maintaining the integrity of the axon-myelin interface as well as for generating and transmitting the action potentials from one node to the other (saltatory conduction).

PATHOLOGICAL ALTERATIONS AND SYMPTOMATOLOGY

The pathological changes occurring in the PNS in response to a disease process are rather limited and comprise of (1) segmental demyelination—focal destruction of myelin with intact axon cylinder, (2) axonal degeneration—destruction of the distal axon with progressive involvement of the proximal portions, leading to "dying back" neuropathy, (3) Wallerian degeneration—degeneration of the axon and myelin distal to the site of an injury, leading to "dying forward" neuropathy, and (4) neuronopathy—the destruction of the cell bodies of motor or sensory neurons leading to motor neuron disease or ganglionopathy, respectively. Besides these, infiltration by inflammatory cells, edema, granulomas, fibrosis, amyloid deposition, tomaculi, and onion bulbs are some of the abnormalities that can be identified by histological studies.

Diseases of the PNS manifest clinically with sensory, motor, reflex, autonomic, and trophic changes. The patterns of impairment aid in the localization of the lesion within the PNS. The symptoms can be classified broadly as positive and negative symptoms. Positive symptoms arise from inappropriate and spontaneous nerve activity, whereas negative symptoms reflect reduced function. Positive symptoms may present earlier in the disease process.

Positive sensory symptoms include paresthesias, dysesthesias, allodynia, and hyperpathia in the involved regions. Negative sensory symptoms include impairment or loss of sensation. Generally, all the sensory modalities are affected; however, in conditions that preferentially affect the small nerve fibers, the temperature sense is impaired, while large nerve fiber involvement leads to a disproportionate loss of the joint position and vibration sensations. In this context, impaired proprioception due to dysfunction of the spinocerebellar fibers leads to ataxia with preserved muscle strength. This is characterized by flinging and stamping movements of legs, which worsen when the visual cues are removed. Wash-basin phenomenon wherein the patient loses balance on closing the eyes, e.g., while washing the face is reported by the patient. In the upper limbs, impairment of proprioceptive sense leads to irregular movements of the digits of the outstretched hands, a phenomenon called as pseudoathetosis. Patients may also sustain painless burns and injuries that get infected easily and heal poorly.

Motor dysfunction manifests with weakness of varying severity, depending upon the acuteness and severity of nerve injury. Muscle stretch reflexes are reduced or lost in disorders affecting the PNS, except in small fiber neuropathies. Skeletal deformities such as pes cavus, hammer toes, talipes equinus, claw hands, and scoliosis reflect the chronicity of the neuropathic process, and usually indicate an onset in childhood. Neuropathic tremors are coarse, irregular, worsen on reaching the target, and have varying amplitude with significant side-to-side oscillation. These tremors are thought to occur due to the loss of input from muscle spindle afferents, and have been described particularly in the setting of myelin-associated glycoprotein (MAG) neuropathy and chronic inflammatory demyelinating polyradiculoneuropathy (CIDP). Fasciculations, cramps, myokymia, neuromyotonia, and other spontaneous muscle activity may be uncommonly present in both acquired and inherited neuropathies. Further, trophic changes that can be seen secondary to impaired sensation and immobility include tight and shiny skin, thickened subcutis, loss of hair, and rigid and curved nails in the affected extremities. Painless loss of digits may occur due to repeated injuries. Chronic neuropathy may lead to an insensate joint, prone to injury, and bone destruction, abnormal bone formation, and subsequent subluxation, dislocation and deformity (Charcot joints).

Deficits arising from impaired functioning of the autonomic nervous system are under-reported and are often overlooked during the bedside evaluation. Features of autonomic insufficiency include orthostatic hypotension, impaired sweating, dry eyes, dry mouth, erectile dysfunction, gut dysmotility, urinary retention or incontinence, constipation and fecal incontinence, among others. These features predominate in small fiber neuropathies. Certain chronic demyelinating and infiltrative neuropathies such as CIDP, Charcot-Marie-Tooth disease (CMT), leprosy, and neurofibromatosis give rise to enlarged nerves which can be detected clinically.[2]

NEUROANATOMICAL POINTS AND THEIR RELEVANCE

The Cervical Plexus

The cervical plexus is formed by the ventral rami of the C1 to C4 spinal roots. These rami divide into ascending and descending parts, which unite to form communicating loops. Several superficial and deep branches arise from these loops. The superficial branches innervate the skin of the head and neck and are organized into ascending and descending groups. The deep branches supply the muscles of the neck and diaphragm and are organized into medial and lateral series **(Table 2)**.

TABLE 2: Summary of the components and branches of the cervical, brachial and lumbosacral plexuses.

Plexus/Nerves	Root values
Cervical plexus	
• Superficial branches	
○ Ascending group	
– Lesser occipital n.	C2
– Greater auricular n.	C2, 3
– Transverse cutaneous n.	C2, 3
○ Descending group	
– Supraclavicular n (medial, lateral and intermediate)	C3, 4
• Deep branches	
○ Medial series	
– N to rectus capitis lateralis	C1
– N to rectus capitis anterior	C1, 2
– N to longus capitis	C1–3
– N to longus colli	C2–4
– Inferior root of ansa cervicalis	C2, 3
– Phrenic n.	C3–5
– Communicating branches to IX and X cranial nerves	C1, 2
○ Lateral series	
– N to sternocleidomastoid	C2–4
– N to trapezius	C2
– N to levator scapulae	C3, 4
– N to scalenus medius	C3, 4
– Communicating branch to XI cranial nerve	C2–4

Continued

Continued

Plexus/Nerves	Root values
Brachial plexus	
• Roots	
○ Long thoracic n.	C5, 6
○ Dorsal scapular n.	C5
○ Branch to phrenic n.	C5
• Trunks	
○ N to subclavius	C5, 6
○ Suprascapular n.	C5, 6
• Cords	
○ Lateral cord	
– Lateral pectoral n.	C5–7
– Musculocutaneous n.	C5–7
– Lateral root of median n.	C6, 7
○ Medial cord	
– Medial pectoral n.	C8, T1
– Medial cutaneous n. of arm	C8, T1
– Medial cutaneous n. of forearm (MABC)	C8, T1
– Ulnar n.	C8, T1
– Medial root of median n.	C8, T1
○ Posterior cord	
– Upper subscapular n.	C6
– Lower subscapular n.	C5, 6
– Thoracodorsal n.	C6–8
– Radial n.	C5–8
– Axillary n.	C5, 6
Lumbosacral plexus	
• Lumbar plexus	
○ Iliohypogastric n.	T12, L1
○ Ilioinguinal n.	L1
○ Genitofemoral n.	L1, 2
○ Lateral femoral cutaneous n.	L2, 3
○ Obturator n.	L2–4
○ Femoral n.	L2–4
○ Lumbosacral trunk	L4
• Sacral plexus	
○ Posterior primary divisions	
– Superior gluteal n.	L4–S1
– Inferior gluteal n.	L5–S2
– Common peroneal n.*	L4–S2
○ Anterior primary divisions	
– Tibial n.*	L4–S3
– Posterior femoral cutaneous n.	S1–3
– Pudendal n.	S1–4

* Components of sciatic n.

Pathological processes affecting the cervical plexus are uncommon. Trauma, including iatrogenic injuries, and mass lesions constitute the etiologies in majority of the cases. The distribution of sensory and motor deficits depends upon the specific branches that are affected. For instance, attempted hanging may cause unilateral or bilateral greater auricular nerve palsy leading to the "numb ear" syndrome. On the other hand, the phrenic nerve is more likely to be affected by lesions in the mediastinum rather than by involvement of the cervical plexus per se.

Brachial Plexus

The brachial plexus extends from the neck to the shoulder and axilla, and is formed by the ventral rami of the C5 to T1 spinal roots, with variable contributions from the C4 and T2 roots. Anatomical variations in the brachial plexus are recognized and they include: (1) prefixed plexus—C4 to C8, (2) postfixed plexus—C6 to T2, (3) expanded plexus—C4 to T2, and (4) contracted plexus—arising from four roots. Anatomically, the ventral rami constitute the "roots" of the brachial plexus, but in clinical parlance, the nervous tissue proximal to the trunks is referred to as roots. The roots lie in between the scalenus anterior and scalenus medius. The roots unite to form the three trunks, the upper, middle, and lower, which in turn divide and unite and give rise to six divisions (three anterior and three posterior) and three cords (medial, lateral, and posterior). The trunks lie in the posterior cervical triangle in relation to the sternocleidomastoid, clavicle, and subclavian artery. While the divisions lie posterior to the clavicle, the cords lie in the axilla, in close relation to the first and second portions of the axillary artery. In the distal axilla, the cords give rise to the terminal nerves, which course through the arm and forearm. Apart from the cords, several nerves also arise directly from the roots and trunks **(Table 2)**. For localization, the brachial plexus is broadly divided into supraclavicular and infraclavicular portions, the former comprising of roots and trunks, and, the latter comprising of cords and terminal nerves. The supraclavicular portion is further subdivided into the upper (C5 and C6 roots/upper trunk), middle (C7 root/middle trunk) and lower (C8 and T1 roots/lower trunk) plexus. This classification is useful at the bedside, since the etiologies, severity and prognosis differ between the supra- and infraclavicular lesions of the brachial plexus **(Box 1)**. **Figure 1** shows the different roots, trunks, divisions, cords, and terminal branches of the brachial plexus along with their relations to the subclavian artery **(Fig. 1)**.

BOX 1 List of important etiologies of brachial plexopathy.

Site-specific brachial plexopathies:
- Supraclavicular:
  - Upper plexus
    - Burner syndrome
    - Rucksack paralysis
    - Classic post-operative paralysis
  - Lower plexus
    - True neurogenic thoracic outlet
    - Median sternotomy
    - Pancoast syndrome
  - Others
    - Avulsions, obstetric palsy
- Infraclavicular:
  - Radiation—lateral cord
  - Midshaft clavicular fracture—medial cord
  - Proximal humerus fracture—axillary n.
  - Shoulder dislocation correction—musculocutaneous n.
  - Compartment syndrome—median n.

Site nonspecific brachial plexopathies:
- Neuralgic amyotrophy
- Borreliosis, Asian tick-borne encephalitis, leprosy, and human immunodeficiency virus
- Primary/secondary neoplasms
- Radiation
- Traumatic/iatrogenic
- Hereditary neuropathy with liability to pressure palsies

Patterns of Neurological Deficits

The patterns of sensorimotor deficits aid in localization within the brachial plexus. Supraclavicular lesions cause segmental impairment in a dermatomal and myotomal distribution, while infraclavicular lesions cause impairment in the distribution of multiple nerves. Thus, the involvement of the lateral cord causes deficits in the distribution of the musculocutaneous and median nerves, the medial cord in the distribution of the ulnar and median nerves, while the posterior cord leads to deficits in the distribution of the subscapular, thoracodorsal, axillary, and radial nerves.

In neoplastic brachial plexopathies, the lower trunk or medial cord is commonly involved, while in radiation-induced plexopathies, paresthesias often occur in the distribution of the lateral cord. Horner syndrome is more common with neoplastic brachial plexopathy rather than with radiation-induced plexopathy. Neuralgic amyotrophy is essentially a "mononeuritis multiplex" with the involvement of one or more nerves of the brachial plexus, commonly the suprascapular, axillary, long thoracic, anterior interosseous, and other terminal nerves. In neurogenic thoracic outlet syndrome, clinically, patients present with greater involvement of T1 than C8; there is thenar muscle wasting, and pain and paresthesias are noted along the medial aspect of the arm, forearm, and hand. Clinical features that strongly correlate with root avulsion are severe pain in an anesthetic limb, Horner syndrome with or without the presence of long-tract signs. The latter arises from concomitant injury to the spinal cord in the setting of severe trauma.[3]

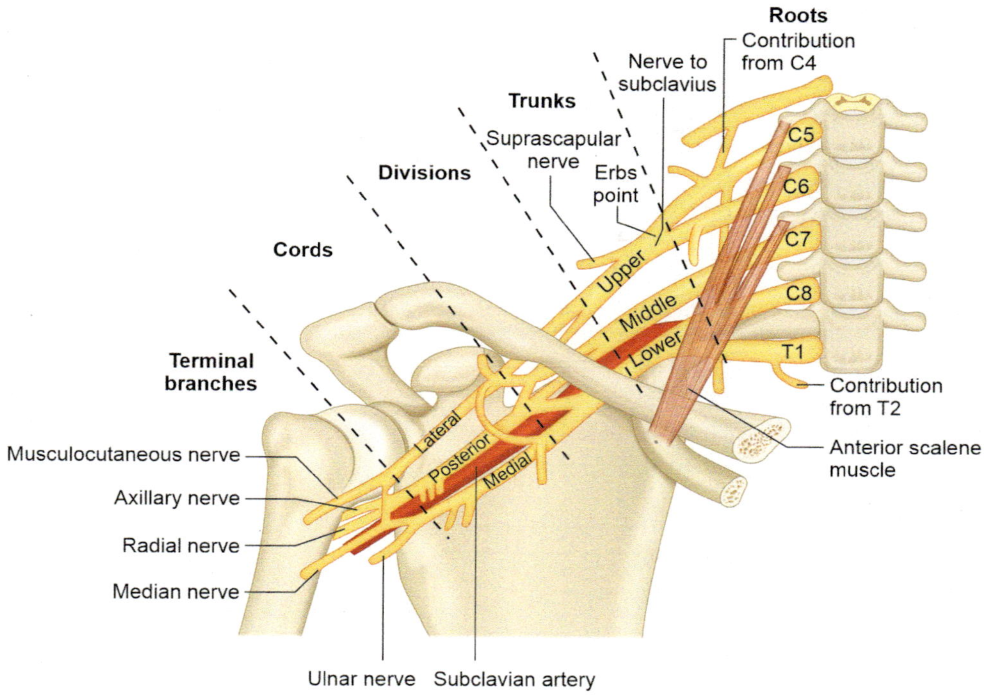

FIG. 1: Schematic diagram showing the different roots, trunks, divisions, cords and terminal branches of the brachial plexus along with their relations to subclavian artery.

Clinical Course

The initial symptom and the subsequent course are important, particularly the circumstances surrounding the onset of symptoms and medical history. In the case of "burner" syndrome, which is common in contact sports, there is a sudden and forceful separation of the shoulder from the head. This leads to traction on the upper plexus. In neuralgic amyotrophy, the clinical course is characterized by pain, followed by the development of weakness and atrophy after a few days to weeks (usually 2–4 weeks), and may be associated with an antecedent event such as infection, trauma, surgery, vaccination, pregnancy, or strenuous unaccustomed exercise (clinical triad: antecedent event, severe pain, and weakness and wasting). Temporal association of the symptoms with back-pack use, trauma or surgery is a valuable pointer for the etiology. In the case of malignancies, the characteristic clinical course is onset with pain followed by weakness, atrophy, and impaired sensation. In radiation-induced plexopathies, paresthesias, rather than pain, may be the presenting symptoms, followed by weakness and a more protracted course.

Painful Brachial Plexopathies

Malignant neoplasms, neuralgic amyotrophy, and burner syndrome are typical examples of painful brachial plexopathies. In neuralgic amyotrophy, pain is severe, often sudden and nocturnal in onset, typically located over the lateral shoulder or periscapular region and worsens with shoulder movement. But the pain may be located anywhere in the upper limb, depending upon the region of the brachial plexus that is predominantly affected. When the brachial plexus is involved by malignant neoplasms due to compression, locoregional infiltration or metastatic deposit, the pain is severe, persistent, burning or boring in nature, and worse at night and often radiates along the medial upper limb. On the other hand, primary nerve tumors such as schwannomas or neurofibromas present as paresthesias and painless masses and they may exhibit "tinel" sign on palpation. In "burner" syndrome, there is abrupt onset of pain and paresthesias in the arm, which are sharp and burning in quality and extend distally, often to the thumb. These symptoms usually subside within a few minutes.

Lumbosacral Plexus

The lumbosacral plexus has two distinct and adjacent components, i.e., the lumbar plexus and sacral plexus. The lumbar plexus comprises of the ventral rami of the L1 to L3 roots, a major portion of the L4 root and a branch from the T12 root. The lumbar plexus is located within the substance of the psoas major muscle posteriorly, in line with the intervertebral foramina. The lumbar roots, immediately on exiting the intervertebral foramina, enter the substance of the psoas major. The branches of the lumbar plexus emerge from the lateral borders and surface of the psoas major **(Table 2)**. The smaller branch from the L4 root unites with the L5 root to form the lumbosacral trunk; this along with the ventral rami of the S1 to S3 roots and a part of the S4 root form the sacral plexus. The sacral plexus is located deep within the pelvic cavity, in front of the piriformis muscle. Anteriorly, it is related to the internal iliac vessels and the

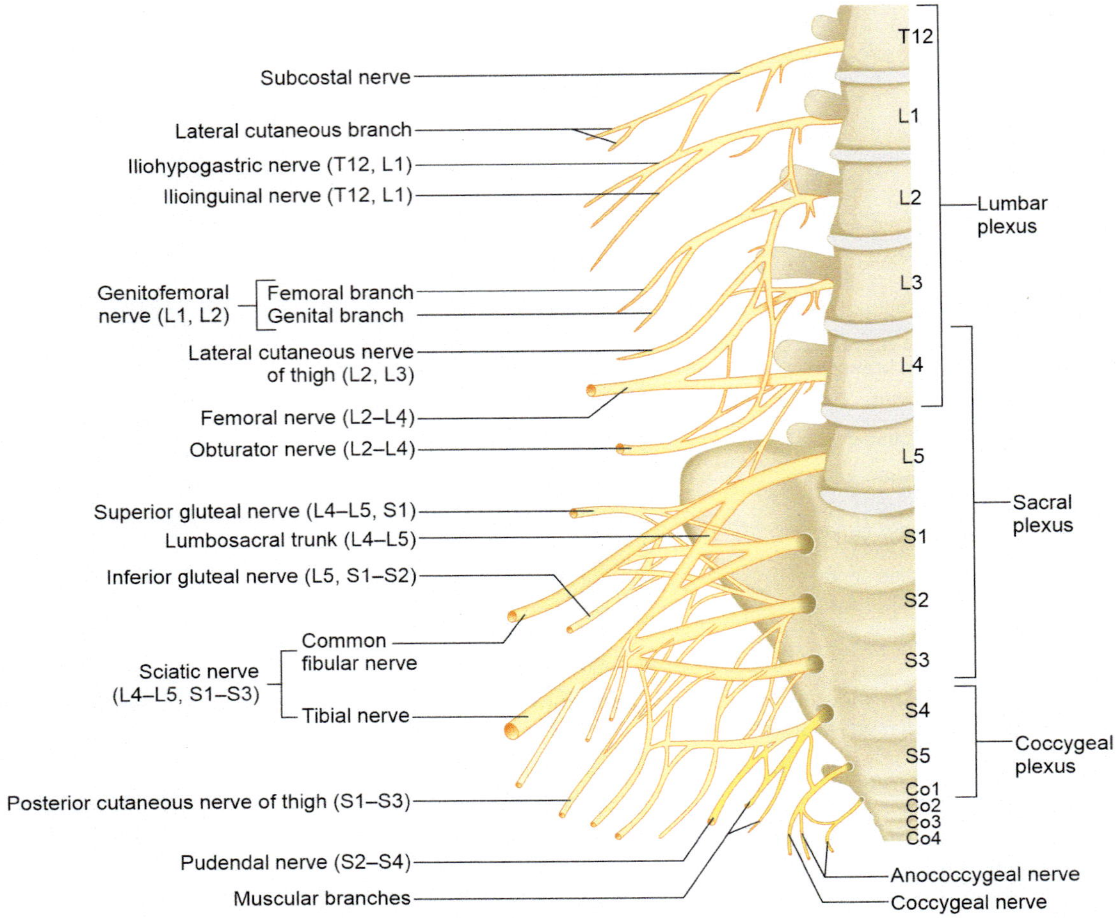

FIG. 2: Schematic diagram showing the different branches of lumbar, sacral and coccygeal plexus with their root values.

ureters. The terminal ileum and sigmoid colon lie anterior to the sacral plexus in the left and right sides, respectively. The rami of the sacral plexus are organized into two bands, i.e., the upper and lower bands. The upper band, comprising the lumbosacral trunk, S1, S2, and a major portion of the S3 roots, becomes the sciatic nerve. The lower band, comprising the remaining smaller portion of S3 and S4 roots, with a small contribution from the S2 root, becomes the pudendal nerve. **Figure 2** shows the different branches of lumbar, sacral, and coccygeal plexus with their nerve roots in a schematic diagram **(Fig. 2)**.

The most common causes of lumbosacral plexopathies are tumors and trauma, apart from diabetes mellitus and nondiabetic plexopathy, which are immune-mediated. In contrast to the brachial plexus, the lumbosacral plexus is fairly well shielded from direct accidental injuries by its deep location. The lumbosacral plexus is less prone to stretch or traction injuries than the brachial plexus. Thus, injuries have to be severe and penetrating to damage the plexus, and these may sometimes be accompanied by damage to other vital structures and the patient may not survive. But the plexus is vulnerable to being involved in disorders that affect the adjacent vascular and other visceral structures such as malignant neoplasms and hematomas. In most of patients with neoplastic plexopathies, the plexopathy occurs in the setting of an already established malignancy; however, in about 15% of patients, plexopathy may be the initial manifestation. Uncommonly, hemorrhage into the iliopsoas muscles may result in compartment syndrome and injury to the lumbar plexus. During labor, the descending fetal head may compress the lumbosacral trunk as it passes over the pelvic brim. Short stature and small pelvic size of the mother, large size of the fetus and instrumental delivery are thought to be the contributing factors **(Box 2)**.

Patterns of Neurological Deficits

Complete lumbosacral plexopathy, leading to weakness, hypo- or areflexia and sensory loss over the entire lower limb, is rare. Lesions of the lumbar plexus manifest with pain and impaired sensation in the anterolateral and medial thigh, and weakness of the hip flexors and adductors and quadriceps. Lesions of the sacral plexus manifest with sensory loss of the posterior thigh, leg, and foot, weakness of hip extensors and knee flexors as well as sphincter involvement. In diabetic plexopathy, there is focal and patchy involvement of proximal and distal portions with/without

BOX 2 List of important etiologies of lumbosacral plexopathy.

- Diabetes mellitus
- Nondiabetic plexopathy: immune-mediated
- *Neoplasms*: Cervix, prostate, colorectum, bladder, kidney, breast, ovary, sarcoma, and lymphoma
- *Trauma*: gunshot wounds, sacroiliac joint separation, fracture of pelvis/acetabulum/femur
- *Surgery*: Pelvic organs and abdominal aorta
- *Retroperitoneal hematoma*: Anticoagulants, hemophilia, femoral vein cannulation, ruptured aneurysms, and lithotripsy
- Radiation
- *Psoas abscess*: Tubercular abscess and pyogenic osteomyelitis
- Herpes virus
- Intravenous heroin
- Idiopathic retroperitoneal fibrosis
- *Intrapartum*: Pressure of fetal head over lumbosacral trunk
- *Others*: Sarcoid and amyloid

dysautonomia. Neoplastic processes commonly involve the lower plexus more commonly, followed by the upper plexus and pan-plexus, less frequently.[4]

Clinical Course

As in the case of the brachial plexus, details regarding the timing of onset of symptoms and their progression are vital. The onset and progression are acute and rapid in case of trauma and iatrogenic injuries following vascular procedures such as femoral catheterization. The course is more gradual (subacute) when the lumbosacral plexus is involved by diabetes, neoplasm, abscess or aneurysm formation, and more chronic in radiation plexopathy. Exercise-induced ischemia of the lumbosacral plexus may occur in patients with high-grade stenosis or occlusion of the arteries supplying the plexus.

The clinical setting in which the deficits occur gives a straightforward clue for the etiology. Diabetic and nondiabetic plexopathies begin focally or asymmetrically. They often involve the proximal and distal leg and may progress to involve the contralateral side. In diabetic plexopathy, the patients experience pain followed by weakness and atrophy. This sequence of insidious onset of the low back, pelvic, or radicular leg pain followed by sensory impairment and weakness is also seen in the setting of cancer, but the course is more protracted over weeks to months. In patients with trauma, the upper plexus is more often involved in gunshot wounds, while the lower plexus is more commonly involved in case of motor vehicle accidents. Other settings for ischemia include aortofemoral or aortoiliac graft surgeries and intra-arterial infusion of chemotherapeutic drugs for pelvic malignancies.

Careful palpation may reveal the presence of a groin mass which may be enlarged inguinal lymph nodes (malignancy) or a hematoma. A pulsatile femoral mass raises the possibility of an aneurysm. The quintet of leg pain, weakness, edema, rectal mass, and hydronephrosis suggests plexopathy due to cancer. A hot and dry foot due to the involvement of the sympathetic trunk in the paravertebral retroperitoneal region has rarely been described as the initial manifestation of a malignant neoplasm. Myokymia is a characteristic feature of radiation plexopathy but is not a very sensitive sign since it is seen in approximately 60% of patients only. Its absence does not exclude radiation plexopathy.

Painful Lumbosacral Plexopathies

Most of the etiologies cause painful plexopathy. In the case of diabetes mellitus, the pain has a sharp or burning quality. Pain in cancer is dull and achy and may be imprecisely localized. It may be radicular in nature and mimic radiculopathy. If the iliopsoas is infiltrated, patients may report difficulty in lying down supine with the affected leg extended. Pain may occur in radiation plexopathy, but it is rarely the presenting symptom and is not usually severe. The diagnosis of a retroperitoneal hematoma should be suspected in any patient who complains of back, groin, thigh, or leg pain; the pain may worsen on leg extension and in fact, the patient prefers to keep the leg flexed and externally rotated to minimize the pain. On the other hand, acute painless ischemic lumbosacral plexopathy, often without signs of limb ischemia may occur with aortic dissection.

Peripheral Nerves

Assessing the patterns of sensory, motor, and autonomic deficits aids in narrowing the differential diagnosis in disorders of the peripheral nerves **(Box 3)**. In polyneuropathy, the sensory and motor deficits are symmetrical and length dependent, i.e., the distal lower limbs that are supplied by the longest axons are first and more severely affected, followed by involvement of the proximal regions in a graded manner. Sensory impairment and paresthesias begin in the distal feet and ascend to the ankles, legs, and knees, at which point the distal fingers become symptomatic. Further progression leads to the involvement of the thighs and forearms and eventually the anterior abdominal wall in an "escutcheon" pattern due to the involvement of the anterior intercostal and lumbar segmental nerves. Likewise, the weakness begins distally in the toe and ankle dorsiflexors. In the upper limbs, the intrinsic hand muscles are involved first. Generally, the extensors are weaker than the flexors.

In mononeuropathy, the sensory loss and weakness are confined to the distribution of a single nerve. In mononeuritis multiplex, multiple individual nerves are involved; thus, the sensory and motor deficits involve multiple body parts sequentially, and when severe/extensive, the deficits may become confluent enough to resemble polyneuropathy. Weakness of proximal muscles early in the disease course raises the possibility of a polyradiculopathy, particularly when combined with hypo- or areflexia.

BOX 3 List of important causes for peripheral neuropathies.

Neuropathies with cranial nerve involvement:
- Diabetes mellitus
- GBS
- Hansen's disease
- HIV/AIDS
- Sjögren
- Lyme disease
- Sarcoidosis
- Diphtheria
- Melkersson–Rosenthal syndrome
- Neoplastic invasion of skull base and meningeal diseases

Neuropathies with predominant upper limb involvement:
- GBS
- Porphyria
- Lead neuropathy
- Diabetes mellitus
- Familial amyloid neuropathy type II
- HMSN

Proximal neuropathies:
- GBS
- Chronic inflammatory demyelinating neuropathy
- Diabetes mellitus
- Porphyria
- Osteosclerotic myeloma and para proteinemias
- Lymphoma
- Diphtheria
- HIV/AIDS
- Lyme disease

Mononeuropathy:
- Compressive/entrapment neuropathies
- Myxedema
- RA
- Amyloidosis
- Acromegaly
- Trauma
- Ischemic neuropathy
- Diabetes mellitus
- Vasculitis
- Leprosy
- Sarcoidosis
- Neoplastic infiltration or compression

Mononeuritis multiplex:
- Diabetes mellitus
- Leprosy
- Vasculitis
- Polyarteritis nodosa
- SLE
- Sjögren's syndrome
- Sarcoidosis
- Amyloidosis
- HIV/AIDS
- CIDP variants
- Hereditary neuropathy with liability to pressure palsies

Length-dependent polyneuropathies:
- Metabolic: Diabetes (most important), obesity
- Endocrine: Hypothyroidism, acromegaly
- Toxic: Alcohol, chemotherapy, OP, heavy metals
- Nutritional deficiency: Vitamin B1, B12, folate, bariatric surgery
- Infections: HIV, Whipple's, leprosy, lyme
- Immune mediated: GBS, CIDP, SLE, RA, sarcoidosis
- Inherited: HMSN/CMT, mitochondrial (NARP)
- Others: Critical illness, amyloid, gout, paraneoplastic, carcinomatous/lymphomatous
- CIAP: One-third (second most common cause after diabetes)

Motor predominant neuropathy:
- GBS
- Diphtheria toxin
- Acute intermittent porphyria
- Lead poisoning
- Dapsone toxicity
- HMSN
- Hypoglycemia

Sensory predominant neuropathy:
- Paraneoplastic (carcinoma/lymphoma)
- Sjögren's syndrome
- Paraproteinemias
- Non-systemic vasculitic neuropathy
- Idiopathic sensory neuronopathy
- Primary biliary cirrhosis
- Crohn's disease
- Chronic gluten enteropathy
- Vitamin E deficiency
- Hereditary sensory neuropathy

(AIDS: acquired immunodeficiency syndrome; CIAP: chronic idiopathic axonal polyneuropathy; CIDP: chronic inflammatory demyelinating polyradiculoneuropathy; CMT: Charcot–Marie–Tooth; GBS: Guillain–Barré syndrome; HIV: human immunodeficiency virus; HMSN: hereditary motor and sensory neuropathy; NARP: neurogenic muscle weakness, ataxia, and retinitis pigmentosa; OP: organophosphorus; RA: rheumatoid arthritis; SLE: systemic lupus erythematosus)

In sensory neuronopathy or ganglionopathy, the dorsal root ganglia that lie on either side of the spinal cord are the primary sites of pathology. There is degeneration of the central projections, i.e., the dorsal spinal roots and the dorsal columns in the spinal cord that contain the spinocerebellar fibers. Clinically, there is a nonlength dependent pattern of involvement with symptoms affecting the scalp, face, oral mucosa, trunk, abdomen, and buttocks, apart from the limbs. Usually, the ganglia of large fibers are commonly affected and lead to impairment or loss of touch, vibration, and joint position sense, along with areflexia. Clinically, this manifests with severe ataxia and pseudoathetosis. Impaired touch in the pharynx affects normal swallowing. When the ganglia of small fibers are affected, the clinical manifestations include burning or stabbing pains and impairment/loss of pain and temperature sense, with normal stretch reflexes. Autonomic ganglia may be simultaneously involved and lead to orthostatic hypotension, gut dysmotility and other features of dysautonomia. The etiologies are limited and include paraneoplastic and systemic autoimmune disorders, infections, and drugs and toxins. Among the neoplasms, small cell lung carcinoma is classically associated with sensory neuronopathy. Others include carcinomas of the breast, stomach, colon, ovaries and prostate, lymphoma, sarcoma, and neuroendocrine tumors. Other paraneoplastic neurological syndromes such as the Lambert-Eaton myasthenic syndrome, limbic encephalitis, and cerebellar degeneration may occur concomitantly. Sjögren's syndrome, and less commonly systemic lupus erythematosus, rheumatoid arthritis, and mixed connective disorders may develop ganglionopathy. In Sjögren's syndrome, the development of facial numbness because of the involvement of the trigeminal ganglia is considered to be typical.

Discerning the onset, duration, and clinical course is a key step in narrowing the etiological diagnosis of neuropathy. Based on the duration of progression, neuropathies can be classified as acute (<4 weeks), subacute (4–8 weeks), and chronic (>8 weeks). Most of the neuropathies have an insidious onset and progressive course. However, acute neuropathies like Guillain-Barré syndrome (GBS) and vasculitic neuropathy may sometimes have a more hyperacute course and evolve over 24–72 hours. Other acute neuropathies include porphyria, toxic neuropathies, diphtheritic polyneuropathy, and critical illness polyneuropathy. Some of the causes of subacute neuropathies include nutritional deficiencies, toxins, paraneoplastic syndromes, malignancies, and systemic connective tissue disorders. Inherited neuropathies and neuropathies that are secondary to metabolic/endocrinological conditions such as diabetes mellitus, present with chronic progressive course. Chronic neuropathies may be further categorized into those that progress over several months to a few years, and those where the neuropathy progresses over several years, such as the inherited neuropathies. Certain disorders like GBS, have a monophasic course; on the other hand, CIDP, hereditary neuropathy with liability to pressure palsies (HNPP), porphyrias, and vasculitis may have a relapsing course. Repeated exposure to toxins may also follow a relapsing course.

The medical history should focus on systemic disorders that are known to cause neuropathy such as diabetes mellitus, hypothyroidism, rheumatological disorders, renal dysfunction, and cancer. There may be multiple mechanisms of neuropathy in the setting of a systemic disorder. For example, cancer can involve the peripheral nerves by direct infiltration, paraneoplastic syndrome, and by the impact of treatment with chemotherapy or radiotherapy. Besides, patients with malignancy are poorly nourished and may have significant weight loss over a relatively short time, making them prone to nutritional deficiency neuropathy and entrapment neuropathy. Personal history should not only encompass dietary habits, but also high-risk sexual behavior and substance abuse, including the intake of alcohol, nicotine, cocaine, and other intravenous drugs of abuse. Occupational exposure to heavy metals, fertilizers, solvents, and other toxins which lead to neuropathy should be enquired into. It is also useful to make a list of medications consumed by the patient, including the "nonprescription" and "over-the-counter" drugs such as vitamins and antibiotics.

At this point, it must be borne in mind that multiple conditions may contribute to neuropathy. Some of the clinically relevant co-occurrences are (1) diabetes mellitus and CIDP, (2) human immunodeficiency virus (HIV) infection and CIDP, and (3) diabetes mellitus and chronic alcohol use. Rarely, an acquired cause (more prevalent in the community) may superimpose on a genetic neuropathy (relatively rare). Apart from the medical history, the surgical history should also be covered. Those that are particularly relevant in the context of neuropathy include bariatric surgery, surgery for entrapment neuropathies (e.g., carpal tunnel syndrome) and orthopedic interventions. A history of clumsiness and lack of an "athletic" build in childhood may raise the possibility of an inherited neuropathy. Further, the presence of foot deformities from childhood and a family history of deformed feet warrants a thorough investigation for inherited neuropathy.[5]

NEUROPHYSIOLOGICAL POINTS AND THEIR RELEVANCE

Electrophysiological testing plays a pivotal role in confirming the clinical diagnosis of neuropathy or plexopathy. Based on the symmetry and patterns of abnormalities, electrodiagnostic testing aids in localizing the lesion within the PNS and identifying subclinical changes, which can also be used for assessing the severity and prognostication, particularly when longitudinal studies are performed. This also guides a clinician to select the appropriate nerve for biopsy, when required.

Nerve conduction studies (NCS) involve percutaneous stimulation of motor and sensory nerves using supramaximal electric current, and recording the corresponding compound muscle action potentials (CMAP) and sensory nerve action potentials (SNAP), respectively. The parameters recorded are the distal latencies, amplitudes, and conduction velocities. In addition, the proximal portions of the PNS can be studied by recording the "late responses" which are the F waves and H reflex. An axonal process is indicated by reduced amplitudes of the recorded potentials. On the other hand, demyelinating lesions affect the large diameter, fast conducting fibers; the slowed conduction is reflected in markedly prolonged distal latency (>130% of the upper limit of normal) and reduced conduction velocity (<75% of the lower limit of normal) as well as delayed (>130% of the upper limit of normal) or absent late responses.

In a patient with polyneuropathy, commensurate with the clinical deficits, a distal-to-proximal gradient is noted on electrophysiological testing also, with the lower limb nerves being affected early and more severely. In the early stages, when the amplitudes are reduced, but still fall within the reference range, comparison with upper limb potentials is useful. The amplitude of the sural nerve is disproportionately reduced as compared to the radial nerve. The sural/radial nerve amplitude ratio (SRAR) of 0.21 has very high sensitivity and specificity for diagnosing axonal polyneuropathy, provided of course that the radial nerve itself is not affected by the disease process. These changes are symmetrical and length dependent; the absence of this would indicate an underlying mononeuritis multiplex resembling a polyneuropathy. In mononeuropathy or mononeuritis multiplex, there is nonuniform, nonlength-dependent asymmetric electrophysiology reflecting the patchy nerve involvement. It is imperative to perform NCS on bilateral limbs to identify asymmetry (>50% difference in amplitudes).

In a patient with demyelinating electrophysiology, NCS parameters may aid in distinguishing inherited from acquired causes. Uniform and diffuse slowing, which is sometimes severe, characterizes inherited neuropathies. While in acquired conditions, the slowing is nonhomogeneous and asymmetric; the multifocal patchy demyelinating process is further supported by conduction blocks and temporal dispersion across nonentrapment sites, whenever present. There are exceptions to this rule, however, and conduction blocks and temporal dispersion are being described in inherited neuropathies also. The classical example is one of X-linked Charcot–Marie–Tooth disease (CMTX) or *GJB1*-associated neuropathy, where the motor conduction is nonuniform and heterogeneous within a single nerve and between multiple nerves, the velocity being more significantly reduced in the median as compared to the ulnar nerve. This interneerve heterogeneity is prominent in females and is hypothesized to be due to the phenomenon of lyonization. On the other hand, demyelination is more severe and uniform in affected males. Exceptionally, temporal dispersion and conduction blocks can also occur due to the presence of rudimentary onion bulbs. NCS of family members may be useful in demyelinating neuropathies, since the slowed conduction velocities are established by 3–5 years of age itself, even if the individual is not symptomatic.

In GBS, the prototype autoimmune disorder of the peripheral nerves, electrophysiological changes are dynamic. They evolve from normal studies during the first few days to abnormal late responses, and subsequently frank demyelination. A proportion of patients have axonal subtype rather than demyelination. Since the NCS parameters vary with the duration of GBS, experts recommend at least two NCS, with the second NCS after 3–8 weeks of onset, for more accurate classification into axonal or demyelinating subtypes. In this context, the newer electrophysiological concept of reversible conduction failure (RCF) or axonal conduction block of the motor nerves has been recently introduced. RCF is considered to be the electrophysiological correlate of a very focal pathology at the node-paranode complex. Reduced amplitude of the distal CMAP may be due to conduction block at the terminal axons. Distinguishing this distal conduction block from axonal degeneration is possible only by serial NCS. This is important for prognostication since axonal GBS has a poor prognosis for complete recovery.

Another peculiar feature of acquired demyelinating neuropathies, is the presence of a "sural sparing" pattern on sensory conduction studies. This ranges from "relative" preservation of the sural nerve amplitude as compared to the median, ulnar, or radial nerves, to the "extreme" pattern of completely absent SNAPs of the upper limb nerves coupled with a normal sural SNAP. This was considered to be specific for a demyelinating subtype of GBS, but has been described in axonal GBS and GBS variants also.

When a patient is suspected to have a plexus lesion, extensive electrophysiological testing including needle electromyogram (EMG) is required. In NCS, examination of the sensory potentials has important implications for localizing the lesion to the post-ganglionic segment and further in identifying the portion of the plexus that is affected. Motor studies are useful in determining the severity of the lesion and in distinguishing axonopathy from uncommon conduction blocks. This also helps to exclude other disorders such as mononeuritis multiplex and multifocal motor neuropathy with conduction blocks that may be mistaken for plexopathy. The examination has to be bilateral, since this may uncover reduced amplitudes of the recorded potentials in the affected side as compared to the normal limb (>50% difference), while the absolute values are still within the set reference ranges.

The brachial plexus and its components innervate the muscles and skin of the upper limbs. The entire plexus or a portion of the plexus may be affected, and certain disorders of the plexus have a regional predilection. Thus, electrophysiological localization helps in narrowing the differential diagnosis. While performing electrophysiological testing of the brachial plexus, only certain nerves are accessible for examination, and they include the median, ulnar, radial, and medial and lateral antebrachial cutaneous nerves. Thus, predominantly only the lower portion of the brachial plexus can be examined by NCS. In this context, needle EMG is invaluable for studying the upper plexus, determining the proximal extent of the lesion, and is a more sensitive indicator of axonal loss as compared to NCS. To begin with, the brachial plexus can be "screened" by performing the sensory conduction studies of the median (first and second digit), ulnar (fifth digit), superficial radial and lateral antebrachial cutaneous nerves **(Fig. 3)**. Depending upon the portion of the brachial plexus that is likely to be affected, a more detailed study protocol can be planned and executed to localize the lesion. **Tables 3 and 4** highlight the abnormalities in motor and sensory nerve conductions studies in lesions affecting different portions of the brachial plexus. The exhaustive review by Ferrante on brachial plexopathies provides the protocols for the electrophysiological assessment of various components of the supraclavicular and infraclavicular plexus.[3]

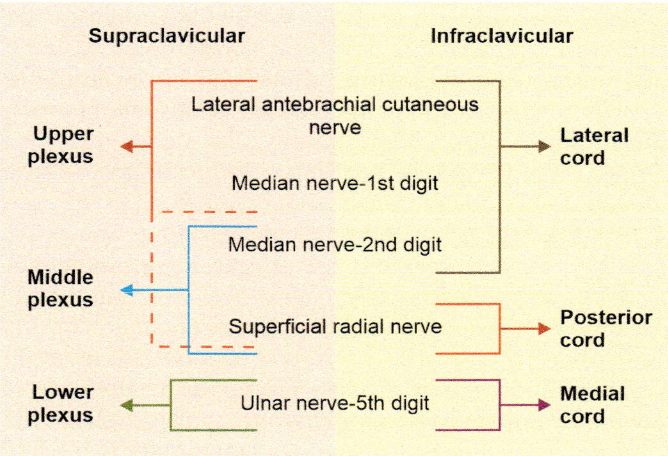

FIG. 3: Nerve conduction studies in a patient with suspected brachial plexopathy and implications for localization.

The lumbosacral plexus innervates the crural muscles, skin of the lower limbs and lower abdomen as well as the sphincters. It is not as ramified as the brachial plexus; nevertheless, electrophysiological testing has its technical difficulties and only a limited number of nerves can be reliably studied by NCS **(Fig. 4)**. Motor conduction studies involve examination of the evoked motor responses from the common peroneal, tibial, and femoral nerves. Sensory studies of the lateral femoral cutaneous, saphenous, superficial peroneal, sural, and medial and lateral plantar nerves are performed. Furthermore, these sensory potentials are technically difficult to record and may be of reduced amplitude or in-excitable, even in normal healthy subjects, especially in old age. As in the case of the brachial plexus, needle EMG plays an important role in assessing the proximal muscles that are innervated by nerves derived directly from the plexus and spinal roots, and thereby distinguishing plexopathy from radiculopathy and sciatic/common peroneal neuropathy.[4]

TABLE 3: Abnormal sensory conduction studies in lesions in different parts of the brachial plexus.

	Trunks			Cords		
Nerves	**Upper**	**Middle**	**Lower**	**Lateral**	**Posterior**	**Medial**
LABC	+ (100%)			+ (100%)		
MABC			+ (100%)			+ (100%)
Median (1st digit)	+ (100%)			+ (100%)		
Median (2nd digit)	+ (20%)	+ (80%)		+ (100%)		
Median (3rd digit)	+ (10%)	+ (70%)	+ (20%)	+ (80%)		+ (20%)
Ulnar (5th digit)			+ (100%)			+ (100%)
Superficial radial	+ (60%)	+ (40%)			+ (100%)	

*Numbers in parentheses indicate the percentage of abnormalities in the tested nerves when lesions occur in the corresponding regions.

TABLE 4: Abnormal motor conduction studies in lesions in different parts of the brachial plexus.

	Trunks			Cords		
Nerves (recording muscle sites)	**Upper**	**Middle**	**Lower**	**Lateral**	**Posterior**	**Medial**
Musculocutaneous (biceps)	+			+		
Axillary (deltoid)	+				+	
Median (APB)			+			+
Ulnar (ADM)			+			+
Ulnar (FDI)			+			+
Radial (EIP)			+		+	
Radial (EDC)					+	
Radial (anconeus)		+			+	

(ADM: abductor digiti minimi; APB: abductor pollicis brevis; EDC: extensor digitorum communis; FDI: first dorsal interosseous; EIP; extensor indicis proprius)

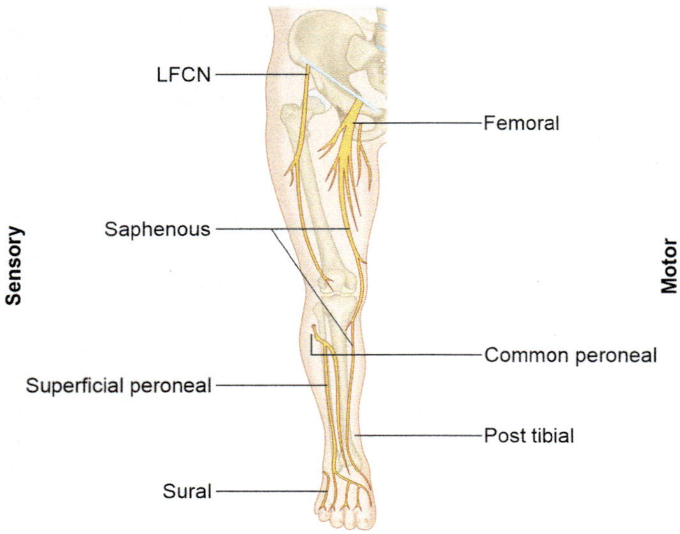

FIG. 4: Nerve conduction studies in lumbosacral plexopathy.
(LFCN: lateral femoral cutaneous nerve)

DISTINGUISHING NEUROPATHY FROM PLEXOPATHY AND RADICULOPATHY

Conundrums arise when a patient presents with focal dysfunction of a limb, and one needs to distinguish mononeuropathy from radiculopathy and mononeuritis multiplex from plexopathy. Careful examination and interpretation of the motor, sensory, and reflex abnormalities aid in this exercise. While examining the muscle power, the aim is to identify weak muscle or muscle groups that have a unique supply by a nerve, but not by the corresponding root, and vice versa, in both proximal and distal segments. For example, in a patient with wrist drop, examining the wrist flexors and brachioradialis distinguishes C7 radiculopathy and radial neuropathy, respectively. It is important to be aware of the dermatomal and nerve pattern of cutaneous innervation. "Splitting" of the fourth digit distinguishes ulnar neuropathy from C8 radiculopathy, where the entire fourth digit is involved. In this context, one must also remember that there are topographical discrepancies between dermatomes and myotomes and generally they are separated from each other, i.e., myotomes often lie under segmentally distant dermatomes.

One looks for the key reflex that aids in localization, apart from examining asymmetry of muscle stretch reflexes. For example, in a patient with foot drop, ankle reflex is lost in S1 radiculopathy, but not in common peroneal neuropathy. One should not only map out the areas of impaired sensation, but also perform maneuvers to elicit positive sensory signs, which are indicative of focal irritation of nerves or roots. Examples include the Spurling maneuver and straight leg raising test which are useful in identifying monoradiculopathies. In addition, the Tinel sign can be elicited over the superficial and vulnerable segments of the peripheral nerves such as the median nerve at wrist and common peroneal nerve as it traverses over the fibular neck.

While distinguishing monoradiculopathies from mononeuropathies, apart from delineating whether the pattern of sensory deficits fit in a dermatomal or nerve distribution, the following points may be taken into consideration: (1) ratio of loss of pain versus loss of touch sensation—in case of neuropathy, the cutaneous area of reduced touch is less than that of reduced pain, (2) the boundaries of impaired sensation are indistinct in the case of root lesions, (3) irritative signs—Spurling maneuver, Tinel sign, etc., (4) weakness and atrophy are prominent in nerve lesions, while muscle stretch reflexes are diminished/ absent in root lesions, and (5) focal or regional autonomic signs—may be present in nerve lesions. In general, weakness and atrophy are less prominent in the case of monoradiculopathies because of overlapping supply. In the context of radiculopathies, one must remember that while radiating pain is a characteristic feature of root involvement, pain due to entrapment of peripheral nerves may also radiate proximally and thus mimic a radicular pain. In this case scenario, signs of local or focal irritation such as the Tinel's sign may be useful.

The presence of sensorimotor deficits in the distribution of multiple spinal roots and peripheral nerves in the upper and lower limbs gives a clue for the involvement of the brachial and lumbosacral plexus, respectively. During clinical and electrophysiological examination, a clinician has to make it a habit to mentally trace the relevant anatomical pathways involved. For example, recording the SNAP from the fifth digit of the upper limbs assesses not only the ulnar nerve, but also the medial cord and lower trunk of the brachial plexus, as well as the C8 spinal nerve and dorsal root ganglion. An example each, of the key steps involved in localizing focal neurological deficits by clinical and electrophysiological examination, in the upper limb and lower limb are provided in **Figures 5 and 6**. In this context, non-neurological conditions such as fibromyalgia, polymyalgia rheumatica, arthropathies, bursitis, tennis elbow, de Quervain's tenosynovitis, trigger finger, cervical spondylosis, rotator cuff injury, avascular necrosis, tendinitis, plantar fasciitis, iliotibial band syndrome, and piriformis syndrome are some of the differential diagnoses that need to be excluded. One should also be aware of "referred" pain of acute visceral disease which occurs in a segmental distribution and closely mimics the pain of nerve root irritation.

OTHER INVESTIGATIONS

Based on the clinical features and abnormalities on electrophysiological testing, one needs to form working hypothesis regarding the localization as well as the possible

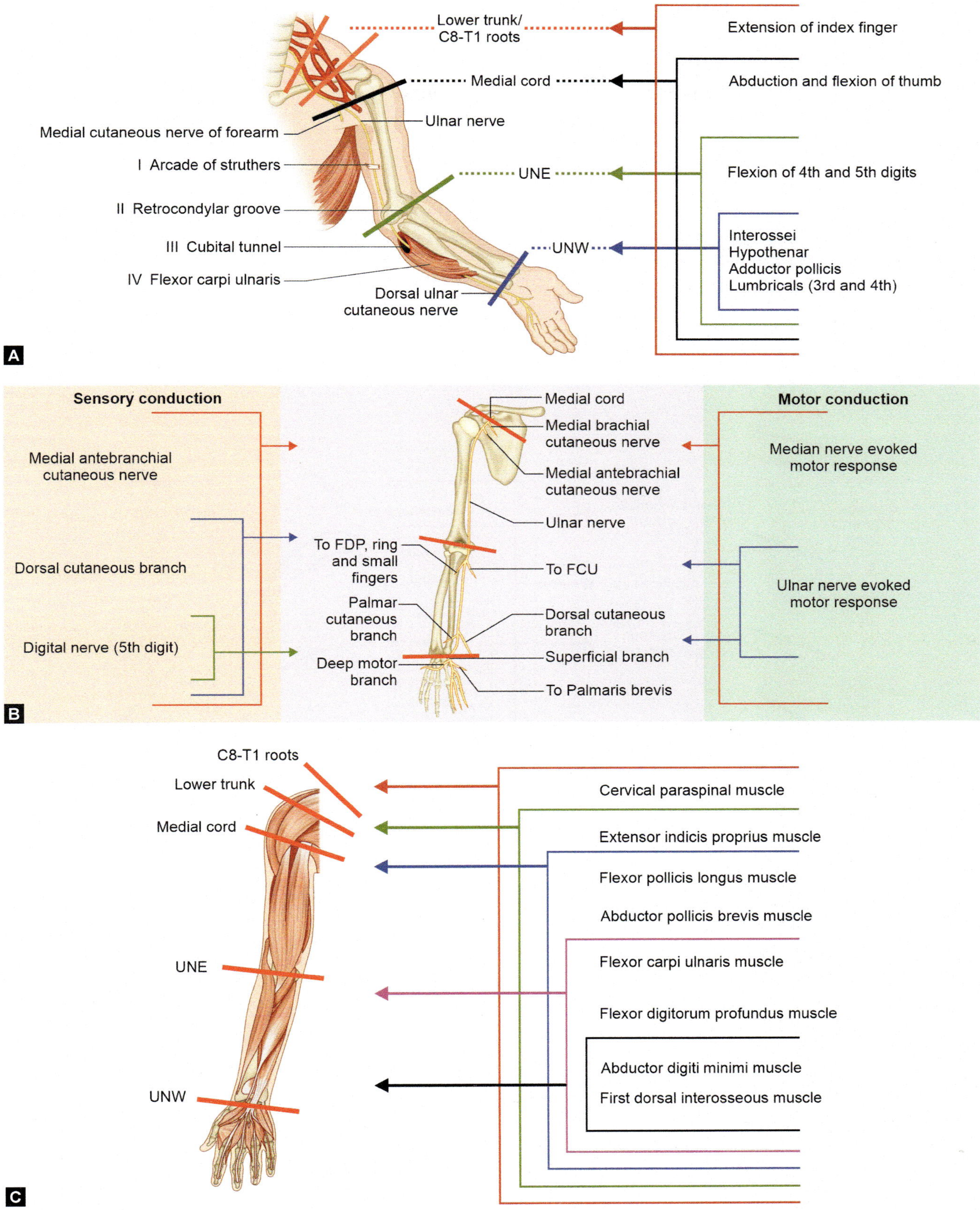

FIGS. 5A TO C: (A) Clinical examination of key muscles for localization in a patient with suspected ulnar neuropathy. (B) Using nerve conduction studies for supporting the clinical localization. (C) Role of needle electromyogram for localization.
(FCU: flexor carpi ulnaris, FDP: flexor digitorum profundus, UNE: ulnar neuropathy at elbow, UNW: ulnar neuropathy at wrist)

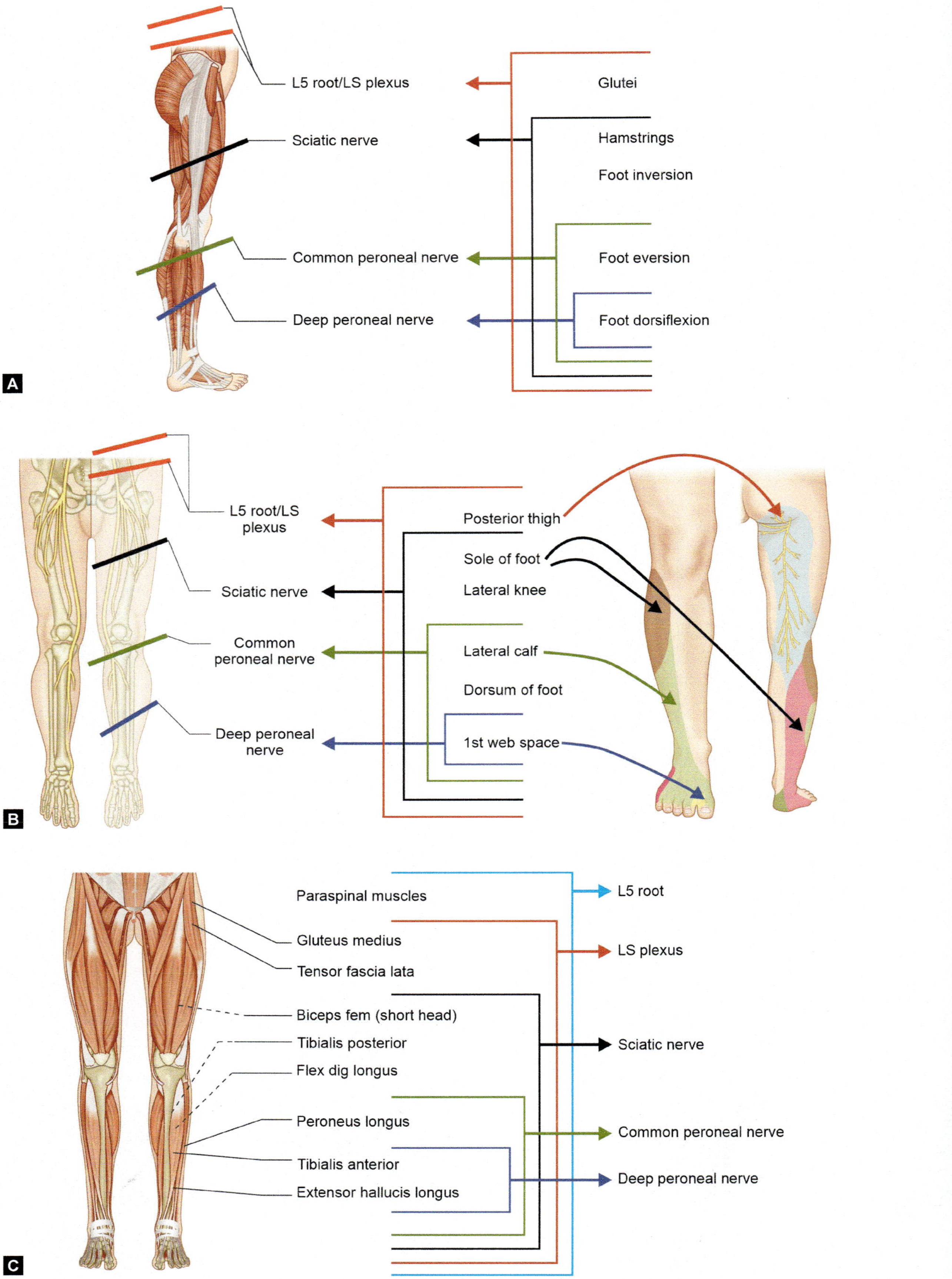

FIGS. 6A TO C: (A) Clinical examination of key muscles for localization in a patient with foot drop. (B) Using nerve conduction studies for supporting the clinical localization. (C) Role of needle electromyogram for localization.

pathology and etiology, so that the appropriate management can be planned. Imaging by high-resolution ultrasound and magnetic resonance imaging (MRI) complements the clinical and electrophysiological examination by providing excellent information regarding the morphological alterations within the plexuses and nerves. Further, a huge armamentarium of tests to identify various immunological, genetic, and neoplastic/paraneoplastic causes is available. These need to be used judiciously to support the clinical diagnosis and exclude the relevant differential diagnosis. Nerve biopsy is performed in selected cases, and is diagnostic in vasculitis, amyloidosis, sarcoidosis, leprosy, neoplasms, and polyglucosan body disease.[6]

CONCLUSION

Integrating the requisite knowledge of anatomy with the physiology and relevant pathology at the bedside, by detailed clinical assessment and other ancillary tests, is essential. This includes understanding the anatomical relationship of the plexuses and nerves with various osseomuscular structures, blood vessels, and other viscera, which has relevance not only in localizing the clinical deficits and but also in deciphering the possible etiologies. The clinical diagnosis and possible etiologies can be supported and confirmed by appropriately performed electrophysiological, imaging, and other laboratory studies.

REFERENCES

1. Trivedi S, Pandit A, Ganguly G, Das SK. Epidemiology of Peripheral Neuropathy: An Indian Perspective. Ann Indian Acad Neurol. 2017;20(3):173-84.
2. Siao P, Kaku M. A clinician's approach to peripheral neuropathy. Semin Neurol. 2019;39(5):519-30.
3. Ferrante MA. Brachial plexopathies: classification, causes, and consequences. Muscle Nerve. 2004;30(5):547-68.
4. Dyck PJ, Thaisetthawatkul P. Lumbosacral plexopathy. Continuum (Minneap Minn). 2014;20(5 Peripheral Nervous System Disorders): 1343-58.
5. Watson JC, Dyck PJ. Peripheral Neuropathy: A Practical Approach to Diagnosis and Symptom Management. Mayo Clin Proc. 2015;90(7):940-51.
6. Willison HJ, Winer JB. Clinical evaluation and investigation of neuropathy. J Neurol Neurosurg Psychiatry. 2003;74(Suppl 2):ii3-ii8.

3

SECTION

Approach to Common Neurological Symptoms

23

CHAPTER

Approach to Transient Loss of Consciousness

William Owen Pickrell, V Preethish Kumar, Inder MS Sawhney

INTRODUCTION

Episodes of transient loss of consciousness (TLOC) are a common presentation in the clinic and emergency department—the lifetime risk of an episode is perhaps as much as 50%.[1] A TLOC is defined as *"a state of real or apparent loss of consciousness with loss of awareness, characterized by amnesia for the period of unconsciousness, abnormal motor control, loss of responsiveness, short duration, and complete recovery"*.[2] It is accepted that this definition of unconsciousness includes loss of arousal and so TLOC is associated with *loss of postural control.* Events with loss of awareness but not loss of posture (e.g., absence seizures or focal seizures with loss of awareness) are therefore, not generally classed as episodes of TLOC.[2]

The causes of TLOC can be broadly classified into *traumatic* (head injury) and *nontraumatic.*[3] We will concentrate on nontraumatic causes of TLOC in this article with the most common nontraumatic causes of TLOC being syncope, epileptic seizures, and dissociative (functional) seizures; together these account for over 90% of TLOC cases **(Table 1)**.[2-4]

MAIN CAUSES OF TRANSIENT LOSS OF CONSCIOUSNESS

Syncope

Syncope is a TLOC caused by cerebral hypoperfusion and is the most common cause of TLOC. Syncope is generally categorized as *reflex, cardiac,* or *orthostatic* depending on the mechanism of cerebral hypoperfusion. *Presyncope* describes the symptoms and signs before unconsciousness.

Reflex Syncope

Reflex or *neurally mediated syncope* is a group of disorders causing syncope through an inappropriate cardiovascular autonomic reflex, although the exact pathophysiology is not fully understood. This reflex may be *vasodepressive* (insufficient sympathetic vasoconstriction causing hypotension), *cardioinhibitory* (parasympathetic mediated bradykinesia or asystole), or a combination of both.[2,3]

Reflex syncope is categorized according to the typical trigger **(Table 1)**. Classically, vasovagal (*vasodilatation* and *vagally* mediated bradycardia) syncope is provoked by emotional stimuli (pain, blood, and fear) and circumstances that decrease central blood volume such as prolonged standing, dehydration, heat, and alcohol. Vasovagal syncope typically starts in the teenage years, and usually decreases in the adult years but may reoccur in older age groups. The first episode of vasovagal syncope is rare after the age of 35 years and so a high index of suspicion should be held for an alternative diagnosis (e.g., cardiac or orthostatic syncope) in this case.[5]

Cardiac Syncope

Cardiac syncope causes cerebral hypoperfusion due to a sudden decrease in cardiac output.[5] It is less common than reflex or orthostatic syncope but carries a significantly higher mortality rate and is perhaps the most worrying cause of TLOC. Cardiac syncope can occur in a *structurally abnormal heart* due to arrhythmias or limited cardiac output or in a *structurally normal heart* due to arrhythmias, which can be congenital or acquired.[6]

Most life-threatening arrhythmias occur in structurally abnormal hearts.[6] Any form of structural heart disease (e.g., previous cardiac ischemia or cardiomyopathy) can result in scar-related ventricular tachycardia which is one of the most common causes of out-of-hospital cardiac arrest.[5,6]

Cardiac disease can limit cardiac output and cause syncope particularly in times of increased demand, e.g., exercise. Common causes include aortic stenosis, obstructive cardiomyopathy, and ischemic heart disease. In the younger patient consider inherited cardiomyopathies such as hypertrophic cardiomyopathy and arrhythmogenic cardiomyopathy.

TABLE1 : Nontraumatic causes of episodes of transient loss of consciousness (TLOC).[3]

Syncope	Reflex (neurally mediated)	• Vasovagal, e.g., standing/pain/fear • Situational (cough/micturition/stretch/sneezing) • Carotid sinus
	Cardiac	• Structurally abnormal heart causing arrhythmias and/or limited cardiac output (valvular disease, ischemia/infarction, hypertrophic cardiomyopathy, cardiac masses, pericardial disease, and congenital abnormalities) • Arrhythmias in a structurally normal heart (sinus node disease, heart block, rarely tachycardias, or inherited cardiac channelopathies)
	Orthostatic	Primary or secondary autonomic failure, drugs, and hypovolemia
Epileptic seizures*	Generalized seizures	Generalized tonic-clonic seizures, tonic seizures, and atonic seizures
	Focal seizures	• Focal to bilateral convulsive seizures • Focal seizures causing ictal arrhythmias and cardiac syncope
Dissociative seizures	Also called functional seizures, psychogenic nonepileptic seizures, and nonepileptic attacks	
Rarer causes	Metabolic	Hypoglycemia. Other metabolic abnormalities can provoke seizures (e.g., hypomagnesemia and hyponatremia)
	Vascular	• Subclavian steal syndrome • Transient ischemic events and strokes (although TLOC is rare and not typical in stroke it can occur occasionally particular in posterior circulation events)
	• Neuroendocrine • Ménierès disease • Intoxication	• Pheochromocytoma, neuroendocrine tumors • Vestibular drop attacks • Alcohol, sedative, psychotropic, and recreational drugs
TLOC mimics	• Cataplexy • Transient focal neurological episodes • Sleep-related	 • Occur in cerebral amyloid angiopathy • Central sleep disorders (narcolepsy and idiopathic hypersomnolence), obstructive sleep apnea, and neurodegenerative disorders

*Seizures causing loss of awareness but not loss of postural tone, e.g., absences or focal seizures with altered awareness are not included here.[3]

Cardiac syncope caused by arrhythmias in a structurally normal heart is rarer than those in a structurally abnormal heart. Bradyarrhythmias are a more common cause of cardiac syncope than tachyarrhythmias. Bradyarrhythmias can be caused by sinus node disease or heart block. Complete heart block is normally straightforward to diagnose when captured on an electrocardiogram (ECG) and is an indication for permanent pacemaker (PPM) insertion. Intermittent complete heart block can be harder to diagnose. Cardiac syncope with complete left bundle branch block or trifascicular block (right bundle branch block, left anterior hemiblock, and first-degree AV block) are also indications for PPM insertion.[6] Remember that certain medications are proarrythmogenic and can cause tachy- or bradyarrhythmias **(Table 2)**.

Hereditary cardiac channelopathies are a rare but important cause of cardiac syncope. Congenital long QT syndrome is the most common hereditary channelopathy and can cause sudden cardiac death through polymorphic ventricular tachycardia (Torsades de pointes) (see on page 8 ECG section in investigations on calculating corrected QT intervals). Syncope frequently occurs during sleep, exercise, or after a startle and typically there is a prolonged corrected QT interval on the ECG. Brugada syndrome has characteristic ECG changes ("pseudo" right bundle branch block and ST elevation in leads V_1–V_3)[5-7] and carries a high risk of cardiac syncope and death. Other inherited cardiac channelopathies include short QT syndrome and catecholaminergic polymorphic ventricular tachycardia.[6] Cardiac syncope due to inherited channelopathies can occasionally mimic epilepsy.[8,9]

TABLE 2: Medications that may increase the risk of syncope through cardiac toxicity or hypotension or increase the risk of seizures through lowering the seizure threshold.[40,41]

Cardiac arrhythmia	Adrenaline, atropine, beta-blockers, clenbuterol, clonidine, cocaine, digoxin, dobutamine, isoprenaline, methyldopa, noradrenaline, organophosphates, reserpine, salbutamol, and verapamil
Cardiac toxicity	Adrenaline, cocaine, isoprenaline, noradrenaline, and tricyclic antidepressants
Systematic hypotension	Clonidine, beta-blockers, doxazosin, isoprenaline, methyldopa, reserpine, sildenafil, tricyclic antidepressants, and verapamil
Lower seizure threshold	Alcohol (withdrawal), amphetamines, antipsychotics, baclofen (acute withdrawal), recreational drugs (cocaine, heroin, phencyclidine, synthetic cannabinoids), tramadol, and other opiates

Orthostatic Syncope

A change in posture causes a rapid shift in blood volume resulting in decreased venous return and blood pressure. Maintaining normal blood pressure with postural changes relies on an adequate blood volume and intact autonomic reflexes that control cardiac function and peripheral resistance.[10] Orthostatic hypotension is defined as a fall in systolic blood pressure (SBP) of 20 mm Hg or more, and/or a drop in diastolic blood pressure (DBP) of 10 mm Hg or more, within 3 minutes of standing.[11]

Orthostatic hypotension can cause presyncope and syncope. The most common cause is a medication that causes vasodilation or hypovolemia **(Table 2)**. Other causes include hypovolemia and autonomic failure. Causes of autonomic failure include neurodegenerative diseases such as Parkinson's disease, Parkinson's plus diseases and primary autonomic failure; diabetes and autonomic neuropathies.[5]

Epileptic Seizures

Epilepsy is an important and common cause of TLOC. Convulsive seizures (generalized tonic-clonic and focal to bilateral convulsive seizures) are the most common type of epileptic seizure causing TLOC although tonic and atonic epileptic seizures can also cause TLOC. The postural tone is normally maintained in absence and focal seizures with or without awareness and so these seizures do not strictly cause TLOC although they can be associated with convulsive seizures and are encountered in TLOC clinics.

The underlying pathophysiology of TLOC in epilepsy is due to the loss of functional connectivity between the areas responsible for consciousness and/or their thalamic connections.[12] Rarely, epileptic seizures can cause ictal arrhythmias and ictal asystole.[13]

Dissociative Seizures

Dissociative seizures (also called functional seizures, psychogenic nonepileptic seizures, or nonepileptic attacks) are a common presentation of a functional neurological disorder.[14] They are an involuntary response to distressing internal or external triggers and are not caused by the excessive or hypersynchronous neuronal discharges that cause epileptic seizures.[15] As with all types of functional neurological disorders, psychological stressors and a history of childhood adversity can increase the risk of dissociative seizures. Psychiatric comorbidities are common, but not essential for the diagnosis. Remember that psychiatric comorbidities are common in neurological disorders such as epilepsy also.[14]

Rarer Causes and TLOC Mimics

Hypoglycemia can cause anxiety, tremor, sweating, dizziness, confusion, seizures, and loss of consciousness. Symptoms may be less pronounced in older people or people with impaired awareness of hypoglycemia. Typically hypoglycemia occurs in people with diabetes due to an imbalance between oral glucose intake and the administration of insulin or other glucose lowering medications. Hypoglycemia causing TLOC in people without diabetes is rare but can occur due to certain medications, alcohol, critical illness, insulinomas, and beta cell disorders.[16] Other electrolyte and metabolic disturbances such as hypomagnesemia, hyponatremia, and hypocalcaemia can cause *provoked* epileptic seizures.

Transient loss of consciousness is extremely rare in *transient ischemic attacks* (TIAs) but may occasionally occur in vertebrobasilar TIAs or *subclavian steal syndrome*.[17,18] If TLOC does occur due to a vertebrobasilar TIA or subclavian steal then it is usually accompanied with brainstem signs such as limb paresis, ataxia, diplopia, and bulbar symptoms.[18]

Rarely, some neuroendocrine disorders can cause TLOC. Pheochromocytoma typically presents with headache, sweating, and tachycardia. It can also cause paroxysmal hypertension, palpitations, sweating, headache, and pallor. It rarely induces orthostatic hypotension and syncope.[19] Neuroendocrine tumors can cause carcinoid syndrome which typically presents with flushing and diarrhea and rarely hypotension leading to syncope.[20]

Ménière's disease is a disorder of the inner ear characterized by episodic vertigo, tinnitus, and hearing loss.[21] It can cause *vestibular drop attacks* (otolithic crisis of Tumarkin) where sudden loss of muscle tone causes sudden falls to the ground.[21,22] The patient can report a sensation of being pushed. Consciousness is normally preserved but occasionally there can also be a brief loss of consciousness.[22]

Cataplexy is a transient, bilateral loss of muscle tone triggered by emotions (e.g., laughter).[23] It is virtually diagnostic for narcolepsy type 1. It is a TLOC mimic as consciousness is preserved.[23]

Transient focal neurological episodes (TFNEs) (amyloid spells) are brief (lasting minutes), normally stereotyped, episodes of cortical dysfunction that occur in cerebral amyloid angiopathy.[24] Symptoms (normally positive or negative sensory or motor disturbances) usually spread and progress and may be caused by cortical spreading depression.[24] They are another TLOC mimic as they do not normally cause TLOC but can resemble focal seizures, TIAs, and migraines.

HISTORY

Obtaining an accurate history is the most important step in obtaining an accurate diagnosis. It is essential to obtain or attempt to obtain a witness history although sometimes this is not possible in an unwitnessed event. An accurate witness history can often be the single most useful piece of information. If it is not possible for a witness to be present in the consultation then they can be contacted by telephone, or in some cases provide a written witness statement. Videos from mobile phones or closed-circuit television (CCTV) footage can be very useful in supplementing the history.[25]

Studies have shown that *how* patients describe their TLOC can be useful when attempting to differentiate between epileptic and dissociative seizures.[26] Patients describing epileptic seizures will try and describe their experiences in detail even though this can be difficult. Patients with dissociative seizures, however, often do not describe the TLOC at all, turning to a witness.[26]

In practice, language issues, cognitive and other communication difficulties are often barriers to obtaining an accurate history. Remember that episodes of TLOC can be frightening for witnesses which may mean that some details are difficult to recollect (duration of TLOC and lateralizing features can be incorrectly recollected).

Diagnosis in the elderly patient can be harder as the presentation of events may differ from those in the younger group. For example, syncopal events may be longer and cause a prolonged postictal period due to increased susceptibility to brain hypoxia and brain injuries. Comorbidities and increased medication may mean that TLOC may be multifactorial.

Key features in the history which can help distinguish between the different etiologies are discussed below and in **Table 3**.

Before the Event

Reflex and orthostatic syncopal events typically have a prodrome (light headedness, feeling warm or cold, clammy, dizziness, sweating, visual blurring, tunnel vision, muffled hearing, or unusual sounds such as whooshing noise). *Presyncope* is a similar prodrome without TLOC. Witnesses may report pallor. Reflex and orthostatic syncope typically occur whilst, or shortly after, standing. *Specific situations* may trigger reflex *syncope (situational syncope)*, these include micturition, defecation, swallowing, pain associated with venepuncture, injury or a procedure, needle phobia, sight of blood, and high intrathoracic pressure associated with coughing, sneezing, or breath holding spells. Benign episodes of syncope typically have *the "3 Ps"* (*p*rovoking factors, *p*rodrome, and *p*osture).

Consider *carotid sinus hypersensitivity,* if TLOC follows head rotation, shaving or is associated with a tight collar.

TABLE 3: Features of the three most common causes of transient loss of consciousness (TLOC).

	Reflex/Orthostatic syncope	Cardiac syncope	Epileptic seizure	Dissociative seizure
Before TLOC	"3 Ps": • *Prodrome* lasting tens of seconds (lightheadedness, nausea, pallor, and sweating) • *Posture*—usually standing • *Provoking factors*—prolonged standing, heat, dehydration, pain, blood, alcohol, micturition, and during or after food	• Can occur without prodrome • Any posture • Sometimes provoked by exercise • Cardiac symptoms (angina, palpitations, and shortness of breath) • Rarely startling stimuli (long QT)	Sometimes triggers, e.g., photosensitivity, and sleep deprivation. Auras, e.g., déjà vu, jamais vu, epigastric sensations, unusual taste, smell, or noise	Sometimes triggers such as stress. Can be situational and occur when the patient is not alone
During TLOC	Usually brief (seconds). Loss of tone. Pallor and sweatiness. Can have a few jerks (<10) and occasional posturing	Usually brief (seconds). Loss of tone. Can have a few jerks (<10) and occasional posturing	Normally, seconds to minutes; eyes normally open; lateral tongue bite; focal features, e.g., head/eye version, unilateral. Cry at seizure onset. Stertorous breathing. Central cyanosis. Stiffness	Normally minutes, can be significantly longer than epileptic seizures. Eyes can be closed or forced eye closure. Pelvic thrusting, waxing and waning of movements. Asynchronous limb movements. Awareness during generalized shaking
After TLOC	Recovery usually quick	Recovery usually quick	Normally prolonged recovery (minutes–hours) with amnesia/confusion. Myalgias and muscle aches reminiscent of delayed onset muscle stiffness after exercise	Postictal crying
Other features	Reflex syncope, onset <35 years old	• History or signs of structural heart disease • Family history of sudden deaths and heart disease • Abnormal ECG	Previous history of focal seizures or other epileptic seizure types, e.g., myoclonus or clinical photosensitivity	Psychiatric comorbidities are common but not essential

Note: Urinary incontinence can occur in any of the above causes of TLOC and is a nondistinguishing feature. *Note* that clinical features can be less distinct in the elderly (see history section).

Cardiac syncope may occur whilst sitting or lying, can be preceded by exertion or exercise and may be associated with palpitations.

Epileptic seizures may occur with any posture (lying or standing). Patients with focal onset-seizures (focal to bilateral convulsive seizures) may describe auras. Auras can be difficult to describe and commonly include epigastric auras and déjà vu in temporal lobe epilepsy, motor auras in frontal lobe seizures and visual symptoms in occipital seizures. Auras not only help in reaching the diagnosis of a seizure but also help in localization. The emission of a cry at the beginning of the episode is very suggestive of an epileptic seizure, vocalization is often associated with frontal lobe seizures.

Dissociative seizures are sometimes associated with stressful situations and commonly occur when the patient is awake and not alone.[27] Sometimes dissociative episodes can be triggered by suggestion which can be useful during electroencephalogram (EEG) recording.[28,29] An aura is sometimes reported before dissociative seizures.[27]

During the Event

Syncopal events are typically brief (seconds to a maximum of a few minutes) as loss of tone results in a fall and a supine position restores adequate cerebral blood flow. If the event lasts longer than 5 minutes then syncope is unlikely. However, syncopal events can be prolonged sometimes, if a sitting/standing position is artificially maintained by well-meaning onlookers. Patients with syncope may suffer from head injury leading to prolonged loss of consciousness. The patient can be pale and sweaty and has reduced or normal tone.

Myoclonic jerks are seen in the majority of patients with syncope because of brain hypoxia (convulsive syncope).[30] This often leads to a misinterpretation of syncope as epileptic seizures (see video: https://www.youtube.com/watch?v=DOHGXoiS_Dk). In a study comparing the semiology of syncope with epileptic seizures, there were typically <10 jerks in syncope and >20 in seizures "10/20" rule. Other differences included less rhythmic jerking and loss of tone in syncope.[31]

In a convulsive *epileptic seizure*, there is usually stiffness (tonic phase) followed by rhythmic limb movements (clonic phase). There may be an unusual cry or moan associated with the onset of the tonic phase due to air being expanded from the diaphragm. The eyes tend to be open and are often rolled up or deviated to one side, there can be apnea or stertorous breathing (snoring or noisy breathing noises) as well as cyanosis. The presence of a lateral tongue bite is specific but not sensitive to convulsive epileptic seizures.[32]

Dissociative seizures are often longer than syncope or epileptic seizures, lasting minutes to even hours in some circumstances. There may be a gradual onset or offset or "waxing and waning" of the movements. There can be asymmetric thrashing movements of limbs and side-to-side movements of the head with a normal tone. Eyes can be closed during dissociative seizures whereas they are normally open during epileptic seizures. Movements during dissociative seizures may not follow the homunculus, e.g., tonic-clonic movements involving the upper and lower limb with sparing of the face. Opisthotonic posturing, variability of movements, and talking or crying during the episode are also pointers toward dissociative seizures. A minority of patients with dissociative seizures have hypokinetic semiology or "swoon events" which resemble syncopal events with a fall to the ground with closed eyes and no limb movements.[33]

We do not find the presence of incontinence useful diagnostically as it can occur in the three main causes of TLOC.

After the Event

Recovery is typically quick after *syncope*. The patient can be orientated in time, space, and person in minutes although in older patients amnesia is common and recovery can be longer.

Epileptic seizures tend to have a longer postictal phase. The length can vary from minutes to hours; prolonged seizures lead to a longer duration of recovery.

The period of recovery after a *dissociative seizure* is variable although a short postictal phase after a prolonged seizure of 15–20 minutes is suggestive of a dissociative seizure.

Previous/Other Events

A significant proportion of patients presenting with an episode of TLOC are likely to have had previous events which can help with diagnosis.[34] Patients presenting with a convulsive epileptic seizure may have non-TLOC epileptic events such as myoclonus or brief focal seizures with or without retained awareness. These may have been subtle and not recognized as seizures and so it can be worth specifically asking about them. In a younger person, ask about morning jerks or spilling things at breakfast time which might represent myoclonus and confirm the diagnosis of juvenile myoclonic epilepsy. Patterns of sunlight through trees as well as flashing lights can represent photosensitivity which is typically associated with generalized epilepsy syndromes. Epileptic seizures tend to be stereotyped whereas dissociative seizures can vary both in semiology and duration.

The frequency of episodes can vary depending on the cause. Most vasovagal episodes are infrequent. Multiple episodes in a young patient over many years suggest a benign etiology. Very frequent episodes over a few days or weeks can occur with dissociative seizures but are also a red flag for a more serious cause, e.g., cardiac syncope.

Medical and Drug History

Other comorbidities are important and can provide clues. A history of structural heart disease, cardiovascular disease, or cardiac arrhythmias increases the risk of cardiac syncope. Patients with Parkinsonism with autonomic dysfunction, diabetes with peripheral neuropathy, and autonomic neuropathies have an increased risk of orthostatic syncope. Medications taken by the patient are relevant as they can increase the risk of syncope through postural hypotension or cardiotoxicity or lower seizure threshold **(Table 2)**.

Significant perinatal events, febrile seizures, moderate or severe head injuries, previous meningitis or encephalitis, and other causes of structural brain disease (e.g., stroke, brain tumors, and hemorrhage) all increase the risk of developing epileptic seizures.

It is important to enquire about *alcohol* and *recreational drug* consumption. Alcohol withdrawal seizures typically occur 6–48 hours after abrupt cessation of chronic alcohol consumption.[35] Rarely, prolonged and/or massive alcohol consumption can provoke epileptic intoxication seizures. Alcohol can also cause metabolic changes including hypoglycemia and hypomagnesemia which can lower the seizure threshold.[35] Many prescription and recreational drugs can lower epileptic seizure threshold including synthetic cannabinoids, opiates (particularly tramadol) amphetamines, cocaine, and MDMA (3,4-methylene-dioxymethamphetamine).[36]

Family History

Any history of sudden or unexplained deaths in the family may be a clue to familial cardiac syndromes that can predispose to cardiac syncope particularly in younger first degree relatives.[6] Reflex syncope also has a familial component with the risk of syncope being increased in relatives.[37]

Having a first-degree relative with epilepsy increases the risk of subsequent epilepsy.[38] A family history of epilepsy might suggest one of the rarer *monogenetic* epilepsy syndromes, e.g., autosomal dominant sleep-related hypermotor epilepsy, autosomal dominant epilepsy with auditory features, or genetic epilepsy with febrile seizures plus.[39]

EXAMINATION

The examination is normal in most cases of TLOC. A cardiovascular examination may reveal evidence of structural heart disease (e.g., heart murmurs, a raised jugular-venous pressure, or peripheral edema). Measure blood pressure in a lying and standard position to check for orthostatic hypotension (see the section on orthostatic syncope above).

The presence of neurocutaneous markers may suggest an underlying neurological abnormality that increases the risk of seizures, e.g., facial angiofibromas or hypomelanotic macules suggestive of tuberous sclerosis. The presence of self-harm scars can be associated with dissociative seizures. Any new focal neurological deficit or optic disc swelling will require urgent brain imaging and raises the possibility of a structural brain problem which can be a risk factor for epileptic seizures.

INVESTIGATIONS

Electrocardiogram

This is probably the single most important investigation and is mandatory for any new case of TLOC.[2,42] The electrocardiogram (ECG) can provide evidence for structural heart disease which increases the risk of cardiac syncope.[6,42,43] These changes include pathological q-waves suggesting previous myocardial infarction or increased QRS voltages associated with left or right ventricular hypertrophy and hypertrophic cardiomyopathy.[43] Other ECG changes associated with an increased risk of cardiac syncope include bundle branch block, trifascicular block, short PR interval and delta waves (Wolff–Parkinson–White syndrome), ST elevation in V_1–V_3 (Brugada syndrome), and long QT interval.[2,43,44]

Remember that machine generated corrected QT intervals (QT_c) can be inaccurate—manually check the QT_c in cases with a high index of suspicion. QT_c is normally calculated using Bazett's formula:

$$QT_c = \frac{QT}{\sqrt{RR}}$$

where the QT and RR intervals are measured in seconds. QT_c > 450 ms (men) or 460 ms (women) are generally considered prolonged.[8]

Brain Imaging

We would recommend brain imaging for most cases of adult-onset TLOC. Urgent brain imaging should be performed when an epileptic seizure is suspected or there are new neurological signs.[45] A magnetic resonance imaging (MRI) brain is more sensitive and specific than computed tomography (CT) imaging and should be the first choice.[46] CT scans can be useful in the acute situation, if there is likely to be a delay in obtaining an MRI scan, or if MRI is contraindicated.[46]

ELECTROENCEPHALOGRAM

The EEG is not always useful and should generally not be performed routinely in cases of suspected *syncope*.[42] Nonspecific EEG changes are common, particularly in older individuals or those taking certain medications and in general EEG findings would not alter a clinical diagnosis of syncope.

EEGs are more useful if an *epileptic seizure* is suspected, particularly in younger people who are more likely to have interictal generalized epileptiform changes which can help diagnose generalized epilepsy and predict further seizures.[47,48] The yield of the EEG in suspected epilepsy can be increased if the EEG is performed as soon as possible after the suspected seizure.[45,47] If the initial EEG is normal then performing serial EEGs or sleep-deprived EEGs can increase diagnostic yield.[48]

We would recommend performing an EEG if *dissociative seizures* are suspected unless the diagnosis is certain. Capturing a typical dissociative seizure on EEG (preferably video EEG) increases diagnostic certainty when communicating the diagnosis. Suggestion techniques can also be used during the EEG procedure to increase yield.[28,29]

Other Investigations

In cases of suspected cardiac syncope, we would strongly recommend early consultation with a cardiologist for advice on further investigations. A transthoracic echocardiogram can be useful to look for signs of structural heart disease. Be wary that a normal 24 hours or 48 hours tape (Holter monitor) does not exclude cardiac syncope if an event is not captured and generally in this case a cardiac event recorder is required.

Ambulatory blood pressure monitoring and tilt table testing can be useful in cases of reflex or orthostatic syncope.[10] For rarer causes of TLOC, other tests such as carotid-sinus massage, fasting glucose testing, and vascular imaging can be useful.

MANAGEMENT

Management depends on the etiology of TLOC. In some cases, the diagnosis of a single witnessed episode of TLOC is certain and appropriate management can be given. In reality, though there are frequently uncertainties, e.g., an unwitnessed event, an event with an unclear witness history or an event with features of more than one diagnosis. In this case, it is appropriate to retain an element of diagnostic uncertainty rather than jump to a definite conclusion that may be incorrect. The diagnosis may become more apparent with further evidence, testing, or the passage of time.

Risk Stratification

Managing diagnostic uncertainty and appropriate risk stratification is therefore important in TLOC. Cardiac syncope carries the highest risk of death amongst the cases of TLOC and prioritizing potential cases of cardiac syncope should be the primary goal in the TLOC clinic.[2,42,49] **Table 4** lists features of high and low-risk syncope that can be used to risk-stratify patients. Urgent cardiological advice should be sought on patients with suspected cardiac syncope.[42]

Convulsive epileptic seizures also carry the risk of injury and death [directly related to seizures as well as sudden unexplained death in epilepsy (SUDEP)]. Noncardiac syncope and dissociative seizures are generally considered more benign although they can also result in significant morbidity, e.g., reflex and orthostatic syncope causing injury particularly in the elderly and iatrogenic harm to patients with dissociative seizures.[50]

TABLE 4: Features that can help risk stratify episodes of syncopal transient loss of consciousness (TLOC).[2]

Higher risk	Lower risk
New onset of chest discomfort, breathlessness, and palpitations before syncope	Typical prodrome lightheadedness, sweating, nausea, blurred vision, and altered hearing
Occurring during exercise or when supine	• Occurring when standing or from sitting to standing • Provoking circumstances, e.g., prolonged standing, hot places, pain, and triggered by cough or micturition
Evidence of structural heart disease and/or abnormal ECG	Absence of structural heart disease and normal ECG
Family history of sudden or unexplained death at a young age, particularly in first-degree relatives	A long history of similar low-risk episodes

Safety and Driving

There are legal driving restrictions after an episode of TLOC in most countries.[51,52] Generally, typical reflex syncope carries few, if any, restrictions but an episode of TLOC due to untreated cardiac syncope or an epileptic seizure will entail a driving restriction. It is important to be familiar with your country's driving regulations for episodes of TLOC and to inform your patient appropriately.[52]

It is important to also inform patients of the potential safety implications of a future episode of TLOC particularly if the diagnosis is uncertain, e.g., informing the line manager in the place of work and avoiding heights and dangerous machinery.

Initial Management of the Common Causes of TLOC

Detailed descriptions of the management of the causes of TLOC are outside the scope of this article but we have covered the important points in the initial management of the common causes of TLOC below.

Reflex and Orthostatic Syncope

There is a strong consensus that education and lifestyle modifications can be useful in reducing the risk of further events.[2] These include increasing oral fluid intake, ensuring adequate dietary salt, avoiding triggers such as prolonged standing in hot environments or specific triggers in situational syncope, and avoiding/reducing medications that can cause hypotension or hypovolemia. Recognizing the prodrome/presyncope, lying down at their onset and activating counter-pressure measures can also be useful.[2] Abdominal binders or compression stockings can be tried for orthostatic syncope in older patients.

If episodes persist, are frequent or cause a significant reduction in quality of life then more specialist treatments are available which include pharmacological therapy (fludrocortisone and midodrine), tilt training and even cardiac pacing for some types of reflex syncope.[2]

Epileptic Seizures

The Medical Research Council Multicentre Trial for Early Epilepsy and Single Seizures found no difference in the quality of life or the risk of longer-term seizure remission when comparing immediate and delayed treatment after a first epileptic seizure.[53] In cases of a first unprovoked epileptic seizure with a low risk of reoccurrence (normal brain imaging, normal EEG, and no focal neurological defects), treatment is therefore not normally required.[47] The patient should be informed to seek medical advice immediately if they have another epileptic seizure so that treatment can be started.

Epilepsy can be diagnosed after a second unprovoked epileptic seizure (at least 24 hours after the first seizure), a first seizure with a high risk of reoccurrence (>60% of reoccurrence over 10 years), or after the diagnosis of an epilepsy syndrome.[54] In this case, treatment with an anti-seizure medication (ASM) is recommended.[45,47] A high risk of seizure occurrence is normally due to a structural brain lesion or problem and/or a significantly abnormal EEG.[54]

Starting an ASM is a significant decision and is not covered in detail in this article.[47] The choice of ASM needs to take into account several factors including epilepsy syndrome/type, comorbidities, potential side effects, childbearing potential, and patient choice.[47] Based on the results of the Standard and New Antiepileptic Drugs (SANAD) trials lamotrigine is commonly started for focal onset epilepsy and valproate (or levetiracetam for women of childbearing age) for generalized epilepsy.[55-58]

As well as a treatment it is important to explain the diagnosis of epilepsy properly which has significant, normally life-changing, implications for the patient. The explanation should be tailored to the patient's needs but could include information on driving, safety at home and work, risks of seizures and SUDEP, first aid information for carers, potential seizure triggers (e.g., sleep deprivation and alcohol), medication side effects, and contact details for the epilepsy team. Supplement oral information with written information and offer appropriate follow-up with the epilepsy team to consolidate information.[45,47]

Dissociative Seizures

It is important to communicate a diagnosis of dissociative seizures clearly, emphasizing that they are a real condition. There are many ways of explaining the mechanism of dissociative seizures that can be useful for the patient. For example explaining that they are a form of involuntary reflex or automatic response that has developed as a response to certain triggers can be helpful.[15] This information can be supplemented with written information and websites.[59-61] Taking time at this stage to communicate the diagnosis effectively can make a significant difference. Offer a follow-up appointment for the patient with dissociative seizures to reduce the sense of rejection that some patients may have at this stage, to address additional questions, and to reiterate explanations.[15] Ideally specific psychological therapies should be offered by specialist neuropsychologists where available.[62]

CASE HISTORIES

Case 1: Hypoglycemic Spells

A 55-year-old woman had a 7-month history of episodic, stereotyped, altered sensorium, and confusional spells characterized by psychomotor slowing, abnormal posturing, and unpurposeful behavior. The attacks lasted from a few minutes to 6 hours with a maximum frequency of 3/day. The attacks did not respond to treatment with carbamazepine and clobazam. MRI of the brain, prolonged video-EEG, and blood biochemistry were normal.

A typical attack was recorded, associated with diffuse slow waves during spontaneous hypoglycemia (1.4 mmol/L). EEG showed nonspecific slowing and abdominal MRI demonstrated an insulinoma **(Figs. 1A and B)**. The patient was cured by resection of the lesion.

Learning Point

Hypoglycemic spells can mimic epileptic seizures.

Case 2: Cardiac Syncope [Adapted from Chadwick, et al. (2010)[9]]

Ms N, a fit and healthy 21-year-old woman had woken her boyfriend in the early hours of the morning because of a sleep-related event. Her body was stiff, her breathing erratic, and she was unresponsive for 2–3 minutes. She did not have tonic-clonic movements or tongue biting. She attended the accident and emergency (A&E) department and her ECG was thought to be unremarkable **(Fig. 2)**. She was then seen in the first seizure clinic. There was uncertainty regarding the cause of TLOC, but it was thought to be a possible seizure arising from sleep. EEG and MRI head were normal. She was seen with the results and there was no recurrence of events. No definite diagnosis could be made and she was advised to a follow-up if she experienced a recurrence. She was found dead in her bed.

Her three brothers had cardiac investigations for the possibility of channelopathy, on the advice of a family friend who was a cardiologist. The investigating cardiologist asked for N's ECG after the first episode **(Fig. 2)**. A diagnosis of long QT3 was made. It was confirmed by a cardiac electrophysiologist who wrote "It is difficult to interpret the A&E ECG and machine has miscalculated the QT and corrected QT (QTc) interval, but there is undoubted QT prolongation. Some QT intervals are almost 600 ms."[9]

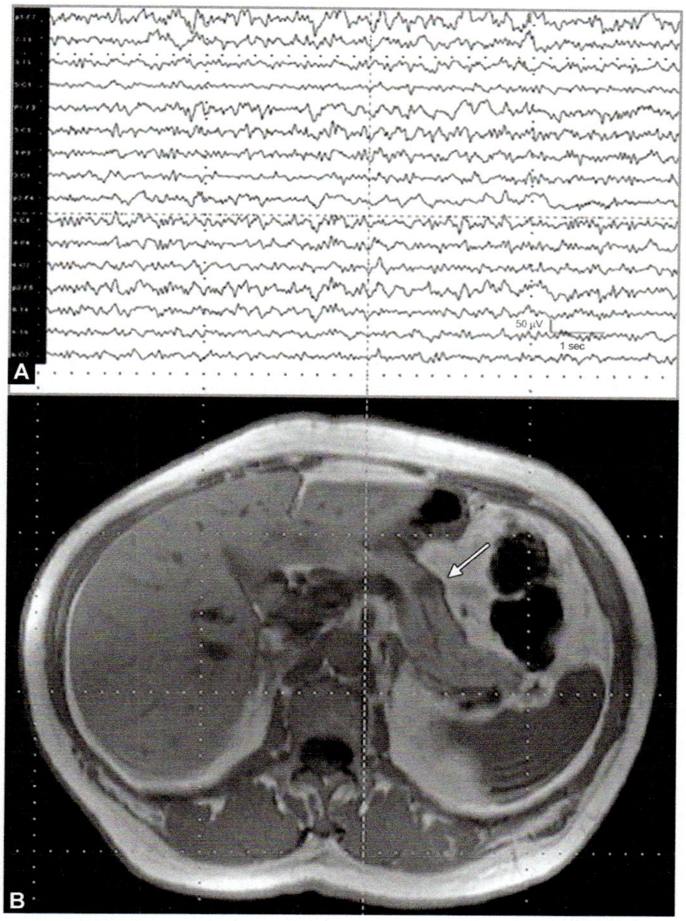

FIGS. 1A AND B: EEG shows nonspecific slowing. Abdominal MRI displays a 1-cm lesion in the pancreatic tail suggestive of insulinoma.

Learning Points

- Electrocardiogram is the most important investigation in cases of TLOC.
- Manually calculate the QTc with Bazett's formula (see ECG section above) in cases of suspected cardiac syncope or indefinite diagnosis.

Case 3: Cardiac Syncope

A 68-year-old retired general practitioner presented with episodes of TLOC without any preictal symptoms. He suffered from hypertension and diabetes, which were well-controlled. Unfortunately, a witness account was not available for the whole episode. A partially observed episode reported loss of consciousness for 5 minutes and postictal confusion for 20–30 minutes. He had a normal ECG and 24-hour cardiac tape. CT scan was normal except for evidence of small vessel disease. EEG showed right temporal slowing and sharp waves. The treating physician made a diagnosis of focal epilepsy with generalization based on prolonged postictal confusion and CT and EEG findings. Within a week of starting carbamazepine, the frequency of seizures increased significantly. After being referred to neurology a repeat video EEG captured an episode and ECG showed intermittent complete heart block.

Learning Points

- If seizures worsen with the use of appropriate ASM, review the diagnosis.
- Carbamazepine can induce heart block in susceptible patients.

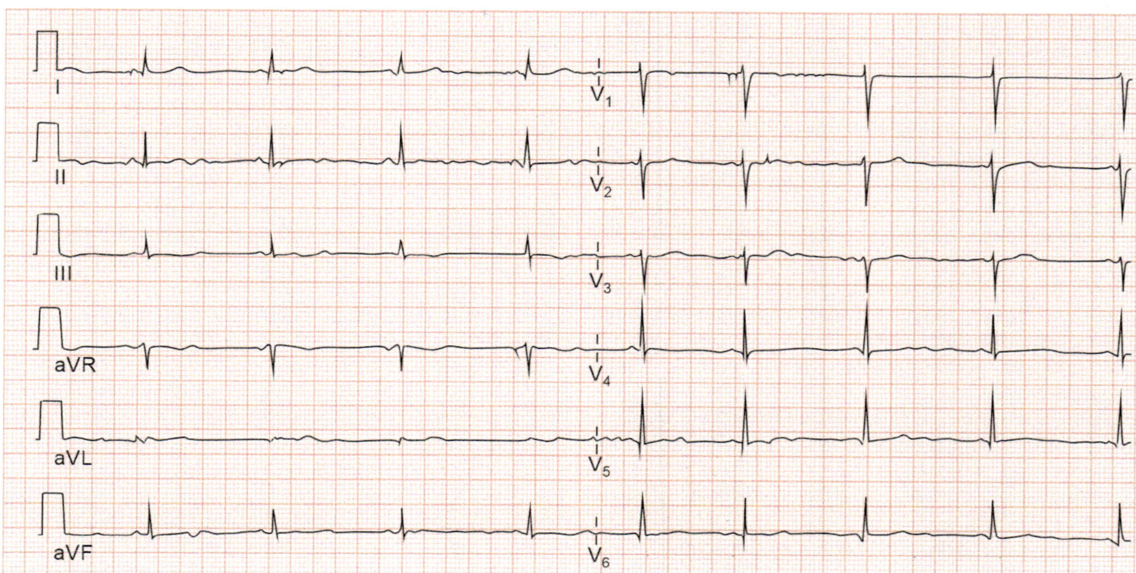

FIG. 2: ECG in the Accident and Emergency (A&E) department after the first episode.[9]

REFERENCES

1. Brignole M, Rivasi G. New insights in diagnostics and therapies in syncope: A novel approach to non-cardiac syncope. Heart. 2021;107(11):864-73.
2. Brignole M, Moya A, de Lange FJ, Deharo JC, Elliott PM, Fanciulli A, et al. 2018 ESC Guidelines for the diagnosis and management of syncope. Eur Heart J. 2018;39(21):1883-948.
3. Thijs R, Dijk J, Wieling W. Reflex Syncope. In: Reuber M, Schachter S (eds). Borderland of Epilepsy Revisited. New York: Oxford University Press; 2013. pp. 17-34.
4. Shorvon S, Guerrini R, Cook M, Lhatoo S. Oxford textbook of epilepsy and epileptic seizures. New York: Oxford University Press; 2012.
5. van Dijk JG, Thijs RD, Benditt DG, Wieling W. A guide to disorders causing transient loss of consciousness: focus on syncope. Nat Rev Neurol. 2009;5(8):438-48.
6. Anderson J, O'Callaghan P, Smith P. Cardiac Syncope. In: Reuber M, Schachter S (eds). Borderland of epilepsy revisited. New York: Oxford University Press; 2013. pp. 35-50.
7. Brugada P, Brugada J. Right bundle branch block, persistent ST segment elevation and sudden cardiac death: A distinct clinical and electrocardiographic syndrome: A multicenter report. J Am Coll Cardiol. 1992;20(6):1391-6.
8. Galtrey CM, Levee V, Arevalo J, Wren D, et al. Long QT syndrome masquerading as epilepsy. Pract Neurol. 2019;19(1):56-61.
9. Chadwick D, Jelen P, Almond S. Life and death diagnosis. Prac Neurol. 2010;10(3):155-9.
10. Thijs RD, Brignole M, Falup-Pecurariu C, Fanciulli A, Freeman R, Guaraldi P, et al. Recommendations for tilt table testing and other provocative cardiovascular autonomic tests in conditions that may cause transient loss of consciousness: Consensus statement of the European Federation of Autonomic Societies (EFAS) endorsed by the American Autonomic Society (AAS) and the European Academy of Neurology (EAN). Clin Auton Res. 2021;31(3):369-84.
11. Low PA, Singer W. Management of neurogenic orthostatic hypotension: an update. Lancet Neurol. 2008;7(5):451-58.
12. Blumenfeld H. Impaired consciousness in epilepsy. Lancet Neurol. 2012;11(9):814-26.
13. Bianco M, Breviario S, Fraccalini T, Ferri R, Biolè C, Destefains P, et al. Epilepsy and syncope - A case report and narrative review of arrhythmias connected to temporal lobe epilepsy. J Electrocardiol. 2022;73:76-8.
14. Hallett M, Aybek S, Dworetzky BA, McWhirter L, Staab JP, Stone J, et al. Functional neurological disorder: new subtypes and shared mechanisms. Lancet Neurol. 2022;21(6):537-50.
15. Reuber M. Dissociative (non-epileptic) seizures: tackling common challenges after the diagnosis. Pract Neurol. 2019;19(4):332-41.
16. Service FJ. Hypoglycemic disorders. N Eng J Med. 1995;332(17): 1144-52.
17. Hennerici M, Klemm C, Rautenberg W. The subclavian steal phenomenon: a common vascular disorder with rare neurologic deficits. Neurology. 1988;38(5):669-73.
18. Savitz SI, Caplan LR. Vertebrobasilar Disease. N Eng J Med. 2005;352(25):2618-26.
19. Ueda T, Oka N, Matsumoto A, Miyazaki H, Ohmura H, Kikuchi T, et al. Pheochromocytoma presenting as recurrent hypotension and syncope. Int Med. 2005;44(3):222-7.
20. Gade AK, Olariu E, Douthit NT. Carcinoid Syndrome: A Review. Cureus. 2020;12(3):e7186.
21. Brevern M. Vertigo and Ataxia. In: Reuber M, Schachter S (eds). Borderland of epilepsy revisited. New York: Oxford University Press; 2013. pp. 74-88.
22. Kutlubaev MA, Pyykko I, Hardy TA. Menière's disease. Pract Neurol. 2021;21(2):137-42.
23. Reading P. Cataplexy. Pract Neurol. 2019;19(1):21-7.
24. Smith EE, Charidimou A, Ayata C, Werring DJ, Greenberg SM. Cerebral amyloid angiopathy–related transient focal neurologic episodes. Neurology. 2021;97(5):231-38.
25. Tatum WO, Hirsch LJ, Gelfand MA, Acton EK, LaFrance WC Jr, Duckrow RB, et al. Assessment of the predictive value of outpatient smartphone videos for diagnosis of epileptic seizures. JAMA Neurol. 2020;77(5):593-600.
26. Reuber M, Monzoni C, Sharrack B, Plug L. Using interactional and linguistic analysis to distinguish between epileptic and psychogenic nonepileptic seizures: A prospective, blinded multirater study. Epilepsy Behav. 2009;16(1):139-44.
27. Benbadis SR. A spell in the epilepsy clinic and a history of "chronic pain" or "fibromyalgia" independently predict a diagnosis of psychogenic seizures. Epilepsy Behav. 2005;6(2):264-65.
28. McGonigal A, Oto M, Russell A, Greene J, Duncan R. Outpatient video EEG recording in the diagnosis of non-epileptic seizures: a randomised controlled trial of simple suggestion techniques. J Neurol Neurosurg Psychiatry. 2002;72(4):549-51.
29. Benbadis SR, Johnson K, Anthony RET, Caines G, Hess G, Jackson C, et al. Induction of psychogenic nonepileptic seizures without placebo. Neurology. 2000;55(12):1904-5.
30. Lempert T, Bauer M, Schmidt D. Syncope: A videometric analysis of 56 episodes of transient cerebral hypoxia. Ann Neurol. 1994;36(2):233-7.
31. Shmuely S, Bauer PR, van Zwet EW, van Dijk JG, Thijs RD. Differentiating motor phenomena in tilt-induced syncope and convulsive seizures. Neurology. 2018;90(15):e1339-e46.
32. Akor F, Liu NM, Besag FM, Ahmad MAS. Value of tongue biting in differentiating between epileptic seizures and syncope. Seizure. 2013;22(4):328.
33. Asadi-Pooya AA, Brigo F, Mesraoua B, Tarrada A, Karakis I, Hosny H, et al. Clinical characteristics of functional (psychogenic nonepileptic) seizures: An international retrospective study. Epilepsy Behav. 2020;111:107197.
34. Firkin AL, Marco DJT, Saya S, Newton MR, O'Brien TJ, Berkovic SF, et al. Mind the gap: Multiple events and lengthy delays before presentation with a "first seizure". Epilepsia. 2015;56(10):1534-41.
35. Samokhvalov A, Keyghobad F, Selby P. Alcohol-related seizure disorders. In: Reuber M, Schachter S (eds). Borderland of epilepsy revisited. New York: Oxford University Press; 2013. pp. 144-54.
36. Wolfe CE, Wood DM, Dines A, Whatley BP, Yates C Heyerdahl F. Seizures as a complication of recreational drug use: Analysis of the Euro-DEN Plus data-set. Neurotoxicology. 2019;73:183-87.
37. Fedorowski A, Pirouzifard M, Sundquist J, Sundquist K, Sutton R, Zöller B. Risk Factors for Syncope Associated With Multigenerational Relatives With a History of Syncope. JAMA Network Open. 2021;4(3):e212521-e21.
38. Peljto AL, Barker-Cummings C, Vasoli VM, Leibson CL, Hauser WA, Buchhalter JR, et al. Familial risk of epilepsy: A population-based study. Brain. 2014;137(3):795-805.
39. Perucca P, Bahlo M, Berkovic SF. The Genetics of Epilepsy. Ann Rev Genomics Hum Genet. 2020;21(1):205-30.
40. Mladěnka P, Applová L, Patočka J, Costa VM, Remiao F, Pourová J, et al. Comprehensive review of cardiovascular toxicity of drugs and related agents. Med Res Rev. 2018;38(4):1332-403.
41. Alldredge BK, Lowenstein DH, Simon RP. Seizures associated with recreational drug abuse. Neurology. 1989;39(8):1037.
42. NICE. (2010). Transient loss of consciousness ('blackouts') in over 16s. [online] Available from https://www.nice.org.uk/guidance/cg109 [Last accessed December 2022].
43. Marsh E, O'Callaghan P, Smith P. The humble electrocardiogram. Pract Neurol. 2008;8(1):46-59.
44. Brugada P, Geelen P. Some electrocardiographic patterns predicting sudden cardiac death that every doctor should recognize. Acta Cardiol. 1997;52(6):473-84.

45. NICE. (2022). Epilepsies in children, young people and adults. [online] Available from https://www.nice.org.uk/guidance/ng217 [Last accessed December, 2022].
46. Duncan JS. Brain imaging in epilepsy. Pract Neurol. 2019;19(5): 438-43.
47. Smith PEM. Initial management of seizure in adults. N Eng J Med. 2021;385(3):251-63.
48. Debicki DB. Electroencephalography after a single unprovoked seizure. Seizure. 2017;49:69-73.
49. Soteriades ES, Evans JC, Larson MG, Chen MH, Chen L, Benjamin EJ, et al. Incidence and Prognosis of Syncope. N Eng J Med. 2002;347(12):878-85.
50. Reuber M, Baker GA, Gill R, Smith DF, Chadwick DW. Failure to recognize psychogenic nonepileptic seizures may cause death. Neurology. 2004;62(5):834-5.
51. DVLA UKDaVLA. (2018). Assessing fitness to drive: a guide for medical professionals. [online] Available from https://www.gov.uk/guidance/assessing-fitness-to-drive-a-guide-for-medical-professionals [LAST accessed December, 2022].
52. Rees J, Cooper P, Cruickshank G, Jenkins N. Eligibility to drive and neurology: the how and the why. Pract Neurol. 2022;22(4):268-73.
53. Kim LG, Johnson TL, Marson AG, Chadwick DW; MRC MESS Study group. Prediction of risk of seizure recurrence after a single seizure and early epilepsy: further results from the MESS trial. Lancet Neurol. 2006;5(4):317-22.
54. Fisher RS, Acevedo C, Arzimanoglou A, Bogacz A, Cross JH, Elger CE, et al. ILAE Official Report: A practical clinical definition of epilepsy. Epilepsia. 2014;55(4):475-82.
55. Marson AG, Al-Kharusi AM, Alwaidh M, Appleton R, Baker GA, Chadwick DW, et al. The SANAD study of effectiveness of carbamazepine, gabapentin, lamotrigine, oxcarbazepine, or topiramate for treatment of partial epilepsy: an unblinded randomised controlled trial. Lancet. 2007;369(9566):1000-15.
56. Marson AG, Al-Kharusi AM, Alwaidh M, Appleton R, Baker GA, Chadwick DW, et al. The SANAD study of effectiveness of valproate, lamotrigine, or topiramate for generalised and unclassifiable epilepsy: an unblinded randomised controlled trial. Lancet. 2007;369(9566):1016-26.
57. Marson A, Burnside G, Appleton R, Smith D, Leach JP, Sills G, et al. The SANAD II study of the effectiveness and cost-effectiveness of valproate versus levetiracetam for newly diagnosed generalised and unclassifiable epilepsy: an open-label, non-inferiority, multicentre, phase 4, randomised controlled trial. Lancet. 2021;397(10282):1375-86.
58. Marson A, Burnside G, Appleton R, Smith D, Leach JP, Sills G, et al. The SANAD II study of the effectiveness and cost-effectiveness of levetiracetam, zonisamide, or lamotrigine for newly diagnosed focal epilepsy: an open-label, non-inferiority, multicentre, phase 4, randomised controlled trial. Lancet. 2021;397(10282): 1363-74.
59. Non-epileptic Attacks [Website with useful information and resources about dissociative seizures]. [online] Available from www.nonepilepticattacks.info [Last accessed December, 2022].
60. Dissociated—the first feature documentary on dissociative seizures (NEAD, PNES) [Documentary on dissociated seizures]. [online] Available from https://www.youtube.com/watch?v=MA1EYAg9y5k [Last accessed December, 2022].
61. FND Guide. (2022) Functional neurological disorder. [online] Available from https://www.neurosymptoms.org/en/symptoms/fnd-symptoms/dissociative-non-epileptic-attacks-blackouts/ [Last accessed December, 2022].
62. Goldstein LH, Robinson EJ, Mellers JDC, Stone J, Carson A, Reuber M, et al. Cognitive behavioural therapy for adults with dissociative seizures (CODES): a pragmatic, multicentre, randomised controlled trial. Lancet Psychiatry. 2020;7(6):491-505.

24

CHAPTER

Approach to Delirium

Neera Chaudhry, Divyani Garg

INTRODUCTION

The term "delirium" is derived from the Latin words, "de" which means "away", and "lira" which means "ridge between furrows," denoting a condition of deviation from the normal state ("delirare") of mind.[1] It is used to describe an acute state of brain dysfunction, characterized by sudden onset of confusion, fluctuating attention, and altered consciousness.[2] It is an extremely common condition in acute and intensive care unit (ICU) settings and denotes a poor prognosis.[3,4] Factors that precipitate delirium are usually multiple and tend to occur outside the brain, although certain central nervous system (CNS) problems such as stroke are known also to trigger delirium.

Delirium has also variously been labeled as "acute brain failure," "acute confusional state," "ICU psychosis," "altered mental status," "acute brain dysfunction," "organic brain syndrome," etc. This wide range of terminologies has led to a negative effect on delirium-related research, creating the need for uniform terminology and definition. Moreover, the term "acute encephalopathy," which denotes the pathophysiological process, is often used interchangeably with delirium, which is used to describe bedside findings.

An interdisciplinary group advocated the use of only two terms to detangle this issue—"acute encephalopathy" and "delirium". Delirium is a clinical syndrome defined using the criteria enlisted in the Diagnostic and Statistical Manual of Mental Disorders, 5th edition (DSM-5).[5] "Acute encephalopathy" refers to the pathobiological state underlying delirium, rather than a clinical syndrome, which if severely disrupted, may lead to coma. It has been proposed to use the umbrella term "delirium disorder" to denote both the above conditions. Another term, called "subsyndromal delirium," refers to a condition in which the patient demonstrates some but not all features of delirium, and therefore does not qualify the diagnostic criteria for delirium, and does not progress to delirium.[6,7]

Delirium has several portentous implications; it leads to an increase in the duration of hospitalization, increased mortality, and caregiver and financial burden.

EPIDEMIOLOGY

The prevalence of delirium is variable and dependent on the setting and the patient population, and the study instrument used for screening and diagnosis. It is frequent in the elderly hospitalized population, with a meta-analysis indicating a prevalence of 23%.[8] In high-risk surgical patients, who have undergone major surgery, the prevalence is >20%.[9] It is also considerably frequent following stroke and may be as high as 25%, based on a meta-analysis. In the acute phase of stroke, this may be 30%.[10] In ventilated patients, the prevalence ranges from 50–70%. In patients in the terminal stages of palliation, this figure is as high as 59–88%. Outside of hospitals, data on community-based prevalence is less robust and is likely to be <2%. Data from India indicates the prevalence of delirium in ICUs to be from 16.1 to 68.2%, and the incidence to be from 8 to 60%.[11] Inpatient mortality among patients with delirium is reported to range from 7 to 30%.

RISK FACTORS

Risk factors for delirium may be identified as "predisposing" and "precipitating" risk factors.[12] "Predisposing factors" are factors preexistent in the patient or the environment that enhance susceptibility to the development of delirium. These include elderly age, underlying dementia, underlying psychiatric illness or depression, use of alcohol or illicit drugs, malnutrition, vision and hearing impairment,[13] and previous history of delirium, etc. These are detailed in **Box 1**. A combination of factors increases risk.

Precipitating factors are acute insults that trigger delirium in the patient. These include conditions like sepsis,

BOX 1 Predisposing factors for delirium.

- Elderly age
- Frailty, malnutrition, and alcohol use
- Depression, other psychiatric illnesses
- Vision and hearing impairment
- Cognitive impairment, dementia, developmental delay, and previous history of delirium

TABLE 1: Precipitating factors for delirium.

Precipitating risk factors	
Infection	Urinary tract infection, respiratory tract infection, and sepsis
Metabolic abnormalities	Hyperglycemia, hypoglycemia, hypernatremia, hyponatremia, hypocalcemia, hypercalcemia, and dehydration
Trauma	Head injury
Stress	Psychological stress
Drugs	Benzodiazepines, L-type calcium channel blockers, antihistaminergic agents, and opiates
Systemic illnesses	Acute renal or hepatic dysfunction
Pain	Pain, urinary retention, and fecal impaction

stroke, acute renal failure, acute hepatic failure, metabolic abnormalities including hypoglycemia or hyperglycemia, hypo- or hypernatremia, etc., and introduction or withdrawal of drugs. These factors are enlisted in **Table 1**.

Metabolic Abnormalities

These are the most frequent cause of delirium, and encompass a wide range of disturbances, including dehydration, hypoxia, hypercarbia, hypoglycemia, hyperglycemia, calcium/magnesium abnormalities, hypo- or hypernatremia or rapid correction, low cardiac output, endocrine disturbances (hyperthyroidism and Cushing syndrome), toxins such as arsenic, bismuth, and mercury, and metabolic disorders such as porphyria.[14] Thiamine deficiency is an important consideration in alcoholics and malnourished patients.[15]

Drugs

The introduction and withdrawal of drugs also constitute a frequent cause of delirium, especially in the elderly population who are on multiple medications routinely. Particularly important are drugs with anticholinergic properties, such as antihistaminic drugs and antidepressants. Long-acting sedative-hypnotics and histaminergic blockers also account for an important group. Corticosteroids may also precipitate delirium, particularly in high doses. Drugs of abuse including alcohol withdrawal, cocaine, and methamphetamine may also precipitate delirium.

Infections

Common infections include urinary and respiratory tract infections and sepsis. CNS infections such as meningitis and encephalitis may also be responsible for delirium.

Stroke

Although any stroke may precipitate delirium, certain areas of involvement have a high predilection. These include involvement of the fusiform gyrus, anterior cingulate or orbitofrontal gyrus, thalamus, and posterior parietal strokes. Other cerebrovascular events that may precipitate delirium include hypertensive encephalopathy, subarachnoid hemorrhage, vasculitis, etc.

Postoperative Delirium

Several factors contribute to the risk of postoperative delirium, which usually sets in at about the third day following surgery and may last for a week or longer.[16] The elderly population is specifically predisposed. Contributory factors include perioperative hypotension, perioperative hypoxia, infections, dyselectrolytemia, drug/anesthetic effects, underlying frailty, malnutrition, or other neurological conditions like Parkinson's disease. Delirium is more frequent after specific procedures, including open-heart or coronary artery bypass surgery (30–40% of patients),[17] orthopedics, and thoracic surgeries. Long-bone fractures, hip replacement, knee replacement, and cataract surgeries may also predispose to delirium, especially in the elderly.

PATHOPHYSIOLOGY

Multiple pathophysiological factors contribute to delirium.[18] In the presence of predisposing factors, such as old age, malnutrition, and frailty, stressors may trigger delirium. In the presence of aging or neurodegeneration, brain networks become susceptible to minor stressors. Neurodegenerative processes lead to exaggeration of the inflammatory response, which may contribute to delirium. Changes in brain vasculature may also contribute. These include an increase in permeability in the blood-brain-barrier, contributing to energy/oxidation stress. Defects in brain bioenergetics may also play a role. These include hypoxia, which may be due to respiratory issues. Hemodynamic failure may lead to microcirculatory failure and tissue hypoxia. Moreover, this process may be compounded by a failure of neurovascular coupling in aging/dementia.

Multiple neurotransmitters have also been postulated to contribute to delirium, including increased dopaminergic state, noradrenaline and glutamate abnormalities, and deficiency of acetylcholine, serotonin, and gamma-aminobutyric acid (GABA) and histamine in the CNS. Mainly, an imbalance in the cholinergic-dopaminergic pathways accounts for delirium. Cholinergic circuits project

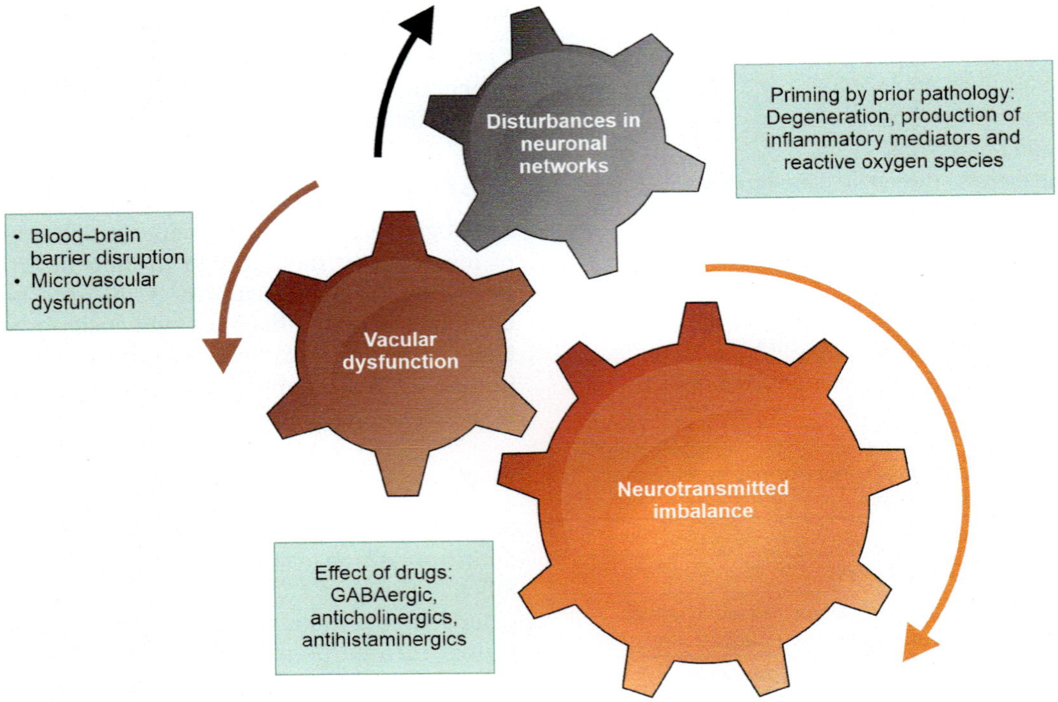

FIG. 1: Proposed pathophysiology of delirium.
(GABA: gamma-aminobutyric acid)

from the pons to the basal forebrain. Cholinergic deficiency decreases input to the frontal cortex.

Anatomical substrates for delirium include the anterior cingulate cortex, which accounts for disturbances in attention; bilateral prefrontal cortex, which controls attention maintenance and executive control, temporoparietal region in shifting attention, upper brainstem, and thalamus. **Figure 1** summarizes the proposed pathophysiology of delirium.

TOOLS FOR ASSESSMENT

A large number of assessment tools are available for delirium. Some serve as screening tools or research tools, while others provide a detailed neuropsychological assessment. Many studies use the DSM-5 criteria for diagnosis and assessment. Above 50 tools are available for the assessment of delirium. Some important tools are described further below.

Confusion Assessment Method

The Confusion Assessment Method (CAM)[19] is based on the 1987 DSM III criteria (revised). These include:

- *Criterion A*: Acute onset and fluctuating course
- *Criterion B*: Lack of attention
- *Criterion C*: Lack of organized thinking
- *Criterion D*: Alternation in level of consciousness

A positive CAM test requires both criteria (A) and (B) to be met, along with either or both criteria (C) and (D). CAM is a popular tool used in clinical studies. The specificity ranges from 0.84 to 1. Another version is the brief CAM (bCAM).[20] Whereas the full CAM make takes 5–10 minutes, bCAM takes around 2 minutes to complete, and has four items. Another variant is the 3D-CAM, which contains 20 items.[21]

4A's Test

The 4A's test (4AT) contains four items and takes around 2 minutes to administer.[22] The four items include alertness, cognition, attention, and presence of acute change or fluctuation in the course. The pooled sensitivity and specificity is 88%.

The 12-item Stanford Proxy Test for Delirium

This is a screening tool for non-ICU patients and can be administered by nurses.[23] It assesses for delirium in the previous eight hours. It has a sensitivity of 0.8 and specificity of 0.9.

Other tools include Richmond Agitation Screening Scale and Recognizing Acute Delirium as part of your routine (RADAR), for screening for delirium among inpatients. In the ICU, delirium assessment tools include the CAM-ICU and the Intensive Care Delirium Screening Checklist (ICDSC).[24]

Delirium Rating Scale-revised-98

This is a revised form of the Delirium Rating Scale.[25] It contains 16 items and is used to distinguish delirium from mimics such as dementia, pseudodementia (depression), and psychosis.

APPROACH TO DELIRIUM

Clinical Approach

It is vital to have a low threshold to diagnose delirium, as nearly two-thirds of patients remain undiagnosed. This is particularly true for the elderly, as they may have a less active form of delirium.

Delirium manifests as acute onset of reduced attention and focus, leading to confusion, memory impairment, and disorganization of thought. Speech tends to be circumlocutory, with repetition, hesitation, and abnormal rate. The sleep-wake cycle is disturbed. Usually, delirium tends to develop over hours to days, with diurnal fluctuations. The nocturnal worsening is known to occur. Patients may also report visual hallucinations and illusions. Associated features such as tremor and myoclonus/asterixis may develop.

The DSM-5 criteria, summarized below, are used to diagnose delirium **(Box 2)**.

Types of Delirium

Based on psychomotor activity, delirium may be classified as hyperactive, hypoactive, or mixed.[26,27]

- *Hyperactive*: Increased psychomotor activity, labile mood, and agitation. Hyperactive type is seen in only 15% of patients. These patients are usually younger and have a more rapid improvement. This type of delirium is usually drug/toxin induced.
- *Hypoactive*: Reduced psychomotor activity, lethargy, or stupor
- *Mixed*: Fluctuation in activity level between hyperactive and hypoactive

Cognitive Abnormalities

Inattention is a hallmark feature of delirium, and patients are easily distracted. Thinking lacks organization. There is a lack of coherence and clarity and a logical sequence of thought. Similarly, speech is circumlocutory with shifts in focus. There may be hesitant and perseverating patterns of speech. Consciousness may be impaired. Patients usually lack alertness and have reduced arousal. A hyperalert state is seen in certain conditions such as delirium tremens.[28] Perceptual dysfunction may occur, with patients having time-lapses, or illusions and visual hallucinations, which are considered to be release phenomena. The latter are vivid and unpleasant to the patient. However, third-person auditory hallucinations are distinctly unusual in delirium. Delusions of persecution and paranoia may also set in. Patients with delirium may also be disoriented to time followed by place, but disorientation to person (particularly self-identity) is preserved. Reduplicative paramnesia may occur. In this phenomenon, the patient is unable to integrate recent observations with remote memories. Hence, they may mistake unfamiliar places to be familiar ones. In another form of reduplicative paramnesia, referred to as Capgras syndrome, relatives are mistaken to be imposters.

In this history, it is also important to attempt to extract any history of infections, drug introduction or withdrawal, any head injury, allergy, malnutrition, and prior history of cognitive impairment.

BOX 2 Diagnosis of delirium according to DSM-5 criteria.

A. Disturbance in attention and awareness (reduced orientation to the environment)

B. Develops over a short period (hours to days), fluctuates in severity throughout the day

C. Additional cognitive deficit (in memory, language, orientation, visuospatial ability, and perception)

D. A and B are not better explained by a preexisting, evolving, or established neurocognitive disorder, severely reduced level of arousal, such as coma

E. Evidence from history, physical examination, or laboratory findings that the disturbance is a direct consequence of another medical condition, substance intoxication or withdrawal, toxin-induced, or due to multiple etiologies

Delirium in the Critically Ill Patient

Delirium affects nearly 50% of patients who are admitted to the ICUs.[4] Despite its frequent occurrence, delirium remains unrecognized to a large extent in ICUs. Specific screening tools designed for application in critically ill patients, such as the CAM-ICU should be employed to detect delirium in ICU populations.[29] The "ABCDEF" bundle, discussed in a later section, is an effective means of reducing the occurrence of delirium.

DIFFERENTIAL DIAGNOSIS

Dementia

Patients with dementia have a longer course of illness. They lack fluctuations in attention typical of delirium. However, delirium and dementia may coexist and overlap, as patients with dementia are susceptible to the development of delirium. This should be suspected in any demented patient who develops acute neurological worsening. Patients with dementia with Lewy bodies (DLB) may have fluctuations in attention and alertness, and visual hallucinations which may resemble delirium. The presence of other features, such as Parkinsonism and rapid eye movement (REM) sleep behavior disorders may provide clues to the diagnosis of DLB. It is important to remember that patients with dementia have two to five times increased risk of developing superimposed delirium.[30]

Wernicke's Aphasia

Patients who have Wernicke's aphasia develop paraphasias and neologisms, and speech is "empty". Attention and perception are usually normal.

Psychiatric Disorders

Delirium may be mimicked by psychiatric disorders, including depression, mania, schizophrenia, dissociative conditions, and Ganser syndrome. Ganser syndrome is a dissociative disorder, in which the patient gives inappropriate or approximate answers. Depression may be mistaken for hypoactive delirium. The typical fluctuation in attention which is typical for delirium is lacking in patients with psychiatric disorders. Hallucinations in patients with schizophrenia are third-person auditory hallucinations with persecutory content, as opposed to hallucinations in delirium which are visual and transient. In persons above the age of 40 years who are premorbidly well, the presence of psychosis or mania should be presumed to be due to delirium, unless otherwise proved.

Subsyndromal Delirium

The term "subsyndromal delirium" is used to refer to patients who present with some of the diagnostic features of delirium. These patients should be approached like patients with full-blown syndrome. Whether the long-term implications of subsyndromal delirium resemble delirium remains unclear from current evidence.

EXAMINATION

Mental Status Examination

The key to examining a patient with delirium is mental status assessment. In mental status assessment, the most important tests include the determination of the level of consciousness and attention. Tests that are commonly used to test attention include:

- Digit span forward and backward
- Recitation of weekdays or months in reverse order
- Continuous performance tasks (patient is instructed to raise a hand when he or she hears a particular letter from a list which is read out) such as the *A* vigilance test
- Spell "WORLD" backward
- Serial 7s or 3s
- Three-step motor response (such as the palm-side-fist test), which also assesses the frontal function.

Impaired attention may not permit further mental status assessment. If possible, an effort should be made to conduct an extended cognitive assessment, including orientation, language, construction, etc.

Physical Examination

The focus of physical examination should be—to decipher predisposing/precipitating factors and assessment of the mental status. The patient should be examined for systemic infections or diseases, focal deficits, signs of meningeal irritation, rise in intracranial pressure, stroke, head injury, etc.

Neurological examination, apart from mental status changes, may reveal the presence of tremor, asterixis, multifocal myoclonus, chorea, dysarthria, etc. Features of catatonia, such as waxy flexibility, carphologia, and increased autonomic activity may also develop.

Investigations

Initial laboratory evaluation is focused on the identification of triggers for delirium. These investigations should be guided by the clinical picture and may include complete blood count, peripheral blood smear, renal function test, liver function test, thyroid function, electrolytes, calcium, blood glucose, etc. Chest X-ray, urine toxicology screen, arterial blood gas, and serum ammonia level should also be done.

Neuroimaging may be required depending on the underlying clinical suspicion, either in the form of computed tomography (CT) or magnetic resonance imaging (MRI) of the brain. If nonconvulsive status epilepticus is a concern, electroencephalography (EEG) should be performed. A sepsis screen may be required in patients with fever and/or leukocytosis.

Electroencephalography in delirium invariably shows abnormalities on serial traces. The most common EEG observation is generalized slowing. In cases of intracranial causes of delirium, such as stroke, focal abnormalities may be detected, including focal slowing, epileptiform discharges, periodic lateralized discharges, and triphasic waves.

Lumbar puncture is not routinely required in patients with delirium, as it usually arises from an underlying medical cause. However, it is important to know that lumbar puncture must be promptly done in patients with suspected meningitis/encephalitis and sometimes, in delirium without a clear cause. It is advisable to conduct neuroimaging before lumbar puncture, particularly if raised intracranial pressure is suspected, and in patients with focal neurological signs.

On rare occasions, in cases with suspected autoimmune/paraneoplastic encephalitis, testing for autoimmune encephalitis antibodies may be indicated.

PREVENTION OF DELIRIUM

A preventive approach is crucial in patients at risk for delirium and all hospitalized patients. Delirium is preventable in nearly 30–40% of patients with appropriate quality care. Early identification and intervention in vulnerable populations, such as the frail elderly,[31] reduce hospital stay and mortality. Programs, such as the Hospital Elder Life Program (HELP), use strategies such as reorientation, reduced use of psychotropic medication, early mobilization, good sleep hygiene, nutrition and hydration, and visual and hearing stimulation. Nocturnal disturbances should be reduced. **Table 2** lists the preventive measures that may be applied to reduce the development of delirium.

TABLE 2: Preventive measures which may reduce the development of delirium.

Setting	Preventive measure
General settings	• Recognizing high-risk populations for delirium • Screening for delirium daily • Orientation to the environment—sensory, auditory, family, etc. • Hydration • Regularizing bowel and bladder habits • Correction of metabolic abnormalities • Pain treatment • Management of sepsis • Mobilization, adequate sleep • Avoid long-acting benzodiazepines • Avoid physical restraints
Intensive care unit settings	• Identification of high-risk population • Avoid long-acting benzodiazepines • Early mobilization • Early removal of devices

MANAGEMENT OF DELIRUM

As delirium constitutes an important problem in all hospitalized patients, it is imperative to recognize and manage it promptly. Management is multilayered as delirium itself is a multifactorial syndrome.[32] These include identification and management of all delirium triggers, normalizing metabolic disturbances, and addressing caretaker concerns. Essentially, management is in three domains, that is, management of the underlying disorder, management of behavioral abnormalities, and environmental adaptations.

Treatment of the Underlying Disorder

Treatment of the underlying condition is crucial. Frequently, multiple factors may require treatment, including infections, metabolic disturbances, hydration status, etc. Urinary retention and constipation should be treated urgently in the elderly population. Any offending drugs should be withdrawn.

Environmental Adaptation

Reduce unfamiliarity in the environment by bringing to the bedside objects which are familiar to the patient, including family photographs, calendars, clocks, etc. Appropriate sensory stimulation (auditory, tactile, and visual) should be provided, taking care to avoid overstimulation. Spectacles and hearing aids should be provided if required by the patient. Use of a nightlight, television set, avoidance of physical restraints, and treatment of pain[33] are other measures. Exposure to unfamiliar persons, including frequent changes in nursing staff, should be avoided.

TABLE 3: The ABCDEF bundle.

ABCDEF bundle component	Intervention/Approach	Risk factor addressed
A	Assess, manage, and prevent pain	Pain
B	Spontaneous breathing trials, spontaneous awake trials	Oversedation, mechanical ventilation
C	Careful sedation, analgesics	Oversedation
D	Assess, manage, and prevent delirium	Vision/hearing impairment, disordered sleep-wake cycle
E	Early mobilization, exercise	Immobility
F	Family engagement	Disorientation

Manipulation and adjustment of the patient's external and interpersonal environment are frequently helpful in the management of confusion and agitation in a patient with delirium. Environmental adjustments include providing a stable environment by avoiding frequent bed changes, not using physical restraints, ensuring exposure to adequate lighting and windows, and using repeated verbal orientation and familiar persons are useful. Delusion and hallucinations should not be contradicted, nor should they be ratified. The use of physical restraints should be avoided to the greatest extent possible, as this is associated with an increased risk of delirium up to three times.[34]

The ABCDEF approach is a bundle of actions or interventions which may be employed to reduce the duration of delirium.[35] This is summarized in **Table 3**.

Pharmacological Measures

The use of drugs in patients with delirium should largely be avoided, due to the risk of worsening of confusion. If needed to make the patient manageable, the lowest and shortest acting medication should be used. Long-acting benzodiazepines should be avoided.[36] Data on the use of antipsychotics in delirium is largely of poor quality in non-ICU settings. In a 2018 Cochrane review, no effect of antipsychotics was observed on the resolution of delirium, symptom severity, or mortality. In 2020, another Cochrane review among terminally ill patients noted that evidence for pharmacotherapy was poor to very poor. Evidence for the use of cholinesterase inhibitors, melatonin, and melatonin receptor agonist ramelteon remains inconsistent.[37] Other drugs studied on a small scale include dexmedetomidine and clonidine. The current consensus, therefore, does not support the use of drugs for the management of the syndrome of delirium. Pragmatically, drugs are used when other measures fail to provide relief. Haloperidol in a low dose (0.25 mg) is used commonly. It is available in various administration formulations and has low anticholinergic properties. Other atypical antipsychotics, including olanzapine, quetiapine, and aripiprazole may similarly be used in small doses.

In ICU settings, haloperidol is frequently used although evidence for its use is not robust. A large, randomized trial, the Modifying the Impact of Neuropsychological Dysfunction-USA (MIND-USA), compared 566 ICU patients given haloperidol, ziprasidone, and placebo, and found no significant differences in the three groups in the primary outcome or any secondary outcome.[38] Another systematic review did not observe any difference in haloperidol, second-generation antipsychotics, or placebo.[39] A small trial found that quetiapine was effective in achieving faster resolution of delirium.[40] Dexmedetomidine is an alpha-2 agonist, which is gaining popularity in ICU settings due to its low predilection to cause respiratory depression and some evidence for reducing delirium.[41-43]

In general, pharmacological therapy has not achieved much success in the management of delirium. One reason may be the heterogeneity associated with delirium, with differing pathophysiological processes playing a role in different patients.

PROGNOSIS

Prognosis in delirium is variable. Correction of the underlying cause often leads to the resolution of the delirious state rapidly. In some patients, delirium may have a prolonged course and last for weeks to months. Persistent delirium at 6 months may be present in 20% of patients, with some features persisting.[44] Persistent delirium is associated with a poorer long-term prognosis. Delirium at discharge is strongly associated with a subsequent increase in mortality. Long-term cognitive impairment has also been strongly associated with delirium. The presence of delirium is a poor prognostic factor among elderly hospitalized patients and increases the risk for mortality, future institutionalization, and worse cognitive and functional outcomes. Hypoactive delirium is associated with poorer outcomes, increased mortality, increased hospital stay, and falls.[45,46]

CONCLUSION

Delirium is an acute confusional state, associated with predisposing and precipitating factors. It is an independent risk factor for adverse outcomes in hospitalized patients, especially in the geriatric age group. Delirium is a result of a combination of predisposing and precipitating factors. Metabolic abnormalities and drugs are the most common underlying cause. Recognition of delirium required a low threshold, as it is often misdiagnosed or underdiagnosed. Several tools are available to diagnose delirium and assess its severity. Management requires treatment of the underlying cause, and environmental manipulation to make the patient comfortable with the environment and provide cognitive stimulation and reorientation. Pharmacological therapy is used in challenging cases and is usually in the form of atypical antipsychotics.

REFERENCES

1. Adamis D, Treloar A, Martin FC, Macdonald AJD. A brief review of the history of delirium as a mental disorder. Hist Psychiatry. 2007;18(72 Pt 4):459-69.
2. Mattison MLP. Delirium. Ann Intern Med. 2020;173(7):ITC49-ITC64.
3. Girard TD, Pandharipande PP, Ely EW. Delirium in the intensive care unit. Crit Care. 2008;12(Suppl 3):S3.
4. Brummel NE, Girard TD. Delirium in the critically ill patient. Handb Clin Neurol. 2019;167:357-75.
5. Regier DA, Kuhl EA, Kupfer DJ. The DSM-5: Classification and criteria changes. World Psychiatry. 2013;12(2):92-8.
6. Sepulveda E, Leonard M, Franco JG, Adamis D, McCarthy G, Dunne C, et al. Subsyndromal delirium compared with delirium, dementia, and subjects without delirium or dementia in elderly general hospital admissions and nursing home residents. Alzheimers Dement (Amst). 2016;7:1-10.
7. Cole MG, Ciampi A, Belzile E, Dubuc-Sarrasin M. Subsyndromal delirium in older people: a systematic review of frequency, risk factors, course and outcomes. Int J Geriatr Psychiatry. 2013;28(8):771-80.
8. Gibb K, Seeley A, Quinn T, Siddiqi N, Shenkin S, Rockwood K, et al. The consistent burden in published estimates of delirium occurrence in medical inpatients over four decades: a systematic review and meta-analysis study. Age Ageing. 2020;49(3):352-60.
9. Watt JA, Goodarzi Z, Veroniki AA, Nincic V, Khan PA, Ghassemi M, et al. Comparative efficacy of interventions for reducing symptoms of depression in people with dementia: systematic review and network meta-analysis. BMJ. 2021;372:n532.
10. Rollo E, Callea A, Brunetti V, Vollono C, Marotta J, Imperatori C, et al. Delirium in acute stroke: A prospective, cross-sectional, cohort study. Eur J Neurol. 2021;28(5):1590-600.
11. Grover S, Kathiravan S, Dua D. Delirium Research in India: A Systematic Review. J Neurosci Rural Pract. 2021;12(2):236-66.
12. Wilson JE, Mart MF, Cunningham C, Shehabi Y, Girard TD, MacLullich AMJ, et al. Delirium. Nat Rev Dis Primers. 2020;6(1):90.
13. Morandi A, Inzitari M, Udina C, Gual N, Mota M, Tassistro E, et al. Visual and Hearing Impairment Are Associated With Delirium in Hospitalized Patients: Results of a Multisite Prevalence Study. J Am Med Dir Assoc. 2021;22(6):1162-67.
14. Laurila JV, Laakkonen ML, Laurila JV, Pitkala KH. Predisposing and precipitating factors for delirium in a frail geriatric population. J Psychosom Res. 2008;65(3):249-54.
15. Truong T, Hetzel F, Stiff KM, Husnain MG. Case of hypoactive delirium precipitated by thiamine deficiency. BMJ Case Rep. 2021;14(3):e239886.
16. Kotekar N, Shenkar A, Nagaraj R. Postoperative cognitive dysfunction - current preventive strategies. Clin Interv Aging. 2018;13:2267-73.
17. Lopez MG, Hughes CG, DeMatteo A, O'Neal JB, McNeil JB, Shotwell MS, et al. Intraoperative Oxidative Damage and Delirium after Cardiac Surgery. Anesthesiology. 2020;132(3):551-61.

18. Maldonado JR. Delirium pathophysiology: An updated hypothesis of the etiology of acute brain failure. Int J Geriatr Psychiatry. 2018;33(11):1428-57.
19. Inouye SK, van Dyck CH, Alessi CA, Balkin S, Siegal AP, Horwitz RI. Clarifying confusion: the confusion assessment method. A new method for detection of delirium. Ann Intern Med. 1990;113(12):941-8.
20. Han JH, Wilson A, Vasilevskis EE, Shintani A, Schnelle JF, Dittus RS, et al. Diagnosing delirium in older emergency department patients: validity and reliability of the delirium triage screen and the brief confusion assessment method. Ann Emerg Med. 2013;62(5): 457-65.
21. Marcantonio ER, Ngo LH, O'Connor M, Jones RN, Crane PK, Metzger ED, et al. 3D-CAM: derivation and validation of a 3-minute diagnostic interview for CAM-defined delirium: a cross-sectional diagnostic test study. Ann Intern Med. 2014;161(8):554-61.
22. Bellelli G, Morandi A, Davis DHJ, Mazzola P, Turco R, Gentile S, et al. Validation of the 4AT, a new instrument for rapid delirium screening: a study in 234 hospitalised older people. Age Ageing. 2014;43(4):496-502.
23. Alosaimi FD, Alghamdi A, Alsuhaibani R, Alhammad G, Albatili A, Albatly L, et al. Validation of the Stanford Proxy Test for Delirium (S-PTD) among critical and noncritical patients. J Psychosom Res. 2018;114:8-14.
24. Gusmao-Flores D, Salluh JIF, Chalhub RÁ, Quarantini LC. The confusion assessment method for the intensive care unit (CAM-ICU) and intensive care delirium screening checklist (ICDSC) for the diagnosis of delirium: a systematic review and meta-analysis of clinical studies. Crit Care. 2012;16(4):R115.
25. Trzepacz PT, Mittal D, Torres R, Kanary K, Norton J, Jimerson N. Validation of the Delirium Rating Scale-revised-98: comparison with the delirium rating scale and the cognitive test for delirium. J Neuropsychiatry Clin Neurosci. 2001;13(2):229-42.
26. Meagher D. Motor subtypes of delirium: past, present and future. Int Rev Psychiatry. 2009;21(1):59-73.
27. Meagher DJ, Leonard M, Donnelly S, Conroy M, Adamis D, Trzepacz PT. A longitudinal study of motor subtypes in delirium: frequency and stability during episodes. J Psychosom Res. 2012;72(3):236-41.
28. Awissi DK, Lebrun G, Coursin DB, Riker RR, Skrobik Y. Alcohol withdrawal and delirium tremens in the critically ill: a systematic review and commentary. Intensive Care Med. 2013;39(1):16-30.
29. Stollings JL, Kotfis K, Chanques G, Pun BT, Pandharipande PP, Ely EW. Delirium in critical illness: clinical manifestations, outcomes, and management. Intensive Care Med. 2021;47(10):1089-103.
30. Morandi A, Bellelli G. Delirium superimposed on dementia. Eur Geriatr Med. 2020;11(1):53-62.
31. Inouye SK. Delirium in hospitalized older patients: recognition and risk factors. J Geriatr Psychiatry Neurol. 1998;11(3):118-25; discussion 157-8.
32. Adeola M, Azad R, Kassie GM, Shirkey B, Taffet G, Liebl M, et al. Multicomponent Interventions Reduce High-Risk Medications for Delirium in Hospitalized Older Adults. J Am Geriatr Soc. 2018;66(8):1638-45.
33. Vaurio LE, Sands LP, Wang Y, Mullen EA, Leung JM. Postoperative delirium: the importance of pain and pain management. Anesth Analg. 2006;102(4):1267-73.
34. Thomann S, Zwakhalen S, Richter D, Bauer S, Hahn S. Restraint use in the acute-care hospital setting: A cross-sectional multi-centre study. Int J Nurs Stud. 2021;114:103807.
35. Marra A, Ely EW, Pandharipande PP, Patel MB. The ABCDEF Bundle in Critical Care. Crit Care Clin. 2017;33(2):225-43.
36. Tune LE, Bylsma FW. Benzodiazepine-induced and anticholinergic-induced delirium in the elderly. Int Psychogeriatr. 1991;3(2): 397-408.
37. de Jonghe A, Korevaar JC, van Munster BC, de Rooij SE. Effectiveness of melatonin treatment on circadian rhythm disturbances in dementia. Are there implications for delirium? A systematic review. Int J Geriatr Psychiatry. 2010;25(12):1201-8.
38. Girard TD, Exline MC, Carson SS, Hough CL, Rock P, Gong MN, et al. Haloperidol and Ziprasidone for Treatment of Delirium in Critical Illness. N Engl J Med. 2018;379(26):2506-16.
39. Nikooie R, Neufeld KJ, Oh ES, Wilson LM, Zhang A, Robinson KA, et al. Antipsychotics for Treating Delirium in Hospitalized Adults: A Systematic Review. Ann Intern Med. 2019;171(7):485-95.
40. Devlin JW, Roberts RJ, Fong JJ, Skrobik Y, Riker RR, Hill NS, et al. Efficacy and safety of quetiapine in critically ill patients with delirium: a prospective, multicenter, randomized, double-blind, placebo-controlled pilot study. Crit Care Med. 2010;38(2):419-27.
41. Riker RR, Shehabi Y, Bokesch PM, Ceraso D, Wisemandle W, Koura F, et al. Dexmedetomidine vs midazolam for sedation of critically ill patients: a randomized trial. JAMA. 2009;301(5):489-99.
42. Shehabi Y, Howe BD, Bellomo R, Arabi YM, Bailey M, Bass FE, et al. Early Sedation with dexmedetomidine in critically ill patients. N Engl J Med. 2019;380(26):2506-17.
43. Reade MC, Eastwood GM, Bellomo R, Bailey M, Bersten A, Cheung B, et al. Effect of dexmedetomidine added to standard care on ventilator-free time in patients with agitated delirium: A randomized clinical trial. JAMA. 2016;315(14):1460-8.
44. Cole MG, Ciampi A, Belzile E, Zhong L. Persistent delirium in older hospital patients: a systematic review of frequency and prognosis. Age Ageing. 2009;38(1):19-26.
45. Gual N, Inzitari M, Carrizo G, Calle A, Udina C, Yuste A, et al. Delirium subtypes and associated characteristics in older patients with exacerbation of chronic conditions. Am J Geriatr Psychiatry. 2018;26(12):1204-12.
46. Peritogiannis V, Bolosi M, Lixouriotis C, Rizos DV. Recent insights on prevalence and corelations of hypoactive delirium. Behav Neurol. 2015;2015:416792.

25

CHAPTER

Approach to Coma

Sarosh M Katrak

INTRODUCTION

In this era of improved resuscitation and support systems, one of the most common problems facing a clinical neurologist is the assessment, diagnosis, and management of a patient in an altered state of consciousness.[1] Assessment of a coma is always a medical emergency. This is a taxing problem, as time is of essence to achieve many goals. Often the history is not available, but the clinician has to make a prompt diagnosis, order relevant investigations, and start appropriate therapy to avoid morbidity and more importantly mortality. A classic example is a subdural hematoma in an elderly patient. If it is not promptly diagnosed and evacuated, there may be a residual neurological deficit, where none should be present.

PATHOPHYSIOLOGY OF CONSCIOUSNESS

Before we dwell on coma, one must understand the normal pathophysiology of consciousness. Consciousness depends on two factors, i.e., arousal and the content of consciousness. Arousal is linked to the ascending reticular formation, a series of neurons in the rostral brainstem, which projects to the diencephalon and cerebral cortex. The content of consciousness, simply put, is awareness of self and environment. It is the exclusive function of the integrated activity of the cortical neurons in both hemispheres. Since both hemispheres are involved, consciousness is not localized to any hemisphere or to one or more lobes of a hemisphere. This results in three states—(1) awake and aware which is the normal level of consciousness, (2) awake but not aware, and (3) not awake and not aware. The last category involves stupor and coma. Hence, in the initial approach to a patient in the intensive care unit (ICU), the clinician should categorize his/her patient into one of these three categories.

When the central nervous system (CNS) is affected by a disease process, the level of consciousness deteriorates.

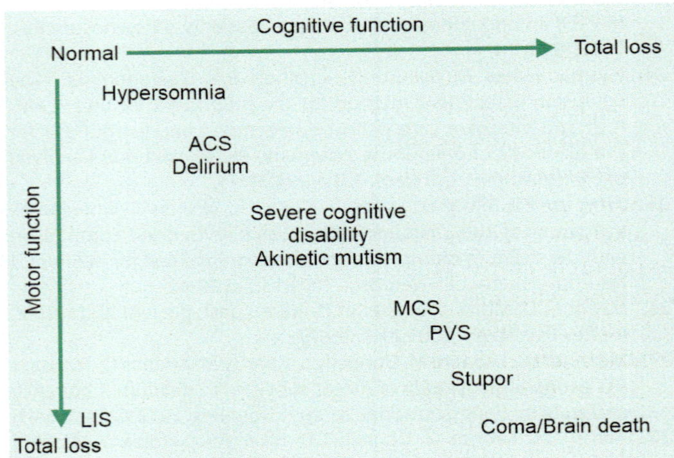

FIG. 1: Cognitive and motor function.
(ACS: acute confusional state; LIS: locked-in state; MCS: minimally conscious state; PVS: persistent vegetative state)

This is assessed by two parameters—cognitive and motor functions **(Fig. 1)**. Hypersomnia, acute confusional state, delirium, and severe cognitive disability/akinetic mutism are a continuum of deterioration in which the patient is awake but not aware. If the disease progresses, the patient deteriorates into a stupor or coma and is not awake and not aware. If the coma is very severe and prolonged, the patient may be brain dead; if severe but not prolonged, he/she may improve partially into a persistent vegetative state (PVS) or a minimally conscious state (MCS), putting them again in the category of awake but not aware.

As mentioned earlier, a normal individual is awake and aware. In **Figure 1**, there is one exception to the rule—the locked-in state (LIS). This condition was described by Plum and Posner in their classic monograph: The Diagnosis of Stupor and Coma in 1966.[2] There is a lesion in the ventral pons sparing the paramedian and lateral tegmentum. This results in severe quadriplegia and anarthria with preserved consciousness, voluntary eye movements, and blinking. Clinically corticospinal, corticobulbar, and corticopontine tract signs are elicited. In the acute phase, such patients have high mortality. If they survive, they are left behind with severe disabilities. It may be of interest to know that in the Count of Monte Cristo, Alexandre Dumas, in 1884, described a character—Monsieur Noirtier as "immovable as a corpse......sight and hearing were the only senses remaining......which gave the impression of a *"corpse with living eyes."* What a beautiful description of a LIS. This state must be distinguished from an akinetic mute state in which the patient is not aware and has no clinical signs, in sharp contrast to the LIS where there are plenty of clinical signs and the patient is appropriately aware. As mentioned earlier, the neurological states in which the patient is awake but not aware are hypersomnia, acute confusional state, delirium, akinetic mutism, PVS, and MCS. The latter two will be discussed later.

Hypersomnia, as the name suggests, is a condition in which the patient sleeps excessively but can be aroused easily with verbal or painful stimuli. Once the stimulus stops, he falls back to sleep. This occurs early when the diencephalon is involved in a disease process.

Acute confusional "state" entails impairment of attention, memory, logical thinking, and lack of recall of part of the day or location. A key feature is prominent distractibility and no coherent conversation. In addition to all these features, a patient with *delirium* has hallucinations and systemic autonomic manifestations, such as tachycardia, tachypnea, hypertension, and sweating. In these states, there is a diffuse cortical involvement and the brain misinterprets all sensory inputs with inappropriate excitement and arousal.

In *akinetic mutism*, the patient appears alert but is silent and immobile. Spontaneous eye opening is present and visual tracking is preserved, but defective. Alertness may be partial. There is a relative paucity of corticospinal signs. The best way to describe this condition is seeming wakefulness without content. The lesions are in the medial frontal lobe, limbic cortex, or diffuse bilateral hemispheric involvement.

In *stupor and coma*, the patient is not awake and not aware. Stupor resembles deep sleep, but the patient responds to vigorous stimulation with limited motor activity. When the stimulation ceases, he/she lapses back into a sleep-like state. Stupor should be differentiated from psychogenic unresponsiveness (PUR). The differentiating features in PUR are resistance to eyelid opening, absence of long tract signs, and optokinetic nystagmus can be elicited. In very difficult cases, ice-cold caloric test will produce nystagmus in PUR, whereas there will be tonic deviation of the eyes to the side of the irrigated ear in stupor. Of course, the electroencephalogram (EEG) will be abnormal in stupor and entirely normal in PUR.

Coma is the focus of this chapter. Coma is a state of unresponsiveness from which the patient cannot be aroused with deep painful stimuli. The eyes are closed but rarely may be open without any fixation or tracking. On deep painful stimulus, the response is reflex flexion of the upper limbs or extension of all four limbs. With further deterioration, there is no motor response with the flaccidity of the limbs. Severe and irreversible coma results in brain death. If the coma is severe but transient, the patient may survive in a PVS, or with a less severe coma, in an MCS.

ETIOLOGIES OF COMA

The etiologies of coma are: (1) large unilateral hemispheric lesion with mass effect; (2) diffuse bilateral hemispheric abnormalities; (3) discrete or diffuse upper brainstem lesion; or (4) cerebellar lesions. In a review of 14 studies between 1981 and 2013, regarding the etiology and outcome of nontraumatic coma, the two most common etiologies were strokes and hypoxic–anoxic encephalopathy. In the African countries, involved in this study, 10–51% of admissions were due to CNS infection, a common feature in developing countries like India.[3] The key components of the pathogenesis of coma are cerebral or cerebellar edema and the resultant herniation of the brain. The main sites of herniation in the supratentorial compartment are transtentorial herniation of the medial part of the temporal lobe—uncal herniation, rostral to caudal herniation of the cerebral hemispheres, and ultimately in the infratentorial compartment, tonsillar herniation through the foramen magnum. It is important to pick up the early signs of central and uncal herniation. In the early stages of central herniation, the patient becomes drowsy with long-cycle Cheyne–Stokes respiration, small but reactive pupils, preserved ciliospinal reflex, intact oculocephalic maneuver (OCM) with mildly impaired upward gaze and localization or flexion response to pain. In the early stages of uncal herniation, the respiration is regular but rapid, an ipsilateral partial third nerve palsy, an early loss of OCM and oculovestibular reflex (OVR), and unilateral or bilateral pyramidal tract signs. The clinician should be alert to these early signs and take appropriate action. If the condition deteriorates, the coma may become irreversible with late signs of central herniation. There is hyperventilation or short-cycle Cheyne–Stokes respiration, fixed mid position/dilated pupils, loss of OCM and OVR, and flexion to extension reflex response to pain or total flaccidity. In the late stages of uncal herniation, there is a total third nerve palsy before the other features merge with those of central herniation.

Coma due to an *infratentorial* lesion may be due to a small discrete brainstem or cerebellar lesion. There are a few distinguishing features that may be overlooked if one is not aware of them.[4] These signs are ataxia just prior to the onset of coma, abnormalities of external ocular movements (EOMs), and very early loss of OCM and OVR. In this context, I would like to stress the "pseudotumoral" presentation of a cerebellar infarct. This is usually a large cerebellar hemispheric infarct, involving the complete posterior inferior cerebellar artery (PICA) territory. Uncommonly, it can be due to a cerebellar hemorrhage. The initial symptoms may be nonspecific to the cerebellum, such as headache and persistent vomiting. Ocular signs are ocular gaze or 6th nerve paresis. As the brainstem gets compressed by the edematous cerebellum, bilateral gaze palsy and/or ocular bobbing occurs. The patient is initially drowsy and deteriorates into a stupor or coma over 1–3 days. The computed tomography (CT) scan may be normal in 25% of cases in the initial stages but the MRI is invariably abnormal. If the patient becomes comatose, 85% will die without surgery. Suboccipital craniectomy is the procedure of choice. Not only is it lifesaving but the results are excellent if it is done before the patient becomes comatose. This is the reason why the treating clinician must be aware of this entity.

The clinician should also be aware of *brainstem depression due to sedative drugs* or intoxication. The danger here lies in the premature diagnosis of brain death. Sedative drugs selectively "paralyses" the median longitudinal fasciculus (MLF) that connects the 6th nerve nucleus to the appropriate part of the 3rd nerve nucleus for conjugate horizontal eye movements. Hence, on eliciting brainstem reflexes, the pupillary and corneal reflexes are preserved out of proportion to the OCM and OVR. In a normal individual, irrigation of both ears with ice-cold water results in upward deviation of the eyes. When the MLF is "paralyzed" by sedative drugs, a horizontal ocular deviation is no longer possible, and vertical ocular deviation does not need the MLF. Thus, ice-cold irrigation of one ear produces upward deviation of the eyes. This test confirms brainstem depression by sedative drugs.

NEUROLOGICAL EXAMINATION

Neurological examination in a comatose patient is limited and essentially consists of good observation and eliciting reflex responses. A structured neurological examination involves observing first the position and posture of the patient and then the respiratory pattern. The respiratory pattern is a good indicator of the level of the brain that is malfunctioning. Diffuse hemispheric dysfunction produces Cheyne–Stokes respiration and midbrain involvement, hyperventilation. The rostral pons may produce a peculiar pattern called apneusis, in which breathing halts briefly in the full inspiration, whereas in the lower pons or upper medullary lesions, the respiration becomes irregular and of uneven depth—ataxic breathing. This pattern often heralds a respiratory arrest. The value of identifying these different types of respiration has probably been overestimated, and assisted ventilation has perhaps made this exercise superfluous. Once this is done, one should rule out a skull or cervical spine fracture and then check for neck stiffness. Look closely for the Battle's sign, which is a discoloration along the course of the posterior auricular artery with ecchymosis near the tip of the mastoid process, indicating a fracture of the base of the skull. The next step is the fundus examination, which may show evidence of hypertension or diabetes. A subhyaloid hemorrhage on fundus examination is practically diagnostic of subarachnoid hemorrhage (SAH). Once this is done, one should judge the level of consciousness, signs of lateralization, and reflexes to establish brainstem activity. The level of consciousness is judged by either the Glasgow Coma Scale (GCS) or the more recent FOUR (Full Outline of UnResponsiveness) score.[5] The FOUR score involves eye responses (0–4), motor responses (0–4), brainstem reflexes (0–4), and respiration (0–4). The main advantage of the FOUR score is in patients who are intubated or have a tracheostomy, as there is no verbal response score.

Lateralizing and motor signs are easily established by good observations at the bedside. Weakness, unilateral grasp reflex, and focal clonic or myoclonic seizure activity establish the abnormal side. The corticospinal tracts are intact if a patient is agitated and plucking or clutching at his clothes. Grimacing to deep painful supraorbital stimulus indicates that the corticobulbar tracts up to the pons are intact. Roving eye movements mean an intact midbrain and pons. Lastly, multifocal myoclonus and orofacial dyskinesia are seen in hypoxic–ischemic and metabolic encephalopathy, respectively.

Brainstem function is judged by the brainstem reflexes—pupillary reaction, the corneal reflex, spontaneous (roving) and reflex (OCM and OVR) eye movements, gag reflex, and respiration. While examining the pupils, note any asymmetry in the position of the two upper eyelids to detect subtle ptosis. It is beyond the scope of this chapter to go into the details of brainstem reflex examination.

CLINICAL CLASSIFICATION OF COMA

Once the neurological assessment is complete, one can categorize the patient into three clinical groups:

1. Coma with focal signs
2. Coma without focal signs but with meningeal signs
3. Coma without focal and meningeal signs

Coma with Focal Signs

The various etiologies are focal trauma, cerebral or cerebellar ischemic or hemorrhagic strokes, neoplasms, or space-occupying lesions (SOLs) such as subdural hematoma, abscess or herpes simplex virus (HSV) encephalitis, and rarely, hypoglycemic hemiplegia. Focal trauma is easily diagnosed by the appearance of the patient and the history of trauma. Strokes usually have associated risk factors such as hypertension, diabetes, or dyslipidemias, and are acute in onset. Neoplasms or SOLs have a subacute or insidious onset and may be associated with signs of the rise of intracranial pressure. Abscesses or HSV encephalitis may have an acute or subacute onset. But are usually associated with fever, headache, and other signs of infection. Rarely, a pitfall in this diagnostic algorithm may be hypoglycemic hemiplegia. Neuroimaging is very useful in this category of patients and shows a variety of abnormalities, which confirm the diagnosis. The exception to the rule is hypoglycemic hemiplegia, where the neuroimaging is normal and the diagnosis is made on the blood glucose levels.

Coma without Focal Signs but with Meningeal Signs

In this category, the main differentiating symptom is fever. With fever, one should consider meningitis/encephalitis be it viral, bacterial, fungal, or protozoal. Without fever, consider SAH. Further investigations such as cerebrospinal fluid (CSF) examination, CT scan, magnetic resonance imaging (MRI), magnetic resonance angiography (MRA), and four-vessel digital subtraction angiography (DSA) aid in arriving at the diagnosis.

Coma without Focal or Meningeal Signs

This is the main category in which general physicians are involved. It includes anoxic-ischemic, metabolic and toxic encephalopathy, nonconvulsive status epilepticus (NCSE), drug intoxication or poisoning, and hypo- or hyperthermic brain damage. Here, neuroimaging may be normal or show nonspecific changes. The EEG is more useful, particularly in NCSE. Anoxic-ischemic encephalopathy is diagnosed because of a history of cardiac arrest and cardiopulmonary resuscitation. The diagnosis of metabolic/toxic encephalopathy is made by the EEG and laboratory investigations. In hypo- or hyperthermic brain damage, there is a prior history of exposure to extremes of temperature.

Nonconvulsive status epilepticus needs a high index of suspicion for diagnosis. In NCSE, motor symptoms may be absent or minimal. The patient may present with mild confusion or even a coma. Negative symptoms such as aphasia, mutism, or amnesia can be the initial presentation. At times, positive symptoms such as tonic eye deviation or nystagmoid jerking of the eyes may lead to the diagnosis. The common underlying etiologies are strokes, SAH, infections, trauma or anoxic-ischemic, and metabolic or toxic encephalopathies (sepsis). Multiagent chemotherapy and β-lactam antibiotics in conjunction with chronic kidney disease can also precipitate NCSE. In a study of EEG monitoring in coma, 8–20% of patients had NCSE. The clinician must have a high index of suspicion for NCSE in any patient with an unexplained alteration in behavior or consciousness. In this situation, an EEG is warranted.

Table 1 outlines all the adverse effects of antibiotics in the ICU. The risk factors for these adverse effects are old age, chronic kidney disease, prior CNS disease, and chronic liver disease for metronidazole. Among the cephalosporins, cefepime is the only one which can produce coma. This happens after 1–10 days of administration and resolves in 2–7 days after stopping the drug. Awareness of this adverse effect of cefepime will prevent a disastrous outcome.

OUTCOME OF COMA

The outcome of a coma depends on many factors—etiology, duration, the presence or absence of the pupillary and corneal reflexes, OCM, OVR, the motor response to pain, or a combination of all the above. Factors predictive of a good outcome are traumatic etiology, a shorter duration of coma, and early return of the pupillary and corneal reflexes. Localization of a painful stimulus and grimacing are good prognostic signs, whereas flaccidity or extensor response to pain eludes to a poor outcome. In a prospective study of 310 patients of nontraumatic coma, Bates et al. found that 25% of patients who were comatose for 6 hours or more had a severe disability or PVS. This increased to 79% of those still in a coma after a week.[6] The chances of regaining independent existence were greater in patients who obeyed commands or moved the limbs appropriately to painful stimuli by 1 day, or had normal EOM, OCM, or OVR. The American Academy of Neurology practice parameters: Prediction of Outcome in Comatose Survivors after Cardiopulmonary Resuscitation concluded that the absence of the pupillary and corneal reflexes and the motor response to pain accurately predicted poor outcomes in these patients.[7]

Persistent Vegetative State

The term persistent vegetative state (PVS) was coined by Jennett and Plum in 1972 to denote patients with severe brain damage in whom the coma had improved to a state of wakefulness without detectable awareness.[8] Thus, the

TABLE 1: Drug-induced seizures and coma.

Antibiotics	Encephalopathy	Seizures	Nonconvulsive status epilepticus	Delirium/psychosis	Coma
Cephalosporins (cefepime)	+		+	+	+
Piperacillin and tazobactam	+	+	+	+	–
Carbapenems	–	++	–	–	–
Quinolones	+	++	+		–
Linezolid	+	–	–	–	–
Metronidazole	+	+	–	–	–

Source: Adapted from Grill MF, Maganti RK. Neurotoxic effects associated with antibiotic use: management considerations. Br J Clin Pharmacol. 2011;72:381-93.

patient is awake but not aware, in fact "partial arousal rather than true awareness".[9] In PVS, sleep-awake cycle and respiration are preserved. The eyes are open but importantly, there is no fixation or tracking. Initially when the patient is emerging from coma, roving eye movements are seen. Motor function is not purposeful and there is no meaningful communication, intellectual thinking, recall, or response to external stimuli.

The use of the word persistent should not be done in haste. Informal guidelines state the word persistent should be used if the patient has been in a vegetative state (VS) for 4 weeks or longer as the chances of awareness decrease considerably as the time spent in VS increases. Secondly, it must also be stressed to the caregivers that longer the patient is in the VS, the more severe is the resultant disability.[9] Lastly, persistent does not imply permanent in every case. In younger patients with traumatic brain injury, delayed improvements have been reported. They may improve to a "minimally conscious state" with further improvements in cognitive functions. However, such cases have been rarely documented. If the PVS persists after 1 year, it is likely to be irreversible.[8]

Minimally Conscious State

The boundaries between PVS and MCS are difficult to define. All the features of PVS are present in MCS with three exceptions. The eyes may open on prodding and there may be ill-sustained tracking. Motor functions may be intermittently purposeful.

EMERGENT THERAPY

The principles of emergent therapy in a comatose patient are:

- Ensure and maintain airway, breathing, and circulation
- Maintain adequate nutrition and supplement vitamins
- Lower intracranial pressure, medically or surgically
- Control seizures and infection
- Maintain fluid, electrolyte, and acid-base balance
- For poisoning, give the specific antidote
- Control agitation and pain
- Protect the eyes

The last point is important as many patients have improved and regained independent or semi-independent existence only to complain of impaired vision due to exposure keratitis. In a comatose patient, the upper eyelid can be pulled down over the eyeball and kept fixed by a 3M or sticky tape or a cello tape. This simple measure will protect the eyes.

CONCLUSION

Coma is a neurological emergency and rapid action is necessary. Knowledge of various terminologies based on the level of consciousness is important. Coma can have a variety of etiologies ranging from metabolic and toxic states to structural lesions placed at the supra- or infratentorial compartments. Clinical examination can give vital clues to the etiology of the coma and also guides therapy. Early and accurate evaluation and therapy can bring satisfactory results.

REFERENCES

1. Bates D. Coma in Clinical Neurology. New York: Churchill Livingstone; 1991. pp. 188-204.
2. Plum F, Poser JB. The diagnosis of stupor and coma. Brain Nerve. 2015;67(3):344-5.
3. Hosting MWB, Franken MD, Meulenbelt J, van Klei WA, de Lange DW. The etiology and outcome of non-traumatic coma in critical care: a systemic review. BMC Anesthesiol. 2015;15:65.
4. Edlow JA, Newman-Toker DE, Savitz SI. Diagnosis and initial management of cerebellar infarction. Lancet Neurol. 2008;7:951-64.
5. Wijdicks EFM, Bamlet WR, Maramattom BV, Manno EM, McClelland RL. Validation of a new coma scale: the FOUR score. Ann Neurol. 2005;58:585-93.
6. Bates D, Caronna JJ, Cartlidge NE, Knill-Jones RP, Levy DE, Shaw DA, et al. A prospective study of non-traumatic coma: methods and results in 310 patients. Ann Neurol. 1977;2:211-20.
7. Wijdicks EF, Hijdra A, Young GB, Bassetti CL, Wiebe S. Practice parameters: prediction of outcome in comatose survivors after cardiopulmonary resuscitation (an evidence-based review): report of the Quality Standards Subcommittee of the American Academy of Neurology). Neurology. 2006;67:203-10.
8. The Multi-society Task Force on PVS. Medical aspects of persistent vegetative state. NEJM. 1994;330:1499-508.
9. Maiese K. (2022). Vegetative state and minimally conscious state. MSD Manual Professional Version. [online] Available from https://www.msdmanuals.com/en-in/professional/neurologic-disorders/coma-and-impaired-consciousness/vegetative-state-and-minimally-conscious-state. [Last accessed March, 2023].

26
CHAPTER

Approach to Mild Cognitive Impairment

Sadanandavalli Retnaswami Chandra

INTRODUCTION

According to Eric Kendel nobel laureate in memory research, we are who we are because of what we learn and remember. Scholars in the BC era who tried to understand this phenomenon are Panini, Patanjali, Charaka, and Baudhayana. Memory is a general term for the mental processes that allow the individual to store information for recall at a later date. Recreation of patterns of the same spatial and temporal sequence, produced by sense organs at a later date, allows us to learn from the past, understand the present, and plan for the future. Memory is evidence that the brain becomes altered by experience. This remarkable property is the basis of thoughts, consciousness, language, and behavior. The human brain achieves this by using the >100 trillion synapses that evolved over a billion years. Memory involves registration, encoding, consolidation, and retrieval. Encoding converts the raw data of information to a brain-compatible format. The content must be processed further to make it available for future storage and retrieved with proper access. Information is held temporarily in the short term, and rehearsal converts it to the long term. Encoding involves the formation of new synaptic connections called memory traces. Storage involves the retention of memory traces by cell and system-level consolidation. Retrieval is accessing the stored memory to change behavior and the conscious experience of remembering. Learning is the result of the above all. The science of memory began with the write-up "In search of the Engram by Lashley". Learning is the modification of behavior by experience. Memory is the retention of that experience (information) over time. One major function of learning and memory is to adapt to the environment, which involves reward and punishment. (DSM 5 ICD 9 cm codes 331.83/10 cm codes-706.7 ICD 11).

WHAT HAPPENS WITH AGE?

Thirty-three stem cells make central nervous system (CNS) by signaling, wiring, perceiving, connecting, inhibiting, completing, and interacting. By the time of 65–80 years, mild insomnia, retrieval defect, fatigue, and inability to attend to several stimuli begin, which is considered normal aging. Moreover, vocabulary and function remain unaltered in normal age-related cognitive change, although performance time may be prolonged. The average adult brain weighs 1,230–1,275 g in females and 1,350–1,410 g in males by 12–15 years. By 80 years, approximately a 20% decrease in the blood flow to the brain and about 233 g of brain weight loss happens. So when a patient claims memory problems but not significant to be classified as dementia, how to differentiate whether it is a subjective cognitive decline (SCD) or normal aging or "just the patient's feeling" is a tough question to answer. When physical frailty is associated with cognitive decline, it is called cognitive frailty (CF). However, at the other end of the spectrum, it is dementia, which makes it important.

WHAT IS THE BENIGN FORGETFULNESS OF AGING?

Subjective sense of decline in memory, impaired performance in standard tests of memory by one SD, and absence of signs of dementia[1] are characteristics of benign forgetfulness. However, mild cognitive impairment (MCI) is a situation characterized by significant cognitive impairment but does not amount to dementia with retained activities of daily living (ADL). Synonyms are dementia prodrome/predementia/cognitive impairment, not dementia (ICD 9 cm codes-331.83/10 cm codes-706.7).

Mild cognitive impairment is of global importance because of suspected dementia ahead but not at this point. Proper recognition and understanding of MCI is a priority. It is considered an intermediary stage between normal aging and dementia, and it is very important to recognize for several reasons. A considerable neuronal loss would have already occurred by the time MCI is diagnosed. Hence, there is an urgent need to recognize preclinical disease for research in preventive treatment options. The decision to evaluate is by personal choice (of the informed patient) in the absence of specific and sensitive markers and a lack of promising therapeutic options. Various biomarkers are identified, but their sensitivity, specificity, or usefulness in predicting dementia is unknown. Therefore, clinical markers are the ideal entry tools in the present scenario.

The possibility of conversion to dementia makes it an important area of concern—the symptomatic predementia[2] MCI is categorized as amnesic MCI (aMCI) and nonamnesic MCI (naMCI). It may have impairments of single domains or multiple domains and may be the amnesic type or nonamnesic type. Single domain amnesic MCI can be prodrome Alzheimer's disease (AD) or depression. Multidomain, in addition, included vascular cognitive decline. The nonamnesic single domain is usually frontotemporal dementia (FTD) and multidomain vascular cognitive decline, corticobasal degeneration (CBD), and diffuse Lewy body dementia (DLBD). The amnesic MCI carries the risk of future AD, and the term prodromal AD is used by IWG (International Working Group).[3]

The cognitive performance decline is more than an age-related change and requires compensatory efforts to remain independent in ADL. The ICD 11 calls it a mild neurocognitive disorder, and DSM-5 also addresses it as the same. Modified criteria proposed by the IWG and the National Institute on Aging and Alzheimer's Association (NIA-AA) include the presence of biomarkers indicative of AD pathophysiology; these criteria are commonly used in clinical practice in Europe for diagnosis and communication to MCI patients.[4]

Mild cognitive impairment is characterized by cognitive impairment that is not severe enough to require help with ADL/instrumental ADL (IADL). MCI is categorized as amnesic or nonamnesic and as single or multidomain based on the number of the affected cognitive domain.[5]

The diagnosis of MCI due to Alzheimer's disease:

- Recommendations from the NIA-AA workgroups on diagnostic guidelines for Alzheimer's disease: Social and occupational functions and ADL remain intact in MCI compared to Dementia.
- Scales formulated are as follows—global deterioration scales 1979, Mayo criteria 1999, key symposium 2004, NIA-AA 2011, DSM V, and the IWG 2013.

Single Domain Amnesic MCI

Memory impaired by 1.5–2 standard deviations below age and gender-matched normal.

Single Domain Nonamnesic MCI

It is characterized by impairment in the nonmemory domain such as executive function, language, or visuospatial skills.

EPIDEMIOLOGY

Mild cognitive impairment prevalence is 10–20% for people aged ≥ 65 years,[6] and this increases with age. The problem lies in not having uniform criteria for diagnosis. Therefore, the reported incidence varies. Other factors possibly involved are lower educational status, poor cognitive reserve, and associated vascular risk factors. Apolipoprotein E4 (APOE-e4) genotype, vitamin D deficiency, sleep-disordered breathing, and prior critical illness are other risk factors.[7]

DEFINITION OF TERMS

In 1997, Petersen et al. defined MCI as a clinical and neuropsychological syndrome characterized by emerging cognitive impairment, i.e., an intermediate state between physiological aging and dementia.[6]

What is Subjective Cognitive Decline?

Subjective cognitive decline initiative working group is an established international consortium to create research criteria for evaluating persons with SCD. Data generated from 2015 to 2017 through the Behavioral Risk Factor Surveillance System (BRFSS) shows an incidence of 11.7% in persons > 65 years and 10.8% in persons between 45 and 65 years. Less with literate whites compared to the illiterate and African Americans. However, it does not imply a diagnosis of cognitive decline by a healthcare professional—a state of self-perceived cognitive decline among cognitively normal individuals. Synonyms are SCI (subjective cognitive impairment) and SCC (subjective cognitive complaint) means everyday cognitive concerns raised by persons without objective evidence of dementia. It is etiologically heterogeneous, and therefore interventions might help some.

Cognitive frailty is the term used for physical frailty plus a Clinical Dementia Rating (CDR) of 0.5, categorized as reversible CF and potentially reversible CF. AD and Tau are more associated with SCD than nonspecific MCI. Brain atrophy, white matter changes, cortical volume loss, and medial temporal volume are possible AD predictors. Functional magnetic resonance imaging (fMRI) shows increased activation of prefrontal cortex (PFC), which is described as compensation, and anterior cingulate and insular regions show decreased activation in fMRI.

What is MCI?

Mayo diagnostic criteria were formulated by Petersen (1997), which were later revised with the following parameters. Memory complaints, normal ADL, normal general cognitive functions, two standard deviations less than normal for age and education, no signs of dementia, and impairment of nonmemory domains. NIA-AA defines MCI due to AD as those symptomatic but nondemented individuals whose underlying pathology in AD[8] is characterized by memory impairment, a longitudinal decline in cognitive function, and a lack of evidence for vascular, traumatic, or other medical causes of cognitive decline. For research purposes, measures of amyloid-beta (Aβ) deposition and neuronal injury can be done but not for routine purposes. The IWG criteria define this as "prodromal AD" or "predementia AD". DSM-5 refers to this stage as "mild neurocognitive disorder.[9]

VASCULAR MILD COGNITIVE IMPAIRMENT

It is a condition that is caused by vascular diseases and in which the patient presents with cognitive deficits not severe enough to fit the criteria for dementia. It is also classified as amnesic and nonamnesic.

It is classified into definite, probable, and possible. Impaired cognitive function in at least one cognitive domain without or with minimal effect on social and occupational function independent of any motor or sensory deficit from a stroke (if present).

Four main categories are defined—(1) amnestic, (2) amnestic plus other domains, (3) nonamnestic single domain, and (4) nonamnestic multiple domains.

- *Probable*: If impaired cognition with imaging evidence of cerebrovascular disease and a temporal association between the onset of stroke and cognitive symptoms, or clear evidence of a temporal association between cognitive impairment and the presence of diffuse, and subcortical cerebrovascular pathology.
- *Possible*: If there is no clear evidence clinically or radiologically.

EVALUATION

If the patient feels they cannot remember as well as before, the following questions are asked:

Does it affect your daily life?

Instrumental activities of daily living asked are:

- Reading map
- Preparing meal
- Shopping groceries
- Making phone calls

Then general health measures like neurological disorders, thyroid conditions, cholesterol, diabetes mellitus, hypertension, smoking, and Framingham combined cardiovascular risk score. After this, screen for depression. Then shall apply Petersen's criteria for the following parameters:

- Subjective memory complaint present, but the limitations are how to confirm. Participant? Informant? (Single questions or questionnaire)
- Normal General cognitive functions, but the issues are? Test selection? Cut-off score? Adjustment for age? Education or prior ability score?
- Objective memory impairment, but the issues are? Test selection, Cut-off score? Adjustment for age? Education or prior ability score?
- Personal ADL should be normal. Here the issues are instrumental or basic? Degree allowed?
- No dementia, but the problem is: can blanket criteria be applied for all?

CLINICAL ASSESSMENT

When a patient reports a cognitive concern, an interview with a reliable informant is very vital. It will help in knowing if the reported impairment represents disease or fear of disease. The trajectory of change in the 24-hour routine concerning baseline function will give important clues. Instead of conveying inferences, they should be encouraged to narrate incidents. Therefore, the reliability of the informant is very important, and we should verify the time spent together, and its context needs to be verified. Patient-centered evaluation is important. Drug history, psychiatric illness endocrine, and notional and metabolic causes which are reversible should be looked into. The neuropsychologist will be able to characterize the profile of impairment better. Slowly evolving change indicates a degenerative cause, but a shorter duration indicates the probable reversible cause.

Tools

Brief screening tools are not very useful.

The commonly used screening tool has 45–60% sensitivity and 65–90% specificity. The mini-cog test combines the Clock Drawing Test with a 3-word recall test and can be performed in ≤3 minutes.[10] The Hindi mental status examination and Montreal Cognitive assessment (MOCA) have a sensitivity of 80–100% and specificity of 50–76%. MOCA is more sensitive than MMSE.

Other tests are the Kokmen short test for mental status, the Free and Cued Selective Reminding Test (FCSRT), the California Verbal Learning Test, the Boston Naming Test, and Appraisal of Guidelines for Research and Evaluation (AGREE) II instrument.

Toronto Cognitive Assessment (TorCA), National Institute for Neurological Disorders and Stroke and Canadian Stroke Network (NINDS-CSN), and FCSRT-recommended testing ADL, and functional assessment, including assessment using the ADL, IADL scale, and functional activities questionnaire (FAQ); and one document of complete neuropsychometric tests are ordered to identify cognitive strengths and weaknesses.

If cognitive dysfunction is quantified and domains and severity assessed, functional impairment should be evaluated in performing tasks, driving, and personal finance. If cognitive impairment is present, but there is no functional impairment, they qualify for MCI. This is found in 6.7% of persons above 60 years (Petersen RC, Lopez o, Armstrong MJ, et al. Practice guidelines update summary MCI Report of guidelines development, dissemination and implementation). In persons above 80 years, it becomes 25.2% (Petersen RC, Lopez O, Armstrong MJ, et al. Practice Guidelines Update Summary MCI Report of guidelines development, dissemination and implementation).

Delirium and depression cause confusion in diagnosis. Delirium is associated with the disturbance of attention, a consciousness of short duration, provoked by infection, metabolic abnormality, or altered sleep-wake cycle. Persons with depression perform poorly on tests; these patients' cognitive test results should be clubbed with validated mood disorder screening. The functional state can be assessed using the FAQ and needs to obtain IAD L[11] using a cut-point of ≥6 points on the FAQ. There is 85% accuracy for differentiating MCI from dementia.[12]

From the information providers, the Informant Questionnaire on Cognitive Decline in the Elderly (IQCODE) can be applied. The Dementia Severity Rating Scale (DSRS) and the AD8 too can be applied. The NIA-AA MCI criteria note that scores on cognitive tests for individuals with MCI are typically 1–1.5 standard deviations below age-adjusted and education-adjusted normative means.[4,13]

Neuroimaging

It helps to rule out other causes such as normal pressure hydrocephalus (NPH), subdural hematoma (SDH), and mass lesions rather than defining MCI. Voxel-based morphometry shows a progressive reduction in hippocampal volume. In those who convert to dementia, nuclear imaging with fluorodeoxyglucose positron emission tomography (PET) shows specific patterns of hypometabolism. In AD, FTD, and DLBD, PET amyloid imaging identifies the presence of amyloid. N-Back task, according to Dumas, showed increased activation with increased cognitive load in cingulum, thalamus, and cerebellar regions, show altered activation in fMRI.[14] Tau PET showing spread to lateral temporal regions probably predicts progression to AD. Biomarkers for other degenerative dementias are not available. Amnesic MCI clubbed with amyloid, Tau information in cerebrospinal fluid (CSF), and imaging can qualify for AD prodrome.[15] Single positron emission computed tomography (SPECT) is used when available. The Imaging Dementia-Evidence for Amyloid Scanning (IDEAS) study demonstrated changes in patient management in 60% of those with MCI after amyloid-PET.

Quantitative Electroencephalography–Positron Emission Tomography

Biological assessment with quantitative electroencephalography (qEEG) showed increased theta. Voxel-based morphometric studies reported gray matter differences in medial temporal, frontal, and smaller hippocampus (Vanden filler). PET studies report decreased cerebral metabolism of glucose in parietotemporal and parahippocampal regions. APOE-e4 allele has more alterations. Higher cortisol was reported by Wolf et al. No change in performance during tasks but observed differences in functional brain activation indicating clinicoimaging discordance.

Event-related Potential

A paradym used in evaluation of event related potentials by Hayers. The phenomenon of negative subsequent is postulated to be the cause of increased activation for failed recall. This is followed by negative subsequent memory in the posterior occipital, superior parietal, and precuneus regions in fMRI. Probably this indicates an altered neural system in SCD for successful memory encoding to maintain normal cognitive functions.

Face-convert Recognition

In face recognition tasks of patients with multidomain MCI–alpha, synchronization underlying and suppression of distracting letters was reduced, believed to be due to the reduced relaxation in the failing brain.

Prediction Error Theory

The brain functions as a statistical optimization engine, making implicit predictions of inputs and actively making inferences instead of passively transmitting. These are projected as a predicted expectation to lateromedial association areas and the PFC. This constant comparison of internally generated prediction and external reality is called predictive coding. Prediction errors lead to mismatch, which is corrected by the dorsal anterior cingulum. This error minimization is poor in SCD and MCI.

Laboratory Parameters

Complete blood count, electrolytes, glucose, calcium, thyroid function, vitamin B12, and folates are recommended to pick up reversible forms of MCI, including infection, renal failure, hypo- or hypermagnesemia, hyperglycemia, hypo- or hypercalcemia, hypo- or hyperthyroidism, liver function, syphilis, Lyme titers (*Borrelia*), and HIV. Aβ 42 and tau protein in CSF are useful to detect potential AD but are routinely recommended.

Outcome Studies

Challenged by heterogeneity in approach, laboratory tests, mode of administration, number of items, response options, domains tested, and intra- and interindividual parameters, differences are all to be addressed. There is probably a complex interaction between SCD and depression-MCI-AD.[16] CSHA (Canadian study of health and aging) MCI with preceding SCD progressed faster. Neither subjective nor objective is normal. Subjective alone SCD, objective alone MCI. Both SCD and objective decline MCI ± dementia. The interrelationship between SCD-MCI-AD seems complex. In the absence of any other findings, SCD alone does not indicate PRE MCI.

Predictors of Progression

Age and gender do not predict. The cognitive scores, hippocampal and parahippocampal volume, and medial temporal lobe atrophy, together can predict conversion by 81%. Olfactory dysfunction MRI/biomarkers/neuropsychology/function loss progressing longitudinally. Decreased Aβ in CSF, due to deposition in the brain. Increased phosphorylated Tau, increased PIB binding. Cortical thickness—anatomically demented patients having NTI—normalized cortical thickness index below the threshold. Widespread atrophy is associated with progression. MMSE remains unaltered if the cognitive reserve is good, so it is not a good predictor.

Spare AD Index

The Baltimore longitudinal study showed a steeper increase of atrophy in those who converted. Progression has a linear correlation with the degree of impairment at presentation, APOE carriers, Hippocampal volume <25% for age and gender, large ventricular volume, abnormal functional imaging characteristics, and low levels of β-amyloid peptide 42 (Aβ42) and elevated levels of tau protein. Positron-emission tomography (PET) with amyloid-binding carbon 11-labeled Pitts—burgh compound B showed amyloid deposition. Acute-phase proteins, cytokines, cholesterol, isoprostanes, homocysteine, reduced levels of Ab1-40, Ab1-42, and Ab1-42/Ab1-40 ratio.[17] Fluid markers are used from CSF and blood-based biomarkers for AD (plasma Aβ and p-tau), and for all-cause neurodegeneration, neurofibrillary tangles are useful.

Causes

Pathophysiological mechanisms are variable. It is Aβ accumulation, extraneurona and neurofibrillary tangles intracellular in AD, Tau in PSP, FTD, CBD, and synuclein in PD and DLBD. Sedentary life, genetics, environmental, nutritional, and vascular factors are all important.

Biomarkers

The Aβ deposition is detected by PET amyloid imaging. Low CSF Aβ increased total and phosphorylated Tau in CSF and FDG PET, showing decreased glucose uptake and volume loss in temporal parietal lobes.

Stable amnesic type, depression, frailty, delirium, comorbidities, APOE4 carrier state, significant atrophy, significant impairment at onset, cerebral voxel-based morphometry changes and white matter hyperintensity (WMH), global atrophy, large ventricles, focal hippocampal atrophy, abnormal brain AB1-42 on PET or CSF analysis, and also abnormal tau on PET or CSF analysis. The likelihood of progression can be measured using biomarkers.

The useful biomarkers are a voxel-based morphometric study of medial temporal lobe volume, FDG PET showing reduced glucose metabolism using 18F-fluorodeoxyglucose, CSF levels of Ab42, phosphorylated and total tau, low neuropsychological scores in MMSE, and ADAS-cog.

The other important factors are APOE-e4, living alone without social interactions, end-organ function loss such as blindness and deafness, depression, high blood pressure, diabetes mellitus, female gender, and age in the eighth decade. Stable MCI is less likely to deteriorate than progressive ones. A small proportion (2%) can even revert to normal. As much as 59% of patients with positive biomarkers convert to AD compared to 4% among MCI persons who are negative.

PATHOLOGY

Mixed pathology is mainly seen. Therefore a synergistic role for inflammation, vascular change, amyloid, neurofibrillary tangles, and alpha-synuclein is likely. Lewy bodies, TDP-43, and hippocampal sclerosis are also seen.

DIAGNOSTIC DILEMMAS

There is no sensitive and specific tool that qualifies definite MCI. Subjective memory complaints are present, but the issue is — is it assessed by the participant or informant? Should it be a single question or questionnaire? Normal general cognitive functions and objective memory impairment are criteria, but issues are test selection, cut-off scores, and adjustment for age, education, or prior ability score. Personal ADL should be normal, but issues are instrumental or basic? Degree allowed? If it is no Dementia — how to prove it? What are the impacts of same criteria for all?

TREATMENT

Treatment options and recommendations reported are inconsistent and do not consider the current diagnostic concepts or the most recent pharmacological and nonpharmacological treatment evidence. Check drugs used like opioids, anticholinergics, antihistamines, hormones, antiepileptics, muscle relaxants, and drugs lowering blood pressure/blood sugar too much should be optimized. Vision, hearing, and sleep apnea to be corrected. Psychiatric symptoms, endocrine features, gait, and peripheral neuropathy, orthostatic hypotension, eye movements, vision, hearing, speech, focal weakness, and ability to stand from a chair are useful for identifying potential contributors to cognitive decline, including stroke, PD, NPH, or neuropathy due to toxins or vitamin deficiency.

Enhancing cognitive reserve, i.e., a concept responsible for reduced susceptibility to impairment due to individual characteristics such as genetics, increased synaptic or neuronal capacity, greater efficiency in engaging brain capacity, or using alternative strategies, is a preventive tool in normal young persons. The cognitive and behavioral problems affect both patients' and caregivers' quality of life. Therefore, there is a need for treatment than just follow-up.

There is compensatory upregulation of choline acetyltransferase in the MCI stage, and therefore there is no rationale to use AChE-I. Donepezil was beneficial for the first 12 months, but it did not last. It was slightly useful in young-onset carriers of APOE-E4 and the Kalow variant of butyrylcholinesterase (BChE-K) genes. Glutamate receptor modulators, antioxidants, anti-inflammatory drugs, nootropics, immunomodulators, mainly amyloid antibodies, secretase inhibitors, and *Ginkgo biloba* are all considered choices (Karakaya et al. 2013). Adverse effects were more in the donepezil group—diarrhea (3.8%), nausea (2.6%), and abnormal dreams (2.6%). A galantamine-memantine N-methyl-D-aspartate antagonist has shown some efficacy. Beta- and gamma-secretase inhibitors and antiamyloid antibodies are not useful. Some improvements were reported with triflusal, a platelet aggregation inhibitor and a nonselective, nonsteroidal anti-inflammatory drug (NSAID). *Ginkgo biloba* showed some improvement in its multiple constituents and their actions:

- Prevention of oxidative stress
- Better mitochondrial function
- Synaptic function and neuronal plasticity
- Control inflammation
- Blood flow

However, cholinesterase inhibitors and memantine are not recommended for MCI treatment. Trials have not established that statins or intensive glycemic control reduces the risk of dementia independent of stroke prevention. Systolic blood pressure and smoking increase leukoaraiosis. Controlling all comorbidities is important. Calcium channel blockers and thiazide diuretics are good in controlling blood pressure fluctuations. Maintaining visual and auditory acuity, gait training and fall prevention, comorbidity control, cognitive retraining, cognitive stimulation, and yoga can be done. Mediterranean diet, aerobic exercises, and social engagement are useful.

Follow-up is important to identify reversible factors. When and how to diagnose and treat MCI is still not certain. Younger nonamnesic MCI less often converts to AD, and such information will be encouraging. Healthy lifestyle behaviors and minimizing risks from polypharmacy are important.

Symptom Modifying and Disease Modifying

Treatment options as such can be as follows:

- Interventions for risk reduction
- Pharmacological interventions
- Nonpharmacological interventions
- Most vital is discontinuing harmful drugs and toxins
- Control systemic comorbidities
- Pharmacotherapy is controversial.
- Mediterranean diet, antioxidants including curcumin and natural agents as well as vitamins, aerobic exercises, cognitive enhancement therapy, counseling for long-term planning for patient and family.[18]
- Physical exercise, yoga, and cognitive enhancement therapy are useful.
- Multidomain Alzheimer Preventive Trial (MAPT) for 3 years is the first trial that evaluated omega-3 fatty acids multidomain lifestyle intervention in a placebo, controlled study. There was no benefit found in this study.
- Finnish Geriatric Intervention Study to Prevent Cognitive Impairment and Disability (FINGER) trial reported improvement at 2 years. Cognitive exercises, control of comorbidities, and diet were the modifications. Neuropsychological scores and executive functions improved in these patients. Yoga improved behavior and caregiver burden in a study conducted by us (Tamil Nadu association of Physcians of India journal).

Diet Souvenaid is a combination of vitamins, omega-3-fatty acids, lipids, and selenium. Eicosapentaenoic acid (EPA) and docosahexaenoic acid (DHA) containing fish oils and antioxidants were found not useful for cognition, depression, and quality of life. Cognitive training, brisk walking for 150 hours a week, and intellectually stimulating activities are useful.

Mild Cognitive Impairment due to Alzheimer's Disease

Cholinesterase inhibitors and anti-inflammatory agents are not recommended. Transdermal nicotine, tesamorelin growth hormone-releasing factor tried with short-term changes.[19]

Mild Cognitive Impairment due to Vascular Cognitive Impairment

Several modifiable risk factors are there which should be addressed. Cholinesterase inhibitors and NMDA antagonists are useful. Aspirin, calcium channel blockers, statin, and vitamin supplementation can be tried.

Mild Cognitive Impairment in Parkinson's Disease

Atomoxetine, an adrenergic reuptake inhibitor, clozapine, serotonin and dopamine, and second-generation tricyclic antidepressant are useful. The guideline was published by the American Academy of Neurology (AAN) (Petersen et al. 2018), and a Spanish MCI consensus document was published by the Spanish Society of Geriatrics and Gerontology (SEGG).

CONCLUSION

In MCI, diagnosis depends on the sensitivity and specificity of the tests used, individualized norms of the test, cut-off scores, norms, and earlier cognitive functioning of the person. No genetic testing or specific disease association is known. Limited efficiency of currently available options in preventing progression is a major limiting factor for investing in evaluating individuals with suspected MCI. Especially when competing causes limiting life expectancy like malignancy and heart diseases are present. While reported MCI conversion to dementia is 5–20% in various studies.[20] There are limitations in clinical diagnosis, neuropsychological, imaging, cut-off scores, and longitudinal versus cross-sectional evaluation. The concept of MCI is appealing from the point of view of early diagnosis and treatment. However, the clinical syndrome is an ill-defined spectrum with multiple domains, heterogeneous etiology, and no definite genotype and is sometimes unstable with our criteria. Therefore the data generated in this condition also carries uncertainty. Uniformity, in assessment tools, is not reached so far. Therefore, promoting a healthy lifestyle, comorbidity control, reducing polypharmacy, and counseling regarding future plans are all that can be done now. However, these patients serve as substrates for research in the future.

REFERENCES

1. Égerházi A, Berecz R, Bartók E, Degrell I. Automated Neuropsychological Test Battery (CANTAB) in mild cognitive impairment and Alzheimer›s disease. Prog Neuropsychopharmacology Biol Psychiatry. 2007;31(3):746-51.
2. Petersen RC, Stevens JC, Ganguli M, Tangalos EG, Cummings JL, DeKosky ST. Practice parameter: Early detection of dementia: mild cognitive impairment (an evidence-based review). Neurology. 2001;56:1133-42.
3. Winblad B, Palmer K, Kivipelto M, Jelic V, Fratiglioni L, Wahlund LO, et al et al. Mild cognitive impairment–beyond controversies, towards a consensus: report of the International Working Group on Mild Cognitive Impairment. J Intern Med. 2004;256(3):240-6.
4. Dubois B, Feldman HH, Jacova C, Cummings JL, Dekosky ST, Barberger-Gateau P, et al. Revising the definition of Alzheimer's disease: A new lexicon. Lancet Neurol. 2010;9(11):1118-27.
5. Yaffe K, Laffan AM, Harrison SL, Redline S, Spira AP, Ensrud KE, et al. Sleep-disordered breathing, hypoxia, and risk of mild cognitive impairment and dementia in older women. JAMA. 2011;306(6): 613-9.
6. Albert MS, DeKosky ST, Dickson D, Dubois B, Feldman HH, Fox NC, et al. The diagnosis of mild cognitive impairment due to Alzheimer's disease: recommendations from the National Institute on Aging-Alzheimer's Association workgroups on diagnostic guidelines for Alzheimer's disease. Alzheimer's Dement. 2011;7(3): 270-9.
7. Kasper S, Bancher C, Eckert A, Förstl H, Frölich L, Hort J, et al. Management of mild cognitive impairment (MCI): the need for national and international guidelines. The World Journal of Biological Psychiatry. 2020;21(8):579-94.
8. Petersen RC. Mild cognitive impairment as a diagnostic entity. J Int Med. 2004;256(3):183-94.
9. Jack Jr CR, Bennett DA, Blennow K, Carrillo MC, Dunn B, Haeberlein SB, et al. NIA-AA research framework: toward a biological definition of Alzheimer's disease. Alzheimer's Dement. 2018;14(4):535-62.
10. Lin JS, O'Connor E, Rossom R, Perdue LA, Burda BU, Thompson M, et al. Screening for Cognitive Impairment in Older Adults: An Evidence Update for the US Preventive Services Task Force. Rockville, MD: Agency for Healthcare Research and Quality; 2013.
11. Pfeffer RI, Kurosaki TT, Harrah CH Jr, Chance JM, Filos S. Measurement of functional activities in older adults in the community. J Gerontol. 1982;37(3):323-9.
12. Teng E, Becker BW, Woo E, Knopman DS, Cummings JL, Lu PH. Utility of the functional activities questionnaire for distinguishing mild cognitive impairment from very mild Alzheimer's disease. Alzheimer's Dis Assoc Disord. 2010;24(4):348-53.
13. Clark CM, Ewbank DC. Performance of the dementia severity rating scale: a caregiver questionnaire for rating severity in Alzheimer's disease. Alzheimer Dis Assoc Disord. 1996;10(1):31-9.
14. Clark CM, Schneider JA, Bedell BJ, Beach TG, Bilker WB, Mintun MA, et al. Use of florbetapir-PET for imaging beta-amyloid pathology. JAMA. 2011;305(3):275-83.
15. Dubois B, Feldman HH, Jacova C, Hampel H, Molinuevo JL, Blennow K, et al. Advancing research diagnostic criteria for Alzheimer's disease: the IWG-2 criteria. Lancet Neurol. 2014;13(6):614Y629.
16. Glodzik-Sobanska L, Reisberg B, De Santi S, Babb JS, Pirraglia E, Rich KE Brys M, et al. Subjective memory complaints: presence, severity and future outcome in normal older subjects. Dement Geriatr Cogn Disord. 2007;24(3):177-84.
17. Song F, Poljak A, Smythe GA, Sachdev P. Plasma biomarkers for mild cognitive impairment and Alzheimer's disease. Brain Res Rev. 2009;61:69–80
18. Kandiah N, Christopher YFC. Strategies for the use of Ginkgo biloba extract, EGb 761 in the treatment and management of mild cognitive impairment in Asia: expert consensus. CNS Neurosci Ther. 2021;27:149-62.
19. Petersen RC, Lopez O, Armstrong MJ, et al. Practice guideline update summary: Mild cognitive impairment: report of the guide- 27. line development, dissemination, and implementation subcommittee of the American Academy of Neurology. Neurology. 2018;90(3):126-135.
20. Farias ST, Mungas D, Reed BR, Harvey D, DeCarli C. Progression of MCI to dementia in clinic vs community-based cohorts. Arch Neurol. 2009;66(9):1151-7.

27 CHAPTER

Approach to Depression and Psychosis in Neurologic Diseases

Parveen Goel

INTRODUCTION

Psychiatric disorders are frequent comorbidities in neurological disorders and they have a detrimental impact on morbidity, mortality, and quality of life. The prevalence of psychiatric illness in neurology patients in a tertiary referral center has been reported to be 51%;[1] among the new neurological outpatients 55% had a current mental disorder, and 65% had, at least, once in their lifetime a psychiatric disorder.[2] Neuropsychiatric symptoms (NPSs) are almost ubiquitous in people with dementia, with prevalence estimates as high as 97%.[3] Despite the wide recognition of the high prevalence, neurologists are not equipped enough to recognize psychiatric disorders, consequently they remain underdiagnosed and undertreated. In the present chapter, we highlight depression, the highly prevalent one, and psychosis, the most serious and debilitating comorbidity in neurological illness. Emerging evidence supports significant connections between depression as well as psychosis and structural and functional brain changes in both primary and neurologic disorders. Furthermore, for management, a recent study has shown that 70% of patients prefer neurologist-prescribing of psychotropics over psychiatric referral.[4] The perceived stigma of psychiatric illness and also the conviction that their symptoms are due to a physical rather than a psychological process makes them resist psychiatric referral. Trimble has defined neuropsychiatry as a discipline that references certain disorders "which, on account of their presentation and pathogenesis, do not fall neatly into one category, and require multidisciplinary ideas for their full understanding".[5]

Neuropsychiatric consultation may be requested for three reasons. The patient presents with neurological symptoms which do not fit with a known neurological illness and there is no organic cause. These are described as functional, e.g., tremors, paralysis, apparent dystonia, dysphonia, and blindness with underlying psychological causes as opposed to organic. The second presentation includes psychiatric symptoms in the context of a known neurological disorder, e.g., depression is a common feature of many neurological disorders, and may be a premorbid feature, a consequence of the illness itself, or a reaction to the diagnosis or the disability. Further, the causes may be drug-related, e.g., levodopa-induced psychosis in Parkinson's disease (PD), depression, and/or psychosis due to antiepileptic drugs in people with epilepsy. In the third type, the patient develops prominent psychiatric symptoms that are the product of an underlying neurological process, e.g., autoimmune encephalitis presenting primarily as psychosis, and multiple sclerosis (MS) presenting as depression.

The present chapter sheds light on depression and psychosis, both of which, classically, constitute a reliable diagnostic challenge in the setting of central nervous system (CNS) illnesses where bidirectionality and high levels of comorbidity continue to prove that the tasks are intertwined and with significant symptom overlap. For example, both, patients with PD and patients with "primary" depressive illness may show symptoms such as bradykinesia, motor retardation, bland expression, apathy, a stooped posture, and sleep difficulties. However, currently, there is no systematic approach to the evaluation and management of psychiatric comorbidities in neurological patients. Simple, cost-effective and quick screening and rating scales for evaluation of these neuropsychiatric comorbidities are also discussed. Timely diagnosis and optimal management of these burdening symptoms are crucial.

DEPRESSION

Depression is a common illness worldwide, with an estimated 3.8% of the population affected, including 5.0% among adults, and 5.7% among adults older than 60 years.[6] Depression is associated with high morbidity and mortality. The World Health Organization (WHO) ranks depression as the single largest contributor to global disability (7.5% of all years lived with disability in 2015).[7] In India, depression is a crucial social issue, as suicide rates have rapidly increased since the year 2000. Alarming still, are the estimates that 75% of people with depression in low- and middle-income countries (LMICs) receive no treatment[8] despite the prolific evidence-based effective treatments available. Barriers to treatment in LMICs include stigma and lack of awareness, limited material and human resources, and insufficient research capacity. Depression significantly impairs the quality of life, independent of the severity of neurological illness. Depression has been targeted as one of the priority conditions covered by the WHO Mental Health Gap Action Programme (mhGAP).[9] The present chapter aims to equip clinicians with the practical skills to identify and manage depression in neurologic diseases effectively.

The Diagnostic Statistical Manual, Fifth Edition (DSM-5)[10] has separated the chapter on "Depressive Disorders" from the chapter on "Bipolar and Related Disorders". The author's aim is also to cover unipolar depression and not depression in the context of bipolar disorder or other psychiatric disorders. The common features of all the disorders listed under "Depressive Disorders" are pervasive and sustained feelings of sad, empty, or irritable mood, accompanied by somatic and cognitive changes that significantly affect the individual's capacity to function. What differ among them are issues of duration, timing, or presumed etiology.

Depressive Disorders

Major Depressive Disorder

Major depressive disorder (MDD) represents the classic condition in this group of disorders. According to DSM-5, the diagnosis requires the presence of five or more of the following nine symptoms for at least 2 weeks, and results in significant distress or impairment in social, occupational, or other areas of functioning: Depressed mood, diminished interest, or pleasure in activities decrease/increase in appetite with subsequent weight loss/gain, insomnia/hypersomnia, psychomotor retardation/agitation, fatigue/adynamia, feelings of guilt and worthlessness, difficulty in concentration and/or decision-making, and suicidal ideas. The symptoms should not be in the context of another medical condition or substance/medication use. There has never been a manic or a hypomanic episode in which case it becomes a bipolar disorder then. The occurrence is not better explained by any psychotic disorder (elaborated later in the chapter).

Postpartum depression, though not recognized as a separate disorder in DSM-5, is identified as a MDD with peripartum onset during pregnancy or within 4 weeks after delivery associated with hormonal changes.

Persistent Depressive Disorder

It is a heterogeneous disorder and subsumes chronic depressive illnesses including dysthymic disorder, recurrent major depression without recovery between episodes, major depressive episodes superimposing on the dysthymic disorder *(double depression)*, and chronic major depression. The DSM-5 diagnostic criteria require that the depressed mood changes be present for at least 2 years with two or more of the following symptoms: change in appetite, insomnia/hypersomnia, fatigue, low self-esteem, poor concentration, and hopelessness.

Disruptive Mood Dysregulation Disorder

This is a unique clinical entity in DSM-5 reserved for children and adolescents from 6 to 18 years, with onset before age 10, presenting with frequent episodes of extreme behavioral dyscontrol with persistent irritability, anger—verbal and/or physical, and temper tantrums present in at least two of three settings (i.e., home, school, and peer group) for at least 12 or more months.

Premenstrual Dysphoric Disorder

Premenstrual dysphoric disorder (PMDD), a severe, often disabling extension of premenstrual syndrome, includes both psychological and physical manifestations. The psychological components include marked affective lability, marked irritability or anger, marked depressed mood, and marked anxiety. The physical components have common gastrointestinal symptoms (nausea, bloating, and abdominal cramps), skin issues (acne), neurologic symptoms (insomnia, headache, and dizziness), and ocular symptoms (vision changes). The potential etiology of PMDD includes combinations of CNS sensitivity to reproductive hormones such as estrogen and progesterone, genetics, and stress.

Substance/Medication-induced Depressive Disorder

This includes prominent and persistent mood disturbances associated with the use of prescription medications, over-the-counter drugs, and illicit drugs. Note, due to the predominance of mood changes, this is different from substance intoxication/withdrawal.

Depressive Disorder due to Another Medical Condition

This diagnosis is made when mood disturbance is the direct pathophysiological consequence of another medical condition. There is generally a temporal association between the onset, exacerbation, or remission of the medical condition and that of the mood disturbance. Also present are features that are atypical of primary mood disorders, e.g., atypical age at onset or course or absence of family history. Etiology is the key factor here, e.g., depression associated with Huntington's disease (HD), PD, traumatic brain injury (TBI), stroke, MS, etc.

Other Specified and Unspecified Depressive Disorders

Other specified and unspecified depressive disorders in DSM-5 include patients who do not meet the full criteria for any of the above diagnostic categories, e.g., there is a short-duration depressive episode, or situations when the clinician chooses not to specify the reason that the criteria are not fully met, e.g., in emergency room settings.

Suicide

At its worst, the most tragic outcome of a depressive episode is suicide. As per the WHO 2019 global health estimates, 703,000 people die by suicide every year; 77% of global suicides occur in LMICs.[11] Worldwide, more than one in every 100 deaths (1.3%) in 2019 was the result of suicide, and India accounted for a share of 2.08% of suicidal deaths across the world.[11] These data are likely underreported due to the stigma attached to suicide and it is even considered illegal in some countries.

Suicidal behavior includes suicidal ideation (contemplations, wishes, and preoccupations with ending one's life), suicide attempts (the act of trying to kill one's self, but survives), and completed suicide (death occurs). Suicidal behavior is most often accompanied by a breakdown in the coping abilities of an individual in the face of acute or chronic stress leading to intense feelings of helplessness, hopelessness, depression, or self-destructive behaviors (parasuicidal behaviors, such as cutting or self-mutilation). All suicidal behavior should be taken seriously, as a prior failed attempt is the single most risk factor for completed suicide in the future. A suicidal gesture should not be invalidated, as it is often a means to signal others to some type of ongoing distress and bids for help. There is considerable ambivalence about life and death in the suicidal person's mind.

Nonetheless, suicides are preventable. WHO's Mental Health Action Plan 2013-2030 includes suicide as one of the priority conditions and the *LIVE LIFE*[12] approach includes evidence-based interventions for preventing suicide **(Box 1)**.

BOX 1	"LIVE LIFE" key evidence-based interventions.[12]

- ***L***imit access to means of suicide
- ***I***nteract with the media on responsible reporting
- ***F***oster life skills in young people
- ***E***arly identify and support everyone affected

Scales for Detecting Depression

Detecting depression among patients with neurologic illness is essential for improving prognosis and quality of life. Classically, depression constitutes a critical diagnostic challenge in a neurological setting due to the overlap of symptoms. For instance, psychomotor retardation, insomnia, loss of appetite, loss of libido, and loss of energy may be obvious recognizable findings in patients with stroke or traumatic brain injuries, but also constitute cardinal symptoms for the diagnosis of depression among patients with primary depressive disorders.

For this reason, the use of depression rating scales in neurological illnesses is often criticized because most of these scales were developed for use in psychiatric populations and include somatic symptoms of depression. The prevalence of depression may, therefore, be overestimated when such scales are used in the neurologic population. Nevertheless, in light of their practical utility and ease of administration, the use of rating scales in the evaluation of depression in neurology practice cannot be dismissed. The screening instruments do not make the diagnosis of depression but help identify patients at risk while also allowing for the follow-up of their symptoms in subsequent visits.

Psychiatric Interviews for Depression in Neurologic Disease

There are semistructured or structured psychiatric interviews to assess the presence of depressive symptoms. Some of the widely used ones include, *Schedules for Clinical Assessment in Neuropsychiatry (SCAN)*,[13] *Quick Structured Clinical Interview for DSM-5 Disorders (QuickSCID-5)*,[14] *Composite International Diagnostic Interview (CIDI)*,[15] and *Mini-International Neuropsychiatric Interview (MINI)*.[16]

Generic Rating Scales for Depression

- *Montgomery-Asberg Depression Rating Scale (MADRS)*:[17] In a 10-item clinician-rated diagnostic questionnaire, each item yields a score of 0–6, the total score range being 0–60. The usual cutoff points are: 0–6—normal/symptom absent, 7-19—mild depression, 20-34—moderate depression, and >34—severe depression. The self-rating version (MADRS-S) has nine items with an overall score range from 0 to 54 points.
- *Center for Epidemiological Studies-Depression (CES-D)*:[18] A 10-item test, self-rated on a 4-point scale as to the frequency with which the patient has experienced depressive symptoms over the past week. The test is useful for both clinical and community samples.
- *Hamilton Depression Rating Scale (HAM-D)*:[19] A 17-item clinician-rated scale was used to rate the severity of depression over the past week. The cut-points are: 0–7—normal, 8-13—mild depression, 14-18—moderate depression, 19-22—severe depression, and >23—very severe depression.
- *Zung Self-Rating Depression Scale (SDS)*:[20] It is a 20-item scale, each item rated from 1 to 4, and with total cut-points as: 20 to 44 normal range, 45 to 59 mildly depressed, 60 to 69 moderately depressed, and ≥70 severely depressed.

- *Beck Depression Inventory-II (BDI-II)*:[21] A 21-item questionnaire, self-rated on a 4-point Likert scale from 0 to 3. Higher scores indicate more severe symptoms. A cut-off score ≥14 indicates at least a mild condition.
- *The Beck Depression Inventory-Fast Screen for Medical Patients (BDI-FS)*:[22] A shortened version of the BDI-II requires less than five minutes, and assesses depression on seven nonsomatic items—sadness, pessimism, past failure, loss of pleasure, self-dislike, self-criticalness, and suicidal ideation, on a 3-point scale. Scores 0–3 indicate minimal depression; 4–6 mild; –9 moderate; and 10–21 indicate severe depression. The scale has been validated for depression in neurological disorders, including MS[23,24] and PD.[25]
- *Hospital Anxiety Depression Scale (HADS)*:[26] It has depression and anxiety subscales, each with 7-items. All items are rated on a four-point scale, score of 0 representing the absence of a symptom and a score 3 representing maximum symptomatology. The score range is 0–21 on each, with higher scores indicating more severe depression or anxiety vis-à-vis.
- *The Geriatric Depression Scale (GDS)*:[27] There is a 30-item version and a shorter 15-item version, both with yes/no responses. The GDS-15 is the preferred choice for older adults due to its brevity and ease of use design. A cut-off score of five for GDS-15 indicates depression.
- *Patient Health Questionnaire (PHQ-9)*:[28] A 9-item self-rated assessment tool scored on a 4-point Likert scale, ranging from 0 = not at all, to 3 = nearly every day. An optimal cut-point of 5/6 indicates depression.
- *The Cornell Dysthymia Rating Scale (CDRS)*:[29] A 20-item clinician-rated inventory to assess milder symptomatology in chronically depressed patients, based on frequency and severity over the previous week. Items are scored from 0 to 4. The total score range is 0–80, where higher scores indicate greater severity of symptoms.

Neurologic Disease-specific Scales for Depression

- *Neurological Disorders Depression Inventory for Epilepsy (NDDI-E)*:[30] An epilepsy-specific, self-rated instrument for identifying and differentiating depression from possible antiseizure medication (ASM) side effects. It comprises six items, scored from four to one. The cut-off score > 15 represents moderate depression. A score > 2 on item 4, i.e., "I'd be better off dead" has been validated for suicidality.[31]
- *The Post Stroke Depression Rating Scale (PSDRS)*:[32] The PSDRS comprises 10 sections, each of which aims to evaluate a specific aspect of the emotional, affective, and vegetative disorders of stroke patients. The PSDRS does not provide a global score but a symptom profile of stroke patients.
- *Depression Intensity Scale Circles (DISC)*:[33] A 6-point ordinal graphic rating scale for the measurement of depression post-TBI.

Several depression rating scales, HAM-D, BDI, HADS, MADRS, GDS, and SDS have been validated and recommended in PD.[34,35]

Pathophysiology of Depression

Depression is a multifactorial disease that involves the complex interplay among genetic, neurobiological, anatomic, cognitive, and environmental aspects. The genome-wide association studies have indicated depression as a polygenic disorder with 30–40% heritability, and nongenetic factors explaining the remaining 60–70% of the variance in susceptibility to MDD. At the *neurobiological level of description* are various explanations:[36] Depleted levels of the monoamines—serotonin, dopamine, and norepinephrine being the most influential one; stress-induced dysfunction of hypothalamic-pituitary-adrenal (HPA) axis leading to elevated cortisol levels; the functional imbalance of the gamma-aminobutyric acid (GABA) and glutamate systems; deficit of neurotrophic support, i.e., brain-derived neurotrophic factor (BDNF) leading to neuronal atrophy, reduction of neurogenesis, and destruction of glia support promoting long-term depression in the hypothalamus; the immune-inflammatory response manifesting as the external phenotype of depressive behavior associated with stress/trauma/infection; recently the role of the microbiota-gut-brain axis that explains the common comorbidity of depression and gastrointestinal diseases; oxidant-antioxidant imbalance; circadian rhythm disturbances; and the reciprocal interaction between oxidative stress and inflammation have all been implicated in the epigenesis of depression, suggesting that depression is clinically and etiologically a heterogeneous disorder with inter-individual variability with respect to stress sensitivity and biological susceptibility to the development and maintenance of depressive symptoms.

At the *anatomical level of description,* the neuroimaging studies in patients with major depression, particularly in those exposed to chronic stress, show atrophy in the cortical and limbic areas, as well as decreased prefrontal cortex and hippocampal volumes.

At the *cognitive level of description,* depressive disorders have been associated with various abnormalities in information processing, broadly distinguishable into "cold" (i.e., emotion-independent)—observable in attention, executive function, and memory, and "hot" (i.e., emotion-dependent)—mood-congruent negative biases in processing of emotional stimuli;[37] and altered reward and punishment processing with hypersensitivity to negative and hyposensitivity to positive feedback.[38]

Neurological Disorders Associated with Depression

Depression in Epilepsy

Epidemiologic studies have shown that one in three people with epilepsy has a lifetime diagnosis of any psychiatric disorder, depression being the most frequent with a pooled prevalence of 23%,[39] and even higher rates at 32% have been reported in a recent community-based study from India.[40] Furthermore, suicides in people with epilepsy are also common, the standardized mortality ratio (SMR) reported as 5.1.[41]

Psychiatric disorders can precede, cooccur, or follow the diagnosis of epilepsy, with substantial evidence for the existence of a bidirectional relationship.[42] Common underlying neurobiological mechanisms operant in both epilepsy and depression, e.g., lesions of mesial temporal structures, and hippocampal volume loss shed light on the reasons for their coexistence and interlinking relationship. Many seizures have NPSs as overpowering and long-lasting consequences of dysregulated reverberating brain circuits.

Psychiatric symptoms in epilepsy may be directly linked to seizure activity and present periictally (preictal, ictal, or postictal) or temporally independent of seizure occurrence (interictally). The *preictal* symptoms of depression may be experienced within 3 days before the seizure, greatest during 24 hours preceding the seizure; *postictal,* when the symptoms of depression start within 3 days after the seizure and can outcast the ictus for up to 2 weeks; and *ictal,* when depressive symptoms are a part of the seizure semiology, e.g., depressed mood may occur as a focal seizure in some patients with temporal lobe epilepsy. The *inter-ictal* depression in epilepsy may present as an atypical pattern, not simply characterized by chronic dysthymic-like features, rather many patients may also present with mood instability and dysphoric symptoms. Blumer[43] coined the term *interictal dysphoric disorder* to refer to an affective-somatoform disorder typical of patients with chronic mesial temporal lobe epilepsy. Furthermore, depression as a part of the *iatrogenic* adverse events of ASMs and surgical treatment of epilepsy has been identified in patients with a current, past, and/or family history of depression.

Comorbid depression among people with epilepsy is associated with lower odds of seizure freedom, diminished quality of life, decreased treatment adherence, increased healthcare utilization leading to a higher economic burden for the patient, family and society as a whole, and increased risk of premature mortality. Psychiatric disorders, including depression, often remain undiagnosed and untreated among people with epilepsy, the depression treatment gap may be as high as 70%.[44,45] This can be potentially reduced by periodic screening in neurology clinics. The NDDIE is a convenient, cost-effective, sensitive and specific screening tool for depression in epilepsy in the clinic environment across a range of geographical and linguistic settings.[30]

Depression in Neurocognitive Disorders

Several patients with cognitive decline and dementia due to Alzheimer's disease (AD) and related conditions like PD, Lewy body disease (LBD), vascular dementia, and frontotemporal degeneration amongst other entities, experience depressive symptoms in greater or lesser grade at some point during the course of the illness. The prevalence of major depression averages around 16% in patients with all-cause neurocognitive disorders and 15% in AD.[46] In frontotemporal dementia (FTD), personality changes are accompanied by depression in 80% of the cases.[47]

Alzheimer's disease is the most frequent type of primary neurodegenerative dementia and one of the leading causes of disability in the elderly. Depression is a symptom of AD but may also represent a trait of the prodromal phase of the disease as well as a risk factor for AD suggesting common neurological pathways. The brain changes associated with depressive episodes that compromise the brain's ability to cope with stress, along with the genetic predisposition may lead to increased vulnerability toward the initiation of a detrimental neurodegenerative cascade. Depression has a strong negative influence on conversion to AD in mild cognitive impairment (MCI) patients. Depression, importantly, contributes to the "cognitive debt" (as opposed to "cognitive reserve") increasing the vulnerability to symptomatic AD.[48] Depression is a modifiable risk factor for Alzheimer's dementia, therefore, early detection and treatment are crucial. Antidepressants have limited efficacy, and the evidence, to date, is mixed. Rather, based on the theoretical rationale of the involvement of cholinergic system in depressive symptoms in Alzheimer's dementia, anti-dementia cholinesterase inhibitors may have a synergistic effect with antidepressants.[49] Recent research has shown the benefit of stronger cholinergic stimulation induced by associating donepezil with the cholinergic precursor choline alphoscerate, leading to higher brain acetylcholine bioavailability that promotes long-term improvement in depression.[50] Adjunctively, psychological treatments and exercise can help ameliorate the suffering of the patient and the burden of the caregivers.

Depression in Traumatic Brain Injury

Individuals with TBI are almost nine times more likely (53%) to have suffered from depression over 12 months post-TBI compared with a 12-month prevalence of all mood disorders at 6% in the general population.[51] TBI is unique among neuropsychiatric disorders because post-traumatic stress disorder (PTSD) can often result from the same traumatic etiology as brain injury. What's more, depression represents a dramatic risk factor for mortality through suicide. Depression is a limiting factor that interferes with rehabilitation and functional independence in the community. Depression also amplifies the cognitive burden after TBI.

Preexisting factors such as personal and family history of mood disorder, history of preinjury psychological trauma, and dysfunctional coping styles can have a cumulative effect with a resulting increase in depression risk post-TBI. Predictors of depression at 3 months post-TBI were found to be: high score on CES-D at 1 month, older age, and lesions on computed tomography brain scan.[52] Early postinjury depression is more likely to be associated with direct injury to the brain tissue in regions that regulate mood, while later postinjury depression is more related to the cognitive and psychosocial sequelae of living with the brain injury.

Despite the prolific psychiatric sequelae after TBI, the majority of patients with TBI and depression do not seek treatment. Untreated depression in TBI has been associated with poor quality of life, and poor psychosocial, functional, and vocational outcomes, following which the caregivers may also develop overwhelming distress and burden. As depression causes morbidity in itself post-TBI, therefore, early detection and treatment are important.

Depression in Movement Disorders

The confluence of studies over the past years has shown that depression may precede motor symptoms over a number of years. About 40–50% of patients with PD have clinically significant depression.[53] Factors that may increase the depression prevalence in PD include the history of depression, younger age, and the progression of the disease itself. Depression may be related to PD-induced genetic alterations, and also the structural changes that include subcortical-cortical neural pathway degeneration, neuronal loss of the substantia nigra, the presence of Lewy body inclusions, and a decline in monoamine neurotransmitter systems. Alternatively, depression may stem from a psychological reaction to PD, the stress and disability of this chronic and progressive disease. The presence of depression in PD also doubles the SMR for suicide than in the general population.[54] Treatment of depression among patients with PD is often successful and leads to improvement in activities of daily living and quality of life over time.

In HD, depression may occur as much as 20 years before motor onset and the depressive symptoms increase in temporal proximity to the clinical onset. Studies suggest that up to 76% of patients with Tourette syndrome experience some kind of mood symptoms, with 13% meeting clinical criteria for depression.[55] Mood symptoms have also been associated with other disorders such as progressive supranuclear palsy, multiple system atrophy, and corticobasal degeneration. Thus, patients with movement disorders should be routinely screened for depression so that adjunctive treatment can be instituted.

Depression in Multiple Sclerosis

Multiple sclerosis is an immune-mediated inflammatory and neurodegenerative demyelinating disease of the CNS. It has an unpredictable disease course which may be relapsing and remitting in some while progressive in others. The intrusiveness and ambiguity associated with MS bring to the fore psychological distress and depression. The pooled prevalence of depression in MS is reported to be 30.5%.[56] Depression in MS is not only reactive to a debilitating disease, but also dependent on structural and functional damage due to MS pathology. The early onset of MS (generally around 20 and 40 years of age) leads to psychosocial disruptions in education, employment, relationships, and life goals at large. Secondary consequences of depression in MS are increased risk of suicide and premature mortality, with SMR almost twice that expected in the general population.[57] The BDI-FS has been validated in MS patients for assessment of depression.[23] Alongside the common treatments that include antidepressants, cognitive behavior therapy (CBT), and rehabilitation through exercise training, bolstering resilience, hope, and grit in people with MS has shown positive results in reducing depression.[58]

Poststroke Depression

Post-stroke depression (PSD) is one of the most frequent and serious neuropsychiatric sequelae of stroke and is strongly associated with high morbidity and mortality. In stroke survivors, PSD represents a huge obstacle to participation in rehabilitation and functional independence, leading to poor quality of life. Approximately, one in three stroke survivors suffer from PSD, and within 2 years, the incidence of PSD a range from 11 to 41%.[59] Much of the burden of stroke and PSD is borne by LMICs. In India, PSD is present in about half of stroke survivors, with a pooled prevalence of 55%.[60] Interestingly, depression itself is a risk factor for stroke, with meta-analysis indicating that depression is associated with a 34–45% increase in stroke risk compared with the general population. There are two different types of PSD—major depression and minor depression; the former is considered as a form of endogenous depression observed in patients with lesions encroaching on the left frontal lobes and the underlying basal ganglia, and the latter, a form of dysthymic (neurotic or reactive) depression with no specific anatomic correlates.

The risk factors for developing PSD include genetic factors that confer vulnerability/resilience, prior medical and psychiatric history, type and severity of the stroke, lesion location, degree of disability, social support, and so on. The patient acceptance of their condition plays a major part in the way that patients experience their illness and can help in achieving greater functional capacity and mobility poststroke rehabilitation.

Migraine and Depression

Persons with migraine have a three to six times elevated risk of depression compared with controls with no history of headaches.[61] Depression affects almost 80% of migraine sufferers at one time or another.[62] Major depression increases the risk for migraine, and migraine increases the risk for major depression, this bidirectional association points to shared etiological factors that include serotonergic dysfunction, hormonal influences, and sensitization of the sensory and emotional neural networks. There is a 40–50% heritable association between migraine and MDD.[63] Further, greater psychiatric comorbidity exists for migraine with aura than without, and is higher in chronic migraine than episodic migraine. Noteworthy is the fact that acute depressive symptomatology is not present during the prodromal phase but emerges only during a migraine attack and at the moment of a forthcoming attack,[64] distinguishing the "trait" lifetime depression in migraine patients and the "state" acute depressive symptoms during a migraine attack. It is important to identify and treat the presence of comorbid depression, which can lead to migraine chronification and make the person refractory to migraine treatment leading to medication overuse and disability.

Management and Treatment of Depression

Psychotherapy

Psychotherapy is especially important in the context of neurological disorders. It is important to provide *psychoeducation* that involves the dissemination of knowledge and education regarding the illness and its treatment, the comorbid conditions, and lifestyle challenges. This helps the patients to understand their symptoms better, e.g., the therapist explains as to what happens in the patient's brain to cause symptoms and what they can do to create new circuits in the brain, thereby encouraging neuroplasticity; and *normalization*, i.e., the person is guided to view the distress as common and understandable.

Cognitive behavior therapy is the dominant force in psychotherapy. With increased focus on evidence-based practice, CBT has continued to evolve, with three overlapping but distinct generations:[65] The first wave of behavior therapy focused upon learning principles of classical and operant conditioning; the traditional second wave CBT based upon *identifying* and cognitively *reframing* and *restructuring* the dysfunctional *automatic thoughts*, *cognitive distortions* and *schemas* to bring about healthy changes in *behavior*; and the third-wave CBT builds upon the first two to be more effective. This is more *process-oriented* emphasizing contextual and experiential change strategies with *psychological (or experiential) acceptance*—acceptance of one's ongoing subjective experience, *mindfulness*—nonjudgmentally becoming aware of the thought processes in the "here and now", *decentering and defusion*—experiencing subjective events and thoughts from a psychological distance as mere mental events rather than as reflections on the world or the self, and *metacognition*—knowledge of one's cognitive processes, being the key constructs.

Pharmacotherapy

Neurologists should be capable of managing mild-to-moderate comorbid depression but referral to mental health specialists is mandatory in severe depression with suicidality. Selective serotonin reuptake inhibitors (SSRIs) and serotonin and norepinephrine reuptake inhibitors (SNRIs) are the preferred first-line medication choices for the treatment of depression. Atypical antidepressants like bupropion and mirtazapine can also be used as first-line treatments in certain patient populations. Benzodiazepines and electroconvulsive therapy (ECT) are frequently used in patients with depression plus catatonic features. SNRIs are used frequently in patients with pain. Bupropion and duloxetine are used in patients with low energy or fatigue. Tricyclic antidepressants and monoamine oxidase inhibitors (MAOIs), because of their adverse effects, are usually reserved for patients who have treatment-resistant depression (TRD). A patient with bipolar depression would be a good candidate for mood stabilizer medications such as lamotrigine. For patients with depression in the context of bipolar spectrum syndrome, an antidepressant may convert the patient to manic or hypomanic symptoms, therefore, accurate diagnosis is important.

Somatic Treatments

Somatic treatments are nonpharmacologic interventions that involve brain stimulation, achieved by different technological methods, e.g., using light, electricity, and magnetism to induce neurochemical changes within specific regions of the brain. These are promising options for patients with TRD.

Electroconvulsive therapy involves brief electrical stimulation of the brain using two electrodes applied to the surface of the head unilaterally or bilaterally under general anesthesia. It is one of the mainstay treatments for drug-resistant psychiatric disorders such as depression and psychosis with efficacy well-established over the decades. There are other novel brain stimulation techniques as well. *Repetitive transcranial magnetic stimulation* (rTMS) is a noninvasive technique of using magnetic stimulation, with a TMS device, to achieve neural stimulation and cortical excitability in specific regions of the brain, e.g., the prefrontal cortex involved in mood regulation. *Vagus nerve stimulation (VNS),* at the outset, was approved for refractory epilepsy in Europe in 1994 and in the US in 1997, with clinical observations of improvement in mood symptoms, as well. In Psychiatry, VNS has evolved as adjunctive therapy for TRD. The procedure involves surgically implanting a small electrical pulse generator in the upper-left side of the chest, which is further connected through the wires to stimulate the vagus nerve in the brain. The electrical pulses are monitored and modified periodically by a neurologist. This procedure modulates signals sent from the vagus nerve to cortico-limbic-thalamic-striatal regions of the brain involved in mood regulation. *Deep brain stimulation* (DBS) is a surgical treatment involving the implantation of a pacemaker-like device that sends electrical impulses to specific parts of the brain. DBS has been approved for treating tremors, dystonia, and PD, and has also shown some promise with TRD. *Transcranial direct current stimulation* applies a low-frequency electrical current over the scalp and can improve symptoms of nontreatment-resistant MDD. *Phototherapy (light therapy)* involves controlled exposure to the intense light of at least 10,000 lux daily for 2–5 weeks, particularly effective for patients with the seasonal affective disorder (SAD). The light influences the hypothalamus, and possibly via altered melatonin production affects circadian and seasonal rhythms.

PSYCHOSIS

Psychosis is a psychiatric condition that arises with considerable frequency in several neurological conditions, and the prevalence varies by the neurologic condition studied. This chapter is intended to educate the neurologist on the psychiatric manifestations of psychosis and its evaluation, diagnosis, and management. How to differentiate a primary psychotic disorder from psychosis secondary to a medical or neurologic condition is also reviewed.

Defining Psychosis

Psychosis is a clinical construct composed of several symptoms implying a change in perception of reality, i.e., impairment in *reality testing*, whereby the person is unable to distinguish the internal experience of the mind and external reality. Historically, Feuchtersleben is credited with first employing the term *psychosis* in 1845, as a synonym for psychopathy.[66] Emil Kraepelin, a German psychiatrist introduced psychotic disorders to neurology, medicine, and the world on the eve of the 20th century and proposed three major types of psychosis: manic-depressive psychosis, paranoia, and *dementia praecox* which is Latin for "premature mental deterioration".[67] Eugen Bleuler followed Kraepelin and coined the term *schizophrenia*, meaning "split mind" (from Greek *schiz-*, or "divide," and *phren*, or "mind").[68] Over the years, the DSM has continuously modified the construct to achieve greater diagnostic precision. In the DSM, 5th Edition, the chapter, "Schizophrenia Spectrum and Other Psychotic Disorders" states that these disorders are defined by abnormalities in one or more of these five domains—(1) hallucinations, (2) delusions, (3) disorganized thinking (speech), (4) grossly disorganized or abnormal motor behavior (including catatonia), and (5) negative symptoms.

The clinical features of psychosis have typically been classified as being *"positive"* or *"negative"*. Positive symptoms are characterized by an excess or distortion of normal function, including hallucinations, delusions, and positive thought disorder (disorganized language output). Negative symptoms are characterized by an absence or lack of normal mental functions in patients, but are present in healthy individuals, e.g., apathy and anhedonia.

To diagnose patients with psychosis, clinicians need to be able to evaluate and assess the aforementioned symptom domains.

Delusions

The DSM-5 defines *delusions* as "fixed false beliefs that are not amenable to change in light of conflicting evidence". Delusions are based on incorrect (false) inferences about reality external to, or about, oneself and held with incorrigible certainty despite every incontrovertible evidence to the contrary. The delusions can be *nonbizarre* or *bizarre*. Nonbizarre delusions derive from a misinterpretation of everyday experiences and, as such, are understandable. For example, being infected by a disease, being followed, or being loved at a distance by someone famous. Bizarre delusions involve phenomena that could never happen in real life and are not understandable to most people in that person's culture, e.g., being cloned by an alien. Another way to classify delusions would be based on the nature of delusions or the themes/content **(Table 1)**.

Furthermore, delusions can be *primary* or *secondary*. Primary delusions are unmediated by thought, understandable and psychologically irreducible, e.g., seeing a man in a crisp black suit as an assassin who is sent to kill the patient. On the other hand, secondary delusions are understandable in the context of preceding affect and experience or some other psychopathologic condition, e.g., a depressed person with delusional guilt.

Delusions are contrasted with *overvalued ideas*, which have strong emotional content and tend to polarize thinking but are still open to reason. Delusions are distinct from *confabulation*, poor memory function may manifest as confabulation. Often inconsistent statements which are neither firm nor fixed may be believed at the moment but soon forgotten, while the persistence of a belief suggests delusion.

Delusional Misidentification Syndromes

Delusional misidentification syndromes (DMSs) are defined by misidentification or impairment in the recognition of one or more people despite the normally functioning sensory recognition pathways **(Table 2)**. Phenomenologically, DMS may be divided into two types—(1) delusional hypoidentification (e.g., Capgras syndrome), or (2) delusional hyperidentification (e.g., Fregoli, intermetamorphosis, subjective doubles syndromes). Misidentification syndromes show a great degree of overlap and at times may evolve into another type. Neuropsychological testing in patients with DMS shows subtle abnormalities in facial recognition with nondominant cerebral compromise. The differential diagnosis is prosopagnosia which is simply a failure to visually recognize familiar faces with a preserved ability to recognize those very familiar people through other sense modalities (e.g., voice and gait), and emotional connection is intact.

Hallucinations

According to DSM-5, "hallucinations are perception-like experiences that occur without an external stimulus".

TABLE 1: Delusional themes.

Delusions	Description	Examples from patients' history
Persecutory delusions	Most common type. The belief that one (or someone close to them) is being plotted against, spied upon, threatened, or harmed	• The food is poisoned • The police are following them
Delusion of theft	The most prevalent delusion in the elderly. The patient believes that one's valuables are being stolen; tends to develop in the context of declarative memory impairments (e.g., Alzheimer's disease)	An 88-year-old woman places her wallet under her pillow as safe-keeping, believing that someone is stealing it
Grandiose delusions/ megalomania	Grandiose beliefs about oneself, one's abilities, wealth, power, knowledge, or fame; these may crystallize into a stable delusional identity	The patient saying that he is known to all the bureaucrats of the country
Referential delusions	Belief that certain gestures, comments, environmental cues, and so forth are directed at oneself	Their lives are depicted on TV or in news stories
Somatic delusions	Irrational beliefs about a person's own body	A 69-year-old female patient believing she is pregnant
Religious delusions	Believing that one is God or an angel, or otherwise deific	• "I am Guru Gobind Singh Ji's son" • "I am Jesus Christ"
Delusion of sin and guilt	The belief that one has committed "the unpardonable sin" or has inflicted great harm on others	They have killed their children
Nihilistic delusions (Cotard's syndrome)	Belief that one (or even one's organs or body parts) or others or the whole world has ceased to exist. A major catastrophe will occur	The patient believes that the right side of his body is rotting
Erotomanic delusions (de Clérambault's syndrome)	Belief that a famous person is in love with them	Bill Clinton is in love with her
Delusions of control/influence	Belief that a person's will, thoughts, or feelings are under the control of external forces, often by means of electronic devices that send signals directly to the brain. • *Thought insertion*: Alien thoughts are being inserted into one's head • *Thought withdrawal*: Outside forces are removing thoughts from one's head • *Thought broadcasting*: The belief that one's thoughts are being broadcast to the outside world so that everyone can hear them	• The government is planting thoughts in their mind • The aliens are stealing their thoughts • Their thoughts are being broadcasted by the TV and radio
Delusions of mind reading	Belief that other people can read their mind or know their thoughts	The neighbor has a device to know his/her thoughts
Delusional parasitosis	Belief that they are infested with insects, lice, or vermin	The patient pulls out worms from his body
Delusions of infidelity/jealousy (Othello syndrome)	Belief that one's spouse or lover is unfaithful	The husband places a recorder by his bedside every night, saying he has the recordings of his wife talk to another man all night
Phantom boarder syndrome	Unseen and unwelcome guests are living in the home	A woman reported to the police that a male intruder has been living on the roof of her house
Incubus syndrome	The patient is visited by demon or phantom lover	The patient believes that he is being sexually approached by an unforeseen lover

They may occur in any sensory modality—auditory, visual, olfactory, gustatory, tactile, nociceptive, thermoceptive, proprioceptive, and others; but auditory hallucinations are most common in schizophrenia and related disorders, while visual hallucinations (VHs) are most common in neurological disorders.

Auditory hallucinations: Typically, auditory hallucinations involve hearing voices, familiar or unfamiliar. The patient may hear one voice or multiple voices, either talking to the patient or talking to each other. The voices may say derogatory things about the patient, such as "You're worthless" or "You're a failure," or the voices may command the patient

TABLE 2: Delusional misidentification syndromes.

Misidentification syndrome	Content
Capgras syndrome	False belief that significant people have been replaced by identical appearing imposters
Fregoli syndrome	Patients believe that a persecutor is capable of changing forms, taking on the appearance of others (the persecutor being accused of changing faces like an actor)
Intermetamorphosis	Patients believe that familiar people and strangers in the environment swap identities while maintaining their original appearance (a variant of Fregoli syndrome)
Subjective doubles syndrome/ heautoscopy/doppelganger	The patient has a twin or second half with the same appearance, but different character traits, living their own life
Lycanthropy (werewolfism)	The patient is episodically transformed into a wolf
Mirror sign	Delusion that one's reflection in a mirror is someone else
TV sign	The patient believes that images/events on television are real, and believed to be occurring in external 3D space
Delusional companion syndrome	The misperception that non-living objects possess consciousness, can think independently, and feel emotions
Clonal pluralization of the self	The patient believes that multiple copies of themselves, psychologically and physically similar, exist
Delusional hermaphroditism	Belief that oneself and a friend of the opposite sex have been incorporated in the same body
Reduplicative paramnesia	A state in which patients believe they are simultaneously in two geographical locations
Nurturing syndrome	Deceased family members believed as still living

to do things—command hallucinations, e.g., "Jump from the terrace", "Go to the next house and kill your boyfriend".

Visual hallucinations: Patients may say they can see dead family members or individuals/faces unknown to them. Patients with neurological conditions often have VH.

Tactile, olfactory, and gustatory hallucinations: Tactile, olfactory, and gustatory hallucinations are unusual in a primary psychotic disorder, and their presence suggests a differential diagnosis of other underlying medical or neurologic causes. Patients with delirium may complain of a sensation of ants crawling on the skin. Olfactory hallucinations of burning or unpleasant smells may be a sign of mesial temporal lobe seizures. 15% of patients with seizures from temporal lobe tumor will have olfactory or gustatory auras.[69]

Hallucinations can also occur transiently when an individual is under extreme physiologic or psychological stress as sensory deprivation, bereavement, severe fatigue, etc. *Hypnagogic* (occur while the person is falling asleep) *and hypnopompic hallucinations* (occur while the person is waking up) can be mistaken for nightmares but are common perceptual phenomena occurring during the sleep transition. Hallucination can also be clinically mistaken for an *illusion*, which is a distorted version of an objective sensory stimulus. Some other perceptual disturbances that should be considered for differential diagnosis of hallucinations are described in **Box 2**.

BOX 2 Perceptual disturbances in the differential diagnosis of hallucinations.

- *Derealization*: One perceives the external world as unreal
- *Depersonalization*: One's own thoughts and feelings seem unreal and the person feels detached from one's own persona
- *Pseudohallucination*: A vivid sensory experience but the individual recognizes that it is not an external stimulus but it is coming from their mind
- *Illusion*: Misperception of a sensory stimulus, e.g., seeing a snake for a rope
- *Palinopsia*: Persistent perception of a visual stimulus after that stimulus is no longer present (afterimages)
- *Synesthesia*: A perceptual condition in which external stimulus in one sensory modality elicits a concurrent sensation in another. For example, the patients says, "I can hear the scenery and see the music"
- *Déjà vu*: Perceiving/experiencing a novel image or scene as one previously witnessed or experienced
- *Deja entendu*: Perceiving/experiencing a novel sound as one previously witnessed or experienced
- *Jamais vu*: Perceiving/experiencing a familiar image or scene as unfamiliar
- *Jamais entendu*: Perceiving/experiencing a familiar sound as unfamiliar
- *Autoscopy*: Seeing one's body from a position outside the (i.e., out-of-body experience)

Disorganized Thinking (Speech)

Different patterns of disruption of speech can occur. **Table 3** lists formal thought disorders and associated speech patterns.

Grossly Disorganized or Abnormal Motor Behavior (Including Catatonia)

Disorganized behavior may manifest in various forms as a disheveled appearance, inappropriate laughing, childlike behavior, or inappropriate and unpredictable agitation. Disorganized behavior may lead to the patient's inability to

TABLE 3: Formal thought disorders.

Thought disorder	Associated speech pattern
Impoverished thought/poverty of speech (laconic speech)	Vague, inadequate
Tangentiality	This is marked by oblique speech in which the patient constantly digresses to irrelevant topics and fails to arrive at the main point. Example: Doctor: "Have you had any trouble sleeping lately?" Patient: "I usually sleep in my bed, but now I'm sleeping on the sofa"
Circumstantiality	Circuitous, indirect speech in which the individual digresses to give nonessential and trivial details before arriving at the main point. This differs from tangentially in that the main point is never lost
Neologisms	The invention of new words or phrases or the use of conventional words in idiosyncratic ways, words not found in even the most comprehensive dictionary. Example, "hangages" for hang together, "goodship" for doing good things
Paraphasias	Unintended utterances with substitution of words at the phonemic level, e.g., hen for pen, or at the semantic level, e.g., car for van
Clang associations	Thoughts associated by the pairing of words that have no relation to one another beyond the fact that they rhyme or sound alike
Perseveration	Repetition of out-of-context words, phrases, or ideas
Stereotypy	Repetition of words or phrases
Echolalia	Mechanical repetition of words and phrases addressed to the patient
Preoccupation	Repeated reference to one major idea
Flight of ideas	A rapid, continuous succession of superficially related thoughts and ideas, manifest as rapid pressurized speech with abrupt shifts in topic
Thought blocking	A sudden disruption of thought or a break in the flow of ideas, and the patient suddenly falls silent with no memory of what he/she was talking about
Derailment (loose associations)	A breakdown in both the logical connection between ideas and the overall sense of goal directedness; the words make sentences, but the sentences do not make sense
Word salad	A complete breakdown of the associational process, so it becomes impossible for the listener to trace any links between successive words and phrases
Concretism	Excessively literal
Stilted speech	Excessively formal, pompous, distant, overpolite
Excessive self-reference	Theme of speech returns to oneself repeatedly and regardless of content of the conversation
Metonyms	Attribution of private meaning to real words
Preoccupation	Repetitive reference to one major idea
Paleological thought	Prelogical thinking with concrete superficial content, excludes logic and reasoning, as occurs in children

complete goal-directed activities, leading to difficulties in performing activities of daily living.

A catatonia is an extreme form of abnormal motor behavior. The DSM-5 diagnostic criteria require the presence of at least three of the following 12 symptoms—stupor, cataplexy, waxy flexibility, mutism, negativism, posturing, mannerism, stereotypy, agitation, grimacing, echolalia, and echopraxia. Catatonia may be associated with another mental disorder or another medical condition or unspecified. The presence of catatonia can cause clinically significant distress or impairment in social, occupational, or other important areas of functioning.

Negative Symptoms

Negative symptoms are more prominently seen in schizophrenia and account for a substantial portion of the disease morbidity. Negative symptoms include diminished emotional expression (flat affect), avolition (lack of voluntary behavior), apathy (lack of motivation), alogia (poverty of speech), anhedonia (decreased ability to experience pleasure), and asociality (lack of interest in social interactions). A predominance of negative symptoms is often associated with poor prognosis.

Cognitive Symptoms

Cognitive symptoms, though *not* listed in DSM-5, are included here, as dysfunction in cognition, metacognition, social cognition, and motivation have a significant impact on patient's functional status which is the key element of recovery and success in daily and community living. Cognition is the mental process of acquiring knowledge and understanding through thought, experience, and the senses. Metacognition refers to the knowledge and regulation of one's cognitive processes. Social cognition includes the ability to identify and interpret social cues (e.g., detecting emotion in faces, and inferring what other people are thinking or feeling). The patient's lack of motivation to engage in the community is part of the negative symptoms of schizophrenia.

Schizophrenia Spectrum and Other Disorders

The disorders under this section of DSM-5, described along a gradient of psychopathology include:

Schizotypal (Personality) Disorder

The DSM-5 diagnostic criteria include five of the following nine symptoms—ideas of reference, excessive social anxiety associated with paranoid fears, odd beliefs or magical thinking (e.g., clairvoyance, telepathy, sixth sense), unusual perceptual experiences and illusions, eccentric behavior or appearance, lack of close friends or confidants, odd thinking and speech, inappropriate affect, and paranoid ideation, leading to significant impairments in personality and interpersonal functioning.

Delusional Disorder

Predominant delusional disorder is the presence of one or more delusions with a duration of one month or longer. Hallucinations are not prominent, and if present are related to the delusional theme. Functioning is not markedly impaired and behavior is not noticeably bizarre.

Brief Psychotic Disorder

One or more of the following psychotic symptoms, i.e., delusions, hallucinations, disorganized speech, and grossly disorganized or catatonic behavior is present for at least one day but less than 1 month, eventually with a complete return to a premorbid level of functioning.

Schizophreniform Disorder

Two or more of the following psychotic symptoms, i.e., delusions, hallucinations, disorganized speech, grossly disorganized or catatonic behavior, and negative symptoms are present for at least 1 month but <6 months.

Schizophrenia

Two or more of the following psychotic symptoms, i.e., delusions, hallucinations, disorganized speech, grossly disorganized or catatonic behavior, and negative symptoms are present for at least 6 months with 1 month of the active phase symptoms and the rest including periods of prodromal or residual symptoms.

Schizoaffective Disorder

The diagnosis of the schizoaffective disorder requires an uninterrupted period of active or residual symptoms of psychosis during which core symptoms of schizophrenia are met (for 2 or more weeks), along with a major mood episode (present for the majority of the total duration of the illness). It is differentiated from affective disorders, such as MDD with psychotic features and bipolar I disorder, where the primary aberration is affective in nature.

Substance/Medication-induced Psychotic Disorder

Presence of delusions and/or hallucinations associated with substance intoxication or withdrawal or exposure to a medication.

Psychotic Disorder due to Another Medical Condition

These are secondary psychotic disorders (discussed in a forthcoming section of this chapter) with prominent delusions or hallucinations attributed to another medical condition.

Unspecified and Other Specified Schizophrenia Spectrum and Other Psychotic Disorders

The unspecified and the specified categories are applied to presentations when the symptoms characteristic of schizophrenia spectrum and other psychotic disorders do not meet the full criteria but cause clinically significant distress or impairment in social, occupational, or other important areas of functioning. The unspecified category is used when there is insufficient information to make a more specific diagnosis, or in situations in which the clinician chooses not to specify the reason that the criteria are not fully met (e.g., emergency room settings). In the specified category, the clinician chooses to specify the reasons with designations such as, persistent auditory hallucinations, delusions with significant overlapping mood episodes, attenuated psychosis syndrome, and delusional symptoms in the partner of an individual with delusional disorder.

Pathophysiology of Psychosis

Emerging evidence supports significant connections between psychosis and structural and functional brain changes in both primary psychotic and neurologic disorders.

Neurotransmitters in psychosis: The neurotransmitter dysfunction in psychosis includes overactivation of dopamine function in the brain, particularly the mesolimbic pathway; dysfunction of the excitatory neurotransmitter, glutamate with decreased function of N-methyl-D-aspartate (NMDA) glutamate receptor; dysfunction of gamma-amino-butyric acid (GABA), an important inhibitory neurotransmitter; and lastly, an imbalance in acetylcholine.

Neurodevelopmental factors in psychosis: Psychosis is due to abnormal synaptic pruning during neurodevelopment, known as the synaptic-pruning hypothesis. Exposure to prenatal environmental insults (e.g., maternal infections, drug toxicity, and nutritional deficiencies), birth complications, postnatal trauma, and various forms of deprivation at critical stages of development is associated with a risk of subsequent psychotic disorders.

Genetic factors in psychosis: Psychosis is a heritable condition, where genes controlling synaptic neurotransmission, particularly genes involving pathways mediated by dopamine and glutamate are associated with psychosis. Chromosome 22q11.2 microdeletion is the most common genetic abnormality associated with a psychotic disorder.

According to the *neuroimaging perspective*, total gray and white matter, as well as whole brain volume is reduced in patients with psychosis compared with those in healthy controls, and ventricular volume is increased.

Autoimmune and inflammatory mechanisms are responsible for the manifestation of psychosis in diseases like systemic lupus erythematosus (SLE) and immune encephalitis (particularly, the autoantibodies of NMDAR type).

Many hypothetical frameworks are possible for VH in neurologic conditions. VHs in psychosis may be due to: The imbalance between top-down and bottom-up aspects of perception, e.g., hallucinations in dementia or PD; chronic deafferentiation causing hyperexcitability to the cortical structures involved in vision, e.g., VH in Charles Bonnet syndrome; misattribution of internal imagery—hallucinations, whatever their modality, result from a failure to correctly attribute internal events as internal due to failures in source monitoring. Peduncular hallucinosis has been postulated to be a release phenomenon related to damage to the ascending reticular activating system. Hallucinations may occur transiently under extreme physiologic or psychological stress.

Scales for Assessment of Psychosis

Psychotic symptoms are challenging to diagnose in the context of cognitive decline. Some of the widely used and recommended scales in the neurological setting are outlined here.

Brief Psychiatric Rating Scale—expanded 24-item version (BPRS, Version 4.0):[70] A clinician-rated scale, designed as a semistructured interview, comprising 24 symptom constructs, each on a 7-point scale ranging from "not present" to "extremely severe". A score on any construct ≥4 represents clinically significant moderate symptoms. The BPRS is a valid transdiagnostic measurement tool, capable of reliably capturing psychopathological symptoms in a wide range of diagnostic categories.[71]

Neuropsychiatric Inventory (NPI):[72] An informant-based scale includes 10 neuropsychiatric domains—delusions, hallucinations, agitation, depression, anxiety, euphoria, apathy, disinhibition, irritability, and aberrant motor activity, and two psychosomatic domains—disturbed sleep and appetite, all rated for frequency from 1 (occasionally, <once/week) to 4 (very frequently—once/day or more) and severity from 1 (mild) to 3 (marked). The total score for each domain is frequency x severity. If the symptom is not present, the score is zero.

Positive and Negative Symptom Scale (PANSS):[73] Comprises 30 distinct items organized into three independent scales—the negative symptoms subscale, the positive subscale, and the general psychopathology subscale. The score range is 30–120 points. The PANSS is considered a gold standard measure of treatment efficacy and is a reliable means of assessing patients chronologically throughout the course of their illness.

Scale for the Assessment of Negative Symptoms (SANS):[74] Measures negative symptoms on a 25 item, 6-point scale. Items are listed under five domains of affective blunting, alogia, avolition/apathy, anhedonia/asociality, and attention.

Since the understanding of negative symptoms has evolved, two next-generation 13-item negative symptom scales have been developed—the *CAINS (Clinical Assessment Interview for Negative Symptoms),*[75] and *BNSS (Brief Negative Symptom Scale).*[76]

Scale for the Assessment of Positive Symptoms (SAPS):[74] Measures positive symptoms on a 34 item, 6-point scale. Items are listed under hallucinations, delusions, bizarre behavior, and positive formal thought disorder. A nine-item SAPS for PD, developed from SAPS has been used in a trial of pimavanserin for PD psychosis.[77]

Several scales have been developed to focus exclusively on psychosis in PD. A recommended selection of the scales includes:[78] The *PD nonmotor symptom scale*[79], subscores of the *MDS-UPDRS-I scale, item 1.2,*[80] the *Parkinson Psychosis Questionnaire (PPQ),*[81] the *SAPS,*[82] and the *Scale for Evaluation of Neuropsychiatric Disorders in PD (SEND-PD).*[83]

Secondary Psychotic Disorders

The acute onset of hallucinations and delusions, especially in elderly patients with no known history of previous psychiatric disorders should prompt a thorough workup for secondary or neurologic causes of psychotic symptoms. When psychotic symptoms develop in association with cognitive impairments due to neurodegenerative conditions like AD, PD, diffuse LBD, frontotemporal lobar degeneration, HD, prion disease, cerebrovascular disease, TBI, human immunodeficiency virus (HIV), and substances/medications, among others, the DSM-5 suggests qualifying the neurocognitive disorder diagnosis with the specifier "with behavioral disturbance (psychosis)" rather than offering a concurrent primary psychotic disorder diagnosis. When hallucinations or delusions predominate the clinical presentation, are not better explained by another mental disorder, are not merely symptoms of delirium, are functionally impairing or distressing, and when there is evidence that their occurrence is pathophysiologically linked to either a neurologic or medical condition or substance abuse or medication, then a diagnosis of, psychotic disorder due to another medical condition, or substance/medication-induced psychotic disorder, respectively, may be made. The following section reviews psychotic symptoms in neurologic conditions that are commonly seen in clinical practice.

Psychosis of Epilepsy

Psychotic disorders represent relatively rare but serious comorbidity of epilepsy. Psychosis develops in 5.6% of people with epilepsy, and the prevalence reaches up to 7% for temporal lobe seizures,[84] this is seven times higher than the frequency of primary psychotic disorders in the general population which ranges between 0.4 and 1%.[85] Also patients with a primary psychotic disorder are at greater risk of developing epilepsy than the general population, suggesting a complex and bidirectional relationship between epilepsy and psychosis.

Psychosis of epilepsy (POE) comprises a group of disorders with distinct phenomenology and etiopathogenic mechanisms that are closely associated with the seizure disorder. Based on the temporal relationship between the psychotic symptoms and the occurrence of seizures, POE can be ictal, postictal, and interictal. In *ictal psychosis*, the psychotic symptoms are the clinical expression of the seizure and occur suddenly and concurrently with epileptic discharges, manifesting with behavioral changes, affective disturbances, fear, anxiety, fluctuation of consciousness, and thought incoherence. Delusions and hallucinations occur but less frequently than in postictal psychosis. Ictal hallucinations are usually brief and stereotyped and include visual and, less frequently, auditory hallucinations. In contrast to "psychotic hallucinations", patients can realize that their hallucinations reflect unreal phenomena. *Postictal psychosis* has a prevalence of 2% in people with epilepsy,[84] and occurs up to 120 hours after the seizure. Various delusions (persecutory, grandiose, somatic, and religious), hallucinations, and affective symptoms (manic or depressive) are the key manifestations of postictal psychosis. Unlike other postictal behavioral symptoms that typically resolve within hours or days, postictal psychosis can last up to 3 months. In *interictal psychosis*, the psychotic episodes are independent of seizures. The clinical features resemble to schizophrenia, however, with subtle clinical differences such as acute onset, more frequent VHs, absence of negative symptoms, and relatively better preserved premorbid personality in epileptic psychosis. The psychosis is less severe and more responsive to pharmacotherapy.

Another manifestation of POE is *Landolt's phenomenon* known as *alternative psychosis*, or *forced normalization*, describing a paradoxical inverse relation between a reduction in seizure burden and the appearance of psychotic symptoms in patients with intractable epilepsy. There is also improvement in EEG activity during periods of abnormal behavior.[86,87] Forced normalization is an uncommon phenomenon with a prevalence estimated at approximately 1% of patients with intractable epilepsy.[88]

Additionally, POE may be the expression of an iatrogenic process to pharmacologic and/or surgical interventions, particularly anterior temporal lobe resections.

An important concern about treating POE is that pharmacological treatments may lower the seizure threshold. Therefore, treatment should be exercised with extreme caution, the drugs of choice being atypical antipsychotics like olanzapine, quetiapine, and risperidone which carry a lesser risk of increasing seizures.

Psychosis in Delirium

Delirium is a severe neuropsychiatric syndrome with psychosis reported in 43%, VHs and delusions being the most common, reported in one-fourth of patients with delirium.[89] Hallucinations and delusions, when present, can be a part of the constellation of symptoms defining delirium, and may be easily mistaken for a psychiatric disorder. It should be remembered that new-onset psychotic symptoms in older adult patients are unlikely to be a primary mental illness, and a search for potentially reversible causes of delirium should be carried out.

The term intensive care unit (ICU) psychosis describes a cluster of psychiatric symptoms in the, particularly, deliriogenic ICU environment characterized by sleep deprivation and sensory overload or monotony. However, the term "ICU psychosis" is a dangerous misnomer because it impedes standardized research and communication, and may reduce the vigilance necessary to promptly investigate and reverse the medical cause of the delirium. The main cause of ICU psychosis is the underlying medical factors. The signs and symptoms of ICU psychosis are consistent with delirium which may be hyperactive, hypoactive, or mixed with different signs and symptoms of both. The novel Confusion Assessment Method for the ICU (CAM-ICU-7) Delirium Severity Assessment Scale is a valid and reliable delirium severity measure among ICU patients.[90] Antipsychotic drugs have no effect on delirium severity, symptom resolution, or mortality reflecting substantial gaps in our understanding of its pathophysiology.

Of note is the association between delirium and dementia with Lewy bodies (DLB) that share certain key features—psychotic symptoms with prominent VHs; fluctuations of cognition and consciousness; and a similar pattern of cognitive deficits with prominent impairments in attention, working memory, and visuoperception present in both delirium and DLB. Therefore, when delirium is resolved, the neurologist should thoroughly evaluate patients for cognitive impairment and other features of DLB.

Psychosis in Alzheimer's Disease

While dementia is classically defined by cognitive impairment, almost all AD patients exhibit a wide range of NPSs, such as aggression, depression, apathy, and alterations in perception (hallucinations) or thought (delusions) that represent the major areas to be probed in the course of diagnostic assessment. A systematic review reported psychosis in 41% of people with AD, 23% had delusions only, 5% had hallucinations only, and 13% had both.[91] Delusions in AD have been described since 1907 with Alois Alzheimer's index case of Auguste Deter, a 51-year-old woman, who presented initially with emotional distress and delusions of infidelity and persecution, followed by cognitive impairment. DMS, when present, are secondary to degeneration of the parietotemporal region affecting face recognition systems.

Among non-AD dementias, psychosis is most prevalent, persistent and intense in DLB (75% prevalence), followed by PD dementia (50%), vascular dementia (15%), and FTD (10%).[92]

Psychosis in Frontotemporal Lobar Degeneration

Patients with behavioral-variant FTD (bvFTD) do not fulfill the DSM diagnostic criteria for a psychiatric disorder more often than patients with other neurodegenerative conditions. In bvFTD, inappropriate behavior can be substantially attributed to a profound loss of social cognition, that is, the ability to read other people's minds and to anticipate their reactions, which is one of the first symptoms to appear. Delusions have been reported to be the presenting NPS in 21% of patients with bvFTD characterized by paranoid, persecutory, and even bizarre content.[93] Delusions of misidentification and grandiosity also occur.

Psychosis in Dementia with Lewy Bodies

Psychotic symptoms in DLB often occur before the onset of cognitive impairment, and the frequency of onset of psychotic symptoms is reported as high as 42%.[94] Three typical forms of prodromal DLB have been proposed—MCI-onset, delirium-onset DLB, and psychiatric-onset DLB.[95] The psychiatric-onset stage is characterized by three principal psychotic features—catatonia, delusions-hallucinations, and depression and/or mania.[96]

Visual hallucinations are common in DLB. Pareidolia, the tendency of perception to impose meaningful interpretations to random ambiguous stimuli, e.g., perceiving images of objects, faces or animals out of cloud formations, out of chipped paint on the roof and walls, etc., is a complex visual illusion in patients with LBDs. Hallucinations, misidentification experiences and delusions have been reported, respectively, in 78%, 56%, and 25% of DLB cases.[97]

Psychosis in Parkinson's Disease

Parkinson's disease psychosis is one of the debilitating nonmotor symptoms with prevalence among untreated patients reported to occur rarely, whereas in treated patients, up to 70% in advanced PD stages.[78] Dopaminergic medication and disease duration seem to play a role in pathogenesis. The psychotic symptoms are generally quite stereotyped and recurrent. VHs are predominant, and are often the heralding symptom of PD dementia. The landscape of psychotic symptoms in PD usually exists on a continuum in which vivid dreams and nightmares in the prodromal phase are followed by minor phenomena (illusions, passage, and presence hallucinations), progressing from hallucinations with retained insight to hallucinations with loss of insight and/or delusions. Hallucinations in nonvisual modalities may occur in the advanced stages of the disease. Unlike the classic symptom of schizophrenia with a predominance of distinct voices with a typical threatening or denigrating character, the auditory hallucinations in PD are mostly indistinct nonthreatening sounds, e.g., a radio playing in the room, or a conversation taking place outside the room.

Delusions occur less often and are paranoid in nature. *Secondary delusions*—false irrational beliefs based on hallucinations, may develop in later disease stages when patients lose insight and may not recognize the misperceptions as unreal anymore. Thus a patient comes to believe that he does have insects on his skin and sprays insect repellant on himself, which he finds useless. Misidentification syndromes—Capgras and/or Fregoli syndrome are also frequently associated with PD dementia.

Psychosis Post-traumatic Brain Injury

The incidence of psychosis post-TBI has been estimated to fall between <1% and 9%, and the mean latency between injury onset and psychotic symptom presentation is ~4 years.[98] The development of psychotic symptoms following TBI has been associated with preinjury substance use, family history of schizophrenia, duration of loss of consciousness, and aphasia syndrome, as well as cortical damage within the frontal and temporal lobes. The most common psychotic symptoms experienced by patients post-TBI include persecutory delusions and auditory hallucinations, whereas negative symptoms (e.g., alogia and flat affect) occur with less frequency than in individuals with schizophrenia without TBI.

Psychosis in Brain Stroke

Poststroke psychosis is a relatively rare phenomenon (depression being the most frequent) affecting approximately 1 in 20 cerebrovascular accident survivors in the postacute stage,[99] and this may increase to approximately 7% over subsequent years.[100] The neural basis of poststroke delusions and hallucinations is still unclear; however, the involvement of a predominantly right-hemispheric cortical pathology, particularly the frontal, temporal and parietal regions, has been described. Rare though, instances of poststroke psychosis with left cortical and/or bilateral subcortical involvement (e.g., psychosis after cerebellar involvement, basal ganglia, or midbrain lesions) have been reported.[101,102] Psychosis occurring due to stroke demonstrates varied clinical characteristics that depend on the location of the stroke within the brain.

Delusional themes in the form of persecutory delusions, delusional jealousy, reduplicative paramnesia, and somatic delusions are the most common after a stroke. Peduncular hallucinosis has been postulated to be a release phenomenon from damage to the ascending reticular system (ARAS) and thalamocortical circuits. Strokes with a direct insult to the primary visual cortex can cause simple VHs (phosphenes or unformed flashes of light) in the hemianopic visual field. Anton's syndrome causes misrepresentation of signals from undamaged visual association cortex areas may result. Sensory aphasia after left hemispheric stroke is a differential diagnosis that may clinically mimic disorganized speech and thoughts seen in psychosis, and must be distinguished from true psychotic symptoms.

Poststroke psychosis is associated with increased illness burden, poor functional outcomes, and high mortality, and should, therefore, be identified and treated promptly.

Psychosis in Other Neurologic Diseases

Psychosis is one of the key features of limbic encephalitis and anti-NMDA encephalitis. It can also be a clinical manifestation of CNS infections, discrete cerebral lesions from a neoplasm or vascular malformation, and a rare presentation in HD.

Treatment of Psychosis in Neurologic Patients

The treatment of neurological patients who develop comorbid hallucinations or delusions is often challenging as many of the treatments for psychosis pose some risk of worsening the underlying neurologic condition. The treatment approaches include psychotherapy, pharmacotherapy, and neuromodulation.

Psychotherapy

Psychological interventions include cognitive-behavioral therapy for psychosis (CBTp), family psychoeducation, and personal therapy. Beck[103] developed CBTp as an evidence-based psychological treatment approach targeted to delusions, hallucinations, negative symptoms, and thought disorder; it is focused more on the coping mechanisms that the patient develops to deal with the psychosis but does not challenge the patient's beliefs as irrational. Social interventions that have been effective thus far include assertive community treatment and vocational training.

Pharmacotherapy

Medications that inhibit dopamine neurotransmission are currently the mainstay of treatment for idiopathic psychotic disorders as well as psychosis secondary to other medical conditions or substances. However, despite the modest efficacy of these medications, the U.S. Food and Drug Administration (FDA) has issued a black box warning against the use of antipsychotics in older patients with dementia, as this efficacy comes at the cost of a substantial adverse effect burden and mortality risk. Overall, the second-generation atypical antipsychotic medications, aripiprazole and risperidone are best recommended, followed by quetiapine and olanzapine. The starting and effective doses of antipsychotics for patients with neurodegenerative diseases are significantly lower than the doses used in primary psychotic disorders.

Pimavanserin, a selective 5-HT_{2A} inverse agonist has been approved by the FDA as effective and safe in the treatment of PD psychosis. Importantly, pimavanserin is the only antipsychotic drug that does not have dopamine-blocking properties. This drug is now being explored for treating individuals with dementia-related psychosis associated with the most common neurodegenerative disorders. The rationale is that 5-HT_{2A} receptor antagonism is a common feature of antipsychotics and is applicable regardless of the associated neuropathology (vascular, plaques, tangle, Lewy bodies, and TDP-43). Clozapine and quetiapine should also be considered in this patient population.

Nonpharmacological Approaches (Neuromodulation)

The noninvasive neurostimulation techniques (ECT, rTMS, and DBS) have a potential role in the treatment of medication-refractory psychosis. For details, refer to the section on Depression—somatic treatments, as already discussed.

CONCLUSION

This chapter examines the conflict of paradigms in the way depression and psychosis are conceptualized—are these neuropsychiatric disorders an understandable psychological reaction to the neurological diagnosis and/or result from psychosocial changes, or the direct result of a biological process of specific underlying neurological impairment. We conclude that depression, as well as psychosis represents a final common pathway emerging from a variety of etiological factors in different individuals. Screening for psychiatric comorbidities is crucial to achieving a holistic approach to patient care. The existing screening and diagnostic tools have been standardized and new disease-specific tools developed and validated for the recognition of these neuropsychiatric comorbidities in neurology practice. Diagnosis and treatment of psychiatric comorbidities in a timely manner can facilitate recovery and improve functional independence in patients with CNS disorders.

REFERENCES

1. Jefferies K, Owino A, Rickards H, Agrawal N. Psychiatric disorders in inpatients on a neurology ward: an estimate of prevalence and usefulness of screening questionnaires. J Neurol Neurosurg Psychiatry. 2007;78:414-6.
2. Fink P, Hansen MS, Søndergaard L, Frydenberg M. Mental illness in new neurological patients. J Neurol Neurosurg Psychiatry. 2003;74:817-9.
3. Steinberg M, Shao H, Zandi P, Lyketsos CG, Welsh-Bohmer KA, Norton MC, et al. Cache County Investigators. Point and 5-year period prevalence of neuropsychiatric symptoms in dementia: the Cache County Study. Int J Geriatr Psychiatry. 2008;23:170-7.
4. Munger Clary HM, Croxton RD, Snively BM, Brenes GA, Lovato J, Sadeghifar F, et al. Neurologist prescribing versus psychiatry referral: Examining patient preferences for anxiety and depression management in a symptomatic epilepsy clinic sample. Epilepsy Behav. 2021;114:107543.
5. Trimble MR. Neuropsychiatry (p. xiv). Chichester, UK: John Wiley & Sons; 1981.
6. World Health Organization (WHO). (2019). Depression. [online] Available from https://www.who.int/news-room/fact-sheets/detail/depression [Last accessed December, 2022].
7. World Health Organization. Depression and Other Common Mental Disorders: Global Health Estimates. Geneva: World Health Organization; 2017.
8. Evans-Lacko S, Aguilar-Gaxiola S, Al-Hamzawi A, Alonso J, Benjet C, Bruffaerts R, et al. Socio-economic variations in the mental health treatment gap for people with anxiety, mood, and substance use disorders: results from the WHO World Mental Health (WMH) surveys. Psychol Med. 2018;48:1560-71.
9. World Health Organization. (2008). mhGAP: Mental Health Gap Action Programme: scaling up care for mental, neurological and substance use disorders. [online] Available from https://apps.who.int/iris/handle/10665/43809 [Last accessed December, 2022].
10. American Psychiatric Association. Diagnostic and Statistical Manual of Mental Disorders: DSM-5, 5th ed. Washington, DC: American Psychiatric Association; 2013.
11. World Health Organization. Suicide worldwide in 2019: Global health estimates. Geneva: World Health Organization; 2021.
12. World Health Organization (WHO). LIVE LIFE: An implementation guide for suicide prevention in countries. Geneva: World Health Organization; 2021.
13. World Health Organization (WHO). Schedules for Clinical Assessment in Neuropsychiatry (SCAN) Version 2.0. Geneva: World Health Organization; 1994.
14. First MB, Williams JBW. Quick Structured Clinical Interview for DSM-5 Disorders (QuickSCID-5). Washington, DC: American Psychiatric Association Publishing; 2021.
15. Wittchen HU. Reliability and validity studies of the WHO-Composite International Diagnostic Interview (CIDI): A critical review. J Psychiatr Res. 1994;28:57-84.
16. Sheehan DV, Lecrubier Y, Sheehan, KH, Amorim P, Janavs J, Weiller E, et al. The Mini International Neuropsychiatric Interview (M.I.N.I.): The development and validation of a structured diagnostic psychiatric interview for DSM-IV and ICD-10. J Clin Psychiatry. 1998;59(Suppl. 20):22-3.
17. Montgomery AS, Asberg M. A new depression scale designed to be sensitive to change. Br J Psychiatry. 1979;134:382-9.
18. Radloff, LS. The CES-D scale: A self-report depression scale for research in the general population. Appl Psychol Meas. 1977;1: 385-401.
19. Hamilton M. Development of a rating scale for primary depressive illness. Br J Soc Clin Psychol. 1967;6:278-96.
20. Zung WW. A Self-rating depression scale. Arch Gen Psychiatry. 1965;12:63-70.
21. Beck AT, Steer RA, Brown GK. Beck Depression Inventory-II. San Antonio, TX: Psychological Corporation; 1996.
22. Beck AT, Steer RA, Brown GK. Manual for the Beck Depression Inventory—Fast Screen for Medical Patients. San Antonio, TX: Psychological Corporation; 2000.
23. Benedict RHB, Fishman I, McClellan MM, Bakshi R, Weinstock-Guttman B. Validity of the Beck Depression Inventory-Fast Screen in multiple sclerosis. Mult Scler. 2003;9:393-6.
24. Strober LB, Arnett PA. Depression in multiple sclerosis: the utility of common self-report instruments and development of a disease-specific measure. J Clin Experiment Neuropsychol. 2015;37: 722-32.
25. Elben S, Dimenshteyn K, Trenado C, Folkerts AK, Ophey A, Sulzer P, et al. Screen fast, screen faster: A pilot study to screen for depressive symptoms using the Beck Depression Inventory Fast Screen in Parkinson's disease with mild cognitive impairment. Front Neurol. 2021;12:640137.
26. Zigmond AS, Snaith RP. The hospital anxiety and depression scale. Acta Psychiatr Scand. 1983;67:361-70.
27. Yesavage JA, Brink TL, Rose TL, Lum O, Huang V, Adey M, et al. Development and validation of a Geriatric Depression Screening Scale: a preliminary report. J Psychiatr Res. 1982;17:37-49.
28. Kroenke K, Spitzer RL, Williams JB. The PHQ-9: validity of a brief depression severity measure. J Gen Intern Med. 2001;16:606-13.
29. Cohen J. Assessment and treatment of dysthymia. The development of the Cornell dysthymia rating scale. Eur Psychiatry. 1997;12: 190-3.
30. Gilliam FG, Barry JJ, Hermann BP, Meador KJ, Vahle V, Kanner AM. Rapid detection of major depression in epilepsy: a multicentre study. Lancet Neurol. 2006;5:399-405.
31. Mula M, McGonigal A, Micoulaud-Franchi J, May TW, Labudda K, Brandt C. Validation of rapid suicidality screening in epilepsy using the NDDIE. Epilepsia. 2016;57:949-55.
32. Gainotti G, Azzoni A, Razzano C, Lanzillotta M, Marra C, Gasparini F. The post-stroke depression rating scale: A test specifically devised to investigate affective disorders of stroke patients. J Clin Exp Neuropsychol. 1997;19:340-56.
33. Turner-Stokes L, Kalmus M, Hirani D, Clegg F. The Depression Intensity Scale Circles (DISCs): a first evaluation of a simple assessment tool for depression in the context of brain injury. J Neurol Neurosurg Psychiatry. 2005;76:1273-8.
34. Torbey E, Pachana NA, Dissanayaka NNW. Depression rating scales in Parkinson's disease: A critical review updating recent literature. J Affect Disord. 2015;184:21624.
35. Schrag A, Barone P, Brown RG, Leentjens AFG, McDonald WM, Starkstein S, et al. Depression rating scales in Parkinson's disease: Critique and recommendations. Mov Disord. 2007;22:1077-92.
36. Li Z, Ruan M, Chen J, Fang Y. Major depressive disorder: Advances in neuroscience research and translational applications. Neuroscience Bull. 2021;36:863-80.
37. Roiser JP, Elliott R, Sahakian BJ. Cognitive mechanisms of treatment in depression. Neuropsychopharmacology. 1012;37:117-36.
38. Roiser JP, Sahakian BJ. Information Processing in Mood Disorders. In: DeRubeis RJ and Strunk DR (Eds). The Oxford Handbook of Mood Disorders. Oxford: Oxford University Press; 2016. pp. 179-89.
39. Fiest KM, Dykeman J, Patten SB, Wiebe S, Kaplan GG, Maxwell CJ, et al. Depression in epilepsy: a systematic review and meta-analysis. Neurology. 2013;80:590-9.
40. Goel P, Singh G, Bansal V, Sharma S, Kumare P, Chaudhry R, et al. Psychiatric comorbidities among people with epilepsy: A population-based assessment in disadvantaged communities. Epilepsy Behav. 2022;137:108965.
41. Mula M, Sander JW. Suicide risk in people with epilepsy taking antiepileptic drugs. Bipolar Disord. 2013;15:622-7.

42. Hesdorffer DC, Ishihara L, Mynepalli L, Webb DJ, Weil J, Hauser WA. Epilepsy, suicidality, and psychiatric disorders: A bidirectional association. Ann Neurol. 2012;72:184-91.
43. Blumer D. Dysphoric disorders and paroxysmal affects: recognition and treatment of epilepsy-related psychiatric disorders. Harv Rev Psychiatry. 2000;8:8-17.
44. Li Q, Chen D, Zhu L, Wang H, Xu D, Tan G, et al. Depression in people with epilepsy in West China: Status, risk factors and treatment gap. Seizure. 2019;66:86-92.
45. Fiest KM, Patten SB, Altura KC, Bulloch AGM, Maxwell CJ, Wiebe S, et al. Patterns and frequency of the treatment of depression in persons with epilepsy. Epilepsy Behav. 2014;39:59-64.
46. Asmer MS, Kirkham J, Newton H, Ismail Z, Elbayoumi H, Leung RH, et al. Meta-analysis of the prevalence of major depressive disorder among older adults with dementia. J Clin Psychiatry. 2018;79:17r11772.
47. Younes K, Miller BL. Neuropsychiatric aspects of frontotemporal dementia. Psychiatr Clin North Am. 2020;43:345-60.
48. Marchant NL, Howard RJ. Cognitive debt and Alzheimer's disease. J Alzheimers Dis. 2015;44:755-70.
49. Agüera-Ortiz L, García-Ramos R, Pérez FJG, López-Álvarez J, Rodríguez JMM, Rodríguez FJO, et al. Depression in Alzheimer's disease: A delphi consensus on etiology, risk factors, and clinical management. Front Psychiatry. 2021;12:638651.
50. Carotenuto A, Fasanaro AM, Manzo V, Amenta F, Traini E. Association between the cholinesterase inhibitor donepezil and the cholinergic precursor choline alphoscerate in the treatment of depression in patients with Alzheimer's disease. J Alzheimers Dis Rep. 2022;6:235-43.
51. Gertler P, Tate RL, Cameron ID. Non-pharmacological interventions for depression in adults and children with traumatic brain injury. Cochrane Database Syst Rev. 2015;2015:CD009871.
52. Levin HS, McCauley SR, Josic CP, Boake C, Brown SA, Goodman HS, et al. Predicting depression following mild traumatic brain injury. Arch Gen Psychiatry. 2005;62:523-8.
53. Reijnders JS, Ehrt U, Weber WE, Aarsland D, Leentjens AFG. A systematic review of prevalence studies of depression in Parkinson's disease. Mov Disord. 2008;23:183-9.
54. Lee T, Lee HB, Ahn MH, Kim J, Kim MS, Chung SJ, et al: Increased suicide risk and clinical correlates of suicide among patients with Parkinson's disease. Parkinsonism Relat Disord. 2016;32:102-7.
55. van Duijn E, Craufurd D, Hubers AA, Giltay EJ, Bonelli R, Rickards H, et al; European Huntington's Disease Network Behavioural Phenotype Working Group. Neuropsychiatric symptoms in a European Huntington's disease cohort (REGISTRY). J Neurol Neurosurg Psychiatry. 2014;85:1411-8.
56. Boeschoten RE, Braamse AMJ, Beekman ATF, Cuijpers P, van Oppen P, Dekker J, et al. Prevalence of depression and anxiety in multiple sclerosis: A systematic review and meta-analysis. J Neurol Sci. 2017;372:331-41.
57. Feinstein A, Pavisian B. Multiple sclerosis and suicide. Mult Scler. 2017;23:923-7.
58. Lee B, Rumrill P, Tansey TN. Examining the role of resilience and hope in grit in multiple sclerosis. Front Neurol. 2022;13:875133.
59. Guo J, Wang J, Sun W, Liu X. The advances of post-stroke depression: 2021 update. J Neurol. 2022;269:1236-49.
60. Patra A, Nitin K, Devi NM, Surya S, Lewis MG, Kamalakannan S. Prevalence of depression among stroke survivors in India: A systematic review and meta-analysis. Front Neurol Neurosci Res.2021;2:100008.
61. Breslau N, Lipton RB, Stewart WF, Schultz LR, Welch KMA. Comorbidity of migraine and depression: investigating potential etiology and prognosis. Neurology. 2003;60:1308-12.
62. Leo RJ, Singh J. Migraine headache and bipolar disorder comorbidity: a systematic review of literature and clinical implications. Scand J Pain. 2016;11:136-45.
63. May A, Schulte LH. Chronic migraine: risk factors, mechanisms and treatment. Nat Rev Neurol. 2016;12:455-64.
64. de Vries Lentsch S, Louter MA, van Oosterhout WPJ, van Zwet EW, van Noorden MS, Terwindt GM. Depressive symptoms during the different phases of a migraine attack: A prospective diary study. J Affect Disord. 2022;297:502-7.
65. Hayes SC. Acceptance and commitment therapy, relational frame theory, and the third wave of behavioral and cognitive therapies. Behav Ther. 2004;35:639-65.
66. von Feuchtersleben E. Lehrbuch der Ärztlichen Seelenkunde. Vienna, Austria: Gerold Verlag; 1845.
67. Kraepelin E. Dementia Praecox and Paraphrenia. RM Barclay, transl. Huntington, NY: Robert E. Kreiger Publishing Co., Inc.; 1999.
68. Bleuler E. (Tarns. J. Zinkin). Dementia Praecox or the Group of Schizophrenias. New York, NY: International Universities Press; 1950.
69. Ronthal M, Venna N, Hunter GJ, Frosch MP. Case records of the Massachusetts General Hospital. Case 15-2016. A 32-year-old man with olfactory hallucinations and paresthesias. N Engl J Med. 2016;374:1966-75.
70. Lukoff D, Nuechterlein KH, Ventura J. Manual for the expanded Brief Psychiatric Rating Scale. Schizophr Bull. 1986;12:594-602.
71. Hofmann AB, Schmid HM, Jabat M, Brackmann N, Noboa V, Bobes J, et al. Utility and validity of the Brief Psychiatric Rating Scale (BPRS) as a transdiagnostic scale. Psychiat Res. 2022;314:114659.
72. Cummings JL, Mega M, Gray K, Rosenberg-Thompson S, Carusi DA, Gornbein J. The Neuropsychiatric Inventory: Comprehensive assessment of psychopathology in dementia. Neurology. 1994;44: 2308-14.
73. Kay SR, Fiszbein A, Opler LA. The positive and negative syndrome scale (PANSS) for schizophrenia. Schizophr Bull. 1987;13:261-76.
74. Andreasen NC. Scale For the Assessment of Negative Symptoms (SANS). Iowa City: University of Iowa; 1984.
75. Kring AM, Raquel, Steven P. The clinical assessment interview for negative symptoms (CAINS): Final development and validation. Am J Psychiatry. 2013;165-72.
76. Kirkpatrick B, Strauss GP, Nguyen L, Fischer BA, Daniel DG, Cienfuegos A, et al. The brief negative symptom scale: psychometric properties. Schizophr Bull. 2011;37:300-5.
77. Cummings J, Isaacson S, Mills R, Williams H, Chi-Burris K, Corbett A, et al. Pimavanserin for patients with Parkinson's disease psychosis: A randomized, placebo-controlled phase 3 trial. Lancet. 2014;383:533Y540.
78. Levin J, Hasan A, Hoglinger GU. Psychosis in Parkinson's disease: Identification, prevention and treatment. J Neural Transm. 2016;123:45-50.
79. Chaudhuri KR, Martinez-Martin P, Brown RG, Sethi K, Stocchi F, Odin P, et al. The metric properties of a novel non-motor symptoms scale for Parkinson's disease: results from an international pilot study. Mov Disord. 2007;22:1901-11.
80. Goetz CG, Fahn S, Martinez-Martin P, Poewe W, Sampaio C, Stebbins GT, et al. Movement Disorder Society-sponsored revision of the Unified Parkinson's Disease Rating Scale (MDS-UPDRS): process, format, and clinimetric testing plan. Mov Disord. 2007;22:41-7.
81. Brandstaedter D, Spieker S, Ulm G, Siebert U, Eichhorn TE, Krieg JC, et al. Development and evaluation of the Parkinson Psychosis Questionnaire a screening-instrument for the early diagnosis of drug-induced psychosis in Parkinson's disease. J Neurol. 2005;252:1060-6.
82. Voss T, Bahr D, Cummings J, Mills R, Ravina B, Williams H. Performance of a shortened Scale for Assessment of Positive Symptoms for Parkinson's disease psychosis. Parkinsonism Relat Disord. 2013;19:295-9.
83. Rodriguez-Violante M, Cervantes-Arriaga A, Vela´zquez-Osuna S, Llorens-Arenas R, Calderón-Fajardo H, Piña-Fuentes D, et al. Independent Validation of the SEND-PD and Correlation with the MDS-UPDRS Part IA. Parkinsons Dis. 2014;2014:260485.

84. Clancy MJ, Clarke MC, Connor DJ, Cannon M, Cotter DR. The prevalence of psychosis in epilepsy; a systematic review and meta-analysis. BMC Psychiatry. 2014;14:75.
85. Hilger E, Zimprich F, Pataraia E, Aull-Watschinger S, Jung R, Baumgartner C, et al. Psychoses in epilepsy: a comparison of postictal and interictal psychoses. Epilepsy Behav. 2016;60: 58-62.
86. Landoldt H. Some clinical electroencephalographical correlations in epileptic psychosis (twilight states). Electroencephalogr Clin Neurophysiol. 1953;5:121.
87. Tellenbach H. Epilepsie als Anfallseiden und als Psychose. Uber alternative psychosen paranoider Pragung bei "forcierter Normalisierung" (Landoldt) des Elektroencephalogramms Epileptischer. Nervarzt. 1965;36:190.
88. Mula M. The Landolt's phenomenon: An update. Epileptologia. 2010;18:39-44.
89. Webster R, Holroyd S. Prevalence of psychotic symptoms in delirium. Psychosomatics. 2000;41:519-22.
90. Khan BA, Perkins AJ, Gao S, Hui SL, Campbell NL, Farber MO, et al. The Confusion Assessment Method for the ICU-7 Delirium Severity Scale: A Novel Delirium Severity Instrument for Use in the ICU. Crit Care Med. 2017;45:851-7.
91. Ropacki SA, Jeste DV. Epidemiology of and risk factors for psychosis of Alzheimer's disease: a review of 55 studies published from 1990 to 2003. Am J Psychiatry. 2005;162:2022-30.
92. Cummings J, Ballard C, Tariot P, Owen R, Foff E, Youakim J, et al. Pimavanserin: Potential treatment for dementia-related psychosis. J Prev Alzheimers Dis. 2018;5:253-8.
93. Sha SJ, Takada LT, Rankin KP, Yokoyama JS, Rutherford NJ, Fong JC, et al. Frontotemporal dementia due to C9ORF72 mutations: clinical and imaging features. Neurology. 2012;79:1002-11.
94. Utsumi K, Fukatsu R, Yamada R, Takamaru Y, Hara Y, Yasumura S. Characteristics of initial symptoms and symptoms at diagnosis in probable dementia with Lewy body disease: Incidence of symptoms and gender differences. Psychogeriatrics. 2020;20: 737-45.
95. McKeith IG, Taylor JP, Thomas A, Donaghy P, Kane J. Revisiting DLB diagnosis: A consideration of prodromal DLB and of the diagnostic overlap with Alzheimer disease. J Geriatric Psychiatry Neurol. 2016;29:249-53.
96. Utsumi K, Fukatsu R, Hara Y, Takamaru Y, Yasumura S. Psychotic features among patients in the prodromal stage of dementia with Lewy bodies during longitudinal observation. J Alzheimer's Dis. 2021;83:1917-27.
97. Nagahama Y, Okina T, Suzuki N, Matsuda M, Fukao K, Murai T. Classification of psychotic symptoms in dementia with Lewy bodies. Am J Geriatr Psychiatry. 2007;15:961-7.
98. David AS, Prince M. Psychosis following head injury: A critical review. J Neurol Neurosurg Psychiatry. 2005;76(Suppl 1):i53-60.
99. Stangeland H, Orgeta V, Bell V. Poststroke psychosis: a systematic review. J Neurol Neurosurg Psychiatry. 2018;89:879-85.
100. Almeida OP, Xiao J. Mortality associated with incident mental health disorders after stroke. Aust N Z J Psychiatry. 2007;41:274-81.
101. Parfianowicz D, Espiridion ED. Chronic post-stroke psychosis with left cortical and bilateral inferior cerebellar involvement. Cureus. 2019;11:e6437.
102. McMurtray A, Tseng B, Diaz N, Chung J, Mehta B, Saito E. Acute psychosis associated with subcortical stroke: Comparison between basal ganglia and mid brain lesions. Case Rep Neurol Med. 2014;2014:428425.
103. Beck AT. Schizophrenia: Cognitive Theory, Research, and Therapy. New York: Guilford Press; 2009.

28

CHAPTER

Approach to Apraxia and Agnosia

Rohan R Mahale, Deepak Menon

APRAXIA

INTRODUCTION

Praxis refers to the ability to perform skilled movements by planning a schema based on stored representations and previously learned movements. The praxis system is composed of component functions associated with particular brain regions that include the frontal and parietal cortex, basal ganglia, and white matter tracts containing projections between these areas. The above brain regions work together to formulate and execute an action. Praxis is predominantly a function of the left hemisphere. The left hemisphere is involved in movements of relatively high complexity, planning and sequencing movements, shifting motor attention, and selecting a motor response from a set of competitors; whereas, the right hemisphere is involved in highly practiced and familiar actions.[1,2] Praxicons or visuokinesthetic motor engrams are the spatiotemporal movement formulas stored in the dominant parietal lobe [inferior parietal lobule (IPL)], which are activated by the visual, auditory, and tactile inputs and aid in the execution of an action. Apart from the praxicon, the parietal lobe (posterior parietal) contains the action semantics about tool action, tool use, and tool-object association. The supplementary motor area in the premotor cortex translates the praxicons into motor programs and relays on to the ipsilateral primary motor cortex and contralateral premotor area through the corpus callosum.[3]

Apraxia is the inability to perform learned, skilled motor acts despite preserved motor and sensory systems, coordination, comprehension, and cooperation. The special features of apraxia include voluntary-automatic dissociation and context dependence. The *voluntary-automatic dissociation* refers to the performance of gestures spontaneously with the inability to perform gestures on command. The execution of the movement improves if the patient focuses on the target of the movement rather than on the movement itself. The context dependence refers to the preserved execution of the movement in a natural context than in the clinical setting. The patient has to explicitly demonstrate the action in the clinical setting, which brings out the executional impairment.[4]

MODELS OF APRAXIA

Before going into the different types of apraxia, we will understand the different models of apraxia. The first apraxia model was proposed by *Liepmann* who suggested that the representation of an action (space-time plan) or "movement formulae" is stored in the left parietal lobe. Whenever there is a need to execute the action, the space-time plan is retrieved from the parietal lobe and, via the left premotor cortex, the information is relayed to the primary motor areas.[3] The information crosses via the corpus callosum to the right premotor areas for the execution of the action by the left hand. The second disconnection model of apraxia was proposed by *Geschwind (1965)*. The verbal command for the movement is comprehended in Wernicke's area and relayed to the ipsilateral motor and premotor areas that control the movement.[5] The third model was proposed by *Heilman and Rothi (1993)*. The knowledge and spatiotemporal representations of learned movements are stored in the left inferior-parietal lobule (angular gyrus and supramarginal gyrus) and relayed to the premotor cortex (including the supplementary motor area) and motor cortex to carry out the action. The damage to anterior regions causes gesture production deficit, whereas the posterior lesion causes impaired movement production and impaired gesture comprehension and discrimination of well- versus ill-formed gestures.[6] The cognitive model of limb praxis was proposed by *Roy and Square* in 1985. Praxis involves two systems namely conceptual and production systems. The "conceptual system" possesses three types of knowledge namely knowledge of the functions of tools and objects, knowledge of actions independent of tools and objects, and knowledge about the organization of single actions into sequences. The "production system" is concerned with the sensorimotor representation of the action and mechanisms for movement control. A deficit in pantomime but not imitation suggests damage to the retrieval of actions from long-term memory. Impaired imitation alone suggests disruption of the translation of visual information into movement. Impairment in pantomime and imitation suggests disturbance at the executive stage of gesture production.[7] Rothi et al. (1991) gave a cognitive neuropsychological model of limb praxis. This model has an *input* that is selective according to the modality (verbal/auditory, visual object, and visual gestural input), action semantics system, action reception lexicon, and action production lexicon.[8] Recently, apraxia is considered a frontotemporoparietal network disorder in the left hemisphere. The dual-stream model comprises *dorsal stream*, which connects the lateral occipitotemporal cortex, superior parietal lobule to the premotor cortex (dorso-dorsal stream) and lateral occipitotemporal cortex, IPL and inferior frontal gyrus (ventrodorsal stream) and *ventral stream*, which connects IPL, superior and middle temporal gyrus, and anterior temporal lobe with the inferior frontal lobe. Abnormalities in copying of meaningless gestures and execution of meaningful gestures are due to dorsal stream involvement, whereas impairment in pantomiming tool action or conceptual error (impaired tool knowledge) is due to ventral stream involvement.[9]

CLINICAL APPROACH

A thorough knowledge of different types of apraxia is required before assessing a patient with apraxia. The localization of different types of apraxia is summarized in **Table 1**.

Types of Apraxia[2,4,10]

The major types of apraxia include ideational and conceptual apraxia, ideomotor apraxia, limb kinetic and constructional apraxia.

Ideomotor Apraxia

It is the most commonly recognized type of apraxia. The patient has difficulty in pantomiming an action to verbal command, inability to imitate the other person's gesture. Patients have temporal and spatial errors, which affect the timing, sequencing, amplitude, configuration, and limb position in space. They use their limb as an object rather than demonstrating how to use the object (body part as object). But the patient's performance significantly improves if they are given the object, they have just been asked to pantomime the action. The visual and tactile feedback from the use of real objects helps in the selection of an appropriate limb posture and finger configuration. Ideomotor apraxia occurs due to damage to the parietal and frontal cortex as well as the white matter connections between these areas. Ideomotor apraxia due to parietal lobe involvement shows spatiotemporal error while pantomiming or using a tool. Patients are unable to orient their arm and hand, impaired trajectory and speed of movement, and impaired gesture identification. Ideomotor apraxia due to frontal lobe involvement shows similar abnormalities except for preserved gesture recognition.

TABLE 1: Localization in apraxia.

Types of apraxia	Brain area
Ideational apraxia	Bilateral parietal lobe
Ideomotor apraxia	Left parietal and frontal cortex and the interconnecting white matter
Conceptual apraxia	Left parietal lobe
Limb-kinetic apraxia	Left supplementary motor area, primary motor cortex
Callosal apraxia	Anterior corpus callosum
Conduction apraxia	Disconnection between verbal, visual input, and parietal lobe
Apraxia of speech	Dominant inferior frontal gyrus, anterior insula
Buccofacial apraxia	Ventral premotor cortex

Ideational Apraxia

It is defined as a disturbance in the conceptual organization of actions. The patient has to perform purposive sequences of actions using various objects in the proper order like preparing a cup of tea. The usage of multiple objects and performing complex sequences place a heavier load on memory and attentional resources. Patients demonstrate inappropriate use of objects and fail in gesture identification and discrimination. For instance, a patient may eat with a toothbrush and brush his teeth with a spoon. They can execute the proper action of brushing their teeth but use the wrong tools.

Conceptual Apraxia

Patients with conceptual apraxia have impairment of tool/object knowledge. They may misuse objects, and have difficulty matching objects and actions. Conceptual apraxia corresponds to a disruption of the conceptual component of the praxis system, i.e., action semantics memory. Patients are unable to name or point to a tool when its function is discussed, make tool-selection error, and perform wrong actions to a given tool but can imitate gestures without spatiotemporal errors.

Limb Kinetic Apraxia

It refers to the loss of coordination between the fine, individuated finger movements needed to perform a skilled task. There is a defect in the final stages of motor processing in the prefrontal regions before the information is relayed to the ipsilateral primary motor cortices causing apraxia in the contralateral limb.

Modality-specific Apraxia

It refers to the differential impairment of gesture production or imitation according to the modality of the testing. These includes:

Conduction Apraxia[11]

Patients with conduction apraxia have superior performance on verbal command than to imitation or very poor performance on verbal command that improved on imitation or when seeing the object. The former is termed visuo-imitative apraxia. Patients with visuo-imitative apraxia may have a defective imitation of meaningless gestures in contrast to the preserved imitation of meaningful gestures or vice-versa.

Constructional Apraxia

It is defined as "the impairment in combinatory or organizing activity in which details must be clearly perceived and in which the relationship among the component parts of the entity must be apprehended". Patients are unable to draw objects spontaneously, copy figures, and build blocks or patterns with sticks. They occur in patients with damage to both the dominant and nondominant hemispheres.

Pantomime Agnosia[12]

Patients have normal gesture production to both imitation and on verbal command, but poor performance in gesture discrimination and identification of examiner pantomime of an action. They can imitate pantomimes but cannot recognize the same.

Tactile Apraxia

Patients with tactile apraxia have a disturbance of transitive hand movements for use of—recognition and interaction with an object, in the presence of preserved intransitive movements (gestures and repetitive movements) and it is seen in parietal lobe lesions.

Other Types of Apraxia

Buccofacial Apraxia

Buccofacial apraxia is an inability to perform skilled nonspeech-related movements involving the muscles of the tongue and face. It can be demonstrated by instructing the patient to cough, click their tongue, blow out a candle, or drink through a straw. The lesion is commonly in the ventral premotor cortex.

Apraxia of Speech

Apraxia of speech refers to a disruption in the precise pattern of orofacial muscular activity during speech production. Patients have slow and effortful speech, errors in the timing of the production of individual syllables, impaired prosody, and difficulty trying to find the right word or sound. The lesion is usually in the dominant inferior frontal gyrus and anterior insular region. Patients with dysarthria have difficulty in pronunciation of single syllable repeatedly (e.g.: pa, pa), whereas patients with apraxia of speech do not have difficulty but they have difficulty in pronunciation of string a number of syllables together (e.g.: pa-ta-ka).

Callosal Apraxia

Callosal apraxia is caused by the lesion in the anterior corpus callosum that usually affects the left upper limb. Patients will have ideomotor or conceptual or dissociative apraxia in the left upper limb.

Crossed Apraxia and Sympathetic Apraxia

Crossed apraxia refers to apraxia involving the right hand due to the right hemispheric lesions and sympathetic apraxia refers to apraxia in the nondominant limb due to the involvement of the anterior left hemisphere.

Neurological Disorders-associated with Apraxia

Apraxia is a diagnostic feature of amnestic Alzheimer's disease (AD), and both ideomotor and ideational apraxia have been reported in amnestic AD. Apraxia is also seen in clinical variants of AD-like posterior cortical atrophy, and logopenic variant of a primary progressive aphasia (PPA). Ideomotor apraxia and apraxia of speech have been reported in a nonfluent variant of PPA, which is included in FTD spectrum disorders.[13] Apraxia is a core clinical feature of the corticobasal syndrome (CBS). Ideomotor and imitation apraxia have been recognized in CBS. ^{18}F-fluorodeoxyglucose-positron emission tomography (FDG-PET) has shown hypometabolism in the angular gyrus in ideomotor apraxia and in the precuneus, posterior cingulate gyrus in imitation apraxia in CBS.[14] A stroke involving the left hemisphere causes apraxia (ideational and ideomotor).

INVESTIGATOR APPROACH

A careful neurological examination must be done in patients with apraxia in order to ensure that the patient's motor symptoms cannot be explained by muscle weakness, spasticity, bradykinesia, ataxia, or sensory loss. To label a patient as apraxic is difficult if the impaired movements result from cognitive disorders involving attention, memory, language comprehension, or executive functions.[15]

The first step in the examination of the patient with apraxia is to ask the patient to *pantomime tool use* (transitive) by issuing a command such as "show me the action how you would hammer in a nail" or "brush your teeth" or "comb your hair", etc. in right and left limb independently. If the patient has persistent difficulty in pantomiming the action despite correction, then it is considered as pathological. When the patient fails to pantomime an action to the examiner's command, then the examiner has to demonstrate the correct action and instruct the patient to *imitate the examiner's pantomime.* In patients with ideational apraxia wherein the conceptual knowledge about the tool is impaired, they have difficulty in pantomiming the action of the tool/object to command but are able to imitate the examiner pantomime.

The second step is asking the patient to demonstrate several *meaningful gestures* (intransitive) such as saluting, waving goodbye, calling someone, etc. and blowing out a candle, drinking through a straw, coughing, etc. Patients with ideational apraxia have difficulty demonstrating meaningful gestures.

The third step is asking the patients to *copy meaningless hand gestures* as demonstrated by the examiner. The meaningless hand gestures are shown in **Figure 1**.

The fourth step is to assess the *gestural knowledge* wherein the examiner demonstrates different transitive and intransitive gestures and asks the patient to identify their function/purpose and discriminate between those that are well and those that are poorly performed.

The fifth step is to assess the *sequential actions* by asking the patient to demonstrate the steps involved in mailing a letter assuming the presence of imaginary tools/objects in front of the patient. The performance of sequential actions is impaired in ideational apraxia.

The sixth step is to assess *conceptual knowledge* by presenting tools or objects and instructing the patients to demonstrate the use of the object. Conceptual knowledge is impaired in ideational/conceptual apraxia.

Lastly, the *testing of fine finger movements* is done by asking the patient to do finger tapping, alternate touching of each finger with the thumb, picking a coin without sliding, etc. This is impaired in limb-kinetic apraxia. The steps in the clinical evaluation of apraxia are summarized in **Table 2**.

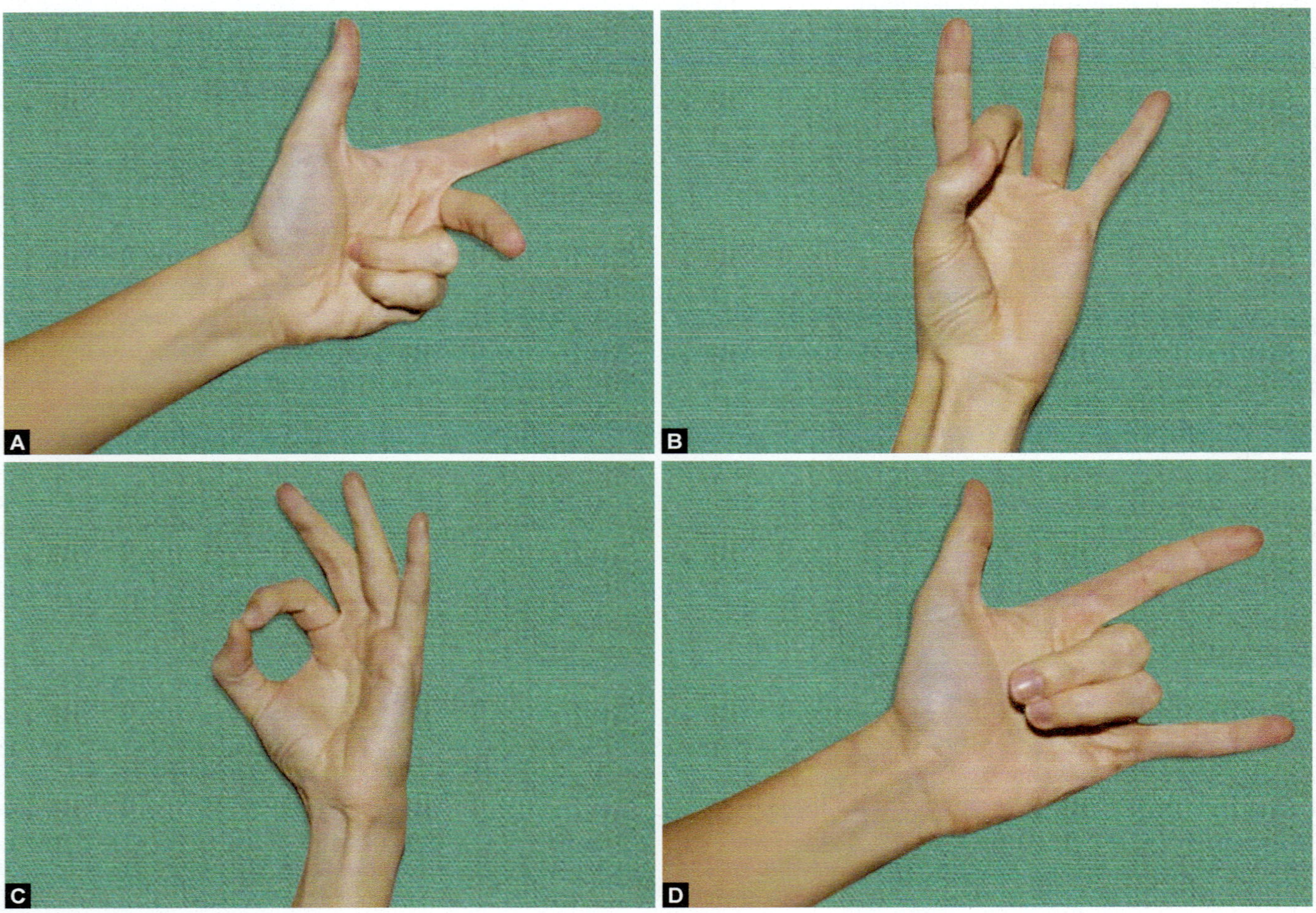

FIGS. 1A TO D: Arbitrary hand postures.

TABLE 2: Clinical differentiation of common types of apraxia.

Steps	Ideational apraxia	Ideomotor apraxia	Conceptual apraxia	Limb-kinetic apraxia
Pantomime a transitive (tool) action	Impaired	Impaired	Impaired	Preserved
Pantomime an intransitive action	Impaired	Impaired	Preserved	Preserved
Imitate meaningful gestures	Preserved	Impaired	Preserved	Preserved
Copy meaningless gestures	Preserved	Impaired	Preserved	Preserved
Identification of meaningful gestures/ gestural knowledge	Impaired	Preserved	Preserved	Preserved
Gesture discrimination	Impaired	Preserved	Preserved	Preserved
Sequential actions	Impaired	Preserved	Impaired	Preserved
Conceptual knowledge—tool selection, tool action knowledge, and pantomime	Impaired	Preserved except tool action pantomime	Impaired	Preserved
Fine finger movements	Preserved	Preserved	Preserved	Impaired
Demonstration of action using tools	Impaired	Preserved	Impaired	Impaired

CONCLUSION

Apraxia is a disorder of praxis wherein there is difficulty in performing learned skilled motor acts. Apractic patients have difficulty in performance of action or object use either due to loss of knowledge of action/tool usage, failure to retrieve from the long-term memory or failure to execute intended action despite having the knowledge of action. Ideomotor apraxia is the most common type of apraxia among the various neurological disorders especially in stroke, dementia, and atypical parkinsonian disorders. Apraxia has a significant effect on the activities of daily living of the patients.

AGNOSIA

INTRODUCTION

The accurate perception of visual, auditory, or tactile stimuli depends on intact registration and higher-order associative streams that can access the preregistered semantic coding relating to the stimulus. Inability to access this semantic knowledge leads to a hollow perception of the stimulus stripped of its essence and meaning, and this forms the basis of agnosia (Gnosis: knowledge). Often, this loss of access is modality specific, such that the patient can unlock the semantic knowledge through an alternate modality. For instance, in visual agnosia, the patient may not identify a bunch of keys by looking at them until he or she hears the jingle, which then immediately leads to an accurate recognition. In simple words, agnosia refers to a disorder of recognition in one sensory modality. Among the various agnosias, visual agnosia is the most frequently encountered and perhaps most disabling to the patient.

The visual pathway originates in the retina and terminates in the primary visual cortex or striate cortex (Brodmann area 17) involved in primary visual information analysis. The retinotopic arrangement means that any damage would essentially result in visual loss in the contralateral visual field. Further higher-order processing takes place in the extrastriate cortices (Brodmann areas 18 and 19) whereby a subsequent ventral stream relays information to the temporal and dorsal stream relays information to the parietal regions.[16]

The existence of a ventral and dorsal stream has been corroborated by clinical situations in which patients have lost either the "what" or the "where" of an object, with selective sparing of the other. For instance, patients with bilateral parieto-occipital lesions were demonstrated to have optic ataxia with preserved object recognition, naming, and matching, while more ventral lesions resulted in agnosia but with preserved hand movement and orientation with respect to the same object.[17] Thus, a lesion in the ventral or "what" pathway leads to classical visual agnosia while that of the dorsal or "what" pathway leads to impairment in the visuospatial and motion attributes of the object. But recent studies have found that these two streams do not work in isolation and, while being parallel, have interconnection both structurally and functionally.

There are conceptual frameworks and models that have been proposed to explain the physiology and pathology behind stimulus perception or the lack thereof, as in agnosia **(Fig. 2)**. Marr's hierarchical model of visual perception in which the visual stimulus progressively attains a primary 2-dimensional sketch followed by a viewer-centered 2 1/2-dimensional sketch and a final object-centered 3-dimensional sketch is commonly invoked to explain visual perception. Once the object-centric view is generated, the semantic concept and the phonological lexicon with regard to the object image have to be accessed and matched, for the patient to recognize and name the object accurately **(Fig. 3)**.[18] Any interruption at any step of this hierarchical process can result in higher-order sensory processing impairment including agnosia as discussed here.

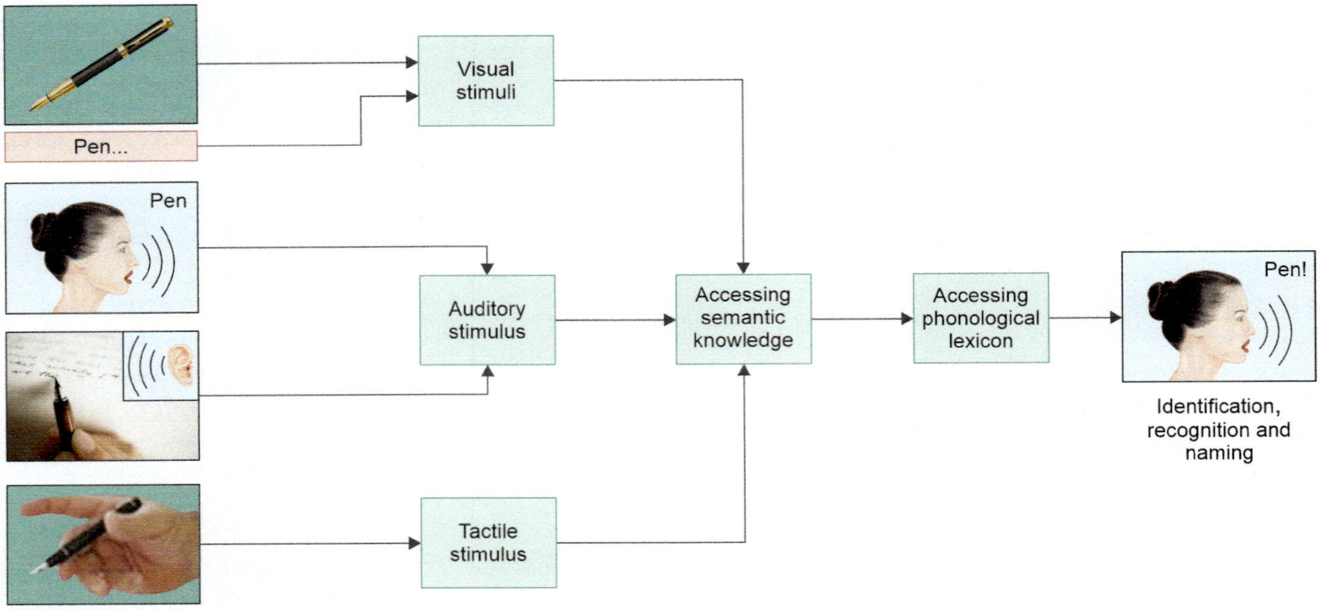

FIG. 2: Conceptual model of "gnosis".

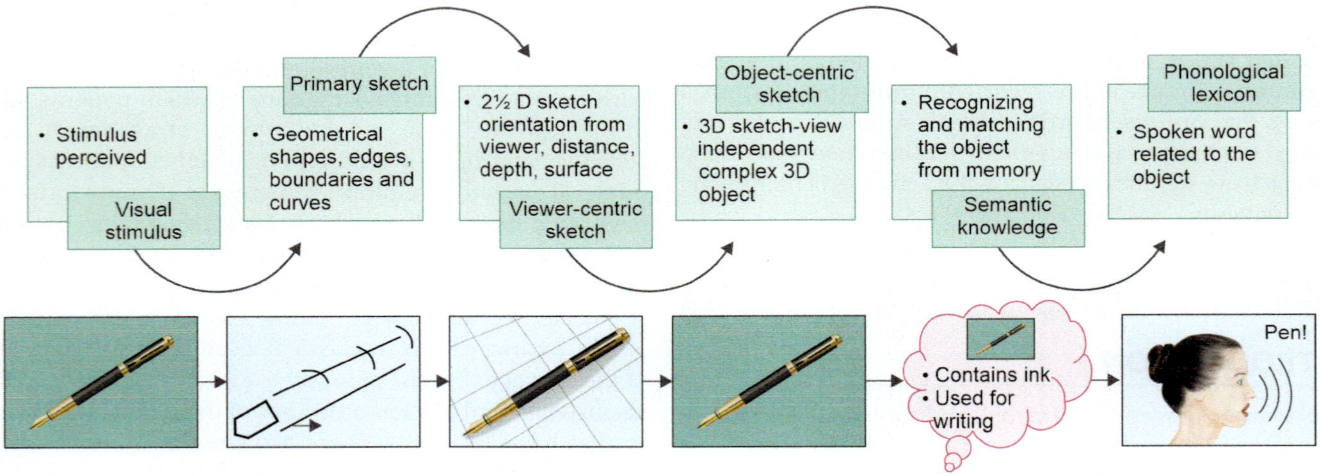

FIG. 3: Hierarchical model of visual recognition of an object.

CLINICAL APPROACH

There are three main types of agnosia, based on the abnormality of a single sensory modality.

1. Visual agnosia
2. Auditory agnosia
3. Tactile agnosia

Visual Agnosia

It refers to the inability to visually recognize objects, faces, pictures, colors despite preserved visual acuity, visual field, color vision, memory, and language. They can recognize the objects in the other sensory modalities. Clues can be obtained by enquiring from the bystanders of the patient's performance of various activities of daily living. The patients have difficulty in differentiating day-to-day items such as a toothbrush, razor, or a comb and may struggle to recognize faces but quickly identify the individual through their voice. Patients can display more difficulties when encountered with a clutter of objects rather than objects in isolation. It must be borne in mind that the mere lack of recognition or difficulty in naming does not equate to agnosia. Other higher-order cognitive disorders such as aphasia or semantic memory loss or defects in vision can lead to similar outcome and the clinical evaluation should be directed keeping in mind the alternate possibilities.

Types of Visual Agnosia

Visual object agnosia: It is a prototypic example of visual agnosia which can be divided into apperceptive and associative agnosia.[19]

- *Apperceptive visual object agnosia*: Patients have difficulty in identifying visually an object as a whole despite preserved ability to identify lines, angles, color, and movement. As the name suggests, the patient has difficulty in the visual perception of an object. Damage to bilateral visual cortices causes apperceptive visual object agnosia. They are unable to copy a figure, match figures, but can draw from memory **(Fig. 4)**.
- *Associative visual object agnosia*: Patients have difficulty in visual recognition of an object despite preserved visual perception. They are unable to name the object, explain the use, or pantomime the action. They can copy figures or draw from the memory but cannot tell what they have drawn or copied. However, they can recognize the object in other sensory modalities **(Fig. 5)**. This is a disconnection syndrome wherein there is disconnection between the occipital and temporal lobe (memory and language).[20,21]

Optic aphasia/optic anomia: Patients are unable to name a visually presented object but able to describe its use and pantomime its action. They can name the objects in other sensory modalities. This is a disconnection syndrome wherein there is disconnection between the occipital and language area.

Prosopagnosia: Patients have inability to name or recognize faces on seeing but can recognize by their voice or mannerism.[22] The semantic knowledge about the person is well preserved. Patients have difficulty in learning new faces. It may be apperceptive prosopagnosia wherein there is abnormality in perception of face or associative prosopagnosia wherein they can perceive the faces but cannot recognize it. The recognition of emotions may or may not be preserved in prosopagnosia. Involvement of inferior occipital lobe (face perception area) and fusiform gyrus (face recognition area) and the disconnection of these areas with the temporal lobe are seen in prosopagnosia.

Simultanagnosia: Patients have the inability to recognize simultaneously multiple objects or multiple features of an object. They can identify individual objects but cannot identify the unifying theme of the scene or picture like missing forest for a tree. Patients with simultanagnosia have reduced focused attention, impaired spatial processing, and reduced spatial window of attention.[23]

Simultanagnosia can be classified into two types:

- *Dorsal simultanagnosia*: Patients are unable to see more than one object at a time. They can identify single object in a picture but once their attention is diverted to the other thing, they can then identify only that thing; other things disappear to them. It is a visual attentional disorder. They have difficulty in reading as it involves viewing more than one word at a time. They often bump into objects that are close together. It is associated with lesions in the bilateral parieto-occipital cortex.[21]
- *Ventral simultanagnosia*: Similar to dorsal simultanagnosia, patients cannot identify more than one object, but they can see more than one object at a time. However,

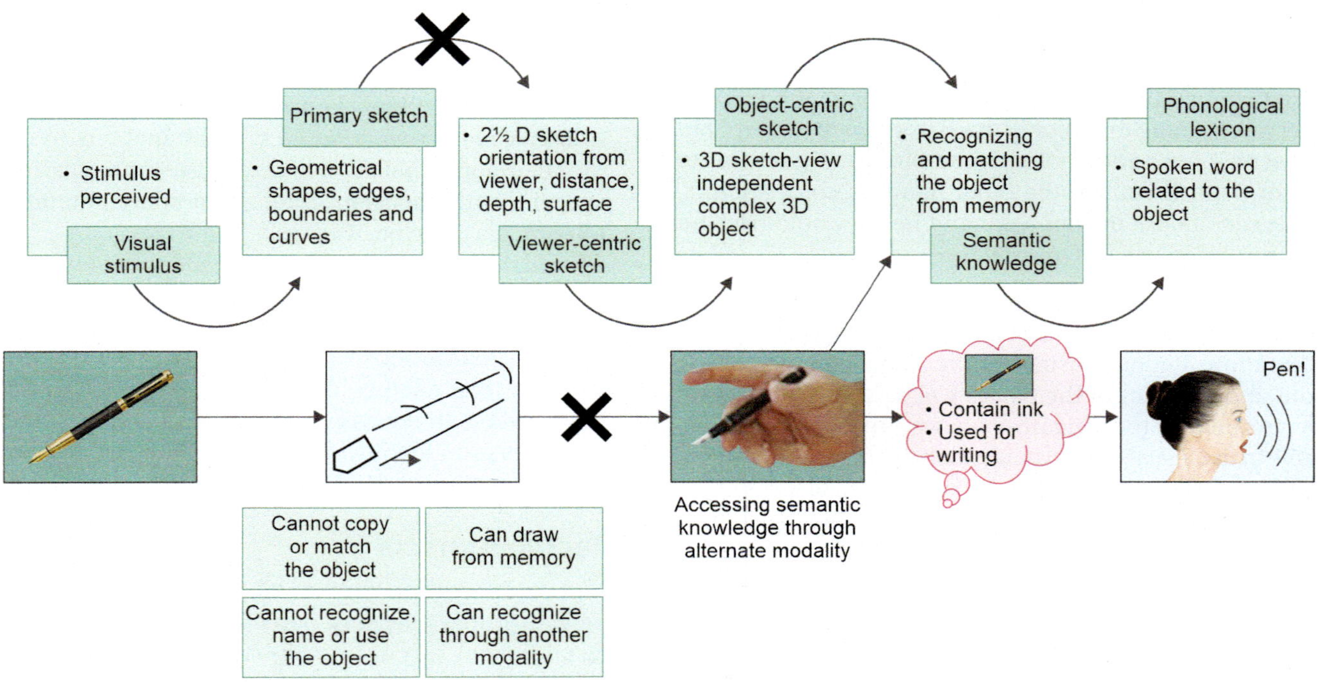

FIG. 4: Conceptual model of apperceptive visual object agnosia.

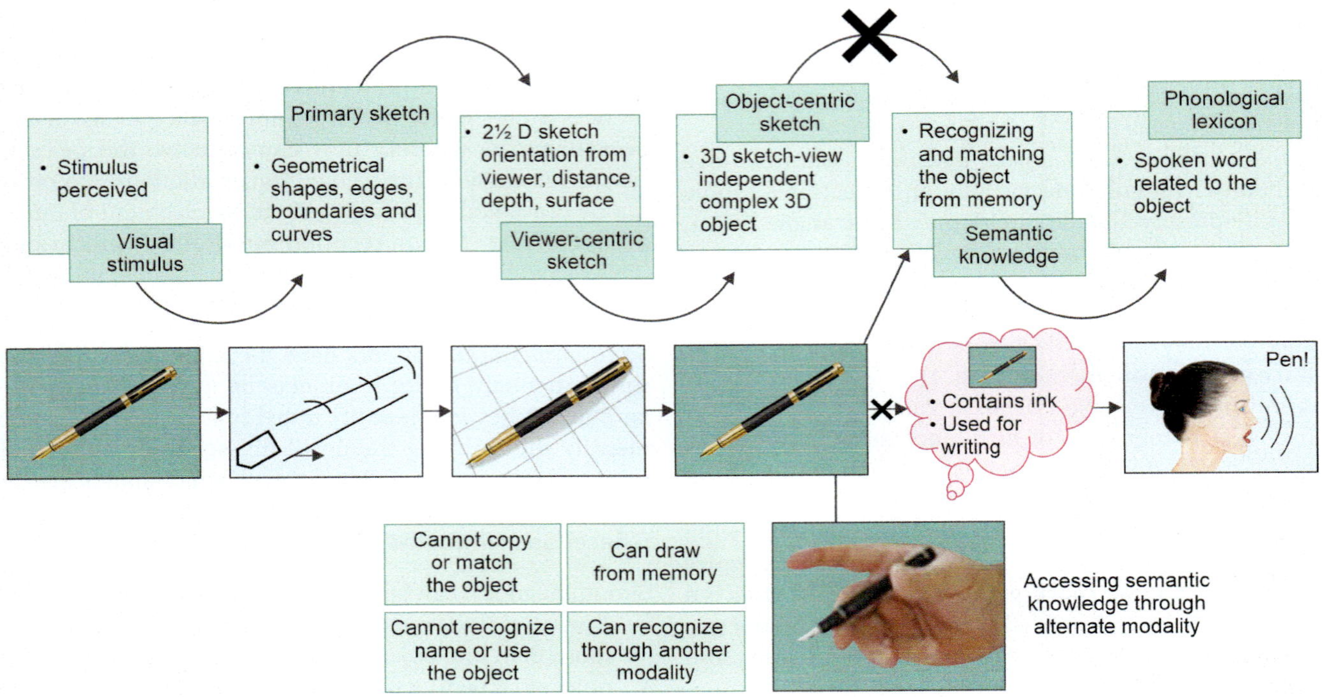

FIG. 5: Conceptual model of associative visual object agnosia.

the patient is unable to name the object correctly. For example, in a picture with moon, stars, etc., patient may identify the moon as a ball and not able to derive the meaning of the whole picture. Lesions in the left inferior occipital area cause ventral simultanagnosia.[21]

Color agnosia: Patients with color agnosia can perceive colors, read the Ishihara plates correctly, but are unable to identify, name, or categorize colors without matching.[21] The color, though perceived and distinguished from others, gets stripped of its meaning rendering "red" unrecognizable as "red". Since the semantic memory about the color is preserved, naming the color of the sky or that of an elephant is preserved but patient struggles to pick the right color to draw or paint them. On the other hand, in color anomia, patient can choose the apt color and hence would have no trouble in coloring a leaf or a red rose.

Topographical agnosia: Patients have inability to orient to surroundings due to their inability to interpret spatial information. Patients usually have good memory of the layout and specifics of the places well known to them, but they are unable to navigate their way through. They are unable to use visual cues to guide them in the right direction. This is seen in lesion in the right posterior cingulate area.[21]

Finger agnosia: Patients are unable to name the fingers of their own hand as well as the that of others. They are not able to show specific fingers of their own hand or examiner hand when instructed. Finger agnosia is a part of Gerstmann syndrome.[21]

Auditory Agnosia

Patients with auditory agnosia can hear the sound, thus differentiating from deafness, but unable to recognize or identify the nature of the sound.[21,24]

Auditory agnosia can be divided into:

- *Auditory verbal agnosia or pure word deafness*: As the name suggests, patients have inability to understand spoken words but can write, read, and speak and have preserved ability to recognize nonverbal sounds. It is the disconnection of both primary auditory cortices from the left hemisphere Wernicke area.
- *Auditory nonverbal agnosia*: It is the inability to comprehend nonverbal sounds and noises, with sparing of speech comprehension. Damage to bilateral temporal lobe causes this type of agnosia.
- *Phonagnosia*: Phonagnosia is the auditory counterpart of prosopagnosia wherein the patients fail to recognize familiar people by their voices. Phonagnosia is seen in temporal lobe lesions.[25]
- *Amusia*: It is inability to recognize the music. Patients have trouble in recognizing the tune, pitch, or familiar melodies or in identifying out-of-tone music. Amusia is seen in temporoparietal lesions.

Tactile Agnosia

Failure to recognize familiar objects by touch despite preserved primary sensory perception constitutes tactile agnosia. Patient can accurately describe the size, shape, weight, and texture of the given object but still fails to recognize it. Astereognosis and agraphesthesia can sometimes be considered as a tactile apperceptive agnosia. But prominently sensory inattention is absent in tactile agnosia. Interesting insights have been gained by asking the patients to draw the object which they cannot recognize tactually by identifying bits and pieces and finally with the patient being able to identify the object through his or her drawing.[26] Tactile agnosia of nondominant limb is seen in anterior corpus callosum lesion.

INVESTIGATOR APPROACH

Before embarking upon an evaluation of the agnosia, the first step would be to rule out an abnormality in primary sensory modality. Visual acuity and visual fields deficits that can alternately explain the symptoms need to be considered and excluded. Other higher cognitive abnormalities in speech, language, memory, and attention should be appropriately looked for.

Visual object agnosia:

- *Naming*: Patient is presented with pictures of familiar objects, figures, or animals and is asked to describe what they see and to name them including their function.
- *Matching of objects and figures*: Patient can be given pictures of objects or figures and can be asked to correctly pick the object from a series of related images. Patients can also be asked to match between dissimilar objects with related function, e.g., pyramids and palm tree.
- *Copying*: Patient is asked to copy line diagrams, figures, or shapes.
- Other tests include Gollin figures, incomplete letter, silhouette identification, and usual/unusual view tests. The Birmingham Object Recognition Battery (BORB) is a 14-point neuropsychological assessment battery for visual object recognition which can be used in research setting.[27]
- *Alternate sensory modality*: In agnosia, the patient's deficits are typically modality specific, and the patient can identify the object through touch, hearing, or smell. Since the semantic knowledge is preserved, the patient would be able to correctly describe the object including its function if asked. For instance, a patient with visual object agnosia may not recognize the key but can accurately describe a key and can even draw a key from memory. **Table 3** summarizes the differences between visual object agnosia from similar higher-order processing disorders.

Color agnosia:

- *Ishihara chart*: Patients with color blindness will not be able to read the numbers depending on the type of color blindness such as red-green or blue-yellow. Patients with achromatopsia will not be able to read the numbers in any of the plates as the whole world appears black, white, or gray. Patients with color agnosia, anomia, or amnesia will be able to read the Ishihara plates correctly.
- *Naming of colors*: The patient can be given colored cards and asked to name the colors and conversely can be asked to point to a particular colored card. Patients can be asked to name the color of a familiar object such as the sky or an elephant which will be preserved in color agnosia, color blindness, or achromatopsia but may be impaired in color anomia and color amnesia.
- *Matching and copying*: The patient should be asked to match or copy the color from a given set of items.
- *Coloring*: The patient is asked about the color of common objects and asked to color appropriately. **Table 4** differentiates color agnosia from related disorders.

Prosopagnosia:

- *Face recognition*: The simple and rudimentary test is the patient's ability to recognize age and culturally familiar and popular faces. The Benton Facial Recognition Test and Cambridge Face Memory Test can be used to test face recognition.[28,29]
- *Face perception*: Patients are asked to differentiate or match between faces. Patients with the apperceptive variant would not be able to match or differentiate between faces while this will be preserved in the associative variant.

Simultanagnosia:

- *Modified single letter cancellation test*: In a modified version of the letter cancellation test, the patient is presented with a sheet of paper on which letters of

TABLE 3: Salient features in object agnosia/optic aphasia/semantic memory impairment.

Test	Apperceptive agnosia	Associative agnosia	Anomia	Semantic memory impairment
Naming	Impaired	Impaired	Impaired	Impaired
Describing its function	Impaired	Impaired	Preserved	Impaired
Matching	Impaired	Preserved	Preserved	Preserved
Copying	Impaired	Preserved	Preserved	Preserved
Recognizing through alternate modality	Preserved	Preserved	Naming impaired—except in optic aphasia/anomia	Impaired
Demonstrating appropriate use	Impaired	Impaired	Preserved	Impaired

TABLE 4: Differentiating features among color identification abnormalities.

Test	Color agnosia	Color blindness	Color anomia	Color achromatopsia	Color amnesia
Ishihara chart	Preserved	Impaired	Preserved	Impaired	Preserved
Color naming	Impaired	Impaired	Impaired	Impaired	Impaired
Matching/copying	Impaired	Impaired	Preserved	Impaired	Preserved
Coloring	Impaired	Impaired	Preserved	Impaired	Impaired

varying sizes are written for instance A. The patient is asked to circle every "A" in the picture. Since the patient has a deficit in visual attention, the patient can only circle the smaller "A" and would miss the larger ones.

- *Global letter made of the focal letter*: The patient is presented with a large alphabet made of smaller alphabets, for instance a large "F" made of small "Es". The patient will not be able to recognize the larger alphabet and can only visualize the E.
- *Global face or object made of focal objects*: The patient may be presented with a painting such as that of a face made up of fruits and asked to describe what he or she sees. The patient with simultanagnosia fails to see the face but can recognize the individual elements.[23]
- *Cookie theft picture or mixed figure test*: The patient is asked to describe all items in a complex scene or that in a picture with multiple overlapping objects. Patients may laboriously struggle through each item in the picture but may not be able to put together the whole theme in the cookie-theft picture or all the individual components in the overlapping mixed figure. The patient with simultanagnosia fails to see the face but can recognize the individual elements.[23]

Tactile agnosia:

- *Test of primary somatosensory function*: Light touch, pinprick, temperature, vibration, joint position, two-point discrimination, and sensory attention should be normal.
- *Object identification*: Patients are asked to identify different objects by palpation. Astereognosis is considered the apperceptive variant of tactile agnosia where a patient cannot identify the size, shape, weight, or texture of an object. In the associative variant, patients can match and even draw the object by touch, which can closely resemble the object, conveying that the perception is normal.[26]

Auditory agnosia:

- *Speech comprehension and repetition*: This will be impaired in pure word deafness or verbal agnosia while preserved in amusia, phonagnosia, and nonverbal agnosia. Preservation of repetition will depend on the variant of agnosia be it apperceptive (resembling Wernicke's aphasia but with preserved reading and writing) or associative.

TABLE 5: Localization in agnosia.

Agnosia	Localization
Apperceptive agnosia	Bilateral occipitotemporal
Associative agnosia	Inferior occipitotemporal
Color agnosia	Dominant inferior occipitotemporal
Auditory agnosia	Bilateral temporal
Tactile agnosia	Either right or left posterior parietotemporal
Prosopagnosia	Bilateral fusiform gyri
Dorsal simultagnosia	Bilateral parieto-occipital
Ventral simultagnosia	Dominant temporo-occipital

- *Nonspeech recognition and repetition*: This will be selectively impaired in nonverbal agnosia. Pitch, rhythm, or timber recognition or identifying familiar melodies—will be selectively impaired in amusia but will also be impaired in nonverbal agnosia.
- *Identification of familiar voices*: In phonagnosia, patients will no longer be able to identify through familiar voices.

Several different etiologies ranging from vascular and degenerative to toxic etiologies such as carbon monoxide poisoning can lead to agnosia. MRI would be the imaging modality of choice. A detailed clinical evaluation including cognitive and neuropsychological assessment is required as an isolated presentation of agnosia is rare. **Table 5** shows the different agnosias and their lesion locations.

CONCLUSION

Agnosia is a disabling dysfunction of higher-order sensory perception, aptly referred to as "mind-blindness" by Lissauer. Without awareness and a bit of clinical inquisitiveness, these can be easily missed and can be brushed aside as a defect of the primary sensory modality which they can superficially resemble. At times, manifesting bizarrely, such as in the "man who mistook his wife for a hat", agnosia provides a window of opportunity to understand the complexities of the human brain. Understanding and counseling regarding the nature of their symptoms can go a long way and is the first step in rehabilitating the patient and their caregivers.

REFERENCES

1. Leiguarda RC, Marsden CD. Limb apraxias: higher-order disorders of sensorimotor integration. Brain. 2000;123:860-79.
2. Gross RG, Grossman M. Update on apraxia. Curr Neurol Neurosci Rep. 2008;8(6):490-6.
3. Heilman KM, Rothi U, Valenstein E. Two forms of ideomotor apraxia. Neurology. 1982;32:342-6.
4. Petreska B, Adriani M, Blanke O, Billard AG. Apraxia: a review. Prog Brain Res. 2007;164:61-83.
5. Geschwind N. The apraxias: neural mechanisms of disorders of learned movement. Am Sci. 1975;63:188-95.
6. Heilman KM, Rothi LJ. Apraxia. In: Heilman KM, Valenstein E (Eds). Clinical Neuropsychology, 3rd edition. New York: Oxford University Press; 1993. pp. 141-63.
7. Roy EA, Square PA. Common considerations in the study of limb, verbal and oral apraxia. In: Roy EA (Ed). Neuropsychological Studies of Apraxia and Related Disorders. North-Holland, Amsterdam: Series Advances in Psychology; 1985. pp. 111-61.
8. Rothi L, Ochipa C, Heilman K. A cognitive neuropsychological model of limb praxis. Cogn Neuropsychol. 1991;8(6):443-58.
9. Dressing A, Kaller CP, Martin M, Nitschke K, Kuemmerer D, Beume LA, et al. Anatomical correlates of recovery in apraxia: A longitudinal lesion-mapping study in stroke patients. Cortex. 2021;142:104-21.
10. Heilman KM. Upper Limb Apraxia. Continuum (Minneap Minn). 2021;27(6):1602-23.
11. Ochipa C, Rothi LJ, Heilman KM. Conduction apraxia. J Neurol Neurosurg Psychiatry. 1994;57(10):1241-4.
12. Niessen E, Fink GR, Weiss PH. Apraxia, pantomime and the parietal cortex. Neuroimage Clin. 2014;5:42-52.
13. Ahmed S, Baker I, Thompson S. Utility of testing for apraxia and associated features in dementia. J Neurol Neurosurg Psychiatry. 2016;87(11):1158-62.
14. Jo S, Oh JS, Cheong EN, Kim HJ, Lee S, Oh M, et al. FDG-PET patterns associated with ideomotor apraxia and imitation apraxia in patients with corticobasal syndrome. Parkinsonism Relat Disord. 2021;88:96-101.
15. Cassidy A. The clinical assessment of apraxia. Pract Neurol. 2016;16:317-22.
16. Milner AD. How do the two visual streams interact with each other? Exp Brain Res. 2017;235(5):1297-308.
17. Martinaud O. Visual agnosia and focal brain injury. Rev Neurol (Paris). 2017;173(7–8):451-60.
18. Kitcher P. Marr's Computational Theory of Vision. Philos Sci. 1988; 55(1):1-24.
19. Greene JDW. Apraxia, agnosias, and higher visual function abnormalities. J Neurol Neurosurg Psychiatry. 2005;76(suppl 5):v25-34.
20. Bartolomeo P. Visual agnosia and imagery after Lissauer. Brain. 2021;144(9):2557-9.
21. Kumar A, Wroten M. (2022). Agnosia. [online] Available from https://www.ncbi.nlm.nih.gov/books/NBK493156/. [Last accessed April, 2023]
22. Lahiri D. Prosopagnosia. Cortex. 2020;132:479.
23. Dalrymple KA, Barton JJS, Kingstone A. A world unglued: simultanagnosia as a spatial restriction of attention. Front Hum Neurosci. 2013;7:145.
24. Slevc LR, Shell AR. Auditory agnosia. Handb Clin Neurol. 2015;129:573-87.
25. Van Lancker DR, Cummings JL, Kreiman J, Dobkin BH. Phonagnosia: a dissociation between familiar and unfamiliar voices. Cortex. 1988;24(2):195-209.
26. Reed CL, Caselli RJ, Farah MJ. Tactile agnosia: Underlying impairment and implications for normal tactile object recognition. Brain. 1996;119(Pt 3):875-88.
27. Riddoch JM, Humphreys GW. Borb: Birmingham Object Recognition Battery. London: Psychology Press; 2022. p. 410.
28. Corrow SL, Dalrymple KA, Barton JJ. Prosopagnosia: current perspectives. Eye Brain. 2016;8:165-75.
29. Albonico A, Malaspina M, Daini R. Italian normative data and validation of two neuropsychological tests of face recognition: Benton Facial Recognition Test and Cambridge Face Memory Test. Neurol Sci. 2017;38(9):1637-43.

29

CHAPTER

Approach to Dysarthrias

Dhananjay Duberakar

INTRODUCTION

Motor speech disorders are syndromes of abnormal articulation, the motor production of speech, without abnormalities of language. Dysarthrias involve the abnormal articulation of sounds or phonemes, and it is a type of motor speech disorder. The pathogenic mechanism in dysarthria is abnormal neuromuscular activation of the speech muscles, affecting the speed, strength, timing, range, or accuracy of movements involving speech.[1] Speech disorders can be mechanical, as in patients with physical disorders of the pharynx and larynx, but dysarthrias are neurogenic, related to dysfunction of the central nervous system, nerves, neuromuscular junction, or muscle, with a contribution of sensory deficits in some cases. Dysarthria not only affects articulation but also phonation, breathing, and prosody (emotional tone) of speech. Anarthria is a total loss of ability to articulate.

Dysarthrias can be analyzed in terms of the brain lesion sites associated with specific patterns of speech impairment. Analysis of dysarthria at the bedside is useful for the localization of neurological lesions and the diagnosis of neurological disorders. An experienced examiner should be able to recognize the major types of dysarthria, rather than referring to "dysarthria" as a single disorder.

NEURAL BASIS OF SPEECH PRODUCTION

In humans, there are four main body systems involved in the production of speech. The respiratory system, laryngeal system, and articulatory system are responsible for the physical manifestations of speech, and the nervous system regulates these systems on both the conscious and the unconscious levels. The production of spoken language involves three major levels of processing: conceptualization, formulation, and articulation. Accordingly, a large portion of the cerebral cortex is involved in simple speech tasks, such as reading a single word or a meaningless syllable. There are three main types of information involved in speech–motor control: auditory, somatosensory, and motor, represented in the temporal, parietal, and frontal lobes of the cerebral cortex, respectively. Additionally medial and lateral prefrontal cortices contribute to the fluent selection and initiation of these speech–motor programs.[2] Activity in these cortical regions is modulated by two loops through subcortical brain regions during speech production: a basal ganglia loop involved in action selection and initiation, and a cerebellar loop involved in generating the finely tuned motor commands that underlie fluent speech. These brain regions and their interconnections, along with additional subcortical nuclei in the thalamus, midbrain, and brainstem, constitute the neural control system responsible for speech production. The DIVA (Directions Into Velocities of Articulators) model and its extension the GODIVA (Gradient Order DIVA) model of speech production provide a computationally and neuroanatomically explicit account of the network of brain regions involved in speech acquisition and production.

The normal speech pattern is achieved through the smooth coordination of respiration, phonation, articulation, resonance, and prosody. Adequate breath support and forced exhalation give way to changes in vocal cord length, position, and vibratory pattern. During exhalation changes in the size and shape of the oral cavity in conjunction with the articulators produce phonemes for speech production. Changes in prosody at the same time attach meanings to phonemes with alterations in pitch, intonation, stress, and rate. Together, these coordinated mechanisms allow us to effectively participate in day-to-day conversation.[1,2]

- *Respiration*: Diaphragm is used to quickly fill the lungs fully, followed by slow, controlled exhalation for speech.
- *Phonation*: Vocal cord use and airflow to produce a voice of varying pitch, loudness, and quality
- *Resonance*: The soft palate is raised and lowered to direct the voice to resonate in the oral and/or nasal cavities to further affect voice quality.

CHAPTER 29

- *Articulation*: Coordination of quick, precise movements of the lips, tongue, mandible, and soft palate for clarity of speech
- *Prosody*: Combination of all elements for a natural flow of conversational speech, with adequate loudness, emphasis, and melodic tone to enhance meaning

APPROACH TO DYSARTHRIA

Normal speech production involves the integration and coordination of five primary physiological subsystems: respiration, phonation, articulation, resonance, and prosody. Lesions along the neuroaxis that produce motor dysfunction of any of these five speech systems may produce dysarthria. Lesions can be unilateral or bilateral and localize to the cerebral cortex, subcortical structures, brainstem, cerebellum, basal ganglia, cranial nerves, upper cervical nerves, or even the neuromuscular junction or muscles.[3] Differentiating among the dysarthrias is not simple as there is much overlap in the semiology of the various types of dysarthria, although certain speech characteristics are often associated with specific types of dysarthria. There have been several attempts in classifying dysarthria since the first attempt by Froeschels in 1943; however, the most seminal contribution in this area has been the Mayo Clinic classification system provided by Darley, Aronson, and Brown (DAB).[4] To this day, their classification system linking brain pathology and speech behavior remains the most utilized classification. The flaccid, spastic, mixed, ataxic, hypokinetic, and hyperkinetic dysarthria are best characterized and will be discussed here.

Flaccid Dysarthria

Flaccid dysarthria or peripheral dysarthria or lower motor neuron (LMN) dysarthria results from damage to the peripheral nervous system. Flaccid paralysis reflects final common pathway damage. Reflexive, automatic, and voluntary movements all are affected, which helps in differentiating this LMN cause from lesions of other parts in the motor system. Flaccid dysarthria is far from being a uniform syndrome. The speech symptoms vary depending upon which particular nerve(s) and/or muscles are primarily affected. The neurology of flaccid dysarthria, therefore, requires a systematic evaluation of several components of the vocal tract, including respiratory, laryngeal, velopharyngeal, and orofacial structures. It is typically caused by damage to cranial nerves V (motor division), VII, X, and XII that supply muscles of articulation.

Flaccid dysarthria commonly seen in bulbar palsy is characterized by excessive hypernasality. Articulation of consonants and/or vowels is imprecise with a slow and labored speech rate. Sometimes rapid weakness with use and recovery with rest suggests neuromuscular junction involvement. Weakness, hypotonia, and diminished reflexes are the main characteristics of flaccid dysarthria; atrophy fasciculations and fibrillations commonly accompany them. Other visible signs that accompany flaccid dysarthria include facial or soft palate droop, or nasal regurgitation with eating (again, if the velum is an affected area). Dysphagia is common, given the shared nature of the muscles for talking and those for chewing and swallowing. It requires evaluation alongside speech difficulties.

Spastic Dysarthria

Spastic dysarthria occurs in patients with bilateral lesions of the motor cortex or corticobulbar tracts, rendering the muscles that govern articulation both weak and spastic. The phonation is typically harsh or "strain-strangle" in vocal quality, with a reduced rate, low pitch, and consonant errors. Patients often have the features of "pseudobulbar palsy," including dysphagia, exaggerated jaw jerk and gag reflexes, and emotional incontinence (pseudobulbar affect, or pathological laughter and crying). On examination, the tongue is protruded and moved from side to side with difficulty. Mouth opening may seem restricted, and speech seems to come from the back of the mouth.

A milder variant of spastic dysarthria, "unilateral upper motor neuron (UMN)" dysarthria, is associated with unilateral UMN lesions.[1] This type of dysarthria has features like those of spastic dysarthria, only in a less severe form. Unilateral UMN dysarthria is one of the most common types of dysarthria, occurring in patients with unilateral strokes.

Amyotrophic lateral sclerosis may cause dysarthria with both spastic and flaccid features.

Ataxic Dysarthria

Ataxic dysarthria is associated with damage to the cerebellar control circuit, which includes the cerebellum and its connections. It is commonly associated with bilateral or generalized cerebellar disease. Lesions in lateral hemispheres or posteromedial and paravermal regions are implicated when focal lesions produce dysarthria. Lesions of the superior cerebellar peduncle or anywhere along frontopontocerebellar pathways may produce ataxic dysarthria.[3] Ataxic dysarthria usually occurs with other cerebellar signs, but occasionally dysarthria is the only sign of cerebellar disease and in these situations, helps in localization.

Characteristic features of ataxic dysarthria are strained voice, monotonicity, and slow rate. Distinguishing features are irregular articulatory errors, equal and excessive stress on syllables, and inappropriate variation of pitch and loudness. Patients with ataxic dysarthria exhibit abnormalities in timing due to impairment in muscular force and incoordination of the muscles of the vocal tract. As the disorder progresses, speech and language errors may increase, causing difficulty in producing intelligible speech. Ataxic dysarthria is described as "slurred speech" having explosive staccato, scanning vocalization, and wavering modulation.[5]

Hypokinetic Dysarthria

Hypokinetic dysarthria is a motor speech disorder most frequently associated with Parkinson's disease.[6] Any process that can damage the basal ganglia control circuit can cause hypokinetic dysarthria. Degenerative conditions account for almost two-third of the cases. Sometimes it is the only presenting symptom of parkinsonism. It is characterized by hypophonia or reduced vocal loudness, monotonous speech with a slow and flat rhythm. Initiation of speech is difficult, resulting in inappropriate silences intermixed, however, with short rushes of speech. Patients often suffer from a lack of respiratory support, as well as phonatory problems which are most characterized by a drop in volume. The rate is variable with wide fluctuations in pitch. It is often associated with other signs of basal ganglia disease.

Hyperkinetic Dysarthria

Speech disorders arising from abnormal activity affecting the cortico-basal ganglia-thalamocortical circuitry causing involuntary movements are broadly classified as hyperkinetic dysarthria.[4,7] It is characterized by abnormal involuntary movements affecting respiratory, phonatory, and articulatory structures affecting communication, deglutition, and quality of life. In hyperkinetic dysarthria, interestingly, affected speech structures exhibit normal strength, speed, and range of motion, though involuntary movements may occur symmetrically, asymmetrically, or unilaterally.[3,4,7] Commonly observed speech patterns in those with hyperkinetic dysarthria include unexpected variations in pitch or loudness, inappropriate pauses, constant or intermittent dysphonia, constant or intermittent hyper- or hyponasality, articulatory imprecision, and slow speaking rate due to frequent or extended pause durations.[8] **Table 1** gives the various types of hyperkinetic dysarthria, while **Table 2** gives a summary of types of dysarthria.

Mixed Dysarthria

Mixed dysarthria is caused by simultaneous damage to two or more primary motor components of the nervous system, such as combined UMN and LMN lesions. Mixed dysarthria is common in patients with multiple sclerosis, motor neuron disease, and severe traumatic brain injury. Speech is very slow and with effort. Articulation is markedly impaired with considerable hypernasality. Pitch is usually low with a strained or strangled vocal quality. Prosody is disrupted by intonation errors and inappropriately shortened sentences. Bulbar involvement in motor neuron disease often presents with dysarthria, hypophonia, drooling of saliva, and progressive swallowing difficulties.

DIFFERENTIAL DIAGNOSIS

Dysarthria and apraxia both are motor speech disorders, and are sometimes difficult to differentiate. Apraxia of speech is a motor programming or planning disorder involving speech production tasks. Automatic and involuntary tasks are usually spared. Subjects are often aware of the errors and make attempts at correcting them. Aphasia is a loss or impairment of language processing, whereas dysarthria is a problem in speech articulation. It is not uncommon for aphasia and dysarthria to coexist. Anarthria is the total loss of ability to articulate.

EVALUATION OF DYSARTHRIA PATIENT

In the evaluation of speech disorders, a speech-language pathologist (SLP) is often consulted to differentiate among the various types of dysarthria and help determine the best treatment strategies. The lack of SLPs in our country puts a lot of burden and responsibility on neurologists for the evaluation of dysarthria. In general, the assessment focuses on the subsystems of speech, including respiration, phonatory, resonance, prosody, and articulation.

Purposes of the motor speech exam:
- Description and problem detection.
- Establish diagnostic possibilities
- Establish a diagnosis
- Determine implications for localization
- Specify severity

Case History

Case history usually consists of hearing, vision, swallowing, and language problems that patients have, followed by

TABLE 1: Hyperkinetic dysarthria types.

Quick	Chorea	Extrapyramidal system	Highly variable pattern of imprecise articulation, episodes of hypernasality, sudden variations in loudness
	Myoclonus		Rhythmic hypernasality phonatory interruptions
	Tourette syndrome		Sudden tic such as grunts, barks, coprolalia
Slow	Athetosis	Extrapyramidal system	No distinct deviation
	Dyskinesia		No distinct deviation
	Dystonia		Prolongations of phonemes, intervals, unsteady rate, loudness
Tremors	Voice tremors	Extrapyramidal system	Rhythmic alterations in pitch, loudness, and voice stoppages

TABLE 2: Summary of types of dysarthria.

	Flaccid	Spastic	Ataxic	Hypokinetic	Hyperkinetic
Pathophysiology	Hypotonia (muscle weakness)	Hypertonia (muscle spasticity)	Hypotonia, dysmetria (impaired movement control)	Hypokinesia (decreased movement)	Hyperkinesia (increased movement)
Articulation	Distorted pressure consonants and vowels slow rate	Imprecise consonants, slow, movements slowed	Distorted vowels, slow articulatory breakdowns, telescoping slow rates	Imprecise consonants, dysfluencies, increased/variable rate	Distorted vowels, irregular articulatory breakdowns, variable rate
Phonation	Hoarse and breathy	Harsh and strained, pitch breaks	Breathy, harsh and strained, voice tremors, pitch breaks	Breathy and harsh, reduced loudness	Breathy and strained, intermittent voice arrests
Prosody	Excess and equal stress, monopitch, monoloudness, prolonged phonemes	Reduced stress, monopitch, monoloudness, short phrases	Excess and equal stress, prolonged phonemes	Reduced stress, monopitch, monoloudness, short rushes of speech	Irregular stress, prolonged silences
Resonance	Hypernasality, nasal emissions	Hypernasality	Intermittent hypo- and hypernasality	Mild hypernasality	Irregular, velopharyngeal incompetence
Respiration	Inhalatory stridor, reduced maximum phonation time	Paradoxical breathing	Excessive loudness variations	Reduced vital capacity	Sudden involuntary inspirations or expirations
Example	ALS	ALS, CP, MS, MSA, PSP	AT, MS, MSA	MSA, PD, PSP	HD, TD

(ALS: amyotrophic lateral sclerosis; AT: ataxia–telangiectasia; CP: cerebral palsy; HD: Huntington's disease; MS: multiple sclerosis; MSA: multiple system atrophy; PD: Parkinson's disease; PSP: progressive supranuclear palsy; TD: tardive dyskinesia)

medication history. Other information includes personal information such as information regarding family, education level, and patients' language proficiency in all language modalities; the patient's communication needs; and the family's expectations for therapy.

Oral Motor Examination

The aim is to assess the accuracy, range, strength, and speed of the lips, tongue, and jaw movements. The oral motor assessment consists of observation of the neck and facial muscle tone during a nonspeech "rest" state by performing the cranial nerve exam (V, VII, IX, X, XII) to identify oral and facial symmetry, tongue movement coordination, speed of movement, range of movement, and strength assessed by performing sequential motion rates and alternating motion rates.

Speech Production Examination

Ask the patient to count (from 1 to 10), and read aloud (word, phrase, sentence). Engage the patient in a brief spontaneous conversation to understand the ability to follow simple and complex instructions, whether there are any changes in pitch, tone, loudness with the conversation, accuracy of speech production, speech rate (i.e., talking too slow or too fast), and speech intelligibility.

ASSESSMENT TOOLS

The accurate diagnosis of the types of dysarthria is important in developing an effective treatment program for patients. Assessment tools used by SLPs could be divided into two types, namely formal and informal assessment tools.[9] The most commonly used formal assessment tool by SLPs is the Frenchay dysarthria assessment (FDA).[10] However, there are other assessment tools used for the diagnosis of dysarthria such as the dysarthria profile, dysarthric speech, and voice handicap index. The informal assessment in terms of the oral motor examination is used alongside the formal assessment.[9] Perceptual assessment (listening to speech characteristics to describe the various dimensions of respiration, phonation, articulation, resonance, and prosody) in order to classify the type and severity of dysarthria is gold standard practice for SLPs.[7] These perceptual judgments are subjective as assessment finding depends on the clinicians' expertise in active listening and analyzing the speech.

MANAGEMENT

The underlying etiology of dysarthria and prognosis for improvement are important considerations when deciding about the treatment plan. Treatment can be restorative (i.e., aimed at improving or restoring impaired function) and/or compensatory (i.e., aimed at compensating for deficits not amenable to retraining). Treatments are grouped into (a) those that directly target the speech-production subsystems, and (b) other treatment options, including communication strategies, environmental modifications, augmentative and alternative communication, and medical/surgical interventions by other specialists. Treatment of respiratory/phonatory deficits includes improving breath support to increase vocal volume. Nonspeech oral motor training is recommended for strengthening muscles and increasing mouth, tongue, and lip range of motion and movement. Changes in loudness and prosody, through intonation and stress patterning tasks, are useful measures. In severe cases, augmentative and alternative communication strategies, such as computerized voice production systems, are useful.

CONCLUSION

Dysarthrias result from a variety of disorders of the articulatory apparatus. Various clinical characteristics can be utilized to scrutinize the types, and anatomical and physiological understanding further helps the identification. A systematic approach to the problem is very informative and clinically rewarding.

REFERENCES

1. Duffy JR. Motor Speech Disorders: Substrates, Differential Diagnosis, and Management. St. Louis: Mosby-Year Book; 1995.
2. Guenther FH. Neural Control of Speech. Cambridge: MIT Press; 2016.
3. Kent RD, Duffy JR, Slama A, Kent JF, Clift A. Clinicoanatomic studies in dysarthria: review, critique, and directions for research. J Speech Lang Hear Res. 2001;44(3):535-51.
4. Darley FL, Aronson AE, Brown JR. Clusters of deviant speech dimensions in the dysarthrias. J Speech Hear Res. 1969;12:462-96.
5. Ogawa K, Yoshihashi H, Suzuki Y, Kamei S, Mizutani T. Clinical study of the responsible lesion for dysarthria in the cerebellum. Intern Med. 2010;49(9):861-4.
6. Moustapha SM, Alain G, Robert E, Bernard T, Mourtalla KM, Lamine G, et al. Pneumophonic coordination impairments in parkinsonian dysarthria: importance of aerodynamic parameters measurements. West Afr J Med. 2012;31(2):129-34.
7. Darley FL, Aronson AE, Brown JR. Differential diagnostic patterns of dysarthria. J Speech Hear Res. 1969;12(2):246-69.
8. Barkmeier-Kraemer JM, Clark HM. Speech–language pathology evaluation and management of hyperkinetic disorders affecting speech and swallowing function. Tremor Other Hyperkinet Mov (NY). 2017;7:489.
9. Collis J, Bloch S. Survey of UK speech and language therapists' assessment and treatment practices for people with progressive dysarthria. Int J Lang Commun Disord. 2012;47(6):725-37.
10. Enderby PM, Palmer R. Frenchay Dysarthria Assessment, 2nd edition. Austin: Pro-Ed, Inc.; 2008.

30

CHAPTER

Approach to Dysphagia

Parul Dubey, Bhawna Sharma

INTRODUCTION

The term dysphagia means "disordered swallowing." Dysphagia can occur across all age groups and in a variety of medical conditions. Dysphagia is a ubiquitous symptom in neurology; therefore, it is important for the neurologist to understand the approach to the evaluation of this significant, yet often overlooked symptom.

This chapter aims at providing a simple understanding of the clinical and investigational approach to dysphagia. Evaluation and management of dysphagia need a multidisciplinary approach including internal medicine, gastroenterology, otolaryngorhinology, neurology, surgery, speech and language therapy, and physiotherapy. Before we embark upon the discussion of the clinical aspects, it is essential to understand the basic anatomy and physiology of normal deglutition and the various pathologies affecting the swallowing process in order to guide a proper evaluation of dysphagia.

NORMAL SWALLOW

Swallowing is an effortless process that develops as early as the 14th or 15th week of gestation. Normal swallow is a precisely coordinated, complex dynamic sensorimotor process involving 26 pairs of muscles of the oropharynx and esophagus and 5 cranial nerves (V, VII, IX, X, and XII), by which food passes from the mouth through the pharynx and eventually into the esophagus.

Swallowing has oral/buccal, pharyngeal, and esophageal phases and involves voluntary and reflexive movements. It is perfectly coordinated with the breathing mechanism as both the processes of deglutition and breathing share the same entrance passage, the pharynx. A failure in this coordination will lead to choking/aspiration of food into the lungs.[1,2]

Oral and Pharyngeal Phases

The oropharynx comprises the tongue, epiglottis, palatine tonsils, hard palate, and soft palate. The voluntary oral phase starts with food manipulation and mastication in the mouth by facial, jaw and tongue muscles and mixing with saliva to form the bolus and deliver it to the pharynx. It is under the control of discrete areas of the motor cortex.

In the oropharyngeal phase, food bolus is reflexively transferred posteriorly to the epiglottis and then to the upper esophageal sphincter (UES). The whole oropharyngeal phase lasts about 0.6–1.0 seconds. When a sufficiently large and adequately prepared cohesive food bolus touches the oropharynx, the tactile receptors in the oropharynx are stimulated and the swallowing reflex is initiated.

Swallowing reflex leads to coordinated sequential processes which ensure that the food/drink enters the esophagus and not into the airway. The tongue blocks the oral cavity to prevent the bolus from going back to the mouth, the soft palate blocks the nasopharynx thereby preventing food from entering the nasal cavity, the vocal folds close to seal the glottis (space between the vocal folds) and the arytenoids tilt forward to touch the base of the epiglottis, and finally hyoid bone and larynx are pulled upward by contraction of the suprahyoid and thyrohyoid muscles. This tucks the larynx under the base of the tongue and the epiglottis tilts backward, flips over, to seal the larynx, covering the entrance to the trachea **(Figs. 1A to C)**. This is the most important step because this prevents the entry of food/drink into the lungs which can be potentially life-threatening.

Breathing is centrally inhibited during the swallow (deglutition apnea). The pharyngeal phase is followed by a prolonged expiration to avert "mist aspiration" (inhalation of air held in the pharynx which is usually saturated with fluid/food particles). After the swallow, structures return to their original position passively supported by the infrahyoid muscles.[1,2]

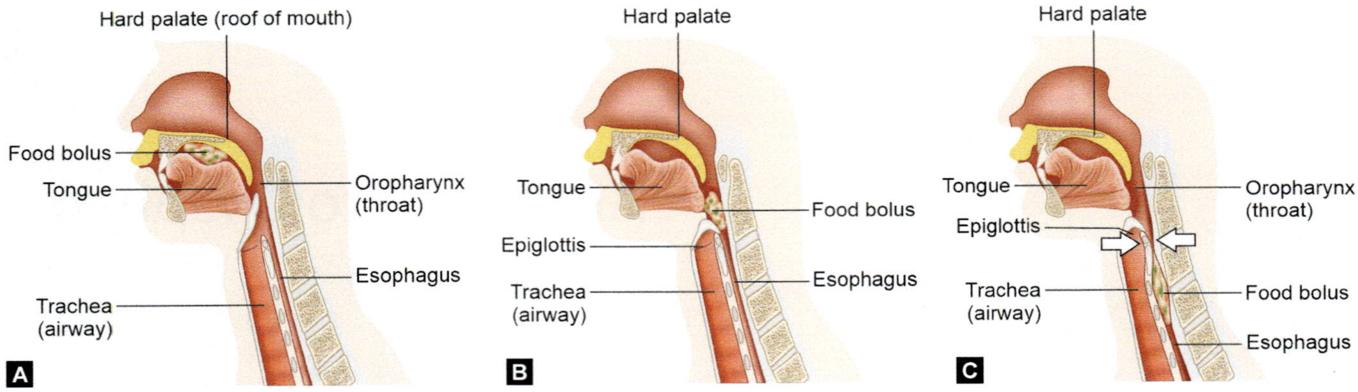

FIGS. 1A TO C: Food bolus passing through the: (A) oral phase, (B) pharyngeal phase, (C) esophageal phase of swallowing.

Source: Modified from Thomas and Keith (2005).

Esophageal Phase

The esophageal phase is slower, may exceed 10 seconds, and is under the dual control of the somatic and autonomic nervous systems. The swallow reflex triggers the esophageal peristaltic movements and relaxes the UES which is formed by inferior pharyngeal constrictor muscles, cricopharyngeus muscle, and proximal part of the esophagus, allowing passage of food to esophagus. The UES is closed at rest by tonic muscle contraction and opens with the pressure of the food bolus, relaxation of cricopharyngeus muscle, and contraction of the suprahyoid and thyrohyoid muscles and pulling the hyolaryngeal complex forward, opening the sphincter. This, combined with the effects of gravity, facilitates food passage down into the stomach. Larynx then moves down to its original position.[2,3]

TABLE 1: Swallowing and cranial nerves.

Steps in the swallowing process	Cranial nerve involved
Bolus preparation	V (motor and sensory)
Bolus propulsion	IX, X, and XII
Palatal elevation	IX, X
Airway protection by apposition of true and false vocal cords and arytenoids against the base of epiglottis (sphincteric action of larynx)	X
Epiglottis inhibits direct contact of the bolus with the laryngeal vestibule	V, VII, C1-C3
Upward and froward movement of hyoid and larynx enhances the airway protection and pulls open the relaxed UES	

Note: Hypoglossal (XII) nerve innervates all intrinsic and extrinsic tongue muscles (except Palatoglossus which is supplied by the XI nerve)

(UES: upper esophageal sphincter)

NEURAL CONTROL OF SWALLOWING

Swallowing is controlled by several cortical areas and brainstem nuclei through the cranial nerves. The swallowing apparatus, oropharyngeal and laryngeal musculature, is under the control of many cranial nerves **(Table 1)**. Sensory information is carried by cranial nerves trigeminal (V), glossopharyngeal (IX), and vagus (X); however, the most potent stimulus for triggering the swallowing reflex is delivered by the superior laryngeal nerve, a branch of the vagus nerve. The motor innervation of the swallowing musculature is provided by five cranial nerves by the release of acetylcholine at neuromuscular junctions **(Table 1)**.[4]

While the swallowing reflex is initiated by the activation of cortical and subcortical areas of the brain, the central pattern generator (CPG) located in the brainstem organizes the sequential activation of motor neurons controlling the oropharyngeal muscles to deliver the bolus from the oropharynx to the esophagus.[5]

The most important cortical areas implicated in swallowing are the anterior insular cortex and frontoparietal operculum, including the inferior part of the sensorimotor cortex and part of the premotor cortex. The corticobulbar connections from these areas project to ipsilateral and contralateral brainstem nuclei of the main cranial nerves involved in swallowing. Magnetoencephalography has shown a predominant left hemispheric activation during the oral phase of swallowing and a predominant right-sided activation during the pharyngeal phase.

The "central pattern generator" (CPG) for swallowing is located in the medulla oblongata and pons and is bilaterally distributed within the reticular formation (RF). CPG corresponds to the area of the nucleus tractus solitarius (NTS) and the nucleus ambiguus (NA). Functionally, there is an afferent component, a complex set of interneurons and an efferent component, which are organized temporally as early, late, or very late neurons which fire sequentially to activate the swallowing musculature. These neurons of the CPG form two units on each side of the brainstem and are arranged as dorsal and ventral groups.[5]

TABLE 2: Neurogenic dysphagia.

Based on localization in the neuraxis	Based on pathomechanisms
Central nervous system: • Cerebral cortex • Subcortical structures • Cerebellum *Peripheral nervous system*: • Cranial nerves • Radicles • Peripheral nerves • Neuromuscular junction • Muscle diseases	*Vascular*: Ischemic or hemorrhagic stroke *Degenerative*: • *Dementia*: Alzheimer's disease (AD), corticobasal degeneration, frontotemporal dementia, Lewy body dementia • Vascular dementia • Basal ganglia disorders • Parkinson's disease, progressive supranuclear palsy (PSP), multiple system atrophy (MSA) • Spinocerebellar ataxia (SCA), Huntington's disease, Wilson's disease *Motor neuron disease (MND)*: Amyotrophic lateral sclerosis (ALS), primary lateral sclerosis *Muscular dystrophies*: Myopathies—Nemaline myopathy, Myotonic dystrophy, Oculopharyngeal dystrophy, Inclusion body myositis *Demyelinating*: • *Central*—multiple sclerosis, acute disseminating encephalomyelitis • *Peripheral*—GBS and CIDP *Inflammatory*: • *Myopathies*: Polymyositis, inclusion body myositis • *Peripheral neuropathies*: Inflammatory systemic neuropathies, diabetic neuropathy • *Mitochondrial*: Myoneuropathies • *Traumatic*: Head injury • *Neoplastic*: Brain tumors • *Congenital*: Cerebral palsy • *Iatrogenic* (medication induced): Tardive dyskinesia and dystonia

(GBS: Guillain–Barré syndrome; CIDP: chronic inflammatory demyelinating polyneuropathy)

Dorsal neurons lie in the NTS and adjacent RF. They receive and integrate both descending inputs from the cerebrum and ascending inputs from cranial nerves V, IX, X carrying sensory information from the oropharynx, larynx, and upper cervical areas. The ventral neurons lie within the RF, adjacent to the NA, which sends signals to the dorsal group (NTS) which in turn sends efferents to the swallowing musculature. NTS modulates swallowing according to bolus size, texture, and temperature. Sensory inputs help to initiate swallowing, modify the threshold for pharyngeal swallow, and alter the level of muscle recruitment during swallowing.

The two hemi-CPGs are closely synchronized and organize coordinated contraction of oropharyngeal muscles bilaterally. Midline crossing fibers connect the two hemi-CPGs. The existence of bilaterally coordinated CPGs can explain the recovery of the swallowing function after a lesion of one CPG.

Subcortical structures, e.g., cerebellum, midbrain (substantia nigra and ventral tegmentum), and basal forebrain (hypothalamus, amygdala, and basal ganglia), have been shown to induce or modulate the swallowing sequence after initial triggering by the cortex or superior laryngeal nerve. This explains dysphagia in basal ganglia disorders caused by marked incoordination of oropharyngeal swallowing.[2,4,5]

Disruption of the anatomical and functional integrity of the extensive swallowing pathways in the central and peripheral nervous system at various levels starting from the cerebral cortex, basal ganglia, brainstem, cranial nerves, cerebellum, peripheral nerves and radicles, and neuromuscular junction to the muscle may cause neurogenic dysphagia (ND) **(Table 2)**.

CLINICAL APPROACH

Dysphagia can be neurological or nonneurological (mechanical or structural) in origin which is to be clinically determined.[6]

To exclude structural causes, evaluation by an otolaryngorhinologist and gastroenterologist is important especially because some structural causes may be initially missed, e.g., tongue base/hypopharynx tumors, upper/lower esophageal sphincter dysfunction, large anterior cervical osteophytes, etc. **(Figs. 2A to D)**.

Causes of dysphagia can be classified based on location—oropharyngeal, esophageal, esophagogastric, and paraesophageal **(Table 3)**.

A detailed history is crucial to a clinical evaluation of dysphagia. Age, sex, occupation, educational/socioeconomic status, level of consciousness, attention, vigilance, and general cognitive status of the patient are noted, which are followed by a focused history **(Box 1)**.

A major point in history that differentiates mechanical from ND is whether the difficulty is more for swallowing

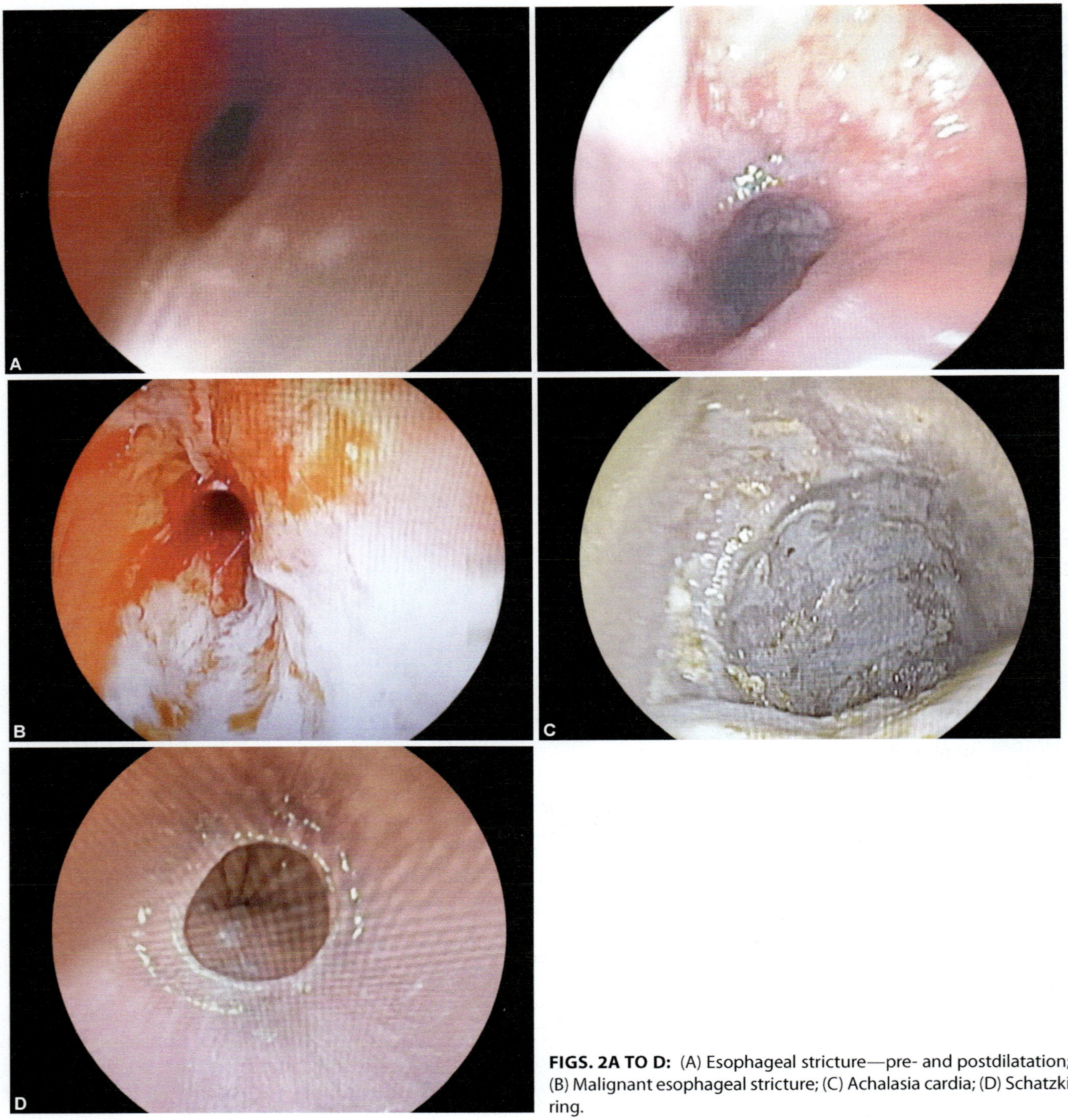

FIGS. 2A TO D: (A) Esophageal stricture—pre- and postdilatation; (B) Malignant esophageal stricture; (C) Achalasia cardia; (D) Schatzki ring.

liquids or solids. A predominant difficulty in swallowing solids compared to liquids generally indicates a mechanical obstruction (diseases of esophagus/base of tongue) while a predominant difficulty in swallowing liquids points toward a neurogenic cause. This is probably because a solid (more cohesive) food bolus is more likely to cause adequate pharyngeal stimulation and triggering of swallow reflex than a liquid bolus which is more difficult to control and may not trigger the swallow reflex.

With oropharyngeal dysphagia (OD), there is difficulty in transferring the bolus from the mouth to the upper esophagus. Patients complain of difficulty in forming the bolus, initiating the swallow, delayed bolus passage, oral stasis of food, coughing, choking, nasopharyngeal

TABLE 3: Types of dysphagia.

Dysphagia	Motor or motility disorder	Mechanical or structural obstruction
Oropharyngeal	• Neurogenic causes (75–85% of OD is due to neurogenic causes) • Upper esophageal sphincter dysfunction	• Head and neck malignancies • Congenital proximal esophageal web • Zenker's diverticulum • Pharyngeal infections • Vertebral osteophytes • Prior head and neck radiation
Esophageal	Diffuse esophageal spasm Achalasia *Secondary motility disorders*: • Connective tissue disorders like scleroderma • Parasitic infections • Pseudo-obstruction related to malignancy • Aging • Diabetes mellitus	• Esophageal carcinoma • Reflux esophagitis • Peptic stricture • Schatzki ring
Esophagogastric	Achalasia	• Gastric carcinoma • Stricture
Paraesophageal Extrinsic esophageal compression by cardiac and vascular structures		• Dysphagia lusoria (any congenital vascular abnormality leading to esophageal dysphagia, e.g., an aberrant right subclavian artery arising from the left side of the aortic arch, double aortic arch or a right aortic arch with left ligamentum arteriosum) • Left atrial enlargement, enlarged thyroid, mediastinal masses, cervical spine disease

BOX 1 History taking in dysphagia.

- Is there a difficulty in swallowing, if yes, in what way?
- Does the food get stuck on swallowing? Can one localize the point of swallowing difficulty—whether food stuck in the throat or chest? (Distal esophageal pathology—sternal notch, proximal—more nonlocalized)
- Is swallowing painful? (Pharyngitis, esophagitis, glossopharyngeal neuralgia, Eagle's syndrome, and pterygoid hamulus bursitis)
- Is there nasal regurgitation of foods and liquids? (Bulbar palsy)
- Is there any choking, throat clearing, coughing, or breathlessness after swallowing? (Indicates aspiration)
- Residues of food in the throat or oral cavity after swallowing?
- Is there a difficulty in chewing? (Jaw muscle weakness as in myasthenia gravis)
- Does the food get accumulated in the cheek? (Facial weakness)
- Is there a difficulty in manipulating the food inside the mouth to make a bolus? (Tongue weakness)
- Is the difficulty more for solids than liquids? (Indicates mechanical obstruction, intrinsic or extrinsic to the esophagus)
- Is the difficulty more for liquids or equal to that of solids? (Indicates a motor/motility disorder)
- Does the swallowing difficulty occur with the first swallow? (Indicates oropharyngeal dysphagia)
- How long has the difficulty been present?
- Is it of acute or subacute onset? (Acute stroke or demyelination, subacute onset inflammatory myopathies, and Guillain–Barré syndrome)
- Is it chronic?
- Is it intermittent? (Indicates motor disorder, Schatzki ring esophageal webs and eosinophilic esophagitis in young)
- Is it static or progressive? (Progressive solid food dysphagia—esophageal stricture or esophageal carcinoma)
- Is it improving? (Resolving reflux esophagitis)
- Is it fluctuating or fatigable? (Neuromuscular junction disorder)
- Time needed for a meal? Does it take longer than 1 second to pass food from the mouth to the esophagus (Oropharyngeal dysphagia)
- Is there any associated heartburn? (Reflux esophagitis, peptic esophageal stricture)

Continued

Continued

- Is there temperature sensitivity to swallowing (Especially cold)? (Dysphagia due to esophageal motility disorders may worsen with cold liquids)
- Is there any associated speech change, symptoms suggesting other cranial nerve involvement, limb weakness or numbness/paresthesiae?
- Is there associated weight loss? (Esophageal carcinoma)
- Is there any associated atypical chest pain, respiratory compromise, hypotension? (May indicate extrinsic esophageal compression by cardiac or vascular structures)
- Is there any change in eating or drinking behavior like avoidance of any particular food consistencies?
- Posture during eating (Improvement in swallowing on head turning to one side—unilateral X or XII palsy)
- Is there a loss of sensation of bolus passage on one side? (IX ± X palsy)
- History of pneumonia, bronchopulmonary infections and infections of undetermined source, dehydration
- *Medications used*: Especially neuroleptic medications
- History of radiation, thyroid disease, neck surgery including anterior discectomy
- Family history (Myotonic dystrophy, oculopharyngeal dystrophy)

regurgitation, change in speech, and may have a history of aspiration pneumonia. Structural pathologies of the oropharynx and diseases of the central nervous system and neuromuscular disorders affect the oropharyngeal phase of swallowing.

Patients with esophageal dysphagia will often complain of food being stuck in the throat/chest at a certain point, however, this is often an unreliable indicator of the actual location of the problem. For example, in case of distal esophageal stricture, patients point to a level lower down, at the level of the sternal notch, more or less corresponding to the site of obstruction while the feeling is not so localized in case of more proximal obstruction. Also, patients may complain of food regurgitation, especially after rushed meals.[7]

Diseases causing narrowing of esophageal lumen typically begin with difficulty in swallowing solids and then may progress eventually to liquids also. On the other hand, esophageal dysmotility disorders (e.g., achalasia) cause difficulty in swallowing liquids or both liquids and solids in the beginning itself. Usually, dysphagia associated with degenerative diseases starts as dysphagia for liquids, but, over time, it becomes mixed, both for liquids and solids.[6-8]

The onset, duration, and course of progression of symptoms, whether dysphagia is acute, subacute, chronic, persistent, intermittent or fluctuating or progressive, can guide toward the etiology.

Acute onset dysphagia suggests stroke and less commonly demyelination while a subacute onset may suggest inflammatory myopathies and Guillain-Barré syndrome. Nonprogressive and long-standing intermittent dysphagia can be due to the lower esophageal mucosal ring (Schatzki's ring) while progressive dysphagia occurs in esophageal strictures and malignancies (associated significant weight loss).[8]

Associated symptoms suggesting other cranial nerve involvement, limb weakness, or sensory abnormalities help in localization of pathology in the neuraxis.

A review of medical records including medications being taken by the patient (especially neuroleptics), any recent dose changes, previous diagnostic or therapeutic interventions, the present diet, or any other comorbidities is indispensable. Standardized questionnaires can be used for systematic history taking.

NEUROGENIC DYSPHAGIA

Neurogenic dysphagia occurs in approximately 400,000–800,000 patients per year due to a multitude of neurological disorders which can be categorized in many ways based on the anatomic localization, etiology, or clinical presentation.[9]

Neurogenic dysphagia predominantly affects the oropharyngeal phase of swallowing, but may occasionally affect the esophageal phase resulting from disorders of esophageal innervation (degeneration of myenteric ganglion cells). ND results from a combination of factors including weakness of the orolingual musculature, failure to form a cohesive food bolus, reduced sensitivity of the pharyngeal receptors, buccolingual apraxia, etc.[9,10]

The reported incidence of dysphagia in specific neurologic diseases is variable **(Box 2)**.

An acute stroke involving the brainstem or one/both the cerebral hemispheres is the most common cause of ND, occurring in 25–42% of cases and does not depend on the site and size of the lesion. Stroke-related dysphagia is most often associated with other cranial nerve involvement and hemiparesis (long tract signs), but occasionally may present as an isolated manifestation as reported in some lacunar infarcts in the periventricular white matter or strategic brainstem location. Dysphagia occurs more commonly in right hemispheric strokes which could be partly attributable to neglect and lack of awareness, predisposing patients to aspiration.

Dysphagia due to brainstem lesions or confluent periventricular infarction may affect predominantly the voluntary initiation of swallowing and spare reflex deglutition. In such cases, symptoms may be confused with Globus hystericus. However, in globus hystericus, a painless, persistent, or intermittent "lump in the throat" is a characteristic symptom but is usually associated with

BOX 2 Percentage of patients having dysphagia in various neurological disorders.

- *Acute stroke*: 65%
- *Parkinson's disease*: 50%
- *Multiple sclerosis*: 31.3%
- *Dementia*: 13–57%
- *Motor neuron disease*: 30–100% (depending on type and stage of disease)
- *Traumatic brain injury*: 60%
- *Dermatomyositis*: 20%
- *Polymyositis*: 30–60%
- *Inclusion body myositis*: 65–86%
- *Patients on prolonged mechanical ventilation*: 60–70%
- *Other less common neurological disorders*: No available data

emotional distress. Patients with globus hystericus have a normal bolus transit time and seldom have actual difficulty with eating or drinking.

Recovery from dysphagia in stroke occurs in 90% of cases in 2 weeks but may persist for >6 months in 8%. Spontaneous recovery, partial or complete, occurs due to the vicarious function of the contralateral CPG. Dysphagia lasting longer than a month is more often associated with right parietal lobe lesions.

In brainstem strokes (Wallenberg's syndrome) or multiple sclerosis, a focal lesion interrupts connections between the NTS and the NA ipsilaterally. After a stroke, patients may present with "silent aspiration," meaning aspiration without cough or other outward clinical signs of aspiration. Silent aspiration should be considered if the patient has other predictors of dysphagia, e.g., a severe neurological deficit, severe dysarthria or aphasia or severe facial palsy.[11]

Dysphagia in basal ganglia disorders is predominantly due to the involvement of pedunculopontine tegmental nucleus (PPTN) and dorsal motor nucleus of the vagus (DMV). Also, CPG dysfunction causes an increased inhibitory output to PPTN and Lewy bodies in the esophageal myenteric plexus contribute to dysphagia in Parkinson disease (PD). Drooling of saliva in Parkinsonism is a result of bradykinesia and incoordination of oropharyngeal musculature rather than an increased production of saliva.

Approximately 80% of patients with PD have dysphagia sometime in the course of the illness which is usually mild enough to have no effect on nutrition. In PD, oral phase (difficulties with lip closure, tongue movements) and pharyngeal phases (food getting stuck in the throat) are affected. 10% of patients have more severe dysphagia correlating with the severity and duration of PD. Tremor and speech disturbance are the main predictors of dysphagia in PD. Parkinsonism plus syndromes such as progressive supranuclear palsy (PSP) and multiple system atrophy (MSA) have more severe dysphagia from the onset.[12]

Spasmodic torticollis also may cause dysphagia which does not correlate with disease duration.

Brainstem lesions cause bulbar and pseudobulbar palsies which affect the oropharyngeal phases. Cerebellar pathology causes incoordination of swallowing muscles but may not be sufficient to cause dysphagia by itself. This is because the cerebellum does not form part of the primary motor swallowing pathway within the brainstem, but coordinated the function of cortical motor swallowing centers and swallowing musculature. In cerebellar disorders, poor coordination of the orofacial musculature may cause inadequate lip seal, difficulties with the timing of the voluntary initiation of swallow reflex, preparation of a cohesive food bolus, and delivery of the bolus to the pharynx.

Isolated peripheral nerve lesions and degeneration of autonomic ganglion cells in the lower two-thirds of esophagus (which result in achalasia) are rare causes of dysphagia. In patients with smooth muscle diseases such as scleroderma, dysphagia may be secondary to gastroesophageal reflux or esophageal dysmotility. Abnormalities of neuromuscular transmission (myasthenia gravis) and muscle diseases (inflammatory or degenerative) may also cause dysphagia.

70–80% of patients on prolonged mechanical ventilation, regardless of the primary illness, present, at least temporarily, with significant dysphagia and aspiration after successful weaning, possibly due to a critical illness polyneuropathy and structural changes caused by artificial airway, e.g., edema of arytenoids which sometimes warrants reintubation.[13]

Sarcopenia refers to age-related changes in head and neck anatomy, and neuromuscular physiology causing reduced functional reserve in older adults, and increasing dysphagia susceptibility in the elderly. Lifetime dysphagia prevalence has been found to be 38% in adults aged 65–94 years.[14]

Complications of ND include malnutrition, dehydration, aspiration (potentially resulting in pneumonia), hospital readmissions, institutionalization, choking, and death. Mortality rates are as high as 50% in adults with known aspirations. Psychosocial consequences of dysphagia include feelings of embarrassment, anxiety, fear of choking, reduced self-esteem, depression, reduced quality of life, social isolation, and physical and economic burden on caregivers.[15]

ASSESSMENT OF DYSPHAGIA

Facies may give clues to diagnosis, e.g., masked facies of PD, Omega sign in PSP, a sardonic smile of Wilson's disease, ptosis in myasthenia, myotonic dystrophy or brainstem pathologies, facial or tongue deviation in stroke, drug-induced orofaciolingual dyskinesia, and so on. Dyskinesia or dystonia of the throat, face, jaw, head, and neck may give clues to an underlying neurological disorder, e.g., Whipple's disease, celiac disease with encephalopathy, and multisystem atrophy.

Assessment of swallowing function starts with a careful examination of the oral cavity using a tongue blade and handheld mirror to assess oral hygiene, structural oromotor problems, local pathologies like ulcers, growths, oral pooling of secretions or food residue, etc.

The patient's voice, its sound and quality, is noted. "Wet voice" may indicate a chronic laryngeal aspiration and a "weak and breathy" voice may suggest a pathology of vocal cords. Voluntary cough may be feeble due to drowsiness or respiratory/laryngeal weakness, while a bovine cough indicates vocal cord paresis. Patients with corticobulbar lesions may have impaired voluntary control of facial movements, cough and respiration while retaining emotional or reflex responses.[4,16]

Position of uvula and rise of palatal and pharyngeal arches on saying "ah" are noted. Unilateral pharyngeal wall paresis causes the paralyzed side to move toward the healthy side. Spastic speech, reduced palatal and pharyngeal movements with brisk jaw jerk, and gag reflex with emotional lability point toward an upper motor neuron involvement (pseudobulbar palsy) while a nasal twang of speech with diminished gag reflex points toward a lower motor neuron involvement (bulbar palsy). The absent gag reflex may or may not correlate with the capacity to swallow. Bedside sensory examination cannot reliably distinguish IX and X nerve lesions but lack of posterior pharyngeal wall sensation has prognostic implications in stroke.

The position of the tongue in the mouth is observed, whether the tongue is flabby and atrophic with fasciculations or is small and spastic. Due to a unilateral XII nerve lesion, the tongue deviates to the healthy side on retraction (unopposed action of styloglossus) and on the affected side on the protrusion (genioglossus).

Loss of integration of swallowing and breathing may cause abnormal respiratory patterns and increase the risk of aspiration; therefore, a simultaneous assessment of breathing is important. Respiratory rate and pattern (stridor in multisystem atrophy, laryngeal dystonia, or respiratory dyskinesia), forced vital capacity (supine and sitting), cough, diaphragm function, blood gases, and chest radiographs are assessed.[17]

By placing the index finger above the thyroid cartilage while swallowing, the normal laryngeal ascent can be assessed. The cartilage should move cephalad against the examiner's finger.

Pulse oximetry is used to assess pulmonary aspiration. Aspiration of food/fluid in the airways causes reflex bronchoconstriction causing ventilation-perfusion mismatch, resulting in oxygen desaturation of arterial blood which can be readily measured with pulse oximetry. Pulse oximetry may predict aspiration in 81.5% of dysphagic stroke patients, but a decline in oxygen saturation of >3% is neither predictive nor sensitive for aspiration. This method is noninvasive, quick, and repeatable but must be interpreted with caution in smokers (high carboxyhemoglobin concentrations may give false negative results) and in those with chronic lung disease.[18]

Bedside swallow evaluations (BSEs) are important in the evaluation of dysphagia which includes: (1) water swallowing tests, (2) multiconsistency tests, and (3) swallow provocation tests. During BSE, swallowing behavior is observed, e.g., multiple swallows per mouthful, reflexive cough, choking, splattering, wet quality of voice, breathlessness, increased respiratory rate, change in breathing pattern after swallowing, etc.[19]

Qualitative water swallow is a good bedside dysphagia screening test. If a patient is conscious, able to sit up and phonate, and has a reasonably strong cough, a bedside water swallow can be done. Water is easily acceptable by the patient as a test drink and is freely available. Swallowing water is also a stringent test for laryngeal closure. The test can be quantified by asking the patient to swallow 50 mL of water in 5 mL aliquots. If the patient is able to take the whole of 50 mL of water without any symptoms, then swallowing is considered normal.[20]

A simple bedside assessment of swallowing speed has been shown to be specific and sensitive (the patient drinks 150 mL of cold tap water while sitting up). A swallowing speed of <10 mL/s suggests dysphagia. Reduced volume per swallow most often is a spontaneous adjustment done by the patient to reduce risk of laryngeal penetration/aspiration. If the patient coughs, has a wet, hoarse voice or chokes or gets breathless, this suggests dysphagia and should be kept nil orally and fed by alternative methods and reassessed later.[20]

Multiconsistency tests such as the "Gugging Swallowing Screen" or the Volume-Viscosity Test evaluate other consistencies besides liquids and, therefore, allow a graded stepwise rating of dysphagia and can help to guide dietary recommendations along with risk assessments.[21]

The "Swallow Provocation Test" exclusively examines the involuntary swallowing reflex and focuses on the pharyngeal phase of deglutition. This may be an alternative in noncooperative patients who cannot take it orally.[22] Various swallowing assessment tools are available to evaluate and quantify dysphagia **(Box 3)**.

But, BSEs are rather considered crude, insensitive indicators of videoscopically defined aspiration. Patients with silent aspiration may be able to swallow without problems during this test. Also, there are wide interobserver variability and a lack of specificity.

Therefore, instrumental assessment of dysphagia, which is more specific and reproducible and gives additional information about swallowing physiology, is increasingly gaining importance.[23] The two most commonly used instrumental techniques are videofluoroscopy and fiberoptic endoscopic evaluation of swallowing. This can objectively define the risk of aspiration and guide more individualized and informed choices about compensatory and rehabilitative strategies for dysphagia. However, from the clinical standpoint, an overemphasis on instrumental assessment for presence or absence of aspiration should be avoided, rather more practically relevant clinical consequences of aspiration like occurrence of chest

BOX 3 Swallowing assessment tools.

- *Swallowing Disturbance Questionnaire*: A self-reported 15-item questionnaire on swallowing disturbances
- *Eating Assessment Tool (EAT-10)*: A self-administered, symptom-specific outcome instrument for dysphagia
- *Dysphagia Outcome and Severity Scale (DOSS)*: A 7-point scale developed to systematically rate the functional severity of dysphagia based on objective assessment
- *Penetration–Aspiration Scale (PAS)*: An 8-point scale based on VFS to describe penetration and aspiration events. This is the most used scale for semiquantitatively assessing the degree of endoscopically and radiologically measured penetration/aspiration

(VFS: videofluoroscopy)

infections, weight loss, amount of oral intake, and a formal observation of eating and drinking should be relied upon.

Videofluoroscopic swallowing study (VFSS) is a radiological assessment and is considered the gold standard for the evaluation of dysphagia. VFSS is a useful tool for determining the presence, severity, and characteristics of dysphagia. VFSS assesses passage of radiopaque barium-coated foods and liquids in lateral and anteroposterior planes to capture all the phases of the swallowing process sequentially from the time the bolus is taken, i.e., oral preparatory, oral, pharyngeal, and esophageal phases. For instance, VFSS findings in PD are—abnormal bolus formation, multiple tongue elevations, delayed swallowed reflex, and prolonged pharyngeal transit time with repetitive swallows to clear the throat. VFSS can determine the degree of swallowing difficulty (mild, moderate, and severe). The disadvantages are use of contrast material and radiation exposure.[23,24]

Flexible endoscopic evaluation of swallowing (FEES) is done with a fiberoptic rhinolaryngoscope passed transnasally which is connected to a camera, light source, and video-recording equipment, enabling direct visualization of bolus flow and the surface anatomy of structures involved in swallowing. FEES captures only the pharyngeal phase of swallowing, but it can identify the exact location of the waste in that phase of swallowing, its quantity, and can determine which maneuvers can be performed to minimize the residue while swallowing.[25]

By definition, "penetration" is the entering of food material into the airway above the level of vocal folds, and "aspiration" is the entering of food below the level of vocal folds. During peak laryngeal excursion, there is a brief (0.5 second) period of "white out" during which the endoscope view is obstructed by soft tissue structures at the point of peak pharyngeal constriction. The presence of aspiration during "white out" is inferred by examining material expectorated from the airway and residue on the subglottic shelf or further inside the trachea after the swallow (word edit). FEES has the advantage of not using radiation and being more easily reproducible.[26]

The FEES and VFSS are considered complementary and combined together have a sensitivity of 80–90% and a specificity of 50% for detecting aspiration in patients with stroke and other ND.[26,27]

The FEES can be done in all adults and is well tolerated. Risks are minimal (<1%) which may include discomfort, epistaxis, vasovagal syncope, self-resolving laryngospasm, gagging, vomiting, and mucosal perforation. The risk of self-limiting epistaxis may increase to 6% in acute stroke patients receiving antithrombotic medications.[27]

Neuroradiology including MRI brain and cervical spine and CT scans of neck and chest and electrophysiological studies including nerve conduction studies, electromyography (EMG), single fiber EMG, etc. guide the etiological evaluation of ND.

Esophageal manometry enables measurements of the intraesophageal pressure gradient and is useful in the evaluation of dysfunction of the cricopharyngeus muscle and abnormalities of esophageal motility.[28]

Other investigations to evaluate dysphagia, which are primarily research tools, include scintigraphy to obtain indices of pharyngeal clearance, ultrasound to evaluate tongue and pharyngeal wall movements, cervical auscultation to detect aspiration, and electrical impedance tomography to measure impedance changes in the neck during swallowing. EMG may be useful to understand the physiology of activation of muscles involved in the oropharyngeal phase of swallowing and also to identify target deglutition muscles for infiltrating with botulinum toxin.[29]

MANAGEMENT OF DYSPHAGIA

The optimal therapy of ND involves multidisciplinary teamwork including neurologist, speech and language therapist, nutritionist, nursing staff, physiotherapists, and occupational therapists. Objective of treatment is to minimize the risk of pulmonary aspiration and to identify a safe diet to maintain sufficient nutrition, hydration, and weight.

Management plan includes restitution, compensation, and adaptation methods. Restitution involves correcting the disturbed swallowing functions. Compensation involves postural and behavioral changes and swallowing maneuvers which the patients may spontaneously assume or may be taught to decrease the chances of aspiration. Adaptation means modifying the type of food to ease nutrition. Dietary modification may help prevent extremely long mealtimes, fatigue, and dread of meals. In addition, specific drugs and/or surgical procedures are available for certain forms of ND. Treatment should be individualized according to the patient's needs and wishes.

Obvious causes such as ill-fitting dentures and oral candidiasis/ulcers should be looked for and treated. Feeding should be encouraged when the patient is alert and fresh with maximum functional ability and should avoid distractions while eating like talking/watching television. Coinciding mealtimes with "on periods" in PD with frequent suctioning of excessive saliva may help.[30]

Drugs may precipitate or aggravate dysphagia, usually in a dose-dependent manner, often reversible after drug discontinuation or dose reduction. Drug-induced dysphagia may be due to a combination of mechanisms. For example, sedatives and hypnotics cause a depressed level of consciousness and rarely a direct inhibition of brainstem neurons, neuroleptic drugs may delay the initiation of swallow reflex, sometimes even without extrapyramidal features, orofacial dyskinesia with dopaminergic agents, xerostomia due to anticholinergics causing inadequate preparation of food bolus, and blocking of acetylcholine release at the neuromuscular junction caused by botulinum toxin (may cause transient dysphagia in 10–28% of patients with spasmodic torticollis who have received the injection in a higher dose and at multiple sites).

Drugs with sedative effects (benzodiazepines and anticonvulsants) should be discontinued or given as a single night dose to ensure conscious and careful swallowing during mealtimes. Dopaminergic medications can help improve swallowing in patients with dysphagia due to PD while decreasing the doses of dopaminergic medications may help the dysphagia aggravated due to drug-induced lingual dyskinesia. Eating may be avoided during peak dose dyskinesia.[31]

Drooling in parkinsonism is primarily due to swallowing difficulties rather than the excessive production of saliva. Anticholinergic medications may help to reduce the secretions (atropine solution poured in the mouth, hyoscine tablets, glycopyrrolate injection/tablet). Beta-blockers may help thicken secretions. But increased viscosity of secretions interferes with bolus preparation and predisposes to mucus plug formation and choking episodes.

Use of fluid thickeners increases the viscosity by increasing the resistance to flow of the bolus and oropharyngeal transit time. The optimum viscosity that ensures safe swallowing is not established. The required fluid thickening is judged subjectively as syrup or yogurt consistency. Very thick fluids are usually unpalatable and rejected by the patients. Dry and sticky foods should be avoided. Soft textures/puréed food can compensate for a poor oral preparation phase and facilitate oral and pharyngeal transport.[32]

Speech and language therapists can help with swallowing therapy. Simple behavioral changes such as slowing down while feeding, helping with feeding, and eating in silence without distractions may help prevent choking.

Exercises to strengthen orofacial musculature, maneuvers to improve poor laryngeal elevation and laryngeal closure during swallowing, and techniques to stimulate the swallow reflex form part of the swallowing therapy. Orofacial muscle exercises improve lip seal, mastication, and tongue movements. Stimulation of the swallow reflex by mechanical, thermal, or gustatory stimuli to trigger swallowing, e.g., cooled drinks that are easier to swallow or repeated application of a small laryngeal mirror dipped in ice to the anterior faucial arch may be useful.[33]

Some patients try to compensate for their swallowing difficulties by taking small, frequent drinks during the meal in order to "wash down" the food bolus. The benefits of postural adjustments are well recognized, e.g., sitting up or head tilt to one side to maximize the effect of gravity, removal of neck restrictions, and control of abnormal movements may be helpful. "Chin tuck" reduces the bolus pharyngeal transit time whereas "chin up" increases the time. Patients with tongue weakness and poor pharyngeal clearance may facilitate swallowing by lying down on one side (at 45° from horizontal) which may be associated with less risk of aspiration than feeding in the upright posture. In those with difficulty in triggering the swallowing reflex, resting the head forward during eating may avoid leaking of the bolus and subsequent aspiration. When impaired tongue movements cause difficulty initiating a swallow, while the pharyngeal phase of swallowing is intact, tilting the head backward helps guide the bolus into the pharynx.[34]

Sufficient evidence is available for Shaker exercise (head-lift exercises while lying) in ND due to various causes, including stroke-related dysphagia, expiratory muscle strength training for Parkinson-related dysphagia, and Mendelsohn maneuver (to some extent) for stroke-related dysphagia.[35] The Mendelsohn maneuver is a technique that helps open the UES and prolong its opening time. The patient has to hold the upward movement of the larynx during swallowing for some seconds. This maneuver is appropriate for patients with pharyngeal residues or deficient opening of the UES. Supraglottic swallow to improve elevation and closure of the larynx involves swallowing while holding breath and then releasing air by coughing. Insufficient evidence exists for procedures of the effortful swallow, the Masako maneuver, super-supraglottic swallow, tongue strengthening, and Lee Silverman Voice Treatment.

Based on a clinical and FEES-directed approach, therapeutic decisions can be taken **(Table 4)**.[36]

TABLE 4: FEES findings in various neurological disorders.

Clinical diagnosis	FEES phenotype	Treatment
Myasthenia gravis	Fatigable swallowing	Cholinesterase inhibitors
Parkinson's disease	Premature spillage	Dopaminergic therapy (Levodopa brings about earlier swallow reflex)
Stroke	Impaired swallowing reflex	Pharyngeal electrical stimulation (triggers sensory remodeling caused by pharyngeal hypesthesia)
Myositis	Residue in piriform sinus	Cricopharyngeal myotomy

(FEES: flexible endoscopic evaluation of swallowing)

Prompt treatment of pulmonary problems, effective coughing techniques, first aid measures (Heimlich maneuver), etc. are all important.

In emergency situations of sepsis or unconsciousness, nasogastric tube (NGT) feeding or intravenous or parenteral feeding has to be started. NGT feeding is indicated in acute stroke, head injury, or unconsciousness due to any cause in which the dysphagia may be transient. Tube feeding should be considered if about 10% or more of the food bolus is aspirated or slow transit of the food bolus, >10 seconds, is seen on videofluoroscopy. In case of easy fatigability of swallowing muscles, patient may initially take orally and can be tube fed later as fatigue sets in. Prolonged NGT feeding is not desirable, it can cause erosion of mucosa, nasopharyngitis, esophageal strictures, epistaxis, and otitis media, etc. Fine bore NGTs deliver feeds at a slow rate and can kink/block easily. NGT does not fully protect against aspiration, 43% of patients aspirated in the first 2 weeks of starting NGT feeding (*Ciocon et al.*). Head-end elevation of bed during and for 1–2 hours after bolus NGT, gastric and intrajejunal feeding reduces the risk of aspiration.[37]

Gastrostomy tube is more suitable for patients with prolonged recovery or degenerative diseases such as Parkinsonism, dementia, or amyotrophic lateral sclerosis (ALS) in which the goal is to feed the patient for prolonged periods. A gastrostomy is more acceptable and also has the advantage of delivering a higher proportion of the diet. In one study, patients who were fed using NGT received 55% of their feeds, whereas those fed with a gastrostomy tube had 93% of their prescribed daily intake.

Gastrostomy can be endoscopic, radiological, or surgical. Enteral feeding can be started a few hours after percutaneous endoscopic gastrostomy (PEG) tube insertion. The volume of feed is usually restricted in the first 24 hours to 1 liter and is given at a rate of 50 mL/h. The volume of feed and the rate of administration are then gradually increased over the next 3–4 days until the patient's daily nutritional needs are met.

It is best to administer bolus gastrostomy feeds during daytime at normal mealtimes in an upright posture. Gastric feed volumes should be gradually increased. A large feed at night in a supine position may lead to esophageal reflux and aspiration. The use of prokinetic agents may help persistent regurgitation or aspiration. Withholding morning gastrostomy feeds usually stimulates the patient's appetite. Transient, self-limiting abdominal pain, and diarrhea may occur in the early postoperative period. The complications may vary from minor (about 20%) such as local pain or skin infections to major, e.g., tube obstruction, wound infection peritonitis, and pneumonia (about 1–3%). However, oral feeding is important for the social and psychological well-being of a patient and should be encouraged as soon as feasible.[38]

In patients who develop gastrointestinal ileus or aspiration after a PEG, enteral nutrition could be established with the intrajejunal feeding of low-residue solutions. However, technically it is easier to insert a gastric rather than an intrajejunal feeding tube. An additional advantage is that bolus gastric tube feeding is more physiological (particularly with respect to insulin secretion) and convenient (intrajejunal feeding should be given continuously rather than intermittently). Direct intrajejunal feeding should probably be reserved for patients with gastroesophageal reflux, hiatus hernia, or recurrent aspiration on PEG.

Despite being nil orally, oropharyngeal secretions may still be responsible for drooling, coughing, and choking, especially in patients with a hyperactive gag reflex as in pseudobulbar palsy. Regular suctioning of secretions by the patient or caregivers is helpful. Salivary duct redirection may help reduce drooling but may not be effective in protecting the airway. Palatal training devices may be useful sometimes. Radiation of salivary glands may help reduce flow of saliva but may also cause xerostomia.

SURGICAL TREATMENT

Oropharyngeal dysphagia due to UES hyperactivity (cricopharyngeus is the main muscle of UES) shows marked improvement with cricopharyngeal myotomy in some patients who have cricopharyngeal dysfunction. It may be effective in ND including stroke, MND, etc. given that patients satisfy two essential conditions which include a demonstration on VFSS of a failure of relaxation of pharyngeal sphincter and a preserved oral phase of swallowing (lip seal, voluntary initiation of swallowing, and propulsive action of tongue). Poor tongue movements (demonstrated on videofluoroscopy by the inability to propel or retrieve the food bolus) are a contraindication to cricopharyngeal myotomy. Patients with absent pharyngeal peristalsis or delayed triggering of the swallow reflex by 10 seconds or more are also unlikely to benefit from this treatment. Cricopharyngeal dysfunction after stroke and traumatic brain injury should be considered after the first 3 months of the disease onset. Chemical myotomy with local botulinum toxin injection is another less invasive alternative to surgery.[39,40]

When to resume oral feeding after tracheostomy is less clear. With an inflated, cuffed tracheostomy tube in situ, oral feeding may not be advised as it may promote aspiration by allowing the secretions to collect above the cuff and impeding laryngeal movements during swallowing. Oral feeding with suitable consistencies may be commenced only when an uncuffed tube is in place and oral secretions are well under control. A videofluoroscopy may be helpful to detect silent aspiration. In dysphagic patients who have a tracheostomy, occlusion of the stoma with a speaking valve during swallowing reduces the risk of pulmonary aspiration presumably by normalizing the pressure in the upper airways.[41]

In intractable aspiration as in bilateral intrinsic laryngeal muscle involvement (brainstem trauma or hemorrhage or hyperactive laryngeal reflexes), invasive measures may be helpful. Teflon injection into vocal cords reduces aspiration risk. Surgical manipulation of arytenoids, epiglottis, and partial or complete closure of larynx in tracheostomized patients or in irreversibly aphonic patients finally a laryngectomy can be done as a drastic measure to prevent aspiration.[42]

CONCLUSION

Swallowing is a fundamental reflex without which our very survival will get jeopardised. This basic function is maintained through an intricate set of neural mechanisms that control the swallowing reflex. Impairment of the swallowing mechanism is a source of much distress to the patient and may be life threatening.

The diagnosis and management of dysphagia requires a multi- pronged approach in unraveling the causes and providing relief to the patient.A thorough and meticulous bedside clinical assessment remains the most practical and handy tool for evaluation and management of dysphagia in day to day practice. An early recognition of the impact and severity of dysphagia clinically, goes a long way in preventing the complications arising due to the disordered swallowing and the resultant morbidity and mortality.

REFERENCES

1. Matsuo K, Palmer JB. Anatomy and physiology of feeding and swallowing: normal and abnormal. Phys Med Rehabil Clin N Am. 2008;19(4):691-707.
2. Sasegbon A, Hamdy S. The anatomy and physiology of normal and abnormal swallowing in oropharyngeal dysphagia. Neurogastroenterol Motil. 2017;29(11):e13100.
3. Shaw SM, Martino R. The normal swallow: muscular and neuro-physiological control. Otolaryngol Clin North Am. 2013;46(6): 937-56.
4. Hughes T, Wiles CM. Neurogenic dysphagia: the role of the neurologist. J Neurol Neurosurg Psychiatr. 1998;64:569-72.
5. Costa MMB. Neural control of swallowing. Arq Gastroenterol. 2018;55(Suppl 1):61-75.
6. Pokieser P, Scharitzer M. The Clinical and Radiological Approach to Dysphagia. In: Ekberg O (Ed). Dysphagia. Medical Radiology. New York: Springer, Cham; 2017.
7. Logemann JA, Larsen K. Oropharyngeal dysphagia: patho-physiology and diagnosis for the anniversary issue of Diseases of the Esophagus. Dis Esophagus. 2012;25(4):299-304.
8. Philpott H, Garg M, Tomic D, Balasubramanian S, Sweis R. Dysphagia: Thinking outside the box. World J Gastroenterol. 2017;23(38):6942-51.
9. Dziewas R, Allescher HD, Aroyo I, Bartolome G, Beilenhoff U, Bohlender J, et al. Diagnosis and treatment of neurogenic dysphagia – S1 guideline of the German Society of Neurology. Neurol Res Pract. 2021;3:23.
10. Panebianco M, Marchese-Ragona R, Masiero S, Restivo DA. Dysphagia in neurological diseases: a literature review. Neurol Sci. 2020;41:3067-73.
11. González-Fernández M, Ottenstein L, Atanelov L, Christian AB. Dysphagia after Stroke: an Overview. Curr Phys Med Rehabil Rep. 2013;1(3):187-96.
12. Suttrup I, Warnecke T. Dysphagia in Parkinson's Disease. Dysphagia. 2016;31(1):24-32.
13. Schefold JC, Berger D, Zürcher P, Lensch M, Perren A, Jakob SM, et al. Dysphagia in Mechanically Ventilated ICU Patients (DYnAMICS): A Prospective Observational Trial. Crit Care Med. 2017;45(12):2061-9.
14. Dellis S, Papadopoulou S, Krikonis K, Zigras F. Sarcopenic Dysphagia. A Narrative Review. J Frailty Sarcopenia Falls. 2018;3(1):1-7.
15. Schindler A, Ginocchio D, Ruoppolo G. What we don't know about dysphagia complications? Rev Laryngol Otol Rhinol (Bord). 2008;129(2):75-8.
16. Vogel AP, Rommel N, Sauer C, Horger M, Krumm P, Himmelbach M, et al. Clinical assessment of dysphagia in neurodegeneration (CADN): development, validity and reliability of a bedside tool for dysphagia assessment. J Neurol. 2017;264(6):1107-17.
17. Matsuo K, Palmer JB. Coordination of Mastication, Swallowing and Breathing. Jpn Dent Sci Rev. 2009;45(1):31-40.
18. Britton D, Roeske A, Ennis SK, Benditt JO, Quinn C, Graville D. Utility of Pulse Oximetry to Detect Aspiration: An Evidence-Based Systematic Review. Dysphagia. 2018;33(3):282-92.
19. Lynch YT, Clark BJ, Macht M, White SD, Taylor H, Wimbish T, et al. The accuracy of the bedside swallowing evaluation for detecting aspiration in survivors of acute respiratory failure. J Crit Care. 2017;39:143-8.
20. Sarve AR, Krishnamurthy R, Balasubramanium RK. The timed water test of swallowing: Reliability, validity, and normative data from Indian population. Int J Health Sci (Qassim). 2021;15(2):14-20.
21. Francesco M, Nicole P, Letizia S, Claudia B, Daniela G, Antonio S, et al. Mixed consistencies in dysphagic patients: A myth to dispel. Dysphagia. 2022;37:116-24.
22. Tejima C, Kikutani T, Takahashi N, Tamura F, Yoshida M. Application of simple swallowing provocation test with fiberoptic endoscopic evaluation of swallowing in a cross-sectional study. BMC Geriatr. 2015;15:48.
23. Birchall O, Bennett M, Lawson N, Cotton SM, Vogel AP. The Role of Instrumental Swallowing Assessment in Adults in Residential Aged Care Homes: A National Modified Delphi Survey Examining Beliefs and Practices. Dysphagia. 2022;37(3):510-22.
24. Rugiu MG. Role of videofluoroscopy in evaluation of neurologic dysphagia. Acta Otorhinolaryngol Ital. 2007;27(6):306-16.
25. Nacci A, Ursino F, La Vela R, Matteucci F, Mallardi V, Fattori B. Fiberoptic endoscopic evaluation of swallowing (FEES): proposal for informed consent. Acta Otorhinolaryngol Ital. 2008;28(4): 206-11.
26. Ozaki K, Kagaya H, Yokoyama M, Saitoh E, Okada S, González-Fernández M, et al. The risk of penetration or aspiration during videofluoroscopic examination of swallowing varies depending on food types. Tohoku J Exp Med. 2010;220(1):41-6.
27. Braun T, Juenemann M, Viard M, Meyer M, Reuter I, Prosiegel M, et al. Adjustment of oral diet based on flexible endoscopic evaluation of swallowing (FEES) in acute stroke patients: a cross-sectional hospital-based registry study. BMC Neurol. 2019;19:282.
28. Wang D, Wang X, Yu Y, Xu X, Wang J, Jia Y, et al. Assessment of esophageal motor disorders using high-resolution mano-metry in esophageal dysphagia with normal endoscopy. J Neurogastroenterol Motil. 2019;25(1):61-7.
29. Audag N, Goubau C, Toussaint M, Reychler G. Screening and evaluation tools of dysphagia in adults with neuromuscular diseases: a systematic review. Ther Adv Chronic Dis. 2019;10: 2040622318821622.
30. Leslie P, Carding PN, Wilson JA. Investigation and management of chronic dysphagia. BMJ. 2003;326(7386):433-6.

31. Schwemmle C, Jungheim M, Miller S, Kühn D, Ptok M. Medikamenteninduzierte Dysphagien: Ein Überblick [Medication-induced dysphagia: A review]. HNO. 2015;63(7):504-10.
32. Cichero JA. Thickening agents used for dysphagia management: effect on bioavailability of water, medication and feelings of satiety. Nutr J. 2013;12:54.
33. Jongprasitkul H, Kitisomprayoonkul W. Effectiveness of Conventional Swallowing Therapy in Acute Stroke Patients with Dysphagia. Rehabil Res Pract. 2020;2020:2907293.
34. Wheeler-Hegland K, Ashford J, Frymark T, McCabe D, Mullen R, Musson N, et al. Evidence-based systematic review: Oropharyngeal dysphagia behavioral treatments. Part II--impact of dysphagia treatment on normal swallow function. J Rehabil Res Dev. 2009;46(2):185-94.
35. Logemann JA, Rademaker A, Pauloski BR, Kelly A, Stangl-McBreen C, Antinoja J, et al. A randomized study comparing the Shaker exercise with traditional therapy: a preliminary study. Dysphagia. 2009;24(4):403-11.
36. Pisegna JM, Murray J. Clinical application of flexible endoscopic evaluation of swallowing in stroke. Semin Speech Lang. 2018;39(1):3-14.
37. Wu C, Zhu X, Zhou X, Li C, Zhang Y, Zhang H, et al. Intermittent tube feeding for stroke patients with dysphagia: a meta-analysis and systematic review. Ann Palliat Med. 2021;10(7):7406-15.
38. Chang WK, Huang HH, Lin HH, Tsai CL. Percutaneous endoscopic gastrostomy versus nasogastric tube feeding: oropharyngeal dysphagia increases risk for pneumonia requiring hospital admission. Nutrients. 2019;11(12):2969.
39. Buchholz DW. Cricopharyngeal myotomy may be effective treatment for selected patients with neurogenic oropharyngeal dysphagia. Dysphagia. 1995;10(4):255-8.
40. Restivo DA, Marchese-Ragona R, Lauria G, Squatrito S, Gullo D, Vigneri R. Botulinum toxin treatment for oropharyngeal dysphagia associated with diabetic neuropathy. Diabetes Care. 2006;29(12):2650-3.
41. Skoretz SA, Anger N, Wellman L, Takai O, Empey A. A systematic review of tracheostomy modifications and swallowing in adults. Dysphagia. 2020;35(6):935-47.
42. Berg HM, Jacobs JB, Persky MS, Cohen NL. Cricopharyngeal myotomy: a review of surgical results in patients with cricopharyngeal achalasia of neurogenic origin. Laryngoscope. 1985;95(11):1337-40.

31 CHAPTER

Approach to Anosmia and Ageusia

Girish Soni, Prachi P Barvalia

INTRODUCTION

Both taste and smell are essential for human survival. They help us detect warning harmful odors from the environment and provide us with many of life's pleasurable experiences such as eating a meal and enjoying the fragrance of a flower. Hence, the inability to smell or taste can have a severe impact on health and quality of life.[1]

There is a heightened sense of taste and smell in pregnancy, to protect the fetus from toxins during its development. Taste is important for determining what to eat, evaluating food for toxicity and nutrients, and influencing digestion. It serves as an endocrine organ by stimulating the secretion of regulatory hormones such as glucagon-like peptide 1 (GLP-1), glucagon, and other peptides. Disorders of smell and taste can be hazardous to humans, causing loss of appetite, unintended weight loss, malnutrition, and poor quality of life. Loss of smell can also lead to depression.

Despite playing such a major role in the quality of life, taste and smell are the least understood and rarely taught topics. For neurologists, it is essential to understand the sense of smell and taste due to the following reasons:

- Olfactory interconnections play a major role in language, memory, and modulating human behavior, relationships, and emotions. Olfaction also plays an important role in appreciating certain tastes. Olfactory subgenome spans 1–2% of total genomic deoxyribonucleic acid (DNA).
- Olfactory dysfunction is a preclinical manifestation of neurodegenerative disorders such as Parkinson's disease (PD) and Alzheimer's disease (AD).[2] In fact, olfactory tests are as effective as single-photon emission computed tomography (SPECT) imaging of the dopamine transporter in detecting PD.[3]
- Recent evidence shows that smell loss and testing can help distinguish idiopathic PD from other parkinsonian syndromes. It can suggest which patients with rapid eye movement (REM) sleep behavior disorder will be more likely to develop PD, and can be predictive of the progression of cognitive impairment and Alzheimer's dementia.
- Not just playing a pivotal role in safety, nutrition, and quality of life, olfaction provides a "health index" or probe for relatively inaccessible brain areas.[4]

The coronavirus disease (COVID-19) pandemic has affected the whole world, and anosmia and ageusia are important manifestations reported by patients infected with COVID-19. The average anosmia incidence rate in India was 30.19% in COVID-19-infected patients.

Though the importance of smell and taste is proven beyond doubt, they are not routinely tested in the neurological examination.

ANATOMY OF OLFACTION AND TASTE

Olfaction

Our olfactory system has two main functions:

1. To detect and identify different environmental odors
2. To detect and identify flavors of our food[2]

Peripheral Connections

Odorant molecules enter the nasal passage via air or by retronasal airflow by chewing and swallowing food. They dissolve in the mucus that covers the olfactory epithelium, which covers the cribriform plate, superior septum, and superior and middle turbinates. The olfactory epithelium is made up of more than 6 million bipolar olfactory receptor cells. The dendrite of each cell lies in the mucus layer, so incoming odor molecules stimulate the bipolar olfactory cells. Bowman's glands produce mucus, and basal cells develop new olfactory cells. New olfactory receptor cells are generated every 30–60 days. About 350 receptor proteins are expressed on the long cilia of the receptor cells, with each cell expressing only one receptor type, which is G protein-coupled receptors. Most olfactory receptors are activated by multiple chemicals. The olfactory receptor cell is unique as it also serves as a first-order neuron, synapsing with glomeruli that are in the outermost region of the olfactory bulb at the base of the brain **(Fig. 1)**.[2] Each glomerulus receives axons from receptor cells that express the same receptor protein, making each of them a functioning representative of a special class of proteins. There is total of six layers in the olfactory bulb: olfactory nerve layer, glomerular layer, external plexiform layer, mitral cell layer, internal plexiform layer, and granule cell layer.[5]

The external plexiform layer is deep to the glomerular layer, mainly comprising (1) secondary dendrites of mitral and tufted cells, which are the primary output neurons of the bulbs, and (2) extensions from granule cells (GABAergic), which are the major interneurons of the olfactory bulb. There are reciprocal synapses occurring between the granule and mitral/tufted cells. Mitral cells can activate granule cells, which in turn inhibit mitral cell activity. Centrifugal fibers from central brain regions synapse on granule cells and selectively alter mitral and tufted cell activity. These central brain areas include olfactory cortex, basal forebrain, ventral pallidum, lateral preoptic, and rostral lateral hypothalamic areas, locus coeruleus, dorsal, and medial raphe nuclei of the midbrain.[2,5]

There is coding for each type of odorant, and brain maps are formed.

Central Connections

The olfactory system, unlike other sensory systems, communicates directly with the cerebral cortex without first relaying in the thalamus. Reciprocal connections occur via the dorsomedial nucleus of the thalamus between primary and secondary olfactory cortical structures **(Flowchart 1)**.

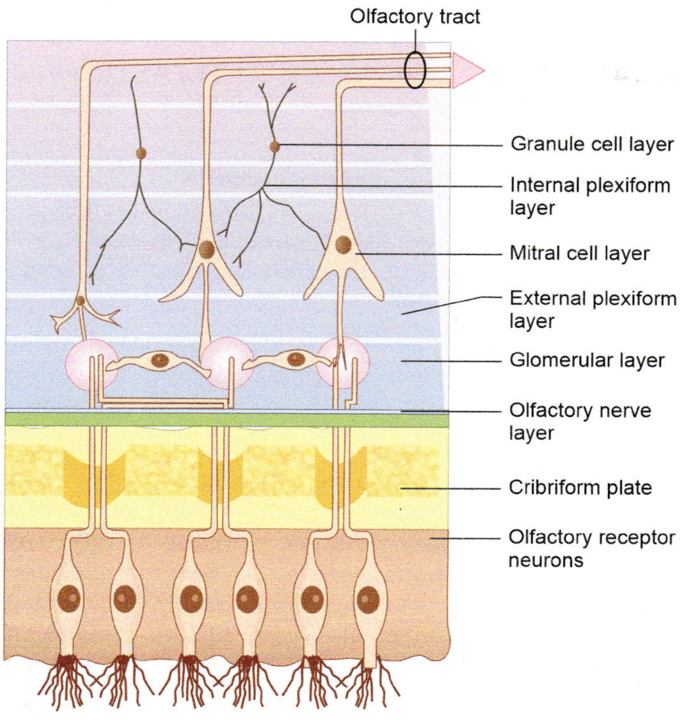

FIG. 1: Major layers of the olfactory bulb.

Processing within the entorhinal cortex (EC) contributes to attention, conditioning, and event and spatial cognition by compressing representations that overlap in time. These are transferred to the hippocampus, where differentiation occurs, and returned to EC.

An adjacent area, the trans-EC, is a major source of incoming fibers to EC that is damaged very early in AD and may contribute to impairment of memory and olfaction in that disorder.[2]

Gustation

There are five basic tastes: sweet, sour, bitter, salty, and umami [savory, monosodium glutamate (MSG)-like].

There are 7,500 taste buds, and each taste bud has 150 receptor cells. Taste buds are modified epithelial cells. They have a turnover time of 10 days. They are widespread on the tongue, palate, oropharynx, larynx, upper esophagus, and intestine. Any taste bud can contain receptors to identify each different taste.

Nerve supply:

- *Lingual nerve*: It is the branch of the third division of the trigeminal nerve: carries somatic sensation from the anterior two-thirds of the tongue.
- *Chorda tympani nerve*: It is the branch of the facial nerve (VII): special taste sensation from the anterior two-third of the tongue.
- *Glossopharyngeal nerve (IX)*: It carries taste sensation and general visceral sensation from the circumvallate and posterior foliate papilla located on the back of the tongue.
- *Greater superficial petrosal division of cranial nerve VII*: Soft palate taste receptors
- *Vagus nerve (X)*: Throat and digestive tract taste receptors

Cranial nerves VII, IX, and X send their axons to the nucleus tractus solitarius, travel to the ventral posterior nucleus of the thalamus via the medial lemniscus, and then travel to the amygdala, anterior insular cortex, and orbital frontal cortex.[2]

CLINICAL APPROACH

A systematic approach is needed to evaluate disorders of smell and taste. Accurate clinical tests are needed to establish an appropriate diagnosis and assess the degree of sensory impairments. It is crucial to know about the etiology of olfactory and gustatory dysfunction for establishing the diagnosis and planning the management. We need to be acquainted with common terminologies **(Table 1)**.[5]

Awareness of the various physiological factors affecting olfaction is also needed **(Box 1)**.[5]

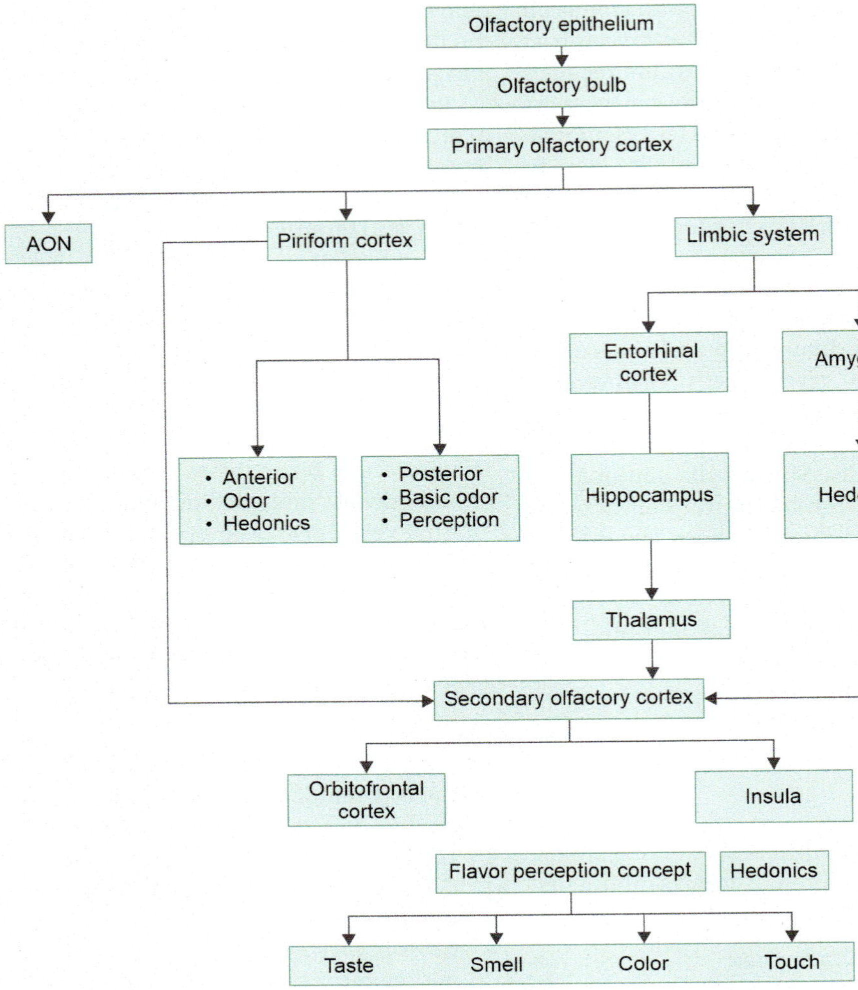

FLOWCHART 1: Central olfactory connections.
(AON: anterior olfactory nucleus)

TABLE 1: Various terminologies and their meaning.

Terminology	Meaning
Anosmia	Complete loss of smell
Hyposmia/microsomia	Less than total loss of smell
Phantosmia	Strange and distorted smell in the absence of a stimuli
Parosmia/dysosmia	Strange and distorted smell when an odorant is smelled
Hyperosmia	Hypersensitivity to odorants
Olfactory agnosia	Inability to identify odors in the presence of an intact olfactory system

BOX 1 Factors affecting smell function.

- Age: 2% population <65 years have chronic impairment of smell. Between 65 and 80 years, dramatically half the population has an impaired ability to smell. In the population older than 85 years, >75% have impaired smell
- Sex: Females are better than men
- Pregnancy
- Smoking

History

Ask questions such as: Is your smell impaired? What odors are affected, and which ones can you still detect? Do you have any altered smells and are they pleasant or unpleasant? Are they triggered, or come spontaneously? Can you identify tastes such as sweet, sour, bitter, and salty? Are you having trouble detecting flavors such as chocolate, vanilla, or strawberry? Have you lost your appetite? Have you lost weight? Take another important history of current medications including vitamins, smoking history, any recent or past head trauma, current or recurrent cold and sinus problems or recurrent allergic rhinitis connected to the onset of altered smell or taste, alcohol abuse, and quality of oral and dental hygiene; enquire about memory disturbances, abnormal movements, cognitive decline. Ask relatives about any change in behavior. Especially in patients with cognitive decline such as diffuse Lewy body disease (DLBD), multiple sclerosis (MS), and AD, symptoms of smell and taste alteration may not be reported directly since patients may not be aware of this problem. Hence, detailed neurological examination is important in these patients.

Sometimes, the altered taste is because of a smell disorder as opposed to a primary taste disorder. If the patient reports that his or her taste of food is impaired and there is no problem in recognizing sweet, sour, bitter, and salt tastes, it is likely that there is a primary smell disorder. It is recommended that a smell test always be performed in every smell- and taste-impaired patient because of the greater likelihood of an abnormality of smell.[2]

Examination

Examination of Smell

Smell testing is neglected in the neurological examination. In a study done by Induraj Kumar, 26.9% of the patients self-reported anosmia before testing. After detailed neurological testing and quantitative evaluation of olfactory dysfunction, the incidence increased to 41.3%. This reflects that anosmia reported by patients is only the tip of an iceberg and that subclinical affection is more than what patients report and is picked up by clinical tests.[6]

Methods to Examine Smell

Examine locally for nasal causes of smell dysfunction before doing a detailed examination.

The smell is tested using non-noxious stimuli. Avoid chemicals like ammonia as they may stimulate the trigeminal nerve instead of the olfactory nerve. Examine each nostril separately while occluding the other. Tell the patient to keep his eyes closed and one nostril occluded, and bring the test substance near the open one. Tell the patient to sniff and indicate whether he smells something. If he can smell something then ask him to identify it. Repeat the same for the other nostril. Compare the two sides. The abnormal side should be examined first. Many substances can be used to test smell (e.g., eucalyptus oil, cloves, coffee, and cinnamon). At the bedside, mouthwash, toothpaste, soap, and similar substances can be used.[5]

In the smell identification test, familiar odorants are presented.

- *University of Pennsylvania smell identification test (UPSIT)*: It is self-administered, and consists of four test booklets with 10 odors in each booklet (40 in total). Each odor has four choices to choose from on the page. The odors are released by using the tip of a pencil that scratches the surface of the odor region of the page. Normative data based on age and sex are available. Its forced-choice design helps identify malingering.
- *Modified sniffin' sticks test*: It employs felt tip pens that present different odorants. The odor identification portion includes 16 sticks (12 odors and 4 blanks). It is more time-consuming.

The perception of smell is enough; accurate identification is not needed. Perceiving the presence of an odor indicates continuity of the olfactory pathways; identification of the odor indicates intact cortical function as well. The perception of smell, even without recognition, excludes anosmia.[5]

Examination of Taste

Four substances are used for testing: sucrose (sweet), sodium chloride (salty), quinine (bitter), and citric acid (sour). The tongue must remain protruded throughout the testing of an individual substance, and the mouth must be rinsed between tests. Bitter should be last because it leaves the most aftertaste. A moist applicator stick may be dipped into a packet of sugar, artificial sweetener, or salt, coated with the test substance, and then placed on one side of the patient's tongue and rubbed around. The patient indicates by raising his hand whether he can identify the substance. He points toward words written on paper to indicate salty, bitter, sweet, or sour taste. Examine the whole of the tongue, as there can be patchy taste loss. Most patients identify the test substance in less than 10 seconds. It is better to apply the substance to the dorsal surface at about the junction of the anterior and middle third of the tongue, as the tip of the tongue has less sensation. Commercially available taste strips are filter paper strips impregnated with sweet, sour, salty, and bitter in different concentrations. They can be used for taste assessment.

Apart from the examination of taste and smell, a thorough evaluation of cranial nerves V, VII, IX, and X, should be done. Oral examination to look for tongue discoloration, coating, furrowing, atrophy, and teeth and gum health should also be inspected. Look for any dryness in the mouth.

Diseases Affecting Olfaction

Olfactory deficits are divided into:

- *Conductive deficits*: Obstruction in the pathway of odorants to contact the olfactory epithelium, such as nasal polyps
- *Sensorineural or neurogenic deficits*: Defects of the receptors or their central connections

Unilateral loss of smell is more significant than bilateral, caused by primarily conductive etiologies. Because the cortical representation of smell in the piriform cortex is bilateral, a unilateral lesion distal to the decussation of the olfactory fibers causes no olfactory impairment.

There are multiple causes of anosmia **(Table 2)**.[2]

Local causes such as rhinitis and polyps cause bilateral anosmia. COVID-19 infection can cause prolonged persistent anosmia. Severe acute respiratory syndrome coronavirus 2 (SARS-CoV-2) enters the human cell by binding angiotensin-converting enzyme 2 (ACE2) receptors, followed by priming of the viral spike protein by the transmembrane protease serine 2 (TMPRSS2). ACE2 and TMPRSS2 are expressed in human olfactory epithelial supporting (sustentacular) cells. Hence, COVID-19 affects the olfactory epithelium and causes anosmia.[7] In COVID-19 patients, ageusia and anosmia are not due to

TABLE 2: Diseases affecting olfaction.

Trauma	Infections	Neurode-generative	Local causes	Genetic	Toxins	Endocrine	Other	Immune mediated
	COVID-19	AD	Rhinosi-nusitis	Kallmann syndrome	Tobacco	Adrenal insufficiency	Anorexia nervosa	Multiple sclerosis
	Upper respiratory infections	PD	Adenoid hypertrophy	22q11 deletion syndrome	Smoking	Diabetes	Congenital	Sjögren's syndrome
	Herpes simplex encephalitis	FTD	Allergies	Asperger syndrome	Alcohol	Cushing's syndrome	Epilepsy	RA
	Leprosy	iRBD	Asthma	Bardet–Biedl syndrome	Chemical exposure	Hypothyroidism	Liver disease	Autoimmune encephalitis
	AIDS/HIV	CBGD		Cystic fibrosis	Medications	Obesity	Renal disease	
		ALS		Down syndrome		Pseudohypo-parathyroidism	Migraine	
		Degenerative ataxias		Turner syndrome			Stroke	
		HD					Narcolepsy cataplexy	
		MSA					Cranial–nasal neoplasms	
		Multi-infarct dementia					Nutritional deficiency	
		DLBD					COPD	
							Psychiatric causes	

(AD: Alzheimer's disease; AIDS: acquired immunodeficiency syndrome; ALS: amyotrophic lateral sclerosis; CBGD: cortical basal ganglionic degeneration; COPD: chronic obstructive pulmonary disease; COVID-19: coronavirus disease; DLBD: diffuse Lewy body disease; FTD: frontotemporal dementia; HD: Huntington's disease; HIV: human immunodeficiency virus; iRBD: idiopathic REM sleep behavior disorder; MSA: multiple system atrophy; PD: Parkinson's disease; RA: rheumatoid arthritis)

nasal obstruction or other rhinitis symptoms but due to the direct damage of the olfactory and gustatory receptors.[7]

Heavy metals such as cadmium, chromium, nickel, and manganese cause anosmia. Intranasal zinc gluconate, which is marketed as a common cold remedy, can cause zinc-induced anosmia syndrome.

Head injury is probably the most common cause of disruption of the olfactory fibers before their decussation. Closed head injury can produce impairment of olfactory recognition, despite relatively preserved olfactory detection due to injury to the orbitofrontal and temporal lobes.

Significant olfactory dysfunction has also been described in AD and minor cognitive impairment (MCI). Olfactory deficits may help discriminate AD from major depression. Olfactory loss in MS patients has been associated with plaque formation in central olfactory brain regions. PD has a relatively early impairment of smell. Hawkes stated that normal olfaction in PD should prompt the review of diagnosis unless the patient is a female with tremor-predominant PD. Braak et al. demonstrated α-synuclein deposition in the olfactory tract and anterior olfactory nucleus on pathological examination of patients even in the earliest stages of PD.[3] Anosmia in suspected progressive supranuclear palsy (PSP) and corticobasal ganglionic degeneration (CBGD) is unusual and should provoke a review of diagnosis. Subjects with anosmia and one apolipoprotein E4 (ApoE4) allele have a fivefold increased risk of AD. Neurodegeneration within the central regions involved in olfaction is the cause of anosmia in PD. About 50% of patients with REM sleep behavior disorder have olfactory dysfunction. In a 4-year prospective study, Postuma and colleagues found that patients with REM sleep behavior disorder who also had olfactory loss had a 65% chance of developing a defined neurodegenerative disease, compared to only 14% who had normal olfaction. Systemic disorders that may affect smell include: Diabetes mellitus, hypothyroidism, chronic liver and kidney diseases, and vitamin B12 and folate deficiencies. More than 50% of patients with diabetes mellitus have a change in their smell and taste probably due to cranial neuropathy.[2]

Congenital anosmia is caused by a cleft palate, absent or hypoplastic olfactory bulbs or tracts. Kallmann syndrome consists of hypogonadotropic hypogonadism and anosmia.[1] Olfactory anomalies may occur in CHARGE (coloboma, heart defects, atresia of choanae, retardation in growth, genital abnormalities, ear malformation) syndrome. Iatrogenic causes such as frontal or temporal lobectomy, rhinoplasty, and radiation therapy can cause anosmia. Olfactory damage is much more common in an anterior hemispheric surgical approach than after the basal interhemispheric approach. Tumors of the olfactory groove (meningiomas), sphenoid wing, pituitary, frontal bone (osteomas), and saccular aneurysm of the circle of Willis can cause compression of olfactory bulb and tract and cause anosmia and Foster Kennedy syndrome, which consists of ipsilateral anosmia, ipsilateral optic atrophy, and contralateral papilledema. Mass lesions of the frontal lobe can cause personality changes and exert pressure on the olfactory system, leading to anosmia. Esthesioneuroblastomas are olfactory neuroblastomas causing anosmia and nasal obstruction.

Parosmia can be seen after a head injury, chronic sinusitis, or viral infection. Olfactory hallucinations can occur in focal seizures with impaired awareness. Olfactory epileptic auras can occur from amygdala lesions or mesial temporal sclerosis (MTS).[2,5]

A recent study in olfaction has found olfactory dysfunction in patients with autoimmune encephalitis. Patients of severe limbic encephalitis and mesial temporal involvement are more likely to get olfactory dysfunction.[8]

Diseases Affecting Taste

Patients with taste complaints will most likely have smell dysfunction due to impaired flavor detection.

The taste system is quite widespread, with three different nerves on each side that subserve taste. Also, complete ageusia is not possible without complete anosmia. See **Table 3** for the varied causes of taste dysfunction. Ageusia can occur due to multiple medications **(Table 4)**. Toxins, and medical diseases such as nutritional deficiency, and renal and liver diseases can cause loss of taste. Local causes such as dental and poor oral hygiene can cause ageusia. Gastroesophageal reflux disorder and endocrine disorders

TABLE 3: Diseases affecting taste.

Local causes	Infections	Head trauma	VII nerve disorders proximal to cauda tympani	Toxins	Endocrine	Other	Immune mediated
Dental causes	Coronavirus disease (COVID-19)		Bell's palsy	Tobacco	Adrenal insufficiency	Nutritional deficiency	Multiple sclerosis
Dental procedures	Candidiasis, gingivitis, periodontitis		Infiltrative lesions of the VII nerve	Smoking	Diabetes	Epilepsy (gustatory aura)	Sjögren's syndrome
				Alcohol	Cushing's syndrome	Migraine headache (gustatory aura)	
				Chemical exposure	Hypothyroidism	Liver disease	
				Medications		Renal disease	
				Radiation		Acid reflux	
						Psychiatric causes	

TABLE 4: Medications affecting olfaction and taste.

Category	Medications affecting both olfaction and taste	Medications affecting olfaction	Medications affecting taste
Antibiotics	• Penicillins • Tetracycline	• Doxycycline • Streptomycin	
Antihistamines		Chlorpheniramine maleate	Diphenhydramine
Anticholinergics	Amitriptyline		
Antiepileptics	Phenytoin		Topiramate, carbamazepine
Angiotensin-converting enzyme inhibitors			Captopril, lisinopril
Antigout			Allopurinol
Cholesterol-lowering drugs	*Statins*: Atorvastatin, pravastatin	Clofibrate	
Chemotherapy	Methotrexate		
Calcium channel blockers	Nifedipine, diltiazem	Amlodipine	
Diuretics			Hydrochlorothiazide, furosemide
Opiates		Codeine, morphine	
Antiarrhythmic			Propranolol, amiodarone
Anti-Parkinsonian agents			Levodopa, selegiline
Nonsteroidal anti-inflammatory			Ibuprofen

can cause ageusia. Bell's palsy can cause mild ageusia because the opposite facial nerve is normal. Facial nerve lesions at the cerebellopontine angle, cisternal segment, geniculate ganglion, and in the facial canal proximal to the chorda tympani nerve can cause taste dysfunction.

INVESTIGATOR APPROACH

Flowchart 2 provides an algorithmic approach for the evaluation of smell dysfunction. Take a detailed history of the onset, duration, and progress of dysfunction. Determine

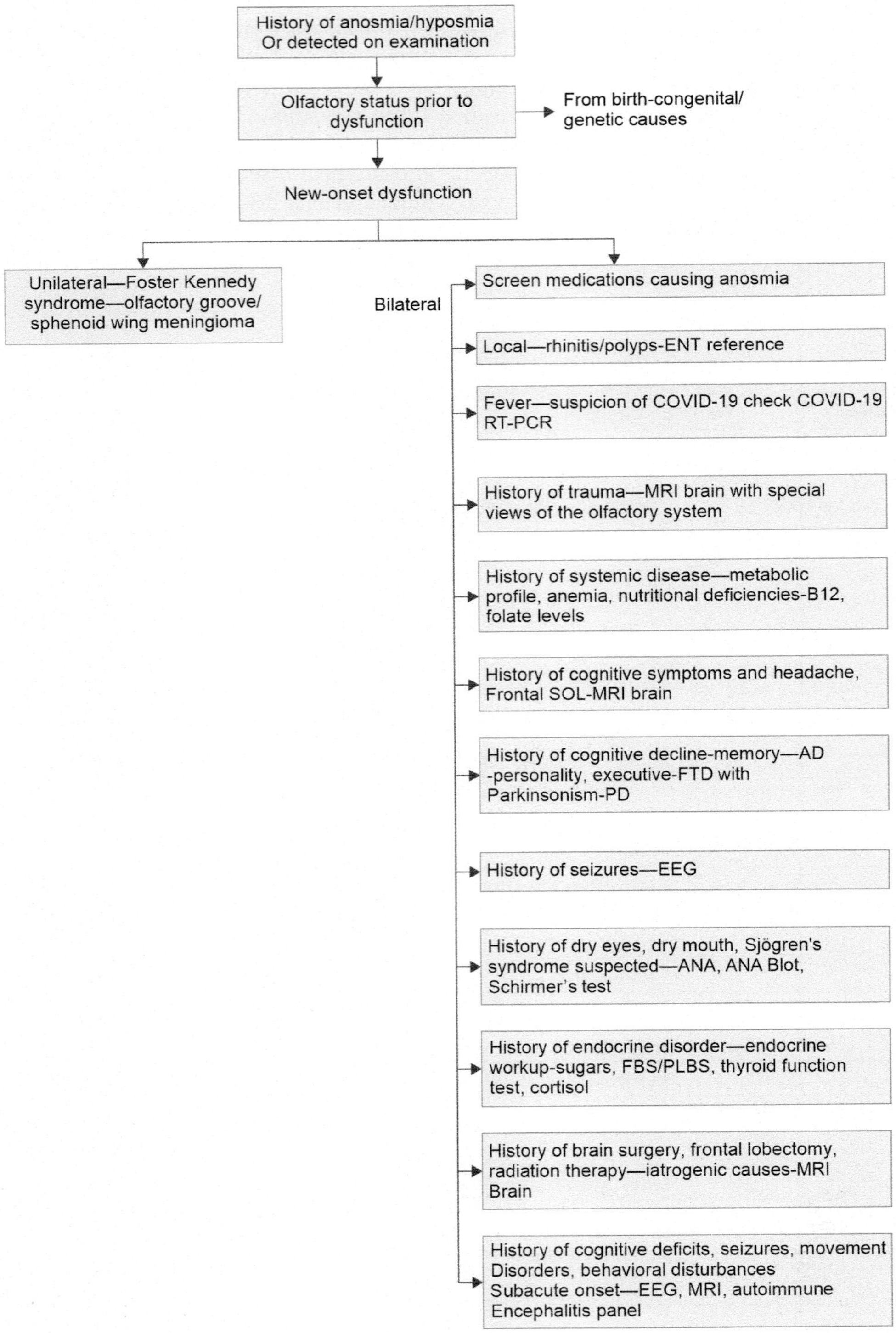

FLOWCHART 2: Algorithm for olfactory dysfunction.

(AD: Alzheimer's disease; ANA: antinuclear antibody; COVID-19: coronavirus disease; EEG: electroencephalogram; ENT: ear, nose, and throat; FBS: fasting blood sugar; FTD: frontotemporal dementia; MRI: magnetic resonance imaging; PD: Parkinson's disease; PLBS: postprandial blood sugar; RT-PCR: reverse transcription polymerase chain reaction; SOL: space-occupying lesion) the status before symptoms. If dysfunction is present from birth, congenital and genetic causes should be looked for. Examine for cleft palate. If it is a new-onset dysfunction, determine the laterality.

Screen all medications thoroughly. Complete blood count (CBC); comprehensive metabolic profile; thyroid-stimulating hormone (TSH); vitamin B12, folate, and methylmalonic acid levels; zinc level; fasting blood sugar; and 2-hour postprandial blood sugar if not a known diabetic should be noted. If there is a history of fever and travel history, COVID-19 reverse transcription polymerase chain reaction (RT-PCR) should be tested. If there is a history of head trauma, magnetic resonance imaging (MRI) of the brain with special views of the olfactory system (cribriform plate, olfactory bulb, medial temporal lobes, and orbital frontal lobes) should be done. If local causes are suspected, a referral to an otolaryngologist should be done. If an autoimmune disorder such as Sjögren's syndrome is suspected, an erythrocyte sedimentation rate and antinuclear and other autoimmune antibodies should be tested, and Schirmer's test should be done. If epilepsy is suspected then electroencephalography (EEG) should be done.[2]

Flowchart 3 provides an algorithmic approach for the evaluation of taste dysfunction. Take a detailed history of the type of taste dysfunction. Always ask for smell dysfunction and examine the same as it can be a cause of taste dysfunction. Thoroughly screen all medications taken by the patient including any exposure to toxins. Do a local oral examination and look for abnormalities on the tongue/teeth and the rest of the oral cavity. Look for oral ulcers, and check nutritional deficiencies by sending B12, folate, CBC, and endocrine workup: check sugars, TSH, and cortisol.

If a history of fever is present, check COVID-19 RT-PCR. Examine all cranial nerves, especially the VII nerve. If an autoimmune disorder such as Sjögren's syndrome is suspected, an erythrocyte sedimentation rate and antinuclear and other autoimmune antibodies should be tested, and Schirmer's test should be done. Psychogenic causes are the diagnosis of exclusion.

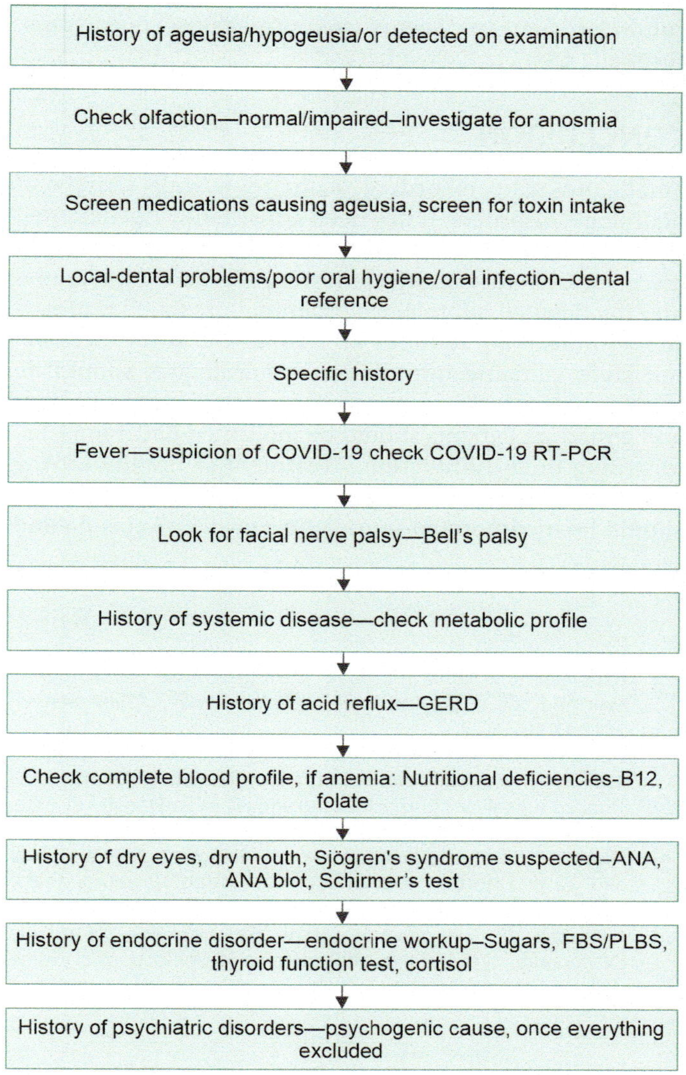

FLOWCHART 3: Algorithm for gustatory dysfunction.
(ANA: antinuclear antibody; COVID-19: coronavirus disease; FBS: fasting blood sugar; GERD: gastroesophageal reflux disease; PLBS: postprandial blood sugar; RT-PCR: reverse transcription polymerase chain reaction)

Management

Patients with impaired smell and taste have a poor quality of life. Counseling and explanation to patients should be done. Home-based care such as installing gas detectors and using deodorants should be done. If there is depression, an antidepressant should be added. Medications causing taste and smell dysfunction should be substituted or stopped. Exposure to toxins should be stopped. Maintaining good oral and nasal hygiene is important. Referral to an ear, nose, and throat (ENT) specialist should be done for suspected local causes. Iron and nutritional deficiencies should be corrected. Identifying and treating the underlying cause are important.

Zinc supplementation has been used to treat age-related taste dysfunction and dysfunction from other causes; however, no benefit was obtained in trials, except in zinc-deficient patients with renal disease.

Modifications can be done in food preparation, e.g., increasing coffee strength.

Patients with hyposmia can detect flavors in much higher concentrations to enjoy their food, by increasing the amount of salt and sugar to compensate for partial loss of flavors. This can worsen diabetes mellitus and hypertension. Hence, artificial sweeteners can be added.

Olfactory training: Patients undergoing olfactory training expose themselves to four different odors twice daily (preferably once in the morning before breakfast and once in the evening before going to bed) for at least 20–30 seconds on each of the four scents separately for at least 24 weeks. Olfactory training includes four 50 mL sniff bottles or jars. Inside each container, 1 mL of an odor solution soaked into cotton pads is kept. Scents used are alcohol, eucalyptus, citronella scent, and clove scent.[9]

CONCLUSION

Smell and taste disorders occur in a wide variety of neurologic disorders. It has been consistently documented in both neurodegenerative and neuroinflammatory diseases. Olfactory and taste testing should be integrated into the detailed neurological examination. Smell testing is self-administered, requires little time, and is inexpensive, but gives valuable information. Neurologists should be acquainted with the various etiologies affecting olfaction and gestation. Patients should be motivated and counseled regarding their dysfunction. Treatment of the underlying cause is important. Olfactory training and food modifications should be incorporated into day-to-day life. Anosmia and ageusia are also important biomarkers for various diseases, such as PD and AD. Olfactory dysfunction has been recently studied in autoimmune disorders such as autoimmune encephalitis. Awareness of the various medications causing olfactory and taste dysfunction is essential as stopping them can cause improvement. It cannot be denied that though highly neglected, smell and taste are extremely essential for having a good quality of life. More research is needed in this field to explore finer tests and pick up early dysfunction before symptoms occur. There is enough evidence now to prove that olfactory epithelium can regenerate. The olfactory system is extraordinarily plastic. This neuroplasticity can be observed at both the cellular and the cognitive levels. With the help of multimodal neuroimaging, we can study these subtle reorganization processes between brain structure and function in olfactory loss and regain, opening up a new horizon and scope for future treatments.[1]

REFERENCES

1. Boesveldt S, Postma EM, Boak D, Welge-Luessen A, Schöpf V, Mainland JD, et al. Anosmia—a clinical review. Chem Senses. 2017;42(7):513-23.
2. DeVere R. Disorders of taste and smell. Continuum (Minneap Minn). 2017;23(2, Selected Topics in Outpatient Neurology):421-46.
3. Tarakad A, Jankovic J. Anosmia and ageusia in Parkinson's disease. Int Rev Neurobiol. 2017;133:541-56.
4. Hawkes CH, Doty RL. Anatomy and physiology of olfaction. Smell and Taste Disorders. Cambridge: Cambridge University Press; 2018. pp. 1-45.
5. Campbell W. The olfactory nerve. DeJong's The Neurologic Examination, 7th edition. Philadelphia: Lippincott Williams & Wilkins; 2013. pp. 137-42.
6. Aanand P, Angral S, Varshney S, Raj R. Incidence of anosmia among COVID-19 patients in India. Indian J Otolaryngol Head Neck Surg. 2022;74(Suppl 2):3427-36.
7. Sudre CH, Keshet A, Graham MS, Joshi AD, Shilo S, Rossman H, et al. 2021. Anosmia, ageusia, and other COVID-19-like symptoms. [online]. Available from: https://www.thelancet.com/action/showPdf?pii=S2589-7500%2821%2900115-1. [Last accessed December, 2022].
8. Morano A, Cerulli Irelli E, Fanella M, Orlando B, Salamone EM, Tinelli E, et al. Olfactory impairment in autoimmune encephalitis: another piece of the puzzle. J Neurol. 2022;269(5):2762-8.
9. Doty RL. Treatments for smell and taste disorders: a critical review. Handb Clin Neurol. 2019;164:455-79.

32

CHAPTER

Approach to Visual Loss

Aastha Takkar, Karthik Vinay Mahesh, Monika Singla, Vivek Lal

INTRODUCTION

Sight is one of the most specialized modalities of the human body, and loss of vision is an extremely alarming symptom for an individual. Evaluation of such a patient requires promptness to mitigate further insults and hasten recovery, wherever feasible. Neurological visual loss (NVL) is the visual impairment caused due to disorder of the brain or the optic nerves instead of the primary eye structures.[1] It is a significant contributor of global burden of blindness or visual impairment. The neuro-ophthalmic causes of vision loss are varied and pose a challenge even to the experienced clinicians because of the myriad of symptoms, signs, pathways, and etiologies involved. Localization of visual loss within the eye or visual pathway is of utmost importance, underscoring the expertise in the knowledge of basic anatomical structures which may be involved in such a patient. A neurologist must be aware of cardinal symptoms and signs which point out to specific structural or etiological diagnosis.[2] This chapter deals with various clinical aspects to be considered in a patient presenting with visual loss.

RELEVANT ANATOMY

The visual pathway begins at retina, the innermost membrane of eye bathed in vitreous humor and consistent of 10 cellular layers. After passing through the most superficial layer of retina, the retinal pigmented epithelium, light rays reach the photoreceptor layer consisting of rods and cones. It is prudent to remember that rods are widely scattered throughout the entire retina except fovea, which is solely occupied by cones.[3] As neither rods nor cones are present at the optic disc, it is perceived as the physiological blind spot on visual field assessment. The absence of rods and concentration of cones at macula lutea make it the point of greatest visual acuity and color perception. The ganglion cell layer (GCL) consists of ganglion cells, the second-order neurons that bridge the photoreceptors, and the lateral geniculate body (LGB). While their cell bodies are located in the GCL, their fibers travel in the retinal nerve fiber layer (RNFL) toward the optic disc, forming the optic nerve and exiting through the lamina cribrosa. These fibers (optic nerve) are myelinated as against the unmyelinated axons of retina. About 5 cm in length, the optic nerve is subdivided into four parts: (1) the intraocular part/optic nerve head (1 mm), (2) the intraorbital part (about 25 mm), (3) the intracanalicular part (about 9 mm), and (4) the intracranial part (12–16 mm). Optic nerves from both sides unite at optic chiasma and then decussate into optic tracts. The chiasma typically lies about 10 mm above the pituitary gland. The nasal fibers of each eye cross the midline to join the temporal fibers of the contralateral eye and hence any deficit beyond this junction gives rise to bilateral deficits. The optic tracts are a compact continuation of the GCL, which move to LGBs carrying visual fibers stimulated from the contralateral visual field **(Figs. 1 and 2)**.[3]

The visual afferents synapse in the LGB on the second-order neurons, which give rise to the optic radiations (Gratiolet radiations, geniculocalcarine tracts, or the inferior longitudinal fasciculus). These represent the visual tracts from the LGB to the primary visual cortex (calcarine area/striate cortex, Brodmann area 17).[4] Another anatomical pearl of localization is the Meyer's loop (loop of Meyer and Archambault), the most anterior extension of the optic radiation in the temporal horns. These represent the second-order axons corresponding to the contralateral upper quadrant originating from the ventrolateral LGB.[5]

The pregeniculate visual pathway has been referred to as anterior visual pathway, and posterior visual pathway is the pathway beyond the LGB **(Fig. 1)**. It is better to refer the visual pathway deficits as pre- and postchiasmal or pre- and postgeniculate in order to provide exact anatomical localization of the lesion.

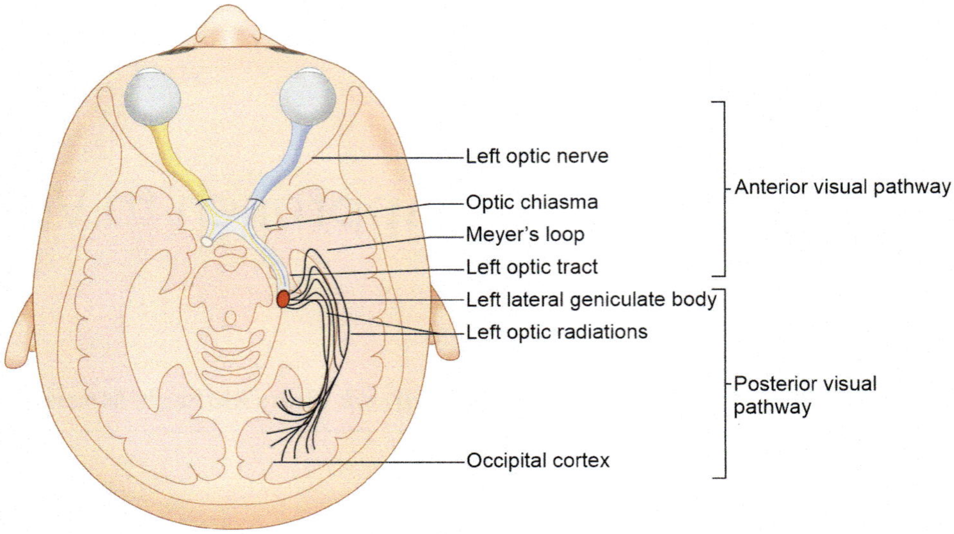

FIG. 1: Showing vital anatomical structures in visual pathway.

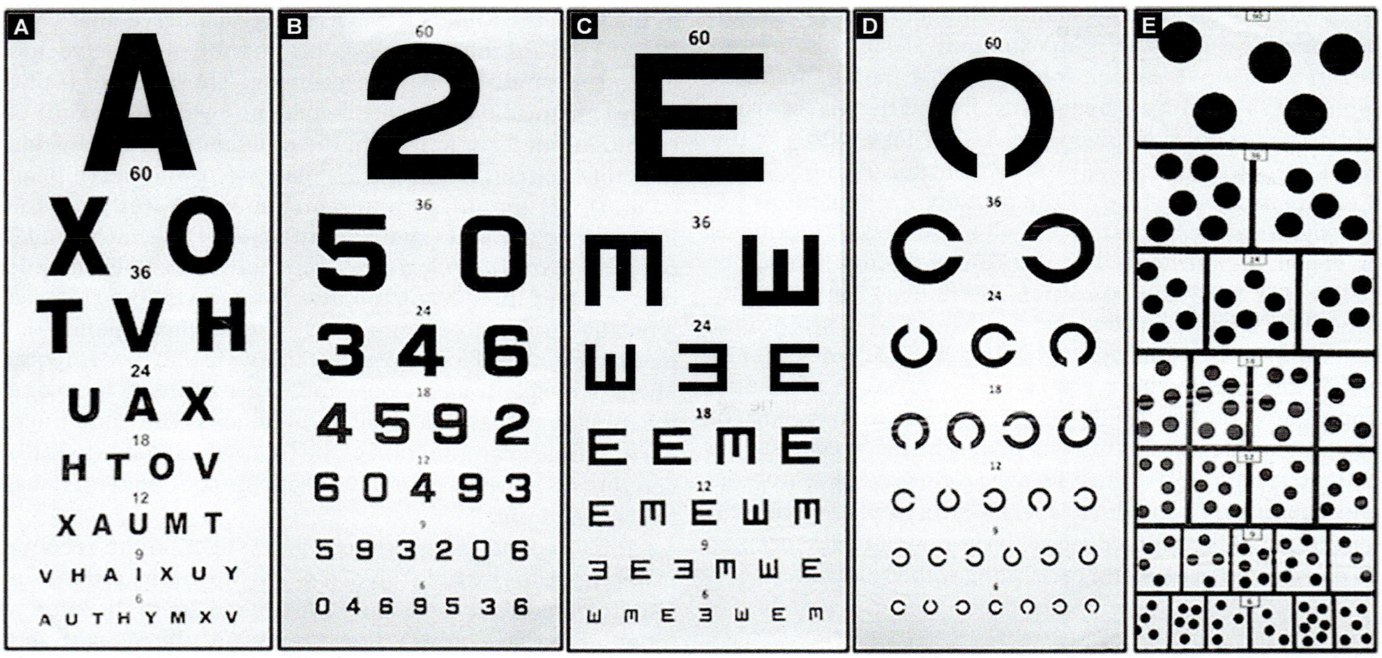

FIGS. 2A TO E: Variations of Snellen's charts available to assess far vision.

CLINICAL APPROACH TO VISION LOSS

History

Detailed history taking is paramount in arriving at a diagnosis. A patient complaining of visual disturbances may have decreased ability to visualize, blurring of vision, cloudy vision, distorted vision, constriction of visual field, and even diplopia. It is prudent to analyze the patient's interpretation of visual loss before proceeding. Initial approach to vision loss should always be focused on delineating the probable substrates. A comprehensive analysis can give vital clues toward exact anatomical localization and also toward probable etiology. **Box 1** shows important questions which should asked to a patient with visual loss.[2,6] Another important step is to localize whether a patient has involvement of pre- or postchiasmal and pre- or postgeniculate visual pathway defect. **Box 2** gives general pointers which may help in identifying as to whether the given patient has the involvement of anterior or posterior visual pathway. Similarly in patients with anterior visual pathway it is important to localize whether the pathology is retinal or in optic nerve. **Table 1** provides a rough guide to differentiate a retinal from an optic nerve pathology.[2]

BOX 1	Questions to be asked to a patient presenting with vision loss.

1. Is the vision loss unilateral or bilateral?
2. Is it acute, subacute, or chronic?
3. Is there any fluctuation of symptoms?
4. Is the visual loss transient or persistent?
5. Is it static or progressive?
6. Are there any visual field defects?
7. Is there any pain?
8. Are there associated symptoms?

Ophthalmological: Periorbital pain, photopsias, macropsias, metamorphopsias, ptosis, proptosis, diplopia, conjunctival congestion

Neurological: Headache, tinnitus, motor or sensory deficits, imbalance, oscillopsia, vertigo, seizures, bowel or bladder symptoms

Systemic: Fever, weight loss, night sweats, photosensitivity, rashes, ulcers, joint pains

Past history: Diabetes, hypertension, hypothyroidism, recent trauma, recent surgery, consumption of medications

BOX 2	General guide to differentiate anterior and posterior visual pathway defects.

- *History*: Unilateral or sequential visual loss favors the optic nerve involvement. Simultaneous severe bilateral visual loss or homonymous hemianopic defects on visual fields suggest posterior visual pathway involvement
- *Light reflexes*: Involvement of pupillary light reflexes or relative afferent pupillary defect is a cardinal sign suggesting involvement of optic nerve/anterior visual pathway. Preservation of pupillary light reflexes despite severe visual loss may suggest posterior visual pathway involvement
- *Color vision*: Although cerebral dyschromatopsia causes color vision deficits in the involved fields, early and profound color desaturation (especially for red color) is a feature of optic nerve involvement
- *Visual field defects*: Visual field defects meeting the vertical meridian favor the posterior visual pathway involvement. The more posterior the cerebral lesion, the more symmetric hemianopic field defects are noted. Congruous homonymic hemianopia is a characteristic of postgeniculate lesions
- *Fundus examination*: While varied fundus abnormalities can be seen in various optic nerve diseases, normal ophthalmoscopic examination is seen in posterior visual pathway defects

Patients' past medical history, history of systemic diseases, family history, and medication and treatment history may often give important clues toward specific neurological etiologies.

Neuro-ophthalmic Examination

When examining a patient with vision loss, it should be borne in mind that each eye should be examined separately initially. The neuro-ophthalmic examination should be systematic and inclusive. Following parameters must be examined in detail.

TABLE 1: General guide to differentiate between retinal and optic nerve diseases.

	Retinal disease	Optic nerve disease
Visual disturbances	• Positive visual phenomenon such as photopsias, macropsias, micropsias, and metamorphopsias • Night blindness/ nyctalopia indicates rod photoreceptor dysfunction. Light intolerance/day blindness or hemeralopia suggests cone photoreceptor dysfunction	• Visual acuity loss or visual field deficit are common complaints • Visual phenomena such as Uhthoff's phenomenon or Pulfrich's phenomenon are common with optic nerve diseases
Color vision	• Visual acuity is equally or more notably impaired than color vision • Acquired blue/ yellow or blue dyschromatopsia is common	• Variable involvement of visual acuity depending upon the etiology. Color vision is often profoundly affected • Acquired red/green dyschromatopsia is common
Visual field abnormalities	Peripheral scotomas, which do not conform to the retinotopic organization	Variable field loss depending upon the etiology (visual field loss meeting horizontal meridian, peripheral field constriction, central or cecocentral scotomas)
Pupillary involvement	RAPD less common unless extensive disease with macular involvement	RAPD is common in patients with asymmetric or unilateral involvement
Specific investigations	Full-field ERG assesses retinal function. The P50 and N95 components of the pattern ERG reflect the macular and RGC	Visual evoked potential abnormalities are observed in optic nerve disorders

(ERG: electroretinogram; RAPD: relative afferent pupillary defect; RGC: retinal ganglion cell)

Visual Acuity

Visual acuity is the measurement of the ability to discriminate two points separated in space at high contrast relative to the background. It is important to determine whether the visual loss is due to a refractive error or not before proceeding further. The patient's visual acuity should be checked with glasses (or with pinhole) in case an underlying refractive defect is present. The *best corrected visual acuity* (BCVA) is recorded to avoid confounding refractory and media errors. Near vision is measured using the Jaeger near vision chart and distant vision by Snellen's or Early Treatment of Diabetic Retinopathy Study (ETDRS) chart.[7,8] It is important that the distance charts are well illuminated and kept at an appropriate distance. **Figures 2A to E** show the various variations of Snellen's charts used for assessment of the visual acuity. Early optic nerve diseases may manifest only as reduction in brightness of images or color desaturation. *Determination of color vision* using pseudoisochromatic color plates is ideal. At least early color desaturation for a bright (red) object should be tested in all patients. Similarly, assessing the *contrast sensitivity* using validated charts may help assess early affection of the optic nerve.[2,9]

External/Anterior Segment Examination

While anterior segment examination is primarily an ophthalmologist's domain, a slit lamp microscopy should be done to visualize cornea, lens, iris anterior chamber, and vitreous in suggestive clinical scenarios. An external examination to assess for conjunctival congestion, lid edema, ptosis, proptosis, exophthalmos, and enophthalmos should be carried out in all patients.

Visual Field Analysis

The field of vision represents the cone of vision with maximum acuity and resolution at the center. The normal field of vision spans around 90° temporally, 50° superiorly and nasally, and 60° inferiorly. The ideal method to qualitatively assess the visual fields is by carrying out perimetry [static threshold perimetry, Humphrey visual field analyzer (HFA)], kinetic (Goldmann perimeter) or the automated octopus perimeter. The HFA is the most commonly used equipment, which also plots the luminance threshold at which the patient detects the static light stimulus. The reliability of results should be adequately assessed before final interpretation.[10] **Figure 3** shows various parameters to be noted on a visual field report for a comprehensive and reliable assessment. Visual field analysis by confrontation method should be done at the least, and the need of perimetry can be tailored as per the patient's clinical profile. The pattern of field defects can help in identifying the anatomical localization of the defect, type of lesion, and sometimes even etiology. A thorough knowledge of the visual pathway is of prime importance before interpreting the visual fields in the said patient. **Figure 4** shows the visual effect of lesions at various anatomical substrates of visual pathway on the visual field. Homonymous field defects can be seen in posterior visual pathway defects, enlarged blind spot can point toward raised intracranial pressure, and altitudinal field defects can be seen in vascular pathologies of the optic nerve head.

Pupillary Examination

The pupils should be tested for shape, size, contour, reactivity to light, and response to accommodation. Demonstration of a *relative afferent pupillary defect (RAPD)/Marcus Gunn pupil* on a swinging flashlight test points toward an anterior visual pathway defect **(Fig. 5)**. RAPD is due to the differential light sensitivity in each eye. The lesions can be in the retinal involvement, optic nerve, and damage to brachium of superior colliculus (RAPD without vision loss). Any damage beyond the LGB does not produce RAPD (posterior visual pathway).[11]

Ophthalmoscopic Examination

Ophthalmoscopic examination requires patience and experience on the part of the examiner. Posterior segment can be analyzed in detail using a direct ophthalmoscope, an indirect ophthalmoscope with a 20 D handheld lens, or by slit lamp biomicroscopy using a 78 or 90 D lens. Direct ophthalmoscopy is the most common technique available to neurologists and can help in identifying lesions of the optic disc and central retina. Pharmacological dilatation (using short-acting parasympathetic antagonists, like tropicamide 1%, or a short-acting sympathomimetic like phenylephrine 2.5%) can be done prior to a detailed fundus examination. The use of red-free filter (green light) for observing the nerve fiber layer details can further be helpful.

While examination of retina may give vital clues in various patients with neurological disorders (retinitis pigmentosa, hypertensive/diabetic retinal changes, neuroretinitis, etc.), in this chapter we will be focusing only on the key optic disc findings.[2]

A normal optic disc is pink or orange in color; it is vertically more than horizontally oval. The normal cup to disc ratio is 0.4:0.7, and spontaneous venous pulsations are usually noted on the disc. The normal arteriovenous (AV) ratio is 2:3. **Figure 6** shows normal optic disc. **Table 2** shows characteristic pathological fundus findings in key neuro-ophthalmic pathologies.

INVESTIGATORY PROFILE

Imaging Modalities

In order to maximize the yield, a clinician must ascertain the basic nature of the neuro-ophthalmic disorder being considered and must localize the lesion before proceeding to the optimal imaging modality. While neuroimaging is one of the most important investigations in the management of NVL, the type of imaging required and special sequences depend on the suspected localization and the etiology. There is no "one size fits all" imaging modality that helps in the diagnosis. Sometimes multiple modal imaging modalities might be required in conjunction with clinical investigations to arrive at a final diagnosis.

Orbital ultrasound (US): The US waves at various acoustic interfaces may a provide real-time display and may particularly be useful in lesions of the globe. B-mode US is often used to provide anatomic and functional information

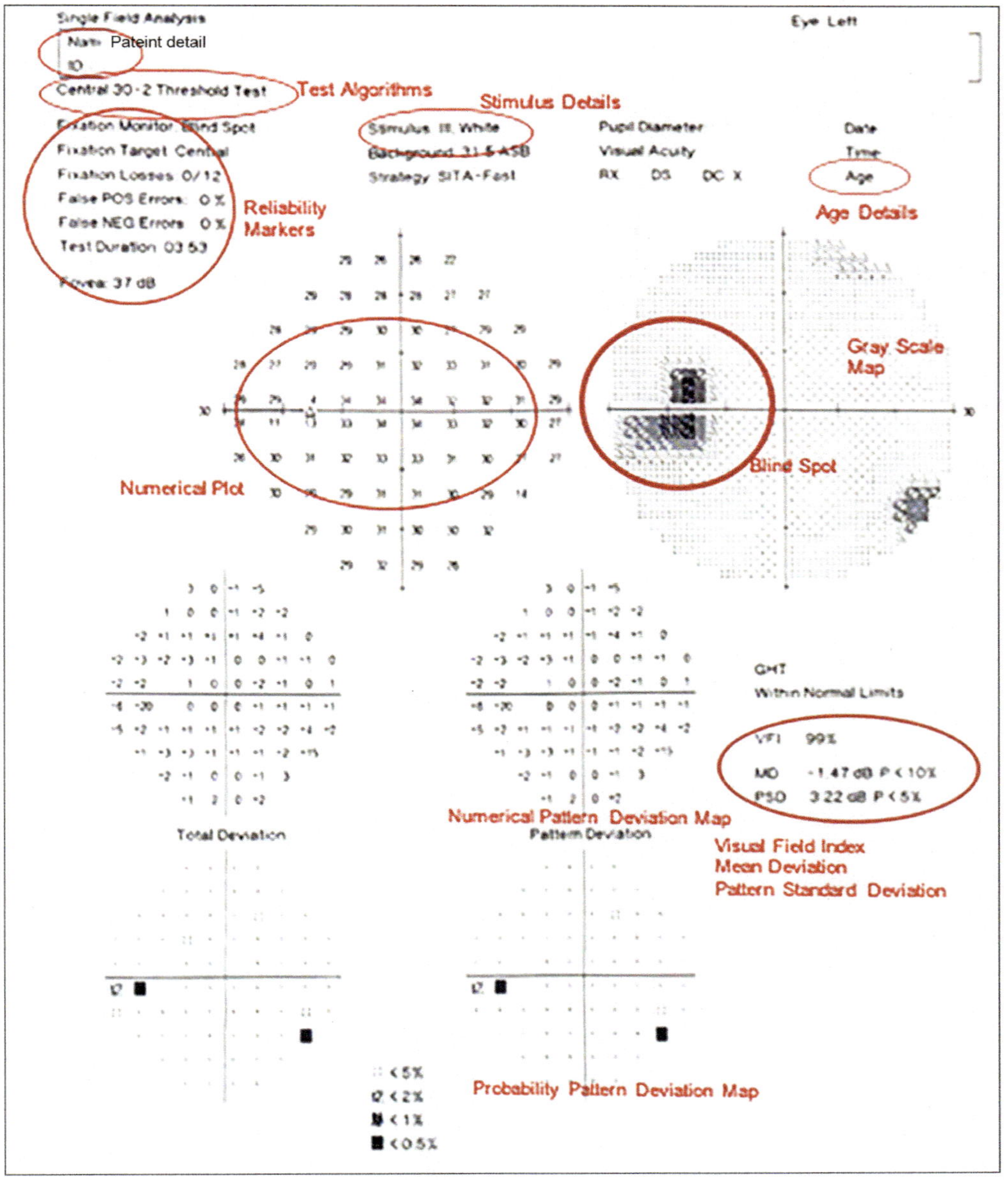

FIG. 3: A 30-2 visual field report carried on a Humphrey visual field analyzer and various important parameters to be noted while analyzing it.

Notes:
- Gray scale is threshold sensitivity value displayed as shades of gray.
- Total deviation represents the difference between a patient's threshold sensitivity and the normal sensitivity of an age-controlled match (from normative database).
- Pattern deviation (PD) represents localized loss at each tested point, after the removal of the effects of any generalized loss.
- Visual field index (VFI) is a metric representing the entire visual field as a single percentage of normal.
- Mean deviation (MD) is a statistical index determining the average difference in visual field sensitivity compared to the mean sensitivity of a normal healthy control.
- Pattern standard deviation (PSD) is an index measuring irregularity by summing the absolute value of the difference between the threshold value for each point and the average visual field sensitivity at each point.

due to its capability in detecting real-time motion. Lesions such as optic nerve drusen, dermoid cyst, cavernous hemangioma, or myocysticercosis of the ocular muscles may show characteristic findings on B-mode orbital US.

Computed tomography (CT) provides a better spatial detail and may enable a better differentiation between soft-tissue densities. CT may provide a better visualization of anterior orbital structures but for structures beyond the orbital apex, magnetic resonance imaging (MRI) of the brain is a more reliable imaging modality.[12] With an exception of hemorrhagic and bony lesions, MRI is a superior modality than CT.[12]

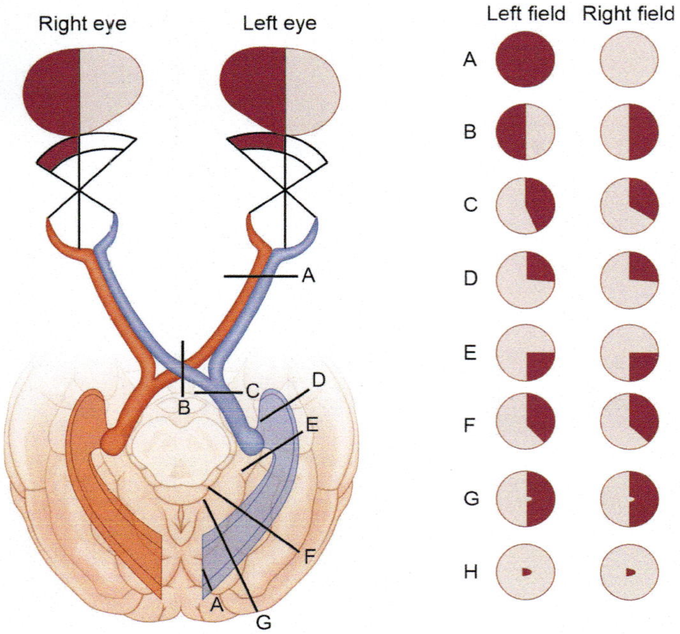

FIG. 4: Visual field defects with lesions in visual pathway. A: Left optic nerve lesion causing loss of vision from the left eye; B: Lesion at optic chiasma causing bitemporal hemianopia; C: Lesion in left optic tract causing right incongruous homonymous hemianopia; D: Lesion at left temporal lobe causing right superior homonymous quadrantanopic defect; E: Lesion at left parietal lobe causing right inferior homonymous quadrantanopic defect; F: Lesion in left optic radiations causing right congruous homonymous hemianopia; G: Lesion at left occipital lobe causing right homonymous macular sparing hemianopia; H: Lesion at the tip of left occipital lobe causing right homonymous scotoma.

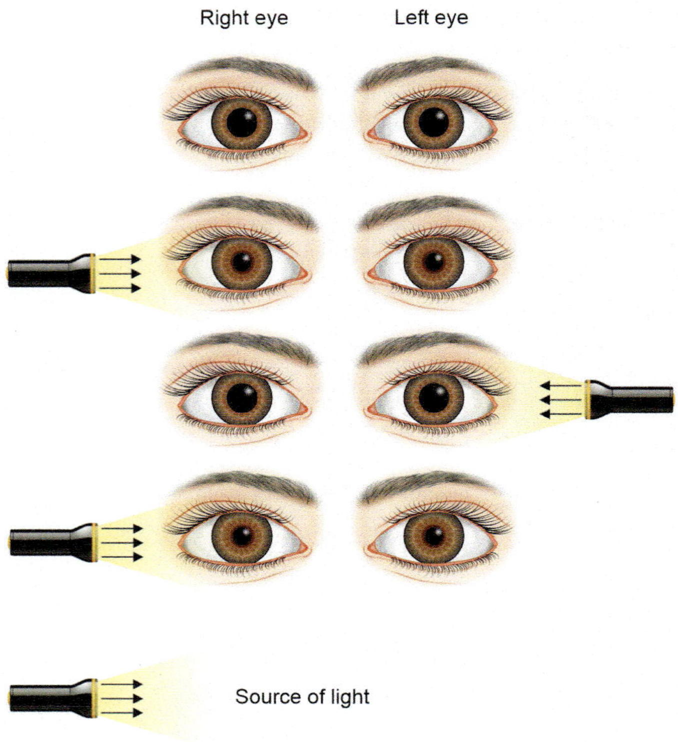

FIG. 5: Relative afferent pupillary defect. Illumination of the normal eye (right) causes constriction of pupils in both eyes due to direct and indirect pupillary reflexes. When the light source is moved toward the affected (left) eye, dilatation of left pupil is noted despite direct illumination due to defect in afferent pathway (optic nerve), along with dilatation of the pupil of the normal eye. Returning the light source toward the right eye again causes constriction in both pupils.

Magnetic resonance imaging: It is an excellent modality for assessing soft tissues such as the optic nerves, optic nerve sheath, chiasma, globes, and the entire visual pathway.

The orbital assessment can be optimized by the use of thin sections of the orbit (<3 mm), with T1 and T2 coronal and axial sections, fat suppression, and the use of short tau inversion recovery (STIR). Gadolinium (Gd)-enhanced images are particularly useful in inflammatory and mitotic lesions. The use of diffusion weighted imaging/apparent diffusion coefficient (DWI/ADC) in optic nerve imaging is limited with only a few studies showing its role in ischemic, demyelinating, or toxic optic neuritis. An additional screening of brain and spine may give other ancillary information and sites of affection in specific clinical scenarios.

The pattern of optic nerve involvement, length of the optic nerve, and the involvement of the chiasma point to specific etiologies. Isolated inflammation of the optic nerve sheath may be seen in optic perineuritis without significant involvement of optic nerve substance.

The signs of raised intracranial pressure such as tortuous optic nerves, scleral indentation, empty sella, and prominent optic nerve sheath can be seen on Gd MRI brain with dedicated optic nerve/orbital sequences. For most posterior visual pathway defects, routine MRI brain sequences, ADC/DWI/susceptibility weighted imaging (SWI) with/without contrast may aid in identifying the site and type of involvement along the visual pathways. Suspected

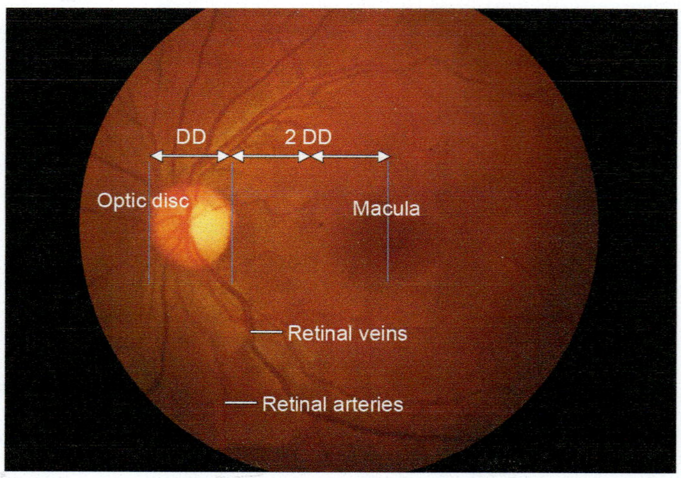

FIG. 6: Optic disc appearance in a healthy individual and in common pathologies.
(DD: disc diameter)

TABLE 2: Pathological fundus findings in various neuro-ophthalmic disorders.

Pathological fundus findings	Comments
Enlarged cup	Cup to disc ratio > 0.7 points toward glaucoma
Narrow AV ratio	Narrowing of AV ratio < 1:3 is seen in hypertension
Absent venous pulsations	Absence of SVPs is one of the early signs of raised intracranial pressure
Disc edema	• Optic neuritis, AION—arteritic and nonarteritic, acute phase of toxic/hereditary optic neuropathy • Disc edema without hemorrhage is seen in optic neuritis. In patients with ION, pale disc edema is seen with peripapillary hemorrhages
Papilledema	Disc edema due to raised intracranial pressure is called papilledema. Hyperemic disc with or without hemorrhages may be seen. Absent SVP and presence of Paton's lines (ophthalmoscopically visible radiating lines due to edema in the underlying retinal nerve fibers)
OA	• OA is recognized by reduction in the number of capillaries observed on optic disc (Kestenbaum index) • Atrophy in the absence of any previous disc swelling or inflammation is termed as primary OA. Disc is chalky white in this condition, and well-demarcated margins with a shallow cup are noted (hereditary/toxic ON) • When OA occurs as a sequel to prior disc edema or papilledema the disc appears dirty or grayish-white with poorly demarcated margins. This is termed as secondary OA and is seen with recurrent or prior optic neuritis, papilledema, etc.
Retinal vascular occlusion	Retinal arterial occlusions (CRAO/BRAO) lead on to attenuated vessels, retinal whitening, and a cherry-red spot in early stages. Retinal vein occlusion (CRVO/BRVO) may cause intraretinal hemorrhage, dilated and tortuous veins, cotton wool spots, macular edema, subretinal fluid, and features suggestive of neovascularization

(AION: anterior ischemic optic neuropathy; AV: arteriovenous; BRAO: branch retinal arterial occlusion; BRVO: branch retinal vein occlusion; CRAO: central retinal arterial occlusion; CRVO: central retinal vein occlusion; ION: ischemic optic neuropathy; OA: optic atrophy; ON: optic neuropathy; SVP: spontaneous venous pulsation)

malignant lesions can be identified by a combination of contrast enhancement, pattern of infiltration, and the use of additional sequences such as magnetic resonance perfusion (MRP), magnetic resonance spectroscopy (MRS), and DWI/ADC. Vascular lesions including infarcts and bleed constitute common posterior visual pathway defects. DWI/ADC are vital sequences for ischemic lesions, and SWI sequences can give important information in patients with central nervous system (CNS) hemorrhage or mineral deposition. Magnetic resonance angiogram/venogram (MRA/MRV) can be helpful in recognizing early atherosclerotic changes, stenosis, aneurysms, AV malformations, and thrombosis.

Electrophysiological Studies

Visual Evoked Potentials

Any damage along the visual pathway may lead to changes in the normal conduction in the form of delayed latencies and decrease in amplitudes.[13] The use of visual evoked potential (VEP) is predominantly for evaluation of demyelinating optic neuropathies; prolongation of latencies is noted. Severe axonal loss due to traumatic or ischemic lesions may lead to decrease in the amplitude of the waves formed. As such VEP can be affected by any lesion in the visual pathway either anterior or posterior. VEP can be prolonged even in subclinical cases without any obvious complains of vision loss in cases of demyelinating disorders, evolving toxic optic neuropathies, degenerative optic neuropathies, etc. Since it is an objective test for integrity of the visual pathway, it can also be used in cases of malingering visual loss.

Cerebrospinal Fluid Analysis

Analysis of cerebrospinal fluid (CSF) provides the assessment of the internal milieu of the brain and spinal cord. As per the revised diagnostic criteria for pseudotumor cerebri, opening CSF pressure of ≥250 mm of water in adults and ≥280 mm of water in nonsedated children is considered to be significantly elevated. Further assessment of inflammatory cells, proteins, sugar, microorganisms, CSF culture, microscopy, enzyme-linked immunosorbent assay (ELISA), and newer techniques such as polymerase chain reaction (PCR), multiplex PCR, and proteomics may increases the diagnostic repertoire for various neuro-ophthalmic conditions.

Specific Ophthalmological Investigations

In the practice of neuro-ophthalmology it is prudent for a neurologist to be aware of some basic investigations, which have traditionally been considered the domain of the ophthalmologists only.

Optical Coherence Tomography

Optical coherence tomography (OCT) is a noninvasive tool to visualize the layers of the retina. It can visualize the peripapillary RNFL (pRNFL) and macular GCL (mGCL) thickness (marker of axonal integrity of optic nerve).[14] It also helps in visualizing the topography of optic nerve head. **Table 3** shows OCT findings in various neuro-ophthalmic conditions.

TABLE 3: Showing findings on OCT in various neuro-ophthalmic disorders.

Pathology	OCT findings
Multiple sclerosis	• Thinning of pRNFL and mGCL/mGCIPL in long-standing/chronic disease • Thickening in pRNFL when optic nerve inflamed in acute stages
NMOSD	Marked thinning in pRNFL and mGCL/mGCIPL compared with MS
Optic disc drusen (pseudo-disc edema)	Seen as signal-poor structure with hyperreflective margin
Idiopathic intracranial hypertension	• May measure and quantify optic disc swelling • Reduction in pRNFL thickness with preserved mGCL/mGCIPL thickness indicates reduction in disc edema without significant axonal loss
Ischemic optic neuropathy	• Thinning of mGCIPL > pRNFL • Acute phase shows increase in thickness due to edema
Compressive optic neuropathy	Early thinning of pRNFL compared with direct examination of fundus. Can pick up subclinical optic nerve compression and the site of compression by relative thinning

(mGCIPL: macular ganglion cell inner plexiform layer; mGCL: macular ganglion cell layer; MS: multiple sclerosis; NMOSD: neuromyelitis optica spectrum disorders; OCT: optical coherence tomography; pRNFL: peripapillary retinal nerve fiber layer)

TABLE 4: FFA findings in various neuro-ophthalmic disorders.

Pathology	FFA findings
Papilledema	Detection of subclinical choroidal folds and identifies disc leakage (which differentiates from pseudopapilledema)
Ischemic optic neuropathy	Filling defects or disc leakage in NA-AION, and delayed choroidal perfusion in A-AION. Sectoral defects may be seen depending upon the extent of vascular hypoperfusion
Leber's hereditary optic neuropathy	Presence of peripapillary telangiectasias and absence of dye leakage in the presence of optic disc edema
Vasculitis	Can detect subclinical branch retinal vessel occlusions and dye leakage suggestive of endothelial damage
Optic neuritis	May demonstrate leakage of dye or perivenous sheathing

(A-AION: arteritic anterior ischemic optic neuropathy; FFA: fundus fluorescein angiography; NA-AION: nonarteritic anterior ischemic optic neuropathy)

Fundus Fluorescein Angiography

Fundus fluorescein angiography (FFA) allows for the direct examination of the retinal vasculature using a fundus camera and a luminescent intravenous dye. It is a dynamic imaging of the retinal blood flow highlighting the perfusion increase or decrease, delayed perfusion, dye leakage due to endothelial damage, and abnormal vasculature.[15] **Table 4** shows FFA findings in various neuro-ophthalmic disorders.

SPECIFIC NEURO-OPHTHALMIC CLINICAL SCENARIOS

In the following part we shall discuss about the specific approach to three common scenarios in neuro-ophthalmology

Patient with Transient Visual Loss

Transient visual loss (TVL) is often a result of transient ischemia. The most common concern in a patient with transient monocular visual loss (TMVL) lasting a few minutes is amaurosis fugax. It represents retinal/choroidal hypoperfusion or intermittent retinal embolization due to carotid occlusive disease.[16]

Another important cause of TMVL associated with headache is retinal migraine. A thorough search for systemic vascular risk factors is warranted under such clinical scenarios.[17]

Transient mono- or binocular visual obscurations (TVOs) occurring on changes in posture, bending, coughing, or straining and lasting for a few seconds may be suggestive of increased intracranial pressure at the optic nerve head.

Transient worsening of vision on exposure to high temperature or after a strenuous exercise may suggest underlying demyelinating optic neuropathy. This phenomenon seen in patients of optic neuritis is known as Uhthoff's phenomenon.[18]

Hypoperfusion in the posterior circulation/basilar artery or posterior cerebral artery territory may lead to transient ischemic episodes of occipital lobes, which are perceived as transient bilateral visual loss (TBVL). Cardioembolic causes and vertebrobasilar ischemia need to be ruled out in suggestive scenarios.[19]

Transient bilateral visual loss can also commonly occur as visual aura in patients of migraine with aura. Typical description involves presence of enlarging scotoma in homonymous visual field, which enlarges slowly over minutes and subsequently disappears. It is surrounded by luminous, jagged, irregular, shimmering edges and is characteristically followed by migraine headache, which is throbbing and hemicranial.[20]

Bilateral transient loss of vision may also arise from other cortical causes like focal occipital seizures in which case the blindness is abrupt in onset and usually lasts for less than a minute.[21]

Posterior reversible encephalopathy may also lead on to cerebral visual loss lasting for hours to days.[22] **Box 3** shows a representative case presenting with TMVL.

BOX 3 Representative case of transient monocular visual loss.

A 36-year-old obese female presented with history of headache and intermittent loss of vision from her right eye for 4 months' duration. The patient reported worsening of headache during early morning hours and was severe enough to wake her up from sleep. The loss of vision was intermittent and, to begin with, was perceived as black scotomas in front of her right eye, which would precipitate on bending or straining. On examination the patient's body mass index was noted to be 35.4 kg/m^2. General physical examination was normal. Best corrected visual acuity was 6/6 both eyes, and visual fields demonstrated enlarged blind spot with mild peripheral constriction. Fundus examination revealed disc edema with hemorrhages. OCT/pRNFL demonstrated an increase in retinal nerve layer thickness **(Figs. 7A to F)**.

Clinical findings suggested papilledema and Gd MRI brain was carried out in order to rule out secondary causes. MRI brain suggested features of increased intracranial pressure (scleral indentation, tortuous bilateral optic nerves, prominent peri optic nerve sheath), and MR venography was normal. Diagnosis of idiopathic intracranial hypertension was confirmed when lumbar puncture revealed an opening pressure of 350 mm H_2O with normal CSF composition. The patient was initiated on acetazolamide (per oral 2 g/day in divided doses) and topiramate (per oral 50 mg/day) after therapeutic CSF tap. The patient showed an immediate improvement and is doing well on 4 months' follow-up.

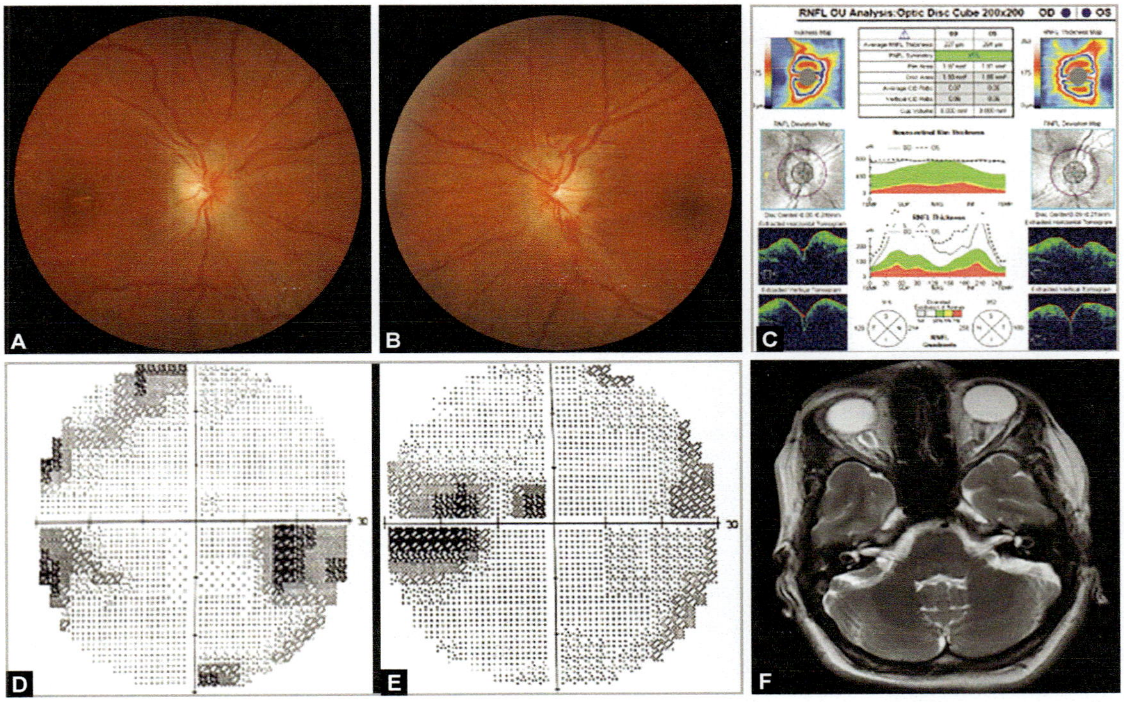

FIGS. 7A TO F: Bilateral papilledema on fundus examination. (A and B) Increased pRNFL on OCT; (C) Enlarged blind spot with peripheral constriction on visual field analysis and MRI brain showing (D and E) scleral indentation, tortuous optic nerves, and (F) prominent optic nerve sheath.

(CSF: cerebrospinal fluid; Gd: gadolinium; MR: magnetic resonance; MRI: magnetic resonance imaging; OCT: optical coherence tomography; pRNFL: peripapillary retinal nerve fiber layer)

Patient with Persistent Monocular Visual Loss

The localization of a persistent monocular visual loss should be prechiasmal visual pathway. A neurologist should be able to differentiate the local ophthalmic causes from the optic nerve pathologies. While it is easy to recognize the anterior chamber abnormalities, retinal pathologies can be intriguingly confusing. The typical features of an optic nerve pathology are (1) RAPD, (2) affection of central field of vision, and (3) swollen or pale optic nerve head. Variable visual field defects or fundus findings may occur depending upon the underlying pathology. **Table 5** gives a general guide to differentiate between various neuro-ophthalmic pathologies. **Box 4** shows a representative case presenting with persistent monocular visual loss.

Patient with Persistent Binocular Visual Loss

Binocular visual loss can be seen in bilateral optic nerve, chiasmal, postchiasmal optic tract, geniculate, postgeniculate optic radiation, or cortical pathologies. The presence of visual field deficits meeting a vertical meridian favor chiasma/retrochiasmal visual pathway defect. Compressive lesions abutting chiasma (such as pituitary adenomas, craniopharyngiomas, meningiomas, or aneurysms) may lead on to bitemporal visual deficits while retrochiasmal lesions produce homonymous hemianopic defects.[23] The more posterior the cerebral lesion, the more symmetric hemianopic field defects are noted. Occipital lobe lesions (usually vascular) lead on to exquisitely congruous homonymous hemianopic defects. It

TABLE 5: Distinctive features of various neuro-ophthalmic disorders leading to mono/binocular visual loss.

Pathology	Clinical profile	Pain	RAPD	Color vision	Visual acuity	Visual field	Fundus	Visual prognosis
Optic neuritis[25]	• Young adults • Females > males	Retrobulbar/pain on eye movement in up to 90% patients	+	Early and prominent color desaturation	Acute-to-subacute visual loss usually worsening to nadir by 1 week	Central field loss	• Disc edema (without hemorrhages) in around 35% • Normal in 65%	Good
AION[26]	• Older (>50 years) • Vascular risk factors present in NA-AION	Infrequent (except in A-AION secondary to GCA	+	May be variably spared	Acute rapid deterioration of vision	Altitudinal visual field loss meeting horizontal meridian	• Disc edema (may be sectoral) with hemorrhages • Small cup–disc ratio	15% risk of involvement of fellow eye within 5 years
Maculopathy[2]	Variable	Rarely painful	–	May cause mild color vision impairment but to a lesser extent as compared to optic nerve pathologies	Visual distortions (metamorphopsias) are common, slow improvement of vision after exposure to bright light, glaring, and photophobia are common	Central scotoma	Macular abnormalities noted	Usually poor but variable depending upon etiology
CSR[27]	• Males (20–50 years) • Variable	Painless	–	Color vision deficits present	Acute-to-subacute visual disturbances. Metamorphopsias common with diminution of central vision	Central visual deficits	Serous fluid accumulation in subretinal space underneath the macula causing relative detachment of retinal layers	• Acute CSR is usually self-limiting. Around 15% may develop chronic complains • High recurrence rate
IIH[28]	Obese young females (20–50 years)	Headache due to increased intracranial pressure; history of migraine common	Rare	Color vision is usually not affected	Vision is affected in patients presenting in advanced stages or in patients with fulminant IIH	Enlarged blind spot and peripheral visual field losses are common	Hyperemic disc edema with/without hemorrhages. Paton's lines may be seen	Usually good with treatment
Toxic/Metabolic/Hereditary optic neuropathy[29]	Variable	Painless	May be present in a patient with asymmetric involvement	Color vision is affected	Significant loss of vision	Central/Cecocentral scotoma	Depends upon the stage of illness. Primary optic atrophy noted in most patients with chronic hereditary optic neuropathy	Poor
Compressive/Infiltrative optic neuropathy[30]	• *Gliomas*: Childhood • *Meningiomas*: 30–40 years • *Lymphomas*: Variable, usually older age	Absent	+	Abnormal	Progressive	• Variable • Infiltration may portend a nodular, irregular, hemorrhagic appearance to the optic disc with yellowish-white infiltrate	Variable	Variable

(A-AION: arteritic anterior ischemic optic neuropathy; AION: anterior ischemic optic neuropathy; CSR: central serous retinopathy; GCA: giant cell arteritis; IIH: idiopathic intracranial hypertension; NA-AION: nonarteritic anterior ischemic optic neuropathy; RAPD: relative afferent pupillary defect)

BOX 4 **Representative case presenting with persistent monocular visual loss.**

A 17-year-old girl presented with sudden-onset loss of vision in her left eye. It was associated with left eye periorbital pain, which increased on eye movements. The patient had a rapid deterioration of vision from her left eye, and on the fourth day the best corrected visual acuity from her left eye was noted to be 6/36. Left eye RAPD could be demonstrated, and left eye color vision was impaired. Visual field was suggestive of central visual loss. The patient's fundus examination was suggestive of left-sided mild disc edema without hemorrhages. Right eye fundus examination was suggestive of mild pallor. Neurological examination was essentially normal except the presence of brisk deep tendon reflexes. Gd MRI brain with fat-suppressed orbital cuts demonstrated inflamed left optic nerve with pericallosal white matter demyelinating plaques. Latency on VEP was prolonged in both eyes (right eye—130 ms/left eye—142 ms). Workup for secondary demyelination including antinuclear antibodies, anti-aquaporin 4, and myelin oligo glycoprotein antibodies, etc., was normal. CSF was normocellular, with mildly raised proteins (52 mg/dL) and normal sugar (46 mg/dL). Oligoclonal bands could be seen in CSF (absent in paired serum sample). The patient was diagnosed as a case of left optic neuritis associated with multiple sclerosis. High-dose intravenous methyl prednisone was started, and the patient improved completely over a duration of next 2 weeks. She was also initiated on oral dimethyl fumarate (240 mg/day in two divided doses) for prevention of future relapses **(Figs. 8A to D)**.

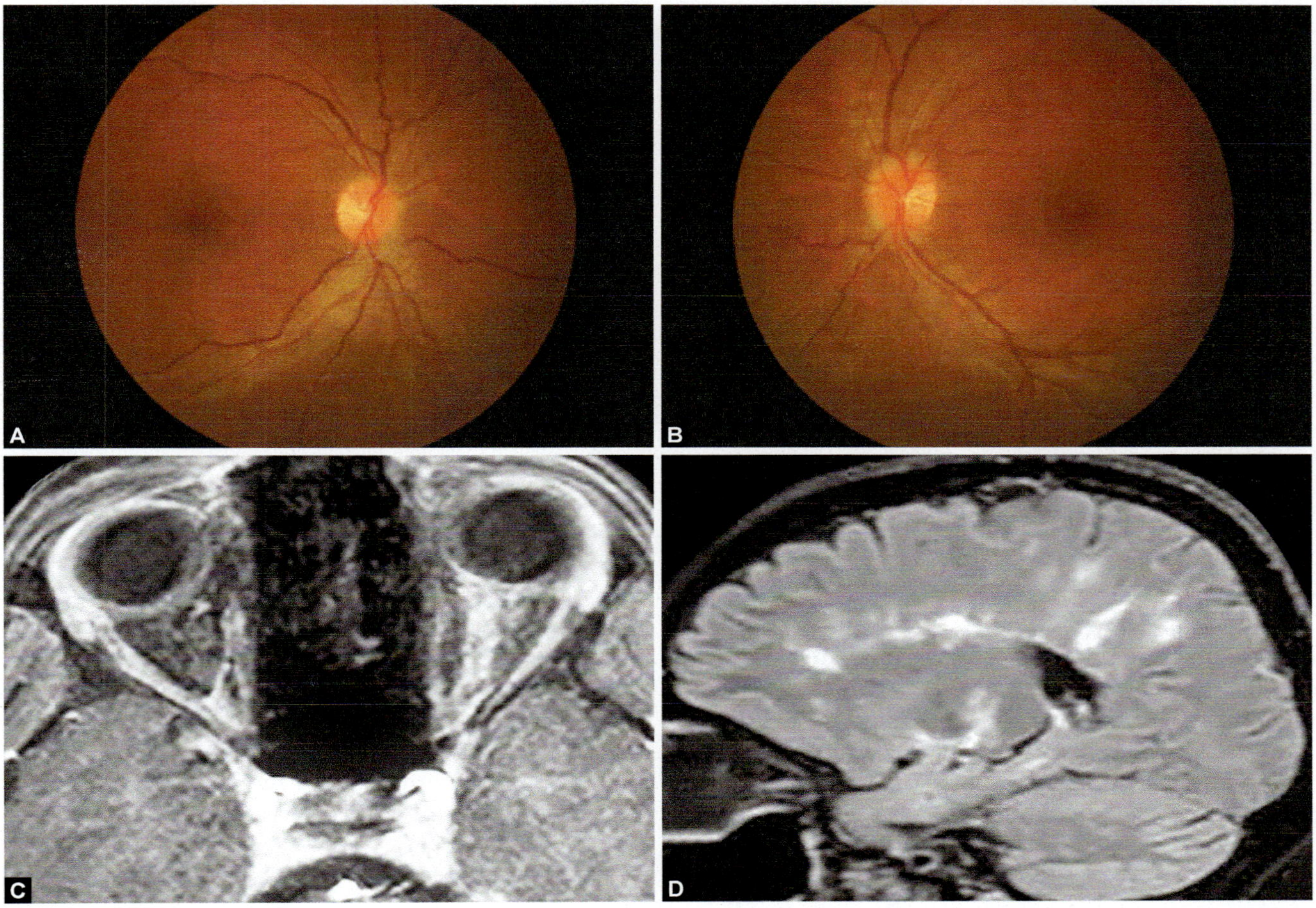

FIGS. 8A TO D: (A) Mild pallor on fundus examination in the right eye and (B) pale disc edema in the left eye; (C) Left optic nerve enhancement; and (D) pericallosal white matter hyperintensities on Gd MRI brain and optic nerves.

(CSF: cerebrospinal fluid; Gd: gadolinium; MRI: magnetic resonance imaging; RAPD: relative afferent pupillary defect; VEP: visual evoked potential)

is important to remember that macular sparing may occur in lesions sparing the posterior-most occipital lobe where macula is represented.[24] The presence of asymmetricity supports a prechiasmal optic nerve pathology. Bilateral symmetrical acute optic neuritis may be difficult to diagnose, but the presence of optic disc edema or pallor may be supportive. Toxic optic, metabolic/nutritional, or hereditary optic neuropathies may present with slowly progressive bilateral visual loss. Increased intracranial pressure may give rise to papilledema and slowly progressive visual field constriction. It is prudent to consider increased intraocular pressure (primary open angle glaucoma) as a differential while diagnosing patients with bilateral optic neuropathies. **Table 5** highlights distinct features of various causes of monocular or binocular visual loss. **Box 5** shows a representative case of binocular visual loss.

BOX 5 Representative case of binocular visual loss.

A 23-year-old female presented with diminution of vision from both eyes for 15 days' duration. The patient was diagnosed with pulmonary tuberculosis 5 months prior to this episode and was taking first-line antitubercular therapy (isoniazid, rifampicin, ethambutol, and pyrazinamide) since then. The patient was on 22 mg/kg body weight dose of ethambutol.

On examination the patient's visual acuity was noted to be counting fingers at 2 m in both eyes. Visual field was suggestive of centrocecal scotomas in both eyes. Fundus examination was suggestive of pale discs on both sides. Gd MRI of optic nerves and brain was suggestive of mild enhancement of both optic nerves with normal brain parenchyma. Blood and CSF workup was within normal range. The patient was diagnosed to be having ethambutol-induced optic neuropathy. Ethambutol was stopped, and the patient was treated with high dose of B-complex vitamins along with vitamin-E (400 mg/day per oral) and pyridoxine (40 mg/day per oral). On 4 months' follow-up the best corrected visual acuity was 6/60 in the right eye and finger counting at 5 m in the left eye **(Figs. 9A to E)**.

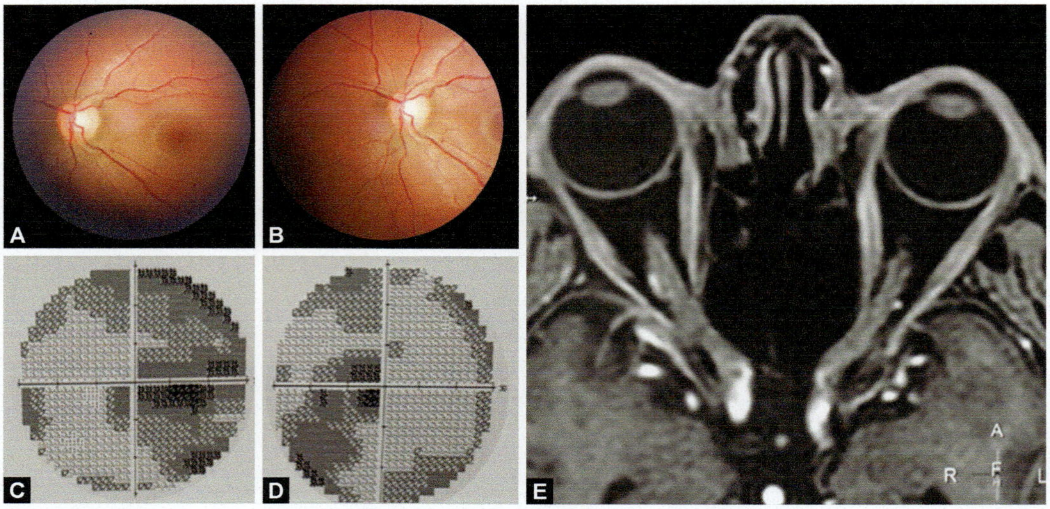

FIGS. 9A TO E: (A and B) Bilateral optic disc pallor; (C and D) Centrocecal scotomas on visual field analysis; (E) Bilateral optic nerve enhancement on Gd MRI of optic nerves.

(CSF: cerebrospinal fluid; Gd: gadolinium; MRI: magnetic resonance imaging)

CONCLUSION

The neuro-ophthalmic causes of vision loss are varied and pose a challenge even to the experienced clinicians because of the myriad of symptoms, signs, pathways, and etiologies involved. Localization of visual loss within the eye or visual pathway is of utmost importance, underscoring the expertise in knowledge of basic anatomical structures which may be involved in such a patient. Once the lesion has been localized to the optic nerve or visual pathways, it is further important to investigate whether the disease is localized or is a part of a discrete neurological or systemic disease. Despite the advances in imaging and investigational techniques, the field of neuro-ophthalmology demands rigorous clinical skills and acumen.

REFERENCES

1. Verma R, Gupta M, Chaudhari TS. Neurogenic vision loss: causes and outcome. An experience from a tertiary center in Northern India. J Neurosci Rural Pract. 2014;5(4):340-8.
2. Newman N, Biousse V. Diagnostic approach to vision loss. Contin Minneap Minn. 2014;20(4 Neuro-ophthalmology):785-815.
3. Salazar JJ, Ramírez AI, de Hoz R, Salobrar-Garcia E, Rojas P, López-Cuenca I, et al. (2019). Anatomy of the human optic nerve: structure and function. [online]. Available from https://eprints.ucm.es/id/eprint/51015/1/Salazar_2019%20IntechOpen%20-%20Anatomy%20of%20the%20human%20optic%20nerve%20-%20Structure%20and%20Funcion.pdf. [Last accessed January, 2023].
4. Peltier J, Travers N, Destrieux C, Velut S. Optic radiations: a microsurgical anatomical study. J Neurosurg. 2006;105(2):294-300.
5. Yogarajah M, Focke NK, Bonelli S, Cercignani M, Acheson J, Parker GJM, et al. Defining Meyer's loop–temporal lobe resections, visual field deficits, and diffusion tensor tractography. Brain. 2009;132(6):1656-68.
6. Madill SA, Riordan-Eva P. Disorders of the anterior visual pathways. J Neurol Neurosurg Psychiatry. 2004;75(suppl 4):iv12-9.
7. Shamir RR, Friedman Y, Joskowicz L, Mimouni M, Blumenthal EZ. Comparison of Snellen and Early Treatment Diabetic Retinopathy Study charts using a computer simulation. Int J Ophthalmol. 2016;9(1):119-23.

8. Sue S. Test distance vision using a Snellen chart. Community Eye Health. 2007;20(63):52.
9. Arden GB, Gucukoglu AG. Grating test of contrast sensitivity in patients with retrobulbar neuritis. Arch Ophthalmol. 1978;96(9):1626-9.
10. Racette L, Fischer M, Bebie H, Holló G, Johnson CA, Matsumoto C. (2018). Chapter 8: Clinical interpretation of a visual field. [online]. Available from https://www.haag-streit.com/fileadmin/Haag-Streit_Diagnostics/perimetry/Visual_Field_Digest/Chapter_8/Visual-Field-Digest_chapter-8.pdf. [Last accessed January, 2023].
11. Rajan RP, Deb AK, Lomte S, Privitera CM, Kannan NB, Ramasamy K, et al. Quantification of relative afferent pupillary defect by an automated pupillometer and its relationship with visual acuity and dimensions of macular lesions in age-related macular degeneration. Indian J Ophthalmol. 2021;69(10):2746-50.
12. Shree R, Bhatkar S, Mahesh KV, Sachdeva J, Goel A, Goyal MK, et al. (2020). Magnetic resonance imaging (MRI) versus computed tomographic scan (CT scan) of brain in evaluation of suspected cavernous sinus syndrome. [online]. Available from https://journals.sagepub.com/doi/abs/10.1177/1971400920970921. [Last accessed January, 2023].
13. Weinstein GW, Odom JV, Cavender S. Visually evoked potentials and electroretinography in neurologic evaluation. Neurol Clin. 1991;9(1):225-42.
14. Bhende M, Shetty S, Parthasarathy MK, Ramya S. Optical coherence tomography: a guide to interpretation of common macular diseases. Indian J Ophthalmol. 2018;66(1):20-35.
15. Littlewood R, Mollan SP, Pepper IM, Hickman SJ. The utility of fundus fluorescein angiography in neuro-ophthalmology. Neuroophthalmology. 2019;43(4):217-34.
16. Pitkänen H, Saarela V. Vasospastic transient monocular visual loss: effect of treatment with different doses of nifedipine. J Neuroophthalmol. 2014;34(4):386-8.
17. Jogi V, Mehta S, Gupta A, Singh P, Lal V. More clinical observations on migraine associated with monocular visual symptoms in an Indian population. Ann Indian Acad Neurol. 2016;19(1):63-8.
18. Pearce JMS. Early observations on optic neuritis and Uhthoff's sign. Eur Neurol. 2010;63(4):243-7.
19. Hoyt WF. Transient bilateral blurring of vision: considerations of an episodic ischemic symptom of vertebral-basilar insufficiency. Arch Ophthalmol. 1963;70(6):746-51.
20. Gobel H. The International Classification of Headache Disorders, 3rd edition. [online]. Available from https://ichd-3.org/. [Last accessed January 2023].
21. Hadjikoutis S, Sawhney IM. Occipital seizures presenting with bilateral visual loss. Neurol India. 2003;51(1):115-6.
22. Bansal S, Bansal R, Goyal MK, Takkar A, Singh R, Singh P, et al. Clinical, etiological, and imaging profile of posterior reversible encephalopathy syndrome: a prospective and follow-up study. Ann Indian Acad Neurol. 2020;23(2):182-8.
23. Rowe FJ, Cheyne CP, García-Fiñana M, Noonan CP, Howard C, Smith J, et al. Detection of visual field loss in pituitary disease: peripheral kinetic versus central static. Neuroophthalmology. 2015;39(3):116.
24. Goodwin D. Homonymous hemianopia: challenges and solutions. Clin Ophthalmol Auckl NZ. 2014;8:1919-27.
25. The clinical profile of optic neuritis: experience of the Optic Neuritis Treatment trial. Arch Ophthalmol. 1991;109(12):1673-8.
26. Hayreh SS. Ischemic optic neuropathy. Indian J Ophthalmol. 2000;48(3):171.
27. Semeraro F, Morescalchi F, Russo A, Gambicorti E, Pilotto A, Parmeggiani F, et al. Central serous chorioretinopathy: pathogenesis and management. Clin Ophthalmol Auckl NZ. 2019;13:2341-52.
28. Takkar A, Lal V. Idiopathic intracranial hypertension: the monster within. Ann Indian Acad Neurol. 2020;23(2):159-66.
29. Sadun AA. Metabolic optic neuropathies. Semin Ophthalmol. 2002;17(1):29-32.
30. Takkar A, Naheed D, Dogra M, Goyal MK, Singh R, Gupta N, et al. Infiltrative optic neuropathies: opening doors to sinister pathologies. Neuroophthalmology. 2017;41(5):279-83.

33

CHAPTER

Approach to Pupillary Disorders

Karthik Vinay Mahesh

INTRODUCTION

Pupils are literally the "windows" to the eyes. The primary function of pupils is to control the amount of light entering the eye, depending upon the illumination. The structure and function are like the aperture in a camera; the aperture size is controlled by adjusting the diaphragm, i.e., the iris. The basic examination of pupils can yield a significant amount of information about the intactness of the afferent and efferent systems of the visual pathways as well as the essential pathways of the autonomic nervous system. In this chapter, we will learn the basic steps in the examination of pupils, normal pupillary reflexes, and approach to a case of anisocoria.

NORMAL PUPIL

The size of the pupil is controlled by the two opposing sympathetic and parasympathetic pathways, which control the radially arranged dilator pupillae (a1 adrenoceptor) and circumferentially arranged sphincter pupillae (m3 cholinoceptors) **(Fig. 1)**.

Sympathetic Pathways[1,2]

The sympathetic pathways originate from the hypothalamus and descend through the spinal cord to the C8–T2 intermediate gray column of Budge and Waller (first-order neurons); from here they synapse with the thoracic

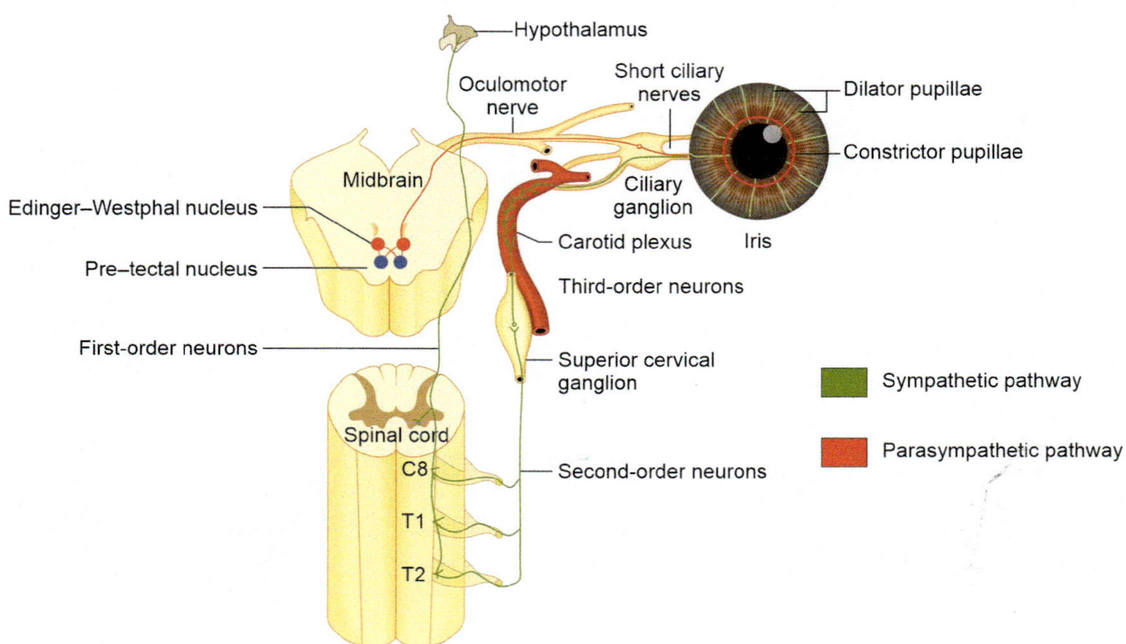

FIG. 1: Figure showing the autonomic pathways of the eye.

sympathetic outlet of stellate ganglion till they synapse in the superior cervical ganglion (second-order neurons). The postsynaptic fibers travel along the internal carotid artery (ICA), forming a plexus around it; they further enter the middle cranial fossa, entering the cavernous sinus through the ophthalmic branch of the trigeminal nerve, further dividing into the nasociliary nerve giving off the long ciliary nerve some branches from the ICA plexus branch into the ciliary ganglion without synapsing and further supplying the iris through short ciliary nerves. They innervate the dilator pupillae from the long ciliary nerve **(Fig. 1)**.

Parasympathetic Pathway[1,2]

The parasympathetic pathway starts in the Edinger–Westphal nucleus (EWN), through the midbrain exits through the oculomotor nerve (III nerve), which then courses through the subarachnoid space where it lies in proximity with the posterior communicating artery (PCOM), basilar artery, and meninges, entering the cavernous sinus and then the orbit. The inferior division of the III nerve branches into the ciliary ganglion where it synapses. The postganglionic fibers innervate the sphincter pupillae and ciliary body (lens accommodation) through short ciliary nerves in the ratio of 1:30.

FUNCTION OF THE PUPIL

The pupil controls the amount of light falling on the retina by the actions of the sphincter and dilator, which reduce and increase the pupillary diameter, respectively. It ensures an appropriate amount of light concerning illumination and the distance of the object in focus from the eye. This is ensured by a series of autonomic reflexes described below.

Light Reflex

The purpose of the reflex is to restrict the amount of light when exposed to increasing luminosity. The reflex starts in the macula (retina) when the light is shone, the retinal ganglion cells transmit these signals along the optic nerve, then chiasma with nasal fibers decussating and going along the optic tracts supplies equally the ipsilateral and contralateral pretectal nuclei at the level of the midbrain **(Fig. 2)**. The pretectal nuclei relay to the ipsilateral and contralateral EWN, the parasympathetic component of the III nerve, which stimulates pupillary constriction.[3] Since the innervation is equal across both EWN, both the pupils constrict equally when light is shone on either eye. The ipsilateral constriction to light is the direct reflex, and the contralateral consensual constriction is the indirect/consensual light reflex.

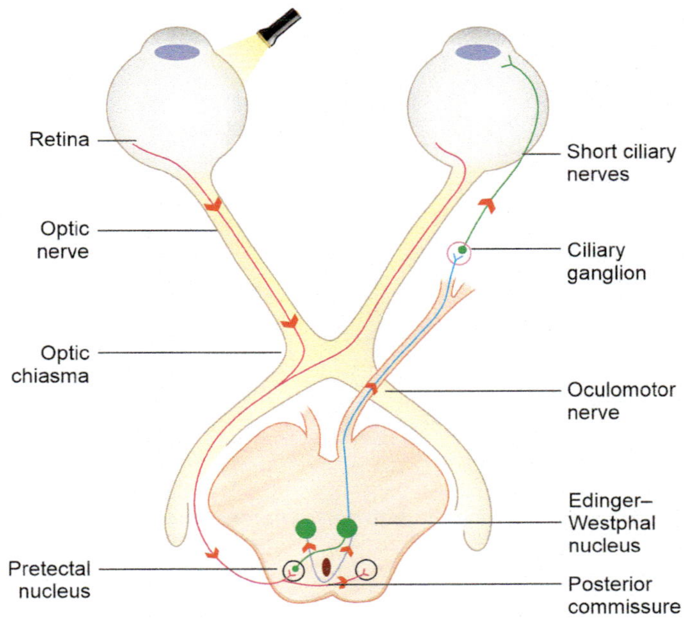

FIG. 2: Figure showing the light reflex pathway.

Pupillary Near Reflex (Accommodation Reflex)

The near reflex is an essential part of stereoscopic vision (depth and solidity of objects). Reflex consists of three components, i.e., convergence, accommodation, and pupillary constriction. When the subject focuses on an object at a distance and then focuses on something nearby, there is convergence of the eyes associated with the relaxation of the ciliary muscles, resulting in increasing lens convexity and finally pupillary constriction. The center for near reflex is in the occipital association areas, likely Brodmann's cortical areas 18 and 19, which mediate the reflex. These areas communicate with the EWN via occipito-mesencephalic pathways, resulting in pupillary constriction and ciliary muscle relaxation increasing lens convexity and through the third motor nucleus cause convergence **(Fig. 3)**. In lesions involving the pretectal nucleus, there is a loss of light reflex, but the near reflex persists (see light-near dissociation) as the ventrally placed accommodation reflex pathways are spared.

Ciliospinal Reflex

The reflex consists of ipsilateral dilation of the pupil to painful stimuli on the ipsilateral side of the neck. Painful stimulation along the side of the neck stimulates the ciliospinal sympathetic center at C8–T2, which through sympathetic connections with the sympathetic fibers of the pupil causes

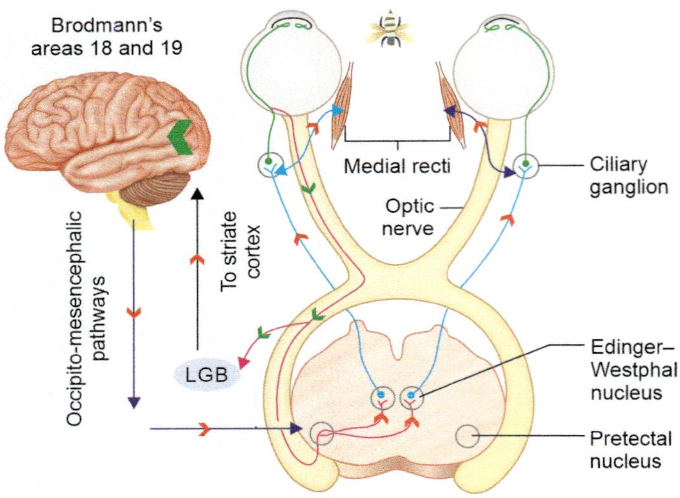

FIG. 3: Figure showing the pathways in the near reflex.
(LGB: lateral geniculate bodies)

reflex dilation of the ipsilateral pupil. It is an important sign to assess the brainstem integrity in a comatose patient.

CLINICAL EVALUATION

The pupils are ideally examined in a dimly lit room as they are in a semidilated state, and the patient looks at a distance to avoid the near pupillary reflex. They should be examined under the following categories:

- *Size*: The normal pupil size is between 2 and 6 mm, and 3–5 mm in ambient light. Children tend to have pupils, and pupil size becomes smaller and irregular with older age. Pupillary diameter >6 mm constitutes mydriasis and <2 mm is called miosis. The diameter is measured with the help of a pupillometer; automated pupilometers can be accurate up to 0.1 mm.
- *Shape*: The shape of the pupil is usually round; asymmetric pupils can be seen as a complication of iridocyclitis, iritis, synechiae formation, and iris trauma. Irregular constriction of the pupil due to segmental iris palsy is seen in postganglionic parasympathetic (ciliary ganglion and short ciliary nerve) damage. A transient segmental spasm of the iris can produce a tadpole-like pupil, which prelude Horner's, Adie's tonic pupil (ATP) or is associated with severe migraine.
- *Equality*: Due to the equal innervation tone of both sympathetic and parasympathetic pathways on both pupils, they are usually equal in size and react symmetrically. Normally, there can be mild asymmetry (anisocoria) up to 1 mm, which can be seen in 15–20% of the normal population. Anything greater than a 2-mm difference is considered significant.
- *Position*: Normal position of the pupil is in the center; any deviation results in corectopia. The causes vary from local eye disorders to neurological syndrome affecting segmental iris innervation like lesions affecting the EWN in the midbrain.
- *Reaction to light*: While examining the light reflex, the patient is asked to focus on a distant object to avoid near reflex, and light is shone from below. The examiner looks at the pupillary constriction on the same side (direct reflex). Again, the light is shone in the same eye but this time the examiner looks at the opposite pupillary constriction (consensual/indirect light reflex). Based on the degree and briskness of pupillary constriction, pupillary light reflex is graded as below:
  - *Pupillary reflex grading*:[4]
    - *4+*: Brisk, large response (normal response)
    - *3+*: Moderate response
    - *2+*: Small and slowed response
    - *1+*: Minimal or just visible response
    - *0*: Unresponsive pupils

The light reflex is the essential reflex that tests the integrity of three different systems: (1) efferent (retina, optic nerve, chiasma), (2) midbrain (EWN, oculomotor nerve nucleus), and (3) afferent systems (III nerve, ciliary ganglion, short ciliary nerves).

Marcus Gunn Pupil

Lesions of the afferent visual pathway produce a relative afferent pupillary defect (RAPD). In disorders affecting the afferent visual pathway, when light is shone on the affected eye after rapidly swinging from the normal eye, there is dilation of the pupil on the affected side instead of constriction.

- *Method*: The swinging flashlight test by Levatin[5] is an improved version of the original Marcus Gunn alternate eye covering-uncovering test for RAPD. The patient is examined in a dim room when he is looking at a distance. The examiner shines a light on one eye at least 5–10 cm away from below for at least 3 seconds and quickly shifts to the opposite eye. This step is repeated a few times (minimum six), shining light for at least 3 seconds on each pupil. The examiner then looks for the pupillary dilation. The Marcus Gunn pupil dilates to consensual light reflex on the normal eye but fails to constrict when directly stimulated by swinging light across **(Fig. 4)**. The degree and briskness of dilation are graded according to Bell's grading **(Table 1)**.[6]

  Relative afferent pupillary defect is a sign of afferent visual pathway defect, i.e., retina (retinal ganglion cells), optic nerve, chiasma, and rarely optic tract, and pretectal lesions can produce RAPD contralateral to the site of the lesion (pretectal lesion can have RAPD with a normal vision.)
- *Near reflex*: As mentioned earlier, this reflex tests three components, i.e., convergence, accommodation, and pupillary constriction. The examiner asks the patient to focus on a distant object and then on a small object in

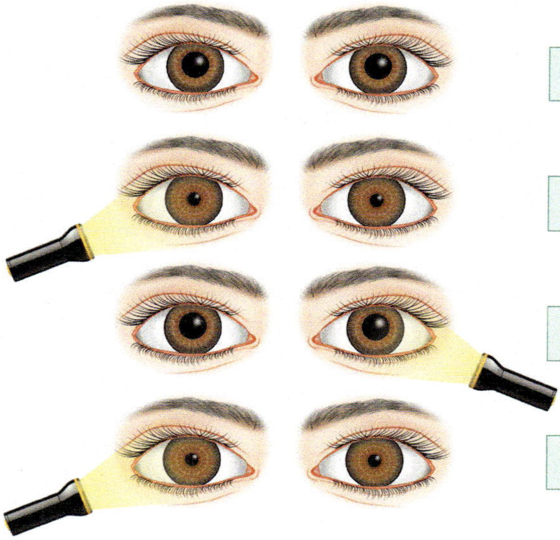

FIG. 4: Figure showing the method of demonstrating RAPD.
(RAPD: relative afferent pupillary defect)

TABLE 1: Grading of relative afferent pupillary defect (RAPD).

Grades	Pupillary response
I	Mild early constriction followed by a greater dilation
II	Pupillary stall followed by a greater dilatation
III	Immediate dilatation
IV	Immediate pupillary dilatation (followed by secondary constriction) following prolonged illumination of a good eye for 6 seconds*
V	Immediate pupillary dilatation with no secondary constriction following prolonged illumination of a good eye for 6 seconds

*Bleaching of the normal eye photoreceptors reduces the afferent stimulation from the normal eye.

front of the eyes (finger/pen). The examiner observes the constriction of pupils and convergence of the eyes. The pupillary constriction is as brisk as the direct light reflex and graded similarly.

- Loss of constriction can be seen in lesions of the parasympathetic pathway.
- Loss of convergence can be due to involvement of the medial rectus/III nerve/cortical lesions affecting the convergence center.
- Convergence insufficiency, partial or complete loss of convergence with mydriasis on attempted near fixation is seen commonly in school-going children, office workers, and those who require prolonged near vision.
- Loss of lens accommodation is seen in presbyopia due to aging.

Hence, a normal pupil examination should ideally be recorded[7] as follows **(Table 2)**.

TABLE 2: Recording of a normal pupil examination.

	Right	Left
Size	4 mm	4 mm
Shape	Round	Round
Light reflex	+3	+3
Near reflex	+3	+3

APPROACH TO PUPILLARY ABNORMALITIES

There are three neurological substrates affecting the pupil size and responses:

1. Autonomic nervous system (sympathetic and parasympathetic)
2. Afferent visual pathway (retina/optic nerve/chiasma)
3. Midbrain tract and nuclei-mediating pupillary reflexes (EW and pretectal nuclei)

Step 1:
History:

- History of onset and progression:
    - *Acute onset*: Trauma, dissection, vascular, toxins/drugs, demyelination
    - *Subacute onset*: Slow-growing tumors/compressive lesions/infections
    - *Chronic*: Congenital/physiological, chronic infections, neurodegenerative
- *Associated symptoms*:
    - *Diplopia/ptosis*: III nerve palsy
    - *Anhidrosis/reverse ptosis*: Horner's syndrome/sympathetic involvement
    - *Myelopathy/upper limb wasting*: Horner's syndrome
    - *Areflexia*: ATP

- *Coma/fever/quadriparesis*: Pontine lesions
- *Hallucinations/confusion/fasciculations*: Toxins/drugs

Step 2:
Identify which is the abnormal pupil in a patient with anisocoria.

- *Smaller* pupil is abnormal when anisocoria *increases in darkness*.
- *Larger* pupil is abnormal when anisocoria *increases in bright light*.
- *If the anisocoria persists equally in both darkness and light without any other neurological abnormalities in the pupillary autonomic and visual pathways, it is likely physiological anisocoria*.

Dilated Pupil

"Pupils dilate as a sympathetic response to fear or anxiety; however, for a neurologist a dilated pupil can just be as anxiety- and fear-provoking in itself." A dilated pupil can be caused by anything as ominous as a transtentorial herniation, an enlarging PCOM aneurysm, or something as benign as an ATP.

A dilated pupil can be seen in lesions affecting these two substrates:

1. *Parasympathetic pathway*:
   - *Preganglionic pathway (III nerve)*: The presence of associated diplopia and ptosis can help in localizing the cause of dilated pupil to III nerve. Sometimes, pupillary dilation may be the only sign of a III nerve palsy, especially for compressive lesions.

     The III nerve carries the pupillary fibers on its periphery. Hence, it is susceptible to extrinsic compression in the subarachnoid space by tumors, aneurysms **(Case 1)**, or an early sign of uncal herniation. The III nerve is also susceptible to vascular insults in diabetes[8,9] and ophthalmoplegic migraine.
   - *Postganglionic pathway*: Damage to ciliary ganglion or short ciliary nerves leads to a *tonic pupil/ATP*. The loss of parasympathetic fibers leads to a mydriatic pupil with attenuation or complete loss of both direct and consensual light reflexes but has a delayed constriction on accommodation. The constriction on accommodation is due to the reinnervation of the few pupillary fibers by most of the remaining ciliary fibers (1:30, pupillary fibers:ciliary fibers).[1] The denervated nerve endings are overly sensitive due to upregulation of the receptors and respond briskly to dilute (0.05–0.125%) pilocarpine[10] (parasympathomimetic), which is diagnostic.

     To best elicit a tonic pupil, the examiner observes pupillary dilation when the patient changes focus to a distant object from near. The tonic pupil redilates slowly whereas the normal pupil dilates briskly **(Fig. 5)**.[7]

     In the chronic phase of the Adie's pupil (little old Adie's), the pupil becomes progressively miotic and may resemble an Argyll Robertson pupil (ARP);[11] however, the *tonicity* of the pupil remains, i.e., the pupils dilate much more slowly than the brisker dilation in an ARP.

     Commonly, ATP is unilateral, commonly seen in young females and idiopathic, and later becomes bilateral. Bilateral ATP at onset is seen in diseases involving the autonomic nervous system **(Table 3)**.[2]
2. *Local iris*:
   - *Damaged iris*: Any local damage to the iris by trauma, inflammation, or ischemia produces a mydriatic pupil, which will have irregular borders and does not constrict with 1% pilocarpine.
   - *Drugs*: A topical mydriatic drug also produces mydriasis, which does not constrict with 1% pilocarpine; however, the pupil margins will be regular in these.

Flowchart 1 shows an approach to a dilated pupil.

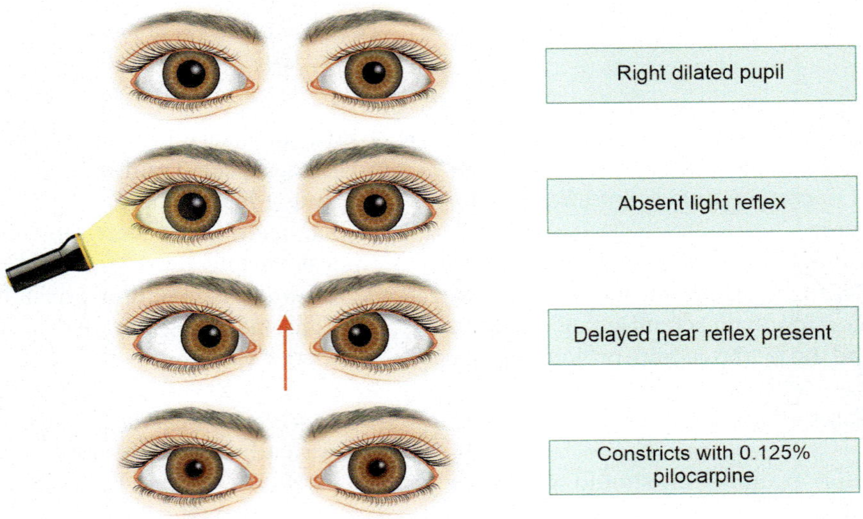

FIG. 5: Adie's tonic pupil.

TABLE 3: Etiologies of Adie's pupils.

Hereditary	Charcot–Marie–Tooth disease, familial dysautonomia
Infections	Neurosyphilis
Paraneoplastic	Lambert–Eaton myasthenic syndrome, Anti-Hu neuropathy
Inflammatory	Sjögren's, chronic inflammatory demyelinating polyneuropathy (CIDP), diabetes, amyloidosis
Degenerative	Shy–Drager syndrome, Ross syndrome*

*Triad of Adie's pupil, segmental hyperhidrosis, and hyporeflexia.

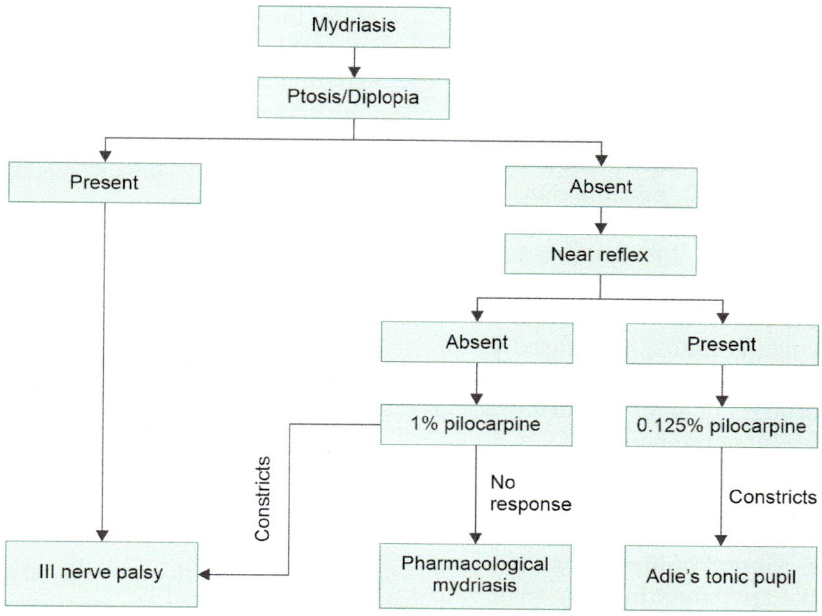

FLOWCHART 1: Algorithm to a dilated pupil.

Representative Case 1

A 42-year-old female presented with a history of worsening headaches for the past 1 week, with acute-onset left eye ptosis and diplopia. On examination, she had left eye minimal ptosis with a dilated and unreactive left pupil **(Fig. 6A)**. Her plain CT head was normal. She underwent a CT angiogram, which was suggestive of a left PCOM aneurysm **(Fig. 6B)**. She later underwent a clipping of the aneurysm.

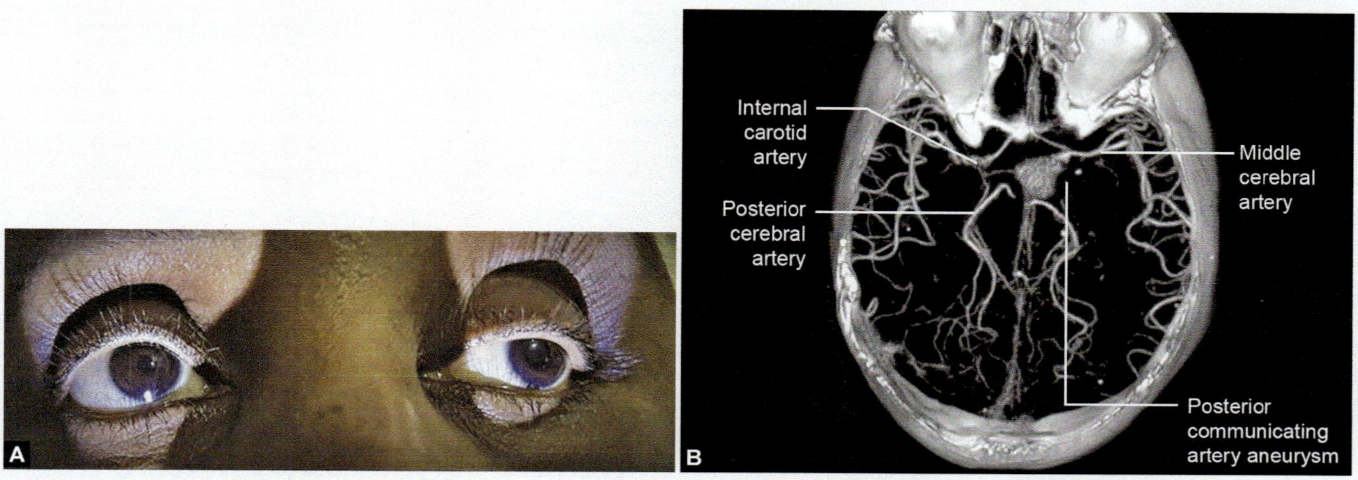

FIGS. 6A AND B: (A) Picture showing left eye ptosis and dilated pupil; (B) CT angiogram showing left PCOM aneurysm.
(CT: computed tomography; PCOM: posterior communicating artery)

Constricted Pupil

A constricted pupil points to pathology in any of these sites:

- *Sympathetic pathway*:
  - *Horner's syndrome*: It is due to a lesion of the sympathetic preganglionic or postganglionic pathway. The syndrome complex consists of a triad of miosis, ptosis, and anhidrosis. Localization of the site of lesion whether first-, second-, or third-order neurons is with the help of associated symptoms and topical tests to differentiate between pre- and postganglionic lesions **(Table 4)**.[12] In case of an irritative lesion of the sympathetic pathway or early compressive lesions, it may cause transient sympathetic stimulation and a reverse Horner's syndrome including mydriasis, exophthalmos, hyperhidrosis, and lid retraction[13] (Pourfour du Petit syndrome).
  - To identify a Horner's pupil, 10% cocaine solution is topically applied and observed for 45 minutes in a dark room. Cocaine blocks the reuptake of norepinephrine, which is tonically released in the intact sympathetic pathway. A normal pupil dilates but a Horner's pupil does not dilate due to the lack of sympathetically released norepinephrine.

    Cocaine is nowadays replaced by 0.5–1% apraclonidine, which is a strong a2 agonist and a weak a1 agonist. In Horner's pupil, there is denervation hypersensitivity to sympathomimetics and even a weak a1 agonist like apraclonidine can dilate and reverse Horner's pupil, whereas it does not have any or minimal effect on normal pupils.[14]

    To differentiate between pre- and postganglionic Horner's syndrome, 1% hydroxy amphetamine is used. This releases norepinephrine from intact postganglionic stores. In preganglionic lesions there is dilation of the pupil because of intact postganglionic fibers, whereas in postganglionic lesions there is no dilation.[15]
- *Light-near dissociation*: Selective damage to the light reflex pathways (retinomesencephalic pathways) with preservation of near reflex pathways (occipital-mesencephalic pathways) produces a constricted pupil, which does not react to light and constricts further (pinpoint pupil) briskly to near reflex, i.e., the light-near dissociation.[16] This phenomenon was commonly seen in neurosyphilis known as an *ARP*. The lesion in an ARP is hypothesized to be in the rostral midbrain sparing the ventral midbrain containing the pathway for accommodation reflex **(Fig. 7)**. Other causes for light-near dissociation are dorsal midbrain syndrome, demyelinating lesions, Wernicke's encephalopathy, and pineal tumors.
- *Local iris*:
  - Topical application of parasympathomimetic can cause significant pinpoint pupils unilaterally; bilateral pinpoint pupils can be seen in morphine or narcotic use and pontine hemorrhage.

Flowchart 2 shows an approach to a constricted pupil.

INVESTIGATORY APPROACH

Ophthalmological Investigations

Slit lamp examination: It helps in a detailed examination of the diseased pupil and in identifying structural lesions of the iris such as synechiae, adhesions, and local iris spasm (a sign of parasympathetic pathway involvement) in ATP.

Topical tests: Topical tests for Horner's (apraclonidine, hydroxy amphetamine) and Adie's pupils (pilocarpine) have been described in earlier sections and help in localization.

TABLE 4: The localization and etiology of Horner's syndrome.

	First order (preganglionic)	Second order (preganglionic)	Third order (postganglionic)
Anatomy	From the hypothalamus descends through the spinal cord till the C8–T2 intermediate gray column of Budge and Waller	Ventral roots from C8–T2, through stellate ganglion till they synapse in the superior cervical ganglion	Plexuses around internal carotid artery (ICA) through the cavernous sinus → ophthalmic division of III nerve → nasociliary division → long ciliary nerve
Associated symptoms	Hypothalamic or brainstem syndrome, myelopathy	Neck pain/swelling, brachial plexopathy, vocal cord or phrenic nerve palsy*	Ipsilateral severe headaches with congestion, flushing, and rhinorrhea
10% cocaine	No dilation of the pupil	No dilation of the pupil	No dilation of the pupil
1% apraclonidine	Dilates pupil	Dilates pupil	Dilates pupil
1% hydroxy amphetamine	Dilates pupil	Dilates pupil	No dilation pupil
Etiology[12]	Lesions affecting the hypothalamus/ brainstem and spinal cord, vascular causes, demyelination, infections, and mitotic lesions	Head and neck neoplasms invading the paraganglionic spaces, cervical rib, thoracic aneurysm, jugular vein thrombosis, neck and chest trauma	Cavernous sinus lesions (neoplasm/ vascular, inflammatory), intracavernous aneurysm, cervical lymphadenopathy

* *Rowland–Payne syndrome*: Horner's syndrome with vocal cord and phrenic nerve palsies.

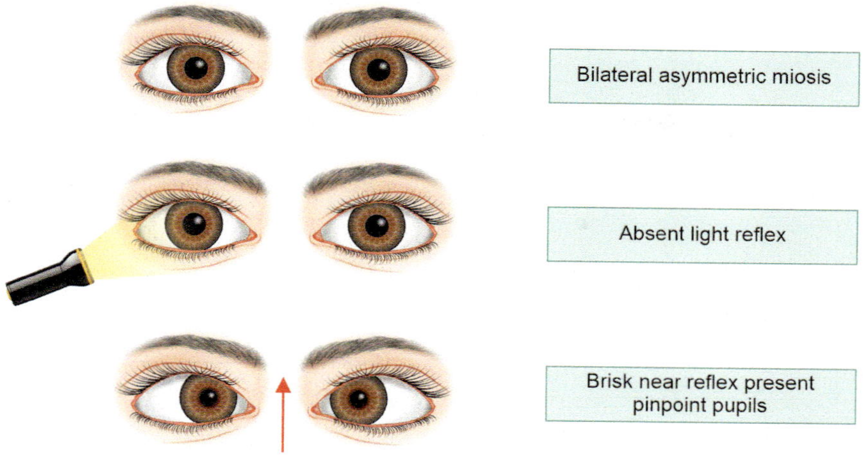

FIG. 7: Demonstration of an Argyll Robertson pupil.

Radiological Investigations

- Contrast-enhanced magnetic resonance imaging (MRI) with dedicated orbital cuts to look at the structures involved in the pupillary pathways. An MR angiogram (MRA) will be required in case a PCOM aneurysm (III nerve palsy) or any carotid aneurysm (Horner's syndrome) is suspected. Once the MRA is negative, if the suspicion is high enough for a vascular abnormality, then a digital subtraction angiography (DSA) can put the doubts to rest.[17] In first-order Horner's syndrome, apart from brain imaging, spinal cord imaging is also a necessity.
- Newer imaging modalities such as constructive interference in steady state (CISS) to look at individual cranial nerves can help identify structural lesions.
- Computed tomography (CT) chest and neck in case of suspected Horner's syndrome with second- and third-order localization **(Case 2)**.

Representative Case 2

A 62-year-old male presented with pain and swelling in the neck for 2 months. He had a prior history of carcinoma epiglottis, which was treated 2 years ago. On examination, he had ipsilateral ptosis, miosis, and reduced sweating (Horner's syndrome) **(Fig. 8A)**; he had hard swelling on the right side of the neck, which was hard and adherent to the underlying soft tissue **(Fig. 8B)**. A contrast-enhanced CT (CECT) of the neck revealed a soft-tissue swelling extending from the epiglottis, involving the cervical lymph nodes, and abutting the right common carotid artery on the same side **(Fig. 8C)**.

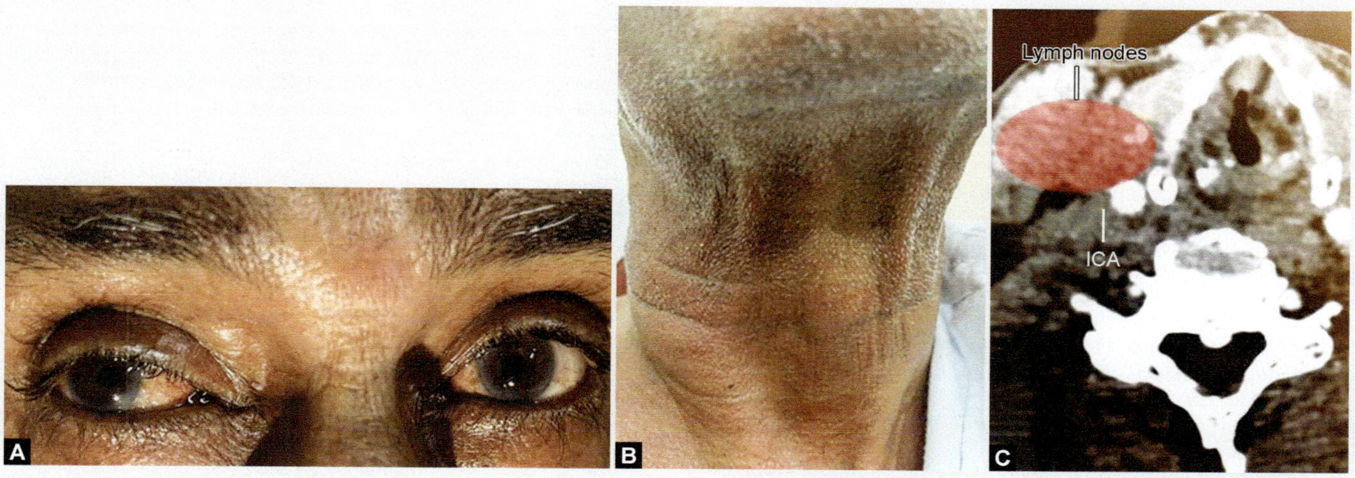

FIGS. 8A TO C: (A) Right eye ptosis with constricted pupil; (B) Hard swelling in the right side of the neck; (C) CECT neck shows lymph nodal mass encroaching the right carotid artery.

(CECT: contrast-enhanced computed tomography; ICA: internal carotid artery)

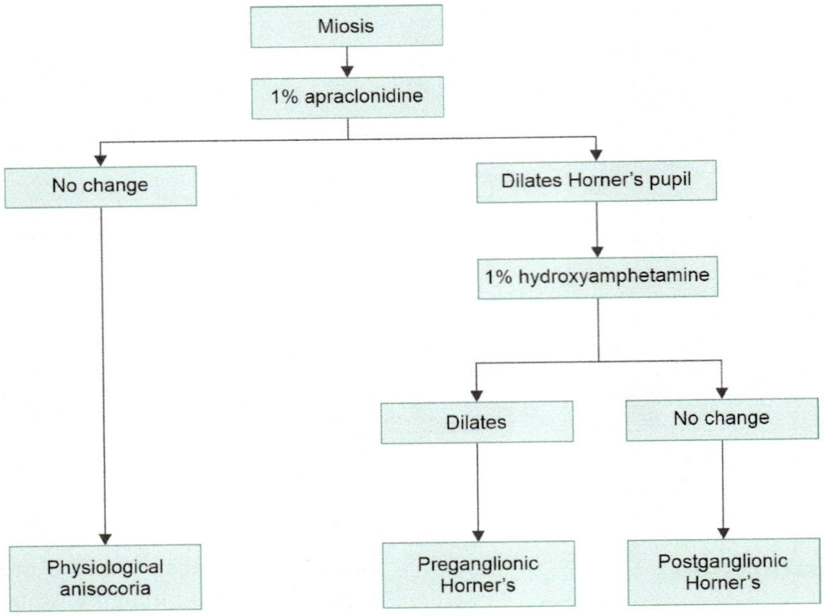

FLOWCHART 2: Algorithm to a constricted pupil.

Serological Investigations

Evaluation for systemic diseases: Diabetes, human immunodeficiency virus (HIV), syphilis, autoimmune disorders, vasculitis, and tumor markers are required, depending on the etiological suspicion **(*see* Tables 3 and 4)**.

CONCLUSION

Pupillary examination though may seem minute and brief, the quanta of information an experienced clinician gets from their examination is vast. A dilated pupil can be the only sign of an impending uncal herniation or a PCOM aneurysm. Finding an ARP points to a possible neurosyphilis. The presence of pinpoint pupils in a comatose patient might indicate a narcotic overdose or a pontine bleed. Localization requires a good grasp of the basic anatomy of the pathways and normal physiology of the reflexes. A well-localized lesion helps in narrowing down the investigations and saves time and resources.

REFERENCES

1. McDougal DH, Gamlin PD. Autonomic control of the eye. Compr Physiol. 2015;5:439.
2. Walsh FB, Hoyt W F. Walsh and Hoyt's Clinical Neuro-Ophthalmology: The Essentials. Philadelphia: Lippincott Williams & Wilkins; 2008.
3. Young MJ, Lund RD. The anatomical substrates subserving the pupillary light reflex in rats: origin of the consensual pupillary response. Neuroscience. 1994;62:481-96.
4. Belliveau AP, Somani AN, Dossani RH. Pupillary Light Reflex. [Updated 2022 Jul 25]. In: StatPearls [Internet]. Treasure Island (FL): StatPearls Publishing; 2022.
5. Levatin P. Pupillary escape in disease of the retina or optic nerve. Arch Ophthalmol. 1959;62:768-79.
6. Bell RA, Waggoner PM, Boyd WM, Akers RE, Yee CE. Clinical grading of relative afferent pupillary defects. Arch Ophthalmol. 1993;111:938-42.
7. James B. The pupils. Ophthalmology: Investigation and Examination Techniques; 1990. pp. 123-7.
8. Kerr FW, Hollowell OW. Location of pupillomotor and accommodation fibers in the oculomotor nerve: experimental observations on paralytic mydriasis. J neurol neurosurg psychiatry. 1964;27: 473-81.
9. Nadeau SE, Trobe JD. Pupil sparing in oculomotor palsy: a brief review. Ann Neurol. 1983;13:143-8.
10. Ramsay DA. Dilute solutions of phenylephrine and pilocarpine in the diagnosis of disordered autonomic innervation of the iris. Observations in normal subjects, and in the syndromes of Horner and Holmes–Adie. J Neurol Sci. 1986;73:125-34.
11. Adie WJ. Pseudo-Argyll Robertson pupils with absent tendon reflexes: a benign disorder simulating tabes dorsalis. Br Med J. 1931;1:928-30.
12. Davagnanam I, Fraser CL, Miszkiel K, Daniel CS, Plant GT. Adult Horner's syndrome: a combined clinical, pharmacological, and imaging algorithm. Eye (Lond). 2013;27(3):291-8.
13. Teeple E, Ferrer EB, Ghia JN, Pallares V. Pourfour du Petit syndrome—hypersympathetic dysfunctional state following a direct nonpenetrating injury to the cervical sympathetic chain and brachial plexus. Anesthesiology. 1981;55:591-2.
14. Koc F, Kavuncu S, Kansu T, Acaroglu G, Firat E. The sensitivity and specificity of 0.5% apraclonidine in the diagnosis of oculosympathetic paresis. Br J Ophthalmol. 2005;89:1442-4.
15. Danesh-Meyer HV, Savino P, Sergot R. The correlation of phenylephrine 1% with hydroxyamphetamine 1% in Horner's syndrome. Br J Ophthalmol. 2004;88:592-3.
16. Thompson HS. Light-near dissociation of the pupil. Ophthalmologica. 1984;189(1-2):21-3.
17. Elmalem VI, Hudgins PA, Bruce BB, Newman NJ, Biousse V. Underdiagnosis of posterior communicating artery aneurysm in noninvasive brain vascular studies. J Neuroophthalmol. 2011;31:103.

34

CHAPTER

Approach to Headache

Sanjay Prakash, K Ravishankar

INTRODUCTION

Although headache is among the most frequent symptoms for which patients see doctors, it remains one of the most misdiagnosed.[1] Misdiagnosis could occur for a number of reasons, including overlapping clinical symptoms across different primary headaches, miscommunication between the patient and the doctor during history-taking, inappropriate investigations, and also a lack of interest in headache disorders among physicians. A long list of primary and secondary headaches further complicates the diagnostic issues.[2] An accurate diagnosis is essential for managing any headache. This chapter outlines an approach for diagnosing headache disorders.

CLASSIFICATION AND EPIDEMIOLOGY OF HEADACHE DISORDERS

There are about 300 different types of headaches identified by the International Classification of Headache Disorders, third edition (ICHD-3).[2] ICHD-3 classifies all headaches as primary, secondary, and cranial neuropathies. Migraine, tension-type headache (TTH), and trigeminal autonomic cephalalgias (TACs) are considered the "big three," and all other primary headaches are clubbed together under the heading, "other primary headache disorders" **(Box 1)**. Secondary headaches are included in groups 5–12 of the classification. Involvement of both intracranial and extracranial structures, the cranium, neck, eyes, nose, sinuses, ears, teeth, mouth, and other facial or cervical structures can also cause secondary headaches.

Epidemiological data assists physicians in choosing the right approach for the presenting symptom. **Table 1**[3–7] shows the prevalence of headache disorders in three different clinical settings. Primary headaches are the most common reason for seeing a doctor. Migraine is the most common reason to consult a physician in both outpatient department (OPD) and emergency settings.[4] The most common headache

BOX 1 International Classification of Headache Disorders, 3rd edition (ICHD-3).

Primary headaches:
- Migraine
- Tension-type headache (TTH)
- Trigeminal autonomic cephalalgias (TACs)
  - Cluster headache (CH)
  - Paroxysmal hemicrania (PH)
  - Short-lasting unilateral neuralgiform headache attacks (SUNHA)
    - Short-lasting unilateral neuralgiform headache attacks with conjunctival injection and tearing (SUNCT)
    - Short-lasting unilateral neuralgiform headache attacks with cranial autonomic symptoms (SUNA)
  - Hemicrania continua (HC)
- *Other primary headache disorders*:
  - Primary cough headache
  - Primary exercise headache
  - Primary headache associated with sexual activity
  - Primary thunderclap headache
  - Cold-stimulus headache
  - External-pressure headache
  - Primary stabbing headache
  - Nummular headache
  - Hypnic headache
  - New daily persistent headache (NDPH)

Secondary headache disorders:
- Headache attributed to trauma or injury to head and/or neck
- Headache attributed to cranial or cervical vascular disorder
- Headache attributed to nonvascular intracranial disorder
- Headache attributed to a substance or its withdrawal
- Headache attributed to infection
- Headache attributed to disorder of homoeostasis
- Headache or facial pain attributed to disorder of the cranium, neck, eyes, ears, nose, sinuses, teeth, mouth, or other facial or cervical structure
- Headache attributed to psychiatric disorder

Painful cranial neuropathies, other facial pains, and other headaches:
- Painful cranial neuropathies and other facial pains
- Other headache disorders

in the general population is TTH. Secondary headaches are less commonly encountered in clinic settings.

DIAGNOSTIC APPROACH FOR HEADACHES

Flowchart 1 provides an overview of the diagnostic approach for headaches.

- *Step 1*: Accurate and detailed history
- *Step 2*: Thorough physical and neurological examinations
- *Step 3*: Recognition of red flags in the history and on physical examinations
- *Step 4*: Investigations based on suspicion and according to red flags
- *Step 5*: Formulating the provisional and final diagnoses

Step 1: History-taking

Overall, 60–75% of headaches seen in clinics are primary headaches.[4,5] The diagnostic approach in a headache patient starts with the exclusion of secondary headaches. Investigations are required for many secondary headaches. The choice of investigations for a particular patient is determined by the identification of red flags. Most red flags are found while taking the history. Physical examination only occasionally provides diagnostic hints. History-taking in headache patients is an art that is acquired by practice and experience.[8]

There is no single, universally accepted sequence of history-taking. However, an orderly approach is more appropriate as there is a long list of secondary headaches. The following points should be included in history-taking:

- *History related to demographic profiles of patients*: Age, gender, history of other diseases (tuberculosis, malignancy, human immunodeficiency virus (HIV), history of trauma, etc.), and possible risk factors (pregnancy, postpartum state, contraceptive pill use, etc.)
- *History of headache characteristics*: Duration of the head pain, pattern or frequency of headache, duration of the attacks, the location, quality, severity, precipitating factors for the headache, etc.
- *History of associated symptoms*: Are there any symptoms other than headaches, such as nausea, vomiting, photophobia, phonophobia, and autonomic features such as lacrimation and rhinorrhea?

TABLE 1: Prevalence of different headache disorders in different settings.

General population[3]		Clinic-based study[4,5]		Emergency setting[6,7]	
Tension-type headache (TTH)	78%	Migraine	60–90%	Migraine	15–90%
Migraine	16%	TTH	3–16%	TTH	2–10%
Fasting	19%	Secondary headaches	3–10%	Secondary headaches	2–20%
Nose/sinus related	15%	Unclassifiable	3–5%	Intracranial disease	1–2%
Head trauma	4%			Unclassified	5–40%
Intracranial disease	0.50%				

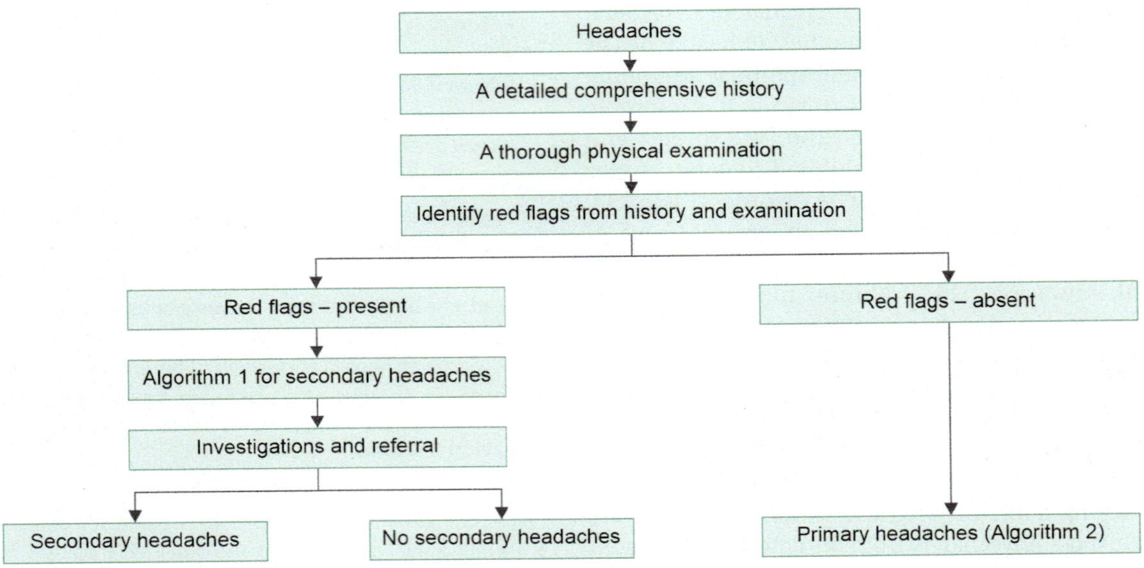

FLOWCHART 1: An overview of the diagnostic approach for headaches.

Pattern or Frequency of Headaches

The mode of onset and progression of headaches are critical in determining whether the headache is primary or secondary. The pattern or frequency of headaches may be gauged based on whether the patient is experiencing (1) the first attack, (2) recurrent attacks, (3) continuous headaches, and/or (4) a recent change in the headache pattern.

A primary headache is largely characterized by recurrent episodic attacks. ICHD-3 specifies the minimum number of attacks required to diagnose primary headaches (2 attacks for migraine with auras, 5 attacks for migraine without auras, and 10 attacks for TTH).[2] It does not consider a diagnosis of any primary headaches in the "first" attack. Unless the headache is severe, patients rarely seek medical attention for their first attack. When the first attack is severe, it is a red flag, suggesting vascular involvement or an acute infective process like meningitis. A sudden severe headache that peaks within 60 seconds is called a thunderclap headache (TCH). It can be a sign of a potentially fatal condition such as subarachnoid hemorrhage (SAH) or reversible cerebral vasoconstriction syndrome (RCVS).[2]

Chronic continuous headaches may have several different patterns. It may be chronic since onset or may evolve from episodic primary headaches. A chronic non-progressive daily headache typically indicates a primary headache. When headaches occur for more than 15 days per month during a 3-month period, it is called chronic daily headache (CDH). Primary CDH includes chronic migraine (CM), chronic TTH (CTTH), hemicrania continua (HC), and new daily persistent headache (NDPH). Patients with HC and NDPH have daily continuous headaches. A headache that has been present on a daily basis since the outset usually indicates NDPH. HC is a type of TACs that is characterized by daily background pain with exacerbations. Progressive worsening of headaches is a red flag, and patients need a detailed assessment. Any recent changes in the headache pattern may indicate the emergence of a new secondary headache over a preexisting headache.

Duration of Individual Attacks

The duration of attacks for several primary headaches has been defined by ICHD-3: TTH usually lasts from 30 minutes to 7 days, migraine lasts from 4 to 72 hours, cluster headache (CH) lasts from 15 to 180 minutes, and paroxysmal hemicrania (PH) lasts from 2 to 30 minutes.[2] Pain in neuralgias and short-lasting unilateral neuralgiform headache attacks (SUNHA) last for a few seconds to a few minutes. In clinical practice, a time limit of 4 hours is an important distinguishing feature between short- and long-lasting headaches. Only four primary headaches last more than 4 hours in a day (long-lasting headaches): migraine, TTH, NDPH, and HC. Patients with NDPH and HC experience daily headaches (a part of CDH), whereas patients with migraine and TTH can have both episodic and chronic headaches.[2]

Location

The location of headaches is described in two ways, depending on sides and sites. The term "side" refers to whether the headache is on the right, left, or both sides of the head. Headaches can be strictly unilateral, side-shifting unilateral, or bilateral. TACs and neuralgias are characterized by strictly unilateral headaches. ICHD-3 mentions "unilateral" location as one of the features of migraine. However, in migraine, unilateral headache is typically side-shifting. Furthermore, more than half of migraine patients experience bilateral headaches.[9] Side-locked headache is unusual in migraine. A headache that is strictly unilateral or localized is a red flag and needs investigation to rule out underlying pathology.

The "sites" of headache are defined as orbital, supra-orbital, frontal, parietal, temporal, occipital, neck, face, teeth, etc. In TACs and a few neuralgias, ICHD-3 defines the sites of pain. Pain that is primarily localized to the eye, neck, or face is a red flag, and patients should be examined and investigated to rule out underlying local pathologies.[10] It is important to note, however, that pain in and around the eyes, neck, sinuses, and face is also seen in migraine and other primary headache patients.

Quality

There are several different terminologies used to describe the types of head pain, such as throbbing, pressing, stabbing, searing, and electric shock-like. An electric shock-like pain is highly suggestive of neuralgias and SUNHA. The pain in CH and PH has been described as excruciating or stabbing. According to ICHD-3, migraine patients experience "throbbing" pain, whereas those with TTH experience "pressing" pain. However, it is important to know that throbbing pain might occur in 40–50% of TTH.[11] Likewise, up to 50% of migraine sufferers may have nonthrobbing pain.[10,11] Therefore, physicians must be careful in diagnosing migraine and TTH based on the quality of the headache.

Severity

The severity of headaches can be graded on the visual analogue scale (VAS) from 0 to 10, where 0 is no pain and 10 is the worst possible pain. The VAS score in CH and other TACs ranges from 8 to 10.[12] The first severe headache with a VAS score of 8–10 is a red flag and suggests the possibility of vascular pathology. Headaches can also be classified as mild, moderate, or severe based on activity restrictions during attacks. Mild headache attacks do not interfere with daily activities, and patients can continue their work as usual. Patients in moderate pain will have to limit their activities. In severe attacks, patients stop performing even routine tasks. Migraine headache attacks are typically moderate to severe. Moreover, migraine headache attacks are aggravated by climbing stairs and by normal physical activity. This will further restrict the activities of patients, and they frequently need bed rest.[13] Headache attacks in TTH are mild to moderate, not aggravated by routine physical activities, and patients rarely require rest during attacks.[13,14]

Restlessness or agitation during attacks is a specific feature of TACs. However, in TACs, restlessness or agitation has specific meanings, and patients should be inquired about this. Agitation means patients will not remain still, and they will engage in some motion-related activities. Walking back and forth, pacing, rolling on the bed, self-inflicted injury, hitting the head against a wall, and rubbing–pressing–holding the aching part are all examples of agitation in TACs.[15]

So, it is critical to understand what patients do during headache attacks. It may give you a diagnostic clue. Patients with migraine typically require rest and cannot continue working, whereas patients with TTH do not require rest and can continue working. Patients with TACs, on the other hand, neither take rest nor work. They become agitated or restless.

Time of the Day

Hypnic headache occurs exclusively during sleep.[2] Nocturnal preponderance is common in CH. Morning headaches could be a sign of increased intracranial pressure, breathing-related disorders, major depressive disorders, or medication overuse headache (MOH).[16,17]

Precipitating or Aggravating Factors

Understanding precipitating factors is critical for headache treatment. In such patients, avoiding triggers may reduce the frequency and severity of headache attacks. A few primary headache disorders, such as primary cough headache, primary exercise headache, primary headache associated with sexual activity, cold-stimulus headache, and external-pressure headache, are diagnosed solely based on precipitating factors. However, a diagnosis of such headaches is made only when secondary causes are ruled out. About 40% of cough headaches are symptomatic. Common secondary causes of cough headaches are Arnold–Chiari malformation, intracranial space-occupying lesions, and vessel-related abnormalities.[2] Likewise, a diagnosis of primary exercise headache and a primary headache associated with sexual activity is made once secondary causes are ruled out.

In the first attack of headache caused by exercise, or sexual activity, or other Valsalva-like activities, SAH, RCVS, and arterial dissection must be ruled out. Physical activities like exertion, exercise, and sexual activity can also cause cardiac cephalalgia. The majority of patients suffering from cardiac cephalalgia have vascular risk factors (elderly age, hypertension, hyperlipidemia, diabetes mellitus, and family history). Cardiac evaluation is necessary for patients who have vascular risk factors and headaches due to physical activities.[2]

Some headaches occur only in a specific position, such as sitting or standing up. Such headaches are known by several different names: positional headache, postural headache, orthostatic headache, and low-pressure headaches. Cerebrospinal fluid (CSF) leak is the most common cause of a postural headache.[18] Other causes of such headaches are postural orthostatic tachycardia syndrome (POTS), neck-tissue abnormalities, brain tumors, and anemia.[19]

Accompanying Features

Migraine patients may have migrainous features and auras. Cranial autonomic features are one of the main features of TACs. The presence of these symptoms is important for diagnosis. Patients should also be asked if they have any local, neurological (other than aura), or systemic features.

Migrainous features: Migrainous symptoms include nausea, vomiting, photophobia, and phonophobia. If none of these symptoms are present, a migraine diagnosis is less likely. However, these features may be found in several other primary and secondary headaches as well. Meningitis can cause a combination of nausea, vomiting, and photophobia. Raised intracranial pressure can cause projectile vomiting. TTH does not cause nausea or vomiting.

Cranial autonomic features: ICHD-3 identifies eight different features that are included as cranial autonomic manifestations: conjunctival injection, lacrimation, nasal congestion, rhinorrhea, eyelid edema, facial sweating, miosis, and ptosis. These features are classically described in TACs.[2] However, it can also be seen sometimes with migraine, particularly when the pain is severe.[20] Rarely, it may also be noted in secondary headaches arising from eyes, nose, sinuses, ears, neck vessels, and other facial structures. A few clinical features of acute angle closure glaucoma may mimic autonomic features of CH or other TACs. Internal carotid artery dissection may cause unilateral headache and cranial autonomic features.[10]

Auras: They affect about one-third of migraineurs.[2] The most common are visual auras. Other types of auras include the sensory, speech-related, motor, brainstem, and retinal. Migraine-like auras may occur in epilepsy, transient ischemic attacks, and psychiatric disorders. Secondary causes of auras should be ruled out if they occur for the first time after the age of 40 years, the symptoms are exclusively negative (e.g., vision loss), and the aura is prolonged or very short.[2]

Neurological features: Migraine with aura is the most common cause of neurologic deficits presenting with a headache.[21] Therefore, any neurological symptom or sign other than typical auras is a red flag. These patients need detailed neurological examinations and investigations.

Local features: Headache and facial pain may arise from extracranial structures such as cranium, neck, eyes, nose, sinuses, ears, teeth, oral cavity, and facial or cervical structures. These structures usually cause localized or side-locked headaches. Pathologies in these structures may also cause some local symptoms and signs. Therefore, all localized pain should be investigated for the presence of symptoms associated with underlying structures.[10]

Systemic features: Secondary headaches, such as those caused by infection, a substance or its withdrawal, a disorder of homeostasis, or arteritis, can cause systemic symptoms such as fever, anorexia, weight loss, generalized body pain, insomnia, irritability, cough, and so on.[21]

Medication History

Nitrates, quinolones, antidepressants, 5-hydroxytryptamine 3 (5HT3) antagonists, and several other drugs are known to cause headaches.[22] The most important thing is to find out if there is a possibility of MOH. MOH is included in ICHD-3 as a secondary headache and makes up for probably the most common secondary headache.[21] In MOH, patients with a preexisting primary headache develop a new type of headache or a significant worsening of their preexisting headache due to frequent use of abortive therapy. The frequency and quantity of use of acute drugs for primary headaches are an important component in diagnosing MOH. Regular consumption of paracetamol, acetylsalicylic acid, and nonsteroidal anti-inflammatory drugs (NSAIDs) on ≥15 days/month for 3 consecutive months in a row or ergotamines, triptans, opioids, and mixture of analgesics on ≥10 days/month for 3 consecutive months in a row indicates the possibility of MOH.[2]

Step 2: Physical Examination

Any new headaches or headaches with red flags require thorough physical and neurological examinations. In other cases, however, the examination can be selective.

Bare minimum examination in each patient: Even if there is no red flag, check every patient's blood pressure, fundi for papilledema, and meningeal signs. Mild (140–159/90–99 mm Hg) or moderate (160–179/100–109 mm Hg) chronic arterial hypertension typically does not cause headache. However, an acute increase in systolic (≥180 mm Hg) and/or diastolic (≥120 mm Hg) blood pressure may cause an acute headache without causing any other physical disabilities.[2] Papilledema may be the sole sign in patients with idiopathic intracranial hypertension (IIH). In aseptic (noninfectious) or subacute-to-chronic meningitis, signs of meningeal inflammation (neck stiffness) may be the only physical finding.

In the elderly: Headache may be the sole presenting symptom of temporal arteritis (TA) and subacute angle closure glaucoma (SACG). A delay in diagnosis of TA and SACG can result in permanent vision loss. Therefore, elderly patients with new headaches should be checked for temporal artery thickening or tenderness, as well as raised intraocular pressure.

Examinations in side-locked headaches: Side-locked headaches can be caused by the involvement of extracranial structures. One of the distinguishing features of headache caused by extracranial structures (group 11, ICHD-3) is that the headache is aggravated by some provocative procedures (either pressure to tissues or some other maneuvers).[2] Pressure can also aggravate a few neuralgias. Therefore, it is recommended that all patients who present with localized or side-locked headaches should undergo provocative procedures to induce headaches. It should be done in an orderly manner to include all structures that may cause side-locked headaches. It is depicted in **Figure 1**. Provocative maneuvers can begin by pressing over the maxillary sinus and can proceed ahead in a semicircular manner to end by testing the neck. In this way, you can induce provocative procedures for headaches due to maxillary sinusitis, ocular inflammation, trochleitis, supraorbital-supratrochlear neuralgia, frontal sinusitis, TA, temporomandibular disorder, ear disorder, occipital neuralgia, and cervical pathology. In selected cases, palpation can be done in the tonsillar fossa (for enlarged styloid—Eagle's syndrome) and teeth (for dental origin pain).[10] Headache patients with orbital pain should be thoroughly examined for visual disturbances, eyelids abnormalities (drooping, swelling), conjunctival injection, ocular palsy, and pain during eye movements.

Referral to other departments: Patients can be referred to eye, ENT, and dental departments for examinations if red flags are indicative of involvement in these areas.

Step 3: Recognition of Red Flags

Red flags noted during history and physical examinations should be assessed for secondary headaches. Traditionally, red flags are described by a mnemonic SNOOP4 (now expanded to SNOOP10).[21] For details on SNOOP10, the readers are encouraged to check the relevant article.[21] Here, we have arranged the red flags in a different format so that algorithm for secondary headaches can be arranged in systemic order **(Table 2)**:

- *Patient-specific*: The mere presence of headaches in this group constitutes a red flag. New-onset headache in an elderly person (>50 years) is a red flag. The prevalence of pathological disorders is about 1% of new-onset headaches in patients under the age of 50 years. The prevalence rises sharply after 50 years of age, with 6% in patients aged 50–74 years and 12% after 75 years.[23]
- *Headache characteristics*: Especially related to the onset, pattern, severity, and site of headaches. A TCH is the most dangerous red flag that requires urgent investigations. NDPH is a primary headache. But several secondary causes mimic NDPH. A diagnosis of TACs and neuralgias is made once secondary causes of all side-locked headaches have been ruled out.
- *Headache precipitating factors*: Valsalva-like activities may aggravate intracranial pressure.
- *Associated symptoms or signs*: Other symptoms (systemic or neurological) that do not meet the migraine aura criteria are red flags.

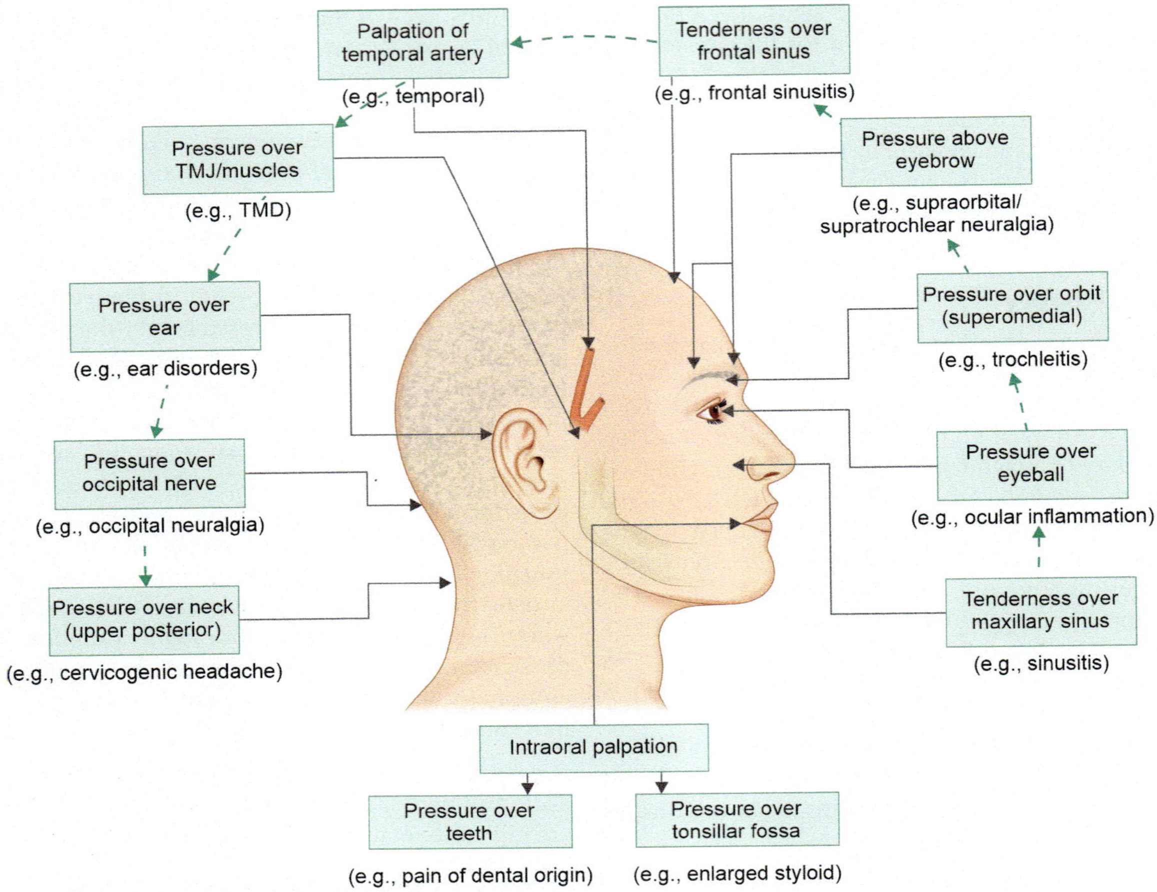

FIG. 1: Provocative procedures to reproduce pain in various secondary headaches and neuralgia.
Source: Reproduced with permission from Prakash S, et al (2016).[10]

TABLE 2: Red flag signs for headaches.

Patient specific	Headache specific	Headache triggers	Associated features
Age > 55 years	*Onset/pattern*: • Sudden/abrupt onset • Gradually progressive • New onset • Recent change in pattern	• Valsalva maneuver • Cough/sneezing • Exertion • Sexual activity • Posture changes	*Local features*: • Artery tenderness • Neck rigidity • Persistent congested eye
Female: • Pregnancy • Postpartum • Recent use of oral contraceptive pills			*System features*: • Fever • Anorexia • Weight loss
History of: • Trauma • Tuberculosis • Tumor • Human immunodeficiency virus (HIV) infection • Immunosuppressant use	*Severity*: • First severe • Worst ever *Sites*: • Localized • Side-locked		*Neurological features*: • Papilledema • Any neurological features not meeting the criteria of migrainous auras

Step 4: Investigations to Confirm or Rule Out Secondary Headaches

The choice of investigations depends on the presence of red flags or provisional diagnoses.[24]

Neuroimaging: Isolated headache with no red flag and fulfilling the ICHD-3 criteria of either TTH or migraine usually does not usually require investigation. TACs, other primary headaches (group 4), and primary neuralgias are diagnosed only if neuroimaging is normal. So, all suspected cases of TACs, other primary headaches, and neuralgias need neuroimaging.

Neuroimaging is required for all patients who have red flags. A computed tomography (CT) scan is preferred in the emergency setting (history of trauma or sudden-onset headache). In all other cases, magnetic resonance imaging (MRI) is a better option. If there is a suspicion of vascular pathology, an MRI of the brain could be supplemented with either MR angiography (MRA) or MR venography (MRV) (TCH, aneurysmal rupture, venous thrombosis, vasculitis, and arterial dissection). As secondary TACs have been reported due to arteriovenous malformation (AVM) or aneurysm, MRA (for both intracranial and extracranial vessels) must be performed in all side-locked headaches. If the patient is suspected of having SAH or RCVS, a digital subtraction angiography (DSA) is performed.[24]

Cerebrospinal fluid examination: It is used as an adjunct to neuroimaging. Its primary role in the acute setting is to rule out infectious or inflammatory processes in the meninges or brain parenchyma. It can also be a help in patients with suspicion of SAH but with a negative CT scan. The presence of red blood cells (RBCs) and xanthochromia in CSF may indicate SAH. Its role in chronic headaches is to rule out headaches caused by CSF pressure abnormalities (IIH and CSF hypotension). The diagnosis of HaNDL syndrome (syndrome of transient headache and neurological deficits with CSF lymphocytosis) is confirmed through disproportionate CSF pleocytosis only.[24]

Other investigations: Patients with red flags may also need other tests. Erythrocyte sedimentation rate (ESR) and C-reactive protein (CRP) should be done in all elderly patients (>50 years). In elderly patients with vascular risk factors, electrocardiogram (ECG) and two-dimensional (2D)-Echo are recommended. Side-locked headaches and facial pain may rarely be linked to lung carcinoma. A chest X-ray should be done in side-locked pain in the elderly.[10] In the case of unexplained morning headaches, a polysomnographic study can be performed to look for sleep apnea and other sleep-related disorders.[17]

Step 5: Formulating a Diagnosis

Red Flags Present: Algorithm for Secondary Headache

The presence of red flags indicates a higher probability of secondary headaches. A typical migraine or TTH does not require any investigations. However, in some circumstance, even migraine or TTH patients with atypical presentation require further evaluation. Migraine or TTH attacks for the first time in the elderly or during pregnancy become red flags. **Flowchart 2, Algorithm 1** provides an approach for secondary headaches based on red flags. The diagnostic approach for secondary headaches depends on the presence of red flags. Here we would discuss a few red flags in detail.

- *TCH*: ICHD-3 criteria for TCH include (1) severe head pain, (2) abrupt onset, reaching maximum intensity in <1 minute, and (3) lasting for >5 minutes.[2] Abrupt onset and severe head pain are two essential features of TCH.

  It should be noted that not all acute headaches or all severe headaches are TCH. It is attributed to vascular intracranial disorders, especially SAH. Other secondary causes of TCH are intracerebral hemorrhage, cerebral venous thrombosis, unruptured vascular malformation, arterial dissection (intra- and extracranial), RCVS, meningitis, colloid cyst of the third ventricle, spontaneous intracranial hypotension (SIH), and acute sinusitis (particularly with barotrauma).[2]

  The priority in TCH patients is to detect SAH. CT scan of the brain is an extremely sensitive test for evaluating SAH and intracranial hemorrhage during the first 6–12 hours of the onset of headache. If a CT scan is negative, a CSF examination is recommended to rule out SAH and meningitis. If both CT and CSF are negative, the search for other causes of TCH begins. MRI of the brain (plain and contrast) combined with MRV and MRA of the cranial and cervical vasculature practically rule out all causes of TCH.[24]
- *New daily headache*: A new or recent onset of daily or continuous headache can be a sign of a number of underlying pathologies, such as SIH, IIH, cerebral venous thrombosis, giant cell arteritis (GCA), cervicogenic headache, chronic meningitis, intracranial neoplasm, cranial artery dissection, sphenoid sinusitis, and chronic subdural hematoma.[24] Initial investigations in all such patients include MRI of the brain (plain and contrast) with MRV and MRA. In patients with suspected SIH, IIH, or chronic meningitis, a lumbar puncture with CSF analysis (including pressure measurement) is recommended.[24]

Red Flags Absent: Algorithm for Primary Headaches

There are about 18 different primary headaches and 6 different neuralgias causing pain in the head. The "appendix" section of ICHD-3 describes a few headaches (epicrania fugax).[2] Once the likelihood of a secondary headache is excluded, diagnosis of a primary headache may be easy. The diagnosis of some rare primary headaches is straightforward if a physician is aware of these disease entities. Therefore, the diagnostic approach for primary headaches should begin with an easy-to-diagnose headache (or straightforward diagnosis) and then move on to a more challenging headache. The algorithm for primary headache **(Flowchart 3, Algorithm 2)** has been organized in this order.

Step 1: Diagnosis by pattern recognition: Epicrania fugax and nummular headache are recognized by their pattern **(Fig. 2)**. An awareness of these headache disorders is enough to make the diagnosis.

- *Nummular headache (coin-shaped headache)*: It is characterized by constant pain at a fixed point on the head, usually in a rounded or coin-shaped area. Patients often outline the boundary of the headache area with a finger.[2]

Red flags	Red flags	Causes	Investigations
Demographic risk factors	Age: More than 50 years	GCA, glaucoma, malignancy, cardiac cephalalgia	ESR, CRP, neuroimaging, ECG, Echo
	Prothrombotic states (e.g., pregnancy, postpartum)	CVT	Neuroimaging, MRV
	Known case of tuberculosis, HIV, malignancy, other systemic disease	Meningitis, ICSOL Other intracranial diseases	Neuroimaging, CSF
	Head or neck trauma Spinal manipulation	SAH, artery dissection	Neuroimaging, CSF, MRA, DSA
Onset pattern	Thunderclap headache	SAH, RCVS, low CSF pressure Valsalva induced (cough, sex) Hypertensive crisis Artery dissection, CVT Pituitary apoplexy	Neuroimaging, CSF, MRA, MRV, DSA
	New daily headache	Low or raised CSF pressure Cerebral venous thrombosis Meningitis, artery dissection	Neuroimaging, CSF, MRA, DSA
	Progressive headache	IIH, ICSOL, CVT, meningitis	Neuroimaging, MRV, CSF
	During night, early morning	Raised ICP, sleep-related disorder, MOH	Neuroimaging, CSF pressure, polysomnography
Location	Headache and/or orbital pain	Glaucoma, painful ophthalmoplegia syndrome	Referral to eye department
	Headache and/or neck pain	Artery dissection, acute setting Cervicogenic headache	Neuroimaging, MRA
Precipitating factors	Valsalva (cough, sex, and exertion)	Chiari malformations Posterior fossa tumor CSF leak	Neuroimaging, CSF, MRA, DSA
	Exercise exertion	As valsalva-related cause Cardiac cephalalgia	Neuroimaging, MRA, DSA, ECG, Echo
	Postural change	CSF-related disorder	Neuroimaging, CSF pressure
Associated features	Local features (related to eye, nose, sinuses, oral cavity)	Related to eye, nose, sinuses, teeth, oral cavity	Referral to other departments
	Systemic features (constitutional features, other system involvement)	PMA, GCA, vasculitis, infective cause, other systemic cause	Extensive biochemical tests, ESR, CRP, CSF, CXR, ANA
	Neurological features (other than auras)	Intracranial pathologies	Neuroimaging, MRV, MRA, CSF

FLOWCHART 2 (ALGORITHM 1): An approach to find out secondary headaches in patients with red flags.

(ANA: antinuclear antibodies; CRP: C-reactive protein; CSF: cerebrospinal fluid; CVT: cortical venous thrombosis; CXR: chest X-ray; DSA: digital subtraction angiography; ECG: electrocardiogram; ESR: erythrocyte sedimentation rate; GCA: giant cell arteritis; ICP: intracranial pressure; ICSOL: intracranial space-occupying lesion; IIH: idiopathic intracranial hypertension; MOH: medication-overuse headaches; MRA: magnetic resonance angiography; MRV: magnetic resonance venography; PMA: polymyalgia rheumatic; RCVS: reversible cerebral vasoconstriction syndrome; SAH: subarachnoid hemorrhage)

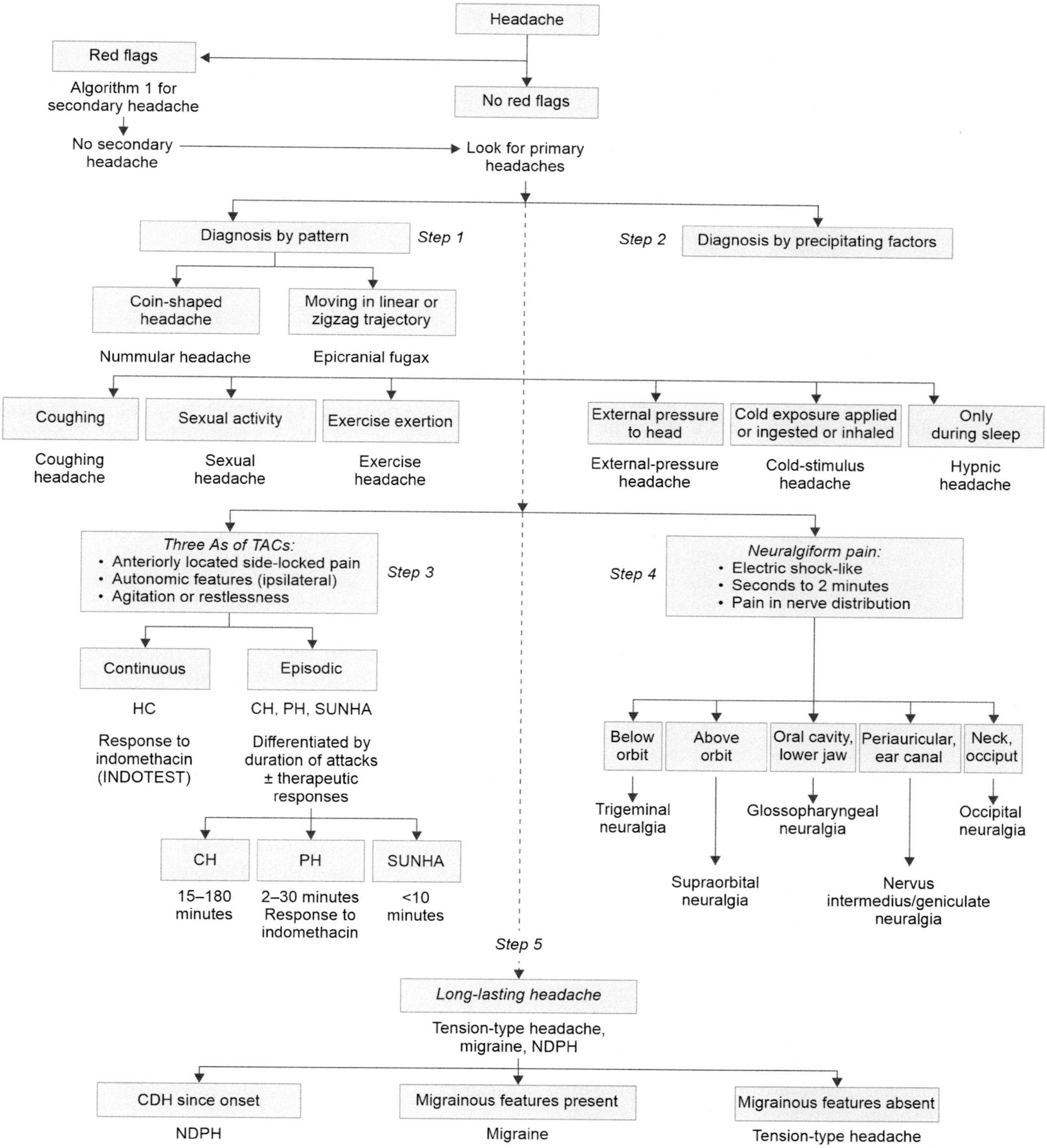

FLOWCHART 3 (ALGORITHM 2): An approach for primary headaches and neuralgias.

(CDH: chronic daily headache; CH: cluster headache; HC: hemicrania continua; NDPH: new daily persistent headache; PH: paroxysmal hemicrania; SUNHA: short-lasting unilateral neuralgiform headache attacks; TACs: trigeminal autonomic cephalgias; TTH: tension-type headache)

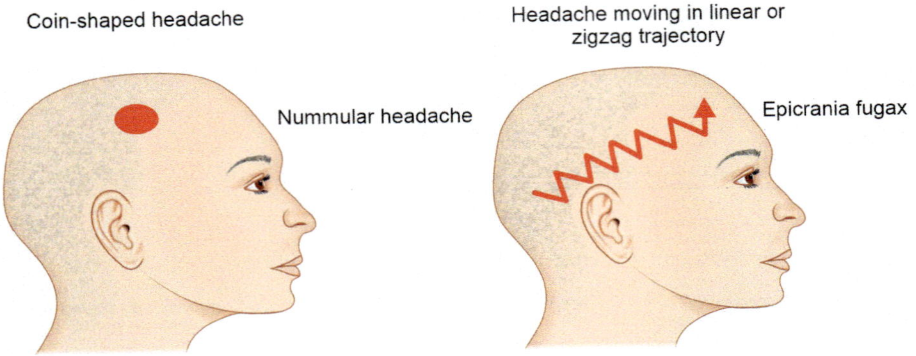

FIG. 2: Diagnosis by pattern.

- *Epicrania fugax*: This condition is characterized by brief (1–15 seconds) pain paroxysms that begin at one point and move in a zigzag or linear pattern on the head. The pain typically moves forward from a posterior hemicranial area toward the ipsilateral forehead, eye, or nose.[2]

Step 2: *Diagnosis by precipitating factors*: Precipitating factors are described in many primary and secondary headaches. However, a few headaches, described in the "other primary headaches" of ICHD-3, have a specific precipitating factor. These headache disorders have "no spontaneous headaches," and headaches are only induced by a specific precipitating factor. An awareness of these headache disorders is enough to make the diagnosis. However, the exclusion of secondary headaches is a must in such headaches. According to ICHD-3 criteria, at least two attacks are required to make a diagnosis of these headache disorders.[2]

- *Primary cough headache*: Headache is specifically brought on by coughing or sometimes by other Valsalva maneuvers, but not by physical exercise. It arises moments after the cough and typically lasts for a few minutes.[2]
- *Primary exercise headache*: This type of headache is caused solely by exercise and occurs during or after strenuous physical activity. Headaches in such patients may last up to 48 hours.[2]
- *Primary headache associated with sexual activity*: It is brought on by sexual activity and starts during sexual activity. The headache begins as a dull bilateral ache as sexual excitement increases and suddenly becomes intense at orgasm. This severe headache may last from 1 minute to 48 hours. There are no spontaneous headaches and no other precipitating factors.
- *Cold-stimulus headache*: Headache is caused by exposure to a cold stimulus (low environmental temperature), the consumption of cold food and beverages, or the inhalation of cold air. It resolves within 10–30 minutes after the removal of the cold stimulus.[2]
- *External-pressure headache*: Headache occurs within 1 hour of sustained external compression of the forehead or scalp by a tight band around the head, hat, helmet, or goggles. Pain is maximal at the site of external compression. The headache resolves within 1 hour after the removal of external compression.[2]

Step 3: *Diagnosis of TACs*: It is easy for experienced physicians as all TACs have a well-defined specific clinical picture. TACs include four different primary headaches: CH, PH, SUNHA, and HC. SUNHA includes two subtypes of headaches: short-lasting unilateral neuralgiform headache with conjunctival injection and tearing (SUNCT), and SUNHA with cranial autonomic symptoms (SUNA). All five TACs share three clinical features **(Fig. 3)**: (1) severe unilateral pain in the trigeminal distribution, (2) ipsilateral cranial autonomic features in the trigeminal distribution, and (3) agitation or restlessness.[2] Individual TACs are identified based on (1) the frequency and duration of attacks and (2) a therapeutic trial using indomethacin. Most of the TACs are episodic, except HC. Hence, if there is suspicion of TACs, first rule out HC, and inquire about the presence of continuous background pain. A therapeutic trial of indomethacin is required to confirm the diagnosis of HC. The frequency and duration of other TACs are: CH (15–180 minutes, 1–8 attacks/day), PH (2–30 minutes, >5 attacks/day), and SUNHA (1 second to 10 minutes, many attacks/day).[2] A positive response to indomethacin favors the diagnosis of PH. Oral indomethacin is usually started to see if there is a response in patients with suspected HC and PH. It may take a few days to show a complete response. However, injectable indomethacin [50 mg intramuscular (IM)] (INDOTEST) can be given for early identification.[25] Unfortunately, injectable preparation of indomethacin is not available in India. **Table 3** provides a comparative view of all TACs.

Step 4: *Diagnosis of neuralgias*: A brief electric shock-like pain (lancinating pain) with an abrupt onset and termination is highly suggestive of neuralgias.[2] Such lancinating pain is not felt in any primary headaches, except SUNHA and primary stabbing headaches. Neuralgias can be either idiopathic (primary) or secondary. Once secondary causes have been ruled out, a diagnosis of primary neuralgia is made. The sites of pain are used to make a diagnosis of various primary neuralgias. Neuralgias are usually triggered by some specific maneuvers.[2,26]

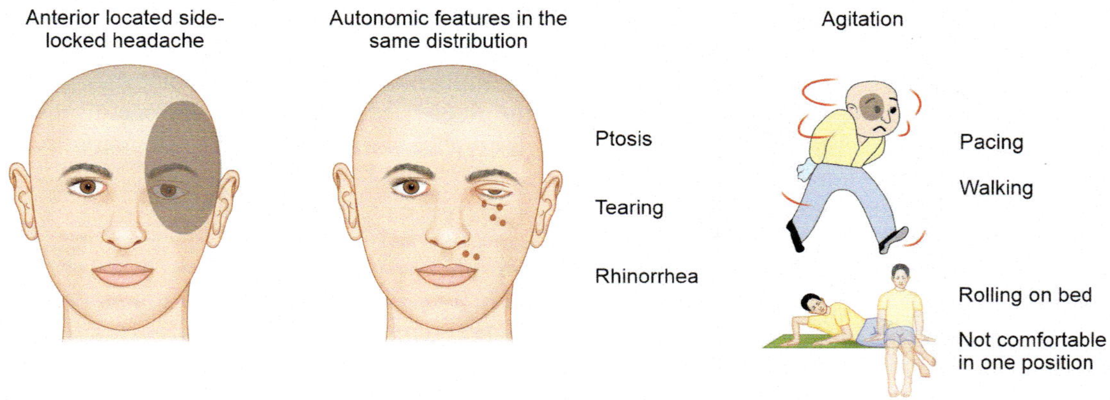

FIG. 3: Clinical features of trigeminal autonomic cephalalgias—3As.

TABLE 3: Comparing the TACs.

Features	CH	PH	SUNHA	HC
Similarities among all TACs				
Pain site	Pain in ophthalmic division of V cranial nerve	Pain in ophthalmic division of V cranial nerve	Pain in ophthalmic division of V cranial nerve	Pain in ophthalmic division of V cranial nerve and hemicranial
Ipsilateral cranial autonomic features	90–95%	90–95%	100%	60–95%
Agitation	Present	Present	±	Present
Differentiating features among TACs				
Pain pattern	Episodic pain	Episodic pain	Episodic pain	Continuous background pain with exacerbations
Duration of attacks/exacerbations	15–180 minutes	2–30 minutes	1 second to 10 minutes	*Exacerbation*: A few seconds to a few days
Frequency of attacks	1/2 to 8/day	>5/day	>1/day	Variable exacerbations
Response to drug	Lithium verapamil	Indomethacin	Lamotrigine or topiramate	Indomethacin

(CH: cluster headache; HC: hemicrania continua; PH: paroxysmal hemicrania; SUNHA: short-lasting unilateral neuralgiform headache attacks; TACs: trigeminal autonomic cephalalgias)

- *Trigeminal neuralgia (TN)*: It usually involves the maxillary division of the trigeminal nerve. The ophthalmic division may rarely be involved in some patients. Ophthalmic TN needs differentiation from SUNCT/SUNA. The points favoring the diagnosis of TN over SUNCT/SUNA are (1) the presence of a refractory period, (2) no or mild cranial autonomic symptoms, (3) easy provocation by stimuli, such as touch, wind, and eating, and (4) a positive response to carbamazepine.[26]
- *Glossopharyngeal neuralgia*: Pain is experienced in the base of the tongue, tonsillar fossa, ear, and/or beneath the angle of the jaw. It is commonly provoked by swallowing, talking, or coughing.[2]
- *Occipital neuralgia*: Pain is felt in the posterior part of the scalp. Attacks may be triggered by pressure on the nerves. Temporary relief in pain by anesthetic block of the nerve favors the diagnosis.[26]
- *Nervus intermedius neuralgia or geniculate neuralgia*: It is characterized by neuralgic pain in the auditory canal and periauricular areas. Attacks may be triggered by pressing the trigger area in the posterior wall of the auditory canal and/or periauricular region.[2,26]
- *Primary stabbing headache*: It is classified under "other primary headaches." However, it is frequently discussed with neuralgia because of its short-lasting attacks. It is characterized by transient and localized stabs (one or a series of stabs) in the head. The points favoring the diagnosis of primary stabbing headache over TN/other neuralgias are as follows: (1) ultrashort duration, more than 80% of attacks last 3 seconds or less, (2) less severe and there is no impact on daily life, (3) no precipitating factors, (4) no refractory period, and (5) response to indomethacin.[2]

Step 5: *Long-lasting headache attacks*: Typically, long-lasting headache means headache lasting for >4 hours a day.[27] This group includes migraine, TTH, NDPH, and HC. By definition, headaches in HC and NDPH are daily and continuous for at least 3 months' duration.[2,27] HC is a type of TAC (discussed above). A daily headache since the onset suggests NDPH. Headaches in migraine and TTH are typically episodic in nature. The presence of aura is highly suggestive of migraine. However, differentiation of TTH from migraine without auras may not be easy. No features are specific to distinguish migraine from TTH or vice versa. A group of symptoms is more helpful in distinguishing one from the other. A mnemonic (POUND) has been suggested to identify migraine.[28] POUND is the acronym for pulsatile headache, one-day headache, unilateral headache, nausea, vomiting, and disabling headache. Features opposed to migraine suggest TTH, i.e., nonpulsatile headache, headache for a few hours (<1 day), bilateral headache, no nausea, and no disabling headache. According to ICHD-3, the duration of headache in TTH varies between 30 minutes and 7 days. However, several studies suggest that most attacks in TTH last for 1–4 hours.[10,11] So, a "one-day" headache is highly suggestive of a migraine. Migraine attacks are typically moderate to severe in intensity, and they get aggravated by routine physical activity. Therefore, a disabling headache, requiring bed rest, is suggestive of a migraine.

CONCLUSION

There are about 18 primary headaches, 6 cranial neuralgias, and more than 250 different types of secondary headaches. However, up to 75% of patients who visit clinics have primary headaches. A diagnosis of primary headache is made based on pattern recognition once the possibility of secondary headaches is ruled out. The diagnosis of secondary headaches depends on the identification of red flags. Stepwise history-taking and physical examination supported by appropriate investigation are required to identify secondary headaches.

REFERENCES

1. Al-Hashel JY, Ahmed SF, Alroughani R, Goadsby PJ. Migraine misdiagnosis as a sinusitis, a delay that can last for many years. J Headache Pain. 2013;14:97.
2. Headache Classification Committee of the International Headache Society (IHS) The International Classification of Headache Disorders, 3rd edition. Cephalalgia. 2018;38(1):1-211.
3. Rasmussen BK, Jensen R, Schroll M, Olesen J. Epidemiology of headache in a general population—a prevalence study. J Clin Epidemiol. 1991;44:1147-57.
4. Tepper SJ, Dahlöf CG, Dowson A, Newman L, Mansbach H, Jones M, et al. Prevalence and diagnosis of migraine in patients consulting their physician with a complaint of headache: data from the Landmark Study. Headache. 2004;44(9):856-64.
5. Guerrero ÁL, Rojo E, Herrero S, Neri MJ, Bautista L, Peñas ML, et al. Characteristics of the first 1,000 headaches in an outpatient headache clinic registry. Headache. 2011;51(2):226-31.
6. Blumenthal HJ, Weisz MA, Kelly KM, Mayer RdL, Blonsky J. Treatment of primary headache in the emergency department. Headache. 2003;43(10):1026-31.
7. Doretti A, Shestaritc I, Ungaro D, Lee JI, Lymperopoulos L, Kokoti L, et al. Headaches in the emergency department—a survey of patients' characteristics, facts, and needs. J Headache Pain. 2019;20(1):1-6.
8. Ravishankar K. The art of history-taking in a headache patient. Ann Indian Acad Neurol. 2012;15(S1):S7-14.
9. Turkdogan D, Cagirici S, Soylemez D, Sur H, Bilge C, Turk U. Characteristic and overlapping features of migraine and tension-type headache. Headache. 2006;46(3):461-8.
10. Prakash S, Rathore C. Side-locked headaches: an algorithm-based approach. J Headache Pain. 2016;17(1):95.
11. Köseoglu E, Nacar ME, Talaslioglu A, Cetinkaya FE. Epidemiological and clinical characteristics of migraine and tension-type headache in 1,146 females in Kayseri, Turkey. Cephalalgia. 2003;23(5):381-8.
12. Prakash S, Patell R. Paroxysmal hemicrania: an update. Curr Pain Headache Rep. 2014;18(4):1-8.
13. Hu XH, Markson LE, Lipton RB, Stewart WF, Berger ML. Burden of migraine in the United States: disability and economic costs. Arch Intern Med. 1999;159(8):813-8.
14. Pryse-Phillips W, Findlay H, Tugwell P, Edmeads J, Murray TJ, Nelson RF. A Canadian population survey on the clinical, epidemiologic, and societal impact of migraine and tension-type headache. Can J Neurol Sci. 1992;19(3):333-9.
15. Torelli P, Manzoni GC. Pain and behavior in cluster headache. A prospective study and review of the literature. Funct Neurol. 2003;18:205-10.
16. Ohayon MM. Prevalence and risk factors of morning headaches in the general population. Arch Intern Med. 2004;164(1):97-102.
17. Göder R, Friege L, Fritzer G, Strenge H, Aldenhoff JB, Hinze-Selch D. Morning headaches in patients with sleep disorders: a systematic polysomnographic study. Sleep Med. 2003;4(5):385-91.
18. Leep Hunderfund AN, Mokri B. Second-half-of-the-day headache as a manifestation of spontaneous CSF leak. J Neurol. 2012; 259(2):306-10.
19. Cook GA Jr, Sandroni P. Management of headache and chronic pain in POTS. Auton Neurosci. 2018;215:37-45.
20. Cortez MM, Millsap L, Brennan KC, Campbell CL. Craniofacial autonomic dysfunction in migraine: implications for treatment and prognosis. J Neuroophthalmol. 2020;40(1):67-73.
21. Do TP, Remmers A, Schytz HW, Schankin C, Nelson SE, Obermann M, et al. Red and orange flags for secondary headaches in clinical practice: SNNOOP10 list. Neurology. 2019;92(3):134-44.
22. Ferrari A, Spaccapelo L, Gallesi D, Sternieri E. Focus on headache as an adverse reaction to drugs. J Headache Pain. 2009;10(4):235-9.
23. Goldstein JN, Camargo CA Jr, Pelletier AJ, Edlow JA. Headache in United States emergency departments: demographics, workup, and frequency of pathological diagnoses. Cephalalgia. 2006;26(6):684-90.
24. Ravishankar K. WHICH headache to investigate, WHEN, and HOW?. Headache. 2016;56(10):1685-97.
25. Antonaci F, Pareja JA, Caminero AB, Sjaastad O. Chronic paroxysmal hemicrania and hemicrania continua. Parenteral indomethacin: the "indotest". Headache. 1998;38(2):122-8.
26. Wilhour D, Nahas SJ. The neuralgias. Curr Neurol Neurosci Rep. 2018;18(10):1-8.
27. Halker RB, Hastriter EV, Dodick DW. Chronic daily headache: an evidence-based and systematic approach to a challenging problem. Neurology. 2011;76(7 Supplement 2):S37-43.
28. Wilson JF. In the clinic. Migraine. Ann Intern Med. 2007;147(9):ITC11-1-ITC11-16.

35

CHAPTER

Approach to Facial Pain

Ashish Kumar Duggal

INTRODUCTION

Facial pain is defined as "pain below the orbitomeatal line, anterior to the pinnae, and above the neck."[1] It is widely prevalent in the community and may affect up to 25% of the population, with almost 11% of patients suffering from chronic facial pain.[2] Patients with orofacial pain may present to different clinicians, including dentists, neurologists, headache physicians, otolaryngologists, and maxillofacial surgeons.[3] Pain in the orofacial region can occur because of the involvement of tissues such as facial skin, oral mucosa, teeth, cranial vessels, masticatory and facial muscles, meninges, cornea, and temporomandibular joint (TMJ).[4,5] The sensory innervation of these facial structures is primarily by the trigeminal nerve supplemented by the glossopharyngeal, vagus, and facial nerves. The sensory input converges on the spinal nucleus of the trigeminal nerve and nucleus of the tractus solitarius. These neurons then project to the thalamus and cortex, and lesions anywhere in the somatosensory pathway can cause facial pain. As a result, the causes of facial pain are myriad, and misdiagnosis and mismanagement are common.

CLASSIFICATION OF FACIAL PAIN

There has been a lot of controversy about the taxonomy of facial pain. There are a considerable number of labels being used for what may, in fact, be the same underlying condition. The International Classification of Headache Disorders (ICHD) does classify facial pains under "headache or facial pain attributed to disorders of the cranium, neck, eyes, ears, nose, sinuses, teeth, mouth, or other facial or cervical structures" and "painful lesions of cranial nerves and other facial pains."[1] However, the ICHD classification of facial pain has limited applicability in patients other than those suffering from headaches, cranial neuralgias, and painful trigeminal neuropathies. The recent International Classification of Orofacial Pain (ICOP), modeled on the ICHD-3 classification, tries to fill the gap and provide a comprehensive overview and diagnostic criteria for the most common conditions causing facial pain **(Table 1)**.[6] ICOP classifies facial pain into six broad categories: pain attributable to disorders of dentoalveolar and anatomically related structures, myofascial orofacial pain (MFOP), TMJ pain, pain attributed to lesion or disease of cranial nerves, pain resembling primary headache disorders, and idiopathic orofacial pain. However, there are some overlapping conditions involving the eyes, ears, sinuses, and neck which can cause facial pain, which does not find a mention in the current ICOP classification.

APPROACH TO A PATIENT WITH FACIAL PAIN

Like all neurological conditions, the clinical evaluation of a patient with facial pain requires a structured approach beginning with a detailed history and examination **(Table 2)**. It is important to distinguish neuralgic pain from neuropathic pain. Neuralgic pain is a paroxysmal, sharp lancinating, or electrical shock-like pain that is maximal at onset, occurring in the distribution of a nerve that is otherwise normal in function.[1,6] Neuropathic pain is caused by a lesion of the central or peripheral somatosensory system. The pain is usually described as continuous aching, burning, or throbbing pain often associated with positive and negative sensory phenomena. Its diagnosis requires the demonstration of a demonstrable disease or lesion in the somatosensory system **(Table 3)**.[1,6] Neurological examination should focus on cranial nerve examination with particular attention to the sensory examination of the face. The importance of a thorough dental evaluation by an experienced dentist cannot be overemphasized. Additionally, the examination should also include cervical spine evaluation (posture and range of motion), palpation of the masticatory and neck muscles, and examination of TMJ (tenderness to palpation, range of motion, joint sounds).

TABLE 1: Classification of orofacial pain.

ICHD classification of facial pains	ICOP classification
11. Headache or facial pain attributed to disorder of the cranium, neck, eyes, ears, nose, sinuses, teeth, mouth, or other facial or cervical structure 11.1 Headache attributed to disorder of cranial bone 11.2 Headache attributed to disorder of the neck 11.2.1 Cervicogenic headache 11.2.2 Headache attributed to retropharyngeal tendonitis 11.2.3 Headache attributed to craniocervical dystonia 11.3 Headache attributed to disorder of the eyes 11.3.1 Headache attributed to acute angle-closure glaucoma 11.3.2 Headache attributed to refractive error 11.3.3 Headache attributed to ocular inflammatory disorder 11.3.4 Trochlear headache 11.4 Headache attributed to disorder of the ears 11.5 Headache attributed to disorder of the nose or paranasal sinuses 11.5.1 Headache attributed to acute rhinosinusitis 11.5.2 Headache attributed to chronic or recurring rhinosinusitis 11.6 Headache attributed to disorder of the teeth 11.7 Headache attributed to TMD 11.8 Head or facial pain attributed to inflammation of the stylohyoid ligament 11.9 Headache or facial pain attributed to other disorders of the cranium, neck, eyes, ears, nose, sinuses, teeth, mouth, or other facial or cervical structure *13. Painful lesions of the cranial nerves and other facial pain* 13.1 Pain attributed to a lesion or disease of the trigeminal nerve 13.1.1 Trigeminal neuralgia 13.1.1.1 Classical trigeminal neuralgia 13.1.1.1.1 Classical trigeminal neuralgia, purely paroxysmal 13.1.1.1.2 Classical trigeminal neuralgia with concomitant continuous pain 13.1.1.2 Secondary trigeminal neuralgia 13.1.1.2.1 Trigeminal neuralgia attributed to MS 13.1.1.2.2 Trigeminal neuralgia attributed to space-occupying lesion 13.1.1.2.3 Trigeminal neuralgia attributed to other causes 13.1.1.3 Idiopathic trigeminal neuralgia 13.1.1.3.1 Idiopathic trigeminal neuralgia, purely paroxysmal 13.1.1.3.2 Idiopathic trigeminal neuralgia with concomitant continuous pain 13.1.2 Painful trigeminal neuropathy 13.1.2.1 Painful trigeminal neuropathy attributed to herpes zoster 13.1.2.2 Trigeminal postherpetic neuralgia 13.1.2.3 Painful post-traumatic trigeminal neuropathy 13.1.2.4 Painful trigeminal neuropathy attributed to other disorders 13.1.2.5 Idiopathic painful trigeminal neuropathy 13.2 Pain attributed to a lesion or disease of the glossopharyngeal nerve 13.2.1 Glossopharyngeal neuralgia 13.2.1.1 Classical glossopharyngeal neuralgia 13.2.1.2 Secondary glossopharyngeal neuralgia	*1. Orofacial pain attributed to disorders of dentoalveolar and anatomically related structures* 1.1 Dental pain 1.1.1 Pulpal pain 1.1.2 Periodontal pain 1.1.3 Gingival pain 1.2 Oral mucosal, salivary gland, and jaw pain 1.2.1 Oral mucosal pain 1.2.2 Salivary gland pain 1.2.3 Jawbone pain *2. Myofascial oral pain* 2.1 Primary myofascial pain 2.1.1 Acute primary myofascial pain 2.1.2 Chronic primary myofascial pain [infrequent, frequent, highly frequent (with or without referral)] 2.2. Secondary myofascial pain 2.2.1 Myofascial pain attributed to tendonitis 2.2.2 Myofascial pain attributed to myositis 2.2.3 Myofascial pain attributed to muscle spasm *3. TMJ pain* 3.1 Primary TMJ pain [acute, chronic—infrequent, frequent, and highly frequent (with or without referral)] 3.2 Secondary TMJ pain 3.2.1. TMJ pain attributed to arthritis (nonsystemic, systemic) 3.2.2 TMJ pain attributed to disc displacement (with reduction ± intermittent locking, without reduction) 3.2.3 TMJ pain attributed to degenerative joint disease 3.2.4 TMJ pain attributed to subluxation *4. Orofacial pain attributed to lesion or disease of the cranial nerves* 4.1 Pain attributed to lesion or disease of the trigeminal nerve 4.1.1 Trigeminal neuralgia 4.1.1.1 Classical trigeminal neuralgia (purely paroxysmal, with concomitant continuous pain) 4.1.1.2 Secondary trigeminal neuralgia 4.1.1.2.1 Trigeminal neuralgia attributed to MS 4.1.1.2.2 Trigeminal neuralgia attributed to space-occupying lesion 4.1.1.2.3 Trigeminal neuralgia attributed to other causes 4.1.1.3 Idiopathic trigeminal neuralgia (purely paroxysmal, with concomitant continuous pain) 4.1.2 Other trigeminal neuropathic pain 4.1.2.1 Trigeminal neuropathic pain attributed to herpes zoster 4.1.2.2 Trigeminal postherpetic neuralgia 4.1.2.3 Post-traumatic trigeminal neuropathic pain 4.1.2.4 Trigeminal neuropathic pain attributed to other disorders 4.1.2.5 Idiopathic trigeminal neuropathic pain 4.2 Pain attributed to lesion or disease of the glossopharyngeal nerve 4.2.1 Glossopharyngeal neuralgia 4.2.1.1 Classical glossopharyngeal neuralgia 4.2.1.2 Secondary glossopharyngeal neuralgia 4.2.1.3 Idiopathic glossopharyngeal neuralgia 4.2.2 Glossopharyngeal neuropathic pain

Continued

Continued

ICHD classification of facial pains	ICOP classification
13.2.1.3 Idiopathic glossopharyngeal neuralgia	4.2.2.1 Glossopharyngeal neuropathic pain attributed to a known cause
13.2.2 Painful glossopharyngeal neuropathy	4.2.2.2 Idiopathic glossopharyngeal neuropathic pain
13.2.2.1 Painful glossopharyngeal neuropathy attributed to a known cause	*5. 5. Orofacial pains resembling presentations of primary headaches*
13.2.2.2 Idiopathic painful glossopharyngeal neuropathy	5.1 Orofacial migraine
13.3 Pain attributed to a lesion or disease of nervus intermedius	5.1.1 Episodic orofacial migraine
13.3.1 Nervus intermedius neuralgia	5.1.2 Chronic orofacial migraine
13.3.1.1 Classical nervus intermedius neuralgia	5.2 Tension-type orofacial pain
13.3.1.2 Secondary nervus intermedius neuralgia	5.3 Trigeminal autonomic orofacial pain
13.3.1.3 Idiopathic nervus intermedius neuralgia	5.3.1 Orofacial cluster attacks
13.3.2 Painful nervus intermedius neuropathy	5.3.1.1 Episodic orofacial cluster attacks
13.3.2.1 Painful nervus intermedius neuropathy attributed to herpes zoster	5.3.1.2 Chronic orofacial cluster attacks
13.3.2.2 Postherpetic neuralgia of nervus intermedius	5.3.2 Paroxysmal hemifacial pain
13.3.2.3 Painful nervus intermedius neuropathy attributed to other disorder	5.3.2.1 Episodic paroxysmal hemifacial pain
13.3.2.4 Idiopathic painful nervus intermedius neuropathy	5.3.2.2 Chronic paroxysmal hemifacial pain
13.4 Occipital neuralgia	5.3.3 SUNFA
13.5 Neck–tongue syndrome	5.3.3.1 Episodic SUNFA
13.6 Painful optic neuritis	5.3.3.2 Chronic SUNFA
13.7 Headache attributed to ischemic ocular motor nerve palsy	5.3.4 Hemifacial continuous pain with autonomic symptoms
13.8 Tolosa–Hunt syndrome	5.4 Neurovascular orofacial pain
13.9 Paratrigeminal oculosympathetic (Raeder's) syndrome	5.4.1 Short-lasting neurovascular orofacial pain
13.10 Recurrent painful ophthalmoplegic neuropathy	5.4.2 Long-lasting neurovascular orofacial pain
13.11 BMS	6. Idiopathic orofacial pain
13.12 PIFP	*6.1 BMS*
13.13 Central neuropathic pain	6.1.1 BMS without somatosensory changes
13.13.1 Central neuropathic pain attributed to MS	6.1.2 BMS with somatosensory changes
13.13.2 CPSP	6.1.3 Probable BMS
	6.2 PIFP
	6.2.1 PIFP without somatosensory changes
	6.2.2 PIFP with somatosensory changes
	6.2.3 Probable PIFP
	6.3 Persistent idiopathic dentoalveolar pain
	6.3.1 Persistent idiopathic dentoalveolar pain without somatosensory changes
	6.3.2 Persistent idiopathic dentoalveolar pain with somatosensory changes
	6.3.3 Probable persistent idiopathic dentoalveolar pain
	6.4 CUFPA facial pain

(BMS: burning mouth syndrome; CPSP: central poststroke pain; CUFPA: constant unilateral facial pain with additional attacks; ICHD: International Classification of Headache Disorders; ICOP: International Classification of Orofacial Pain; MS: multiple sclerosis; PIFP: persistent idiopathic facial pain; SUNFA: short-lasting unilateral neuralgiform facial pain attacks with cranial autonomic symptoms; TMD: temporomandibular disorder; TMJ: temporomandibular joint)

In the next sections, we will discuss the clinical manifestations and approaches to common conditions causing facial pain.

OROFACIAL PAIN ATTRIBUTABLE TO DISORDERS OF DENTOALVEOLAR AND ANATOMICALLY RELATED STRUCTURES

The disorders in this category primarily belong to the domain of dentists and maxillofacial surgeons. In general, the pain is nociceptive and/or inflammatory in nature and usually acute.[6] Occasionally, because of the natural history of the underlying condition, the pain may be reported as episodic or less commonly chronic if the underlying disorder is not treated properly. Some of the neuralgic, neuropathic, and orofacial presentations of headache disorders such as neurovascular orofacial pain (NVOP) can cause tooth pain, resulting in misdiagnosis and mismanagement with multiple tooth extractions. Salivary gland disorders such as tumors and duct blockage can elicit pain in the distribution of trigeminal nerve V (CN V).[7] The pain is characteristically intermittent and occurs just before eating, which can again

TABLE 2: Approach to a patient with orofacial pain.

Clinical features to be assessed	Comments
Localization of pain	Is the pain unilateral or bilateral? Is the pain side-locked or change sides? *Distribution of pain*: (Use a pain drawing for accurate assessment) Localized to one nerve, division of nerve or its named sensory branches—indicating neuralgia or isolated neuropathic pain Diffuse pain radiates beyond the single cranial nerve—indicating a central or multiple cranial nerve pain syndrome
Quality of pain	Paroxysmal, continuous, or discontinuous pain with superimposed paroxysms Duration of each episode Time taken to reach peak intensity for each episode
Severity of pain	Assessed on the visual analog scale
Character of pain	Dull, aching, throbbing, pulsating, sharp, stinging, prickling, burning, or electrical
Associated sensory and motor symptoms of trigeminal neuropathy	*Presence of sensory loss*: Hypoalgesia, hypoesthesia Loss of taste sensation, altered taste sensation Paresthesia or dysesthesias Allodynia hyperesthesia Conductive hearing loss and otitis media indicate weakness of tensor veli palatini muscle innervated by V3 division Cold-induced visual blurring due to episodic corneal edema Accidental tongue bites *Palpebromandibular synkinesia*: Jaw protrusion and deviation may be triggered by eye blinking
Triggers	Is the pain spontaneous or triggerable? Triggering factors: Chewing, shaving, brushing or flossing the teeth, washing the face, smiling, applying facial cosmetics, exposure to wind or cool breeze, swallowing, coughing, speaking, yawning, touching the neck or external auditory canal, presence of latency and refractory period
Aggravating and relieving factors	Effect of hot, cold, or sweet food Prolonged chewing, eating, clenching, bruxing habits
Temporal profile	Is the pain daily, episodic? Does the pain occur in clusters followed by remissions? Duration of remissions if any Progression of pain (intensity and frequency) over time
Associated autonomic phenomenon	Conjunctival congestion, lacrimation, rhinorrhea Facial cheek swelling Periorbital edema
Other associated phenomena	Nausea, vomiting, photophobia, phonophobia Locking or clicking of temporomandibular joint Crepitus in the temporomandibular joint Deviation of the mandible on jaw opening Dry eyes, dry mouth Weakness or difficulty with chewing Altered taste sensation, loss of taste
Neurological symptoms	*Vision loss, amaurosis fugax*: Optic neuritis, giant cell arteritis *Double vision*: Idiopathic orbital inflammation, Tolosa–Hunt syndrome Conjunctival congestion, lacrimation, and proptosis may indicate orbital myositis, cavernous sinus syndrome *Hearing loss*: Cerebellopontine angle tumor *Neck stiffness, Kernig sign*: Meningitis-associated trigeminal neuropathy *Horner syndrome*: Raeder syndrome, arterial dissection *Associated hemiparesis*: Central poststroke pain
Associated headache and neck pain	History of migraine, tension-type headache, chronic widespread pain, fibromyalgia
Preceding identifiable insult	Dental extractions, trauma, rash (herpes zoster)
Impact of pain	Sleep, mood, concentration, fatigue quality of life

TABLE 3: Neuralgic pain versus neuropathic pain.

	Neuralgic pain	Neuropathic pain
Definition	Pain occurs in the distribution of a nerve(s) with normal function	Pain occurs due to a lesion or disease of the somatosensory system
Quality of pain	Paroxysmal >> continuous Paroxysmal pain is lancinating, shock-like pain, typically maximum at the onset	Continuous >> paroxysmal Continuous steady aching, burning, or throbbing pain with superimposed shock-like pain
Sensory symptoms	Minimal sensory loss may be present	Sensory loss is present Associated hyperesthesia, paresthesia, and dysesthesia
Allodynia	Present but triggers a shock-like pain	Present but triggers a steady pain
Triggers	Localized punctate trigger areas present in or out of the pain area, intraoral triggers are more likely in trigeminal neuralgia (TN)	Allodynic areas are much larger, and non-noxious stimulus over a large area may provoke pain
Pathology	Demyelination at the nerve root	Damage to the nerve root, nerve, nucleus, or the tract

lead to misdiagnosis as trigeminal neuralgia (TN) or giant cell arteritis (GCA). However, salivary gland disorders are associated with tenderness of the involved salivary gland, and appropriate imaging techniques usually lead to the correct diagnosis.[8]

FACIAL PAIN DUE TO TEMPOROMANDIBULAR DISORDERS

Temporomandibular disorders (TMDs) are probably the most common nondental causes of facial pain. Pain associated with TMD is almost twice as prevalent in females as compared to males and peaks in the age group of 20–45 years.[9] Generalized pain conditions such as fibromyalgia, tension-type headache (TTH), low backache, and irritable bowel syndrome are frequently comorbid.[10] TMDs are further classified into masticatory (MFOP) and TMJ disorders.

Myofascial Orofacial Pain

Myofascial orofacial pain is often described as a deep aching diffuse pain with referral to the temporal area, TMJ, ear, angle, and ramus of the mandible and teeth. The pain is often described as weight or pressure feeling on the side of the face, though some patients may describe it as throbbing or needles being poked in the face.[7] It is modified (increased or decreased) by jaw movement, chewing, teeth grinding, or clenching. It may be intermittent occurring episodically or unremitting and continuous.[6,7] The episodes usually last more than 30 minutes, and patients may have several episodes in a single day.[6] There may be associated functional impairment in the form of difficulty in moving the lower jaw while chewing, wide yawning, etc. Pain may also radiate to the head and thus classify as a headache attributable to TMD.[1] Patients may complain of pain early in the morning, which is probably related to bruxism at night. The examination should focus on the reproduction of familiar pain through provocative procedures—standardized palpation and/or maximum jaw opening (assisted or unassisted). On palpation, there may be a pain at the site of palpation (tender point), or it may spread to other parts of the muscle being palpated.[11] On the other hand, trigger point refers to pain being felt at a site beyond the anatomical boundary of muscle (myofascial pain with referral). Trigger point palpation may be associated with a twitch response from the patient. While palpating, the force and duration should be standardized—1 kg for 2 seconds to establish pain on palpation and 1 kg for 5 seconds to establish pain spread or referral. Jaw function should be assessed by maximum unassisted jaw opening, which may be decreased in patients with MFOP (<40 mm).[11]

International Classification of Orofacial Pain has classified MFOP as primary or secondary **(Flowchart 1)**.[6] Secondary myofascial pain is caused by an underlying disorder causing infection, inflammation, or muscle spasm of the masticatory muscles.[6] Myositis of masticatory muscle may occur acutely because of trauma or infection or chronically in association with systemic autoimmune disorders. Acute myositis is often associated with erythema, edema, and warmth over the affected muscle. Serum creatinine kinase and autoimmune profile should be done if autoimmune myositis is suspected. Muscle spasms may present with sudden involuntary tonic contraction of masticatory muscles with acute painful malocclusion.[6]

An important differential diagnosis of MFOP is GCA. Jaw claudication in GCA needs to be differentiated from jaw pain in MFOP. Unlike GCA, jaw pain in MFOP starts immediately after eating without a latency, seen characteristically in jaw claudication.[12] Additional differentiating features are the limitation of jaw opening and tenderness of the masticatory muscles, which are present in MFOP.

Temporomandibular Joint Disorders

Temporomandibular joint disorders, though very common in the general population, can also cause facial pain as well as headache. Malocclusion as a result of ill-fitting dentures

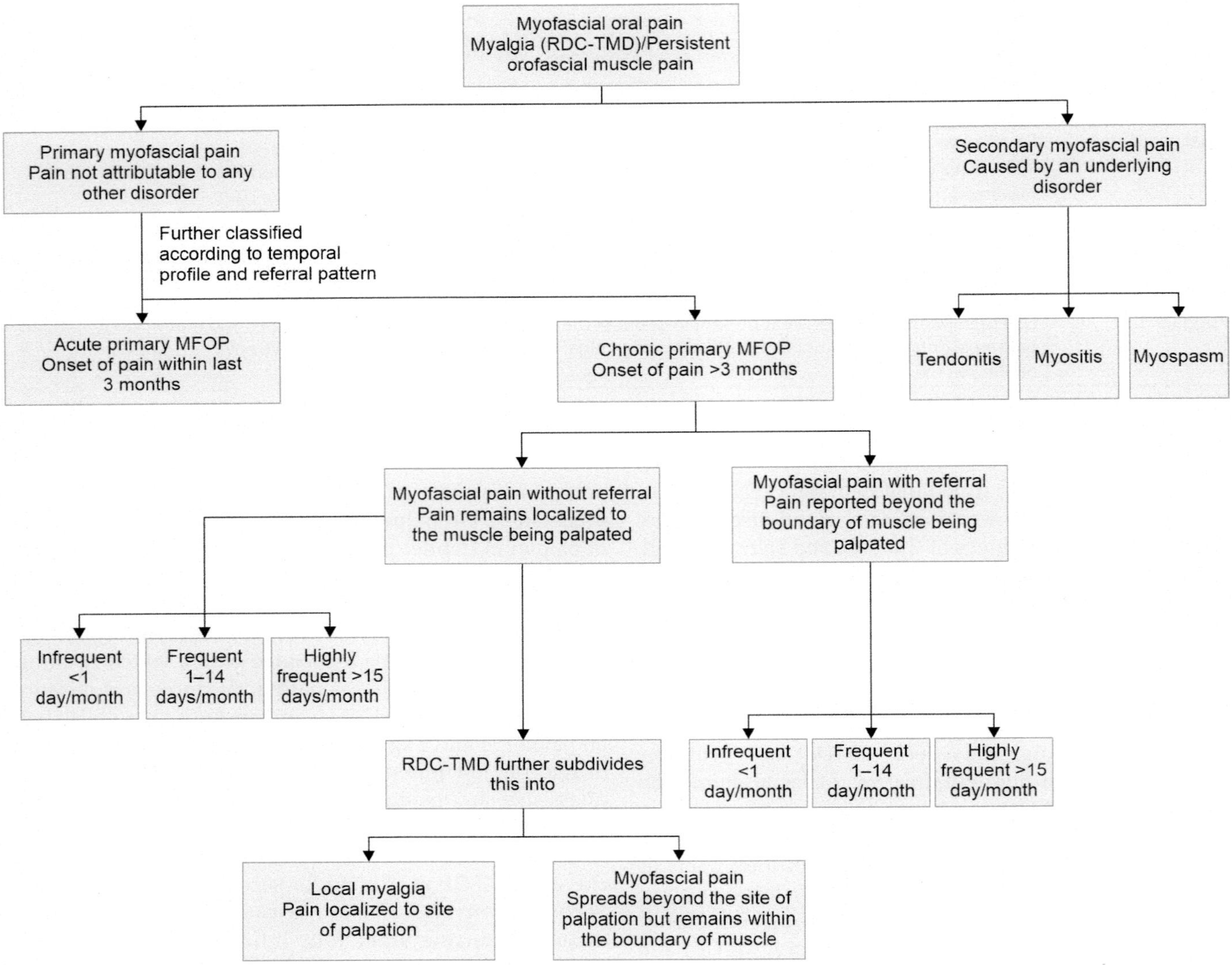

FLOWCHART 1: Classification of MFOP.
(MFOP: myofascial orofacial pain; RDC-TMD: research diagnostic criteria for temporomandibular disorders)

or loss of molar teeth, and teeth clenching, can lead to distortion and degenerative changes in the TMJ.[13] Pain is usually localized in the preauricular region with radiation to the temporal area and face. Pain is moderate to intense and often present at rest, may fluctuate during the day with exacerbations during jaw movements. There may be a sharp component with referral to the ear.[14] Pain may be episodic with variable frequency or unremitting. Patients may report clicking noises or crepitus on jaw movements. Some patients may complain of deviation of mandible to the affected side on jaw opening or locking of the jaw in the opening or closing position. Patients may complain of associated tinnitus, earaches, headaches, and dizziness—Costen's syndrome.[15] Examination reveals tenderness over the joint, crepitus on opening the mouth, and limitation of the jaw opening (normal > 40 mm).[11] To test for tenderness of the TMJ, the examiner can palpate the joint from its posterior aspect by placing the finger in the external auditory meatus and then pressing forward.[11] This maneuver should be able to replicate the familiar pain in the patient. Like MFOP, TMJ pain is also classified into primary and secondary forms **(Flowchart 2)**.[6] The TMJ pain is classified as primary TMJ pain [arthralgia in research diagnostic criteria for TMD (RDC-TMD criteria)] when no specific etiology or cause can be identified. The underlying etiologies for secondary TMJ pain can be arthritis, disc displacements (DDs), degenerative joint disease (DJD), and subluxation. It should be noted that these TMJ conditions—DD and DJD—are very common in the general population and may not necessarily be associated with pain.[10] Magnetic resonance imaging (MRI) can be used to substantiate the clinical diagnosis of joint disease and rule out other pathological conditions.[11] Appropriate investigations to determine the cause of arthritis such as rheumatoid factor, anticyclic citrullinated peptide

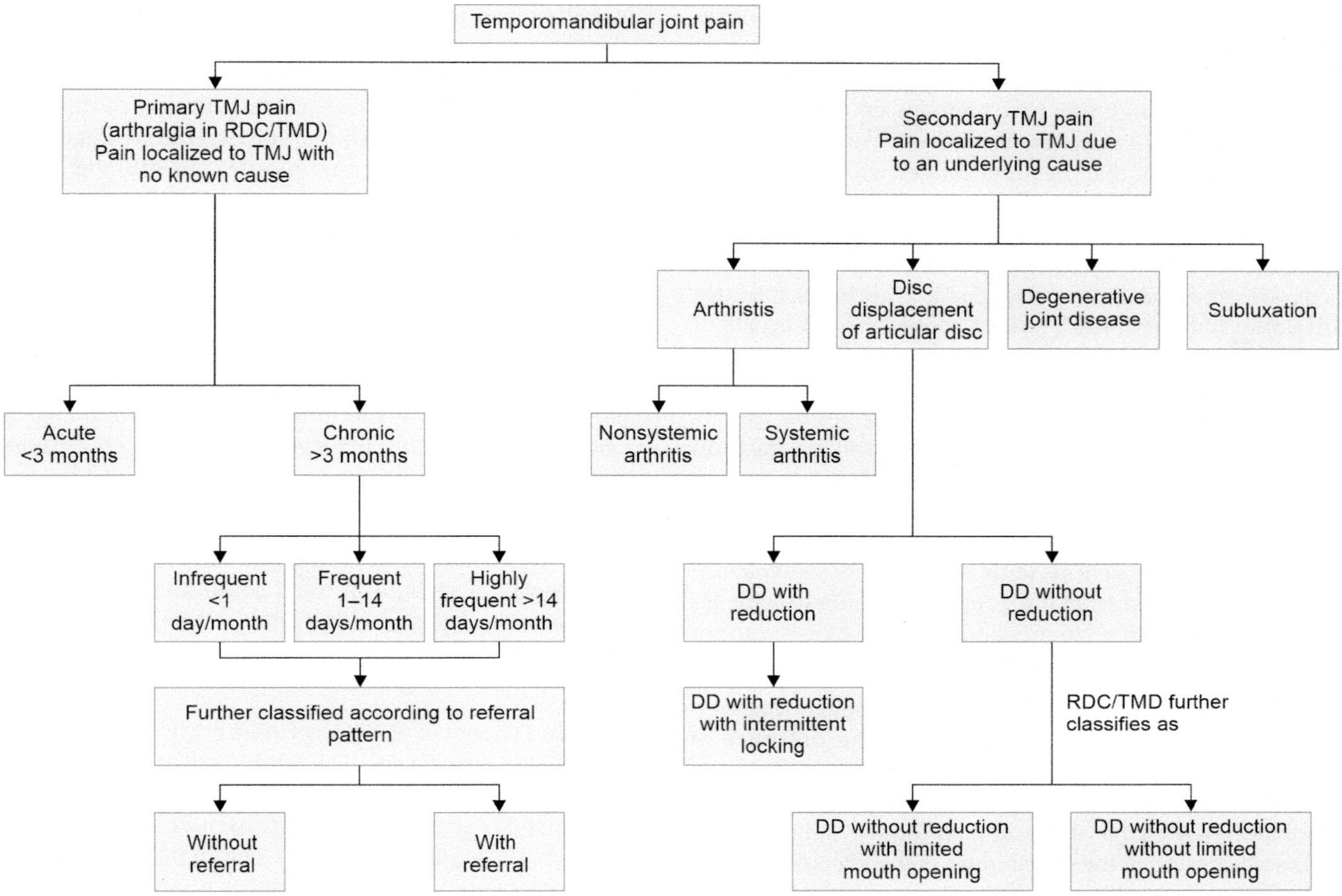

FLOWCHART 2: Classification of TMJ disorders.

(DD: disc displacement; RDC/TMD: research diagnostic criteria for temporomandibular disorders; TMJ: temporomandibular joint)

antibodies, antinuclear antibodies (ANA), and uric acid may also be needed.[11]

Treatment of most cases of TMD is through self-management with education, physiotherapy, and cognitive behavior therapy forming the cornerstone of therapy in most cases.[16] Physical strategies such as stretching and relaxation oral splints have been used with modest efficacy [number needed to treat (NNT) of 3–4 for MFOP and 5–6 for TMJ arthralgia].[14] Pharmacological therapies include simple analgesics, tricyclic antidepressants (amitriptyline), and gabapentin with variable success. Surgical procedures such as arthrocentesis and arthroscopy should be used only in cases of functional limitation.[14]

CRANIAL NEURALGIAS

Cranial neuralgias are one of the most debilitating forms of pain that are known to mankind. *TN* is the most common cranial neuralgia. Its prevalence is estimated to be between 5 and 29 per 100, 1,000 person-years.[17,18] Females are almost twice as likely to be affected as compared to males with a peak age of onset in the fifth decade.[19] TN classically manifests as paroxysmal stereotyped attacks of intense sharp electric shock-like sensation or stabbing pain in the distribution of one or more divisions of the trigeminal nerve.

Location: The pain is strictly localized to the distribution of CN V in contrast to short-lasting unilateral neuralgiform headache attacks (SUNHA) in which extratrigeminal spread may be seen.[1] Pain most commonly involves the V2 and V3 subdivisions. Isolated involvement of V1 is seen in <5% of patients.[19] A single division (V2 or V3) is involved in 36% of cases, and two divisions (V2 and V3) are involved in 35%, with all three divisions involved in 17% of cases.[20] TN is classically unilateral. It may become bilateral over time in 4% of cases,[19] though simultaneous onset on both sides is rare and should raise suspicion of multiple sclerosis (MS).

Quality: Pain in TN is paroxysmal, which is maximal at onset, and there may be associated facial muscle spasms due to the severity of pain—tic douloureux. The pain can be variably described as shooting, piercing, stabbing, or electric shock-like in nature. It is extremely severe, rated as 9–10 on the visual analog scale (VAS) by the patients.[21]

Temporal pattern: The individual attacks have a rapid onset and abrupt cessation, with each attack lasting from 10 seconds to 2 minutes.[1] The paroxysms are brief, lasting only a few seconds, though this may be followed by a lingering postshock pain that may last for a few minutes (<2). The duration of attacks may become longer with time, and a minority of patients may report that attacks last for up to 4–5 minutes. The paroxysms may recur in rapid succession, sometimes with a refractory period. These repetitive paroxysms may occur in cycles lasting up to 60 minutes with some patients (40%) having more than 10 cycles of paroxysmal pain per day.[19] The refractory period is a key diagnostic feature of TN, which helps differentiate TN from other ultrashort facial pains. The refractory period usually lasts 2–3 minutes but its presence and duration may depend on the severity and duration of the preceding paroxysm.[19] TN patients very rarely have nocturnal attacks. Classically, patients with TN may go into remissions of variable duration (lasting weeks to years) with subsequent relapses.[19] However, most cases have a progressive course with an increasing frequency of attacks and increasing resistance to pharmacotherapy and surgical treatment.

Triggers: Almost all patients with TN experience triggered pain. In fact, ICOP and ICHD-3 require the presence of triggered attacks as an essential criterion for the diagnosis of TN.[1,6] There may be a short period of latency between the stimulation of a trigger area and pain onset.[22] Trigger areas are usually located in the distribution of the affected division and are often located near the midline, particularly around the lips and in the gingivae.[23] Trigger zones can sometimes be demonstrated on physical examination, though demonstrating these zones may be difficult.[1,6] The triggering stimuli are usually innocuous and include talking (76%), chewing (74%), touch (65%), temperature (cold 48%, heat 1%), wind, and shaving.[24] It should be noted that trigger-like areas may be detected in about 9% of other causes of orofacial pain such as SUNHA, so the presence of trigger zones is suggestive but not pathognomonic of TN.[25] Notably triggering factors (such as noise, light, and stress) are distinct from trigger areas. These also are nonspecific and may be seen in other orofacial pain syndromes.

Autonomic symptoms (AS): They are usually mild and most often seen in V1 distribution TN.[19] The presence of AS, especially when prominent, is more suggestive of SUNHA.

Concomitant continuous pain: In almost 50% of patients with TN, there may be a concomitant continuous pain of variable duration and severity in addition to paroxysmal pain (atypical TN, TN type 2). It is usually milder than paroxysmal pain with a median intensity of 4.6 on VAS. Usually, the concomitant continuous pain starts after the onset of paroxysmal pain with a median lag of 1.5 years. In about 18% of patients, the persistent pain may be present before the onset of paroxysmal pain—pre-TN.[26] This pain is usually a dull, continuous aching pain localized in the jaw that can often be mistaken for dental pain and lead to unnecessary dental procedures. The duration of this pain can also be variable.[27] In some patients, it may linger as a postparoxysm pain for a few minutes. In other patients (~50%), continuous pain is present throughout the day, while 21% of patients have pain for more than half of the day.[27] Sensory abnormalities are more common in patients with continuous pain (48%) as compared to those with purely paroxysmal pain.[22] In almost half of the patients, the continuous pain can also be triggered by innocuous stimuli such as wind and talking. Central sensitization of the central trigeminal processing is the most likely pathophysiological mechanism responsible for the concomitant continuous pain in TN.[22]

Associated sensory and motor signs: Sensory disturbances such as hypoesthesia are rare but may occur in some patients particularly late in the disease and can be more readily detected by employing sophisticated examination techniques.[1,6,19] Thus, the presence of sensory abnormalities does not rule out a diagnosis of TN.[1,6]

Diagnosis: Diagnosis of TN is primarily clinical according to diagnostic criteria for TN published by ICHD-3 and ICOP, which are listed in **Box 1**.[6] TN has been classified as classical TN (caused by neurovascular compression), secondary TN (caused by MS or cerebellopontine angle tumor, arteriovenous malformation), and idiopathic. Although bilateral pain, isolated involvement of V1 division, sensory loss, and younger age of onset are indicators of secondary TN, it is difficult to clinically differentiate primary from secondary TN.[6] Therefore, all patients with TN should undergo imaging with a high-resolution MRI with thin cuts through the region of the trigeminal ganglion with heavily T2-weighted images with contrast and three-dimensional (3D) time-of-flight magnetic resonance angiography (MRA) to look for neurovascular compression and rule out secondary causes.[28] Mere contact of a vessel with CN V is insufficient to diagnose neurovascular compression.[6] Diagnosis of primary TN requires the presence of morphological changes such as dislocation, distortion, atrophy, or compression of the nerve at its origin in the pons either on imaging or during surgery **(Flowchart 3)**. Differential diagnosis includes trigeminal neuropathic pain, dental pain, SUNHA [SUNHA with conjunctival injection and tearing (SUNCT)/SUNHA with cranial autonomic symptoms (SUNA)], primary stabbing headache, first bite syndrome, and persistent idiopathic facial pain (PIFP). **Table 4** lists the differentiating features of common differential diagnoses of facial pain. It is important to note that in patients with pre-TN, thermal stimuli may trigger a throbbing type of pain, thus mimicking dental pain. Since

BOX 1 Diagnostic criteria for trigeminal neuralgia.

4.1.1 Trigeminal neuralgia

A. Recurrent paroxysms of unilateral facial pain in the distribution(s) of one or more divisions of the trigeminal nerve, with no radiation beyond 1 and fulfilling criteria B and C

B. Pain has all the following characteristics:
   1. Lasting from a fraction of a second to 2 minutes
   2. Severe intensity
   3. Electric shock-like, shooting, stabbing or sharp in quality

C. Precipitated by innocuous stimuli within the affected trigeminal distribution

D. Not better accounted for by another ICOP or ICHD-3 diagnosis

4.1.1.1 Classical trigeminal neuralgia

A. Recurrent paroxysms of unilateral pain fulfilling criteria for trigeminal neuralgia

B. Demonstration on MRI or during surgery of neurovascular compression (not simply contact), with morphological changes 1 in the trigeminal nerve root

4.1.1.1.1 Classical trigeminal neuralgia, purely paroxysmal: Pain-free between attacks in the affected trigeminal distribution

4.1.1.1.2 Classical trigeminal neuralgia with concomitant continuous pain: Concomitant continuous or near-continuous pain between attacks in the ipsilateral trigeminal distribution

4.1.1.2 Secondary trigeminal neuralgia

A. Recurrent paroxysms of unilateral pain fulfilling criteria for 4.1.1 trigeminal neuralgia, either purely paroxysmal or associated with concomitant continuous or near-continuous pain

B. An underlying disease has been demonstrated that is known to be able to cause, and explain, the neuralgia 2

C. Not better accounted for by another ICOP or ICHD-3 diagnosis

4.1.1.3 Idiopathic trigeminal neuralgia

A. Recurrent paroxysms of unilateral pain fulfilling criteria for 4.1.1 trigeminal neuralgia, either purely paroxysmal or associated with concomitant continuous or near-continuous pain

B. Neither 4.1.1.1 classical trigeminal neuralgia nor 4.1.1.2 secondary trigeminal neuralgia has been confirmed by adequate investigations

C. Not better accounted for by another ICHD-3 or ICOP diagnosis

(ICHD: International Classification of Headache Disorders; ICOP: International Classification of Orofacial Pain; MI: magnetic resonance imaging)

dental pain is much more common than TN, a careful dental evaluation should be done. A trial of carbamazepine should be given if no abnormality is found since pre-TN responds to carbamazepine.[29]

Treatment of TN is initially pharmacological, with carbamazepine and oxcarbazepine being the first-line agents **(Table 5)**.[28] TN patients have an excellent response to carbamazepine and oxcarbazepine, though the response may not be sustained over time. At least in the early course of TN, periodic attempts should be made to withdraw after a sustained pain-free interval of 3–6 months.[21] Surgical management includes microvascular decompression, rhizotomy, radiosurgery, and peripheral neurectomy. Surgical management in refractory TN patients with MS can provide short-term improvement in symptoms.[21] Some patients may have a double crush mechanism, i.e., a demyelinating lesion and neurovascular compression.[30] Phenytoin, lidocaine, and sumatriptan may be used as rescue therapy while the prophylactic medicines are being titrated.[31]

Cluster Tic Syndrome

Cluster tic syndrome is a combination of cluster headache (CH) and coexistent TN. There are three types of pain: paroxysmal short-lasting pain resembling TN, pain resembling CH of variable length (15–180 minutes) with the autonomic phenomenon, and a combination of both pains often provoked by trigger points and neck movements.[32]

Glossopharyngeal Neuralgia

Glossopharyngeal neuralgia (GN) is defined as paroxysmal pain in areas innervated by the glossopharyngeal nerve and the auricular and pharyngeal branches of the vagus nerve. Although GN is much rarer than TN, the quality of pain and the temporal profile are quite similar. The pain involves the ear, throat, tonsillar fossa, base of the tongue, or beneath the angle of the jaw.[1,6] GN may be associated with bradycardia and syncope due to the triggering of cardioinhibitory impulses by afferent vagal pain impulses.[33] Pain is triggered by chewing, talking, drinking, and swallowing.[33] Similar to TN, there may be a deep interictal burning type of pain or a globus or a foreign body sensation in the throat. Treatment is mainly medical, but the threshold for surgical management is lower in cases with syncope. Secondary GN can be caused by MS, regional infectious or inflammatory processes, cerebellopontine or pontine lesions, and tonsillar carcinoma.[6]

Nervus Intermedius Neuralgia

Nervus intermedius neuralgia (NIN) is characterized by pain deep in the ear with a trigger point in the posterior wall of the auditory canal. The pain is usually paroxysmal sharp and stabbing but may be of gradual onset and persistent nature.[34]

Other Trigeminal Neuropathic Pain/ Painful Trigeminal Neuropathy (PTN)

Facial pain in the distribution of one or more branches of CN V can be a result of a disorder associated with neural damage. Trigeminal neuropathy (TNO) can initially be associated with positive symptoms (paresthesia, dysesthesias, and pain), and as the disorder underlying it progresses and neurons are destroyed negative symptoms (sensory loss and motor weakness) become prominent. The primary pain is usually continuous or near continuous and is

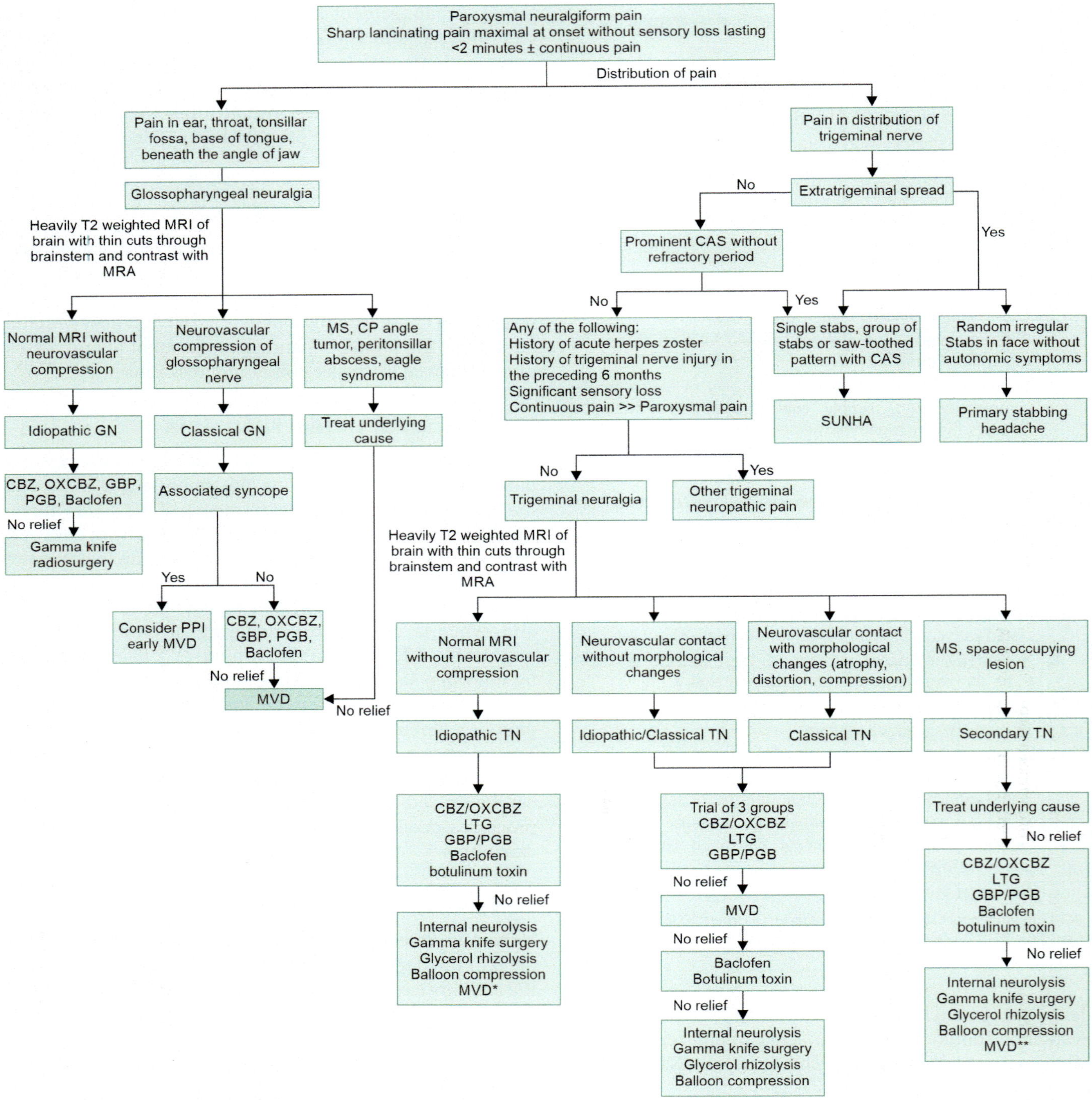

* MVD appears effective in idiopathic TN without neurovascular contact.

** MVD may be considered in secondary cases, if the underlying cause is optimally treated and there is evidence of neurovascular contact.

FLOWCHART 3: Algorithm for management of paroxysmal pain.

(CAS: cranial autonomic symptoms; CBZ: carbamazepine; CP: cerebellopontine; GBP: gabapentin; GN: glossopharyngeal neuralgia; LTG: lamotrigine; MRA: magnetic resonance angiography; MRI: magnetic resonance imaging; MS: multiple sclerosis; MVD: microvascular decompression; OXCBZ: oxcarbazepine; PGB: pregabalin; PPI: permanent pacemaker; SUNHA: short-lasting unilateral neuralgiform headache attacks; TN: trigeminal neuralgia)

TABLE 4: Differential diagnosis of facial pain.

	TN	TN with concomitant continuous pain	TMD	Trigeminal neuropathic pain	SUNHA	Facial cluster	NVOP	PIFP	BMS	PDAP
Age of onset	50–60	50–60	20–40	45–50	50–60	30–40	40–50	40–50	50–60	40–50
Gender (F:M)	2:1	2:1	2:1	F > M	2:1	1:5	1:3	F >> M	5:1	F >> M
Pain										
Location Intraoral/facial	IO + F	IO + F	F	IO + F	F	IO + F	IO	F	IO	F
Trigeminal division involved	II, III > I	II, III > I	III	Depends on cause	I = II > III	II/III	II/III	Spreads	Spreads	Spreads
Extratrigeminal spread	No	No	Yes	No	Yes	Yes	Yes	Yes	No	No
Paroxysmal/ continuous	P	P >> C	C	C + P	P	P	C	C	C	C
Laterality	Uni	Uni	Uni > B/L	Uni >> B/L	Uni	Uni	Uni > B/L	Uni > B/L	B/L	Uni
Side locked	Yes	Yes	No	Yes	Yes	Yes	No	No	No	No
Duration	1–120 seconds	Variable	Hours to days	Hours to days	1–600 seconds	15–180 minutes	1 hour to 4 days	Hours to days	Hours to days	Hours to days
Frequency	Variable (10–100/day)	Multiple + chronic	Chronic	Chronic	40–100/day	1–8/day	Episodic 1/day	Chronic	Chronic	Chronic
Quality	Stabs/ electrical	Stabs/electrical + aching	Pressure-like	Burning/ squeezing/pins and needles	Burning/ stabbing	Tearing/ stabbing	Throbbing/ toothache-like	Aching/burning/ throbbing	Burning	Deep pressure-like
Severity	Very severe	Very severe + moderate	Moderate	Moderate	Very severe	Very severe	Moderate	Moderate	Moderate	Moderate
Remissions	Yes	Less common	Yes	No	Yes	Yes	Yes	No (rare)	No (rare)	No (rare)
Wakens during sleep (%)	10	10	20	40		50	35	Rare	Rare	Rare
Autonomic signs	Rare	Rare	No	No	Yes	Yes	May occur	No	No	No
Triggers/ provoking factors	Cutaneous Non-nociceptive trigger	Cutaneous Non-nociceptive trigger	Jaw movement Clenching	Touch (allodynia)	Spontaneous >> trigger	Smells Alcohol Hypoxia	Cold stimuli	None	None	None
Relieving factors	Keeping still	Keeping still	Rest Decrease mouth opening	Avoid touch	Nil	Oxygen	Rest	None	Sucking lozenges	None

(B/L: bilateral; BMS: burning mouth syndrome; C: continuous; F: facial; IO: intraoral; NVOP: neurovascular orofacial pain; P: paroxysmal; PDAP: persistent dentoalveolar pain; PIFP: persistent idiopathic facial pain; SUNHA: short-lasting unilateral neuralgiform headaches; TMD: temporomandibular disorders; TN: trigeminal neuralgia)

TABLE 5: Treatment of trigeminal neuralgia.

Prophylactic therapy								
Drug	**Initial dose**	**Titration**	**Usual dose**	**Frequency**	**Tapering**	**Adverse effects**	**Level of evidence**	**Comments**
Carbamazepine	200 mg	200 mg every 3 days	200–1,200 mg	Two to four times per day	200 mg every 7 days	Dizziness, drowsiness, fatigue, ataxia, diplopia, nausea, cognitive slowing, hyponatremia leukopenia, thrombocytopenia, skin reactions, abnormal liver function tests	A	NNT = 1.9 Initial efficacy ~ 70–100% Later ~ 50%
Oxcarbazepine	300 mg	300 mg every 3 days	300–1,800 mg	Four times per day	300 mg every 7 days	Dizziness, drowsiness, fatigue, nausea, ataxia, hyponatremia, skin reaction	A	Similar in efficacy to CBZ Initial efficacy ~ 88% Better tolerated than CBZ
Lamotrigine	25 mg	25 mg for 2 weeks, 50 mg for 1 week, then increase by 50 mg every week	25–400 mg	Two times per day	50 mg every 7 days	Dizziness, drowsiness, fatigue, headache, gastrointestinal symptoms, irritability, sleep disorders, tremor, cognitive slowing, rash	A	NNT = 2.1 Evidence of efficacy as an add-on therapy
Baclofen	15 mg	15 mg every 7 days	15–90 mg	Three times per day	15 mg every 7 days	Confusion, dizziness, drowsiness, gastrointestinal symptoms, euphoria, hallucinations	A	NNT = 1.4
Gabapentin	300 mg	300 mg every 3 days	300–3,600 mg	Three times per day	300 mg every 7 days	Dizziness, confusion, fatigue, ataxia, increased risk of infection, gastrointestinal symptoms, weight gain; use cautiously with opioids	B	NNT for PHN = 3.9 Possibly effective in TN Used as an adjunct
Pregabalin	150 mg	150 mg every 7 days	150–600 mg	Two times per day	100 mg every 7 days	Dizziness, confusion, ataxia, increased risk of infection, gastrointestinal symptoms, weight gain	C	
Topiramate	25 mg	25 mg/week	100–200 mg	Twice a day	25 mg/week	Cognitive impairment, weight loss, sedation, paresthesia, fatigue, dizziness, depression, and mood problems, kidney stones, acute myopia, and secondary angle-closure glaucoma	C	
Botulinum toxin type A	25–195 units	NA	25–195 units	Every 12 weeks	NA	Transient facial asymmetry, transient bruising at injection site, transient drooling and difficulty in chewing	B	50% responder rate = 77%

Continued

Continued

Rescue therapy					
Drug	**Route**	**Dose**	**Duration of action**	**Level of evidence**	**Adverse events**
Lidocaine	IV infusion	5 mg/kg/h for 1 hour	~24 hours	Moderate 52% reduction in pain score at 24 hours	Somnolence requires continuous cardiac monitoring with ECG and frequent blood pressure checks
	Nasal	8% lidocaine (0.2 mL) for V2 TN	5 hours	High Complete relief in 40%	Stinging, burning, or numbness in nose
	Oral	8% lidocaine (0.2 mL) rubbed into trigger zone	2.8 hours	Moderate Complete relief in 46%	Stinging, burning, or numbness
Sumatriptan	SC	3–6 mg	1–20 hours	High Complete pain free in 50%	Mild elevation in blood pressure, fatigue, nausea
	Oral	50 mg once a day for 1 week (following SC sumatriptan)	1 week	Low Maintained analgesia for 1 week	Chest pain, fatigue, malaise, sensation of tightness, vertigo
Phenytoin	IV infusion	15–18 mg/kg over 1 hour	1–20 days	Low Case reports	Cardiac conduction disorder, purple glove syndrome, edema, discoloration, and pain distal to injection site

Surgical therapy										
Procedure	**Efficacy (pain-free %)**	**Mortality**	**Morbidity**							
			Facial sensory changes	Corneal hy-poesthesia	Hearing loss	Motor weakness	Cranial nerve palsy	Meningitis	CSF leak	Anesthesia dolorosa
Microvascular decompression	Overall: 62–89% 2 years: 81% 5 years: 76% 10 years: 70%	0.3–0.4%	3%	0.3%	1.8%	0	4.1%	0.4%	0.02%	0.3%
Stereotactic radiosurgery	30–66%	0	16%	0	0	0	0.2	0	0	0
Radiofrequency thermocoagulation	26–82% 2 years: 68% 5 years: 48%	0	19%	6.6%	0.1%	6.2%	0.8%	0.02%	0.1%	0.6%
Balloon compression	55–80% 2 years: 79%	0	15%	0.7%	0	4.5%	1.6%	5.7%	0	0.1%
Glycerol rhizolysis	19–58% 2 years: 63% 5 years: 45%	0	40%	6.6%	0.3%	1.7%	0	0	0	0.7%
Internal neurolysis	72%	0	96%	0	0	0	0	0	3.8%	3.9%

(CBZ: carbamazepine; ECG: electrocardiogram; IV: intravenous; NA: not applicable; NNT: number needed to treat; PHN: postherpetic neuralgia; SC: subcutaneous; TN: trigeminal neuralgia) commonly described as burning, squeezing, or likened to pins and needles.[35] There may be associated superimposed paroxysms, but they are not the predominant pain type. Some conditions such as MS and cerebellopontine angle tumors can cause neuropathic pain or neuralgic pain. In such cases differentiation is made based on clinical characteristics—the quality of spontaneous pain, evoked pain, and presence of sensory deficits **(Table 3)**.

Clinical evaluation should focus on identifying the sensory and motor abnormalities associated with the involvement of CN V and other cranial nerves **(Table 2)**. The importance of assessing the corneal reflex in a suspected case of TNO cannot be overemphasized. In addition to neuroimaging with an MRI focusing on the CN V (MRI with and without gadolinium contrast with attention to the skull base, and extension to the upper cervical spinal cord), a blink reflex can also provide useful information about the pathology of CN V and its central connections.[35] TNO can be caused by several diseases including traumatic, vascular, inflammatory, demyelinating, infectious, and neoplastic disorders **(Box 2)**.[35]

BOX 2 Causes of TN.

Trauma:
- *Accidental*: Blunt, closed, and penetrating head injury, basilar skull fracture
- Surgical (for cerebellopontine angle tumors, MVD for TN)
- Dental (especially at third molar), denture trauma at the mental foramen
- Chemical (glycerol rhizotomy)
- Radiation

Inflammatory/autoimmune:
- Undifferentiated and mixed connective tissue disease
- Progressive systemic scleroderma
- Sjögren syndrome
- Sarcoidosis
- *Multiple sclerosis*: May cause both TN and TNO

Vascular:
- Pontomedullary ischemia or hemorrhage (CNS mimic)
- Vascular malformation

Neoplastic:
- Intra- or extracranial compression (meningioma, trigeminal or vestibular schwannoma, nasopharyngeal carcinoma)
- Perineural spread (adenoid cystic carcinoma, squamous cell carcinoma, lymphoma)
- Metastasis (breast and lung carcinoma, melanoma)
- Carcinomatous meningitis (breast and lung carcinoma, melanoma, lymphoma)

Infectious:
- *Leprosy*: Can cause TN and painful TNO
- *Varicella zoster virus*: Acute herpes zoster and postherpetic neuralgia
- Herpes simplex virus
- Lyme disease
- Syphilis
- Fungi (actinomycosis)

Degenerative:
- *TISN*: Paroxysmal pain ± ongoing pain with sensory loss

Toxic–metabolic:
- Stilbamidine, trichloroethylene, oxaliplatin, diabetes mellitus
- Idiopathic trigeminal neuropathy

Others:
- Amyloidosis, pseudotumor cerebri

(CNS: central nervous system; MVD: microvascular decompression; TISN: trigeminal isolated sensory neuropathy; TN: trigeminal neuralgia; TNO: trigeminal neuropathy)

Trigeminal Neuropathic Pain Attributed to Herpes Zoster

This is a unilateral facial pain most often in the distribution of V1 division associated with clinical or laboratory evidence of varicella-zoster virus reactivation. The pain of herpes zoster is typically a constant multimodal pain with burning, shooting, stabbing, aching, tingling, pricking, and itching components. Pain often precedes the vesicular eruption, though on occasions, there may not be any vesicular eruptions—zoster sine herpete. Pain associated with acute herpes zoster persists for 3 months.[36] If it persists for more than 3 months, it is labeled as postherpetic neuralgia (PHN).[1,6,36] The character of pain is similar to the pain seen in acute herpes zoster, and itching may be a prominent feature of PHN.[37] Although named as neuralgia, it is actually a neuropathy of neuronopathy involving the CN V.[6] Mostly pain develops with the onset of rash, but rarely it may develop later after the rash has healed. Risk factors for PHN include advanced age, severe prodromal pain, severe acute pain, and severe rash.[38] Treatment is primarily medical with amitriptyline, gabapentin, pregabalin, and topical lidocaine.[39]

Post-traumatic Trigeminal Neuropathic Pain

Post-traumatic trigeminal neuropathic (PTTN) pain (anesthesia dolorosa) is unilateral or bilateral facial pain caused by trauma to the trigeminal nerve or its branches with or without clinical signs of trigeminal nerve dysfunction. To diagnose PTTN, there should be a history of injury to the CN V and laboratory evidence of trigeminal nerve dysfunction.[1,6] If there is no electrophysiological or imaging evidence of CN V dysfunction, then a diagnosis of probable PTTN can be made.[6] Associated somatosensory signs (positive or negative) are usually present in the affected area. Pain may be constant, often associated with superimposed paroxysms. A similar condition may be seen due to the involvement of the glossopharyngeal nerve.[6] Differentiation needs to be made from persistent idiopathic dentoalveolar pain (PIDAP). Unlike PTTN, there is no temporal relationship with injury in PIDAP, and the pain and somatosensory changes do not follow neuroanatomically defined areas.[1,6]

OROFACIAL PAIN RESEMBLING PRIMARY HEADACHES

There is a significant overlap between primary headache disorders and facial pain. The trigeminocervical complex plays an important role in the pathophysiology of migraine and trigeminal autonomic cephalalgias (TAC) and pain in these conditions can be referred to the face including the lower part of the face. So, some patients with headaches can have additional facial pain.[6] Another group is of patients whose headaches have been replaced by facial pain, the so-called relocated migraine.[40] Finally, there are headache naïve patients who develop de novo orofacial pain attacks that resemble one of the primary headaches **(Fig. 1)**. Some migraine patients (~8.9%) may have pain in the malar region and upper and lower teeth in addition to the headache.[41] Those having facial pain tend to have significantly more AS as compared to those with a pure headache. Isolated facial migraine however is rare (~0.2%).[42] The clinical features and diagnostic criteria of facial migraine are otherwise similar to migraine.[6] There may be episodic or chronic pain occurring exclusively in the orofacial region with characteristics similar to TTH—tension-type orofacial pain. This however is distinct from MFOP, which is characterized by pain and tenderness in the masticatory muscles.[6] At present, there is insufficient evidence to establish any relationship between the two entities. TACs are characterized by pain in the distribution of CN V, usually the V1 division, and the pain is primarily periorbital along with prominent AS. So, by definition, the periorbital region is in the face, making TACs an important cause of orofacial pain. CH is characterized by severe, strictly unilateral, side-locked headache and/or orofacial pain lasting 15–180 minutes with AS and/or restlessness.[1] CH has two subtypes—upper CH (periorbital pain radiates to the forehead, temporal, and parietal regions) and lower CH (periorbital pain radiates to teeth, jaws, and neck). Lower CH patients have more AS compared to upper CH.[43] Less

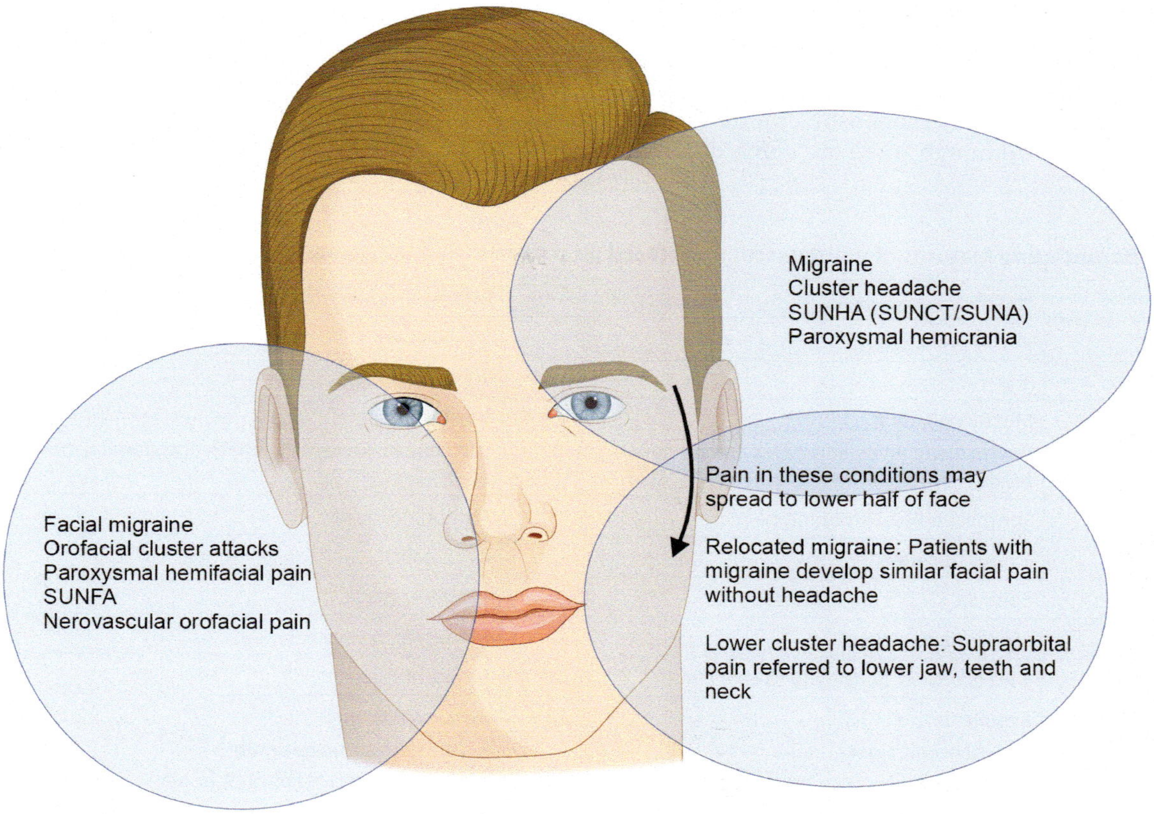

FIG. 1: Overlap of primary headache disorders and facial pain.

(SUNA: short-lasting unilateral neuralgiform headache attacks with cranial autonomic symptoms; SUNCT: short-lasting unilateral neuralgiform headache attacks with conjunctival injection and tearing; SUNFA: short-lasting unilateral neuralgiform facial attacks with autonomic signs; SUNHA: short-lasting unilateral neuralgiform headache attacks) commonly, patients with CH can have orofacial pain without the headache, which can resemble a toothache leading to dental extractions.[44] Notably, AS may be less prominent in patients with facial cluster attacks. Paroxysmal hemifacial pain is the facial counterpart of paroxysmal hemicrania.[6] Finally, short-lasting unilateral neuralgiform facial pain attacks with cranial AS (SUNFA) refer to facial pain attacks which resemble SUNHA.[6] SUNHA is a close differential diagnosis of TN with significant overlap in pathophysiology and clinical features, and it may be difficult to differentiate between the two conditions. While an extension of pain to the lower face may occur in hemicrania continua (HC), an isolated facial equivalent of HC has not yet been described.[6]

Neurovascular Orofacial Pain

Neurovascular orofacial pain (NVOP) is characterized by intraoral pain of variable duration (1 hour to 4 days), often accompanied by toothache-like or pulsating pain with mild migrainous symptoms or AS.[6] The autonomic/migrainous symptoms are mild and do not fulfill the criteria for facial migraine or TACs.[6] It is more commonly unilateral but can be bilateral.[45] The pain is moderately severe (6–9 on VAS) and may wake the patient from sleep. The pain primarily affects the alveolar process or the mucosa, but referral may occur to the perioral (lip, chin), infraorbital, and periauricular areas.[46] It may be episodic (1/3) or chronic (2/3) in nature.[2] The pain may be exaggerated by physical activity, and cold allodynia is characteristically present. Diagnostic criteria for NVOP are listed in **Box 3**.[6] Although there are some differences between migraine and NVOP **(Table 6)**, the treatment of NVOP is similar to that of migraine.

BOX 3 Diagnostic criteria for neurovascular orofacial pain.

5.4 Neurovascular orofacial pain

A. At least five attacks of unilateral intraoral pain 1 of variable duration, without head pain, fulfilling criteria B–D

B. Pain has both of the following characteristics:
   1. Moderate or severe intensity
   2. Either or both of the following qualities:
      a) Toothache-like
      b) Pulsating

C. Pain is accompanied by at least one of the following:
   1. Ipsilateral lacrimation and/or conjunctival injection
   2. Ipsilateral rhinorrhea and/or nasal congestion
   3. Ipsilateral cheek swelling
   4. Photophobia and/or phonophobia
   5. Nausea and/or vomiting

D. Pain is unexplained by any local cause, and clinical and radiographic examinations are normal

E. Not better accounted for by another ICOP or ICHD-3 diagnosis.

(ICHD: International Classification of Headache Disorders; ICOP: International Classification of Orofacial Pain)

Idiopathic Orofacial Pain

Idiopathic orofacial pain is a term used for diseases characterized by intraoral or facial pain that does not

TABLE 6: Differentiating features of neurovascular orofacial pain (NVOP) and migraine.

	NVOP	Migraine
Age of onset	40–50 years	20–40 years
Male:female	1:3	1:2
Location	Mostly unilateral *Pain in teeth*: Alveolar process and mucosa of multiple teeth, may radiate to the face	Mostly unilateral In forehead, lower face (cheek and maxilla), nose, jaw, and teeth
Character of pain	Toothache-like, throbbing pain	Throbbing, deep
Duration	1 hour to 4 days	4–72 hours
Time course	Episodic (2/3) > chronic (1/3)	Mostly episodic
Pain intensity	Moderate to severe	Moderate to severe
Precipitating factors	*Cold allodynia*: Sensitivity to cold stimuli	Stress, hunger, etc.
Associated signs	*Requires one of*: • Autonomic signs • Nausea and/or vomiting • Photophobia and/or phonophobia	*Requires one of*: • Nausea and/or vomiting • Photophobia and phonophobia

TABLE 7: Causes of secondary burning mouth syndrome.

Cause	Comments and investigations
Candidiasis	
Lichen planus	
Herpetic infections	
Xerostomia	
Drugs	Angiotensin-converting enzyme inhibitors Anticholinergic medications
• Sjögren syndrome • Systematic lupus erythematosus • Rheumatoid arthritis	• ANA, anti SS-A, anti SS-B • Rheumatoid factor • Anti-CCP
• Nutritional deficiencies—vitamin B12. • Folate, iron deficiency	• Serum vitamin B12 • Serum folate • Hemoglobin, serum ferritin, serum iron profile
Untreated diabetes	Blood sugar, HbA1c
Thyroid abnormalities	Thyroid function tests

(ANA: antinuclear antibodies; CCP: cyclic citrullinated peptide; HbA1c: glycated hemoglobin; SS: Sjögren syndrome)

follow the distribution of a particular branch or division of CN V, is poorly localized, and has a dull, pressing, or burning character. In general, no underlying etiology can be identified for these disorders.[6]

Burning Mouth Syndrome

Burning mouth syndrome (BMS) (stomatodynia, glossodynia) is characterized by a chronic intraoral burning or dysesthetic sensation felt superficially in the oral mucosa.[6] Pain is most commonly felt bilaterally and symmetrically in the tip of the tongue but can also be present on the dorsum and lateral aspect of the tongue, anterior aspect of the hard palate, and labial mucosa of lips. The pain does not follow peripheral nerve distribution, which helps in differentiating from pre-TN.[47] Approximately 50% of patients have a spontaneous onset; rest may identify a trigger such as infection, dental procedure, or medication use. The pain usually occurs daily, and is continuous, though its severity may fluctuate, often worsening over the day. In some patients, it may be intermittent but should last for >2 hours per day.[6] The pain in BMS is usually provoked by stress and eating spicy foods, but in others distraction and eating or drinking may relieve the pain. The severity of pain is variable, varying from mild discomfort to the worst possible pain. Some patients may complain of dry mouth, taste disturbance, hyposalivation, and thirst. Several local and systemic conditions affecting the oral mucosa can sometimes cause similar symptoms (previously secondary BMS), which should be ruled out by appropriate investigations **(Table 7)**.[48] The pathophysiology of BMS is not clear, but recent evidence has shown that it is an intraoral small fiber neuropathy with abnormal brainstem reflex responses. There is significant comorbidity with depression and anxiety, which is more likely the result of BMS. Management consists of patient education, avoidance of spicy foods, and sucking sugar-free lozenges. Pharmacological therapy in the form of alpha lipoic acid, capsaicin, clonazepam (topical or systematic), gabapentin, and pregabalin have been tried with variable success.[47] Less than 5% of patients may undergo spontaneous remission. Pramipexole has also been used in BMS with the premise that the number of unoccupied D2 dopamine receptors is increased in chronic painful conditions.[49]

Persistent Idiopathic Facial Pain/Atypical Facial Pain

Persistent idiopathic facial pain is a chronic daily persistent facial pain that occurs in the absence of any clinical neurological deficit or preceding causative event.[6] The pain is poorly localized and does not follow the distribution of a peripheral nerve. The pain predominantly starts unilaterally in the cheeks (nasolabial fold) and upper jaw but may become bilateral and radiate or spread to a wider area in the craniocervical pattern in a nondermatomal fashion. Although sensory loss is not demonstratable, some patients may complain of paresthesias in the form of "concrete poured on the face and moving around." Quantitative sensory testing may reveal somatosensory changes. The pain may be spontaneous in onset or may be triggered by minor surgical or otolaryngologic procedures. The pain is variably described as aching, burning, throbbing, and often stabbing. Severity is also variable, varying from mild to severe (mean VAS score = 7). The severity of pain may fluctuate with exacerbations related to stress, but paroxysmal neuralgic pain is not seen.[40] The present theory for the pathogenesis of PIFP is a disproportionate reaction of the somatosensory system to a mild injury. Rarely persistent facial pain may be caused by lesions such as nasopharyngeal carcinoma or apical lung carcinoma, thereby requiring close observation while managing such patients.[40] Treatment is primarily cognitive behavioral therapy supplemented by tricyclic antidepressants and serotonin-norepinephrine reuptake inhibitors.[40]

Persistent Idiopathic Dentoalveolar Pain/Atypical Odontalgia/Phantom Tooth Pain

Persistent idiopathic dentoalveolar pain is a pain localized to the dentoalveolar site of a molar or premolar tooth. It starts in localized dentoalveolar tissue but may move from one tooth to another. With progression, pain may spread to a wider area including the face. The pain may be described as deep or superficial, often as a pressure-like quality. It is moderately severe and occurs daily with exacerbations often related to stress.[6] Treatment is similar to PIFP.

Constant Unilateral Facial Pain with Additional Attacks

Constant unilateral facial pain with additional attacks (CUFPA) is a recently described pain syndrome characterized by constant (unremitting), dull, side-locked facial pain of mild-to-moderate intensity, accompanied by distinct attacks of moderate-to-severe pain in the same location lasting 10–30 minutes. There are no typical autonomic and/or migrainoid features accompanying either the constant pain or the additional pain attacks.[50]

Central Facial Pain

Central facial pain can be caused by the involvement of the central somatosensory pathways as in MS and stroke.[1] MS can cause both TN and central facial pain due to demyelinating lesions involving the central connections of CN V. The central pain in MS may be continuous pain often associated with sensory disturbances. A stroke in the brainstem affecting the central connections of CN V and the thalamus can also cause facial pain.[51] According to ICHD-3, the onset of pain must be within 3 months of the stroke, though cases with delayed onset have been reported.[1] The pain is usually continuous and often described as burning, aching, pricking, or lacerating. Burning pain is more common in brainstem lesions, while thalamic lesions cause lacerating pain.[52] Associated sensory symptoms (paresthesias, dysesthesias) and sensory loss are common. Most poststroke pain would involve other areas of the body as well, and isolated facial pain is most commonly seen in brainstem lesions involving the medulla.[52] Pharmacological treatment is primarily with amitriptyline, lamotrigine, gabapentin, and pregabalin.[51]

Facial Pain Associated with Vascular Disorders

Giant Cell Arteritis

Giant cell arteritis is an important differential diagnosis of facial pain in patients >50 years of age. The pain is commonly temporal and preauricular in location; it can be more widespread and even involve the tongue. In jaw claudication, pain typically begins with latency after heavy chewing and is localized to the masticatory muscles. In some cases, trismus like a symptom, rather than fatigue or pain, may occur. Prompt treatment with steroids is necessary for this vision-threatening condition.[12]

Carotidynia

Carotidynia is an obsolete term coined by Temple Fay to designate a special type of cervicofacial pain that could be elicited by pressure on the common carotid artery in patients with atypical facial pain.[52] ICHD-3 recognizes that noninflammatory disorders of cervical arteries can cause craniofacial pain but has removed the term carotidynia because it was not considered a distinct clinical entity but a syndrome encompassing varieties of causes of pain in the cervicofacial region.[1] Dissection of the carotid artery is the most important cause of pain in the neck radiating to the cheek or periorbital region along with ipsilateral Horner syndrome. Other causes of a similar syndrome include aneurysms, carotid body tumor, large vessel vasculitis, fibromuscular dysplasia, and various inflammatory or neoplastic processes involving the neck. Of note, *transient perivascular inflammation of the carotid artery (TIPIC)* is characterized by acute pounding, sharp or dull pain in the neck that may radiate to the jaw and face along with the tenderness of the carotid artery.[52] This is usually a self-limiting condition lasting for a few days to months. During the attack, pain may be aggravated by head movement, chewing, and swallowing. The disease is thought to be related to swelling or inflammation of the tissue surrounding carotid bifurcation, which is often visible on MRI/computed tomography (CT). Treatment is mainly supportive in the form of analgesics, and steroids can decrease pain in severe cases.[52]

CONCLUSION

Facial pain is a common complaint with a wide differential diagnosis that can have a significant social and psychological impact on the quality of life of the patient. Accurate diagnosis and management require a good history and meticulous examination. An attempt should be made to differentiate neuralgia; neuropathic, headache-related facial pain; and idiopathic pain **(Flowchart 4)**. A pain drawing by the patient can be of enormous value in delineating the cause of pain. The importance of a dental examination and imaging cannot be overemphasized. Neuroimaging should focus on the lower cranial nerves and brainstem to identify any secondary lesions. Finally, the management of facial pain requires a holistic and multidisciplinary approach with a biopsychological model in association with medical and surgical management.

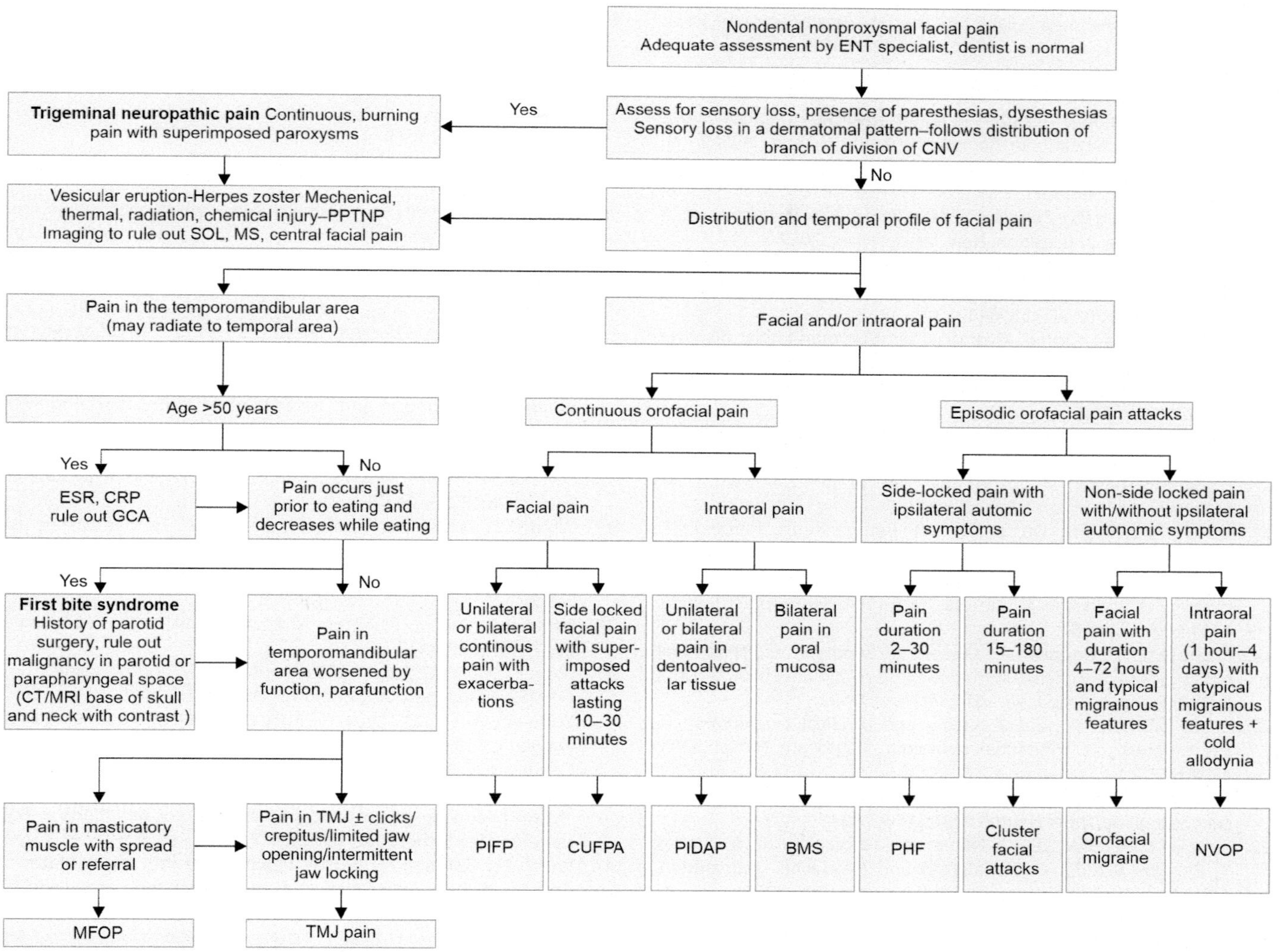

FLOWCHART 4: Approach to nondental facial pain.

(BMS: burning mouth syndrome; CNV: cranial nerve V; CRP: C-reactive protein; CT: computed tomography; CUFPA: continuous unilateral facial pain with attacks; ENT: ear, nose, and throat; ESR: erythrocyte sedimentation rate; GCA: giant cell arteritis; MFOP: myofascial orofacial pain; MRI: magnetic resonance imaging; MS: multiple sclerosis; NVOP: neurovascular orofacial pain; PHF: paroxysmal hemifacial pain; PIDAP: persistent idiopathic dentoalveolar pain; PIFP: persistent idiopathic facial pain; PTNP: post-traumatic trigeminal neuropathic pain; SOL: space-occupying lesion; TMJ: temporomandibular joint)

REFERENCES

1. Headache Classification Committee of the International Headache Society (IHS). The International Classification of Headache Disorders, 3rd edition. Cephalalgia. 2018;38:1-211.
2. Benoliel R, Birman N, Eliav E, Sharav Y. The International Classification of Headache Disorders: accurate diagnosis of orofacial pain? Cephalalgia. 2008;28:752-62.
3. Bell GW, Smith GL, Rodgers JM, Flynn RW, Malone CH. Patient choice of primary care practitioner for orofacial symptoms. Br Dent J. 2008;204:669-73.
4. Matthews B, Sessle BJ. Peripheral mechanisms of orofacial pain. In: Sessle BJ, Lavigne GJ, Lund JP (Eds). Orofacial Pain, 2nd edition. Batavia: Quintessence Publishing Co. Inc.; 2020. pp. 27-43.
5. Sessle BJ. Acute and chronic craniofacial pain: brainstem mechanisms of nociceptive transmission and neuroplasticity, and their clinical correlates. Crit Rev Oral Biol Med. 2000;11(1):57-91.
6. International Classification of Orofacial Pain, 1st edition (ICOP). Cephalalgia. 2020;40(2):129-221.
7. Shephard MK, Macgregor EA, Zakrzewska JM. Orofacial pain: a guide for the headache physician. Headache. 2014;54(1):22-39.
8. Zakrzewska JM. Differential diagnosis of facial pain and guidelines for management. Br J Anaesth. 2013;111(1):95-104.
9. Maixner W, Diatchenko L, Dubner R, Fillingim RB, Greenspan JD, Knott C, et al. Orofacial pain prospective evaluation and risk assessment study—the OPPERA study. J Pain. 2011;12(11 suppl):T4-11.e1-2.
10. Gauer RL, Semidey MJ. Diagnosis and treatment of temporomandibular disorders. Am Fam Physician. 2015;91(6):378-86.
11. Schiffman E, Ohrbach R, Truelove E, Look J, Anderson G, Goulet JP, et al; International RDC/TMD Consortium Network, International association for Dental Research; Orofacial Pain Special Interest Group, International Association for the Study of Pain. Diagnostic criteria for temporomandibular disorders (DC/TMD) for clinical and research applications: recommendations of the International RDC/TMD Consortium Network and Orofacial Pain Special Interest Group. J Oral Facial Pain Headache. 2014;28(1):6-27.

12. Smith JH, Swanson JW. Giant cell arteritis. Headache. 2014;54(8): 1273-89.
13. Gesch D, Bernhardt O, Kocher T, John U, Hensel E, Alte D. Association of malocclusion and functional occlusion with signs of temporomandibular disorders in adults: results of the population-based study of health in Pomerania. Angle Orthod. 2004;74(4): 512-20.
14. Sessle BJ, Baad-Hansen L, Exposto F, Svensson P. Orofacial pain. In: Lynch ME, Craig KD, Peng PW (Eds). Clinical Pain Management: A Practical Guide, 2nd edition. New Jersey: Wiley; 2022.
15. Caio B, Ana Beatriz M, Mirto P. Updated review Costen's syndrome: clinical relationship between dentistry and medicine. Adv Dent Oral Health. 2020;12(5):555846.
16. Schindler H, Svensson P. Myofascial temporomandibular disorder pain. In: Turp JC, Sommer C, Hugger A (Eds). The Puzzle of Orofacial Pain: Pain and Headache. Basel: Karger Publishers; 2007. pp. 91-123.
17. MacDonald BK, Cockerell OC, Sander JW, Shorvon SD. The incidence and lifetime prevalence of neurological disorders in a prospective community-based study in the UK. Brain. 2000;123(Pt 4): 665-76.
18. Katusic S, Williams DB, Beard CM, Bergstralh EJ, Kurland LT. Epidemiology and clinical features of idiopathic trigeminal neuralgia and glossopharyngeal neuralgia: similarities and differences, Rochester, Minnesota, 1945-1984. Neuroepidemiology. 1991;10(5-6):276-81.
19. Maarbjerg S, Gozalov A, Olesen J, Bendtsen L. Trigeminal neuralgia—a prospective systematic study of clinical characteristics in 158 patients. Headache. 2014;54(10):1574-82.
20. Casey KF. Role of patient history and physical examination in the diagnosis of trigeminal neuralgia. Neurosurg Focus. 2005; 18(5):E1.
21. Lambru G, Zakrzewska J, Matharu M. Trigeminal neuralgia: a practical guide. Pract Neurol. 2021;21:392-402.
22. Benoliel R, Heir GM, Eliav E. Neuropathic orofacial pain. In: Sharav Y, Benoliel R (Eds). Orofacial Pain and Headache, 2nd edition. Chicago, Illinois: Quintessence Publishing Co., Inc.; 2015.
23. Cheshire WP Jr. Cranial neuralgias. Continuum (Minneap Minn). 2015;21(4 Headache):1072-85.
24. David Bowsher. Trigeminal neuralgia: a symptomatic study of 126 successive patients with and without previous interventions. Pain Clinic. 2000;12(2):93-101.
25. Sato J, Saitoh T, Notani K, Fukuda H, Kaneyama K, Segami N. Diagnostic significance of carbamazepine and trigger zones in trigeminal neuralgia. Oral Surg Oral Med Oral Pathol Oral Radiol Endod. 2004;97(1):18-22.
26. Wright E, Evans J. Oral pre-trigeminal neuralgia pain: clinical differential diagnosis and descriptive study results. Cranio. 2014;32(3):193-8.
27. Maarbjerg S, Gozalov A, Olesen J, Bendtsen L. Concomitant persistent pain in classical trigeminal neuralgia—evidence for different subtypes. Headache. 2014;54:1173-83.
28. Bendtsen L, Zakrzewska JM, Abbott J, Braschinsky M, Di Stefano G, Donnet A, et al. European Academy of Neurology guideline on trigeminal neuralgia. Eur J Neurol. 2019;26(6):831-49.
29. Benoliel R, Heir GM, Eliav E. Neuropathic orofacial pain. In: Sharav Y, Benoliel R (Eds). Orofacial Pain and Headache. Missouri: Mosby; 2008. pp. 255-94.
30. Truini A, Prosperini L, Calistri V, Fiorelli M, Pozzilli C, Millefiorini E, et al. A dual concurrent mechanism explains trigeminal neuralgia in patients with multiple sclerosis. Neurology. 2016;86:2094-9.
31. Moore D, Chong MS, Shetty A, Zakrzewska JM. A systematic review of rescue analgesic strategies in acute exacerbations of primary trigeminal neuralgia. Br J Anaesth. 2019;123(2):e385-96.
32. Alberca R, Ochoa JJ. Cluster tic syndrome. Neurology. 1994;44(6): 996-9.
33. Rushton JG, Stevens JC, Miller RH. Glossopharyngeal (vagoglossopharyngeal) neuralgia: a study of 217 cases. Arch Neurol. 1981;38(4):201-5.
34. Bruyn GW. Nervus intermedius neuralgia (Hunt). Cephalalgia. 1984;4(1):71-8.
35. Smith JH, Cutrer FM. Numbness matters: a clinical review of trigeminal neuropathy. Cephalalgia. 2011;31(10):1131-44.
36. Dworkin RH, Gnann JW Jr, Oaklander AL, Raja SN, Schmader KE, Whitley RJ. Diagnosis and assessment of pain associated with herpes zoster and postherpetic neuralgia. J Pain. 2008;9(1 Suppl 1): S37-44.
37. Dworkin RH, Portenoy RK. Pain and its persistence in herpes zoster. Pain. 1996;67(2-3):241-51.
38. Whitley RJ, Weiss HL, Soong SJ, Gnann JW. Herpes zoster: risk categories for persistent pain. J Infect Dis. 1999 Jan;179(1):9-15.
39. Johnson RW, Rice AS. Clinical practice. Postherpetic neuralgia. N Engl J Med. 2014;371(16):1526-33.
40. Benoliel R, Gaul C. Persistent idiopathic facial pain. Cephalalgia. 2017;37(7):680-91.
41. Eross E, Dodick D, Eross M. The sinus, allergy, and migraine study (SAMS). Headache. 2007;47(2):213-24.
42. Yoon MS, Mueller D, Hansen N, Poitz F, Slomke M, Dommes P, et al. Prevalence of facial pain in migraine: a population-based study. Cephalalgia. 2010;30(1):92-6.
43. Cademartiri C, Torelli P, Cologno D, Manzoni GC. Upper and lower cluster headache: clinical and pathogenetic observations in 608 patients. Headache. 2002;42(7):630-7.
44. Rozen TD, Fishman RS. Cluster headache in the United States of America: demographics, clinical characteristics, triggers, suicidality, and personal burden. Headache. 2012;52(1):99-113.
45. Benoliel R, Sharav Y, Eliav E. Neurovascular orofacial pain. J Am Dent Assoc. 2010;141(9):1094-6.
46. Benoliel R, Elishoov H, Sharav Y. Orofacial pain with vascular-type features. Oral Surg Oral Med Oral Pathol Oral Radiol Endod. 1997;84(5):506-12.
47. Klasser GD, Grushka M, Su N. Burning mouth syndrome. Oral Maxillofac Surg Clin North Am. 2016;28(3):381-96.
48. Zakrzewska JM. Multidimensionality of chronic pain of the oral cavity and face. J Headache Pain. 2013;14(1):37.
49. Cárcamo Fonfría A, Gómez-Vicente L, Pedraza MI, Cuadrado-Pérez ML, Guerrero Peral AL, Porta-Etessam J. Burning mouth syndrome: clinical description, pathophysiological approach, and a new therapeutic option. Neurologia. 2017;32:219.
50. Ziegeler C, May A. Facial presentations of migraine, TACs, and other paroxysmal facial pain syndromes. Neurology. 2019;93(12):e1138-47.
51. Klit H, Finnerup NB, Jensen TS. Central poststroke pain: clinical characteristics, pathophysiology, and management. Lancet Neurol. 2009;8(9):857-68.
52. Andersen G, Vestergaard K, Ingeman-Nielsen M, Jensen TS. Incidence of central poststroke pain. Pain. 1995;61(2):187-193.

36

CHAPTER

Approach to Ataxia

Vaibhav Mathur, Pettarusp M Wadia

INTRODUCTION

The term "*Ataxia*" has a Greek origin, which literally means the absence of order.[1] In modern clinical neurology, the term ataxia denotes disturbance in the coordination of movement and balance and is associated with dysfunction of the cerebellum or its afferent/efferent connections. This causes errors in the "rate, range, force, and direction" of movements.[2]

Ataxia is a neurological sign, not a disease by itself, and can be a manifestation of cerebellar dysfunction, or impaired vestibular or proprioceptive afferent input to the cerebellum. Underlying etiologies can range from nutritional causes and transient parainfectious processes to progressive degenerative and genetic ataxias. Identifying the cause can be clinically challenging. In this chapter, we aim to provide a stepwise approach to identify the possible causes.

The evaluation of ataxia constitutes a detailed history, thorough neurological examination, and appropriate investigations. The history must include the onset, duration and progression of symptoms, family history, notification of recent infections, seizures, head injury, and possible exposure to heavy metals, gases, solvents, or medications. Moreover, it is important to enquire regarding associated headaches, vomiting, photophobia, vertigo, and altered mental status.

CLASSIFICATION OF ATAXIA

Ataxia, based on localization, can be classified into three broad types **(Table 1)**:[3]

1. Sensory ataxia due to small- or large-fiber neuropathy/neuronopathy/dorsal column affection
2. Vestibular ataxia due to dysfunction of semicircular canals and/or otolith organs, or their efferent connections
3. Cerebellar ataxia due to altered cerebellar pathways

Additionally, gait is also affected in diseases involving the fronto-ponto-cerebellar fibers en route to synapse in the pontine nuclei and is called as frontal ataxia or preferably gait apraxia. Often, patients exhibit signs and symptoms of more than one type of ataxia, but the classification is primarily based on the major contributing type. Their distinguishing features are summarized in **Table 1**. In the most part of this chapter, we will focus mainly on an approach to the diagnosis of cerebellar ataxias.

TABLE 1: Summary of clinical differences among major types of ataxia.

	Cerebellar	Vestibular	Sensory
History	• Imbalance while walking, swaying to both sides, more in narrow passages, uneven grounds, stairs, and high heels • Clumsiness of limb movements, spillage of contents on pouring, eating • Speech issues • Head nodding • Transient double vision on quickly turning the head • Cognitive affection possible	• Prominent vertigo, dizziness, and vomiting • Positional vertigo • Associated tinnitus, hearing deficits, positional vertigo • Swaying to one side • Imbalance more on closing eyes	• Gait imbalance, with associated features of tingling, numbness, paresthesia, and distal foot weakness • Feeling of walking on cotton wool • Aggravation of imbalance in dark, washbasin sign • Spared speech and upper limbs

Continued

Continued

	Cerebellar	Vestibular	Sensory
Clinical examination	• Gaze-evoked nystagmus • Vertical nystagmus • Hypermetric/hypometric saccades, saccadic intrusions in primary gaze or pursuit • Scanning/staccato slow slurred speech • Dysdiadochokinesia • Intention tremors • Finger chase, finger–nose–finger, nose finger tests positive • Tandem gait for truncal/gait ataxia • Wide-based stance • Rarely false positive head impulse test[4,5]	• Rinne's, Weber's, Hennebert's test • HINTS examination: Head impulse test, nystagmus, and skew deviation (can differentiate peripheral and central causes) • Romberg test • Fukuda (Unterberger) test • Dix–Hallpike maneuver	• High steppage gait, stomping/feet slapping gait • Cautious gait • Impaired vibration and joint position sense • Positive Romberg sign • Pseudoathetosis possible in upper limbs • Hyporeflexia (DTRs may be retained in the dorsal column or nonlength-dependent dorsal root ganglion pathologies)
Causes	See **Tables 6 to 8**	• Peripheral causes (benign paroxysmal positional vertigo, labyrinthitis, vestibular migraine, acoustic neuroma) • Central causes (multiple sclerosis, progressive supranuclear palsy, multiple system atrophy, stroke, migraine, cerebellar disorders)[6]	See **Table 2**
Investigations	• Specific blood tests • MRI imaging • CSF testing • Genetic testing	• Pure tone audiometry • Caloric tests • MRI brain	• Nerve conduction studies • Vitamin B12, VDRL testing • MRI spine • CSF testing

(CSF: cerebrospinal fluid; DTR: deep tendon reflex; MRI: magnetic resonance imaging; VDRL: venereal disease research laboratory)

SENSORY ATAXIA

Abnormal gait can be caused by sensory disturbance, and its characteristics are related to the location of the lesion. Disorders might affect the sensory conduction from peripheral nerves/nerve roots, dorsal root ganglion, spinal roots, dorsal column, and even cerebellar, thalamic, and sensory cortical connections **(Fig. 1)**.

Patients with sensory ataxia present with gait disturbance due to misplaced and/or mistimed foot placement, with significant worsening of unsteadiness with visual deprivation (while overhead removal of clothes, during face wash in a basin, or in dim light). They may lift their legs to a very high position (high-stepping gait), might put their feet down in a stomping fashion, or slap their feet on the ground while walking. Peripheral nerve affection may have additional tingling, numbness neuropathic pain, and/or distal motor weakness, while diseases affecting dorsal root ganglion and dorsal column would have ataxia, proprioceptive and vibration sense deficits out of proportion to temperature, pain, and motor deficits. The discordance between the sensory ataxia and loss of reflexes but normal sensory nerve conduction studies should make one consider the involvement of the dorsal root ganglion or the sensory roots suspicious of a sensory neuronopathy. Causes of sensory neuronopathy include paraproteinemias, Sjögren's syndrome, paraneoplastic disorders, infective causes such as HIV, human T-cell lymphotropic virus (HTLV), and hepatitis C virus (HCV), and pyridoxine toxicity, while chronic immune sensory polyradiculopathy (CISP) involves sensory roots. Selective involvement of small sensory fibers (for pain and temperature sensations) rarely causes ataxia. The presence of spasticity and brisk knee jerks in the setting of sensory ataxia suggests upper motor neuron involvement (e.g., myeloneuropathy).[6-8]

Based on progression, sensory ataxia can be acute, subacute, or chronic; while on an etiological basis, it can be inherited or acquired. Common inherited causes of sensory ataxia are Friedreich's ataxia (FA), ataxia with vitamin E deficiency (AVED), abetalipoproteinemia, spinocerebellar ataxia (SCA) with neuropathy, mitochondrial neuropathies such as sensory ataxic neuropathy, dysarthria, and ophthalmoparesis (SANDO). Acquired causes such as diabetes, vitamin deficiencies, chronic infections, immune-mediated neuropathies, and drug-induced neuropathies are suspected in appropriate cases **(Table 2)**.

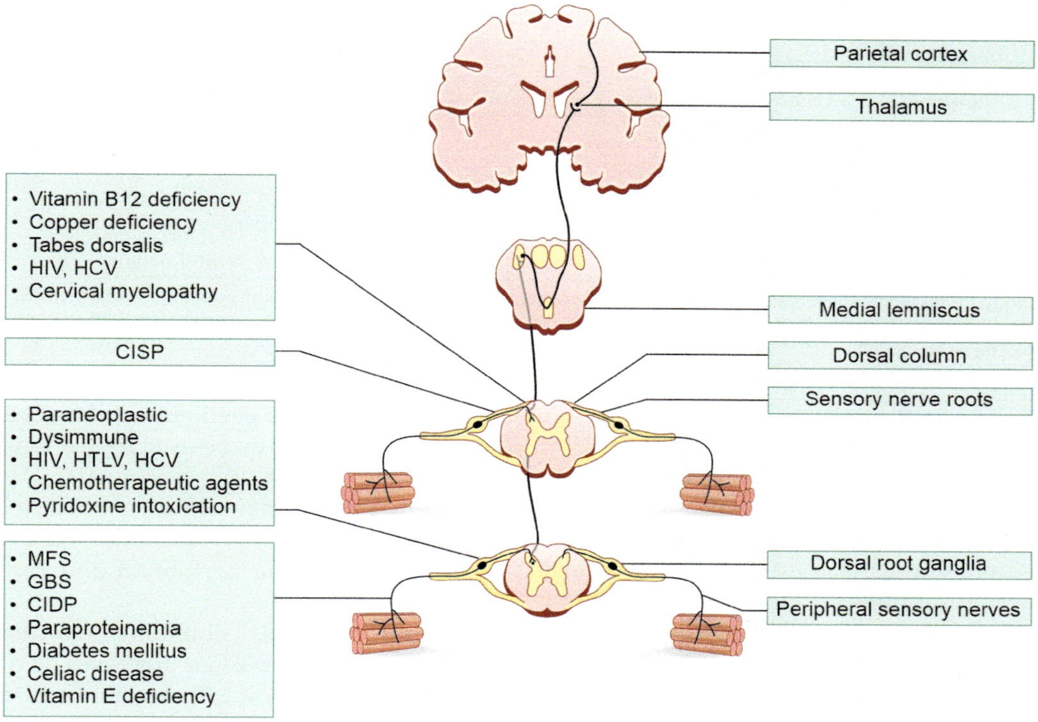

FIG. 1: Various lesion sites of sensory ataxic disorders.[9]

(CIDP: chronic inflammatory demyelinating polyneuropathy; CISP: chronic immune sensory polyradiculopathy; HTLV: human T-cell lymphotropic virus; HCV: hepatitis C virus; MFS: Miller Fisher syndrome; GBS: Guillain–Barré syndrome)

TABLE 2: Common causes of sensory ataxia.[10]

Site of involvement	Onset	Etiology	Ancillary investigations
Peripheral nerve/ nerve root	Acute	• Miller Fisher syndrome (MFS) • Sensory variant GBS • Diphtheric neuropathy	• NCS, antiganglioside antibodies, cerebrospinal fluid (CSF) • Throat culture
	Subacute	• Lyme's disease • Neurosarcoidosis	• Lyme's serology • CSF, NCS, serum ACE, PET scan
	Chronic	• CIDP • Paraproteinemia • Diabetes mellitus • Celiac disease • Vitamin E deficiency • Drug/toxin induced • Hereditary neuropathies (CMT—early onset, CANVAS—late onset) • Mitochondrial ataxia disorders	• NCS, CSF • Protein electrophoresis, anti-MAG • HbA1c, fasting blood sugar • Anti-tTG antibodies • Serum vitamin E levels • Arsenic, mercury levels • Family history, nerve biopsy, genetic testing • Muscle biopsy, mitochondrial genetics
Dorsal root ganglion[11]	Subacute	• HIV, HTLV-1, HCV infection • Paraneoplastic (Ca lung, Ca colon, neuroendocrine tumors) • Pyridoxine intoxication • Chemotherapeutic agents • Thalidomide • Organophosphate exposure • Paraneoplastic (breast and ovarian cancer)	• Serology • Anti-Hu, anti-CRMP-5, imaging • History of exposure • History of exposure • History of exposure • History of exposure • Relevant imaging
	Chronic	• Sjögren's syndrome • Friedreich's ataxia, SCA (additional cerebellar ataxia)	• ANA ENA (anti-SS-A/SS-B), lip biopsy, RF • NCS, genetic testing

Continued

Continued

Site of involvement	Onset	Etiology	Ancillary investigations
Spinal root	Chronic	Chronic immune sensory polyradiculopathy (CISP)	NCS, SSEP, CSF, and MRI
Dorsal column	Chronic	• Vitamin B12 deficiency • Copper deficiency • Tabes dorsalis • HIV, HCV • Cervical myelopathy	• Serum B12, Schilling's test • Serum copper and ceruloplasmin level • Syphilis serology • Serology • Neuroimaging

(ANA: antinuclear antibody; CIDP: chronic inflammatory demyelinating polyneuropathy; CMT: Charcot–Marie–Tooth disease; CANVAS: cerebellar ataxia, neuropathy, and vestibular areflexia syndrome; GBS: Guillain–Barré syndrome; HTLV: human T-cell lymphotropic virus; MAG: myelin-associated glycoprotein; MRI: magnetic resonance imaging; NCS: nerve conduction studies; PET: positron emission tomography; SSEP: somatosensory evoked potentials; tTG: tissue transglutaminase)

VESTIBULAR ATAXIA

The vestibular system plays role in the maintenance of equilibrium through three reflex mechanisms:

1. *Vestibulo-ocular reflexes (VORs)*: VOR helps to maintain images onto fovea during head turning, the eyes move proportionally in the opposite direction to maintain fixation. The horizontal canals respond to angular motion, while saccule and utricle to linear acceleration and gravity. The cerebellum is involved in the central modulation and regulation of vestibular function, wherein flocculus helps VOR adaptations and modulus adjusts the duration of VOR responses preventing under or overshooting the target. The anterior superior vermis of the cerebellum controls the vestibulospinal reflex, gait, and truncal stability.[12]
2. *Vestibulospinal reflex (VSR)*: It maintains body position in relation to head movements and involves lateral/medial vestibulospinal tract and reticulospinal tracts.
3. *Vestibulocollic reflex*: This reflex maintains neck musculature in relation to head position. For example, when the head is turned to the right, the right sterno-cleidomastoid (SCM) relaxes and the opposite side contracts.

Symptoms of Vestibular Dysfunction

Patients may describe spinning, whirling, rotational sensations, tilting, sinking, free-falling, or rising, and all these symptoms defined as true "vertigo" imply a higher likelihood of a vestibular process. Ataxic symptoms, if any, are more prominent ipsilateral to the affected ear. Such symptoms are quite uncommon in presyncope. Dizziness and lightheadedness, nausea, yawning, visible pallor observed by others, diaphoresis, and a feeling as though one is about to pass out are much more characteristic of cardiovascular causes of dizziness. Dizziness accompanied by imbalance and uncoordinated limb movements is more suggestive of cerebellar dysfunction **(Table 3)**.[13]

Clinical Evaluation of Vestibular Dysfunction[19]

- The vestibular system examination begins with a hearing test. A finger rub testing in each ear sequentially and then simultaneously is good enough for gross evaluation. A tuning fork can then be used for the Rinne's and Weber test.[20]
- HINTS examination (head impulse test, nystagmus, and test for skew) is a standard examination method for differentiating peripheral and central vestibular dysfunction.
- Head thrust test is commonly performed wherein the patient is asked to fixate their eyes on a target (usually the examiner's nose). The examiner does a quick head turn of around 20° to throw the eyes out of the fixated target, which would be countered by a normal VOR. A displacement off target to the affected side followed by a catch-up saccade suggests vestibular dysfunction.[21]
- End-gaze nystagmus is a tell-tale sign; the corrective phase is faster toward the normal side in vestibular dysfunction. A slow-motion recording in a phone camera helps. Peripheral nystagmus may have a torsional component, is fatigable, and stops as patients fixate their eyes on a target. Conversely, vertical nystagmus is always due to a central cause. People with vestibular dysfunction generally get some dizzy symptoms when following a target to the affected side.
- Skew deviation can be clinically determined by a cover–uncover test, and vertical misalignment (skew) is suggestive of a central cause.
- Dix–Hallpike maneuver is classically described to detect a posterior canal benign paroxysmal positional vertigo (BPPV). It causes nystagmus and precipitates dizziness with the head hanging down or when switching to the upright position from lying down.
- Dynamic visual acuity testing is performed as patients read from a Snellen's chart to check their best baseline visual acuity. Now after a head-shaking test, that visual acuity is checked again. If there is a new impairment or dizziness, it is likely to be due to vestibular dysfunction.[22]
- A sharpened Romberg test or a tandem stance test is also a useful test for vestibular dysfunction. The patient is asked to stand toe to heel, with arms crossed, and eyes closed. The balance system is dependent on our visual and sensorimotor inputs to the vestibular system, which is both taken out with closed eyes and crossed arms, and balance entirely depends on the vestibular system. There is a consistent sway or fall onto the affected side

TABLE 3: Common disorders with vertigo and dizziness with/without ataxia.[14-16]

	Symptom description	Onset	Duration	Associated features	Likely diagnosis
Vestibular disorders	Spinning, rotating, whirling, tilting, or floating sensations	Abrupt	5–60 seconds	Nystagmus with Dix–Hallpike test	Benign paroxysmal positional vertigo
		Abrupt or evolving over 30 minutes	Days to weeks	Worse with head motion, nausea, abnormal head impulse test to affected side	Vestibular neuritis, labyrinthitis
		Insidious, occasionally abrupt	Continuous symptoms	Positive Romberg sign, dynamic visual acuity reduced	Bilateral vestibulopathy
Hemodynamic disorders[17]	Near-faintness, "about to pass out," "lightheadedness"	Abrupt, usually on standing	Minutes, ends up as syncope or abates, may be recurrent on standing	Pallor, diaphoresis, symptoms relieved by lying flat; abnormal orthostatic heart rate/blood pressure	Orthostatic dizziness (orthostatic intolerance or hypotension)
Central nervous system disorders	Spinning, tilting, rocking, floating sensations	Abrupt/ gradual, or discrete spells, varying intensity	• Brief quick • Spins, or in spells, light induced vertigo/dizziness, motion sensitivity	• Migraine headache history, periodic, pulsatile pain, photophobia or phonophobia • Examination usually normal	Vestibular migraine
	Vertigo, poor equilibrium, ataxia	Abrupt, transient	Sudden onset, resolves in 5–20 minutes	Transient nystagmus and ataxia but resolve in minute	Transient ischemic attack
		Abrupt persistent	Continues, some gradual improvement over days to months	• Poor gait balance • Gaze-evoked nystagmus, transient diplopia on head turns, dysarthria, possibly hemiataxia and other CNS signs	Posterior circulation stroke[18]
		Insidious	Continuous in degenerative and lesion-based cerebellar diseases	Balance worsens with fatigue, alcohol, sedation. Gaze-evoked or vertical nystagmus; limb and truncal ataxia, dysarthria, abnormal pursuit, and saccadic eye movements	Dizziness due to cerebellar affection

(CNS: central nervous system)

in unilateral peripheral vestibular dysfunction. With bilateral dysfunction, there is imbalance and shaking with a tendency to fall to either side.

- In the "Fukuda stepping test," the patient is asked to march with their eyes closed and arms straightforward. In unilateral vestibular dysfunction, there is a tendency to turn to the side of vestibular dysfunction.[23]

CEREBELLUM AND ITS CONNECTIONS

The cerebellum and its afferent and efferent connections, the vestibular system, and the proprioceptive sensory pathway **(Fig. 2)** can be all involved in causing ataxia. Hence, an understanding of these anatomical connections helps with localization.

Anatomically speaking, cerebellum constitutes of "the cortex", "central white matter", and "deep nuclei".

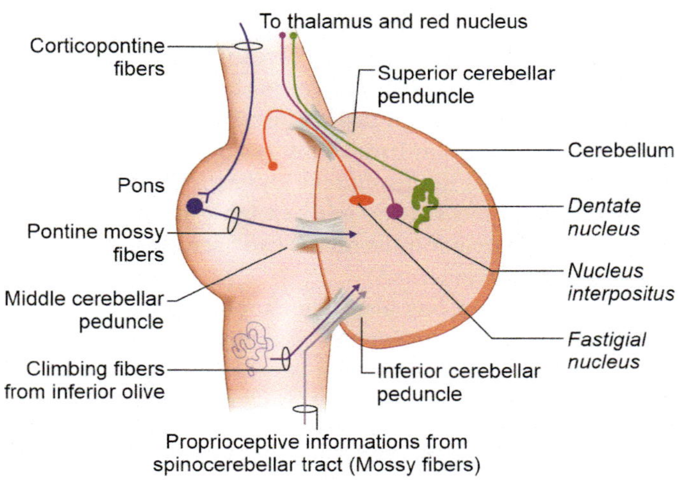

FIG. 2: Cerebellar connections and tracts.

TABLE 4: Functional circuity and connections of the cerebellum.

	Structures involved	Connections[26]	Function	Dysfunction
Archicerebellum	Flocculonodular lobe and fastigial nucleus	*Input*: • Vestibular/reticular nuclei and vestibulocerebellar tracts *Output*: • Fastigial nucleus → (via ICP) vestibulospinal tract, reticulospinal tracts	Maintenance of balance (equilibrium), posture, and coordination of eye movements	Disequilibrium, vertigo, and gait ataxia
Paleocerebellum	Vermis, paravermis, fastigial/emboliform nucleus	*Input*: • Dorsal spinocerebellar tracts (via ICP) • Ventral spinocerebellar tract and rubrocerebellar tracts (via SCP) *Output*: • Globose nucleus + emboliform nucleus + fastigial nucleus → via SCP rubrospinal tract	Controls the tone and posture of the trunk and proximal limb muscles through the vermal–cerebellar pathway	Dysarthria, gait, and truncal ataxia, relatively spared limbs
Neocerebellum	Cerebellar hemisphere (except pyramid and uvula) and dentate nucleus	*Input*: • Cortico-pontocerebellar fibers from pontine nuclei, cerebral cortex (via MCP) *Output*: • Cerebral cortex → corticopontine fibers → dentate nucleus → via SCP → cerebello-rubro-thalamo-cortical fibers	Controls the highly skilled muscle coordination and trajectory, speed, and force of movements	Ataxia of intended limb movements

(SCP: superior cerebellar peduncle; MCP: middle cerebral peduncle; ICP: inferior cerebral peduncle)

The cerebellar cortex has three-layered architecture comprising an external "molecular layer", containing outer stellate and inner basket cells; a "middle layer", with Purkinje cells; and an internal "granular layer", where granular cells are located. The deep cerebellar nuclei (the dentate, emboliform, globose, and fastigial) are the output cells of the cerebellar cortex. The cerebellar circuitry **(Table 4)** modifies inputs from the central nervous system (CNS) and sends efferent signals back to various areas of the brain and spine.[2]

A *functional/phylogenetic classification* separates the cerebellum **(Fig. 3)** into archicerebellum/vestibulocerebellum, paleocerebellum or spinocerebellum, and neocerebellum or cerebrocerebellum. Dysfunction of the lower vermis (vestibulocerebellum) results in truncal ataxia. Spinocerebellar lesions (upper vermis and anterior parts of hemispheres) lead to the unsteadiness of gait and stance, while irregular, jerky limb movements suggest neocerebellar damage (cerebellar hemispheres). Dysarthric speech, which is slow, segmented speech with variable intonation, and disturbances of ocular movements can accompany ataxia of gait and limb movements.[24,25]

The cerebellum has also been topographically recognized to have three anterior–posterior divisions: the anterior lobe (lobules I–V) is separated from the posterior lobe by the primary fissure, and the posterior lobe (lobules VI–IX) is separated from the flocculonodular lobe (lobule X) by the posterolateral fissure.[27]

1. The anterior lobe and lobule VIII represent sensorimotor cerebellum.
2. Lobules VI and VII of the posterior lobes form the cognitive cerebellum
3. The posterior vermis is the limbic cerebellum

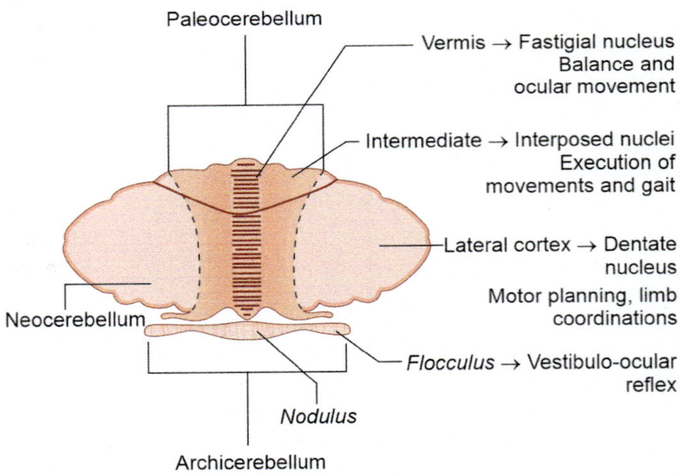

FIG. 3: Functional parts of the cerebellum.

Classification of Cerebellar Ataxia

Ataxia can be classified in various ways—on anatomic involvement; focal or generalized; the age of onset, the tempo of onset, and clinical course; or acquired or inherited.

Anatomical/Structural Basis

The first step while taking a history of ataxia is to distinguish between focal cerebellar disease (tumor, abscess, ischemia, hemorrhage, focal demyelination) and nonfocal disorders (cerebellitis, genetic and neurodegenerative ataxias). A more definite distinction between focal and nonfocal cerebellar disorders is later achieved with neuroimaging [magnetic resonance imaging (MRI) is preferable to computed

TABLE 5: Ataxia localization in posterior circulation strokes.[29,31]

Vascular territory (Fig. 4)	Anatomical location	Stroke syndrome	Clinical findings
Posterior inferior cerebellar artery (PICA)	Inferior posterior cerebellar hemisphere, inferior vermis, lateral medulla	Lateral medullary syndrome/Wallenberg syndrome	Vertigo, nausea, vomiting, ipsilateral facial numbness, contralateral hemisensory loss, Horner's syndrome, dysphagia, and hemiataxia
Superior cerebellar artery (CA)	Dorsolateral upper brainstem, cerebellum, and superior cerebellar peduncle	Superior CA syndrome	Ipsilateral limb ataxia, vertigo, nystagmus, dysarthria
Anterior inferior cerebellar artery (AICA)	Ipsilateral labyrinth, lateral pontine tegmentum	Lateral pontine syndrome	Ipsilateral ataxia, hearing loss, tinnitus, Horner's syndrome, and contralateral hemisensory affection
Top of the basilar	Midbrain, thalamus, mesial temporal lobes and occipital lobes	Top of the basilar syndrome	Somnolence, convergence, nystagmus, skew deviation, and vertical gaze paresis
Mid-basilar	Lateral and medial pontine perforators	Lateral/medial mid-pontine syndrome	Ipsilateral ataxia, opposite gaze deviation, contralateral weakness (medial pontine), and ipsilateral facial numbness (lateral pontine)
Proximal basilar	Bilateral lower pons	Locked-in syndrome	Quadriplegia, horizontal gaze paresis, bifacial paresis, only vertical eye movements preserved
Vertebral artery (VA)	Medulla and cervical spinal cord	Medial medullary syndrome	Contralateral arm/leg weakness, ipsilateral tongue paresis

tomography (CT) as it provides high resolution detailing of cerebellum and brainstem at different planes].[28]

Focal cerebellar disorders: An acute disease onset, with or without headache, vomiting, or impaired awareness, associated with unilateral symptoms, strongly favors a focal cerebellar affection. Stroke **(Table 5)**, demyelination, and neoplasms are likely to produce focal symptoms. The additional sensorimotor examination further helps localization. Even affection of cerebellar peduncles with or without involving the brainstem and cerebellum can have focal clinical signs.[29] Conversely, the presence of surrounding brain edema, multifocal lesions, and involved crossing fibers (cerebellar diaschisis) may mislead clinical localization.[30]

Strokes causing ataxic hemiparesis:[29] Ataxic hemiparesis refers to weakness and ataxia on the same side of the body. The syndrome is usually caused by lacunar infarction in the contralateral posterior limb of the internal capsule, pons, corona radiata, lateral part of the thalamus, cerebellum or in the frontal cortex (anterior cerebral artery territory).

Nonfocal cerebellar disorders: Disorders which symmetrically affect cerebellar hemispheres are likely to produce bilateral clinical findings and need to be then evaluated on basis of age of illness onset, progression, associated movement disorders and surrogate investigations.

Based on the Onset and Progression of the Illness (Table 6)[32,33]

Acute-onset ataxia: Ataxias developing over minutes to a few days mostly result from an ischemic or hemorrhagic stroke, demyelination, or infection affecting the cerebellum and/or its connections. Moreover, some disorders such as

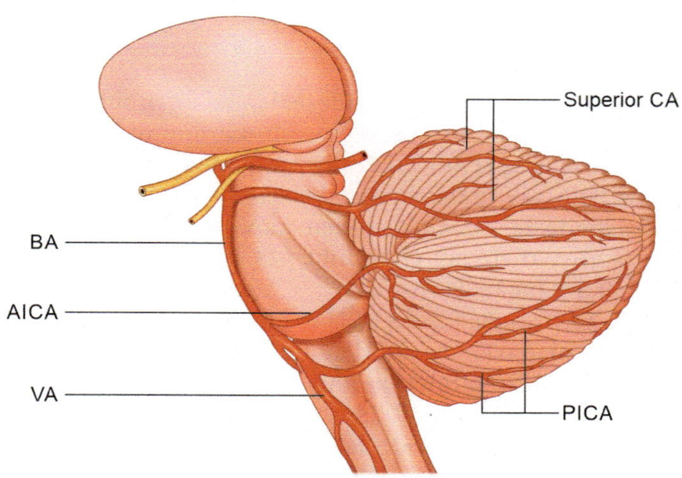

FIG. 4: The posterior circulation and cerebellum.
(AICA: anterior inferior cerebellar artery; BA: basilar artery; PICA: posterior inferior cerebellar artery; CA: cerebellar artery; VA: vertebral artery)

viral cerebellar encephalitis,[34] Miller Fisher syndrome,[35] paraneoplastic cerebellar degeneration,[36] transmissible spongiform encephalopathy (prion disease), and Wernicke's encephalopathy can have a rapidly progressive course after onset.

Subacute-onset ataxia: Ataxia gradually developing over weeks to months results mostly from infectious, immunological causes, or vitamin-deficient states.

Chronic progressive ataxia: Ataxia with an insidious onset, followed by a slowly progressive clinical course, as in genetic and neurodegenerative causes, however, reversible, and treatable etiologies should be actively sought.

TABLE 6: Causes of ataxia according to onset.

Acute causes	Subacute causes	Chronic causes	Episodic ataxias
Vascular (posterior circulation stroke)	Paraneoplastic cerebellar degeneration (anti-Yo/Hu/Tr/Ri)[39,40]	Genetic ataxia (AD, AR, FXTAS)	Genetic episodic ataxia (EA1 to EA8)
Ethanol intoxication	Creutzfeldt–Jakob disease	Alcoholic cerebellar degeneration[41]	GLUT1 deficiency
Medication induced (phenytoin, phenobarbital carbamazepine, lithium)	Autoimmune causes (antiglutamic acid decarboxylase ataxia, opsoclonus–myoclonus ataxia, anti-NMDA/CASPR2/DPPX)[40]	Phenytoin cerebellar degeneration[42]	Multiple sclerosis
Toxins (mercury, thallium, toluene)	Vitamin B12 deficiency (subacute combined degeneration)	Ataxia associated with gluten sensitivity, Whipple's disease	Mitochondrial diseases (POLG, MELAS, etc.)
Demyelination (multiple sclerosis, acute disseminated encephalomyelitis)	Superficial siderosis	Mitochondrial disorders (MERRF, NARP, MILS, or KSS syndrome)[43]	Basilar migraine, benign paroxysmal vertigo
Infective (viral cerebellitis, cerebellar abscess, basilar meningitis)	Brain malignancy	Multiple system atrophy	Psychogenic ataxia
Wernicke encephalopathy/thiamine deficiency		Idiopathic late-onset cerebellar ataxia	

(AD/AR: autosomal dominant/recessive; CASPR2: contactin-associated protein 2; DPPX: dipeptidyl peptidase-like protein 6; FXTAS: fragile X-associated tremor/ataxia syndrome; EA: episodic ataxia; GLUT1: glucose transporter type 1 deficiency syndrome; KSS: Kearns–Sayre syndrome; MELAS: mitochondrial encephalopathy, lactic acidosis, and stroke-like events; MERRF: myoclonic epilepsy with ragged-red fibers; MILS: maternally inherited Leigh syndrome; NARP: neuropathy ataxia and retinitis pigmentosa; NMDA: N-methyl-D-aspartate)

Episodic ataxia: Ataxia is manifested in an intermittent and transient fashion, mostly seen with a group of inherited episodic ataxias (EAs), clinically presenting as episodes of ataxia with gait imbalance and slurred speech, occurring spontaneously, or with sudden movement, excitement, or exercise. There are eight subtypes of EA described.[37,38] (Details in Chapter 88: Ataxias)

The EA1 results from a KCNA1 mutation, with recurrent episodes of ataxia, dysarthria, and coarse tremors, which last for seconds to minutes and are followed by interictal myokymia. While EA2 is a calcium channelopathy (CACNA1A), ataxic episodes last hours to days, with interictal nystagmus and associated migraine in half the cases.

Based on the Age of Onset

Ataxia presenting in infancy reflects a congenital or developmental cause, often genetic. Early onset ataxia is considered when the onset is before 20 years of age and is usually genetic [autosomal recessive (AR) or mitochondrial inheritance], even without an elicitable family history. Conversely, third and fourth decades onward, dominant ataxias (including the SCAs) are commonly the cause. However, considerable variation in onset age is not unexpected, FA can have a late onset (with intact or even brisk reflexes) and some SCAs have very young onset forms (associated with large CAG repeat expansions). Cerebellar ataxia with neuropathy and vestibular areflexia syndrome (CANVAS), despite recessive inheritance, presents unusually late (in middle age).[44]

Early onset ataxias:[45]

- *Ataxia due to structural defects*: Ataxia can be a result of disorders causing brainstem or cerebellar hypoplasia and/or malformations. The yield of neuroimaging in a child with global developmental delay/intellectual disability increases in presence of microcephaly, headaches suspicious of raised intracranial pressure, abnormal general examination (features typical of a syndrome), acquired nystagmus, acquired ocular malalignment, and asymmetric motor findings. The imaging modality of choice is MRI. Examples include Dandy–Walker malformation, Joubert syndrome, cerebellar hypoplasia, pontocerebellar hypoplasia, etc.[46,47]
- *Nonprogressive ataxia*: It is common in children with developmental delay. The ataxia is not congenital in the strict sense because it is preceded by hypotonia and delayed motor and language milestones. Patients have an increased prevalence of nystagmus, strabismus, epilepsy, autism, and microcephaly. Besides the subnormal fine and/or gross motor skills, the movement and coordination issues become noticeable between 3 and 7 years of age. With increasing age, ataxia persists, however, becomes less functionally significant as compared to behavioral and cognitive impairment.[48]
- *Chronic progressive ataxias*: *Hereditary ataxias* are common in children. AR ataxias [FA, ataxia telangiectasia (AT), AVED, apraxia with oculomotor apraxia, etc.] usually present before 25 years of age, while dominantly inherited ataxias (SCAs), in most cases, are adulthood

onset. Neuroimaging is vital in the evaluation of chronic progressive ataxias. While MRI may not provide a specific diagnosis, however, the affection of white versus gray matter or vermis versus cerebellar hemispheres may direct subsequent biochemical, metabolic, or genetic investigations.[45]

- *Common structural causes* include pediatric posterior fossa tumors such as pilocytic astrocytomas, medulloblastomas, ependymomas, and diffuse intrinsic pontine gliomas. *Leukodystrophies* such as Krabbe disease, and *inborn errors of metabolism* disorders such as juvenile forms of GM2 gangliosidoses, and sulfatide lipidoses (metachromatic leukodystrophy) can present with cerebellar ataxia and should be considered. Besides, Joubert syndrome, X-linked adrenoleukodystrophy, Wilson disease, Niemann–Pick type C, and childhood ataxia with CNS hypomyelination/vanishing white matter disease are other considerations in this age group as well.[49,50] *Vitamin B-12 deficiency* occasionally presents with chronic sensory ataxia in childhood, often related to loss of proprioception.

Adulthood-onset ataxias:

- *Adult-onset hereditary ataxias*: The SCAs constitute of a genetically heterogeneous group of autosomal dominant ataxia disorders, characterized by loss of balance and coordination accompanied by slurred speech; onset is most often in adult life. As an exception, childhood-onset occurs in some SCAs such as SCA5, SCA13, SCA21, SCA25, SCA29, and SCA47.[51] While SCA6, SCA12, and SCA31 might typically have an average onset in the sixth decade.[52]
- *Immune-mediated ataxias*: Subacute progressive ataxias in adults need evaluation for autoimmune causes. Adults are mostly affected due to antibodies to intracellular, synaptic antigens such as glutamic acid decarboxylase (GAD), amphiphysin, or to cell surface receptors such as N-methyl-D-aspartate (NMDA), contactin-associated protein 2 (CASPR2), and dipeptidyl peptidase-like protein 6 (DPPX). Moreover, the presence of encephalopathy and myoclonus warrants testing for anti-thyroid peroxidase (anti-TPO) antibodies.[40,53,54]
- *Ataxia associated with deficiencies and toxicity*: Adult-onset acquired ataxia can occur because of a deficiency of vitamin B1, vitamin B12, or vitamin E. Moreover, alcohol-related cerebellar degeneration, drug-induced ataxias (phenytoin, amiodarone, lithium, cytarabine, etc.), and heavy metal poisoning (mercury, lead, and thallium) also need evaluation in appropriate settings.[55]

Ataxias in older adults:

- *Multiple system atrophy–cerebellar subtype (MSA-C)*:[56,57] MSA-C is characterized by late-onset (>30 years age) progressive cerebellar ataxia, parkinsonism, autonomic dysfunction (orthostatic hypotension; impotence; and urinary frequency, urgency, and incontinence), and pyramidal signs. In the initial stages, patients might present with relatively isolated cerebellar ataxia. Therefore, for patients with cerebellar ataxia onset later in life, history and examination should target for signs of parkinsonism, dysautonomia, upper motor neuron signs, and for rapid eye movement sleep behavior disorder, inspiratory stridor and obstructive sleep apnea. Further investigations include MRI brain (hot cross bun sign), autonomic tests, and sleep studies.
- *Idiopathic late-onset cerebellar ataxia (ILOCA)*:[57] ILOCA has a slower progression as compared to multiple system atrophy, and it usually does not compromise the lifespan. Pure late-onset cerebellar ataxia without any evidence of parkinsonism or autonomic dysfunction within 5 years of ataxia onset is likely to follow a benign clinical course and given a diagnosis of ILOCA.
- *Fragile X-associated tremor/ataxia syndrome (FXTAS)*:[58] FXTAS is a neurodegenerative disorder caused due to triplet repeat expansion (CGG repeats) in the *FMR1* gene on chromosome X. Onset is usually late, the sixth-early seventh decade in men. The constellation includes gait ataxia, intention tremors, frontal executive dysfunction, mild parkinsonism, peripheral neuropathy, cognitive–psychiatric symptoms, hypogonadism, and autonomic dysfunction, with T2 hyperintensity at the middle cerebral peduncle. Women, if affected, have the mild phenotype.
- *Lesion-related*: Structural cause of ataxia in older adults is mostly due to a stroke, infection, neoplasm, or metastases.
- *Immune-mediated ataxias*: Paraneoplastic cerebellar degeneration is suspected in patients with the subacute onset and rapid progression of ataxia, defined as progression to severe ataxia in <12 weeks.[59] Antibodies are directed to intracellular antigens such as Hu (ANNA-1), Ri (ANNA-2), Yo (PCA-1), Tr, mGluR1, CV2 (CRMP5), ZIC4, and VGCC, which have high tumor association. The clinical features of various onconeural antibodies vary; however, additional peripheral neuropathy, cognitive deficits, dysautonomia, and hearing loss are pointers to paraneoplastic causes **(Table 7)**.[39,60] Besides MRI brain and cerebrospinal fluid (CSF) testing for pleocytosis, a careful and recurrent search for the primary tumor is required with CT of the chest, abdomen, and pelvis, or whole-body fluorodeoxyglucose positron emission tomography (PET)/CT.[61]

Based on Etiology

Holmes was the first to distinguish spinocerebellar degeneration, cerebellar cortex degeneration, and olivopontocerebellar atrophy.[64] Later, Harding[1] classified ataxia as congenital, hereditary, and nonhereditary, which still is an accepted etiological subdivision:

1. Sporadic acquired ataxias, due to exogenous or endogenous nongenetic causes
2. Hereditary ataxias
3. Nonhereditary degenerative ataxias

TABLE 7: Clinical clues to immune-mediated ataxias.[39,40,53,60]

	Antibodies linked	Clinical clues
Cerebellar affection due to another disease/condition		
Gluten ataxia[62,63]	Antigliadin, anti-TG6 antibodies	40–50 years onset, subacute-chronic, gait > limb ataxia, MRI—vermian involvement, CSF-OCB in 50%, associated neuropathy, cortical myoclonus. GI symptoms, gluten sensitivity, associated diabetes, and thyroid dysfunction
Postinfectious cerebellitis		Young children, usually after viral infection (varicella, EBV, coxsackie, influenza A, B, etc.). Acute-onset gait ataxia associated with meningeal signs, irritability, altered mentation, CSF pleocytosis, and MRI mostly normal
Miller Fisher syndrome	GQ1b Ab	Acute-onset ataxia, areflexia, and ophthalmoplegia subtype of GBS
Opsoclonus–myoclonus ataxia syndrome (OMAS)	Anti-Ri Ab (common in paraneoplastic OMAS)	• Can be paraneoplastic, postinfectious, or idiopathic • Children commonly affected, associated with neuroblastoma. Chaotic multiplanar eye movements, with action myoclonus and ataxia. Subacute vertigo and high-CSF protein and leukocytes in 50% idiopathic OMAS, while encephalopathy more common in paraneoplastic OMAS. Postinfectious OMAS is self-limiting
Paraneoplastic cerebellar degeneration	Anti-Yo	Breast and ovarian cancer. Associated brainstem encephalitis, neuropathy
	Anti-Hu	Small cell lung cancer. Encephalomyelitis, limbic encephalitis, and sensory neuropathy
	Anti-CV2	Thymoma, small cell lung cancer. Chorea, cognitive decline, neuropathy, optic neuritis, and myelitis
	Anti-Ri	Breast cancer. Limbic or brainstem encephalitis, myelitis, and opsoclonus
	Anti-Tr	Hodgkin's lymphoma, encephalopathy, or neuropathy
	Anti-Zic4	Small cell lung cancer. Ataxia, parkinsonism
	Anti-PCA2	Small-cell lung cancer. Limbic/brainstem encephalitis, myelitis, neuropathy, LEMS
	Anti-VGCC	Small-cell lung cancer, associated LEMS or limbic encephalitis
	Anti-GFAP	Diverse neoplasms, meningoencephalomyelitis, epilepsy, cognitive–psychiatric problems, and ataxia
Cerebellar affection not triggered by another disease or condition		
Anti-GAD ataxia	Anti-GAD[65]	Truncal ataxia, nystagmus, and dysarthria typically in females >60 years of age; history of brainstem/cerebellar dysfunction or persistent vertigo before permanent ataxia in some patients. Associated autoimmune diseases, e.g., diabetes type 1 and thyroiditis. Overlap with stiff person syndrome, limbic encephalitis, and temporal lobe epilepsy
Primary autoimmune cerebellar ataxia[60]	Anti-DPPX	Limbic encephalitis, diarrhea, weight loss, dysautonomia, ataxia, pyramidal signs, sensory symptoms, and cognitive issues
	Anti-LGI1	Limbic encephalitis, ataxia, hyponatremia, and faciobrachial dystonia
	Anti-CASPR2	Mostly males >65 years of age, limbic encephalitis, peripheral nerve hyperexcitability syndrome, ataxia (rarely paroxysmal/episodic ataxia), sleep dysfunction. 20% have thymoma
Antibodies likely pathogenic unreported to be pathogenic	Anti-NMDAR	More in children, around 50% of affected girls have ovarian teratoma. Behavioral changes, psychiatric disorders, facial dyskinesias, cognitive affection, seizures, and dysautonomia
Unreported to be pathogenic	Anti-mGluR1	Isolated ataxia, dysgeusia present in half, and lymphoma association
	Anti-TPO	
Others	Anti-SS-A, SS-B	
	Anti-PKCγ	Reported in a few patients with neoplasm
	Anti-Ca/ARHGAP26	Reported in a few patients with neoplasm
	Anti-SOX1	Reported in a few patients with neoplasm
	Anti-CARP VIII	Reported in a few patients with neoplasm
	Anti-Homer3	Reported in a few patients with neoplasm
	Anti-Sj/ITPR-1	Unknown

Continued

Continued

	Antibodies linked	Clinical clues
Others	Anti-Septin-5	Unknown
	Anti-neurochondrin	Unknown
	Anti-Nb/AP3B2	Unknown

(Ab: antibody; CASPR2: contactin-associated protein 2; CSF-OCB: cerebrospinal fluid–oligoclonal band; DPPX: dipeptidyl peptidase-like protein 6; GAD: glutamic acid decarboxylase; GBS: Guillain–Barré syndrome; GI: gastrointestinal; LEMS: Lambert–Eaton myasthenic syndrome; NMDAR: N-methyl-D-aspartate receptor)

Sporadic acquired ataxias: Sporadic ataxia remains a temporary diagnosis for adults before a definitive etiology is found. Despite an intensive laboratory workup and neuroimaging facilities, sporadic adult-onset ataxia often remains a diagnostic challenge.[55]

Hereditary ataxias (detailed description in Chapter 88 on Ataxias):

- *Autosomal dominant*: Autosomal dominant cerebellar ataxias (ADCAs) frequently represent SCAs. Numerous new SCA loci are being rapidly discovered and nomenclature has extended from SCA-1 to SCA-48 till date. The clinical features of SCA overlap, and distinguishing the subtypes of SCA with clinical manifestations is difficult.[51,65] However, some characteristics point toward a specific type of SCA. A detailed description of SCA has been undertaken in Chapter 88.
- *Autosomal recessive*:[66,67] The AR cerebellar ataxias are a heterogeneous group of disorders presenting often in childhood or adolescence, having complex, mixed neurological syndromes including sensory with/without motor peripheral neuropathy, spasticity, or posterior column degeneration in addition to ataxia. Moreover, ataxia may be associated with hyperkinetic movement disorders such as dystonia, chorea, myoclonus, and tremors, occurring in about one-third of such patients.[68] Some noteworthy AR ataxias are:
  - *Friedreich's ataxia* is the most common AR ataxia syndrome resulting from >90 GAA trinucleotide expansion in the *FRDA* gene. The disease is marked by gait ataxia, axonal neuropathy, areflexia with extensor plantar, cardiomyopathy, and diabetes mellitus.[69,70]
  - *Ataxia with vitamin E deficiency* is progressive but treatable ataxia mimicking FA. Onset is usually early childhood, with retinitis pigmentosa, dystonia, and low vitamin E levels, requiring lifetime supplementation.[71-73]
  - *Ataxia telangiectasia* is another progressive childhood-onset movement disorder characterized by ataxia with hyperkinetic movements such as chorea, athetosis, and dystonia and association with immunodeficiency (low IgA levels), susceptibility to recurrent infections, leukemias, and later telangiectasias visible at conjunctiva, pinna, and cheeks.[74,75]
  - *Ataxia with oculomotor apraxia 1 (AOA-1)*: AR ataxia caused by APTX genetic mutation, manifesting in 2–18 years, as ataxia with choreoathetosis, oculomotor apraxia, sensory neuropathy, hyporeflexia, and cognitive impairment[76,77]
  - *Ataxia with oculomotor apraxia 2 (AOA-2)*: Another progressive ataxia syndrome, less prevalent than AOA-1, due to SETX mutation, presenting at 13–18 years in association with areflexia, and oculomotor apraxia and diffuse cerebellar atrophy[78,79]
  - *Autosomal recessive cerebellar ataxia-1 (ARCA1)*: Uncommon disorder due to SYNE1 mutation having late age of onset, presenting as pure cerebellar ataxia, cognitive affection, and occasional pyramidal signs, pes cavus, scoliosis, and cerebellar atrophy.[38,80,81]
  - *Autosomal recessive cerebellar ataxia-2 (ARCA2)*: Relatively childhood-onset ataxia due to CABC1 mutation, having exercise intolerance, epilepsy, myoclonus, cognitive impairment, cerebellar atrophy, occasional stroke-like cerebral lesions.[82,83]
  - *Cerebrotendinous xanthomatosis (CTX)* is a rare, AR lipid storage disorder, where neurological symptoms outset around 15–20 years of age, resulting in a spastic–ataxic phenotype over time. Congenital/juvenile cataracts, xanthomas at the Achilles' tendon, extensor tendons of elbows, hand, and knees are associated features.[84,85]
- *X-linked ataxia*: The most common X-linked ataxia is FXTAS,[58] caused by CGG repeat expansions within the *FMR1* gene as discussed earlier. A longer repeat expansion of the *FMR1* gene, however, causes anticipation, resulting in a premature ovarian failure in the patients' daughters and mental retardation in patients' grandsons, making these questions important in family history.[86]
- *Mitochondrial ataxia*:[87,88] Mitochondrial disorders are a group of heterogeneous diseases, characterized by defects in any of the multiple mitochondrial metabolic pathways, involving the cellular oxidative phosphorylation, and are caused by mitochondrial DNA (mtDNA) or nuclear DNA (nDNA) mutations while displaying maternal and Mendelian inheritance. There exists a predilection for the affection of multiple energy-demanding tissues, such as the CNS, peripheral nervous system (PNS), eyes, inner ears, heart, gastrointestinal and endocrine system, kidneys, as well as bone marrow.[89] Given the heteroplasmy, wide variations exist in onset age, and systems involved among family members.

Ataxia in mitochondrial disorders can be pure cerebellar, sensory, or spinocerebellar, and is observed in both pediatric and adult populations. Common disorders to be considered are listed in **Table 8**.

TABLE 8: Common mitochondrial ataxias.

Mutation	Mitochondrial syndrome		Cerebellar ataxia	Sensory ataxia	Spinocerebellar ataxia	Clinical clues
mtDNA point mutations	MERRF		✓			Childhood-onset, myoclonus, GTCS, muscle weakness, dementia
	NARP			✓		Childhood-onset, sensory neuropathy, ataxia, and visual issues (pigmentary retinopathy)
	MELAS		✓			2–40 years onset, • Stroke-like episodes, due to focal, asymmetric brain lesions not corresponding to defined vascular territories • Decreased NAA signals, lactate peak at spectroscopy • Encephalopathy, marked by seizure and/or dementia • Myopathy with ragged-red fibers
	"LHON plus"		✓			Bilateral, painless, subacute visual failure, rarely associated with ataxia
	KSS spectrum	KSS	✓			<20 years onset, PEO and pigmentary retinopathy, cardiac conduction defects, ataxia, and/or elevated CSF protein
		Pearson syndrome	✓			
		CPEO	✓			
nDNA mutations	Maternally inherited Leigh syndrome (MILS)		✓			Symmetrical basal ganglia lesions
	IOSCA				✓	Infancy onset, severe spinocerebellar ataxia, muscle hypotonia, hyporeflexia, and athetosis
	POLG1 spectrum[90]	SANDO		✓		A heterogeneous spectrum of neurological and musculoskeletal disorders, with ataxia, either sensory/cerebellar/spinocerebellar, as the main or additional feature
		MIRAS			✓	
		MEMSA			✓	
		AD-CPEO			✓	
	LBSL		✓			Infancy onset, severe leukodystrophy with cerebellar, brainstem, and spinal cord involvement and/or cardiomyopathy, lactic acidosis, and hepatocerebral syndrome
	ADOA plus			✓		Bilateral, symmetric progressive visual loss in the first decade of life. Subsequently, ataxia and axonal sensorimotor polyneuropathy
	Primary CoQ deficiency		✓			*Five clinical phenotypes*: 1. Isolated myopathic form 2. Steroid-resistant nephrotic syndrome, deafness, and retinopathy 3. Mitochondrial encephalomyopathy form 4. Severe infantile multisystem form 5. Pure isolated ataxic form

(ADOA: autosomal dominant optic atrophy; CPEO: chronic progressive external ophthalmoplegia; IOSCA: infantile onset spinocerebellar ataxia; KSS: Kearns–Sayre syndrome; LHON: Leber's hereditary optic neuropathy; LBSL: leukoencephalopathy with brainstem and spinal cord involvement and lactate elevation; MELAS: mitochondrial encephalopathy, lactic acidosis, and stroke-like events; MEMSA: myoclonic epilepsy myopathy sensory ataxia; MERRF: myoclonic epilepsy with ragged-red fibers; MILS: maternally inherited Leigh syndrome; MIRAS: mitochondrial recessive ataxia syndrome; NARP: neuropathy ataxia and retinitis pigmentosa)

CLINICAL FEATURES OF ATAXIA

A thorough history of symptoms provides clues to the type of ataxia (e.g., cerebellar, vestibular, or sensory ataxia), the affected parts of the body (e.g., pan-cerebellar ataxia, isolated gait ataxia), associated manifestations, and the possible etiology.

Symptoms of Ataxia

The most common symptom in ataxia is often an imbalance of gait. Initially, patients might have difficulty in traversing narrow passages, maintaining balance on uneven grounds, or requiring holding rails while going up and downstairs, difficulty running, trouble walking in high heels, or veering toward one side and falls.[91] Vertigo and dizziness are more associated with lesions of the vestibulocerebellar, vestibulospinal, or cerebellar ocular motor systems.

Besides, instability while sitting and standing, hand movement incoordination, intention tremors, slurred speech, problems with buttoning clothes, loss of hand dexterity, and change in handwriting can also be the presenting complaints. In the early stages, patients may complain of transient and mild double vision, especially on quickly turning their heads. Furthermore, patients may experience surroundings moving to-and-fro horizontally or vertically (oscillopsia); difficulty looking up, especially when lying down (e.g., people doing bench press might have difficulty looking at the weight bar); difficulty reading road signs in a moving car; or looking down a long grocery list.

Moreover, questions regarding symptoms of peripheral neuropathy, parkinsonism, sleep dysfunction, autonomic symptoms, seizures, and hearing loss guide toward specific differentials.

Signs of Cerebellar Ataxia

Examination in an ataxic patient is focused on eliciting unilateral or bilateral cerebellar signs and evaluating affection of eyes, speech, limbs, balance, gait, cognition, and additional rigidity/spasticity or neuropathic or autonomic features. Sensory ataxia and vestibular signs need to be ruled out.

Expected ocular signs comprise manifestations of ocular instability, saccadic and smooth pursuit abnormalities, impaired VOR, and ocular misalignment **(Table 9)**. Ataxic dysarthria results from the affection of the superior paravermal region, and the intermediate and lateral cerebellar

TABLE 9: Ocular examination in ataxia.[97,98]

Parameters to be assessed	Clinical maneuvers used	Possible findings to look for
Eye movements, fundus and vision	*Oculomotor tests*: Ocular stability and gaze holding[99]	• *Gaze-evoked nystagmus* is the most common finding • *Rebound nystagmus* • *Downbeat nystagmus*: Seen in bilateral floccular, craniocervical junction, or bilateral medial longitudinal fasciculi affection, and in spinocerebellar ataxia (SCA) type 6 (SCA6)[42] • *Periodic alternating nystagmus*: A spontaneous, primary-position, horizontal-jerk nystagmus changing direction approximately every 2 minutes[100] • *Positional nystagmus*: Seen in vestibular vertigo or cerebellar nodulus lesions • *Head-shaking nystagmus*: Ipsilesional head-shaking nystagmus is possible in cerebellar strokes[101]
	Saccadic testing[102]	• *Saccadic dysmetria* (hyper- or hypometric saccades) • *Saccadic lateropulsion*: Observed with Wallenberg syndrome, however, can be seen with cerebellar dysfunction too[103] • *Saccadic intrusions in fixed gaze*: Square-wave jerks (SWJ), macro square-wave jerks, macro-saccadic oscillations, ocular flutter, opsoclonus • SWJ is especially seen in FA, PSP, and SCAs • *Slow saccades*: Classically described in SCA-2[104,105]
	Smooth pursuit testing	*Impaired smooth pursuit*: Not specific to cerebellar lesions but helps in detecting a subtle cerebellar syndrome. Jerky pursuits and saccadic intrusions may be seen
	Head impulse test	*Impaired VOR*: VOR might show impaired gain (decrease or increase) and direction (i.e., horizontal head thrust inducing vertical slow phase)[106]
	Ocular alignment testing	• *Alternating skew deviation*: Skew deviation is a nonparalytic vertical ocular misalignment. Alternating skew deviation, seen in cerebellar disorders, refers to skew changing with horizontal eye position, the abducting eye being the higher[107] • *Esotropia*[108]

Continued

Continued

Parameters to be assessed	Clinical maneuvers used	Possible findings to look for
Specific disease-related clinical findings	Ophthalmoplegia and/or ptosis	Can be seen in sensory ataxic neuropathy, dysarthria, and ophthalmoparesis (SANDO) and ataxia associated with mitochondrial genome mutations[90]
	Oculomotor apraxia	Develop in ataxia telangiectasia and in ataxia with oculomotor apraxia type 2 and occasionally type 1
	Papilledema	In presence of raised ICP and space-occupying lesions
	Cherry red spot and retinitis pigmentosa	Storage and mitochondrial disorders
	Optic atrophy	Mitochondrial diseases (LHON plus)
	Cataracts	Cerebrotendinous xanthomatosis, Marinesco–Sjögren syndrome

(FA: Friedreich's ataxia; LHON: Leber's hereditary optic neuropathy; PSP: progressive supranuclear palsy; VOR: vestibulo-ocular reflex)

cortex. Appendicular signs such as dysdiadochokinesia, dysmetria, grasping deficits, and dyssynergia are primarily due to the "decomposition of movements" where multijoint movements are broken down into a series of single joint movements and dysfunctional force perception and proprioceptive sense during active movements. Hypotonia is difficult to assess but is observed in acute conditions with extensive damage. Gait in cerebellar disorders is staggering and wide-based resulting from impaired inter-joint intra-limb coordination and increased compensatory antagonist muscle co-contraction **(Table 10)**.

The role of the cerebellum in cognition, behavior, and affect has been lately well accepted. Current evidence suggests that cognitive and limbic regions are in the posterior lobe (lobule VI, lobule VIIA with Crus I and Crus II, and lobule VIIB).[92] Cerebellar cognitive deficits include impairments in executive function, visual-spatial processing, linguistic dysfunction, and affective dysregulation as defined in Schmahmann's syndrome.

ATAXIA EVALUATION SCALES

The International Cooperative Ataxia Rating Scale (ICARS),[93] the Scale for the Assessment and Rating of Ataxia (SARA),[94] and the Friedreich's Ataxia Rating Scale (FARS)[95] were developed for research purposes in inherited ataxias to monitor the natural history and therapeutic response. However, they can also be used in the evaluation of acquired ataxias to help gauge a patient's functional disability and activities of daily living. The Brief Ataxia Rating Scale (BARS)[96] is less time-consuming than these rating scales yet captures key ataxia measures and is useful in clinical practice.

STEPS TO APPROACH AND EVALUATE A PATIENT OF ATAXIA (FLOWCHART 1)[9,112-114]

1. *History*: The first step in ataxia evaluation is to take a detailed clinical history, past history of illness and drugs, family history, followed by targeted neurological and systemic physical examination, and relevant investigations. The understanding of the onset and temporal course of illness is pivotal for determining the underlying etiology. While a chronic progressive evolution over months to years, without trauma or toxin exposure, with family history (not necessary) would suggest a genetic ataxia, an acute or subacute onset would point toward an acquired cause. Additional features such as headache, fever, or an associated autoimmune disorder should prompt the consideration of acquired etiologies. One should attempt to exclude acquired and treatable causes of ataxia.[55,115] Questioning for previous toxin exposure, traumatic injuries, and signs and symptoms suggestive of infectious, vascular, or metastatic disease needs to be done.
2. *Examination*: To assess for cerebellar, sensory, or vestibular signs and narrow down the differentials as per the localization **(Table 1)**. Additionally, associated features to look for are motor neuron involvement, polyneuropathy, extrapyramidal affection, eye movement abnormalities such as oculomotor apraxia, cognitive affection, and multisystemic involvement, which can guide toward a particular diagnosis **(Table 11)**.
3. *Investigations*: Neuroimaging, preferably with MRI, is an essential tool to evaluate the presence of cerebellar atrophy or signal anomalies, to search for associated atrophy of brainstem and peduncles, to rule out space-occupying lesions, and to look for changes suggestive of specific diseases **(Table 12)**. Electromyography and nerve conduction studies can prove the presence of clinically suspected or subclinical neuropathy and provide evidence of associated myopathy. Specific testing for antibodies involved in paraneoplastic or autoimmune cerebellar degeneration may be useful for patients with a subacute progression, older age at onset, and absence of family history. Also, degenerative causes like MSA-C are diagnosed clinically with supportive imaging, and additional features of dysautonomia.[56,129] Advanced workup includes dopamine transporter scan (TRODaT, F-Dopa PET), anal sphincter electromyography (EMG),

TABLE 10: Other bedside findings in cerebellar ataxia.[97,98]

Speech and swallowing	Repeat syllables, words, and sentences	• *Dysdiadochokinesia of speech*: Jerky, explosive, slurred, labored • Slow, monotonous, *scanned* speech • *Staccato speech* • *Cerebellar mutism* (seen after removal of posterior fossa tumors in children)
Appendicular ataxia	• Finger-to-nose test • Finger–nose–finger test • Finger chase	• *Dysmetria and dyssynergia*: Clumsiness in reaching and grasping an object. Grasping involves the transport of the hand toward the object (hand transport) and shaping of the fingers is required for object size/shape (grasp formation), both of which are affected in cerebellar disorders • Associated *intention tremors and kinetic tremors*, which are irregular tremors, affecting the proximal more than distal muscles, and mostly in the line of gravity
	Rapid alternating movements	*Dysdiadochokinesia*: Rapid alternating movements tested by pronation–supination of the forearm at elbow joint. Irregularities in rate or range of movements
	Stewart–Holmes maneuver	*Rebound phenomenon*: Elicited by asking the patient attempt to move a limb against resistance. On sudden removal of this resistance, the limb normally moves a short distance in the desired direction and then rebounds (i.e., jerks back in the opposite direction). Holmes suggested this rebound phenomenon is—(1) present in normal limbs, (2) exaggerated in spastic limbs, and (3) absent in limbs affected by cerebellar disease[109]
	Tone abnormalities	• *Hypotonia*: A fundamental abnormality in cerebellar motor dysfunction[110] • Rarely, *hypertonia* (cerebellar fits/spasms due to extensor tone disinhibition) is observed in posterior fossa tumors, Chiari malformations, and cerebellar strokes (sparing the nuclei)
	Heel to shin test	For the decomposition of movements and *dysmetria* of lower limbs
	Handwriting and Archimedes' spirals	Irregular *megalographic writing*, kinetic tremors, and *dysmetric spirals*
Balance and gait	• Quality of sitting • Standing in a natural position, feet together • Regular gait/walking capacities • Tandem gait	• *Titubation*: 3–7 Hz postural sway of head/neck • *Truncal ataxia* • *Wide-based* gait • Clumsy, staggering movements • *Gait Variability* • *Impaired tandem gait*
Cognition and affect	Cerebellar cognitive affective syndrome (CCAS)[111]	• *Executive dysfunction* • *Short-term memory impairments* • *Visuospatial deficits* • *Expressive language deficits* • *Blunt affect*
Autonomic system	• Postural fall in blood pressure • Impaired heart rate (HR) variability with standing, deep breathing, and during Valsalva maneuver • Tilt table testing	• *Exaggerated postural fall of SBP >30 mm Hg and/or DBP >15 mm Hg* • HR rise of <10/minute; on standing, <1.0 RR interval ratio at 30th:15th beat, <1.20 Valsalva ratio

(DBP: diastolic blood pressure; SBP: systolic blood pressure)

and metaiodobenzylguanidine (MIBG) scans for detection and documentation of the above.[130,131]

4. *Clinical differentials*: Once acquired causes appear less likely, a genetic etiology may be considered, especially in case of early onset, chronic progressive ataxias with a positive family history. However, sporadic cases can occur with AR and mitochondrial inheritance, de novo mutations, genetic anticipation, incomplete penetrance, variability in disease expression, paternity error, gonadic mosaicism, or incomplete phenotyping of family members. If AR inheritance is suspected, the next step is to assess if the clinical spectrum fits a well-described disorder. Again, the age of onset and associated neurological features guide the diagnosis.

While there is no generalization, presentation in infancy should raise suspicion of AT or autosomal recessive spastic ataxia of Charlevoix-Saguenay (ARSACS). Childhood or teenage onset suggests the

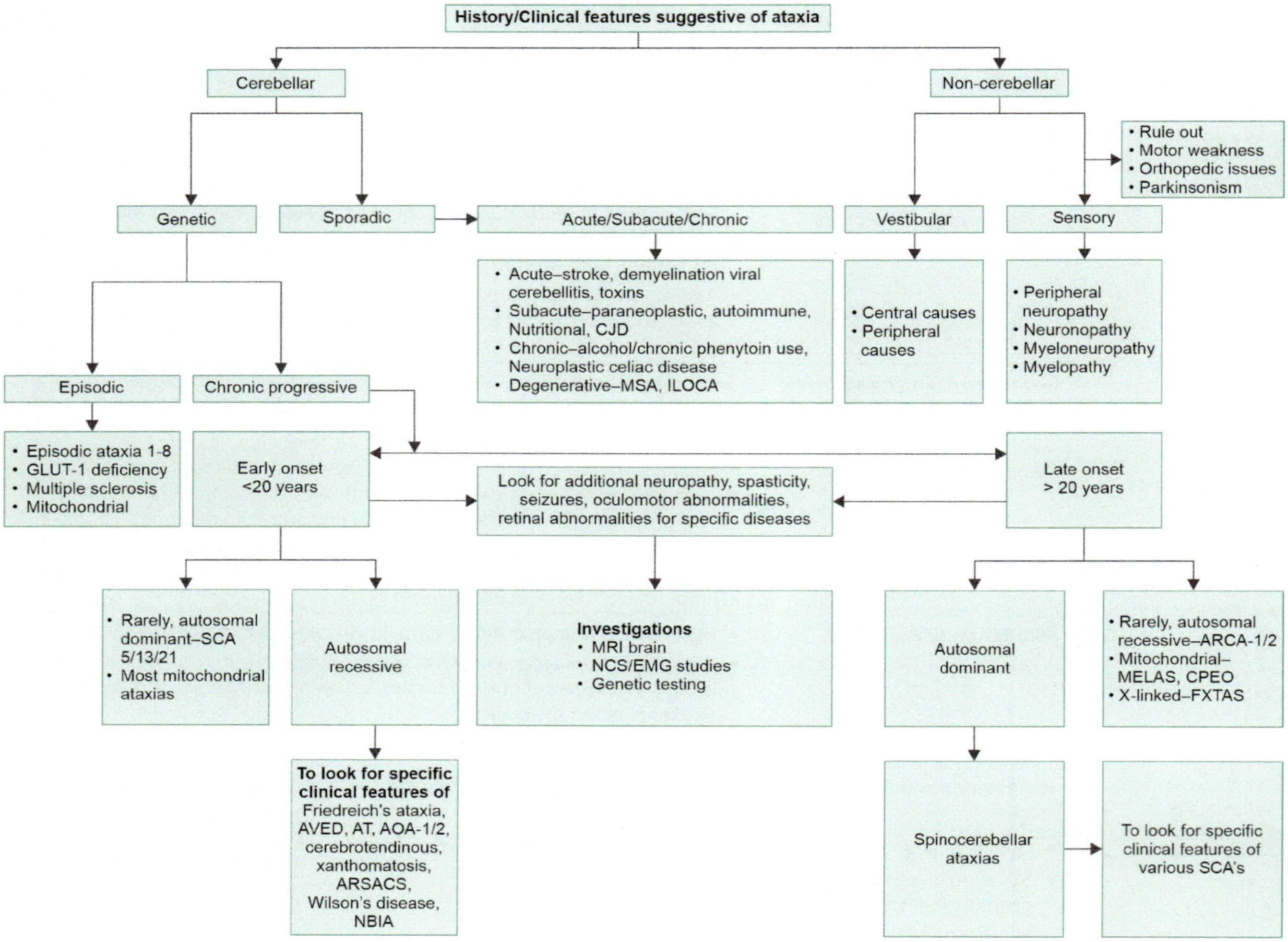

FLOWCHART 1: Clinical approach to ataxia.

(ARCA: autosomal recessive cerebellar ataxia; AVED: ataxia with vitamin E deficiency; CJD: Creutzfeldt–Jacob disease; EMG: electromyography; FXTAS: fragile X-associated tremor/ataxia syndrome; ILOCA: idiopathic late-onset cerebellar ataxia; MELAS: mitochondrial encephalopathy, lactic acidosis, and stroke-like events; MSA: multiple system atrophy; NCS: nerve conduction study; SCA: spinocerebellar ataxia)

TABLE 11: Ataxia in combination with other features.

			Associated features
Cerebellar ataxia with neuropathy	With sensory neuronopathy	*Early onset*: • Friedreich's ataxia (FA)[69,70]	Teenage onset, areflexia, Babinski sign, Pes cavus, scoliosis, square-wave jerks, late dysarthria, cervical cord atrophy, absence of cerebellar atrophy, hypertrophic cardiomyopathy, and diabetes
		• Ataxia with vitamin E deficiency (AVED)[71-73]	High prevalence around Mediterranean sea, close mimic of FA (dorsal column involvement, areflexia, skeletal deformities, teenage onset, spinal cord atrophy, occasional cerebellar atrophy), head titubation, retinitis pigmentosa, low-serum vitamin E
		• SANDO[90,116]	Ptosis, myoclonus, epilepsy along with sensory ataxia, dysarthria, and ophthalmoplegia
		Late onset: • SCA2[117]	Cerebellar ataxia, peripheral neuronopathy, and characteristic slow saccades
	With sensorimotor axonal neuropathy	Ataxia telangiectasia[74,75]	First-decade chorea–dystonia, recurrent infections, telangiectasia, elevated AFP susceptibility to lymphoma, leukemia
		Ataxia with oculomotor apraxia-1 (AOA-1)[76,77]	Prevalent in Japan, first decade, oculomotor apraxia, chorea–dystonia, low albumin, high-creatine kinase, cholesterol
		Ataxia with oculomotor apraxia-2 (AOA-2)[78,79]	Second to third decade, oculomotor apraxia, chorea–dystonia, hypogonadism, elevated AFP

Continued

Continued

			Associated features
Cerebellar ataxia with spasticity (spastic ataxia)[118]	Childhood onset	• ARSACS • AVED • SPAX-1/4/5 • Early onset cerebellar ataxia with retained reflexes	First-decade ataxia with lower limb spasticity, late sensorimotor neuropathy, retinal nerve fibers thickening Onset first to second decade preserved tendon reflexes, less severe course than Friedreich's
	Adult onset	SPG-7[119]	Complicated HSP phenotype with predominant ataxia with or without spasticity
		• SCA-1 (Chapter 88) • Adult-onset Alexander disease • Cerebrotendinous xanthomatosis (CTX)[85]	• 25% adulthood onset, ataxia, slowly progressive bulbar, pseudobulbar syndrome, spastic paraparesis, palatal myoclonus • Spasticity, cognitive decline, tendon xanthomas, chronic diarrhea, premature atherosclerosis premature cataract
	Variable onset	SCA-3 (Chapter 88) SPAX-2/7	
Cerebellar ataxia with diagnostic eye movement abnormalities	Vertical gaze palsy	Niemann–Pick disease[120]	• First to third decade onset, hepatosplenomegaly, dystonia, and cognitive decline
	Horizontal gaze palsy	Gaucher's disease type 3[121]	• Gaucher type 3 patients have seizures, pancytopenia, hepatosplenomegaly, and/or bone affection. Horizontal saccades decelerate earlier, while vertical saccades follow. Additionally, posterior segment abnormalities of the eye might be seen too
	Slow saccades	SCA-2[104]	
	Oculomotor apraxia	AOA-1, AOA-2, AOA-4, AT	
Cerebellar ataxia with dystonia[122]	Infancy/ childhood onset	• AT, AOA-1/2/4 • Wilson's disease • NBIA—PLA2G6 • DYT—TUBB4A • Biotin-thiamine-responsive basal ganglia degeneration (BTRBGD) • GLUT-1 deficiency • Glutaric aciduria • FA, AVED	• KF rings, Wing beating tremors • Truncal hypotonia, spasticity, mental retardation, and seizures • Pyramidal/Bulbar signs, oculogyric crisis • Infantile onset, reversible basal ganglia affection, responsive to biotin and thiamine supplementation • Episodic ataxia, exercise-induced dystonia, events associated with low CSF sugar, crisscross gait
	Adulthood onset	• Niemann–Pick disease type C • POLG disorders • SCA-3 (rarely 1/2/6)	
	Late onset	MSA	
Cerebellar ataxia with myoclonus/ seizures[123,124]	*Genetic early onset:* Progressive myoclonic ataxia (PMA)	Lafora disease	Childhood-onset, stimulus sensitive myoclonus, cognitive affection, inclusion bodies on skin biopsy (Lafora bodies)
		• Unverricht–Lundborg disease • MERRF • Sialidosis type-1	
		NCL (neuronal ceroid lipofuscinosis)	NCL has visual deficits and cognitive affection along with seizures and ataxia, NCL-6 can be adolescence/adulthood onset
		Ramsay–Hunt syndrome	Early onset cerebellar ataxia with myoclonus

Continued

Continued

			Associated features
Cerebellar ataxia with myoclonus/ seizures[123,124]	Genetic adulthood onset	• DRPLA • SCA-14 • Mitochondrial (MERRF/ MELAS)	Chorea, seizures, myoclonus, and dementia
	Nongenetic	Celiac disease[63]	GI symptoms, epilepsy, myopathy, neuropathy, gluten encephalopathy, and occipital calcifications
		• CJD • MSA	
Cerebellar ataxia with vestibular/ sensory ataxia	Childhood/ adult onset	POLG ataxia[90]	Cerebellar and sensory ataxia, dysarthria, ophthalmoplegia, myoclonus, epilepsy, myopathy, migraine, signal abnormalities in the cerebellum and thalamus
	Late adulthood onset	CANVAS[125]	Cerebellar, vestibular, and sensory ataxic component, abnormal visually enhanced vestibulo-ocular reflex (VVOR), anterior and dorsal vermis atrophy, chronic dry cough
Cerebellar ataxia with retinal degeneration	Retinitis pigmentosa[126]	• Refsum's disease • Abetalipoproteinemia (posterior fundus) • AVED • NCL	Ichthyosis, night blindness, myeloneuropathy
	Cherry red spot[127]	Sialidosis type 1	Second to third decade onset, also called "cherry red spot myoclonus" syndrome, associated with ataxia, hyperreflexia, and loss of vision
	Macular degeneration	Spinocerebellar ataxia-7	
	Retinal dystrophy	Cockayne syndrome[128]	• *Type 1 (classic)*: Moderate symptoms, childhood • *Type 2* is severe and early in onset • *Type 3* is mild and present with adolescence/early adulthood ataxic phenotype

(AVED: ataxia with vitamin E deficiency; ARSACS: autosomal recessive spastic ataxia of Charlevoix-Saguenay; CANVAS: cerebellar ataxia neuropathy vestibular areflexia syndrome; HSP: hereditary spastic paraplegia; MELAS: mitochondrial encephalopathy, lactic acidosis, and stroke-like events; MERRF: myoclonic epilepsy with ragged-red fibers; MSA: multiple system atrophy; SANDO: sensory ataxic neuropathy, dysarthria, and ophthalmoparesis)

TABLE 12: MRI findings peculiar of specific ataxias.

Diagnostic findings	MSA-C, SCA-2/3	Hot cross bun **(Fig. 5A)**, pontine atrophy
	FXTAS	MCP sign
	Aceruloplasminemia	Decreased dentate, red nuclei, basal ganglia T2 signal
	Superficial siderosis	Hemosiderin deposition around the brainstem, cerebellar atrophy
	Sporadic CJD **(Fig. 5B)**	Striatal hyperintensity, cortical ribboning
	ARSACS	Hypointense pontine strips, superior vermis atrophy, thinning of posterior mid-body of corpus callosum
	SPG7	High-dentate nuclei signal
	CTX **(Fig. 5C)**	MCP hyperintensity, dentate hyperintensity, white matter and cerebellar hyperintensity
	Wernicke's encephalopathy	T2 hyperintensity in mamillary bodies, periaqueductal gray and paraventricular thalamus
	Adult-onset Alexander disease	Medullary and upper cervical cord atrophy, Tadpole sign
Suggestive findings	Friedreich's ataxia	Upper cervical cord atrophy, and cerebellar atrophy late in course
	AT, AOA-1, -2	Cerebellar atrophy
	AD-SCA	Cerebellar and pontine atrophy
	POLG ataxia, ataxia with gluten sensitivity	Bilateral inferior olivary T2 hyperintensity

(AD: autosomal dominant; AT: ataxia telangiectasia; AOA-1, -2: ataxia with oculomotor apraxia; CTX: cerebrotendinous xanthomatosis; CJD: Creutzfeldt–Jacob disease; FXTAS: fragile X-associated tremor/ataxia syndrome; SCA: spinocerebellar ataxia)

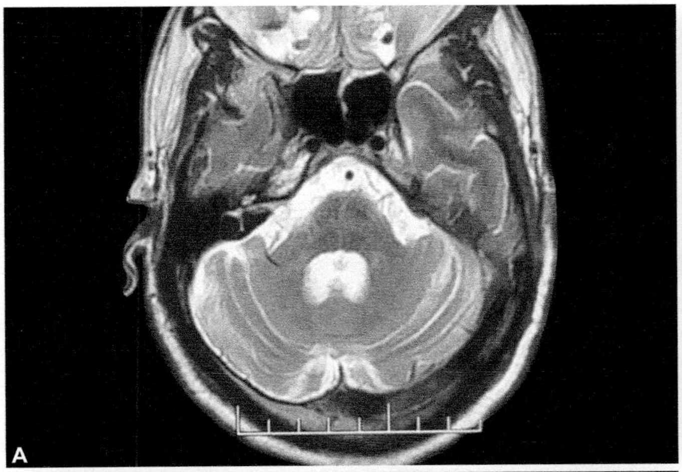

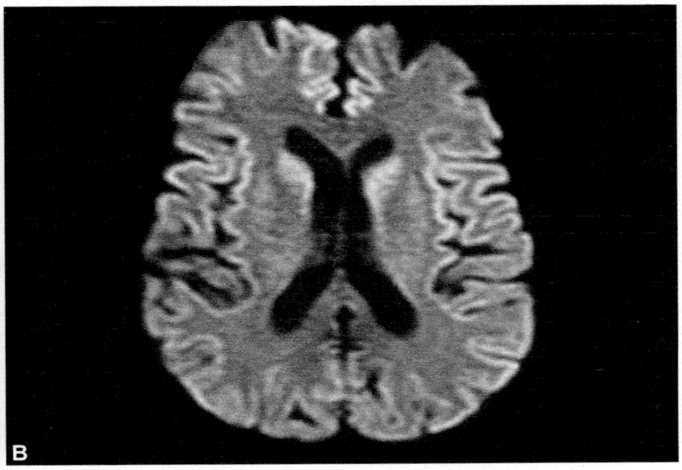

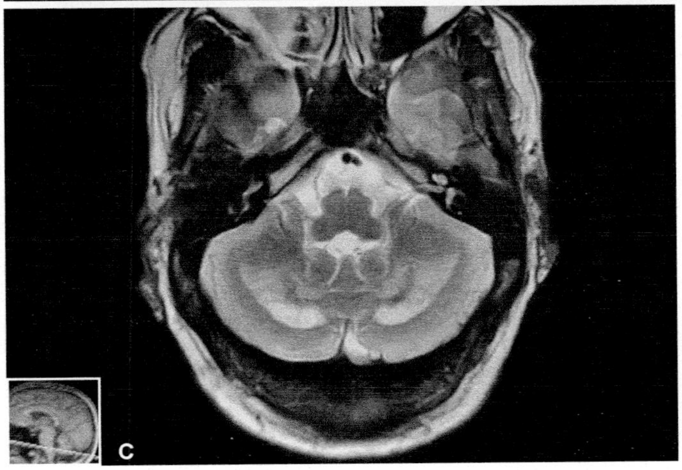

FIGS. 5A TO C: A few typical imaging findings. (A) Hot cross bun sign MSA-C and some SCA's; (B) Striatal hyperintensity and cortical ribboning in CJD; (C) Dentate hyperintensity in CTX.

(CJD: Creutzfeldt–Jacob disease; CTX: cerebrotendinous xanthomatosis; MSA-C: multiple system atrophy–cerebellar subtype; SCA: spinocerebellar ataxia)

possibility of FA, ataxia with oculomotor apraxia 1 and 2, and POLG-related disorders. Finally, ataxia with onset in adulthood is evocative of autosomal dominant SCAs (less likely AR cerebellar ataxia 1 and 3, late-onset FA, and spastic paraplegia). Finally, differentials for late-onset ataxia without family history would be MSA and ILOCA.

5. *Genetic testing*: Once the clinical assessment is complete, genetic testing is indicated to confirm the mutated gene. Initial testing should include searching for the FA-associated trinucleotide repeat expansion (*FXN* gene) considering the high prevalence of this mutation, and the heterogeneous clinical phenotype. Moreover, clinicians may consider testing for another specific gene through Sanger sequencing or multiplex ligation-dependent probe amplification (MLPA) with high clinical suspicion. Finally, a panel for the dominantly inherited CAG repeat expansion SCAs may also be considered as part of the initial assessment if family history is inconclusive, considering the high prevalence of these mutations and their incomplete coverage through the next-generation sequencing methods.
6. *Whole exome and genome sequencing*: After excluding the repeat-related ataxias, whole-exome sequencing can be very useful in determining sequence alterations. Limitations of whole-exome sequencing for ataxia being not sensitive to large chromosomal deletions or duplications (such as in SCA20), or mitochondrial genome mutations, or repeat expansions in the noncoding regions. The highest yield is obtained for patients with early onset ataxia and positive family history and consanguinity among parents. Once genetic testing identifies a pathogenic mutation, specialized genetic counseling for the patient and his or her relatives is essential along with symptom management and disease treatment when available.

CONCLUSION

Ataxia may be cerebellar, sensory, or vestibular. Other neurologic disorders that can give rise to similar problems with gait and dexterity (e.g., nerve and muscle disorders, spinal cord diseases, and basal ganglia diseases), however, can usually be distinguished with a careful history and clinical examination.

The causes of cerebellar ataxia are many and frequently present as a diagnostic challenge. This requires a systematic evaluation, where acquired causes of ataxia should be first considered, followed by genetic and degenerative forms. Age of onset, focal or generalized presentation, time course, and family history are important points when making the differential diagnosis. If genetic ataxia is suspected, pathologic repeat expansions in genes should be determined first, followed by an assessment of sequence alterations. Among late-onset cerebellar ataxias, multiple system atrophy is the most common and needs to be kept in mind in cases with sporadic cerebellar ataxia. Treatable causes such as autoimmune cerebellar disorders, drug-induced ataxias, nutritional and vascular causes need to be evaluated in all cases.

REFERENCES

1. Harding AE. Classification of the hereditary ataxias and paraplegias. Lancet. 1983;321(8334):1151-5.
2. Singh R; IntechOpen. (2021). Cerebellum: Its Anatomy, Functions and Diseases. Neurodegenerative Diseases—Molecular Mechanisms and Current Therapeutic Approaches. [online] Available from https://www.intechopen.com/books/9157. [Last accessed April, 2023].
3. Zhang Q, Zhou X, Li Y, Yang X, Abbasi QH. Clinical recognition of sensory ataxia and cerebellar ataxia. Front Hum Neurosci. 2021;15:639871.
4. Park HK, Kim JS, Strupp M, Zee DS. Isolated floccular infarction: impaired vestibular responses to horizontal head impulse. J Neurol. 2013;260(6):1576-82.
5. Kremmyda O, Kirchner H, Glasauer S, Brandt T, Jahn K, Strupp M. False-positive head-impulse test in cerebellar ataxia. Front Neurol. 2012;3:162.
6. Barohn RJ, Amato AA. Pattern-recognition approach to neuropathy and neuronopathy. Neurol Clin. 2013;31(2):343-61.
7. Thomann KH, Dul MW. Abnormal gait in neurologic disease. Optom Clin. 1996;5(3–4):181-92.
8. Missaoui B, Thoumie P. Balance training in ataxic neuropathies. Effects on balance and gait parameters. Gait Posture. 2013;38(3):471-6.
9. Chhetri SK, Gow D, Shaunak S, Varma A. Clinical assessment of the sensory ataxias; diagnostic algorithm with illustrative cases. Pract Neurol. 2014;14(4):242-51.
10. Mathis S, Duval F, Soulages A, Solé G, le Masson G. The ataxic neuropathies. J Neurol. 2021;268(10):3675-89.
11. Amato AA, Ropper AH. Sensory Ganglionopathy. N Eng J Med. 2020;383(17):1657-62.
12. Ito M. Cerebellar Control of the Vestibulo-Ocular Reflex--Around the Flocculus Hypothesis. Annu Rev Neurosci. 1982;5(1):275-97.
13. Wieling W, Thijs RD, van Dijk N, Wilde AAM, Benditt DG, van Dijk JG. Symptoms and signs of syncope: a review of the link between physiology and clinical clues. Brain. 2009;132(10):2630-42.
14. Eggers SDZ. Episodic Spontaneous Dizziness. Continuum (Minneap Minn). 2021;27(2):369-401.
15. Fife TD. Approach to the history and evaluation of vertigo and dizziness. Continuum (Minneap Minn). 2021;27(2):306-29.
16. Kerber KA. Episodic positional dizziness. Continuum (Minneap Minn). 2021;27(2):348-68.
17. Stewart JM, Clarke D. "He's Dizzy When He Stands Up": An Introduction to Initial Orthostatic Hypotension. J Pediatr. 2011;158(3):499-504.
18. Kim SH, Kim HJ, Kim JS. Isolated vestibular syndromes due to brainstem and cerebellar lesions. J Neurol. 2017;264(S1):63-9.
19. Muncie HL, Sirmans SM, James E. Dizziness: Approach to Evaluation and Management. Am Fam Physician. 2017;95(3):154-62.
20. Said Mogutham NN, Abdullah JM, Idris Z, Ghani ARI, Abdul Halim S, Naesarajoo JJJ, et al. Examination approach to the dizzy and swaying patient. Malays J Med Sci. 2020;27(6):89-101.
21. Edlow JA, Newman-Toker DE, Savitz SI. Diagnosis and initial management of cerebellar infarction. Lancet Neurol. 2008;7(10): 951-64.
22. Peters BT, Mulavara AP, Cohen HS, Sangi-Haghpeykar H, Bloomberg JJ. Dynamic visual acuity testing for screening patients with vestibular impairments. J Vestib Res. 2012;22(2-3):145-51.
23. Fukuda T. The Stepping Test: Two Phases of the Labyrinthine Reflex. Acta Otolaryngol. 1959;50(1-2):95-108.
24. Diener HC, Dichgans J. Pathophysiology of cerebellar ataxia. Mov Disord. 1992;7(2):95-109.
25. Bastian AJ, Martin TA, Keating JG, Thach WT. Cerebellar ataxia: abnormal control of interaction torques across multiple joints. J Neurophysiol. 1996;76(1):492-509.
26. Sajja Srinivasa Siva Naga R. Anatomy of cerebellum. In: Bozzetto Ambrosi P (Ed). Spinocerebellar Ataxia - Concepts, Particularities and Generalities. London: IntechOpen; 2022.
27. Stoodley CJ, Schmahmann JD. Evidence for topographic organization in the cerebellum of motor control versus cognitive and affective processing. Cortex. 2010;46(7):831-44.
28. Wullner U, Klockgether T, Petersen D, Naegele T, Dichgans J. Magnetic resonance imaging in hereditary and idiopathic ataxia. Neurology. 1993;43(2):318-25.
29. Luijckx GJ, Spaans F, Boiten J, Lodder J. Ataxic hemiparesis caused by infarction of the cerebral peduncle. Cerebrovasc Dis. 1997;7(3):183-4.
30. McKenna C, Fellus J, Barrett AM. False localizing signs in traumatic brain injury. Brain Inj. 2009;23(7-8):597-601.
31. Manto MU. Cerebellar Disorders. Cambridge, UK: Cambridge University Press; 2010.
32. Vadhanan P, Kumar P. Anesthetic management of a patient with spinocerebellar degeneration. J Anaesthesiol Clin Pharmacol. 2011;27(2):249-52.
33. Yasen, J. (2014). Ataxia, acute or subacute. In A. Ettinger & D. Weisbrot (Eds.), Neurologic Differential Diagnosis: A Case-Based Approach (pp. 45-54). Cambridge: Cambridge University Press.
34. Klockgether T, Döller G, Wüllner U, Petersen D, Dichgans J. Cerebellar encephalitis in adults. J Neurol. 1993;240(1):17-20.
35. Berlit P, Rakicky J. The Miller Fisher syndrome. Review of the literature. J Clin Neuroophthalmol. 1992;12(1):57-63.
36. Dalmau J, Gultekin HS, Posner JB. Paraneoplastic neurologic syndromes: Pathogenesis and physiopathology. Brain Pathol. 2006;9(2):275-84.
37. Wu H, Lau W, Chan TY, Chen SP, Ko C. Differentiating episodic ataxia type 2 from migraine: a case report. Hong Kong Med J. 2020;26(6):526-7.
38. Sesh S, Radhakrishnan A. Episodic ataxia in a child with senataxin mutation. Neurol India. 2018;66(3):842-4.
39. Balint B, Vincent A, Meinck HM, Irani SR, Bhatia KP. Movement disorders with neuronal antibodies: syndromic approach, genetic parallels and pathophysiology. Brain. 2018;141(1):13-36.
40. Gövert F, Leypoldt F, Junker R, Wandinger KP, Deuschl G, Bhatia KP, et al. Antibody-related movement disorders – a comprehensive review of phenotype-autoantibody correlations and a guide to testing. Neurol Res Pract. 2020;2(1):6.
41. Shanmugarajah PD, Hoggard N, Currie S, Aeschlimann DP, Aeschlimann PC, Gleeson DC, et al. Alcohol-related cerebellar degeneration: not all down to toxicity? Cerebellum Ataxias. 2016;3:17.
42. Shanmugarajah P, Hoggard N, Howell S, Dennis G, Reuber M, Grunewald R, et al. Phenytoin and cerebellar ataxia: not all down to toxicity? J Neurol Neurosurg Psychiatry. 2013;84(11):e2.6-e2.
43. Finsterer J. Mitochondrial ataxias. Can J Neurol Sci. 2009;36(5): 543-53.

44. Cortese A, Simone R, Sullivan R, Vandrovcova J, Tariq H, Yau WY, et al. Biallelic expansion of an intronic repeat in RFC1 is a common cause of late-onset ataxia. Nat Genet. 2019;51(4):649-58.
45. Singer HS, Mink JW, Gilbert DL, Jankovic J. Ataxia. Movement Disorders in Childhood. New York: Elsevier; 2015. pp. 263-300.
46. Musselman KE, Stoyanov CT, Marasigan R, Jenkins ME, Konczak J, Morton SM, et al. Prevalence of ataxia in children: a systematic review. Neurology. 2014;82(1):80-9.
47. Moeschler JB, Shevell M, Moeschler JB, Shevell M, Saul RA, Chen E, et al. Comprehensive evaluation of the child with intellectual disability or global developmental delays. Pediatrics. 2014;134(3):e903-18.
48. Bertini E, Zanni G, Boltshauser E. Nonprogressive congenital ataxias. Handb Clin Neurol. 2018;155:91-103.
49. Manto M, Marmolino D. Cerebellar ataxias. Curr Opin Neurol. 2009;22(4):419-29.
50. Brusse E, Maat-Kievit JA, van Swieten JC. Diagnosis and management of early- and late-onset cerebellar ataxia. Clin Genet. 2007;71(1):12-24.
51. Klockgether T, Mariotti C, Paulson HL. Spinocerebellar ataxia. Nat Rev Dis Primers. 2019;5(1):24.
52. Zhuchenko O, Bailey J, Bonnen P, Ashizawa T, Stockton DW, Amos C, et al. Autosomal dominant cerebellar ataxia (SCA6) associated with small polyglutamine expansions in the α1A-voltage-dependent calcium channel. Nat Genet. 1997;15(1):62-9.
53. Demarquay G, Honnorat J. Clinical presentation of immune-mediated cerebellar ataxia. Rev Neurol (Paris). 2011;167(5):408-17.
54. Prüss H. Autoantibodies in neurological disease. Nat Rev Immunol. 2021;21(12):798-813.
55. Klockgether T. Sporadic ataxia with adult onset: classification and diagnostic criteria. Lancet Neurol. 2010;9(1):94-104.
56. Wenning GK, Stankovic I, Vignatelli L, Fanciulli A, Calandra-Buonaura G, Seppi K, et al. The Movement Disorder Society Criteria for the Diagnosis of Multiple System Atrophy. Movement Disorders. 2022;37(6):1131-48.
57. Fanciulli A, Wenning GK. Multiple-System Atrophy. N Engl J Med. 2015;372(3):249-63.
58. Leehey MA. Fragile X-Associated Tremor/Ataxia Syndrome. J Invest Med. 2009;57(8):830-6.
59. Graus F. Recommended diagnostic criteria for paraneoplastic neurological syndromes. J Neurol Neurosurg Psychiatry. 2004;75(8):1135-40.
60. Hadjivassiliou M, Graus F, Honnorat J, Jarius S, Titulaer M, Manto M, et al. Diagnostic Criteria for Primary Autoimmune Cerebellar Ataxia—Guidelines from an International Task Force on Immune-Mediated Cerebellar Ataxias. Cerebellum. 2020;19(4):605-10.
61. Linke R, Schroeder M, Helmberger T, Voltz R. Antibody-positive paraneoplastic neurologic syndromes: Value of CT and PET for tumor diagnosis. Neurology. 2004;63(2):282-6.
62. Pengiran Tengah DSNA. Neurological complications of coeliac disease. Postgrad Med J. 2002;78(921):393-8.
63. Vinagre-Aragón A, Zis P, Grunewald R, Hadjivassiliou M. Movement Disorders Related to Gluten Sensitivity: A Systematic Review. Nutrients. 2018;10(8):1034.
64. Holmes G. An attempt to classify cerebellar disease, with a note on Marie's hereditary cerebellar ataxia. Brain. 1908;30(4):545-67.
65. Kim JS, Cho JW. Hereditary Cerebellar Ataxias: A Korean Perspective. J Mov Disord. 2015;8(2):67-75.
66. Beaudin M, Matilla-Dueñas A, Soong BW, Pedroso JL, Barsottini OG, Mitoma H, et al. The classification of autosomal recessive cerebellar ataxias: a consensus statement from the Society for Research on the Cerebellum and Ataxias Task Force. Cerebellum. 2019;18(6):1098-125.
67. Beaudin M, Klein CJ, Rouleau GA, Dupré N. Systematic review of autosomal recessive ataxias and proposal for a classification. Cerebellum Ataxias. 2017;4(1):3.
68. Pearson TS. More than ataxia: Hyperkinetic Movement Disorders in Childhood Autosomal Recessive Ataxia Syndromes. Tremor Other Hyperkinet Mov (N Y). 2016;6:368.
69. Dürr A, Cossee M, Agid Y, Campuzano V, Mignard C, Penet C, et al. Clinical and Genetic Abnormalities in Patients with Friedreich's Ataxia. N Engl J Med. 1996;335(16):1169-75.
70. Campuzano V, Montermini L, Moltò MD, Pianese L, Cossée M, Cavalcanti F, et al. Friedreich's Ataxia: Autosomal Recessive Disease Caused by an Intronic GAA Triplet Repeat Expansion. Science (1979). 1996;271(5254):1423-7.
71. Yokota T, Shiojiri T, Gotoda T, Arita M, Arai H, Ohga T, et al. Friedreich-like ataxia with retinitis pigmentosa caused by the His101Gln mutation of the ?-Tocopherol transfer protein gene. Ann Neurol. 1997;41(6):826-32.
72. Euch-Fayache G El, Bouhlal Y, Amouri R, Feki M, Hentati F. Molecular, clinical and peripheral neuropathy study of Tunisian patients with ataxia with vitamin E deficiency. Brain. 2014;137(2):402-10.
73. Ouahchi K, Arita M, Kayden H, Hentati F, Hamida M ben, Sokol R, et al. Ataxia with isolated vitamin E deficiency is caused by mutations in the α-tocopherol transfer protein. Nat Genet. 1995;9(2):141-5.
74. Wright J, Teraoka S, Onengut S, Tolun A, Gatti RA, Ochs HD, et al. A high frequency of distinct ATM gene mutations in ataxia-telangiectasia. Am J Hum Genet. 1996;59(4):839-46.
75. Levy A, Lang AE. Ataxia-telangiectasia: A review of movement disorders, clinical features, and genotype correlations. Mov Disord. 2018;33(8):1238-47.
76. Date H, Onodera O, Tanaka H, Iwabuchi K, Uekawa K, Igarashi S, et al. Early-onset ataxia with ocular motor apraxia and hypoalbuminemia is caused by mutations in a new HIT superfamily gene. Nat Genet. 2001;29(2):184-8.
77. Moreira MC, Barbot C, Tachi N, Kozuka N, Uchida E, Gibson T, et al. The gene mutated in ataxia-ocular apraxia 1 encodes the new HIT/Zn-finger protein aprataxin. Nat Genet. 2001;29(2):189-93.
78. Le Ber I, Bouslam N, Rivaud-Péchoux S, Guimarães J, Benomar A, Chamayou C, et al. Frequency and phenotypic spectrum of ataxia with oculomotor apraxia 2: a clinical and genetic study in 18 patients. Brain. 2004;127(4):759-67.
79. Moreira MC, Klur S, Watanabe M, Németh AH, Ber I le, Moniz JC, et al. Senataxin, the ortholog of a yeast RNA helicase, is mutant in ataxia-ocular apraxia 2. Nat Genet. 2004;36(3):225-7.
80. Izumi Y, Miyamoto R, Morino H, Yoshizawa A, Nishinaka K, Udaka F, et al. Cerebellar ataxia with SYNE1 mutation accompanying motor neuron disease. Neurology. 2013;80(6):600-1.
81. Gros-Louis F, Dupré N, Dion P, Fox MA, Laurent S, Verreault S, et al. Mutations in SYNE1 lead to a newly discovered form of autosomal recessive cerebellar ataxia. Nat Genet. 2007;39(1):80-5.
82. Lagier-Tourenne C, Tazir M, López LC, Quinzii CM, Assoum M, Drouot N, et al. ADCK3, an Ancestral Kinase, Is Mutated in a Form of Recessive Ataxia Associated with Coenzyme Q10 Deficiency. Am J Hum Genet. 2008;82(3):661-72.
83. Mollet J, Delahodde A, Serre V, Chretien D, Schlemmer D, Lombes A, et al. CABC1 Gene Mutations Cause Ubiquinone Deficiency with Cerebellar Ataxia and Seizures. Am J Hum Genet. 2008;82(3):623-30.
84. Nie S, Chen G, Cao X, Zhang Y. Cerebrotendinous xanthomatosis: a comprehensive review of pathogenesis, clinical manifestations, diagnosis, and management. Orphanet J Rare Dis. 2014;9(1):179.
85. Wong JC, Walsh K, Hayden D, Eichler FS. Natural history of neurological abnormalities in cerebrotendinous xanthomatosis. J Inherit Metab Dis. 2018;41(4):647-56.
86. Hagerman PJ, Hagerman RJ. Fragile X-associated tremor/ataxia syndrome—an older face of the fragile X gene. Nat Clin Pract Neurol. 2007;3(2):107-12.
87. Lopriore P, Ricciarini V, Siciliano G, Mancuso M, Montano V. Mitochondrial Ataxias: Molecular Classification and Clinical Heterogeneity. Neurol Int. 2022;14(2):337-56.

88. Zeviani M, Simonati A, Bindoff LA. Ataxia in mitochondrial disorders. Handb Clin Neurol. 2012;103:359-72.
89. Zeviani M, Carelli V. Mitochondrial disorders. Curr Opin Neurol. 2007;20(5):564-71.
90. van Goethem G, Martin JJ, Dermaut B, Löfgren A, Wibail A, Ververken D, et al. Recessive POLG mutations presenting with sensory and ataxic neuropathy in compound heterozygote patients with progressive external ophthalmoplegia. Neuromuscul Disord. 2003;13(2):133-42.
91. Luo L, Wang J, Lo RY, Figueroa KP, Pulst SM, Kuo PH, et al. The initial symptom and motor progression in spinocerebellar ataxias. Cerebellum. 2017;16(3):615-22.
92. Stoodley CJ, Valera EM, Schmahmann JD. Functional topography of the cerebellum for motor and cognitive tasks: an fMRI study. Neuroimage. 2012;59(2):1560-70.
93. Trouillas P, Takayanagi T, Hallett M, Currier RD, Subramony SH, Wessel K, et al. International Cooperative Ataxia Rating Scale for pharmacological assessment of the cerebellar syndrome. J Neurol Sci. 1997;145(2):205-11.
94. Schmitz-Hubsch T, du Montcel ST, Baliko L, Berciano J, Boesch S, Depondt C, et al. Scale for the assessment and rating of ataxia: Development of a new clinical scale. Neurology. 2006;66(11): 1717-20.
95. Subramony SH, May W, Lynch D, Gomez C, Fischbeck K, Hallett M, et al. Measuring Friedreich ataxia: Interrater reliability of a neurologic rating scale. Neurology. 2005;64(7):1261-2.
96. Schmahmann JD, Gardner R, MacMore J, Vangel MG. Development of a brief ataxia rating scale (BARS) based on a modified form of the ICARS. Mov Disord. 2009;24(12):1820-8.
97. Bodranghien F, Bastian A, Casali C, Hallett M, Louis ED, Manto M, et al. Consensus Paper: Revisiting the Symptoms and Signs of Cerebellar Syndrome. Cerebellum. 2016;15(3):369-91.
98. Marsden JF. Cerebellar ataxia. Handb Clin Neurol. 2018;159:261-81.
99. Kheradmand A, Zee DS. Cerebellum and ocular motor control. Front Neurol. 2011;2:53.
100. Waespe W, Cohen B, Raphan T. Dynamic modification of the vestibulo-ocular reflex by the nodulus and uvula. Science. 1985;228(4696):199-202.
101. Huh YE, Kim JS. Patterns of spontaneous and head-shaking nystagmus in cerebellar infarction: imaging correlations. Brain. 2011;134(Pt 12):3662-71.
102. Termsarasab P, Thammongkolchai T, Rucker JC, Frucht SJ. The diagnostic value of saccades in movement disorder patients: a practical guide and review. J Clin Mov Disord. 2015;2(1):14.
103. Helmchen C, Straube A, Büttner U. Saccadic lateropulsion in Wallenberg's syndrome may be caused by a functional lesion of the fastigial nucleus. J Neurol. 1994;241(7):421-6.
104. Wadia NH, Swami RK. A new form of heredo-familial spinocerebellar degeneration with slow eye movements (nine families). Brain. 1971;94(2):359-74.
105. Ying SH, Horn AKE, Geiner S, Wadia NH, Büttner-Ennever JA. Selective, circuit-wide sparing of floccular connections in hereditary olivopontine cerebellar atrophy with slow saccades. Prog Brain Res. 2008;171:583-6.
106. Thurston SE, Leigh RJ, Abel LA, Dell'Osso LF. Hyperactive vestibulo-ocular reflex in cerebellar degeneration: pathogenesis and treatment. Neurology. 1987;37(1):53-7.
107. Colen CB, Ketko A, George E, van Stavern GP. Periodic alternating nystagmus and periodic alternating skew deviation in spino-cerebellar ataxia type 6. J Neuroophthalmol. 2008;28(4):287-8.
108. Hüfner K, Frenzel C, Kremmyda O, Adrion C, Bardins S, Glasauer S, et al. Esophoria or esotropia in adulthood: a sign of cerebellar dysfunction? J Neurol. 2015;262(3):585-92.
109. Angel RW. The rebound phenomenon of gordon holmes. Arch Neurol. 1977;34(4):250.
110. Holmes G. The cerebellum of man. Brain. 1939;62(1):1-30.
111. Hoche F, Guell X, Vangel MG, Sherman JC, Schmahmann JD. The cerebellar cognitive affective/Schmahmann syndrome scale. Brain. 2018;141(1):248-70.
112. Chakor R, Bharote H. Inherited ataxia with slow saccades. J Postgrad Med. 2012;58(4):318.
113. Coarelli G, Wirth T, Tranchant C, Koenig M, Durr A, Anheim M. The inherited cerebellar ataxias: an update. J Neurol. 2023;270(1): 208-22.
114. Brandsma R, Verschuuren-Bemelmans CC, Amrom D, Barisic N, Baxter P, Bertini E, et al. A clinical diagnostic algorithm for early onset cerebellar ataxia. Eur J Paediatr Neurol. 2019;23(5):692-706.
115. Stezin A, Pal PK. Treatable Ataxias: How to Find the Needle in the Haystack? J Mov Disord. 2022;15(3):206-26.
116. Winterthun S, Ferrari G, He L, Taylor RW, Zeviani M, Turnbull DM, et al. Autosomal recessive mitochondrial ataxic syndrome due to mitochondrial polymerase mutations. Neurology. 2005;64(7):1204-8.
117. Pelosi L, Iodice R, Antenora A, Kilfoyle D, Mulroy E, Rodrigues M, et al. Spinocerebellar ataxia type 2-neuronopathy or neuropathy? Muscle Nerve. 2019;60(3):271-8.
118. Bereznyakova O, Dupré N. Spastic ataxias. Handb Clin Neurol. 2018;155:191-203.
119. Yahikozawa H, Yoshida K, Sato S, Hanyu N, Doi H, Miyatake S, et al. Predominant cerebellar phenotype in spastic paraplegia 7 (SPG7). Hum Genome Var. 2015;2(1):15012.
120. Gupta DK, Blanco-Palmero VA, Chung WK, Kuo SH. Abnormal vertical eye movements as a clue for diagnosis of Niemann-Pick type C. Tremor Other Hyperkinet Mov (N Y). 2018;8:560.
121. Hopf S, Pfeiffer N, Liesenfeld M, Mengel KE, Hennermann JB, Schmidtmann I, et al. A comprehensive monocentric ophthalmic study with Gaucher disease type 3 patients: vitreoretinal lesions, retinal atrophy and characterization of abnormal saccades. Orphanet J Rare Dis. 2019;14(1):257.
122. Rossi M, Balint B, Millar Vernetti P, Bhatia KP, Merello M. Genetic dystonia-ataxia syndromes: Clinical spectrum, diagnostic approach, and treatment options. Mov Disord Clin Pract. 2018;5(4):373-82.
123. van der Veen S, Zutt R, Elting JWJ, Becker CE, de Koning TJ, Tijssen MAJ. Progressive myoclonus ataxia: Time for a new definition? Mov Disord. 2018;33(8):1281-6.
124. Rossi M, van der Veen S, Merello M, Tijssen MAJ, van de Warrenburg B. Myoclonus-ataxia syndromes: A diagnostic approach. Mov Disord Clin Pract. 2021;8(1):9-24.
125. Szmulewicz DJ, Roberts L, McLean CA, MacDougall HG, Halmagyi GM, Storey E. Proposed diagnostic criteria for cerebellar ataxia with neuropathy and vestibular areflexia syndrome (CANVAS). Neurol Clin Pract. 2016;6(1):61-8.
126. Tuck RR, McLeod JG. Retinitis pigmentosa, ataxia, and peripheral neuropathy. J Neurol Neurosurg Psychiatry. 1983;46(3):206-13.
127. Nemeth AH, Downes SM. Disorders of Vision. Practical Guide to Neurogenetics. London: Elsevier; 2009. pp. 49-74.
128. Rapin I, Weidenheim K, Lindenbaum Y, Rosenbaum P, Merchant SN, Krishna S, et al. Cockayne syndrome in adults: Review with clinical and pathologic study of a new case. J Child Neurol. 2006;21(11):991-1006.
129. Pellecchia MT, Stankovic I, Fanciulli A, Krismer F, Meissner WG, Palma JA, et al. Can autonomic testing and imaging contribute to the early diagnosis of multiple system atrophy? A systematic review and recommendations by the Movement Disorder Society Multiple System Atrophy Study Group. Mov Disord Clin Pract. 2020;7(7):750-62.
130. Vodušek DB. How to diagnose MSA early: the role of sphincter EMG. J Neural Transm. 2005;112(12):1657-68.
131. Skowronek C, Zange L, Lipp A. Cardiac 123I-MIBG scintigraphy in neurodegenerative Parkinson syndromes: Performance and pitfalls in clinical practice. Front Neurol. 2019;10:152.

37
CHAPTER

Approach to Tremor

Roopa Rajan, Divya M Radhakrishnan

INTRODUCTION

Tremor is a common movement disorder characterized by the involuntary rhythmic oscillatory movement of a body part. It is among the most common movement disorders with an estimated prevalence of over 1.33% worldwide. The prevalence of tremors increases markedly with age, and in the oldest age groups up to 10–20% of the population may have tremors. Tremors can affect body parts ranging from the head, jaw, voice, tongue, upper limbs, lower limbs, and trunk. It can be a significantly disabling symptom for patients, affecting their functional abilities and day-to-day activities in many ways. In this chapter, we will discuss the important tremor syndromes, their clinical features, and an approach to diagnosis.

CLINICAL APPROACH

Diagnosis of tremor is predominantly a clinical exercise, although some investigations may aid in identifying the type of tremor and its etiology. Currently, tremor is classified according to the 2017 Movement Disorder Society consensus statement on the classification of tremors.[1] According to this classification system, a 2-axis approach is used to describe tremor: At one level, it classifies tremor according to its clinical features (axis 1) and subsequently according to the etiology (axis 2). Clinical features, including the age at onset, temporal onset and progression, family history, and past medical history, may provide clues to the etiology of tremor. Response to alcohol can be elicited in history; over two-thirds of patients with essential tremor (ET) report a reduction in tremor severity after taking alcohol; however, this is not specific to ET as other hyperkinetic movement disorders such as dystonic tremor or myoclonus-dystonia may respond as well. Tremor is focal when only one body region is involved, segmental when two or more contiguous body regions are involved either in the upper or in the lower body, and generalized when both the upper and lower body regions are involved. A tremor present on only one side of the body is called hemi-tremor, as may be seen in early Parkinson's disease (PD).

The activation condition of tremor is one of the most important clues to the diagnosis. Broadly, tremors may be classified as rest or action tremors **(Flowchart 1)**. Rest tremors appear in a limb that is at rest and fully supported against gravity, such as the arms hanging on the arms of a chair or the head while lying down. Action tremors may be divided further into kinetic, postural, or isometric tremors. Kinetic tremors occur while the limb is in active movement or during the performance of several activities. A simple kinetic tremor occurs equally throughout the action while intention tremors are apparent toward the end of a goal-directed activity, such as reaching out to a target. Task-specific tremor occurs only on performing specific tasks; a classical example is primary writing tremor. Postural tremors occur when the hand or body part is held against gravity without active movement; these may be position independent, occurring in any posture or position-dependent, where the tremor is obvious only when the hand is held in a specific posture; for instance, the wing-beating position or semipronation of the forearm may bring forth tremors that were not apparent in other postures. Isometric tremor occurs when the limb contracts against a fixed resistance; orthostatic tremor is an example.

The frequency of tremor is another important finding to assess. Although it is not possible to identify the exact frequency by clinical observation alone, it is possible to classify as "slow frequency," "high frequency," and "irregular frequency" by inspection of tremor.[2] Further confirmation of tremor frequency requires electrophysiological analysis, as detailed in the subsequent sections. Generally, tremors that are <4 Hz in frequency are known as low-frequency tremors and those >12 Hz are considered high-frequency tremors. Most pathological tremors occur at a frequency of 4–8 Hz. There are certain notable exceptions, such as myorhythmia or palatal tremor, which occur at frequencies lower than

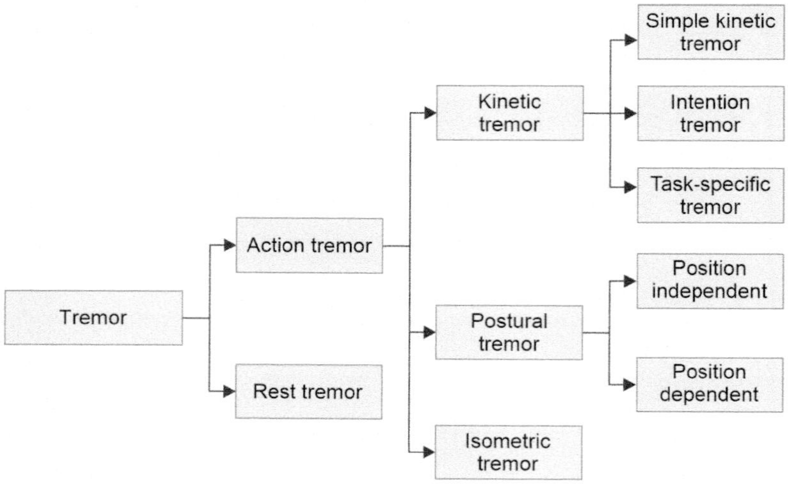

FLOWCHART 1: Activation conditions of tremor.

4 Hz. Primary orthostatic tremor has a frequency range of 13–18 Hz. Physiological tremors and exaggerated physiological tremors have frequencies ranging from 8 to 12 Hz. Cortical myoclonic tremor may often have a frequency of >8 Hz. Dystonic tremor is known for its variability in frequency, often showing slow, fast, and jerky tremors in the same limb. Variability in tremor frequency and/or amplitude is also an important sign of functional or psychogenic tremor.

Having assessed the tremor characteristics, the examination proceeds to look for associated signs. These may include signs of systemic illness such as hepatomegaly, splenomegaly, or neurocutaneous markers such as Kayser–Fleischer ring that point toward specific diagnoses. Apart from these, it is essential to pick up coexisting movement disorder phenomenologies such as dystonia, ataxia, bradykinesia, rigidity, or postural instability. These may be very subtle, such as questionable dystonia or mild ataxia, but are important to characterize tremor. To accurately identify these and other tremor characteristics, it is important to examine the patient head to foot and observe for tremors with the affected body part at several postures or tasks. Specifically, the upper face, lower face, tongue, voice, head, trunk, and limbs need to be examined. Voice tremor may be brought out by asking the patient to speak and say "aah" or "eeee." Head tremors should be examined with the patient lying down (rest) and while sitting up or walking. The direction of the head tremor may be horizontal (no-no) or vertical (yes-yes). The latter often suggests titubation, a tremor of cerebellar origin. The multidirectional nature of head tremor may suggest a functional origin. The hands should be examined at rest, with arms outstretched and elbows extended, arms abducted with elbows flexed and fingertips pointing toward each other (wing-beating) position, during finger–nose testing, and while performing tasks such as writing and pouring. Gradually pronating and supinating the outstretched arms may reveal the presence of a null point; this is a specific position of the limb at which the tremor nearly disappears. The null point can also be elicited for head tremors by gradually rotating the head from one side to the other. The presence of a null point suggests a dystonic tremor, and it usually coincides with the position of maximal dystonic contractions.

An additional feature on clinical examination that may help to distinguish among tremors is spiral drawing, especially for patients with upper limb tremors. The patient is asked to draw an Archimedes spiral on plain paper or trace between the lines of a printed spiral. Patients with PD draw small spirals where the distance between the lines reduces as they advance, resulting in crisscrossing or converging lines **(Figs. 1A to D)**. Cerebellar ataxia results in progressively increasing widths of the loops. ET and dystonic tremor spirals show tremor-related fluctuations or wobbles. The presence of tremor-related fluctuations more in a particular direction, known as a spiral axis, is considered a feature of ET.

Generally, no additional investigations are required for axis-1 (phenomenological) classification of tremor; however, in certain specific situations electrophysiological tests may be helpful. Combined surface electromyography (EMG)–accelerometry is the gold standard electrophysiological investigation for objective evaluation and confirmation of tremor characteristics. It may be helpful for the diagnosis of tremors such as orthostatic tremor or functional tremor. Currently, orthostatic tremor is the only tremor disorder for which electrophysiology is mandatory for diagnosis. Presynaptic dopaminergic imaging may help make a diagnosis of tremor associated with parkinsonism. Uncommonly, serum and tissue biomarkers may be useful such as thyroid function tests in a patient with exaggerated physiological tremor.

Taking into consideration the history, tremor characteristics, associated signs and symptoms, and additional laboratory tests (in selected situations) a phenomenological diagnosis of tremor can be formulated.[3] Broadly, the phenomenological diagnosis would be that of an isolated tremor syndrome, or a combined tremor syndrome.

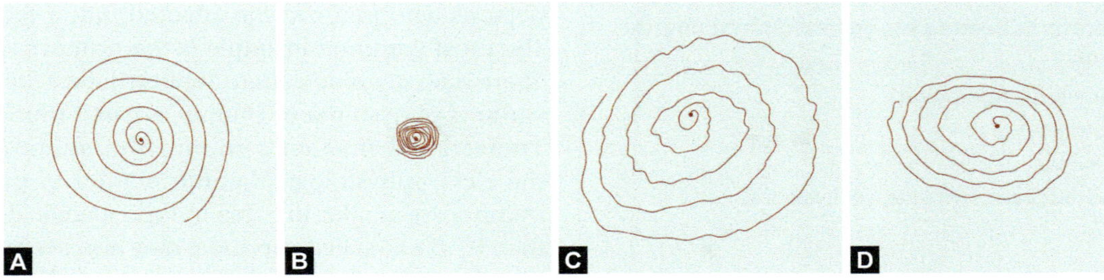

FIGS. 1A TO D: Freehand spiral drawing specimens from (A) healthy volunteer, (B) Parkinson's disease—note the small size of the spiral and decreasing widths of spiral loops, (C) essential tremor—note that the tremor-related fluctuations are more prominent at 2 O'clock and 7 O'clock positions, a feature known as spiral axis, and (D) dystonic tremor.

TABLE 1: Common tremor syndromes.

Isolated tremor	Combined tremor
Essential tremor	Dystonic tremor
Essential tremor plus	Tremor associated with dystonia
Physiological tremor	Parkinsonism-associated tremors
Exaggerated physiological tremor	Intention tremor
Isolated focal tremor	Holmes tremor
Isolated segmental postural/ action tremor	Symptomatic palatal tremor
Isolated rest tremor	Myorhythmia
Isolated task/position-specific tremor	Neuropathic tremor
Essential palatal tremor	Functional tremor
Orthostatic tremor	
Functional tremor	

Tremor is the only clinical feature in isolated tremor, for instance, ET. In combined tremors, there are additional neurological or systemic signs, e.g., dystonic tremors or tremors associated with parkinsonism. It has been noted that certain combinations of neurological signs and symptoms coexist frequently and, therefore, certain tremor syndromes have been predefined **(Table 1)**. The commonly encountered tremor syndromes include the ET syndrome, task- and position-specific tremors, and tremors with prominent additional signs such as dystonic tremors, parkinsonism-associated tremors, intention tremors, and Holmes tremor.

Isolated Tremor Syndromes

Essential tremor is an isolated tremor syndrome of bilateral upper limb action tremor, which is present for at least 3 years, with or without a tremor in other locations such as the head, voice, or lower limbs, in the absence of other neurological signs such as dystonia, ataxia, or parkinsonism.[4] Very often, patients with a tremor that looks like an ET may also have some additional subtle neurological signs of uncertain significance, such as tandem gait impairment, questionable dystonic posturing, or memory impairment. When such subtle signs are present along with the characteristic tremor of ET, the syndrome is classified as ET plus. ET with rest tremor is also considered ET plus. There are certain important exclusion criteria for ET and ET plus isolated focal tremors such as those of the voice or the head without upper limb involvement are not considered ET. Orthostatic tremor with the frequency of >12 Hz is not considered ET, so also task- and position-specific tremors. Sudden onset and stepwise deterioration are exclusion criteria for ET. Alcohol responsiveness is no more considered a necessary feature to diagnose ET. Tremors of the head, voice, tongue, face, or upper limbs which do not meet the criteria for ET may be classified as isolated segmental, postural, or kinetic tremor syndrome. Although the characterization of ET and ET plus helps in deep phenotyping and picking up subtle signs, it is debated whether these two entities represent different tremor disorders or subtypes of the same disease. Naturally, as there are no objective measures to confirm subtle signs of dystonia, ataxia, etc. The inter-rater agreement for a diagnosis of ET or ET plus is modest. With increasing usage of the current classification system, it has become apparent that subtle signs of some sort may be present in the majority of patients with an ET syndrome, making "pure" ET less common than ET plus.

Physiological tremor is seen in all normal healthy individuals. This is a fine, postural tremor with the frequency of 8–12 Hz. It is usually not visible to the naked eye and does not cause any functional limitations. Physiological tremor is thought to be due to mechanical oscillations of the limb or body part and conducted effects of the cardioballistic impulse. The frequency of physiological tremor is lower in childhood, increases to 12 Hz by mid second decade, and decreases slightly at about the age of 60 years. Certain situations such as stress, anxiety, fatigue, consumption of caffeine, and lack of sleep can cause exaggerated or enhanced physiological tremor. Several medications such as beta agonists, valproic acid, lithium, and others may also increase physiological tremor **(Box 1)**. Other conditions that can exaggerate the physiological tremor include thyrotoxicosis, hypoglycemia, and pheochromocytoma. Enhanced physiological tremor is a mechanical reflex tremor, i.e., it is not generated by a central oscillator,

BOX 1	Medications causing exaggerated physiological tremor.

- Salbutamol, salmeterol, formoterol
- Valproate, lamotrigine
- Thyroxine, adrenaline
- SSRIs/SNRIs (escitalopram, sertraline, venlafaxine)
- Amitriptyline
- Lithium
- Amiodarone, procainamide, mexiletine
- Cyclosporine, tacrolimus
- Amphetamine

(SNRI: serotonin and norepinephrine reuptake inhibitor; SSRI: selective serotonin reuptake inhibitor)

rather is due to an exaggeration of the mechanical limb oscillations and addition of a muscular contraction component, possibly mediated by enhanced stretch and other reflexes. Generally, the tremor is of low amplitude and does not cause significant functional disability. However, in individuals in whom tremor is interfering with their functional abilities, beta blockers may help reduce the severity of the physiological tremor. Physiological tremor and exaggerated physiological tremor can be confirmed on electrophysiological testing by demonstrating a shift in the frequency peak to the left after loading weight (see subsequent sections). It is important to recognize physiological and exaggerated physiological tremors as most often the causes are potentially reversible.[5]

Other isolated tremor syndromes include isolated rest tremor syndrome, isolated focal tremors including isolated voice tremor, head tremor, jaw tremor, rabbit syndrome, etc. Jaw tremor and rabbit syndrome are often manifestations of drug-induced or tardive tremors. A palatal tremor is a rhythmic movement of the soft palate at 0.5–5 Hz. Essential palatal tremor is attributed to the contraction of the tensor veli palatini, and apart from tremor, there are no other neurological abnormalities. Patients often present with the symptom of an ear click, and investigations including magnetic resonance imaging (MRI) of the inferior olive are normal. The etiology of essential palatal tremor is not known, but a functional origin has been considered. On the other hand, patients with symptomatic palatal tremor present with a low-frequency tremor of the soft palate without an ear click. This tremor is due to the involvement of the levator veli palatini and other muscles innervated by the brainstem nuclei. In addition to the soft palate, facial muscles and eye movements may be affected. Symptomatic palatal tremor is usually seen in combination with ataxia and is due to lesions in the dentato-olivary pathway. Symptomatic palatal tremor is usually a combined tremor syndrome and most often occurs with lesions in the Guillain–Mollaret triangle. Inferior olivary hypertrophy may be observed on MRI.

Isolated task- and position-specific tremors occur only during performing a specific task or assuming a specific posture. These are usually focal tremors and are seen in persons who perform the affected motor task repetitively. The most common example is the primary writing tremor. There is an ongoing debate about whether these tremors are variants of dystonia or unique isolated tremor syndromes. Transcranial magnetic stimulation studies suggest that the electrophysiological abnormalities in primary writing tremors are similar to those in task-specific dystonia, rather than ET. Task-specific tremors may also occur in the hand or mouth in musicians, sports persons, hairdressers, etc.

Orthostatic tremor is a generalized, 13–18 Hz, isolated tremor syndrome. These tremors occur in the leg only when standing, usually after a latency of a few seconds of standing. Often, orthostatic tremors may be more palpable than visible. They may also be audible by the auscultation of the thigh or calf muscles, resulting in a buzzing/revving sound—the so-called helicopter sign. Surface EMG confirmation is required for the diagnosis of orthostatic tremor. Electrophysiologically, this tremor is characterized by a high-frequency, highly coherent tremor. Patients with orthostatic tremor who have additional features such as parkinsonism, ataxia, or dementia are classified as having primary orthostatic tremor plus. Pseudo-orthostatic tremor is a slower orthostatic tremor with the frequency of <13 Hz, usually associated with additional neurological signs and encountered in the setting of diseases, such as PD or spinocerebellar ataxia. Orthostatic myoclonus is another differential of orthostatic tremor, which can be confirmed on electrophysiological analysis.

Combined Tremor Syndromes

Parkinsonian tremor is one of the most common forms of combined tremor syndrome. Typically, the tremor in PD is a rest tremor, which becomes less in amplitude with voluntary movement. A tremor in PD most often appears in the distal upper limb and then gradually progresses proximally to involve the other limbs. Isolated jaw tremor is uncommon in PD, although it may occur along with tremors in other body parts. Over two-thirds of patients with PD present with tremors and they usually have a better prognosis compared to the akinetic rigid phenotype. Rest tremor is not the only form of tremor in PD; action as well as postural tremor may occur in addition to the rest tremor. The postural tremor in PD may be a reemergent tremor, i.e., the tremor disappears for a few seconds on assuming a new posture and reappears after a latent period, at the same frequency as the rest tremor. Non-reemergent postural and action tremors may also be seen. According to the current classification, regardless of the activation condition of the tremor, these are classified as tremors associated with parkinsonism. Typically, the tremor is a 4–7 Hz, pill-rolling rest tremor. Early in the course of PD, when patients present with only tremor, the diagnosis of PD may be unclear. In such situations, a response to levodopa may help to make a diagnosis of PD tremor. Presynaptic dopaminergic imaging using a dopamine active transporter single-photon emission computed tomography

(DAT-SPECT) or fluorodopa positron emission tomography (PET) may be useful in distinguishing tremor-dominant PD from ET.

Dystonic tremor syndromes are another common cause of combined tremor, where tremor and dystonia are prominent neurological signs.[6] Dystonic tremor is diagnosed when tremor and dystonia occur in the same body part. When tremor and dystonia occur in different body parts, it is known as tremor associated with dystonia. In the setting of established dystonia, the diagnosis of dystonic tremor may be obvious; however, in patients with subtle dystonia there may be a diagnostic uncertainty between dystonic tremor and an ET syndrome, especially ET plus. The presence of a sensory trick, task, or position sensitivity and the presence of mirror dystonia may be features that may help to distinguish dystonic tremor from ET plus. Dystonic tremors may be irregular with variable frequency and a jerky, myoclonic-like character. The null point is a certain specific position of the body part in which the tremor disappears or is minimal in amplitude compared to other positions. The null point, which is noted in up to 30% of patients with dystonic tremor, can be brought about by rotating the extended arm 180° in the outstretched position. For head tremors, it can be assessed by rotating the head from one side to the other slowly and observing for a specific position when the tremor is minimal.

Other types of combined tremors include intention tremor syndromes, which are due to lesions in the cerebellum and its connections. Here, the tremor generator is thought to be the cerebellum, and it is usually characterized by a <5 Hz intention tremor. Holmes tremor or cerebellar outflow tract tremor is a specific type of tremor characterized by rest and postural tremors with a prominent proximal component, along with intention tremor. It is often of a low frequency <5 Hz and lesions anywhere in the dentato-rubro-thalamic tract or other motor pathways connected to it. Myorhythmia is a slow, 2–4 Hz, rhythmic, rest or action tremor of the cranial or limb muscles seen in association with the brainstem, midbrain, or cerebellar signs. It is a rare tremor and is usually associated with diagnosable etiology. Functional or psychogenic tremors may present as rest, postural, or action tremors. These are characterized by distractibility, change in frequency with entrainment, or coactivation of agonist and antagonist muscles. Additional features, such as inconsistency of symptoms, abrupt onset, fluctuation in the distribution, frequency or activation characteristics, and other functional neurological symptoms or signs may be present. Although other additional psychiatric features, such as depression or anxiety may be present in some patients, these are not required for a diagnosis of functional tremor. Entrainment can be demonstrated clinically by asking the patient to tap an uninvolved body part at a frequency different from that of the tremulous limb. In functional tremor, the tremor attains the frequency of the tapping rhythm. Coactivation can also be demonstrated clinically by demonstrating an increased tone during passive movement of the limb, and once the increased tone disappears, the tremor also disappears. Electrophysiological analysis may help diagnose functional tremor by demonstrating entrainment, distractibility, and coactivation of agonists and antagonists.[7] A neuropathic tremor is a form of postural tremor that is seen in patients with coexisting peripheral neuropathy, predominantly demyelinating neuropathies such as chronic inflammatory demyelinating neuropathy or hereditary sensory motor neuropathy. Patients who do not fit into any of the established syndromes may require longitudinal observation to clarify the tremor syndrome, and are classified as indeterminate tremor.

Etiologically tremor may be divided into acquired, genetically defined, or idiopathic tremor. Idiopathic tremors may be familiar or sporadic. Acquired tremors would include tremors due to structural lesions, drug-induced or tardive tremors, and tremors secondary to metabolic disorders such as hyperthyroidism. Although the criteria for many tremor syndromes are well laid out, some such as ET plus require the identification of features like subtle dystonia. This may result in significant inter-rater disagreement in the classification of tremors.[8] To objectively quantify tremor, several rating scales are available. These include the Fahn–Tolosa–Marin tremor rating scale, Tremor Research Group essential tremor rating scale (TETRAS), Bain and Findley scale, etc.

INVESTIGATIONS

Electrophysiological tremor analysis is the gold standard method to objectively measure tremor. Combined accelerometry–surface EMG is widely used to measure tremor, although other transducers such as gyroscopes and digitizing tablets may also be used. Transducer-based measurements help to identify the frequency, amplitude (or surrogate measures thereof, such as with an accelerometer), and coherence characteristics of tremor.[9] These are generally derived after the Fourier transformation of the spectral recording. Coherence is a measure of how in-phase tremors in two body parts are; orthostatic tremor is the most coherent tremor. After analysis of accelerometry–surface EMG recordings, one can determine the location of the tremor generator or oscillator.[10] Briefly, in physiological tremor while the accelerometer shows a peak between 8 and 12 Hz, there is no corresponding EMG peak, suggesting that the mechanical oscillations of the limb rather than muscle contractions are responsible for the tremor. In exaggerated physiological tremor, a similar frequency peak is noted in the accelerometer and surface EMG leads, suggesting a muscular component to the tremor. In both physiological tremor and exaggerated physiological tremor, loading 500 g weight on the affected limb causes the tremor peak to shift to the left, i.e., decrease in frequency. If both the accelerometer and EMG spectra show corresponding peaks, which do not shift to the left after loading weight, this confirms the presence of a central oscillator mechanism for

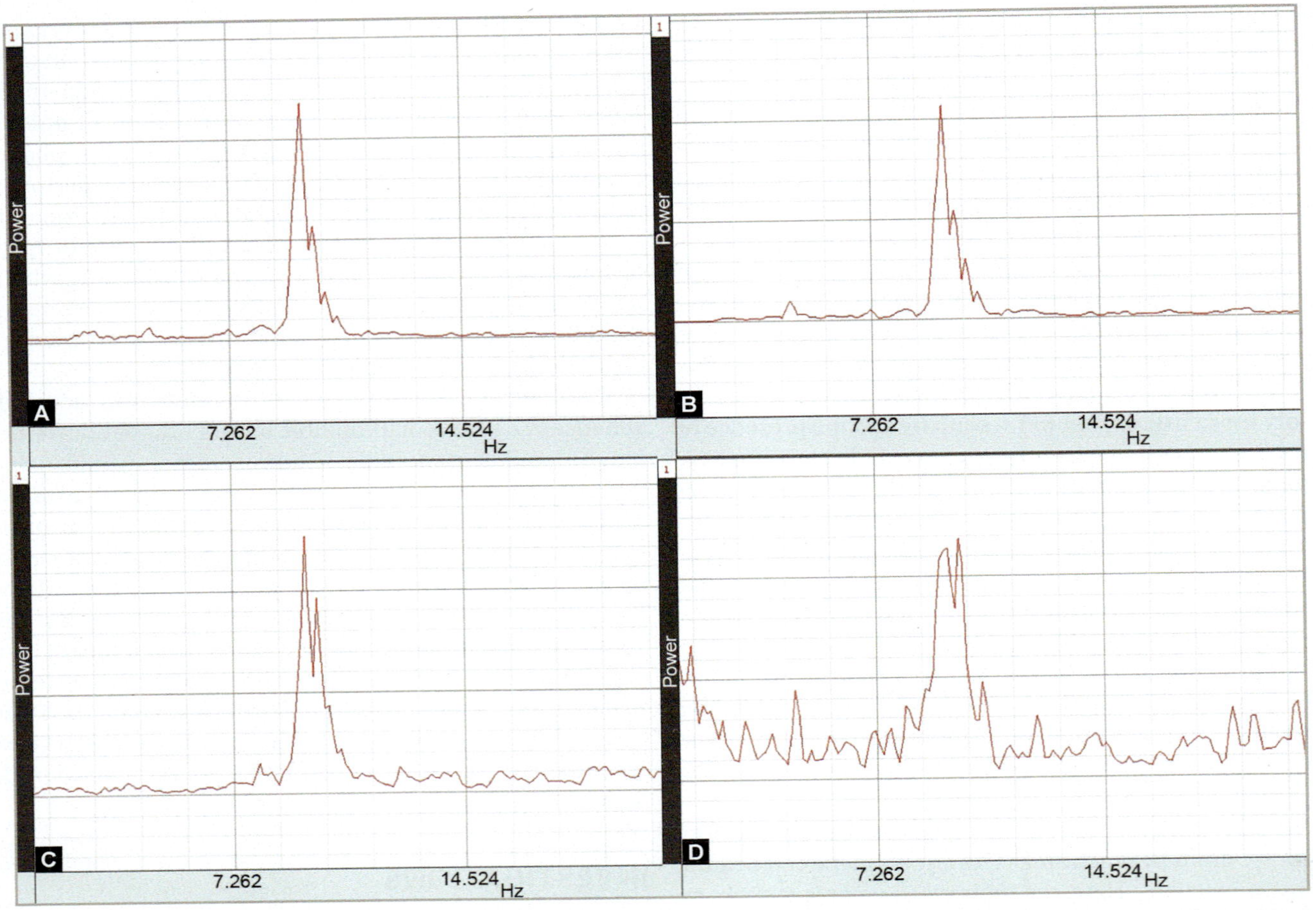

FIGS. 2A TO D: Accelerometry recordings showing a single well-defined peak at 8 Hz in the outstretched arm (A) with no change in frequency on loading weight; (B) The lower panels showing corresponding peaks on EMG, in posture without load and (C) after loading 500 g weight; (D) Consistent tremor peaks without change in frequency on loading weight suggest the presence of a central oscillator.

tremor **(Figs. 2A to D)**. The central oscillator may be the cerebellum, basal ganglia, or other parts of the distributed motor network. Although considered the gold standard, there are certain limitations to accelerometry–surface EMG tremor analysis. It is a time-consuming technique requiring considerable technical skills to perform and interpret. Uniaxial or biaxial accelerometers, unless placed accurately according to the direction or plane of movement of a tremor, can miss measuring tremor. Triaxial accelerometers are preferred to address this problem. Gravitational artefacts may impair the accuracy of the readings. To overcome some of these limitations, alternate transducer-based methods are being explored, such as at-home activity monitors and digitizing tablets. Spiral drawings on paper or acquired on digitizing tablets may be a source of valuable information on upper limb action tremor. The electrophysiological analysis is mandatory for the diagnosis of orthostatic tremor and may support the diagnosis of functional tremor.

Additional investigations for the etiology of tremor include thyroid function tests, parathormone levels, and medication screen for causes of exaggerated physiological tremor. Brain imaging is often helpful in ruling out degenerative, neurometabolic, or other diseases such as spinocerebellar ataxia, Wilson's disease, tumors, strokes, and demyelination. DAT-SPECT or ^{18}F-fluoro-dihydroxyphenylalanine (^{18}F-DOPA) PET may be used to demonstrate a presynaptic dopaminergic deficiency in early parkinsonism.

CONCLUSION

Tremor is one of the most common movement disorders encountered in a neurology clinic. Most tremor syndromes are diagnosed clinically, with electrophysiology or other tests required in specific situations. A thorough understanding of the characteristics of tremors and a systematic approach to examination will help classify tremor accurately and guide management.

REFERENCES

1. Bhatia KP, Bain P, Bajaj N, Elble RJ, Hallett M, Louis ED, et al; Tremor Task Force of the International Parkinson and Movement Disorder Society. Consensus statement on the classification of tremors. from the task force on tremor of the International Parkinson and Movement Disorder Society. Mov Disord. 2018;33(1):75-87.
2. Erro R, Reich SG. Rare tremors and tremors occurring in other neurological disorders. J Neurol Sci. 2022;435:120200.
3. Lenka A, Jankovic J. Tremor syndromes: an updated review. Front Neurol. 2021;12:684835.
4. Welton T, Cardoso F, Carr JA, Chan LL, Deuschl G, Jankovic J, et al. Essential tremor. Nat Rev Dis Primers. 2021;7(1):83.
5. Sharma S, Pandey S. Approach to a tremor patient. Ann Indian Acad Neurol. 2016;19(4):433-43.
6. Bhidayasiri R. Differential diagnosis of common tremor syndromes. Postgrad Med J. 2005;81:756-62.
7. Deuschl G, Raethjen J, Lindemann M, Krack P. The pathophysiology of tremor. Muscle Nerve. 2001;24(6):716-35.
8. Rajan R, Pandey S, Anandapadmanabhan R, Srivastava AK. Interrater and intrarater agreement on the 2018 consensus statement on classification of tremors. Mov Disord. 2018;33(12):1966-7.
9. Haubenberger D, Abbruzzese G, Bain PG, Bajaj N, Benito-León J, Bhatia KP, et al. Transducer-based evaluation of tremor. Mov Disord. 2016;31(9):1327-36.
10. Vial F, Kassavetis P, Merchant S, Haubenberger D, Hallett M. How to do an electrophysiological study of tremor. Clin Neurophysiol Pract. 2019;4:134-42.

38

CHAPTER

Approach to Hypokinesia

Charulata Savant Sankhla, Ruta Savaj, Sahil Patel

INTRODUCTION

Movement disorders are clinically divided into hypokinetic or hyperkinetic disorders or both. Hypokinesia is the reverse of the term hyperkinesia. It occurs when you have too little movement, and hyperkinesia occurs when you have too many involuntary movements.

Hypokinesia is a type of movement disorder when movements have a "decreased amplitude" or in simple terms movements are not as big as you would expect them to be and are dominated by a poverty of movement or slowness of the movement. The important clinical feature of hypokinesia is the absence of weakness or paralysis.

Hypokinesia is seen in parkinsonian syndromes **(Table 1)**. But it can also be a symptom of other conditions such as depression, schizophrenia and strokes.

TABLE 1: Classification of parkinsonian syndromes.

Parkinsonian syndrome	Features
Parkinson's disease (sporadic and familial)	
Atypical parkinsonism	• Progressive supranuclear palsy (PSP) • Multisystem atrophy (MSA) • Corticobasal syndrome (CBS) • Dementia with lewy bodies (DLB)
Secondary parkinsonism	• Vascular parkinsonism • Drugs/toxins induced • Postinfectious • Metabolic • Tumor/trauma • Normal pressure hydrocephalus
Heredodegenerative parkinsonism	• Spinocerebellar ataxia • Lubag disease • Wilson's disease • Neurodegeneration with brain iron accumulation (NBIA) • Huntington's disease

Hypokinesia is related to akinesia, which means the absence of movement, and bradykinesia, which means slowness of movement. The three terms are often characterized together and referred to under the umbrella of term bradykinesia. These movement disorders are often equated with Parkinson's disease (PD) when associated with tremors, rigidity, and balance issues.

CLINICAL SYMPTOMS AND SIGNS

Hypokinesia often presents with symptoms with overall reduced speed of activities of daily living. These include difficulty in getting out of a chair or car, difficulty in turning in the bed, and difficulty in starting and stopping, which can be a manifestation of hypokinesia. This can cause start hesitation, difficulty in turning, reaching a target while walking, or freezing. Difficulty in stopping can cause festination.

CLINICAL EXAMINATION

Clinical examination is performed with the patient at rest, posture holding, execution of tasks, and walking.

Examination at Rest

Observe the patient while taking the history sitting comfortably. The extremities should be supported. While talking to the patient most patients have spontaneous gestures. The individuals move their hands or often cross their legs, and shake their legs. They often smile while chatting. In hypokinetic disorders there is a loss of these normal gestures and spontaneous movements. There is a scarceness in the movements. The face lacks expression with a reduced rate of blinking, termed as hypomimia. This can be often misinterpreted as depression by relatives. It is often seen on clinical examination as an expressionless face, parted lips, and decreased blinking frequency.[1]

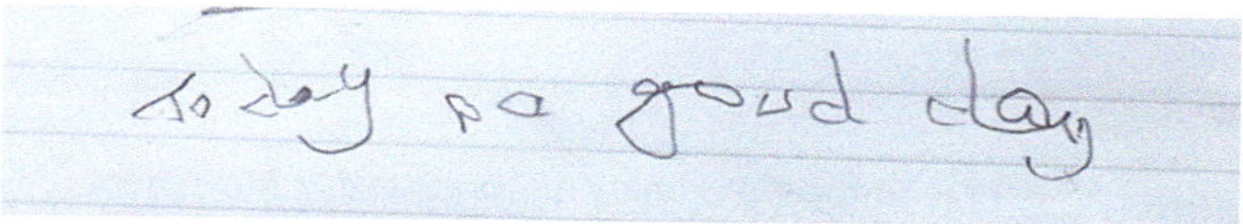

FIG. 1: Micrographia in Parkinson's disease (PD).

Posture Holding

Posture holding may interrupt the rest tremor transiently, only to emerge a few seconds later. This is termed a re-emergent tremor and is seen in association with hypokinesia in PD.

Execution of Tasks

Hypokinesia can interrupt many tasks. Handwriting in bradykinesia is small and crowded **(Fig. 1)**. Spiral drawings are small and cramped. Finger tapping is slow and of smaller amplitude with a decrement of the amplitude with repetition. This is opposed to bradykinesia due to pyramidal tract involvement where the amplitude of repetitive finger tapping remains the same. This is also seen on foot tapping.

Bulbar dysfunction occurs in the form of dysarthria, hypophonia, dysphagia, sialorrhea, and masticatory issues. This represents orofacial-laryngeal bradykinesia and rigidity. Speech becomes slurred and loses its volume (monotonic and hypophonic dysarthria). Stuttering and palilalia (involuntary repetition of a phrase with increasing rapidity) may also be seen. Chewing becomes laborious, and choking while swallowing may occur. Excessive salivation and drooling may also occur, which is due to the slowness of spontaneous swallowing, necessitating the use of a tissue or handkerchief. Dysphagia may also occur, which is often subclinical in the early stages.[1]

Gradual slowing of activities of daily living occurs. Handwriting often becomes smaller (micrographia). Writing speed decreases, and eventually the writing becomes illegible. Clumsiness or reduced dexterity in dressing, buttoning/unbuttoning, feeding, and handling utensils is often noted. Hygiene, including showering or bathing, becomes slower.[1]

PATHOPHYSIOLOGY OF HYPOKINESIA

The basal ganglia (BG) are made up of putamen, caudate, globus pallidus interna (GPi) and externa (GPe), substantia nigra (SN) pars compacta (SNc) and reticularis (SNr), and subthalamic nucleus (STN). The caudate and putamen form the striatum, and the putamen and globus pallidus form the lentiform nucleus. GPi is structurally and functionally homologous with SNr.

Functional Organization of the Basal Ganglia

The striatum receives excitatory input from virtually all of the cerebral cortex, thalamus, SN, locus coeruleus, raphe nuclei, hippocampus, and amygdala. The corticostriatal projections have a roughly topographic organization. However, a single cortical area projects divergently to multiple striatal zones, resulting in the convergence of several functionally related cortical areas to overlap. Thus, there is a significant convergence and divergence of the corticostriatal tracts.[2,3]

The glutamatergic cortical input terminates on the heads of the dendritic spines, and the dopaminergic input from SNc terminates on the shafts of the dendritic spines of medium spiny neurons. Five types of G protein-coupled dopamine receptors have been described (D1–D5): the D1 family (excitatory) includes D1 and D5 receptors, and the D2 family (inhibitory) includes D2, D3, and D4 receptors.[4] GABAergic striatal inhibitory interneurons receive excitatory input from the cerebral cortex and inhibit the medium spiny neurons. Medium spiny striatal neurons are GABAergic and can be divided into two types. One contains gamma-aminobutyric acid (GABA), dynorphin, and substance P, which primarily expresses D1 receptors and projects to the GPi/SNr. The other contains GABA and enkephalin, which primarily expresses D2 receptors and projects to the GPe.[5] STN receives inhibitory GABAergic input from the GPe. The STN output is glutamatergic and directed to the GPe and GPi/SNr. The output from GPi/SNr is GABAergic inhibitory and directed to the thalamus, which in turn projects to the frontal lobes.[2,3] A part of the output from GPi/SNr also goes to the pedunculopontine nucleus (PPN). The BG motor output has a somatotopic organization. The GPi represents the neck and the structures below it, and the SNr represents the head and the eyes. This separate representation is maintained throughout the BG such that an individual GPi neuron sends output via the thalamus to just one area of the cortex.[5]

The BG have widespread input and output connections as well as dense internuclear connections. These can be separated into three major divisions: (i) sensorimotor, (ii) associative, and (iii) limbic **(Table 2)**.[2,3]

Basal Ganglia Circuits

Direct Pathway

Excitatory neurons from the cortex synapse on putaminal neurons, which in turn send inhibitory projection to the GPi/SNr, resulting in disinhibition of the thalamus leading to excitatory thalamocortical pathway enhancing the cortical activity. Thus, this functions to maintain the ongoing motor activity.[5]

Indirect Pathway

Excitatory neurons from the cortex synapse on putaminal neurons, which in turn send inhibitory projection to the GPe. The GPe sends inhibitory projection to the STN. The result is a disinhibition of the STN, which sends an excitatory signal to GPi/SNr, resulting in inhibition of the thalamus

TABLE 2: Basal ganglia connections.

Division	Afferent connections	BG nucleus	Efferent connections	Function
Sensorimotor	Motor cortex	Putamen	Premotor and primary motor cortex, supplementary motor area	Movement
Associative	Frontal, parietal, temporal, and occipital cortex	Dorsal caudate	Prefrontal cortex	Cognition
Limbic	Hippocampus, amygdala, cingulate cortex, temporal cortex, orbitofrontal cortex	Ventral striatum	Anterior cingulate cortex, medial orbitofrontal cortex	• Emotion • Motivation

leading to cortical inhibition. Thus, this functions to inhibit ongoing motor activity.[5]

Hyperdirect Pathway

There is some evidence of a hyperdirect pathway from the cerebral cortex to the STN and then to the thalamus.[5]

Thus, the BG aim to moderate motor activity rather than control it. The relative activities in the direct and indirect pathways serve to balance the scale of movement.

In *PD*, the death of neurons in the SNc results in decreased activity in the direct pathway and increased activity in the indirect pathway leading to increased firing in the STN and GPi, causing hypokinesia/bradykinesia.[6]

PARKINSON'S DISEASE

Parkinson's disease was first described by James Parkinson in 1817 in his monograph, The Shaking Palsy. The dopamine deficiency was then described by Hornykiewicz in 1959.[7]

Parkinson's disease shows a gradual increase in prevalence after the age of 50 years. There is a steep increase in prevalence after the age of 60 years. PD can be divided based on the age of onset into:[8]

- *Juvenile-onset PD (JOPD)*: Childhood or adolescence
- *Young-onset PD (YOPD)*: Between 21 and 40 years of age
- *Late-onset PD (LOPD)*: >60 years of age

Pathology

Parkinson's disease is characterized by neuronal loss and gliosis in the BG system, especially the SN. There is a widespread presence of Lewy bodies. These are cytoplasmic inclusions having a dense eosinophilic core and pale halo and contain hyperphosphorylated neurofilament proteins, lipids, iron, ubiquitin, and alpha-synuclein. Lewy body pathology is also found in the brainstem, intermediolateral gray column of the spinal cord, and myenteric intestinal and cardiac plexus.[9]

Braak introduced a staging system to demonstrate the progression of neurodegenerative changes as follows:[10]

- *Stage 1*: Olfactory bulb and dorsal motor nucleus of the vagus nerve
- *Stage 2*: Medulla oblongata and pontine tegmentum
- *Stage 3*: Amygdala and SN
- *Stage 4*: Temporal cortex
- *Stages 5 and 6*: Neocortex

Physiology

Parkinson's disease patients are unable to produce an initial agonist burst to exert a force, which results in insufficient effort to reach the desired target while performing fast single-joint movements. Thus, the movement is performed by a sequence of small amplitude movements by repeated agonist and antagonist electromyography (EMG) muscle bursts. Prolonged continuous discharge on EMG is also seen. The patient can perform a movement of a larger amplitude than the first burst if he wishes. Smaller size movements than appropriate are used to perform a motor task as seen in many studies. This indicates that bradykinesia is produced from an inappropriate grading of the dynamic muscle forces, the so-called scaling effect. The majority of the studies show movement preparation is prolonged due to delay in muscle activation and slowing of simple reaction time. Hence, the addition of vocal or visual stimuli improved the reaction time in PD patients.[11]

Genetics

Table 3 lists the common genes associated with PD.

Clinical Features

Motor Abnormalities

Usually, PD has a gradual and asymmetrical onset and progression and usually remains asymmetrical till the advanced stages. The symptoms often go unnoticed by the patient and relatives for a few months, especially when they are on the nondominant side. Based on clinical features, there are two motor phenotypes: (1) "Tremor dominant" with slow progression and favorable long-term prognosis, and (2) "Postural instability gait difficulty" (PIGD) with rapid progression and associated with nonmotor symptoms; (3) "Mixed" with features of both.[8]

The most common presentation is with a unilateral rest tremor in the hand. This is the typical parkinsonian tremor, which occurs at a frequency of 4–5 Hz and is observed with hands resting on the thighs or in the lap. It can also be noted in the lips, chin, jaw, face, and legs. Postural tremors and reemergent tremors also occur after keeping hands outstretched or in a wing-beating position. Kinetic tremors are less common in PD.[1,12,13] The rest and reemergent tremors are related to dopamine deficiency while the action-postural tremor is related to serotonergic deficiency.[8,14]

TABLE 3: Common genes associated with PD and their mode of inheritance and age of onset.[10,11]

	Gene	Inheritance	Locus	Onset
PARK1	*SNCA*	AD	4q21	Late
PARK2	*PARKIN*	AR	6q25	Early
PARK3	Unknown	AD	2p13	Late
PARK4	*SNCA*	AD	4q21	Early
PARK5	*UCHL1*	AD	4p14	Late
PARK6	*PINK1*	AR	1p35	Early
PARK7	*DJ-1*	AR	1p36	Early
PARK8	*LRRK2*	AD	12q12	Late
PARK9	*ATP13A2*	AR	1p36	Early
PARK10	Unknown	?	1p32	Late
PARK11	*GIGYF2*	AD	2q36	Late
PARK12	Unknown	?	Xq21-q25	Late
PARK13	*OMI/HTRA2*	AD	2p13	Late
PARK14	*PLA2G6*	AR	22q13.1	Early
PARK15	*FBXO7*	AR	22q12	Early
PARK16	Unknown	?	1q32	Late
PARK17	*VPS35*	AD	16q11.2	Late
PARK18	*EIF4G1*	AD	3q27.1	Late
PARK19	*DNAJC6*	AR	1p31.3	Early
PARK20	*SYNJ1*	AR	21q22.11	Early
PARK21	*DNAJC13*	AD	3q22	Late
PARK22	*CHCHD2*	AD	7p11.2	Late
PARK23	*VPS13C*	AR	15q22.2	Early

(AD: autosomal dominant; AR: autosomal recessive; PD: Parkinson's disease)

Clinical features of bradykinesia have been described earlier. Bradykinesia and rigidity are often detectable, early in the course of the disease, on the symptomatic side. Gradually, bradykinesia becomes generalized, leading to difficulty in performing axial movements such as turning in bed or getting out of a chair

The rigidity can be noted as increased muscle tone in both flexor and extensor muscles and is present throughout the passive range of movement across the joint. It can be of lead pipe or cogwheel type. The rigidity can be brought out by reinforcing maneuvers (Froment sign).[1]

Musculoskeletal problems like a painful/frozen shoulder are one of the most common early symptoms of PD, possibly related to decreased arm swing and secondary joint changes or shoulder muscle rigidity. Skeletal deformities are also seen such as anterocollis, scoliosis (usually away from the side of onset of symptoms), Pisa sign (lateral bending of the trunk), and camptocormia (severe flexion of the thoracolumbar spine >45°). Striatal limb deformities such as a striatal hand (flexion at the metacarpophalangeal joints, extension at the proximal interphalangeal joints, flexion at the distal interphalangeal joints, adduction of all fingers, and opposition of the thumb to the index finger) or foot (hammertoe-like deformity with the extension of the great toe) also occur.[1,15,16]

Patients also develop neck and truncal rigidity (axial rigidity). They develop a stooped posture with flexion of the neck (dropped head), trunk, elbows, and knees. The gait and balance are also affected, and unprovoked falls may occur. The patient walks with short, shuffling steps with a narrow base, flexed knees and elbows, and reduced arm swing. Turning needs multiple steps (turning en bloc). Later, there is a tendency to advance more rapidly with shorter and shorter steps (festination). When this occurs, the patient can only stop with the help of a nearby wall or an unobstructed fall. Sometimes, the patient may have a sudden and transient inability to move (freezing/motor block). In the beginning, this occurs with the initiation of walking (start hesitation) or when turning (particularly in enclosed spaces), or attempts to walk through an enclosed area or a narrow passage such as a doorway or walking in or out of an elevator. Prominent freezing with poor postural stability results in frequent provoked falls. Later, impaired postural reflexes may cause unprovoked falls.[1,15,16]

The Movement Disorder Society (MDS)-Unified PD Rating Scale (UPDRS) is used to quantitate the various motor symptoms and signs of PD and to chart the course of the disease. The modified Hoehn and Yahr staging outlines the milestones in the progression of the illness from mild unilateral symptoms through the end-stage nonambulatory state.[17]

Nonmotor Abnormalities

Nonmotor features can precede motor abnormalities by months to years.

Depression, apathy, and anxiety are common problems and often overlooked. Patients become withdrawn, passive, and less motivated to socialize and often develop bradyphrenia (slowness of thought processes), anhedonia, and inattentiveness. Cognitive and behavioral dysfunctions are also common. Executive dysfunction with diminished working memory, planning, and organization is seen. Patients may eventually develop dementia with disease progression.[1,18]

Autonomic dysfunction is common and may be the presenting feature. Constipation and postprandial bloating may occur as a result of gastroparesis or ileus. Urinary complaints such as frequency, urgency, nocturia, and the sensation of incomplete bladder emptying are also common. Orthostatic hypotension may lead to postural giddiness or falls, and antiparkinsonian drugs often aggravate the problem. Erectile dysfunction and impotence are less common.[1,18]

Rapid eye movement (REM) sleep behavior disorder (RBD) characterized by increased violent dream content and accompanied by talking, shouting, swearing, punching, hitting, kicking, jumping, or other such dream enactments may be seen as an early clinical feature and now considered a preparkinsonian state. These are potentially injurious to the self as well as to the bed partner. Restless leg syndrome and periodic leg movements of sleep are common.[1,19,20]

Fatigue and lack of energy are common and complex symptoms of PD. Patients may have poorly explained sensory complaints such as numbness, tingling, aching, pains, akathisias, and anosmia.[21]

Diplopia may occur during reading secondary to impaired convergence. Oculogyric crises, which are sudden episodes of involuntary ocular deviation (most often up and to the side) in the absence of neuroleptic drug exposure, are occasionally seen in young PD. Saccadic pursuit and hypometric saccades can be found in PD. Impairment of visual acuity, contrast sensitivity, and color and motor perception is also found.[22-24]

In a patient presenting with signs and symptoms of parkinsonism, if you find the following red flags then you should consider the diagnosis of atypical/secondary parkinsonism.

Red flags in Parkinson's disease, which suggest atypical parkinsonism:[25]

- Early or prominent dementia
- Symmetrical signs (exception is corticobasal degeneration)
- Bulbar dysfunction
- Early gaze palsies
- Early gait disorder
- Falls within the first year
- Wheelchair dependence within 5 years
- Early autonomic failure
- Sleep apnea
- Inspiratory stridor
- Apraxia
- Alien limb
- Cortical sensory loss

Atypical Parkinsonism

- Progressive supranuclear palsy (PSP)
- Multisystem atrophy (MSA)
- Corticobasal syndrome (CBS)
- Dementia with Lewy bodies (DLB)

Progressive supranuclear palsy and CBS are tauopathies while MSA and DLB are synucleinopathies. The first case of MSA was described in 1900 as olivopontocerebellar atrophy;[26] later in 1960 it was labelled as "Shy-Drager syndrome"[27] and in 1969 was named "MSA" by Graham and Oppenheimer. Steele, Richardson and Olszewski described PSP in 1964.[28]

Rebeiz and colleagues in 1968 reported patients with asymmetric parkinsonism, apraxia and posturing, and a unique pathology involving the cortex as well as the BG, cerebellum and with neuronal achromasia. They referred to this as corticodentatonigral degeneration with neuronal achromasia, which was later termed as corticobasal degeneration and now as a CBS.[29]

Pathology

Most atypical parkinsonism are proteinopathies, and these abnormal proteins are accumulated in the cytoplasm of the neuron, which leads to the following:

- Causes disruption of axonal flow of neuron
- Causes synaptic dysfunction
- *Causes impairment of cell organelles function*: Mitochondrial dysfunction, increased burden on endoplasmic retinaculum

Mitochondrial dysfunction will cause oxidative stress and release of free radicals, along with the formation of protein adducts, which damages the membrane.

This will activate mitochondrial caspases, leading to apoptosis and cell death.[30]

Synucleinopathy

Synucleinopathy includes PD, MSA, and diffuse Lewy body dementia.

They have characteristic symptoms such as RBD and autonomic dysfunction before the onset of parkinsonism and may appear even more than 10 years before the onset of parkinsonism, especially in MSA.

In MSA, major pathology is synuclein deposit in the cytoplasm of oligodendrocytes.

Tauopathy

Tauopathy includes PSP, CBS, frontotemporal degeneration, and Alzheimer's disease. In a normal cell, a gene called *MAPT* on chromosome 17 produces tau protein, which is required for normal microtubular function.

Hyperphosphorylation of tau leads to its abnormal accumulation inside the cytoplasm, and it will hamper the microtubular function and axoplasmic flow.

In PSP at autopsy, the midbrain is atrophied, and the sylvian aqueduct is dilated. The SN is depigmented and appears orange and shrunken. The locus coeruleus may show some depigmentation, but this is less prominent than in PD. Frontal lobes, STN, and superior cerebellar peduncle may also show atrophy. Other pathological findings include neuronal loss, gliosis, neurofibrillary tangles, and granulovacuolar degeneration in neurons of the brainstem. There are tufted astrocytes in the motor cortex and the striatum, and the typical neuronal lesion is the globose neurofibrillary tangle, made up of hyperphosphorylated four-repeat tau protein filaments.[31]

In CBS, patients have gross brain atrophy. Tau-positive neuronal and glial lesions, especially gray and white matter astrocytic plaques and thread-like lesions, and neuronal loss in the cortex and SN are typical microscopic changes **(Figs. 2A and B)**. The inclusions are formed of hyperphosphorylated four-repeat tau **(Table 4)**. Overlap with other conditions including Alzheimer's disease, PSP, PD, frontotemporal dementia and parkinsonism (FTDP), and hippocampal sclerosis is seen.[32]

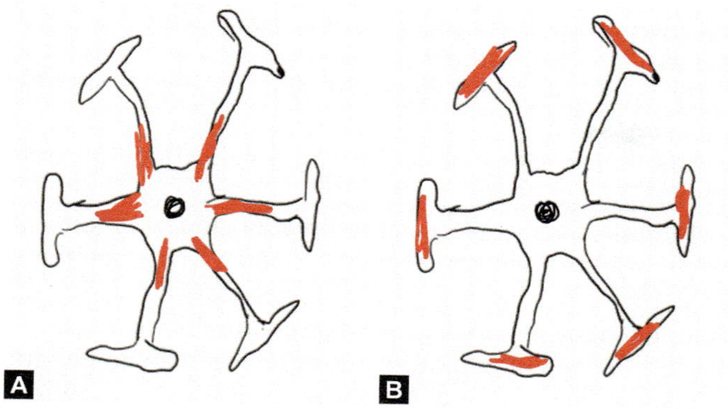

FIGS. 2A AND B: (A) Astrocyte of PSP: Red color is accumulated tau giving it tufted appearance; (B) Astrocyte of CBD: Here tau is accumulated in the foot process, forming astrocytic plaque.
(CBD: corticobasal degeneration; PSP: progressive supranuclear palsy)

TABLE 4: Pathological features to differentiate PSP and CBD.

Cell type	PSP	CBD
Neuron	Filamentous deposition, can form globose neurofibrillary tangle	Ballooned neurons with phosphorylated neuro-filaments, tau, ubiquitin
Astrocyte	Tufted astrocyte	Astrocytic plaque in the foot process
Oligoden-drocyte	Coiled body	Coiled body

(CBD: corticobasal degeneration; PSP: progressive supranuclear palsy)

Progressive Supranuclear Palsy

The typical age of onset is the sixth decade of life.

Features are symmetrical parkinsonism, supranuclear gaze palsy, symmetric akinetic-rigid syndrome, postural instability, and falls.

Supranuclear gaze palsy: In PSP voluntary control from the cortex to the oculomotor complex is affected, so most of the voluntary eye movements are affected including saccades, fixation, pursuits, vergence, etc.

The earliest finding is loss of vertical optokinetic nystagmus; saccades are affected more when you are moving the tape in the upward direction than in the downward direction.[24]

Normal vestibulo-ocular reflex helps in differentiating it from a nuclear lesion.

Clinical Signs of PSP[33]

- *Face*: Procerus sign/omega sign (due to excessive contraction of corrugator muscle)
  - Reptilian facies
- *Eye*: Blepharospasm/eyelid apraxia (both opening and closing apraxia is seen; opening is much more common)
  - Prominent upper sclera
  - Square wave jerks
  - Slow saccades
  - Broken pursuit
  - Downgaze palsy more than upgaze palsy (downgaze palsy is more specific)
- Early dysphagia and silent aspiration
- Extended neck, axial rigidity more than appendicular rigidity
- *Dirty tie sign*: Because of the inability to look down, patients tend to soil their shirts while eating.
- Tremor is rarely seen; if present, it is symmetrical.
- *Gunslinger's gait*: Patients of PSP keep their upper limbs flexed and hands toward their body.
- *Rocket sign*: While getting up from a chair because of axial stiffness, they get up suddenly without bending forward and tend to fall back into the chair because of loss of balance.
- *Applause sign*: PSP is very commonly associated with frontal lobar dysfunction; so patients will have executive dysfunction and other frontal lobar signs early without significant memory impairment; while asking patients to clap thrice, due to disinhibition they will keep on clapping.
- *Frequent falls*: Multiple reasons have been identified:
  - Disinhibition in PSP can lead to falls.
  - In contrast to PD, patients with PSP tend to have a more broad-based gait with knee extension, and instead of turning en bloc they tend to pivot on their toes and sometimes even cross their legs, which contributes to frequent falls.
  - Freezing of gait
- Pseudobulbar affect and depression are common features.
- Lack of response to levodopa

PSP Variants[34]

- Classical PSP or PSP-RS
- PSP-F (frontal)
- PSP-CBS
- PSP-speech and language predominant
- PSP-P
- PSP-progressive gait freezing predominant
- PSP-postural instability predominant
- PSP-oculomotor

PSP Mimics

- Spinocerebellar ataxia
- Whipple's disease
- Prion disease
- Autoimmune encephalitis associated with sleep disorders (REM, rapid onset)
- Nieman pick type C

Magnetic Resonance Imaging (MRI) Findings of PSP

- *Axial view*: Morning glory sign and mickey mouse sign
- *Sagittal view*: Hummingbird sign, reduced midbrain to pons ratio (<0.12)
- Abnormal magnetic resonance Parkinsonism index[35]

All these MRI signs are due to predominant tectal atrophy of the midbrain and sparing of the pons.

Corticobasal Syndrome

The age of onset is usually 60–64 years.[34] CBS has asymmetrical rigidity and bradykinesia. Patients can have hemidystonia, an alien limb phenomenon (feeling that the body part does not belong to him).

Clinical Features (Box 1)

Some patients with CBS do make movements with a limb that seem foreign to them, but they often have an overflow phenomenon in which movement in one limb triggers an involuntary movement in another.

Resting tremor is very rare, but action tremor, often combined with myoclonus, is common. Supranuclear gaze palsies are rare and can occur late in the disease.

Magnetic resonance imaging shows asymmetrical cortical atrophy, especially in the parieto-occipital cortex.

Multisystem Atrophy

The age of onset is 30–55 years, with a mean age of 54 years.[34] Clinical features include parkinsonism with predominant autonomic dysfunction with or without dystonia/ataxia. It is mainly divided into two types: MSA-P (parkinsonism) and MSA-C (cerebellar).

MSA-P

In addition to autonomic dysfunction, the patients have bradykinesia and rigidity and develop symmetrical akinetic rigid syndrome later. They may present with anterocollis, and axial dystonia can cause Pisa syndrome (the leaning of the body toward one side).

The main pathology here is striatonigral degeneration

MSA-C

Along with autonomic dysfunction they have predominant cerebellar signs such as scanning speech, square wave jerks, hypometric saccade, ataxia, and wide-based gait **(Box 2)**.

The main pathology seems to be olivopontocerebellar degeneration.

Other than these clinical features, MSA patients can have stridor and RBD.

Attempts to treat MSA rather than just the symptoms of MSA have so far been unsuccessful. As with PD, new attempts at treating MSA have focused on detoxifying misfolded α-synuclein to prevent disease progression.[36]

Clinical tests of autonomic dysfunction may be helpful in diagnosis or treatment. Testing of cardiovascular reflexes such as heart rate variability at rest and during forced respiration, as well as blood pressure changes during head-up tilt, may help establish a clinical diagnosis of MSA. A lack of responsiveness of growth hormone to clonidine challenges and denervation on rectal sphincter EMG are also characteristic findings.

MRI Findings

In MSA-P, predominant BG involvement with atrophy shows T2 hyperintensity in dorsolateral putamen known as the putaminal rim sign. In MSA-C, predominant pontine and cerebellar involvement gives a hot-cross bun sign. But these are not exclusively seen in MSA.

Metaiodobenzylguanidine (MIBG) Scan

It can help differentiate between preganglionic and postganglionic autonomic affection.

In idiopathic PD there is postganglionic autonomic fiber damage while in MSA there is preganglionic autonomic fiber damage. MIBG scan checks for postganglionic cardiac autonomic denervation. It is abnormal in idiopathic PD while normal in MSA.[37]

Single-photon Emission Computed Tomography (SPECT)/Positron Emission Tomography (PET) Scan

PET scan with [^{11}C]methylpiperidin-4-yl propionate (PMP) that images subcortical acetylcholinesterase (AChE)

BOX 1 Clinical features of corticobasal syndrome.

Cortical features:
- Early dementia
- Cortical myoclonus
- Alien limb
- Ideomotor apraxia
- Cortical sensory loss
- Hemiparesis
- Primary progressive aphasia

Brainstem features:
- Bulbar palsy
- Gaze: Impaired convergence

Extrapyramidal features:
- Bradykinesia
- Rigidity
- Dystonia of limb

BOX 2 Clinical features of cerebellar multisystem atrophy.

Autonomic dysfunction:
- Orthostatic hypotension/hypertension
- Urinary incontinence
- Erectile dysfunction
- Anhidrosis

Cerebellar:
- Nystagmus
- Square wave jerks
- Ataxia
- Wide-based gait

Extrapyramidal:
- Bradykinesia
- Rigidity
- Anterocolis and Pisa syndrome

activity is significantly more decreased in MSA-P and PSP than in PD, reflecting greater impairment in the pontine cholinergic neurons (PPN); this may account for the greater gait disturbances in the early stages of these two disorders compared to PD.[38] In SPECT scan same areas show significant hypoperfusion.

Role of Dopamine Transporter Scan in Diagnosing Parkinsonism

In the dopamine transporter (DAT) scan, ioflupane 123 is injected and its uptake by the dopaminergic transporter is assessed.

It helps differentiate between:
- Drug-induced parkinsonism and PD
- Diffuse Lewy body dementia and Alzheimer's disease[38]

However, it cannot differentiate between PD and atypical parkinsonism.

CONCLUSION

Movement disorders are broadly classified according to the abnormal speed of movements into hypokinesia, which means reduced movement, and hyperkinesia, which means increased movements. The terms hypokinesia, bradykinesia, and akinesia are arbitrarily used to describe parkinsonism across the literature. Hypokinesia is a clinical feature of PD, atypical parkinsonism, and secondary and heredodegenerative disorders. Hypokinesia is seen in pyramidal and psychiatric disorders. While sequence effect is a feature of PD, it is absent in pyramidal and psychiatric disorders. Pathophysiology shows delayed muscle activation, slower simple reaction time, and disinhibition of STN nucleus resulting in inhibiting thalamocortical pathway leading to cortical inhibition. Clinical symptoms include hypomimia, hypophonia, and slowness of activities of daily living.

REFERENCES

1. Jankovic J. Parkinson's disease: clinical features and diagnosis. J Neurol Neurosurg Psychiatry. 2008;79(4):368-76.
2. Alexander GE, DeLong MR, Strick PL. Parallel organization of functionally segregated circuits linking basal ganglia and cortex. Annu Rev Neurosci. 1986;9:357-81.
3. Alexander GE, Crutcher MD. Functional architecture of basal ganglia circuits: neural substrates of parallel processing. Trends Neurosci. 1990;13(7):266-71.
4. Sibley DR, Monsma FJ. Molecular biology of dopamine receptors. Trends Pharmacol Sci. 1992;13:61-9.
5. Obeso JA, Rodríguez-Oroz MC, Benitez-Temino B, Blesa FJ, Guridi J, Marin C, et al. Functional organization of the basal ganglia: therapeutic implications for Parkinson's disease. Mov Disord. 2008;23(S3):S548-59.
6. Rodriguez-Oroz MC, Jahanshahi M, Krack P, Litvan I, Macias R, Bezard E, et al. Initial clinical manifestations of Parkinson's disease: features and pathophysiological mechanisms. Lancet Neurol. 2009;8(12):1128-39.
7. Obeso JA, Stamelou M, Goetz CG, Poewe W, Lang AE, Weintraub D, et al. Past, present, and future of Parkinson's disease: a special essay on the 200th anniversary of The Shaking Palsy. Mov Disord. 2017;32(9):1264-310.
8. Thenganatt MA, Jankovic J. Parkinson disease subtypes. JAMA Neurol. 2014;71(4):499.
9. Jellinger KA. Neuropathology of sporadic Parkinson's disease: evaluation and changes of concepts. Mov Disord. 2012;27(1):8-30.
10. Goedert M, Spillantini MG, Del Tredici K, Braak H. 100 years of Lewy pathology. Nat Rev Neurol. 2013;9(1):13-24.
11. Stelmach GE, Worringham CJ, Strand EA. Movement preparation in Parkinson's disease. The use of advance information. Brain J Neurol. 1986;109(Pt 6):1179-94.
12. Jankovic J, Schwartz K, Ondo W. Reemergent tremor of Parkinson's disease. J Neurol Neurosurg Psychiatry. 1999;67(5):646-50.
13. Jankovic J. How do I examine for reemergent tremor? Mov Disord Clin Pract. 2016;3(2):216-7.
14. Jankovic J. Parkinson's disease tremors and serotonin. Brain J Neurol. 2018;141(3):624-6.
15. Jankovic J. Camptocormia, head drop, and other bent spine syndromes: heterogeneous etiology and pathogenesis of parkinsonian deformities. Mov Disord. 2010;25(5):527-8.
16. Wijemanne S, Jankovic J. Hand, foot, and spine deformities in parkinsonian disorders. J Neural Transm. 2019;126(3):253-64.
17. Goetz CG, Tilley BC, Shaftman SR, Stebbins GT, Fahn S, Martinez-Martin P, et al. Movement Disorder Society-sponsored revision of the Unified Parkinson's Disease Rating Scale (MDS-UPDRS): scale presentation and clinimetric testing results: MDS-UPDRS: clinimetric assessment. Mov Disord. 2008;23(15):2129-70.
18. Zesiewicz TA, Sullivan KL, Hauser RA. Nonmotor symptoms of Parkinson's disease. Expert Rev Neurother. 2006;6(12):1811-22.
19. Schenck CH, Bundlie SR, Mahowald MW. Delayed emergence of a parkinsonian disorder in 38% of 29 older men initially diagnosed with idiopathic rapid eye movement sleep behavior disorder. Neurology. 1996;46(2):388-93.
20. Borek LL, Kohn R, Friedman JH. Phenomenology of dreams in Parkinson's disease. Mov Disord. 2007;22(2):198-202.
21. Patel N, Jankovic J, Hallett M. Sensory aspects of movement disorders. Lancet Neurol. 2014;13(1):100-12.
22. Archibald NK, Clarke MP, Mosimann UP, Burn DJ. Visual symptoms in Parkinson's disease and Parkinson's disease dementia. Mov Disord. 2011;26(13):2387-95.
23. Sankhla CS. Visual symptoms in Parkinson's disease. Neurol India. 2019;67(1):56.
24. Waln O, Jankovic J. Neuro-ophthalmology of movement disorders. Expert Rev Ophthalmol. 2018;13(5):283-92.
25. McFarland NR, Hess CW. Recognizing atypical parkinsonisms: "red flags" and therapeutic approaches. Semin Neurol. 2017;37(2):215-27.
26. Lantos PL. The definition of multiple system atrophy: a review of recent developments. J Neuropathol Exp Neurol. 1998;57(12):1099-111.
27. Shy GM, Drager GA. A neurological syndrome associated with orthostatic hypotension: a clinical–pathologic study. Arch Neurol. 1960;2:511-27.
28. Steele JC, Richardson JC, Olszewski J. Progressive supranuclear palsy: a heterogeneous degeneration involving the brain stem, basal ganglia and cerebellum with vertical gaze and pseudobulbar palsy, nuchal dystonia, and dementia. Arch Neurol. 1964;10(4):333-59.
29. Rebeiz JJ, Kolodny EH, Richardson EP. Corticodentatonigral degeneration with neuronal achromasia. Arch Neurol. 1968;18(1):20-33.

30. Chu CT. Mechanisms of selective autophagy and mitophagy: implications for neurodegenerative diseases. Neurobiol Dis. 2019;122:23-34.
31. Dickson DW, Ahmed Z, Algom AA, Tsuboi Y, Josephs KA. Neuropathology of variants of progressive supranuclear palsy. Curr Opin Neurol. 2010;23(4):394-400.
32. Kouri N, Whitwell JL, Josephs KA, Rademakers R, Dickson DW. Corticobasal degeneration: a pathologically distinct 4R tauopathy. Nat Rev Neurol. 2011;7(5):263-72.
33. Höglinger GU, Respondek G, Stamelou M, Kurz C, Josephs KA, Lang AE, et al. Clinical diagnosis of progressive supranuclear palsy: the movement disorder society criteria: MDS clinical diagnostic criteria for PSP. Mov Disord. 2017;32(6):853-64.
34. Stamelou M, Quinn NP, Bhatia KP. "Atypical" atypical parkinsonism: new genetic conditions presenting with features of progressive supranuclear palsy, corticobasal degeneration, or multiple system atrophy—a diagnostic guide. Mov Disord. 2013;28(9):1184-99.
35. Sankhla CS, Patil KB, Sawant N, Gupta S. Diagnostic accuracy of magnetic resonance Parkinsonism index in differentiating progressive supranuclear palsy from Parkinson's disease and controls in Indian patients. Neurol India. 2016;64(2):239.
36. Koga S, Dickson DW. Recent advances in neuropathology, biomarkers, and therapeutic approach of multiple system atrophy. J Neurol Neurosurg Psychiatry. 2018;89(2):175-84.
37. Sakuramoto H, Fujita H, Suzuki K, Matsubara T, Watanabe Y, Hamaguchi M, et al. Combination of midbrain-to-pontine ratio and cardiac MIBG scintigraphy to differentiate Parkinson's disease from multiple system atrophy and progressive supranuclear palsy. Clin Park Relat Disord. 2020;2:20-4.
38. Isaacson SH, Fisher S, Gupta F, Hermanowicz N, Kremens DE, Lew MF, et al. Clinical utility of DaTscan™ imaging in the evaluation of patients with parkinsonism: a US perspective. Expert Rev Neurother. 2017;17(3):219-25.

39

CHAPTER

Approach to Chorea, Athetosis, Ballismus, and Dystonia

Jacky Ganguly, Hrishikesh Kumar

INTRODUCTION

This chapter deals with four hyperkinetic movement disorders namely, chorea, athetosis, ballismus, and dystonia. These are common and seen frequently in clinical practice. A sound clinical approach is important in the evaluation of these diseases. This chapter deals with the definitions, clinical presentations, differential diagnoses, and investigative aspects of these diseases.

CHOREA

Chorea consists of discrete involuntary movements or movement fragments that are nonrhythmic, nonpatterned, fleeting, semipurposeful, and flow randomly from one part of the body to another.[1] However, movements can be brisk and abrupt (e.g., Sydenham's chorea, lupus chorea) or slower and flowing [e.g., Huntington's disease (HD)]. The patient often appears fidgety and clumsy. Two important terminologies regarding chorea are parakinesia and motor impersistence.[2] Parakinesia is the phenomenon of integrating the choreic movements into normal movements, whereas motor impersistence is the inability to do sustained movements. This can be demonstrated by the inability to maintain tongue protrusion (lizard's tongue or "Jack-in-the-box" tongue) and handgrip (milkmaid's grip).

Clinical Approach to Chorea

Chorea should be approached clinically according to the age of onset (childhood- or adult-onset), mode of onset (acute or insidious), and the type of disease course (remitting, continuous or paroxysmal). Sydenham's chorea is the most common cause of chorea in childhood, whereas the most common cause of chronic progressive chorea in adults is HD.[1] Considering mode of onset, acute onset of chorea can be the manifestation of stroke, metabolic abnormalities such as nonketotic hyperglycemia, or chorea gravidarum. The subacute course can indicate metabolic (e.g., uremia), infective, or autoimmune, or paraneoplastic etiology. Drug-induced chorea can be acute, subacute, or gradual onset such as levodopa-induced dyskinesia or tardive dyskinesia. Insidious onset and the slowly progressive course usually suggest underlying neurodegenerative disorders like HD. Remitting chorea commonly indicates vascular or metabolic etiology. Paroxysmal chorea can be kinesigenic (e.g., *PRRT2* mediated), nonkinesigenic (e.g., *MR1* mediated), or exercise-induced (e.g., *GLUT1* mediated).[3] Recurrent chorea can also be seen in chorea gravidarum and Sydenham's chorea.

Next, it should be determined whether the chorea is hereditary or acquired in nature. Hereditary choreas can be inherited as autosomal dominant (AD), autosomal recessive (AR), and X-linked (XL) manner.[4] **Tables 1 and 2** summarizes common causes and key clinical features of childhood-onset and adult-onset hereditary choreas. **Flowchart 1** shows the approach to HD Phenocopy syndromes.[5] **Table 3** summarizes common acquired causes of chorea.

The predilection of chorea for specific body regions often provides a clue to the diagnosis.[1] Upper facial or forehead chorea is classically seen in HD. Lower facial chorea and associated feeding dystonia are classically seen in chorea-acanthocytosis. Orofacial involvement is also prominent in tardive dyskinesia, edentulous dyskinesia, neuroferritinopathy, pantothenate kinase-associated neurodegeneration (PKAN), Lesch–Nyhan syndrome, anti-N-methyl-D-aspartate receptor (anti-NMDAR) encephalitis and postpump chorea. In children, choreoathetosis, hypotonia, affective changes, and pseudobulbar signs (CHAP syndrome) are seen in hypoxia commonly associated with cardiac surgery.[6] Predominant lower limb chorea is seen in diphasic dyskinesia of Parkinson's disease (PD). Hemichorea is commonly associated with stroke or hyperglycemic state.

TABLE 1: Causes of childhood-onset hereditary chorea.

Disorder	Gene	Mode of inheritance
Benign hereditary chorea (BHC)	*NKX2-1*	AD
ADCY5 related	*ADCY5*	AD
PDE10A related	*PDE10A*	AD or AR
Ataxia telangiectasia (AT)	*ATM*	AR
• Ataxia with oculomotor • Apraxia types 1 and 2 (AOA1, AOA2)	*APTX, SETX*	AR
Hereditary epileptic-dyskinetic encephalopathies	*GNAO1, GRIN1, FOXG1, FRRS1L, IRF2BPL*	AR

(AD: autosomal dominant; AR: autosomal recessive)

TABLE 2: Causes of adult-onset hereditary chorea.

Disorder	Gene	Mode of inheritance
Huntington's disease (HD)	*HTT*	AD
C9orf72 expansions	*C9orf72*	AD
Spinocerebellar ataxia 17 (SCA17)	*TBP*	AD
Huntington disease-like 1 (HDL1)	*PRNP*	AD
Huntington disease-like 2 (HDL2)	*JPH3*	AD
Neuroferritinopathy	*FTL*	AD
Dentatorubral-pallidoluysian atrophy (DRPLA)	*ATN1*	AD
Aceruloplasminemia	*CP*	AR
Chorea-acanthocytosis	*VPS13A*	AR
McLeod syndrome	*XK*	XL

(AD: autosomal dominant; AR: autosomal recessive)

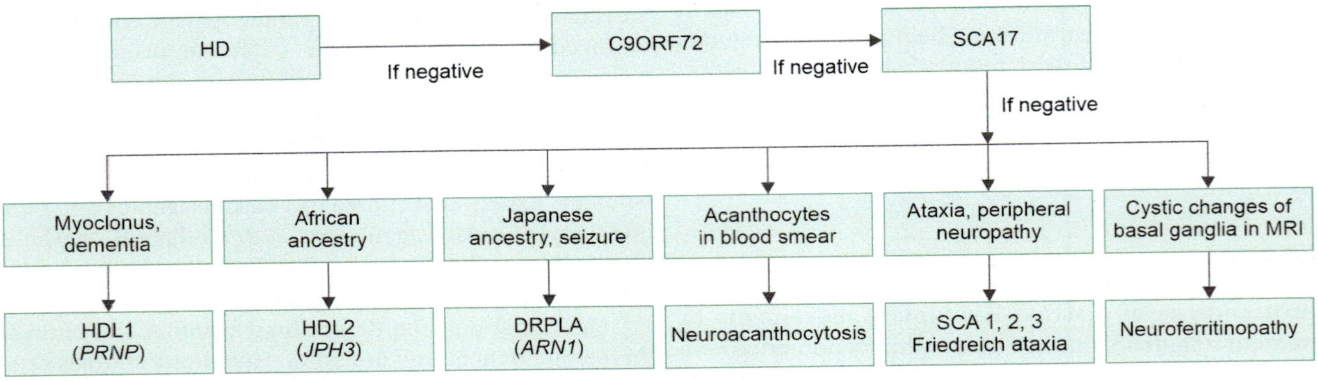

FLOWCHART 1: Approach to Huntington's disease (HD) phenocopy syndromes.

TABLE 3: Causes of acquired chorea.

Endocrine/Metabolic	Hyperthyroidism, hyperglycemia, hyper-/hyponatremia, hypocalcemia, hypomagnesemia, uremia, non-Wilsonian hepatolenticular degeneration, kernicterus
Vascular	Stroke, small vessel disease
Drugs/toxins	Acute drug-induced chorea, tardive chorea, alcohol, CO poisoning
Nutritional	Vitamin B1 and B12 deficiency
Infectious/parainfectious	Sydenham's chorea, variant Creutzfeldt–Jakob disease (vCJD), HIV
Hematological	Polycythemia vera, essential thrombocythemia
Autoimmune/paraneoplastic	• SLE, antiphospholipid antibody syndrome (APLA), Behçet's disease, Sjögren syndrome, celiac disease, anti-NMDAR, anti-neurexin-3 alpha, anti-IgLON5, anti-D2R, anti-GABA-AR, anti-LG1, anti-Caspr2, anti-PDE10A encephalitis • Anti-CV2/CRMP5, anti-Hu encephalitis
Demyelinating	Acute disseminated encephalomyelitis (ADEM), multiple sclerosis, central pontine, and extrapontine myelinolysis
Hypoxia	Cardiac arrest, hypothermia, postpump chorea
Others	Chorea gravidarum

(HIV: human immunodeficiency virus; NMDAR: N-methyl-D-aspartate receptor; SLE: systemic lupus erythematosus)

TABLE 4: Clinical pearls for chorea.

Chorea with neuropsychiatric symptoms	HD, chorea-acanthocytosis, McLeod syndrome, SCA17, HDL2, DRPLA, PKAN, Wilson disease, Chorea gravidarum, APLA
Chorea with self-mutilation behavior	Lesch–Nyhan syndrome, chorea-acanthocytosis
Chorea with seizures	Chorea-acanthocytosis, McLeod syndrome, SCA17, DRPLA, HDL1, juvenile HD
Chorea with epileptic encephalopathies	*GNAO1, GRIN1, FOXG1, FRRS1L, IRF2BPL*
Chorea with tics	HD, chorea-acanthocytosis
Chorea with ataxia	SCA17, DRPLA, AT, AOA1, AOA2
Chorea with dystonia	HD, HDL2, SCA17, chorea-acanthocytosis, DRPLA, neuroferritinopathy
Chorea with facio-bucco-lingual dystonia	Chorea-acanthocytosis, McLeod syndrome, tardive dyskinesia, PKAN, Lesch–Nyhan syndrome, aceruloplasminemia, neuroferritinopathy, Wilson's disease, Lubag disease
Chorea with myoclonus	HDL1, DRPLA
Chorea with saccadic apraxia and head thrusts to initiate a saccade	HD, AT, AOA1 and 2
Chorea with axial hypotonia, violent head drops	Chorea-acanthocytosis
Chorea with axial hypotonia, nocturnal ballistic bouts	*ADCY5* dyskinesia
Chorea with peripheral neuropathy	Chorea-acanthocytosis, McLeod syndrome, AT, AOA1, AOA2
Chorea with frontotemporal dementia/amyotrophic lateral sclerosis (FTD-ALS) spectrum	*C9orf72* disorder
Chorea with prominent parasomnia	Anti-IgLON5 disease
Chorea with systemic signs	• Cardiomyopathy, atrial fibrillation, hepatosplenomegaly: McLeod syndrome • Arthritis, photosensitive malar rash: Lupus • Anemia, diabetes mellitus, retinal degeneration: Aceruloplasminemia • Thyroid and lung dysfunction: Benign hereditary chorea

(ALPA: antiphospholipid antibody syndrome; DRPLA: dentatorubral-pallidoluysian atrophy; HD: Huntington's disease; HDL2: Huntington disease-like 2; PKAN: pantothenate kinase-associated neurodegeneration; SCA17: spinocerebellar ataxia 17)

Next, associated neurological and systemic signs should be looked for. **Table 4** summarizes clinical pearls for chorea.

Investigation

Most of the treatable causes of chorea are of acute or subacute onset, while a protracted course is seen in neurodegenerative disorders such as HD or HD phenocopies. Screening for thyroid, renal, and liver dysfunction, and dyselectrolytemia should be done along with testing of erythrocyte sedimentation rate, fresh blood acanthocyte, and magnetic resonance imaging (MRI) brain. Autoimmune panels including antinuclear, antiphospholipid, anti-double-stranded DNA, anticardiolipin antibody, lupus anticoagulant, anti-NMDA, anti-IgLON5, and anti-CV2 should be screened, especially in subacute onset cases.[7] As Sydenham's chorea and HD are the two most common choreas in children and adults, these two disorders should be tested for and excluded before proceeding to other diagnostic pathways. If HD genetics comes negative, *C9orf72* and SCA17 in white individuals and HDL2 in black African ancestry should be screened.[5] *PRRT2, MR1, KCNMA1,* and *SLC2A1/GLUT1* genetics should be tested in paroxysmal choreas.[3]

Magnetic resonance imaging brain often helps in the etiological diagnosis of choreic syndromes. Caudate atrophy is seen in HD and chorea-acanthocytosis. Cerebellar atrophy is seen in SCA17 and dentatorubral-pallidoluysian atrophy (DRPLA). T1 hyperintensity in putamen is seen in nonketotic hyperglycemia and acquired hepatocerebral degeneration.[8] PDE10A mutations are associated with bilateral striatal T2 hyperintensities.[9] Thalamic pulvinar T2, and fluid attenuated inversion recovery (FLAIR) hyperintensities are seen in variant Creutzfeldt–Jakob disease (vCJD). The distinctive pattern of iron deposition in T2 and SWI sequences suggests neurodegeneration with brain iron accumulation (NBIA) including PKAN, neuroferritinopathy, and aceruloplasminemia. Additional cystic changes in basal ganglia are classically seen in neuroferritinopathy.[10]

ATHETOSIS

Athetosis is defined as an involuntary movement with writhing, nonrhythmic, nonforceful, *slow sinuous* continuously flowing quality that prevents the maintenance of a sustained posture. It commonly involves distal extremities. The term athetosis is rarely used in isolation nowadays.

It often accompanies either chorea (*choreoathetosis*) or dystonia. However, in contrast to dystonia, pure athetosis is nonsustained. Chorea also often evolves into athetosis and vice versa. Athetosis is commonly seen in children with cerebral palsy (CP).[11] Athetoid CP is usually not associated with significant cognitive impairment or epilepsy, in contrast to other varieties of CP. Dystonia-athetosis or choreoathetosis can be seen as one of the poststroke movement disorders. Choreoathetosis has been reported in thyrotoxicosis, hypernatremia, hypoxia, phenytoin toxicity, cerebral folate deficiency, Wernicke's encephalopathy, glutaric aciduria, Lesch–Nyhan syndrome, acute organophosphate poisoning, congenital disorders of glycosylation, anti-N-methyl-D-aspartate (anti-NMDA) encephalitis, ADCY5 dyskinesia, LRRK2 mutation along with parkinsonism, in HD, in paroxysmal kinesigenic dyskinesia and can be drug-induced (e.g., antipsychotics, levodopa).[12-21] Dystonia-athetosis has been documented in FOXG1 mutation-related Rett phenotype and parkinsonism and in Rasmussen's encephalitis.[22,23] Choreoathetoid-dystonic movements can also be associated with syringomyelia and prion disease.

Athetosis should be differentiated from *pseudoathetosis* which is characterized by abnormal writhing movements of the digits, occurring with the eyes closed due to proprioceptive deficit.[24] Pseudoathetosis can result from lesions located anywhere in sensory pathways, including peripheral nerve, the posterior column of the spinal cord, thalamus, and parietal cortex.

BALLISMUS

Ballismus represents large amplitude, intermittent, *flinging* movement present unilaterally involving proximal body parts. Ischemic or hemorrhagic stroke and nonketotic hyperglycemia (diabetic striatopathy) are the two most common causes of hemiballismus, commonly associated with hemichorea. Because of the vascular insult to the unilateral subthalamic nucleus (STN) or other basal ganglia nuclei affecting the firing pattern of globus pallidus internus (GPi), ballismus is commonly unilateral (hemi), affecting contralateral to the affected side.[25] These movements can often be violent. Ballismus forms part of the spectrum of chorea, however, it is larger in amplitude and more forceful, involving more proximal musculature compared to chorea.

Hemichorea-hemiballismus (HCHB) can be the presenting feature of type 1 diabetes mellitus in adolescence and can recur during infections. Brain MRI typically shows T1 hyperintensities **(Fig. 1)** in the contralateral striatum in cases with hyperglycemic hemiballismus.[26] Other reported causes include central nervous system (CNS) infection (e.g., toxoplasmosis, tuberculosis, neurosyphilis, and cryptococcosis), post-COVID-19 vaccination, CNS vasculitis, neurolupus, antiphospholipid antibody syndrome (APLA), multiple sclerosis, mass lesion (cyst, neoplasm), drug-induced (e.g., neuroleptics, levodopa, phenytoin, and oral contraceptives) and paraneoplastic (anti-Yo).[25,27,28] Brief

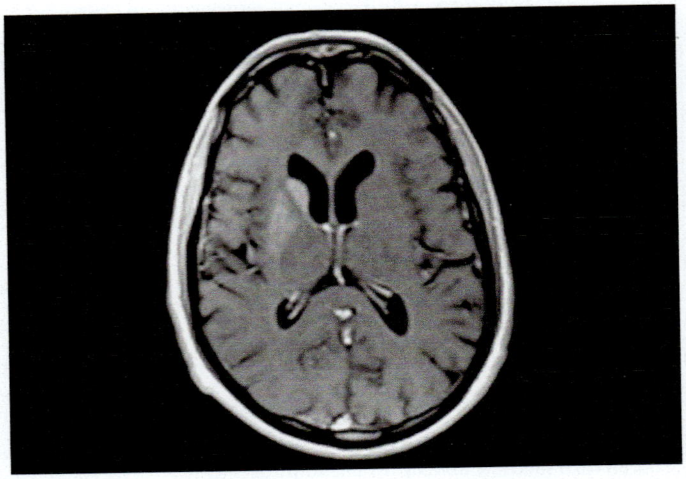

FIG. 1: T1 hyperintensity of right basal ganglia in hemichorea-hemiballismus.

episodes of HCHB can be a manifestation of limb shaking transient ischemic attack from the carotid or vertebrobasilar territory.[29]

Biballism or *paraballism* is rare where bilateral involvement is seen. It has been reported in bilateral basal ganglia vascular lesion, drug-induced (e.g., oral contraceptive pills and lamotrigine), multiple sclerosis, and nonketotic hyperglycemia.[30,31]

DYSTONIA

Dystonia is characterized by involuntary movements or postures due to *sustained* or *intermittent* muscle contractions. The movements are typically *patterned* leading to twisting and repetitive muscle contractions. Contractions of the dystonic muscles often lead to an oscillatory movement (*dystonic tremor* or *dynamic dystonia*) being exacerbated while attempting to maintain primary posture.[32]

Some characteristics of dystonia are: (1) *Presence of null point*, where the dystonic tremor is being relieved by allowing the abnormal dystonic posture to fully develop; (2) *Overflow*, when unintentional muscle contraction involves an anatomically distinct area from the primary dystonic movement; (3) *Mirror dystonia*, a posturing of similar character appears in the more severely affected side when movements or actions are performed by contralateral side; and (4) *Presence of tricks or geste antagoniste*, those are voluntary actions targeted to the affected area to correct or alleviate the abnormal dystonic posture. Tricks can be motor, sensory, forcible, and imaginary.[33]

Clinical Approach to Dystonia

Albanese et al. have classified dystonia in axis 1 (clinical characteristics) and axis 2 (etiology).[34] Axis 1 consists of the age of onset infancy, childhood, adolescence, early adulthood, late adulthood), body distribution (focal, segmental, multifocal, generalized, hemidystonia), temporal pattern (static or progressive disease course, variability such as persistent, action-specific, diurnal, and paroxysmal) and associated features (isolated, combined with other movement disorders, or neurological manifestations). **Table 5** summarizes combined dystonia syndromes where dystonia is associated with other movement disorders.

Axis 2 involves nervous system pathology and classifying it as inherited, acquired, or idiopathic. **Tables 6 and 7** shows major inherited causes of dystonia and clinical pearls to suspect them. Perinatal insult, brain injury, stroke, neoplastic/paraneoplastic, toxin or drug, and infection are common *acquired* causes. Sudden onset, rapid progression, lower limb onset in adults, craniocervical onset in childhood, fixed spasm, hemidystonia, onset in infancy, and presence of other neurological or systemic signs indicate secondary dystonia.

Among all these causes, Wilson's disease (WD) is the most common cause of early-onset dystonia in the Indian subcontinent. WD is an AR disorder due to *ATP7B* gene mutation, resulting in defective copper metabolism, primarily affecting the liver and brain. The most common ATP7B mutation detected in India is p.C271X. Positive family history can be found in 50% of Indian WD cases because of the high rate of consanguinity.[35] Neuropsychiatric and hepatic manifestations dominate the clinical picture, whereas osseomuscular presentation is also prevalent in India. Dystonia-parkinsonism is the most common neurological manifestation. Craniofacial dystonia with atypical "vacuous smile" is characteristic. Kayser–Fleischer (KF) ring is seen in 97–100% neurologic WD cases, while 14–87% in hepatic WD. Psychiatric features include mania, depression, bipolar affective disorder, suicidal ideation, and schizophrenia-like illnesses. "Modified Leipzig score" is an easily administered screening tool to diagnose WD in the Indian subcontinent.[36] It consists of KF rings, serum ceruloplasmin, 24-hour urinary copper, Coomb's negative hemolytic anemia with liver disorder, genetic mutation, liver biopsy, neurobehavioral symptoms, MRI brain, and family history of WD.

Investigation

Wilson's disease screening with serum ceruloplasmin and 24-hour urinary copper should be tested in any case of early onset dystonia. Similarly, a levodopa trial often helps to identify dopa-responsive dystonia (DRD) spectrum and juvenile PD like PARK2 in the case of younger onset dystonia. MRI brain is the next step of investigation as it can provide helpful radiological clues in dystonia, such as, "face of the

TABLE 5: Combined dystonia syndromes.

Dystonia + Parkinsonism	• *Primary genetic dystonia*: DYT 3 or Lubag (*TAF1*), DYT 5 and dopa-responsive dystonia (DRD) spectrum (*GTPCH1/TH/SPR*), DYT 12 or rapid-onset dystonia-parkinsonism (*ATP1A3*), DYT 16 or early onset dystonia-parkinsonism (*PRKRA*) • *Secondary dystonia as a part of other movement disorders*: Wilson's disease, juvenile genetic Parkinson's disease (*Parkin/PINK1/DJ1*), neurodegeneration with brain iron accumulation such as PKAN, PLAN (*PLA2G6*), Kufor–Rakeb (*ATP13A2*), Huntington's disease (Westphal variant), SCA3 (*ATXN3*), SPG11 • *Associated with classic akinetic-rigid syndromes*: Corticobasal syndrome (CBS), progressive supranuclear palsy (PSP), multiple system atrophy (MSA)
Dystonia + Myoclonus	DYT 11 (*SGCE*), DYT 24 (*ANO3*), mitochondrial (*POLG*), tyrosine hydroxylase deficiency (*TH*), corticobasal syndrome, multiple system atrophy
Dystonia + Ataxia	SCA1 (*ATXN1*), SCA2 (*ATXN2*), SCA3 (*ATXN3*), SCA6 (*CACNA1A*), SCA17 (*TBP*), AT (*ATM*), AOA1 (*APTX*), AOA2 (*SETX*), Niemann–Pick type C (*NPC1,2*), mitochondrial (*POLG*), PLAN (*PLA2G6*), DYT4 (*TUBB4*), Friedreich ataxia (*FXN*), ataxia with vitamin E deficiency or AVED (*TTPA*), SPG7, GLUT1 deficiency (*SLC2A1*)
Dystonia + Chorea	DYT 4 (*TUBB4*), AT (*ATM*), AOA1 (*APTX*), AOA2 (*SETX*), Huntington's disease, SCA17 (*TBP*), Lesch–Nyhan syndrome (*HPRT*), ADCY5 dyskinesia, chorea-acanthocytosis (*VPS13A*)

TABLE 6: Major inherited dystonia syndromes.

Mode of inheritance	Dystonia syndromes
Autosomal dominant	• DYT1 (*TOR1A*), DYT4 (*TUBB4*), DYT5 or Segawa variant (*GTPCH1*) • DYT6 (*THAP1*), DYT11 or myoclonus-dystonia (*SGCE*), DYT12 or rapid onset dystonia-parkinsonism (*ATP1A3*), neuroferritinopathy (*FTL1*), Huntington's disease, spinocerebellar ataxia type 3 or SCA3 (*ATXN3*)
Autosomal recessive	Wilson disease (*ATP7B*), neurodegeneration with brain iron accumulation like PKAN (*PANK2*) and PLAN (*PLA2G6*), juvenile Parkinson's disease like PARK2 (*parkin*), Niemann–Pick type C (NPC), ataxia telangiectasia (*ATM*), GM2 gangliosidosis (HEXA, HEXB), glutaric aciduria (*GCDH*), methylmalonic aciduria
X-linked recessive	DYT3 or Lubag (*TAF1*), Lesch–Nyhan syndrome (*HPRT*), Mohr–Tranebjaerg syndrome (*TIMM8A*)
Mitochondrial	Leigh syndrome, myoclonic epilepsy with ragged red fibers or MERRF (*MT-TK*), Leber's hereditary optic neuropathy or LHON, *POLG* mediated

TABLE 7: Clinical pearls for dystonia.

Ethnic clues for dystonia	• *Ashkenazi Jews*: DYT1 (*TOR1A*) • *Middle east*: Kufor–Rakeb (*ATP13A2*), Woodhouse–Sakati (*DCAF17*) • *Filipino*: DYT3 (*TAF1*) • *Portuguese*: SCA3 (*ATXN3*) • *Amish–Mennonites*: DYT6 (*THAP1*)
Dystonia with alopecia	Woodhouse–Sakati (*DCAF17*)
Dystonia with deafness	Mohr–Tranebjaerg syndrome or deafness-dystonia-optic neuropathy (DDON) syndrome (*TIMM8A*), Woodhouse–Sakati (*DCAF17*), mitochondrial, Waardenburg syndrome
Dystonia with prominent orobulbar involvement	Pantothenate kinase-associated neurodegeneration (PKAN), neuroacanthocytosis, Lesch–Nyhan syndrome, DYT12 (*ATP1A3*), DYT4 (*TUBB4*), DYT6 (*THAP1*), DYT28 (*KMT2B*)
Feeding dystonia	Neuroacanthocytosis
Dystonia with a cherry-red spot	GM1 and GM2 gangliosidosis
Dystonia with optic atrophy	DDON syndrome (*TIMM8A*), SPG7, mitochondrial membrane protein-associated neurodegeneration (MPAN), metachromatic leukodystrophy, methylmalonic aciduria
Dystonia with retinitis pigmentosa	PKAN, mitochondrial, SCA7, metachromatic leukodystrophy
Dystonia with ectopic lentis	Homocystinuria
Dystonia with KF ring	Wilson's disease (*ATP7B*)
Dystonia with oculomotor apraxia	Ataxia-telangiectasia (AT), ataxia with oculomotor apraxia (AOA), corticobasal syndrome
Dystonia with vertical gaze palsy	Niemann–Pick type C (NPC), Kufor–Rakeb syndrome (KRS), SPG7, *PLA2G6* associated neurodegeneration (PLAN), PSP, 18p deletion syndrome
Dystonia with gelastic cataplexy	Niemann–Pick type C
Early onset dystonia with macrocephaly	Glutaric aciduria type 1, megalencephalic leukoencephalopathy with subcortical cysts
Dystonia with facial-faucial-finger minipolymyoclonus	Kufor–Rakeb (*ATP13A2*)
Dystonia with facial dysmorphism	18p deletion syndrome (round face), homocystinuria
Dystonia with peripheral neuropathy	SCA3, SCA1, SCA2, NPC, AT, AOA, metachromatic leukodystrophy, chorea-acanthocytosis, Friedreich ataxia, mitochondrial (POLG), Tay–Sachs, MPAN
Dystonia with "praying mantis sign"	Pantothenate kinase-associated neurodegeneration
Dystonia with self-mutilation	Lesch–Nyhan syndrome
Dystonia with unilateral or asymmetric arm posturing	DYT12 (*ATP1A3*)
Prominent cervical onset dystonia	• Early onset—DYT6 (*THAP1*) • Late-onset—DYT23 (*CIZ1*), DYT25 (*GNAL*) • Early onset or late onset, with postural tremor—DYT24 (*ANO3*)
Dystonia with atypical gait	• Hobby horse—DYT4 (*TUBB4*) • Phasic knee bending—DYT3 (XDP, *TAF1*) • Rubber man gait—chorea-acanthocytosis (*VPS13A*) • Cock walk—manganese intoxication • Dystonic pseudo foot drop—PARK2 (*Parkin*) • Dromedary gait—early-onset generalized dystonia (especially DYT1)

giant panda" sign in Wilson's disease, T1 hyperintensity of basal ganglia in manganese toxicity, "eye of the tiger" sign in PKAN, "nigral halo" sign in beta-propeller protein-associated neurodegeneration (BPAN), "split pallidum" sign in mitochondrial membrane protein-associated neurodegeneration (MPAN)[10] **(Fig. 2)**, enlarged Sylvian fissure with "batwing" appearance in glutaric aciduria type 1, caudate atrophy in HD and chorea-acanthocytosis and T1 hyper-/T2 hypo-intensity of the thalamus in Tay–Sachs (GM2 gangliosidosis).[37] Subsequently, genetic testing should be done, combining the clinical and radiological clues.

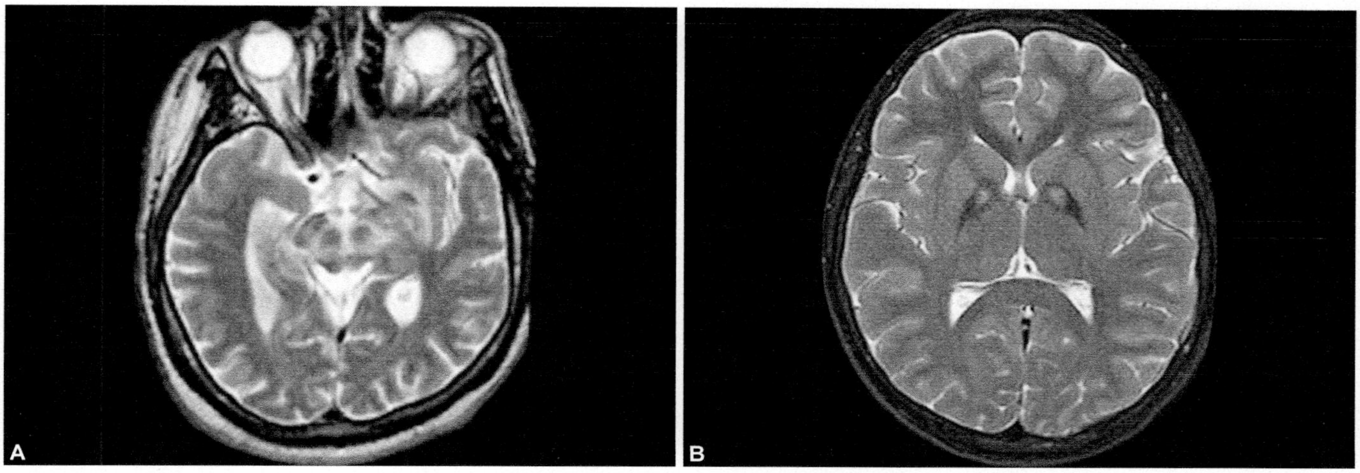

FIGS. 2A AND B: "Face of the giant panda" sign in Wilson's disease (A); "Eye of the tiger" sign in PKAN (B).

PSEUDODYSTONIA

Pseudodystonia describes abnormal postures, repetitive movements, or both, where clinical, imaging, laboratory, or electrophysiological studies provide a definite explanation of symptoms that is not compatible with dystonia.[38] Pseudodystonia can be classified into four main groups—(1) Pseudodystonia in *non-neurological disorders of the musculoskeletal system* (congenital muscular torticollis, posterior fossa or neck mass, subluxation and joint deformities, contractures, Sandifer's syndrome, congenital Klippel-Feil syndrome); (2) Pseudodystonia in *disorders of the sensory pathway* (parietal lobe damage, myeloneuropathy); (3) Pseudodystonia in *disorders of the motor pathway* (Stiff-person syndrome, myotonia, neuromyotonia, spasms, tetanus, peripheral nerve hyperexcitability); (4) *Compensatory postures* in other neurological disorders (head tilt due to vestibulopathy, trochlear/abducens nerve palsy).[38]

CONCLUSION

A variety of hyperkinetic movement disorders have been discussed in this chapter. As can be seen, their clinical presentations are varied and the differential diagnosis is wide. A systematic approach to the clinical and investigative approach is important in managing these disorders.

REFERENCES

1. Mestre TA. Chorea. Continuum (Minneap Minn). 2016;22:1186-207.
2. Bhidayasiri R, Truong DD. Chorea and related disorders. Postgrad Med J. 2004;80(947):527-34.
3. Harvey S, King MD, Gorman KM. Paroxysmal Movement Disorders. Front Neurol. 2021;12:659064.
4. Martinez-Ramirez D, Walker RH, Rodríguez-Violante M, Gatto EM; Rare Movement Disorders Study Group of International Parkinson's Disease. Review of Hereditary and Acquired Rare Choreas. Tremor Other Hyperkinet Mov (N Y). 2020;10:24.
5. Schneider SA, Bird T. Huntington's Disease, Huntington's Disease Look-Alikes, and Benign Hereditary Chorea: What's New? Mov Disord Clin Pract. 2016;3(4):342-54.
6. Baizabal-Carvallo JF, Cardoso F. Chorea in children: etiology, diagnostic approach and management. J Neural Transm (Vienna). 2020;127(10):1323-42.
7. Kyle K, Bordelon Y, Venna N, Linnoila J. Autoimmune and Paraneoplastic Chorea: A Review of the Literature. Front Neurol. 2022;13:829076.
8. Batty R. A review of pathologies associated with high T1W signal intensity in the basal ganglia on Magnetic Resonance Imaging. Pol J Radiol. 2014;79:126-30.
9. Mencacci NE, Kamsteeg EJ, Nakashima K, R'Bibo L, Lynch DS, Balint B, et al. De Novo Mutations in PDE10A Cause Childhood-Onset Chorea with Bilateral Striatal Lesions. Am J Hum Genet. 2016;98(4):763-71.
10. Lee JH, Yun JY, Gregory A, Hogarth P, Hayflick SJ. Brain MRI Pattern Recognition in Neurodegeneration With Brain Iron Accumulation. Front Neurol. 2020;11:1024.
11. Morris JGL, Grattan-Smith P, Jankelowitz SK, Fung VSC, Clouston PD, Hayes MW. Athetosis II: The syndrome of mild athetoid cerebral palsy. Movement Disorders. 2002;17(6):1281-7.
12. Marks P, Anderson J, Vincent R. Choreo-athetosis with severe thyrotoxicosis. Postgrad Med J. 1979;55(649):830-1.
13. Mann TP. Transient choreo-athetosis following hypernatremia. Dev Med Child Neurol. 1969;11(5):637-40.
14. McLellan DL, Swash M. Choreo-athetosis and Encephalopathy Induced by Phenytoin. BMJ. 1974;2(5912):204-5.
15. Gordon N. Cerebral folate deficiency. Dev Med Child Neurol. 2009;51(3):180-2.
16. Mostile G, Barone R, Nicoletti A, Rizzo R, Martinelli D, Sturiale L, et al. Hyperkinetic movement disorders in congenital disorders of glycosylation. Eur J Neurol. 2019;26(9):1226-34.

17. Brandt NJ, Brandt S, Christensen E, Gregersen N, Rasmussen K. Glutaric aciduria in progressive choreo-athetosis. Clin Genet. 2008;13(1):77-80.
18. Duan BC, Weng WC, Lin KL, D, Wong LC, Li ST, Hsu MH, et al. Variations of movement disorders in anti-N-methyl-D-aspartate receptor encephalitis. Medicine (Baltimore). 2016;95(37):e4365.
19. Borroni B, Cotelli MS, Marchina E, Filosto M, Premi E, Padovani A. Choreo-athetosis in LRRK2 R1441C mutation: Expanding the clinical phenotype. Clin Neurol Neurosurg. 2013;115(10):2217-8.
20. Mrcp JJ, Joubert PH, van der Spuy M, van Graan E. Acute organophosphate poisoning presenting with choreo-athetosis. J Toxicol Clin Toxicol. 1984;22(2):187-91.
21. Vijiaratnam N, Bhatia KP, Lang AE, Raskind WH, Espay AJ. ADCY5-related Dyskinesia: Improving Clinical Detection of an Evolving Disorder. Mov Disord Clin Pract. 2019;6(7):512-20.
22. Méneret A, Mignot C, An I, Habert MO, Jacquette A, Vidailhet M, et al. Generalized dystonia, athetosis, and parkinsonism associated with FOXG1 mutation. Mov Disord. 2012;27(1):160-1.
23. Frucht S. Dystonia, athetosis, and epilepsia partialis continua in a patient with late-onset Rasmussen's encephalitis. Mov Disord. 2002;17(3):609-12.
24. Bhidayasiri R, Tarsy D. Pseudoathetosis. In: Bhidayasiri R, Tarsy D (Eds). Movement Disorders: A Video Atlas (Current Clinical Neurology). Totowa, NJ: Humana Press; 2012. pp. 178-80.
25. Hawley JS, Weiner WJ. Hemiballismus: current concepts and review. Parkinsonism Relat Disord. 2012;18(2):125-9.
26. Chua CB, Sun CK, Hsu CW, Tai YC, Liang CY, Tsai IT. "Diabetic striatopathy": clinical presentations, controversy, pathogenesis, treatments, and outcomes. Sci Rep. 2020;10(1):1594.
27. Dimal NPM, Santos NJC, Reyes NGD, Astejada MN, Jamora RDG. Hemichorea-Hemiballismus as a Presentation of Cerebritis from Intracranial Toxoplasmosis and Tuberculosis. Tremor Hyperkinet Mov (N Y). 2021;11:2.
28. Goldstein L, Djaldetti R, Benninger F. Anti-Yo, chorea and hemiballismus: A case report. J Clin Neurosci. 2017;42:113-4.
29. Alonso JV, del Pozo FJF, Simón JC, Valenzuela S, Perez Gomez F, Lopera E. Limb-Shaking TIA Presenting as Hemichorea–Hemiballismus: TIA Chameleons Diagnostic Challenge in the Emergency Department. J Stroke Cerebrovasc Dis 2015;24(11): e327-31.
30. Caparros-Lefebvre D, Deleume JF, Bradai N, Petit H. Biballism caused by bilateral infarction in the substantia nigra. Mov Disord. 1994;9(1):108-10.
31. Boughammoura-Bouatay A, Chebel S, Younes-Mhenni S, Frih-Ayed M. Biballism due to non-ketotic hyperglycaemia. Diabetes Metab. 2008;34(6):617-9.
32. Grütz K, Klein C. Dystonia updates: definition, nomenclature, clinical classification, and etiology. J Neural Transm (Vienna). 2021;128(4):395-404.
33. Batla A. Dystonia: A review. Neurol India. 2018;66(7):S48-S58.
34. Albanese A, Bhatia K, Bressman SB, Delong MR, Fahn S, Fung VS, et al. Phenomenology and classification of dystonia: A consensus update. Mov Disord. 2013;28(7):863-73.
35. Kumar N, Prashant L, Goyal V. Wilson's Disease update: An Indian perspective. Ann Indian Acad Neurol. 2021;24(5):652-63.
36. Nagral A, Sarma MS, Matthai J, Kukkle PL, Devarbhavi H, Sinha S, et al. Wilson's Disease: Clinical Practice Guidelines of the Indian National Association for Study of the Liver, the Indian Society of Pediatric Gastroenterology, Hepatology and Nutrition, and the Movement Disorders Society of India. J Clin Exp Hepatol. 2019;9(1):74-98.
37. Paprocka J, Machnikowska-Sokołowska M, Gruszczyńska K, Emich-Widera E. Neuroimaging of Basal Ganglia in Neurometabolic Diseases in Children. Brain Sci. 2020;10(11):849.
38. Berlot R, Bhatia KP, Kojović M. Pseudodystonia: A new perspective on an old phenomenon. Parkinsonism Relat Disord. 2019;62:44-50.

40
CHAPTER

Approach to Gait Disorders

Koustubh Bavdhankar, Shruti Agrawal, Neeraj Jain, Pankaj A Agarwal

INTRODUCTION

Animals have evolved from quadrupedalism to bipedalism and gained free use of hands while standing upright. The ability to stand upright is further evolved into complex tasks like walking and running.

Every person has a distinct style of walking. The manner of walking is called gait. The cerebral cortex integrates inputs from sensory systems like proprioceptive, visual, and vestibular and additionally receives inputs from the basal ganglia, cerebellum, and brainstem, which enables a person to walk efficiently. Normal gait requires coordination of the nervous system at all levels and requires a sound musculoskeletal and cardiovascular system. Gait is also influenced by age, gender, mood, and personality. Weakness due to stroke, cerebellar ataxia, sensory ataxia, parkinsonism, subcortical vascular encephalopathy, and executive dysfunction secondary to dementia are some of the most common neurological causes of gait disorders, while knee and hip osteoarthritis are the most common causes of gait dysfunction.[1] Many congenital and psychomotor conditions in the perinatal period may manifest as delayed onset of gait disorder. Gait disorders may lead to falls, leading to injuries and can cause great disability and distress due to hampered personal independence in the affected individuals.[2] Analyzing gait is a complex but high-yielding part of the neurological examination as it gives an insight into the localization of the illness across the neurological axis. Many gait disorders are treatable to an extent, for instance, dopaminergic therapy and gait training in Parkinson's disease and cerebrospinal fluid (CSF) shunt in normal pressure hydrocephalus (NPH). The use of assistive devices and physiotherapy may potentially improve the quality of life of the affected individuals.

ANATOMY OF GAIT

Studies in lower quadruped animals[3] show that brainstem and cerebellar locomotor regions stimulate the ventromedial spinal cord through descending reticulospinal pathways to modulate central and peripheral muscle tone leading to the adoption and maintenance of upright posture. Descending pontomedullary reticular projections activate a network of spinal interneurons leading to patterned and repetitive stepping movements. The propriospinal network connects motor neurons of the trunk and limbs leading to coordinated movements. Locomotion in humans is maintained by similar mechanisms. However, it is noted that the spinal cord alone cannot generate rhythmic stepping movements and brainstem and higher gait involvement is necessary for walking.[4] Innervation from frontal motor regions to pontomedullary reticular formation is required for accurate foot movements, as they modulate the postural responses required for stepping. All the sensory information regarding the external surroundings, body, and limb orientation concerning surroundings is integrated by the parietal cortex. The cerebellum adjusts the rate, rhythm, amplitude, and force of stepping. The anterior and flocculonodular lobes maintain truncal posture and balance via projections to the medial brainstem efferent system. Though the anatomy of gait is known to a great extent, the exact means by which it controls automatic and voluntary aspects of walking remain unknown.[5]

REQUIREMENTS FOR NORMAL GAIT

Equilibrium, which means ability to assume upright posture and to maintain balance, and locomotion, which includes initiation and maintenance of rhythmic stepping, are the two processes required for walking.

- *Righting reflexes*: To make a stance to initiate a walk, humans must assume a vertical position from sitting or lying down position, which is achieved by righting reflex. These reflexes are triggered by any one of the vestibular, visual, tactile, and proprioceptive stimuli.[6] Loss of righting reactions causes the inability to rise.
- *Supporting reactions*: Maintenance of upright posture by contraction of antigravity muscles is achieved

with supportive reactions.[6] The vertical posture is constantly threatened by inherent body sways, voluntary movements of the body, or external perturbations. The human body provides resistance to sway by stabilizing joints which are passively maintained by the elasticity of ligaments, tendons, and muscles to some extent, but active muscle contractions which are maintained by integration of visual, vestibular, and proprioceptive inputs and experience and foreknowledge play a major role in the maintenance of balance.[7] Loss of supportive reactions causes the inability to stand.

- *Anticipatory postural reflexes*: Feed-forward reflexes which are anticipatory reflexes before limb movements and feedback reflexes which are postural adjustments during body movements.
- *Reactive postural responses*: Maintenance of balance is achieved by reactive postural responses when the center of gravity shifts beyond a certain point in a standing patient.
- *Rescue reactions*: They are activated when anticipatory postural reflexes and reactive postural responses are failed. Nature of these reactions is dictated by the circumstances in which they are called upon.
- *Protective reactions*: If the subject is unable to prevent disequilibrium and falls, protective reactions come into action to break the fall like outstretching the arm to protect the torso from injury.

Disturbance in anticipatory postural reactions, reactive postural responses, rescue reactions, and postural reactions causes an inability to maintain an upright posture.

When equilibrium is maintained, locomotion can begin. It can be divided into gait initiation and stepping. For gait initiation center of gravity first shifts laterally and then forward which is achieved by redistribution of contraction in posturally active muscles. It is then followed by the gait cycle.[8]

Gait cycle: Gait is divided into eight phases denoting changes in one leg from initial contact to the ground to the time it contacts the ground again while walking. If movements of the right foot are taken into account, as seen in **Figure 1**.

Stance phase:

- *Initial contact (heel strike)*—occurs when the heel of the right foot contacts the ground.
- *Loading response (initial double limb support)*—occurs after initial contact of the right foot to the ground until the left foot is taken off the ground. During the loading response, bodyweight is transferred onto the supporting limb (i.e., from left leg to right leg)
- *Mid-stance (single limb support)*—from the elevation of the left leg until both ankles are aligned in the coronal plane.
- *Terminal stance (single limb support)*—begins when the heel of the right leg rises from the ground and continues until the heel of the left leg touches the ground.
- *Preswing (second double limb support)*—from initial contact of the left heel to ground to just before the elevation of the right leg off ground.

Swing phase:

- *Initial swing (toe-off)*—from elevation of right leg to point of maximal knee flexion
- *Mid-swing (foot clearance)*—following right knee flexion to the point where the tibia is vertical
- *Terminal swing (tibia vertical)*—from the point where the tibia is vertical to just before initial contact (heel strike of right leg)[1,9,10]

Table 1 contains a glossary of terms used in the gait cycle.

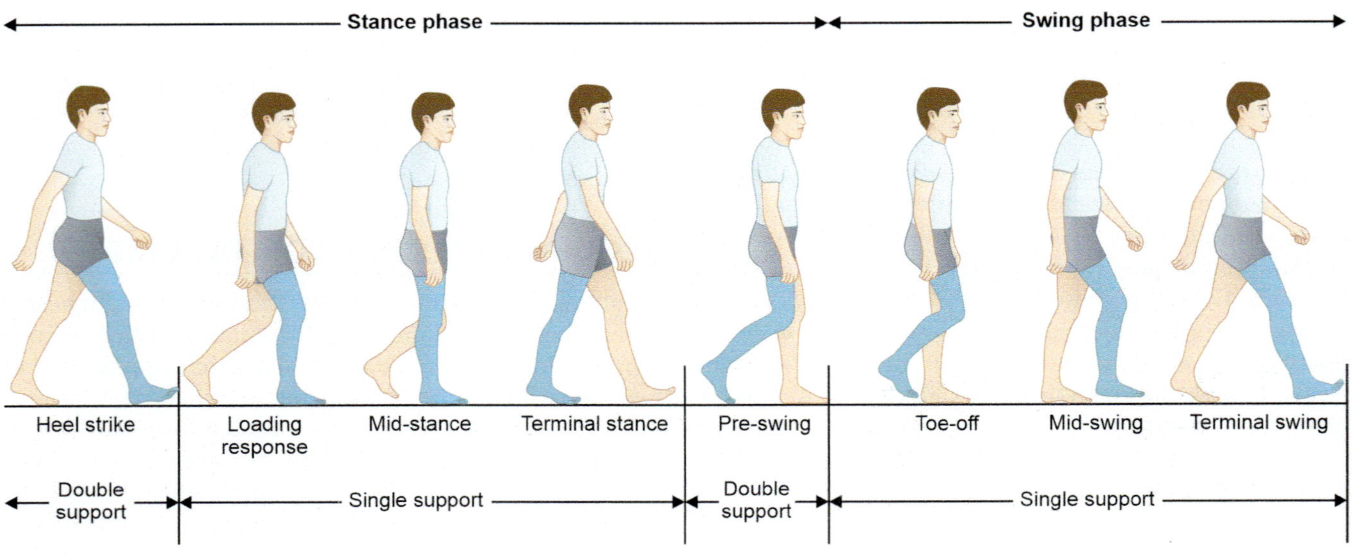

FIG. 1: Gait cycle.

Source: Modified from Pirker W, et al (2017).[1]

TABLE 1: Commonly used terms in the "gait cycle."

Term	Meaning
Cadence	Number of steps in unit time
Step length	Distance covered during the swing phase of a given step
Stride length	Distance covered during one gait cycle
Step width	Distance between two feet at a perpendicular axis to the walking direction of a given step
Step height	Maximum distance between forefoot and ground during swing phase
Symmetry	The ratio between step length of 2 legs
Coordination	Timing of leg activation with respect to other leg in the gait cycle

CLINICAL APPROACH TO GAIT DISORDERS

As with any other neurological case, the approach to gait disorders should be done in a structured manner. A detailed history followed by a detailed neurological examination including a gait examination is required for anatomical localization and correct diagnosis. Also, an examination of the musculoskeletal system and general physical examination is required to rule out all non-neurological causes of impaired gait.

History

- *Onset and progression of complaints*—often provide insight into the etiology of the disease. A hyperacute history static or improving course of difficulty while walking might provide a clue to a vascular etiology such as acute ischemic or hemorrhagic stroke. However, a very chronic history might lead us to a degenerative etiology. A stepwise manner of progression may indicate vascular parkinsonism.

  An episodic history without periodicity of gait disturbance may indicate paroxysmal dyskinesias. But pseudoperiodicity can also be noted with freezing of gait (FOG) or claudication. Also, functional gait disorders may have an acute onset and fluctuating course.

  A long and progressive history of asymmetric parkinsonism with a lack of red flags and a good response to levodopa therapy may suggest idiopathic Parkinson's disease (IPD). However, an insidious onset of gait complaints with early falls or autonomic involvement in a parkinsonian patient might point toward Parkinson plus syndromes such as progressive supranuclear palsy (PSP) and multisystem atrophy, respectively.
- *Weakness*: Many patients attribute all kinds of gait complaints to weakness. However, an examination does not show any weakness. Here, a detailed history helps in identifying the cause of gait complaints.

  A patient presenting with dragging of the foot along the ground with tripping and falls may have hemiplegia with spastic equinovarus deformity or may have foot drop causing weakness of dorsiflexion with a high stepping gait. Whereas weakness of ankle plantarflexion causes shallow stepped gait. Weakness of foot evertors causes difficulty while walking on uneven surfaces and repeated twisting of the ankle. Weakness of knee extension presents as recurrent buckling of the knee while standing or walking downstairs. Weakness of knee and hip flexion causes difficulty lifting leg while putting it onto next step while climbing upstairs. Difficulty while getting up from the chair and sitting position indicates weakness of extensors at proximal and semidistal joints. Truncal weakness may present as difficulty while sitting up from lying down position and turning in bed. Also, patients may complain of fatigue while walking in any kind of weakness, which indicates extra effort required in presence of weakness.[5,9,10]
- *Stiffness*: Patient complains of tightness or stiffness of legs in spasticity, rigidity, or dystonia. Patients having spastic paraparesis or hemiparesis drag their feet while walking and they trip and fall even due to the smallest surface irregularities. While taking history for tone, it is important to note circumstances in which stiffness is noted by the patient.[9,11] Patients having dystonia usually present with complaints of leg stiffness only while walking and might have a normal tone on neurological examination. Primary dystonia of the foot may present with stiffness in the legs and signs of the striatal toe or toe walking may be noticed only on walking or running during the later course of the disease. In adults, patients with parkinsonism may have a similar presentation.[5]
- *Slowness*: Slowness while walking may be a deceiving symptom. It can be seen in normal elderly people. However, slowness of gait concerning age-matched controls is an early indicator of dementia in elderly patients.[12,13] It is present in Parkinson's disease due to bradykinesia and in advanced stages, it may have shuffling and festinating gait as the patient takes multiple short steps during walking. The patient may present with an inability to initiate gait or difficulty while navigating obstacles as feet get glued to the floor, suggestive of FOG. Ataxic patients walk slowly to avoid falls due to imbalance. Also, leg stiffness, weakness, or musculoskeletal causes such as pain and deformity may lead to slowness.[11]
- *Imbalance*: It is predominantly seen in cerebellar, sensory, vestibular ataxias, or neurodegenerative disorders. Unsteadiness, staggering, swaying to both sides, and inability to walk in a straight line are the complaints seen in patients with cerebellar ataxia. They tend to have severe imbalance while changing pace or direction of walking suddenly or while taking sudden turns and while walking on uneven surfaces. Patients with sensory ataxia report imbalance, which is exaggerated while walking in dark, or after the closure of their eyes while taking bath or washing their face as they are not able to visually compensate in absence of joint position sense. They are

not able to feel the texture of the ground and report the sensation of walking on cotton wool. Deficits of chronic vestibulopathy are unmasked in presence of visual or proprioceptive deficits. In chronic vestibulopathies, the patient complains of imbalance while walking in places with many moving objects like crowded places. However, acute vestibulopathy is associated with vertigo, severe imbalance, and sometimes vomiting. Acute problems in maintaining balance are also seen in lesions of vascular etiology involving the cerebellum, basal ganglia, and thalamus. NPH may present with a wide-based gait associated with difficulty performing the dual task, turning backward or walking backward.[1,5,14]

- *Falls*: It can be classified as collapsing, tripping, or freezing.
  - *Collapsing*—when muscle tone is lost, and the patient falls onto himself.

    It can be seen with akinetic seizures, negative myoclonus, or syncope.
  - *Toppling*: When muscle tone is maintained during the fall. Falls are due to lost postural reflexes. The patient falls like a wooden log.
    - In PSP, the patient usually falls backward while standing still and while getting up from a chair.
    - In IPD, patients have falls during the late course of the disease, which can be seen while turning suddenly.
  - *Tripping*: When feet do not clear the ground, the patient falls forward injuring knees or on outstretched hands.

    It can be seen with foot drop, spasticity associated with pyramidal disorders, or due to rigidity secondary to parkinsonism.

    It can also be seen due to inattention, cognitive impairment, or poor vision.
  - *Other causes of falls*:
    - In cerebellar ataxias, falls are secondary to imbalance and unsteadiness of movements—the patient may fall to sides, front, or back.
    - In the weakness of semidistal and proximal muscles, falls may be due to buckling or sudden giveaway of lower limb tone.
    - Due to FOG, feet do not move in concordance with the patient's body and remain glued to the ground causing the patient to fall forward.
    - Imbalance and falls while performing dual tasks are seen in cortical and subcortical dysfunction.
    - *Bizarre falls*: Falls secondary to bizarre postures and gait that are inconsistent in the pattern. They are commonly seen in functional movement disorders. Patients typically do not get injured.[15-17]
- *Other associated symptoms*:
  - *Sensory complaints*: A pattern of sensory complaints provides a clue for anatomical localization.
    - Paresthesia and negative sensory complaints in distal lower limbs indicate polyneuropathy.
    - Radicular pain and band-like sensation may be present in compressive myelopathy.
    - Radiating pain is present in radiculopathy.
    - Intermittent throbbing pain is seen in vascular and neurogenic claudication.
    - Pain aggravated by joint movement is seen in musculoskeletal diseases.
  - *Urinary complaints*: Urinary urgency, frequency, urge incontinence, and feeling of incomplete evacuation with spasticity in lower limbs are seen in lesions of the spinal cord.

    Urinating and defecating at inappropriate places may be seen in parasagittal frontal lobe lesions. Acute onset of bladder complaints may be seen with anterior cerebral artery territory infarcts or may have a subacute or chronic course in hydrocephalus or tumors.
  - *Cognitive impairment*: It is associated with a slow gait. When gait disturbance is associated with urinary complaints and cognitive dysfunction, NPH should be considered.

    When gait disturbances are associated with visual hallucinations, parkinsonism, and fluctuations of symptoms, dementia with Lewy bodies should be thought of.[1,5,18]
- *Medical history*:
  - Prior or current respiratory, cardiac, or psychiatric illness
  - Psychoactive medications
  - Medication history
  - Intoxication
  - Family history of neurological or psychiatric illness

Examination of Posture and Gait

- *Getting up from a sitting position*: The patient should be examined while getting up from a sitting position from a chair without arms. Patients with proximal weakness tend to lean forward while getting up from a sitting position. Patients with frontal lobe and higher-level gait disorders (HLGDs) use faulty strategies while getting up. They might not align their feet with their body and tend to lean back while getting up and may sustain a fall while getting up from a sitting position. This is particularly seen in PSP where the person tries to get up suddenly from the chair while leaning backward and sustains a fall while doing so. It is described as a rocket sign. In the case of ataxia, patient may sway and take multiple attempts to get up.[5,8]
- *Standing*:
  - *Stance base*: It indicates the distance between two feet. It is to be observed while standing from a sitting position, standing, as well as while walking. The stance base is typically widened in sensory as well as cerebellar ataxia but can be seen in patients with HLGDs. Increased distance between two feet helps to

maintain better balance as it allows a wider room for the displacement of the center of gravity. Short-based gait is seen in parkinsonism.

- *Trunk posture*: In normal persons, it is upright in a standing position.
  - *IPD*: Stooped posture with forward flexion of the trunk
  - Extended posture of the neck is seen in PSP.
  - *Forward flexion of the neck*—is seen in disorders with neck extensor weakness like motor neuron disease (MND), myasthenia gravis, and polymyositis.
  - Truncal dystonia in the form of antecollis as well as laterocollis is seen in multiple system atrophy (MSA), PD and anti-IgLON5 ab disease.
  - Body may tilt toward one side—vascular lesions of thalamus, lateral medullary syndrome, and vestibulopathies.
  - Exaggerated lumbar lordosis—proximal myopathies and stiff person syndrome
  - Lastly, local causes such as scoliosis, lumbar spondylosis, hip pain, and limb length discrepancy may lead to abnormal trunk posture.
- *Sways*: Abnormal sways are seen in chorea and ataxia.
- *Romberg test*: Abnormal in sensory ataxia
- *Pull test*: While performing the test, the patient is explained that a tug of pull will be given from his back and he should try to maintain his balance and avoid falling. Then the patient should be made to stand upright and not allowed to lean forward. Then the patient is pulled backward by holding his shoulders briskly and forcefully. The examiner should stand against a wall to be able to catch the patient in case he falls but the patient should be allowed to have enough room for recovery and at least three steps backward should be observed. If the patient recovers within two steps, the test is considered normal. But if the patient takes more than two steps to recover or falls irrespective of the number of steps, it is considered to be a positive test and indicates poor postural responses.[19,20]

- *Walking*:[5,11]
  - *Initiation*: Gait initiation difficulty may range from very mild signs in the form of few short shuffling steps during initiation of gait to FOG during which the patient feels that his feet are stuck to the ground, however, his body continues to move forward leading to the displacement of the center of gravity backward, and the patient falls forward. Gait initiation difficulty is usually associated with HLGDs.
  - Speed of gait may vary with many factors. As young individuals walk at a greater pace whereas older individuals tend to walk at a slower pace. However, excessively slow gait in elderly individuals is an early indicator of the development of dementia. Pathological slow gait is seen in ataxia, spasticity, weakness, or local pain; however, pattern of gait differs with each cause.
  - *Stance base*: Wide-based stance is seen in patients with imbalance which is predominantly seen in ataxia patients. And the narrow base is observed in hypokinetic disorders.
  - *Step length*: A shorter step length is seen with hypokinetic disorders. It also can be seen in patients with weakness, or imbalance due to ataxia or pain. A long-step length is observed in patients with hyperkinesia, dyskinesia, and imbalance due to vestibular causes.

    Short-step length on one side is observed in asymmetric hypokinesia or weakness seen in IPD and hemiparesis, respectively. Variability in step length can be seen in cortical gait disorders.
  - *Cadence*: It can be defined as the number of steps in unit time. It increases in patients with parkinsonism and imbalance due to vestibular causes. However, it is reduced in gait disorders due to weakness, spasticity, and ataxia.
  - *Trajectory or path of step*: A low trajectory of steps is seen in parkinsonism, and a high-steppage gait is seen in distal weakness while walking. A circumduction gait is seen in patients with unilateral spastic weakness in which leg extension and plantar flexion are seen. However, when present in both legs, it is called a scissoring gait. As spasticity is velocity dependent, spastic gait aggravates during running. Equine gait is another type of stiff gait in which the patient uses hip flexion to walk as the limb has extensor posturing with plantar flexion.

    When the gait is affected by involuntary movements, it is called dyskinetic gait.

    A silly walk is seen in levodopa-induced parkinsonism. Cock-walk is seen in manganese toxicity or pantothenate kinase-associated neurodegeneration which leads to dystonia due to dysfunction of globus pallidus. During cock-walk, patient stands in an erect position with flexed elbows and walks on toes with feet lifted high in the air. In generalized dystonia, a dromedary gait can be seen. Lordosis due to dystonia causes protrusion of the buttocks with high steppage.

    A bouncing gait is seen in negative and positive myoclonus.
  - *Associated truncal and arm movements*: Proximal weakness leads to exaggerated lateral truncal sways and hip elevation. When quadriceps muscles are weak, a typical pattern is observed in which a step on a weak leg leads to hyperextension of the knee and a sudden movement of the trunk is seen. Arm swing associated with walking is lost in parkinsonism. Also, chorea and dystonia seen in IPD, levodopa-induced dyskinesias, and tardive syndromes get exaggerated while walking and should not be missed.

- *Turning while walking*: Turning requires more precise balance than while walking. Gait abnormalities may first be noticed in patients while turning. Slow turns are noted in patients with parkinsonism and cerebrovascular disease. A wide base of gait while turning is seen during ataxia.
- *Challenging tasks*:
  - *Dual tasks*: Patients with cortical gait disorders show FOG or increased instability when asked to perform a cognitive task such as counting numbers backward or calculating while walking.
  - *Navigating narrow passages*: Patients with HLGDs show difficulty while navigating narrow passages.

- *General examination*: A thorough neurological examination should be done to note the involvement of various neurological axes such as change in tone, weakness, sensory deficits, ataxia, or abnormal higher mental function. Also, the spinal column should be observed in standing position for any deformities and spinal tenderness should be ruled out which might give rise to abnormal posture. The presence of a tuft of hair along the spinal cord is an indicator of spina bifida and should not be missed. Also, the range of movements at all the joints of lower limbs should be examined to rule out contractures. Limb discrepancy, if any, should be noted.

  Finally, an examination of the cardiovascular and respiratory systems is important as these play an important role in sustaining prolonged physical activity required to maintain gait.
- *Gait patterns*: Gait disorders can be classified based on phenomenology or hierarchical classification **(Flowchart 1)**.

Hierarchical classification: Hughlings Jackson divided the nervous system into three levels.[21] The anterior horn cell was considered "lower level"; the basal ganglia and motor cortex as "middle level"; and the prefrontal cortex as "higher level." David Marsden, Philip Thompson, and John Nutt adopted this simple classification for gait disorders.[8,22] As gait is a sensory motor function, the sensory system was also included in the system.

The lower-level motor system produced the force for locomotion and balance, while the lower-level sensory system provided the sensory information for the correct orientation of the person with the surface he/she is walking on. The middle level adjusted the force required for a bipedal stance, balance, and locomotion. The higher-level function coordinates between sensory information received and organize motor programs desired for action to be carried out.[22]

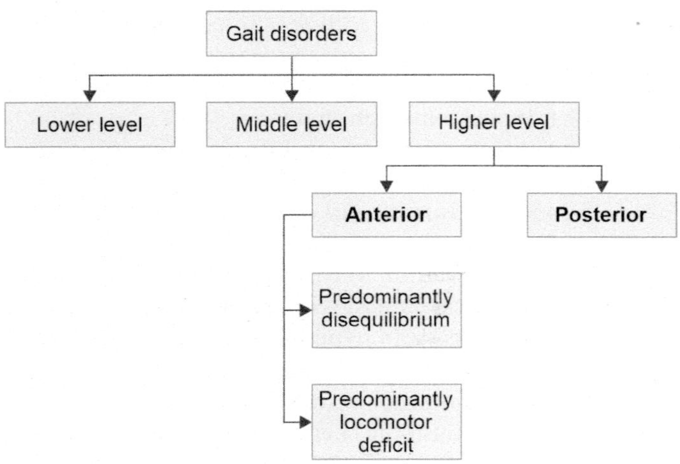

FLOWCHART 1: Classification of gait disorders.

Lower-level gait disorders: Lower-level gait disorders are due to sensory loss including loss of joint position, touch sensation, visual or vestibular sensation, or due to motor weakness. **Table 2** shows the history and examination findings of "lower-level" gait disorders.[11]

Middle-level gait disorders: They arise from—(1) pyramidal tracts causing spasticity, (2) parkinsonism causing hypokinetic gait, (3) affection of cerebellum and its connections causing ataxic gait, and (4) hyperkinetic movement disorders. **Table 3** shows history and examination findings of "lower-level" gait disorders.[5,19]

An adult patient presenting as hemidystonia or isolated leg dystonia points toward a structural cause. It is usually associated with early falls due to the loss of postural reflexes.[5]

Mixed movement disorders: Athetoid cerebral palsy presents in childhood with involvement of multiple neuraxis including pyramidal system, cerebellar trunk, and limb ataxia and dystonia. It is a close differential of primary torsion dystonia, having similar age of onset. Patients with athetoid cerebral palsy have a history suggestive of perinatal hypoxic injury such as perinatal hypotonia, poor cry, and delayed developmental milestones. Poor balance at early age, spasticity, and ataxia favor athetoid CP.

Orthostatic tremor: It has a typical 16-Hz frequency and affects leg and trunk muscles while standing, and causes a severe subjective sense of imbalance, which is relieved by sitting down or walking. So, patients try to shuffle while standing at one place. However, they rarely fall. The tremors are rarely seen but better palpated. Local ultrasonography (USG) and surface electromyography (EMG) assist with the diagnosis.[23]

Action myoclonus: It usually presents in posthypoxia patients called the Lance–Adams syndrome. Myoclonus is induced by action and associated with "negative" myoclonus—causing a "bouncing" gait due to asterixis of thigh muscles before falling. Patients have a severe disability due to multiple falls and can remain in wheelchair.[5]

Higher-level gait disorders: The HLGD consists of multiple patterns of gait disorders, without disproportionately little neurological signs—such as sensory deficits and loss of joint and position and vibration sense, weakness, hypertonia,

TABLE 2: History and examination findings of "lower-level" gait disorders.

	Myopathic	Neuropathic motor	Quadriceps gait	Sensory ataxia	Vestibular
History and examination	Slowly progressive, usually proximal, symmetrical, pure motor weakness	Acute or chronic onset, distal, weakness of ankle dorsiflexion causing foot drop	Recurrent buckling of the knee while walking (predominantly downstairs) or standing	High-steppage gait with slapping sound, slow steps under visual guidance, worsening on uneven surfaces	*Acute onset*: Nystagmus, vertigo, nausea, sway to one side aggravated by eye closure, the patient tries to lie still
Mechanism	Pelvic instability secondary to weakness, exaggerated pelvic rotation	Common peroneal, sciatic nerve palsy, L5 radiculopathy	Femoral neuropathy causes weakness of knee extension—associated with diabetes mellitus, PMA, inclusion body myositis	Large proprioceptive nerves, posterior root, dorsal root ganglion or dorsal column affection—loss of proprioceptive signals from L/L	Disequilibrium due to vestibular dysfunction (Fukuda and star walking test positive)
Gait	Waddling gait, Trendelenburg sign	High-steppage gait/ drag to gait	Quadriceps gait	Ataxic gait	—
Getting up from sitting	Uses support, Gower sign	Difficulty due to ankle imbalance	Difficulty due to knee extension	Normal	Severe imbalance
Stance base	Narrow	Narrow	Narrow	Wide	Normal/wide
Trunk posture	Exaggerated lumbar lordosis due to weakness of hip extensors	Normal	Normal	Stooped	Normal, leaning, tilting to the side of the lesion (cerebellum and lateral medullary syndrome)
Sway while standing	Absent	Absent	Absent	Present	+ (to the side of the lesion, exaggerate by eye closure)
Romberg	Absent	Negative	Negative	Positive	Negative
Pull test	Negative	Negative	Negative	Negative	Negative
Gait initiation	Normal	Normal	Normal	Normal	Normal
Speed	Normal/slowed	Normal/slowed	Normal/slowed	Reduced	Increased
Stance base	Narrow	Narrow	Narrow	Wide	Normal/increased
Step length, step height	Normal/reduced	Decreased/increased	Decreased/decreased	Normal/increased	Normal/increased
Cadence	Normal/reduced	Normal/reduced	Normal/reduced	Reduced	Increased
Arm movements	Normal/reduced	Normal	Normal	Normal	Normal
Turning	Normal	Normal	Normal	Minimal effect	This may increase with neck movements
Dual tasks	No worsening	No worsening	No worsening	No worsening	No worsening

(PMA: progressive muscular atrophy)

ataxia, and parkinsonism.[22] Also sometimes HLGD may begin as a middle-level disorder and progress to become higher-level. An example of such progression is Parkinson's disease in which initial slowing of gait, which is responsive to L-Dopa, is considered a middle-level gait disorder; however, postural instability and freezing, which are unresponsive to L-Dopa, are HLGD.[5]

Higher-level gait disorder can be classified into two categories: anterior (frontal) and posterior (parieto-temporo-occipital), which are analogous to the simple classification of aphasias as anterior Broca's and posterior Wernicke's aphasia. Anterior HLGD is the more common of the two. The frontal/anterior pattern is characterized by FOG, small steps, and postural instability.[22] Elbe postulated that dysfunction in corticobasal ganglia loops causes HLGD. He described four prominent features of the same. First, the performance of the patient differed from time to time based upon mood of the patient, environment, and other variables, in contrast to lower- and middle-level disorders in which performance remained constant. Second, FOG or start and turn hesitation was common. Third, postural synergies were inappropriate or bizarre, and rescue reactions were inappropriate. Fourth, rescue reactions were inappropriate or not present. And the fifth feature, which was not written but implied, was

TABLE 3: History and examination findings of "middle-level" gait disorders.

	Spastic gait					
	Unilateral	**Bilateral**	**Cerebellar ataxia**	**Hypokinetic**	**Choreic**	**Dystonic**
History and examination	Weakness and stiffness in U/L and L/L of one side (spastic hemiparesis)	Stiffness and weakness in B/L lower limbs (spastic paraparesis) may be seen in spastic cerebral palsy, hereditary spastic paraplegia, and myelopathies	• Loss of truncal balance, increased body sway, and sway while walking—in central cerebellar lesions • In hemispheric lesions—walks like a drunken person	The slowness of activity of daily living, stooped posture, and short shuffling steps—Response to levodopa is a marker of middle-level gait disorder	Abnormal, involuntary, semi-purposive movements with flowing quality with motor persistence	Sustained or intermittent muscle contractions causing abnormal repetitive movements or postures
Mechanism	Lateral flexion of the trunk toward the unaffected side and hyperextension of the hip on the same side leads to the swinging of the paralyzed leg, dragging toe of the weak leg	Circumduction of both legs leading to scissoring	• Due to pathology of the anterior lobe and vermis—wide-based stance—legs extended, and hips slightly flexed to avoid truncal sways • In hemispheric lesions, steps with irregular timing, length, and direction	With stooped posture, patients try to catch their center of gravity and to avoid disequilibrium, they take multiple small steps	Random movements of chorea increase during walking—dance-like appearance with excess legs and arm movements	• Most difficult to analyze gait patterns • Plantar flexion and inversion are the most common patterns
Gait	Circumduction gait	Scissors gait	Lurching/staggering quality of gait	Parkinsonian gait	Stuttering, lurching, or stumbling gait	Dystonic gait
Getting up from sitting	Difficulty due to weakness on one side	Difficulty due to weakness in both legs	Impaired due to truncal and gait ataxia	Difficulty due to postural instability	Clumsiness due to chorea	Variable, depending on the site of leg dystonia
Stance base	Slightly wide	Narrow	Wide	Narrow	Wide-based, variable	Variable
Trunk posture	The body is supported on an unaffected leg	Normal or hyperextension may be present	Sway/veering +	Stooped flexion at knees, trunk, shoulders, and neck	–	Action-induced dystonia may be present while walking
Sway while standing	Absent	Absent	3-Hz anteroposterior rhythmic swaying of trunk and neck is seen in anterior cerebellar lobar atrophy (titubation)—multidirectional sway with severe disequilibrium with relatively preserved limb movements is seen in flocculonodular lobar pathology	Absent	Present due to chorea (dance-like quality)	May present in later stages
Romberg	Negative	Negative	Negative	Negative	Negative	Negative
Pull test	Impaired (postural instability)	Impaired	Negative	Positive	Negative	Variable
Gait initiation	Normal	Normal	Normal	Start hesitation—rapid short shuffling steps	Normal	Normal

Continued

Continued

	Spastic gait					
	Unilateral	**Bilateral**	**Cerebellar ataxia**	**Hypokinetic**	**Choreic**	**Dystonic**
Speed	Slow	Slow	Normal/ slow; variable (hemispheric lesions)	Reduced	Slow	Slow
Stance base	Wide	Narrow	Wide; variable (hemispheric lesions)	Narrow	Wide and variable	Variable
Step length/ height	Asymmetric Reduced on the normal side	Decreased/ decreased	Normal/increased; variable (hemispheric lesions)	Reduced	Variable length and timing	Variable
Cadence	Reduced	Reduced	Reduced; variable (hemispheric lesions)	Decreased, increases if festination +	Normal/increased	Normal/ decreased
Trajectory of steps	Circumduction on affected side	Bilateral circumduction	Irregular; variable (hemispheric lesions)	Short shuffling steps	Variable	Variable
Arm movements	Reduced on affected side	Compensatory increase	Normal	Asymmetrically reduced	Increased	Dystonic movements, may be present in generalized dystonia
Turning	Difficulty due to spasticity	Difficulty due to spasticity	Veers away	Difficulties ++	Normal	Difficulties ++
Dual tasks	Normal/mild decompensation	Normal/mild decompensation	Normal	Decompensation +	Decompensation +	Decompensation +
Other findings	–	–	Midline cerebellar signs +, Falls—less prevalent	• Upper limb tremors + while walking, interruption in gait is present due to freezing • Poor response to L-Dopa in later stages marks higher-level gait disorder	• Equilibrium is maintained till late stages in HD but impaired causing multiple falls in Sydenham's and chorea gravidarum • Haloperidol reduces chorea but no gait improvement	• May mimic spastic paraparesis seen in dopa-responsive dystonia in childhood due to brisk reflexes—diurnal variation with sleep benefit • Striatal toe may be misinterpreted as a Babinski response

gait and balance dysfunction which could not be explained by lower- or middle-level neurological dysfunction.[24] The anterior or frontal HLGD includes gait disorders secondary to parkinsonian syndromes, NPH, subcortical vascular pathologies, and many other frontal lobar pathologies.

Frontal HLGD can further be classified into disequilibrium subtype and locomotor subtype.[25,26] Disequilibrium can be seen in patients with PSP and other frontal lesions. The locomotor subtype manifests as start and turn hesitation which is seen in various parkinsonian syndromes and when no pathological correlation is found, it is called as primary progressive FOG.[27] Although these subtypes initially affect predominantly their respective domains, with disease progression, a mixed clinical picture with the affection of equilibrium as well as locomotion is seen in advanced disease.

Posterior HLGD is characterized by abnormalities in the special domains leading to distortions of environment and body maps or sense of postural vertical is disturbed. "Pusher syndrome" is the characteristic example of this phenomenon, in which the patient pushes toward the lesioned side to try to correct the perceived deviation from the vertical.[28] It is seen in parietal and thalamic infarcts. Also, elderly patients with MRI suggestive of parietal and occipital white matter lesions have impaired motility due to affection of sensory function required for gait and balance.[29]

Along with neurological deficits, HLGD also include patients' *adaptations* to their deficits. A "cautious" gait is characterized by short steps, en bloc turns, or a slightly widened base which can be seen in a normal person while navigating a slippery surface. Cautious gait may, therefore, be a first clue to HLGD which was adapted by the patient to compensate for his or her deficits in equilibrium. An extreme form of this adaptation includes an "overly cautious" gait in which patients hold on to walls or hold a hand of a relative, and refuse to walk further. This fear of falling is often disproportionate to the deficit the patient has. "Reckless gait" is a maladaptive behavior to HLGD, in which the patient has a lack of insight and impulsivity, which leads to multiple falls as the subject is not aware of his neurological deficit.[22]

Psychogenic gait disorders: Patients present with acute onset complaints which show variability, inconsistency, incongruity with known organic disease gait patterns, a lack of economy of gait, transient fluctuations while walking and inappropriate slowness, an abnormal posture with postural adjustments with each step, the excessive body sways without any falls and injuries or weakness in both lower limbs which improve with distraction and have a sudden, rapid, and complete improvement.[30]

MANAGEMENT

The management of gait disorders should follow the clinical approach for the diagnosis of gait disorders. The first step is to *identify the disorder which leads to compensatory changes* in the gait. The second step involves *management of destabilization factors* such as stiffness or hyperkinesis which may be caused by spasticity, dystonia, or myoclonus respectively. The Third step involves *treatment of the primary etiology*, i.e., L-Dopa for parkinsonism, or CSF shunting for NPH, and the fourth and last step is *rehabilitation*. A detailed review of these management strategies is outside the scope of this article and can be obtained from other sources.

CONCLUSION

Gait disorders are a fascinating subject area that encompasses the vast breadth of various neurological diseases, arising as they do from a myriad of anatomical regions of the central and peripheral nervous system, not to mention the non-neurological causes, which are also very important to keep in mind. A thorough and systematic clinical approach to this vexatious clinical problem, as outlined above, will serve the astute clinician well in accurately diagnosing and managing disorders of gait.

REFERENCES

1. Pirker W, Katzenschlager R. Gait disorders in adults and the elderly: A clinical guide. Wien Klin Wochenschr. 2017;129(3-4):81-95.
2. Sudarsky L. Gait disorders: prevalence, morbidity, and etiology. Adv Neurol. 2001;87:111-7.
3. Takakusaki K. Neurophysiology of gait: from the spinal cord to the frontal lobe. Mov Disord. 2013;28(11):1483-91.
4. Bussel B, Roby-Brami A, Azouvi P, Biraben A, Yakovleff A, Held JP. Myoclonus in a patient with spinal cord transection: possible involvement of the spinal stepping generator. Brain. 1988;111:1235-45.
5. Jankovic J, Mazziotta JC, Pomeroy SL, Newman NJ. Bradley and Daroff's Neurology in Clinical Practice, volume 2, 8th edition. Philadelphia, PA: Elsevier Saunders; 2022. pp. 334-45.
6. Magnus R. Physiology of posture. Lancet. 1926;2:531-6, 585-8.
7. Davidoff RA. Skeletal muscle tone and the misunderstood stretch reflex. Neurology. 1992;42:951-63.
8. Nutt JG, Marsden CD, Thompson PD. Human walking and higher-level gait disorders, particularly in the elderly. Neurology. 1993;43(2):268-79.
9. Ružička E, Jankovic JJ. Disorders of gait. In: Jankovic JJ, Tolosa E (Eds). Parkinson's disease and movement disorders, 4th edition. Philadelphia: Lippincott, Williams and Wilkins; 2002. pp. 409-29.
10. Lim MR, Huang RC, Wu A, Girardi FP, Cammisa FP Jr. Evaluation of the elderly patient with an abnormal gait. J Am Acad Orthop Surg. 2007;15(2):107-17.
11. Snijders AH, van de Warrenburg BP, Giladi N, Bloem BR. Neurological gait disorders in elderly people: clinical approach and classification. Lancet Neurol. 2007;6:63-74.
12. Mielke MM, Roberts RO, Savica R, Cha R, Drubach DI, Christianson T, et al. Assessing the temporal relationship between cognition and gait: slow gait predicts cognitive decline in the Mayo Clinic Study of Aging. J Gerontol A Biol Sci Med Sci. 2013;68(8):929-37.
13. Verghese J, Annweiler C, Ayers E, Barzilai N, Beauchet O, Bennett DA, et al. Motoric cognitive risk syndrome: multicountry prevalence and dementia risk. Neurology. 2014;83(8):718-26.
14. Wuehr M, Schniepp R, Schlick C, Huth S, Pradhan C, Dieterich M, et al. Sensory loss and walking speed related factors for gait alterations in patients with peripheral neuropathy. Gait Posture. 2014;39(3):852-8.
15. Voermans NC, Snijders AH, Schoon Y, Bloem BR. Why old people fall (and how to stop them). Pract Neurol. 2007;7(3):158-71.
16. Boers I, Gerschlager W, Stalenhoef PA, Bloem BR. Falls in the elderly. II. Strategies for prevention. Wien Klin Wochenschr. 2001;113 (11-12):398-407.
17. Bloem BR, Boers I, Cramer M, Westendorp RG, Gerschlager W. Falls in the elderly. I. Identification of risk factors. Wien Klin Wochenschr. 2001;113(10):352-62.
18. Kuhtz-Buschbeck JP, Johnk K, Mader S, Stolze H, Mehdorn M. Analysis of gait in cervical myelopathy. Gait Posture. 1999;9(3):184-9.
19. Fasano A, Bloem BR. Gait disorders. Continuum (Minneap Minn). 2013;19(5 Movement Disorders):1344-82.
20. Hunt AL, Sethi KD. The pull test: a history. Mov Disord. 2006;21: 894-99.
21. Walshe FMR. Contributions of John Hughlings Jackson to neurology. Arch Neurol. 1961;5:119-131.
22. Nutt JG. Higher-level gait disorders: An open frontier. Mov Disord. 2013;28:1560-5.
23. Hassan A, Ahlskog JE, Matsumoto JY, Milber JM, Bower JH, Wilkinson JR. Orthostatic tremor: Clinical, electrophysiologic, and treatment findings in 184 patients. Neurology. 2016;86(5):458-64.
24. Elble RJ. Gait and dementia: moving beyond the notion of gait apraxia. J Neural Transm. 2007;114:1253-8.
25. Baezner H, Hennerici M. From trepidant abasia to motor network failure—gait disorders as a consequence of subcortical vascular

encephalopathy (SVE): review of historical and contemporary concepts. J Neurol Sci. 2005;229-230:81-8.
26. Liston R, Mickelborough J, Bene J, Tallis R. A new classification of higher level gait disorders in patients with cerebral multi-infarct states. Age Ageing. 2003;32:252-8.
27. Factor SA, Jennings DL, Molho ES, Marek KL. The natural history of the syndrome of primary progressive freezing gait. Arch Neurol. 2002;59:1778-83.
28. Karnath HO. Pusher syndrome—a frequent but little-known disturbance of body orientation perception. J Neurol. 2007;254:415-24.
29. Benson RR, Guttmann CR, Wei X, Warfield SK, Hall C, Schmidt JA, et al. Older people with impaired mobility have specific loci of periventricular abnormality on MRI. Neurology. 2002;58:48-55.
30. Sokol LL, Espay AJ. Clinical signs in functional (psychogenic) gait disorders: a brief survey. J Clin Mov Disord. 2016;3:3.

41

CHAPTER

Approach to Hemiplegia and Monoplegia

Jain RS, Jitesh Agrawal

INTRODUCTION

Hemiplegia and monoplegia are common in clinical practice and hence, it is important to develop a sound clinical approach to this presentation. Hemiplegia and monoplegia are motor system manifestations having good anatomical localization.

DEFINITIONS

The word "plegia" is derived from a Greek word meaning "to strike," and refers to severe or complete loss of motor function and word "paresis" is used for partial loss.[1] Hemiplegia involves the arm, leg, and sometimes face on one side of the body mostly attributable to a lesion of the contralateral corticospinal system. Monoplegia refers to paralysis of all the muscles of one leg or arm (this excludes paralysis of muscles supplied by a single nerve or motor root).

NEUROANATOMY

Motor activity is initiated by voluntary effort. Projections from premotor frontal lobe to motor cortex activate pyramidal tract. Sensory inputs convert into planning in premotor cortex which has projections to motor/prefrontal/parietal and supplementary motor cortices and also to basal ganglia, thalamus, and spinal cord.

The terms pyramidal, corticospinal, and upper motor neuron are not synonymous.[1] The pyramidal tract is constituted by the fibers coursing longitudinally in the pyramid of the medulla oblongata. The medullary pyramid contains nearly 1 million axons while there only 25,000–30,000 Betz cells located in fifth layer of the precentral convolution (primary motor cortex, Brodmann area 4).[2] Thus, there are contributions from Brodmann areas 4, 6, 3, 1, 2, 5, and 7 other than Betz cells for the formation of pyramidal tract. Pyramidal tract after the origin traverses the subcortical white matter (corona radiata) and descends through internal capsule to brainstem (cerebral peduncle, basis pontis, and medulla) as corticobulbar tracts and to spinal cord as corticospinal tracts. Majority of the fibers cross in the brainstem (mainly at the level of lower medulla) and continue as corticobulbar or lateral corticospinal tracts. Fibers for upper limb cross first. Some fibers continue uncrossed as anterior (ventral) corticospinal tract supplying ipsilateral axial muscles and some cross before supplying contralateral motor neurons **(Fig. 1)**.

The homunculus pattern of topography of body is represented upside down in primary motor cortex ("little man" as suggested by Wilder Penfield) **(Fig. 2)**.[3,4] The somatotopic organization of corticospinal fibers has clinical relevance. The discrete cortical-subcortical lesion will produce weakness restricted to arm and hand or leg and foot. Corticospinal tract converges and descends through posterior limb of internal capsule with fibers from face located anteriorly, hand and arm occupying central position, and foot and leg located posteriorly. Thus a small lesion in internal capsule will produce hemiplegia with almost equal affection of face, arm, hand, leg, and foot. In cerebral peduncle, corticospinal fibers occupy the middle portion of peduncle with fibers for facial nuclei situated most medially. In basis pontis, the descending motor tracts separate into bundles interspersed with pontocerebellar neurons and their cerebellopetal fibers. Therefore pontine lacunar infarct will result in selective weakness of face and hand with dysarthria, or of the leg. The descending pontine bundles devoid of corticopontine fibers reunite to form medullary pyramid. The brachial-crural pattern may persist in pyramids and is reconstituted in the lateral columns of the spinal cord though the separation at cervical, thoracic, lumbar, and sacral levels is not very discrete.

Basal ganglia act as a modulator while cerebellum behaves as both—monitor and modulator of motor activity.[5]

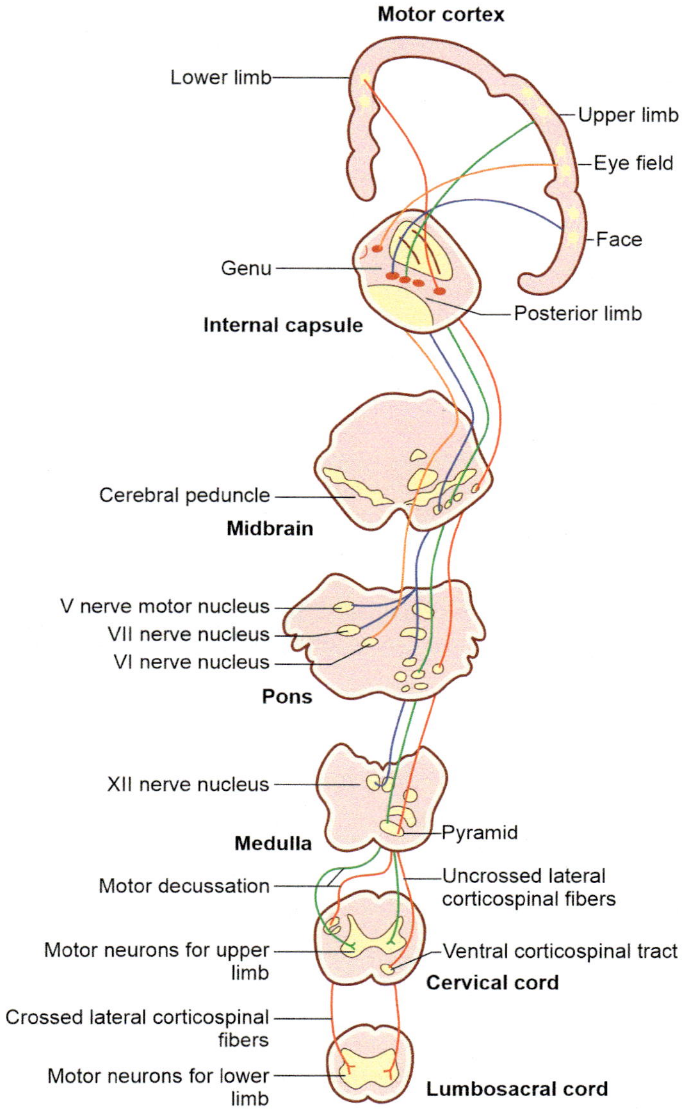

FIG. 1: Corticobulbar and corticospinal tracts. (Blue: Corticobulbar fibers connection CN V, VII, and XII nuclei; Orange: Frontal eyefield fibers connecting CN VI nuclei; Green: Corticospinal tract for upper limb; Red: Corticospinal tract for lower limb)

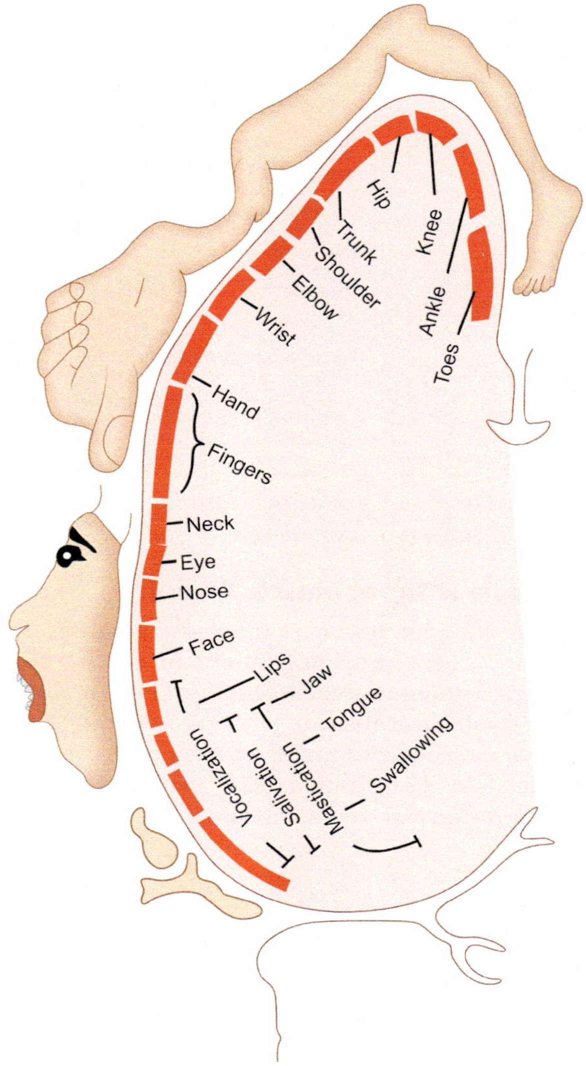

FIG. 2: The motor homunculus in motor cotex ("little man" as suggested by Wilder Penfield).

HEMIPLEGIA

Hemiplegia results from affection of contralateral corticospinal pathways except in rare circumstances. Diseases localized to the cerebral cortex, cerebral white matter (corona radiata), internal capsule, and upper brainstem usually manifest themselves by weakness of the contralateral leg, arm, and lower face. The brainstem lesions can manifest as "crossed hemiplegia" **(Tables 1 and 2)**.[1,5,6]

In some situations, an ipsilateral hemiplegia may be caused by a lesion in the corticospinal tract of the cervical spinal cord though generally the pathologic process is large enough to produce bilateral signs. A hemiparesis sparing the face, if combined with ipsilateral loss of vibration and position sense and contralateral loss of pain and temperature, signifies disease of the spinal cord on the side of the hemiparesis (Brown-Séquard syndrome).

MUSCLE ATROPHY

Hemiplegia

There may be disuse atrophy in an upper motor neuron lesion. However, when the motor cortex and adjacent parts of the parietal lobe are damaged in infancy or childhood, normal development of the musculoskeletal system may be impaired in the affected limbs. The limbs and even the trunk are smaller on affected side. This is not seen beyond puberty as most of the skeletal growth has occurred by that time. In hemiplegia caused by spinal cord lesions, muscles at the level of the lesion may atrophy as a result of damage to anterior horn cells or ventral roots.

TABLE 1: Anatomical localization.

Site of lesion	Symptoms	Signs
Motor cortex	Variable weakness of contralateral face, arm, and leg	Weakness often associated with incoordination, aphasia, apraxia, neglect
Internal capsule	Almost equal affection of contralateral face, arm, and leg	Sensory loss associated
Basal ganglia	Contralateral weakness with incoordination	Weakness often without sensory impairment
Thalamus	Mild or no weakness	Sensory impairment significant
Brainstem	Contralateral or ipsilateral weakness	Associated crossed sensory impairment, cranial nerve affection, ataxia
Spinal cord	Restricted lesions rarely produce hemiparesis	Mostly bilateral signs

Monoplegia

The presence or absence of muscle atrophy may help in the differential diagnosis of monoplegia.[7]

Monoplegia without Muscle Atrophy

A cerebral vascular lesion is the most common cause followed by a localized brain tumor or abscess for the monoplegia without muscular atrophy. Other pathologies such as a small cortical lesion in the motor strip, multiple sclerosis, and spinal cord tumor, early in their course, may cause weakness of one limb, usually the leg. Atrophy may not appear for several weeks in acute diseases of the lower motor neuron.

Monoplegia with Muscle Atrophy

This is more frequent than monoplegia without muscle atrophy. Long-continued disuse of one limb may lead to atrophy, but it is usually of lesser degree than atrophy caused by lower motor neuron disease (denervation atrophy). The lesion can be localized (in nerves, spinal roots, or spinal cord) by the pattern of weakness, associated neurologic symptoms and signs, and investigations including MRI of the spine, cerebrospinal fluid (CSF) analysis, and neurophysiological studies.

A complete atrophic brachial monoplegia is uncommon; when present in an infant, it suggests birth injury; in a child, poliomyelitis; and in an adult, syringomyelia, amyotrophic lateral sclerosis (ALS), or a brachial plexus lesion. Atrophic crural monoplegia is more frequent than atrophic brachial monoplegia and may be caused by a lesion of the lumbosacral spinal cord or plexus.

PATHOPHYSIOLOGY OF HEMIPLEGIA

Hemiplegia can be due to organic and nonorganic causes. The most common cause is cerebral lesions including cortical, subcortical, or both.

Cortical lesions: A small cortical lesion results in focal weakness while hemiplegia requires a large cortical involvement. Seizures can produce hemiplegia either as ictal phenomenon where EEG may demonstrate slow wave activity and PLEDS or as postictal Todd's paralysis which is transient contralateral weakness maximally lasting up to 36 hours. Alternating hemiplegia of childhood and hemiconvulsion, hemiplegia, and epilepsy (HHE) syndrome may also account for hemiplegia.

Subcortical lesions: Following account for hemiplegia—
- Infarction
- Hemorrhage
- Leukoencephalopathies: Multiple sclerosis and progressive multifocal leukoencephalopathy

Cortical and subcortical lesions both producing hemiplegia are:
- Infarction
- Hemorrhage: Intraparenchymal/intraventricular/subarachnoid/subdural/epidural hemorrhage
- Infection
- Tumors
- Autoimmune: Demyelinating/acute disseminated encephalomyelitis/neurosarcoidosis

PATHOPHYSIOLOGY OF MONOPLEGIA

Monoplegia may be produced by cerebral, brainstem, spinal, and peripheral lesions.
- *Cerebral lesions*: Monoplegia is less frequently produced though cortical lesion may result in monoplegia.
    - Infarction:
        - Middle cerebral artery branch—contralateral arm weakness
        - Anterior cerebral artery branch—contralateral leg weakness
    - Transient ischemic attack
    - Migraine
    - Seizure
    - Multiple sclerosis
    - Tumors
    - Infections

TABLE 2: Common brainstem syndromes.

Anatomical site	Syndrome	Cranial nerves affected	Other structures affected	Clinical features	Etiology
Midbrain					
Base	Weber	III	CST	Oculomotor palsy with crossed hemiplegia	Vascular occlusion, tumor, aneurysm
Tegmentum	Claude	III	Red nucleus, SCP after decussation	Oculomotor palsy with contralateral cerebellar ataxia and tremor	Vascular occlusion, tumor, aneurysm
Tegmentum	Benedikt	III	Red nucleus, CST, and SCP after decussation	Oculomotor palsy with contralateral cerebellar ataxia, tremor, and corticospinal signs, may have choreoathetosis	Infarct, hemorrhage, tuberculoma, tumor
Base	Top of the basilar	III	Occipital and medial temporal lobes, cerebral peduncle, thalamus	Oculomotor palsy, contralateral hemiplegia and sensory deficit, cortical blindness, memory impairment	Infarct
Tectum	Nothnagel	Uni/bilateral III	SCP	Ocular palsies (IV), paralysis of gaze, nystagmus, and ataxia	Tumor
Dorsal	Parinaud	-	Supranuclear mechanism for upward gaze and other structures in periaqueductal gray matter	Paralysis of upward gaze and accommodation; fixed pupils	Pinealoma and other lesions of dorsal midbrain, hydrocephalus
Pons					
Base (ventral)	Millard–Gubler	VII and often VI	CST	Facial and abducens palsy and contralateral hemiplegia	Infarct, tumor
Base (ventral)	Raymond–Foville	VII	CST, PPRF	Ipsilateral facial and horizontal gaze palsy with contralateral hemiplegia	Infarct, tumor
Ventral	Clumsy hand	VII	CST	Contralateral hemiplegia, dysarthria, often with facial weakness	Infarct, tumor
Ventral	Raymond's (Yelloly, Landry)	VI	CST	Abducens palsy and contralateral hemiplegia	Infarct

Continued

Continued

Anatomical site	Syndrome	Cranial nerves affected	Other structures affected	Clinical features	Etiology
Medulla					
Tegmentum	Avellis	X	STT; sometimes descending pupillary fibers, with Bernard–Horner syndrome	Paralysis of soft palate and vocal cord with contralateral hemianesthesia	Infarct, tumor
Tegmentum	Jackson syndrome	X, XII	CST	Avellis syndrome + ipsilateral tongue paralysis, contralateral hemiplegia	Infarct, tumor
Lateral tegmentum	Wallenberg syndrome	Spinal V, IX, X, XI	Lateral STT, descending pupillodilator fibers, spinocerebellar and olivocerebellar tracts	Ipsilateral V, IX, X, XI palsy, Horner syndrome, and cerebellar ataxia; contralateral loss of pain and temperature sense	Occlusion of vertebral or posterior-inferior cerebellar artery
Medial tegmentum	Dejerine's anterior bulbar (pyramid hypoglossal)	XII	CST, medial lemniscus	Contralateral hemiplegia sparing face and loss of vibration and position sense, ipsilateral tongue paralysis	Infarct
Lower tegmentum	Schmidt's (vagoaccessory)	X and XI nuclei/ fibers	-	Ipsilateral paralysis of soft palate, pharynx, larynx, SCM, and trapezius (partial)	
Medial and lateral tegmentum	Babinski–Nageotte (hemimedullary)	V spinal, X, XII (+/–)	CST, solitary, ICP, sympathetic, medial lemniscus	Medial and lateral medullary features	Multiple infarcts
Tegmentum	Céstan–Chenais	X	CST, ICP, sympathetics, medial lemniscus	Ipsilateral paralysis of soft palate, pharynx, and larynx, cerebellar ataxia, Horner's, contralateral hemiplegia with loss of vibration and position sense	Infarcts

(CST: corticospinal tract; ICP: inferior cerebellar peduncle; PPRF: paramedian pontine reticular formation; SCM: sternocleidomastoid; SCP: superior cerebellar peduncle; STT: spinothalamic tract)

- *Brainstem lesions*: Seldom produce monoplegia
- *Spinal lesions*: Lower limb monoplegia is more commonly seen with spinal lesions.
    - Tumors or other mass lesions
    - Immune and inflammatory diseases
    - Stroke
- *Peripheral lesions*: Anterior horn cell, nerve, nerve root, or plexus lesion can sometimes produce monoplegia.
    - Amyotrophic lateral sclerosis
    - Focal spinal muscular atrophy (SMA)
    - Pressure palsies:
        - Hereditary neuropathy with predisposition to pressure palsies
        - Pressure palsies in polyneuropathy

ETIOLOGY

The underlying etiology of common symptoms such as hemiplegia and monoplegia is varied depending upon age group, onset, duration, and progression of weakness.

Causes of Hemiplegia

The most common cause of hemiplegia is ischemic or hemorrhagic brain stroke followed by trauma (brain contusion, epidural, and subdural hemorrhage). Other important causes in order of frequency are brain tumor, demyelinating disease, brain abscess, and the vascular complications of meningoencephalitis. Hysteria (conversion disorder) is another common cause of hemiplegia. Migraineurs can manifest with alternating transient hemiparesis.

Causes of hemiplegia depending on onset are as follows:
- *Acute onset*: Acute onset hemiplegia can be due to organic and nonorganic causes.
    - Organic
    - Nonorganic
- Insidious onset, slowly progressive

Causes of Acute Onset Hemiplegia

- *Organic*:
    - Stroke: Ischemic and hemorrhagic
    - Trauma: Contusion, epidural/subdural hemorrhage
    - Cerebral venous sinus thrombosis: Venous infarct
    - Infection: Meningitis, encephalitis [herpes simplex encephalitis (HSE)], brain abscess, granulomatous infections [tubercular meningitis (TBM)-vasculitis—middle cerebral artery), dengue, falciparum malaria
    - Space occupying lesion: Bleeding in tumor
    - Demyelinating disorders: Acute disseminated encephalomyelitis (ADEM) and multiple sclerosis (MS)
    - Seizure: Todd's paralysis, at stroke onset [embolic and cerebral venous sinus thrombosis (CVST)]
    - Metabolic derangements: Hyponatremia, hypo- or hyperglycemia
- *Nonorganic*: Functional or psychogenic—conversion reaction and malingering

Causes of Insidious Onset, Slowly Progressive Hemiplegia

- *Space occupying lesion*: Brain (metastasis and glioma), cervical spinal cord
- *Chronic infections/inflammation*: Central nervous system (CNS) tuberculosis (tuberculoma), neurosarcoidosis, hydatid cyst
- *Motor neuron disease (MND)*: Mill's hemiplegic variant

Causes of Monoplegia

The causes of monoplegia can be classified depending on onset and limb affected, and may be organic or nonorganic in nature.
- Acute onset:
    - Upper limb:
        - Organic
        - Nonorganic
    - Lower limb:
        - Organic
        - Nonorganic
- *Insidious onset, slowly progressive*
    - Upper limb
    - Lower limb

Causes of Acute Onset Monoplegia Involving the Upper Limb

Selective lesions of parietal lobe, cervical spinal cord, multiple cervical nerve roots, or brachial plexus can produce acute onset monoplegia of the upper limb.
- *Organic*:
    - Stroke: Superior division of middle cerebral artery territory and unpaired anterior cerebral artery
    - Trauma: Parietal lobe, and multiple cervical nerve roots/brachial plexus
    - Infection: Parietal lobe granuloma and abscess
    - Postinfectious: Brachial plexitis
    - Demyelinating: Multiple sclerosis
- *Nonorganic*: Functional or psychogenic

Causes of Acute Onset Monoplegia Involving the Lower Limb

Selective lesions of frontal lobe, lumbosacral spinal cord, and multiple lumbosacral nerve roots/plexus can produce acute onset monoplegia of the lower limb.
- *Organic:*
    - Stroke: Anterior cerebral artery territory
    - Cerebral venous sinus thrombosis: Superior sagittal sinus
    - Infection: Frontal lobe granuloma and abscess
    - Trauma: Frontal lobe, and multiple lumbosacral nerve roots/plexus
    - Demyelinating: Multiple sclerosis
    - Metabolic: Diabetic lumbosacral plexopathy
- *Nonorganic*: Functional or psychogenic

Causes of Insidious Onset, Slowly Progressive Monoplegia Involving Upper Limb

- *Space occupying lesion*: Parietal lobe, cervical spinal cord, brachial plexus
- *Compressive lesion*: Large disc prolapse in cervical spinal cord region
- *Chronic infection*: Tuberculosis of brain (parietal lobe) or spinal cord (cervical region)

Causes of Insidious Onset, Slowly Progressive Monoplegia Involving Lower Limb

- *Space occupying lesion*: Frontal lobe, thoracic, or lumbar spinal cord
- *Chronic infection*: Tuberculosis of brain (frontal lobe) or spinal cord (thoracic or lumbar) tuberculosis
- *Metabolic*: Diabetic lumbosacral plexopathy

INVESTIGATIONS

A systematic approach during history and examination guides to plan the relevant investigations to determine anatomical site with extent of lesion and possible etiology.

LEARNING POINTS

- The terms pyramidal, corticospinal, and upper motor neuron are not synonymous.
- Pyramidal tract fibers receive contributions from Brodmann areas 4, 6, 3, 1, 2, 5, and 7 as the number of Betz cells is much less than the axons in medullary pyramids
- The homunculus pattern of topography of body is represented upside down in primary motor cortex.
- The body parts capable of most delicate movements have the largest cortical representation.
- "Crossed paralysis" is characteristic of brainstem lesion.
- Topographic separation of motor fibers at cervical, thoracic, lumbar, and sacral levels is not as discrete as shown in schematic diagrams of the spinal cord.
- Ipsilateral hemiplegia may be caused by a lesion in the corticospinal tract of the cervical spinal cord.
- Lower limb monoplegia is more commonly seen with spinal lesions and atrophic crural monoplegia is more frequent than atrophic brachial monoplegia.

REFERENCES

1. Ropper AH, Samuels MA, Klein JP, Prasad S (Eds). Paralysis and weakness. Adams and Victor's Principles of Neurology, 11th edition. New York; McGraw-Hill Education; 56-75, 2019.
2. Judaš M, Cepanec M, Sedmak G. Brodmann's map of the human cerebral cortex—or Brodmann's maps? Translat Neurosci. 2012;3: 67-74.
3. Schott GD. Penfield's homunculus: a note on cerebral cartography. J Neurol Neurosurg Psychiatry. 1993;56(4):329-33.
4. Sembulingam K, Sembulingam P. Essentials of Medical Physiology, 6th edition. New Delhi: Jaypee Brothers Medical Publishers; 2012. p. 890.
5. Murray EL, Misulis KE. Hemiplegia and monoplegia. In: Daroff RB, Bradley WG (Eds). Bradley and Daroff's Neurology in Clinical Practice, 8th edition. Philadelphia, PA: Elsevier/Saunders; 345-55, 2021.
6. Campbell WW, Barohn RJ. Brainstem and multiple cranial nerve syndromes. DeJong's The Neurologic Examination, 8th edition. Philadelphia: JB Lippincott Company; 2020.
7. Kumar S, Kaul S. (2017). Approach to a patient with hemiplegia and monoplegia. [online]. Available from http://www.apiindia.org/pdf/progress_in_medicine_2017/mu_27.pdf [Last accessed August, 2022].

42

CHAPTER

Approach to Paraplegias

Sarika Patil, Kaumil Kothari

INTRODUCTION

Paraplegias are devastating illness with poor outcome and significant infirmity. Prompt clinical diagnosis and treatment are of foremost importance to prevent disability. Systemic approach is needed to make an accurate localization and to arrive at etiological diagnosis. Advances of magnetic resonance imaging (MRI) have revolutionized the diagnosis of paraplegias to the extent that specific diagnosis is often made with MRI alone but not all paraplegias are associated with MRI lesions. Clinical history and examination should be used in conjunction with MRI and other investigations to establish a diagnosis. Paraplegias can occur from lesions anywhere in cerebrum, brainstem, spinal cord, or peripheral nerves. In this review, we will see clinical-anatomic background of spinal cord which will provide the framework for localization, clinical and investigational approach to paraplegias.

TABLE 1: Clinical clues toward different localizations of paraplegias.

Parasagittal lesion	Myelopathy	Peripheral neuropathy
• Paratonic rigidity • Cortical type bladder • No postvoid urinary volume • Cognitive impairment • Signs of raised intracranial tension	• Sensory level on trunk • Urinary retention • Spinal tract crossed findings (e.g., unilateral pyramidal signs with contralateral spinothalamic findings) • Spinal tract-specific sensory findings (e.g., suspended sensory loss, dissociated sensory loss)	• Graded sensory loss • No vibration level on vertebral column • All modalities of sensation affected at same level • No Lhermitte sign • Absent reflexes

CLINICAL APPROACH

Diagnostic Approach to Paraplegia

Paraplegia comes from Greek language para + plessein means "strike at side". Paraplegia is sensory motor weakness of both lower limbs. When a patient of paraplegia is encountered, we need to confirm whether the patient is having neurological condition or another illness simulating paraplegia, e.g., fracture of hip or pelvis or polyarthritis. Also we need to confirm whether paraplegia is the result of involvement of brain, spinal cord, peripheral nervous system or muscles.

Complete paralysis of both **(Table 1)** lower limbs is paraplegia whereas partial paralysis is called paraparesis. Depending upon part of nervous system involved and resulting tone, paraplegia is of two types—(1) spastic paraplegia and (2) flaccid paraplegia.

Spastic Paraplegia

Weakness of both lower limbs is associated with increased tone. It occurs due to upper motor neuron (UMN) diseases. Clinically along with increased tone, the patient can have exaggerated deep tendon reflexes, extensor plantar response with or without clonus. Further, it is divided into two types: (1) paraplegia in extension and (2) paraplegia in flexion.

1. *Paraplegia in extension*: It occurs in initial stages or partial transection of spinal cord due to involvement of pyramidal tracts. This causes more hypertonia in extensor group of muscles resulting both lower limb extension. Pyramidal signs such as exaggerated deep tendon reflexes, clonus, and bladder precipitancy are more prominent compared to paraplegia in flexion.

2. *Paraplegia in flexion*: It occurs as disease progresses further or with complete transection of spinal cord. Along with pyramidal, extrapyramidal tracts also gets involved which leads to more hypertonia in flexor group of muscles resulting in flexed posture of limbs.

Flaccid Paraplegia

Weakness is associated with decreased tone and contractility of muscles. It occurs due to lower motor neuron (LMN) diseases. Other clinical features are absent deep tendon reflexes, atrophy of muscles, and flexor plantar response with or without fasciculations.

Localization of the lesion in cord can be determined by careful history examination combined with knowledge of anatomy of spinal cord.

ANATOMY OF SPINAL CORD

Understanding the neuroanatomic structure of the spinal cord is very important in localization of its various disorders. Localizing a lesion to the spinal cord as opposed to brain or peripheral nerve is more important than localizing within the spinal cord. It is an essential skill for any neurologist to localize a lesion within the spinal cord and it helps in formulating differential diagnosis and targeted investigations. The arrangement of the gray matter within the white matter which contains the tracts and its arterial supply and venous drainage make it a fascinating but complex structure.

Spinal cord is a central nervous system structure that arises from the inferior medulla and terminates between L1 and L2 vertebra and is housed in the spinal canal of the vertebral column. The spinal cord is bathed within the cerebrospinal fluid (CSF) which also runs in the central canal.

The cervical and lumbar enlargements are related to the increased number of neurons supplying the extremities. Motor nerve roots exit ventrally while sensory nerve roots exit dorsally to form the mixed spinal nerve.

The growth of the spinal cord lags behind the growth of the vertebral column hence the numerical cord level is one segment greater (higher) than the vertebral level in upper cervical area, two segments in lower cervical and thoracic and three segments in lumbar areas. The clinical importance lies in the actual level of the spinal cord while assessing the vibration level over the vertebral bodies.

The exit of the nerve roots varies as there are seven cervical vertebra and eight cervical nerve roots. Hence, the nerve roots exit through the foramen above the like numbered vertebra from C1 to C7, while the C8 root exits below C7 and then each successive root exits below the like numbered vertebra. Thus, the root compression for the C5-C6 disc protrusion will be C6 while the root compressed in a L4-L5 disc would be L4.

The lumbar and sacral roots descend in the spinal canal vertically to reach the respective vertebral foramen for exit and form the cauda equina.

The spinal cord is a structure which is organized segmentally and somatotopically. The arrangement is due to economy of space and it transmits sensory, motor, and autonomic information at each spinal level. A segment of spinal cord refers to the section where a pair of sensory and motor nerves attach, but there is no internal demarcation to separate each segment.

The central gray matter contains the ventral and dorsal horns which are the anterior and posterior columns. The ventral horns contain alpha and gamma motor neurons with the interneurons. These motor neurons innervate the muscles of each segment and the deep tendon reflexes help localization at a particular level. The intermediate gray area between ventral and dorsal roots is the region of autonomic preganglionic cells. The sensory afferent fibers enter the cord in the dorsal root and the cell body lies in the dorsal root ganglion.

The white matter of the spinal cord surrounds the gray matter. Descending motor pathways of corticospinal tract run in the lateral and anterior corticospinal tracts. The fibers are arranged somatotopically in the tract, with the cervical representation medially and sacral laterally. These motor pathways synapse with the anterior horn cell. The anterior horn cells innervate the muscles via motor nerve root. The gamma motor neuron innervates the muscle spindle responsible for the tone. The elicitation of UMN signs at any particular level with normal signs above that level helps localize the higher-most (cranial most) level of pyramidal involvement. Other descending motor tracts are extrapyramidal tract and convey involuntary information (rubrospinal, vestibulospinal, and others).

Sensations of pinprick, temperature, and touch are carried via the spinothalamic tract which lies anterolaterally in the cord. The neurons synapse in the dorsal horn, then ascend for two to three vertebral segments and then cross the midline. Like the corticospinal tract, the cervical representation is medial and sacral is lateral in the spinothalamic tract. Proprioception and vibration sense are carried by the dorsal column where the medial tracts carry sensation from the sacral region and the lateral most tracts carry sensations from the cervical region. Thus, a hemisection of the spinal cord would carry the descending motor tracts from opposite cerebral hemisphere, spinothalamic tracts from the opposite side, and dorsal column from the same side.

Vascular Supply

The anterior spinal artery supplies the anterior two-thirds of the spinal cord (including the corticospinal tract) and a pair of posterior spinal arteries supply posterior one-third (including the dorsal column). These major vessels are reinforced by the radiculomedullary arteries which supply the spinal cord at different levels at which they enter the spinal canal. Artery of Adamkiewicz is the radiculomedullary artery that anastomoses with anterior spinal artery between T9 and T12 in most individuals and supplies anterior spinal cord in the lower thoracic region up to the conus medullaris.

The clinical import of the arterial supply is that spinal cord infarctions occur due to thrombosis of the anterior spinal artery and spare the dorsal column (hence proprioception and vibration are preserved). The spinal cord infarction is most common at the "watershed" region between the cranial and caudal reinforcements of the anterior spinal artery, which is the lower thoracic cord.

DIAGNOSTIC APPROACH TO MYELOPATHIES

The most common cause for paraplegia is myelopathies. The following steps are useful guide toward identification and localization of a lesion within the spinal cord **(Fig. 1)**.

Step 1: Confirmation of Spinal Cord Dysfunction

Clue to spinal cord lesions from history:
- Sensory level on trunk
- Tight band around the trunk or torso
- Urinary retention, bowel, and/or sexual dysfunction
- Lhermitte or Uhthoff phenomenon
- Neurogenic claudication suggests cauda equina involvement rather than lower cord lesion
- Stiffness in legs

Clue to spinal cord lesions from examination:
- Upper motor neuron signs (spasticity, hyperreflexia, clonus, pyramidal weakness, and extensor plantar response)
- Inverted biceps or brachioradialis/supinator reflex
- Spinal/neurogenic shock
- Involvement of multiple contiguous dermatomes

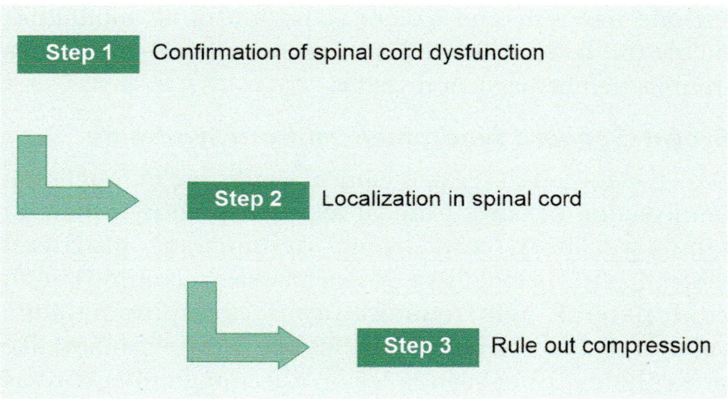

FIG. 1: Steps in diagnostic approach to myelopathies.

- Spinal tract crossed findings (e.g., unilateral pyramidal signs with contralateral spinothalamic findings)
- Spinal tract-specific sensory findings (e.g., suspended sensory loss and dissociated sensory loss)
- Various spinal cord syndromes (discussed later)

Signs consistent with but not diagnostic of myelopathy:
- Glove-and-stocking sensory loss (consider peripheral neuropathy)
- Hyporeflexia/hypotonia (consider peripheral neuropathy)
- Unilateral or bilateral UMN signs (consider brain or brainstem disorders)

Signs suggesting alternative diagnosis:
- Spasms, rather than spasticity (consider stiff-person syndrome)
- Paratonic rigidity (consider frontal lobe disorder)
- Cognitive impairment (consider frontal lobe or diffuse brain disorder)
- Dysarthria and dysphagia (consider brainstem disorder, such as motor neuron disease)

Step 2: Localization in Spinal Cord

Localization of lesion in spinal cord is very essential for physicians, it helps with differential diagnosis and targeted investigation. Certain pattern of signs may lead to the diagnosis of a spinal cord syndrome.

Step 2A: Longitudinal Localization

The longitudinal localization of the spinal cord depends on the level of affection of the spinal cord. Each level has specific clinical pointers which help localize.

Foramen Magnum Syndrome

The important clinical features include downbeat nystagmus, cerebellar ataxia, and suboccipital pain radiating to the neck and papilledema. The weakness and spasticity are seen in characteristic distribution, either hemiplegia cruciate (crossed spasticity of one upper limb and another lower limb) or Elsberg phenomenon[1] (one upper limb becomes weak followed by ipsilateral lower limb, then contralateral lower limb is affected, and finally contralateral lower limb in a U-shaped manner).

This is due to the peculiar decussation of upper limb fibers which cross cranial to the lower limb fibers and not at the same level.

High Cervical Cord Level

There is quadriparesis with diaphragmatic weakness.

Characteristic features include Lhermitte's sign[2] (flexion of neck causes a shock-like sensation running down the spine) (Lhermitte's sign is actually a symptom) and involvement of the spinal accessory nerve with weakness of the trapezius and sternocleidomastoid.

Typical sensory loss pattern is called the Balaclava helmet or Dejerine or onion-skin facial sensory loss. There is loss of pain and temperature over the lateral face with sparing of the central face. This is due to the rostral-caudal somatotopic arrangement of the spinal nucleus of the Fifth nerve in the cervical spinal cord. The perioral area is represented rostrally and lateral face caudally.

Myelopathic hand is a deformity of the upper limbs in which there is inability to adduct and extend the little finger. This indicates a spinal cord lesion above C6. Distal hand muscles wasting and weakness is a false localizing sign as the distal muscles are represented by lower cervical dermatomes, while it indicates a lesion in the upper cervical cord. The reason for this peculiar involvement is debated. According to one school of thought, it is due to venous congestion while others consider it an arterial watershed zone.

Lower Cervical and Thoracic Cord Lesion

The lesions of these regions behave the most like typical "myelopathies" that is there are LMN signs at the level of the lesion and UMN signs below it. There is presence of Horner's syndrome whenever the sympathetic tract is involved. The sympathetic nerves arise from the intermediolateral nucleus in the gray matter from the T1 to L3 spinal segments.

Lesions above D6 result in mass reflex or autonomic dysreflexia.[3] The symptoms include hypertension, bradycardia, profuse sweating of the face and neck, and severe headache. The most common cause is blockage of urinary catheter, but it can be triggered by distention of other viscera, urologic procedures, stroking of the skin, and rarely by application of heat or cold and decubitus ulcer. The mechanism is related to lack of inhibition of the impulses travelling via the spinothalamic tract and posterior columns by the higher cortical centers. This lack of inhibition is especially marked in lesions above D6 and it results in significant increase in impulses from the sympathetic system. There is facilitation of impulses along the whole sympathetic chain causing a mass reflex.

Inverted reflexes are the contraction of muscles other than the expected ones. In the inverted supinator reflex, there is finger flexion instead of biceps contraction which indicates the lesion at C5-C6 level. Inverted triceps cause flexion of the elbow instead of extension localizing the lesion to C7.

Lesion at or above D10 causes Beevor's sign[4] which is contraction of umbilicus upward on flexion of the trunk.

Conus Medullaris and Cauda Equina Lesions

The most distal bulbous part of the spinal cord is called the conus medullaris, typically between the first and second lumbar vertebrae. Cauda equina is the collection of nerve roots distal to this end of the spinal cord. Hence, conus medullaris syndrome indicates compression of a part of the spinal cord, while cauda equina syndrome is the compression of spinal roots.

TABLE 2: Differences between conus medullaris and cauda equina.

	Conus medullaris	Cauda equina
Onset	Sudden and bilateral	Gradual and unilateral
Spontaneous pain	Less severe, symmetrical in perineum	Often very prominent and severe, asymmetrical, and radicular
Motor findings	Not severe, symmetrical	Severe asymmetrical
Sensory findings	Saddle distribution, bilateral, symmetrical	Saddle distribution, more asymmetrical, dermatomal sensory loss in lower limb
Reflex changes	Epiconus-knee jerk present ankle jerk absent *Conus*: Both knee and ankle jerk are present	Both knee jerk and ankle jerk absent
Male sexual function	Impaired early	Impairment less severe

Table 2 summarizes the differences between conus medullaris and cauda equina syndrome.

Step 2B: Transverse Localization (Spinal Cord Syndromes)

White matter of spinal cord has peculiar arrangement of ascending and descending long tracts and short inter and intrasegmental tracts. Because of the anatomy of the spinal cord, selective injury to the spinal cord can generate characteristic clinical syndromes diagnostic of myelopathy and some of these specific syndromes are associated with peculiar etiologies.

Syndrome of Complete Cord Transection

Complete transverse myelopathy causes total loss of function below the level of the lesion. Clinical features include paralysis and loss of sensation of all modalities below the level of the lesion. Common etiology includes trauma, hemorrhage, or myelitis.

Brown–Sequard Syndrome/Hemicord Syndrome

Brown–Sequard described clinical syndrome of functional hemisection of cord. Clinical features include ipsilateral motor weakness (corticospinal dysfunction), ipsilateral vibratory/proprioceptive loss (posterior column), and contralateral pain/temperature loss (spinothalamic column) below the level of the lesion. Brown–Sequard like presentation is not seen in lesion affecting lumbar cord as only few spinothalamic fibers cross to opposite side at this level. This syndrome is common with extramedullary tumor compression than with trauma or intramedullary lesions.

Brown Sequard plus syndrome is associated with additional findings involving the eyes, bowel, or bladder.

Dorsal Column Syndrome

Clinically, there is impairment of vibration and proprioceptive sensation with sparing of pain temperature sensation and motor strength. Classic *Lhermitte sign* described above can be seen with dorsal column syndrome. Common etiology includes syphilitic spinal cord disease (tabes dorsalis), posterior spinal artery infarction, multiple sclerosis (MS), partial cord trauma, and after platinum-based chemotherapy.

Posterolateral Column Syndrome

This syndrome is due to simultaneous affection of lateral corticospinal and dorsal column. Clinical features are motor weakness, spasticity, and prominent loss of vibratory and position sense with relative preservation of pain and temperature. Various causes include vitamin B12 deficiency, copper deficiency, human immunodeficiency virus (HIV)-associated vacuolar myelopathy, adrenomyeloneuropathy, and human T-lymphotropic virus (HTLV)-associated myelopathy.

Central Cord Syndrome

It is one of the recurrent cord syndrome in which there is affection of the central aspect of the spinal cord, with relative sparing of the periphery. Patient develops suspended sensory loss with segmental weakness at the involved level due to anterior horn gray matter affection. Classically described with syringomyelia, it is also seen with intramedullary tumors, neuromyelitis optica or with hyperextension injury.

Anterior Cord Syndrome

This syndrome develops due to infarct in the territory of anterior spinal artery. There is dysfunction of the entire spinal cord, except for the posterior columns. Affected patients develop paraparesis with dissociated sensory loss (affection of pain temperature sensation with sparing of vibration and proprioception).

Anterior Horn Syndrome

It is characterized by loss of anterior horn cells only. Clinically affected patients show LMN type weakness with preservation of all sensory modalities. Etiologies include degenerative diseases such as spinal muscular atrophy, Kennedy disease, monomelic amyotrophy, and infective diseases such as West Nile virus myelitis and poliomyelitis.

Step 3: Rule Out Compression

Structural or compressive causes of myelopathy need to be diagnosed early as timely intervention can improve or at least, arrest symptoms **(Tables 3 and 4)**.

TABLE 3: Differentiating features between compressive and noncompressive myelopathy.

	Compressive myelopathy	Non compressive myelopathy
Level of lesion	Clear LMN signs above UMN signs	No clear level
Sensory level	Upper level of sensory loss, girdle-like sensation present	No clear upper sensory level
Long tract affection	Nonselective	Selective tractopathies, e.g., pyramidal and postcolumn
Bone deformity, bony tenderness	Present	Absent

(LMN: lower motor neuron; UMN: upper motor neuron)

TABLE 4: Clinical differences between extramedullary and intramedullary cord lesions.

Clinical features	Extramedullary	Intramedullary
Spontaneous pain	Radicular type, severe pain	Burning, funicular type
Sensory deficit	No dissociation of sensation	Dissociation of sensation
UMN/long tract sign	Prominent, early	Late, mild
Saddle sensory loss	Early and marked	Less marked and late
Sensory loss	Ascending loss (lower limb fibers are placed outer)	Descending loss
Brown–Sequard syndrome	Common	Less common
Lhermitte symptoms	Less common	Common
Urinary symptoms	Late	Early and common
Trophic changes	Not marked	More marked
Spinal subarachnoid block and CSF changes	Early marked	Less marked, late

(CSF: cerebrospinal fluid; UMN: upper motor neuron)

INVESTIGATIONAL APPROACH

Investigations for paraplegias depend on the localization. In case of cerebral localization, MRI of the brain is indispensable. Gadolinium contrast should be used whenever a focal lesion apart from ischemic stroke or hemorrhage is identified.

Peripheral nervous system localization would entail a nerve conduction and electromyography study. These studies are also useful in evaluation of lumbar radiculopathies and cauda equina syndrome. Systemic inflammatory workup may be necessary if an immune cause is suspected. A nerve-muscle biopsy may rarely be required if a myopathy (inflammatory or degenerative) is suspected.

After localizing the lesion to the spinal cord, it is important to order the correct set of tests to confirm the etiology. The spinal cord can be affected by diverse etiologies and their segregation is important.

Magnetic Resonance Imaging

Hyperintense intramedullary signal at T2-weighted imaging is a common and important indicator of myelopathy 'on' (not at) MRI. It may indicate edema, ischemia, cavitation, and breakdown of blood-spinal cord barrier or myelomalacia.[5]

Extrinsic compression of the spinal cord includes myelopathy secondary to intervertebral disc disease (the most common cause of compressive myelopathy, ligamentum flavum hypertrophy, vertebral body compression fracture, malignancy, or infection of the surrounding spinal cord amongst others). The signal in these disorders is usually adjacent to the causative lesion or seen focally; however, sometimes a compressive lesion can lead to a long-segment myelopathy. Pancake-like enhancement is seen at the site of maximal stenosis strongly suggests cervical stenosis as the cause of myelopathy. It is due to focal disruption of the blood-spinal cord barrier.[6]

Demyelinating disease forms a large chunk of spinal cord lesions. The primary etiologies include MS, neuromyelitis optica spectrum disorders (NMOSD), transverse myelitis, and acute demyelinating encephalomyelitis (ADEM). In all demyelinating disorders, it is essential to perform imaging of the brain.

In MS, the cervical spinal cord is affected most commonly. Lesions are short segment (< 1–1.5 vertebral segments longitudinally), peripheral and affecting less than half the cross-section of the spinal cord.[7] Cord swelling and contrast enhancement can be seen in acute setting, however, the cord swelling is less than that seen in NMOSD.

The spinal cord lesion in NMOSD is usually long segment (>3 vertebral segments) [called longitudinally extensive transverse myelitis (LETM)], involves central gray matter of the spinal cord, and frequently extends up to the medulla.[8] Bright spotty lesions, which indicate T2 lesions as bright as CSF and corresponding T1 hypointensity, are highly specific for NMOSD.[9] Cord expansion and complete cross-sectional involvement of the cord are also seen more commonly in NMOSD.

Acute demyelinating encephalomyelitis is seen more commonly in pediatric population. The spinal cord MRI lesions are seen more commonly in the thoracic spinal cord, they are poorly marginated and larger in cross-sectional area and vertical extent than in MS. MRI may show involvement of the brain with multifocal-enhancing lesions.[10]

Acute transverse myelitis is a diagnosis of exclusion. Spinal cord involvement is typically long segment, seen in the upper cord, with >50% cross-sectional area affected with central prominence and contrast enhancement.[11]

Immune-mediated causes of myelopathy include systemic lupus erythematosus, neurosarcoidosis, and Sjögren disease. Primary diagnosis rests on history and ancillary investigations. MRI shows a long-segment nonexpansile T2 hyperintensity. Neurosarcoid has a few characteristic features including dorsal cord involvement, leptomeningeal enhancement, and crescentic posterior subpial enhancement called trident sign.[12]

Ischemic myelopathy is hyperacute in onset and >70% of the patients have backache. Anterior spinal artery syndrome is more common than posterior spinal artery syndrome. The anterior spinal artery infarct produces a T2 hyperintensity in the anterior horns and surrounding white matter, forming the "owl's eye" sign.[13] Diffusion-weighted imaging of the spinal cord is not routinely performed and it needs to be asked for whenever the clinical suspicion is high. Venous infarction is uncommon but venous congestion secondary to spinal dural arteriovenous fistula (DAVF) can be seen.[14] It causes T2 hyperintensity in the spinal cord with cord enlargement. Dilated perimedullary veins can be seen as multiple flow voids along the surface of the spinal cord.

Infectious myelopathy in our subcontinent is most commonly a compressive myelopathy secondary to tuberculosis of the spine (Pott's spine). It involves the paradiscal regions of vertebral bodies with tubercular abscess extending into the spinal canal and compressing the spinal cord.[15] A few viral infections such as West Nile virus cause predominant affection of the anterior horn cells causing a polioclastic illness. Other bacterial and fungal myelopathies are indistinguishable from demyelinating causes and CSF as well as laboratory parameters help in their evaluation.

Human immunodeficiency virus myelopathy is characterized by symmetric nonenhancing T2 hyperintensity in posterior columns. It is secondary to vacuolization within the white matter of the cord and thus is called vacuolar myelopathy.[16] In patients infected with HIV, there can be clinical evidence of myelopathy with a normal MRI.

Intramedullary or extramedullary neoplastic lesions are common causes of myelopathy. Extramedullary neoplastic lesions cause compressive myelopathy. Intramedullary lesions can be seen as T2 hyperintensity in the spinal cord. Historical details are very important in neoplastic lesions as they present with insidious and progressive symptoms. Imaging features pointing toward neoplastic lesion include cord expansion, focal or nodular enhancement, cystic changes, and hemorrhage. Common neoplastic lesions include astrocytoma, ependymoma, and hemangioblastoma which are intramedullary tumors. Extramedullary tumors include neurofibroma, meningioma, or metastasis.[17]

Metabolic disorders include many diseases including vitamin deficiency states, leukodystrophies, mitochondrial diseases, and genetic syndromes. Metabolic disorders predominantly involve specific tracts (like dorsal column and lateral column) and hence are referred as tractopathies. Involvement of the bilateral dorsal columns in an inverted V configuration is seen in subacute combined degeneration (SACD) secondary to vitamin B12 deficiency, and can also be seen in copper deficiency, zinc toxicity, and nitrous oxide toxicity.[18,19]

Postradiation myelopathy can be seen after a variable latent period and presents as a long-segment T2 hyperintensity with variable enhancement with gadolinium.[20] In chronic stages, it may show spinal cord atrophy or cystic necrosis.

Cerebrospinal Fluid Examination

Cerebrospinal fluid examination can give important clues toward the etiology of paraplegias. It can show albuminocytological dissociation in acute polyradiculoneuropathies (Guillain–Barré syndrome). CSF examination is of utmost importance in infective causes and culture can isolate the offending organism and antibiotic sensitivity pattern can guide treatment decisions.

In demyelinating disorders, presence of CSF oligoclonal bands and CSF IgG synthesis can point toward MS or ADEM. However, a cellular CSF with lymphocytic predominance and high proteins may be seen in all demyelinating and inflammatory conditions. In metastatic lesions, CSF may show atypical cells.

Froin's syndrome is the combination of elevated protein in CSF (>500 mg/dL), xanthochromia, and hypercoagulated CSF. It is seen in spinal tumors, severe disc disease, or infections. This characteristic CSF picture is due to stagnation of CSF causing passive and/or active diffusive processes.

Blood Work

The importance of blood investigations lies in the systemic disorders causing paraplegias. Immune markers in the blood can confirm the suspicion of an autoimmune disorder. NMO and myelin oligodendrocyte glycoprotein (MOG) antibodies are tested from the serum. Low serum vitamin levels are a validation for vitamin deficiency myelopathies. Infective causes may show concomitant sepsis.

Digital Subtraction Angiography

Spinal digital subtraction angiography (DSA) is the most important confirmatory test for a spinal DAVF or arteriovenous malformation (AVM). A cranial feeder may also cause a spinal DAVF hence bilateral vertebral artery runs are also mandatory.

ETIOLOGICAL APPROACH

Speed of symptom onset—the lesions of spinal cord can be differentiated on the basis of the speed of onset. Hyperacute causes include infarction and hemorrhage. Acute causes include demyelinating disorders (NMO, MS, etc.), autoimmune disorders, and infectious causes. Subacute causes include the ones with acute onset as well as metabolic and vascular malformations. Chronic myelopathies include hereditary, neoplastic, and paraneoplastic causes.

CONCLUSION

Paraplegias are common but serious neurological illnesses with similar presentations and varied etiologies. Localization in paraplegias ranges from cerebrum to spinal cord as well as peripheral nervous system. Systematic approach to history taking is a skill which develops with experience. The importance of examination in paraplegias cannot be stressed enough. A clear understanding of the neuroanatomic organization of the spinal cord is important while evaluating paraplegias. Examination helps to narrow the differential diagnosis to a probable few. The various spinal cord syndromes discussed point to a specific localization. MRI is the most important investigation providing a clue to the diagnosis. Localizing the part to be scanned is very important as the pathology of cervical or dorsal cord is often missed if only the lumbosacral region is scanned. It is equally important to use gadolinium-enhanced contrast scanning to delineate various etiologies. MRI may not provide the answer always and other investigations are even more important in such scenarios. The prognosis depends on the etiology and often the patient is left with a significant disability. Further advances in rehabilitation will help reduce the disability.

REFERENCES

1. Elsberg CA. (1925) Tumors of the spinal cord and the symptoms of irritation and compression of the spinal cord and nerve roots. Pathology, symptomatology, diagnosis and treatment. Ann Surg. 1926;83(1):155-6.
2. Walton JN, John N . Brain's Diseases of the Nervous System, 8th edition. Oxford: Oxford University Press; 1977.
3. Cowan H, Lakra C, Desai M. Autonomic dysreflexia in spinal cord injury. BMJ. 2020;371:m3596.
4. Tashiro K. Charles Edward Beevor (1854-1908). J Neurol. 2001;258:635-6.
5. Lee MJ, Aronberg R, Manganaro MS, Ibrahim M, Parmar HA. Diagnostic approach to intrinsic abnormality of spinal cord signal intensity. Radiographics. 2019;39(6):1824-39.
6. Grayev AM, Kissane J, Kanekar S. Imaging approach to the cord T2 hyperintensity (myelopathy). Radiol Clin North Am. 2014;52(2):427-46.
7. Filippi M, Rocca MA. MR imaging of multiple sclerosis. Radiology. 2011;259(3):659-81.
8. Jarius S, Wildemann B, Paul F. Neuromyelitis optica: Clinical features, immunopathogenesis and treatment. Clin Exp Immunol. 2014;176(2):149-64.

9. Yonezu T, Ito S, Mori M, Ogawa Y, Makino T, Uzawa A, et al. "Bright spotty lesions" on spinal magnetic resonance imaging differentiate neuromyelitis optica from multiple sclerosis. Mult Scler. 2014;20(3):331-7.
10. Rossi A. Imaging of acute disseminated encephalomyelitis. Neuroimaging Clin N Am. 2008;18(1):149-61.
11. Jacob A, Weinshenker BG. An approach to the diagnosis of acute transverse myelitis. Semin Neurol. 2008;28(1):105-20.
12. Zalewski NL, Krecke KN, Weinshenker BG, Aksamit AJ, Conway BL, McKeon A, et al. Central canal enhancement and the trident sign in spinal cord sarcoidosis. Neurology. 2016;87(7):743-4.
13. Vargas MI, Gariani J, Sztajzel R, Barnaure-Nachbar I, Delattre BM, Lovblad Ko, et al. Spinal cord ischemia: practical imaging tips, pearls, and pitfalls. Am J Neuroradiol. 2015;36(5):825-30.
14. Krings T, Geibprasert S. Spinal dural arteriovenous fistulas. Am J Neuroradiol. 2009;30(4):639-48.
15. Garg RK, Somvanshi DS. Spinal tuberculosis: a review. J Spinal Cord Med. 2011;34(5):440-54.
16. Candy S, Chang G, Andronikou S. Acute myelopathy or cauda equina syndrome in HIV-positive adults in a tuberculosis endemic setting: MRI, clinical and pathologic findings. Am J Neuroradiol. 2014;35(8):1634-41.
17. Samartzis D, Gillis CC, Shih P, O'Toole JE, Fessler RG. Intramedullary Spinal Cord Tumors. I. Epidemiology, Pathophysiology, and Diagnosis. Global Spine J. 2015;5(5):425-35.
18. Narra R, Mandapalli A, Jukuri N, Guddanti P. "Inverted V sign" in Sub-acute Combined Degeneration of Cord. J Clin Diagn Res. 2015;9(5):TJ01.
19. Kumar A, Singh AK. Teaching NeuroImage: Inverted V sign in subacute combined degeneration of spinal cord. Neurology. 2009;72(1):e4.
20. Khan M, Ambady P, Kimbrough D, Shoemaker T, Terezakis S, Blakeley J, et al. Radiation-induced myelitis: Initial and follow-up MRI and clinical features in patients at a single tertiary care institution during 20 years. Am J Neuroradiol. 2018;39(8): 1576-81.

43

CHAPTER

Approach to Lower Motor Neuron Weakness

Rajesh Benny

INTRODUCTION

Weakness is one of the common presentations of diseases involving the neuromuscular system. When measured objectively using the medical research council (MRC) scoring, weakness can result from diseases involving the entire neuroaxis, ranging from the motor cortex to the distal-most muscle. Most of the lower motor neuron weaknesses tend to be proximal and symmetric; however, they can present asymmetrically and distally also.

IS THE WEAKNESS DUE TO UPPER MOTOR NEURON OR LOWER MOTOR NEURON?

Clinical features of upper motor neuron (UMN) and lower motor neuron (LMN) are given in **Table 1**.

TABLE 1: Clinical features of upper motor neuron (UMN) and lower motor neuron (LMN).

Clinical features	UMN	LMN
Pattern of motor weakness	Pyramidal distribution of weakness. In the upper limbs, there is preferential weakness of shoulder abductors, elbow extensors, forearm supinators, and wrist extensors. In the lower limbs, there is preferential weakness of hip abductors, knee flexors, ankle dorsiflexors, and evertors	Depending on the anatomical site of lesion (see description after this table in the section: Lesions involving the LMN)
Tone	Increased	Reduced or normal
Deep tendon reflexes	Brisk	Absent or normal
Extensor plantar reflex	Yes	No
Superficial reflexes	Absent	Present
Atrophy	No or mild (disuse atrophy)	Yes, severe
Hypertrophy	No	Yes (muscular dystrophies, congenital myotonias)
Fasciculations	No	Yes
Sensory abnormality	Hemisensory/level on the trunk/dissociate anesthesia/suspended sensory loss	Depending on the anatomical site of lesion (see description after this table in the section: Lesions involving the LMN)
Respiratory muscle involvement	Rare; only in lesions involving the medulla	Common; may be early at some anatomic sites (e.g., NM junction, AHC)

(AHC: anterior horn cell; NM: neuromuscular)

LESIONS INVOLVING THE UPPER MOTOR NEURON

Stroke is one of the most common causes of motor weakness. Most strokes present with hemiparesis, ataxia, associated cranial nerve or sensory involvement, and evidence of pyramidal dysfunction.

Pathologies involving the spinal cord also present with motor weakness. But, most present with paraparesis or quadriparesis with evidence of pyramidal dysfunction, sensory level on the trunk and early bladder, or bowel involvement. The presence of a dissociated pattern of sensory loss (involvement of the spinothalamic tract but sparing of the posterior column) also points toward the spinal cord as the site of motor weakness (typically seen in those with intramedullary lesions like syrinx).

LESIONS INVOLVING THE LOWER MOTOR NEURON

Lower motor neuron pattern of weakness can occur due to lesions at various sites of the neuroaxis.

Anterior Horn Cell

Anterior horn cell (AHC) lesions usually present with an asymmetric, pure motor weakness with wasting and fasciculations. The weakness can start distally or proximally. Weakness involves the limb muscles, cranial musculature [extraocular muscles (EOMs) are spared], and paraspinal muscles. AHC can present as an isolated LMN abnormality [polio, spinal muscular atrophy (SMA)] or a combination of LMN and UMN [amyotrophic lateral sclerosis (ALS)]. The presence of LMN and UMN features in the same myotome is pathognomonic of ALS. There may be differential wasting (split hand sign) **(Figs. 1A and B)**.

However, there are exceptions. SMA (caused due to genetic abnormality of the survival motor neuron 1 gene) is characterized by symmetric weakness in a limb-girdle pattern. SMA type IV (adult-onset) mimics limb-girdle muscular dystrophy (LGMD). Bulbospinal muscular atrophy (Kennedy's disease) is an X-linked CAG repeat disorder that along with the other typical LMN AHC features also has prominent muscle cramps, tremors, paresthesia, autonomic abnormality (sweat dysfunction), and systemic involvement (gynecomastia, endocrine abnormality).[2]

ROOT

Radiculopathies usually present with pain, sensory loss, weakness (which is asymmetric), and reflex loss in root distribution. Knowledge of the sensory distribution of the root (dermatome) and pointer muscles helps to localize the involved root. Most abnormalities of the root are due to compression of the cervical or lumbosacral (LS) roots due to prolapsed intervertebral disk. Multiple root involvement can be seen with herpes zoster or arachnoiditis involving the cauda equina roots (tuberculous, carcinomatous, etc.). Root lesions can be associated with UMN features (radiculomyelopathy; due to compression) and can also present with symmetric, generalized weakness [as in acute and chronic inflammatory demyelinating polyradiculoneuropathy (AIDP and CIDP)]. Various maneuvers can be done at the bedside to demonstrate the involvement of the roots in these mixed lesions like the straight leg raising test (SLR) for the lower limb and the Spurling test[3] for demonstrating radiculopathy in the upper limb.

Plexus

Lesions involving the brachial or LS plexus are rare causes of limb weakness, and generally tend to be unilateral with simultaneous involvement of multiple nerves. This results in an asymmetric limb weakness with the involvement of multiple muscles and sensory loss in a peripheral nerve pattern. Most plexus lesions tend to be painful. Pain may be worse at night and in the supine position.

Brachial plexopathy is more common than LS plexopathy. Brachial plexopathy can be caused by trauma or

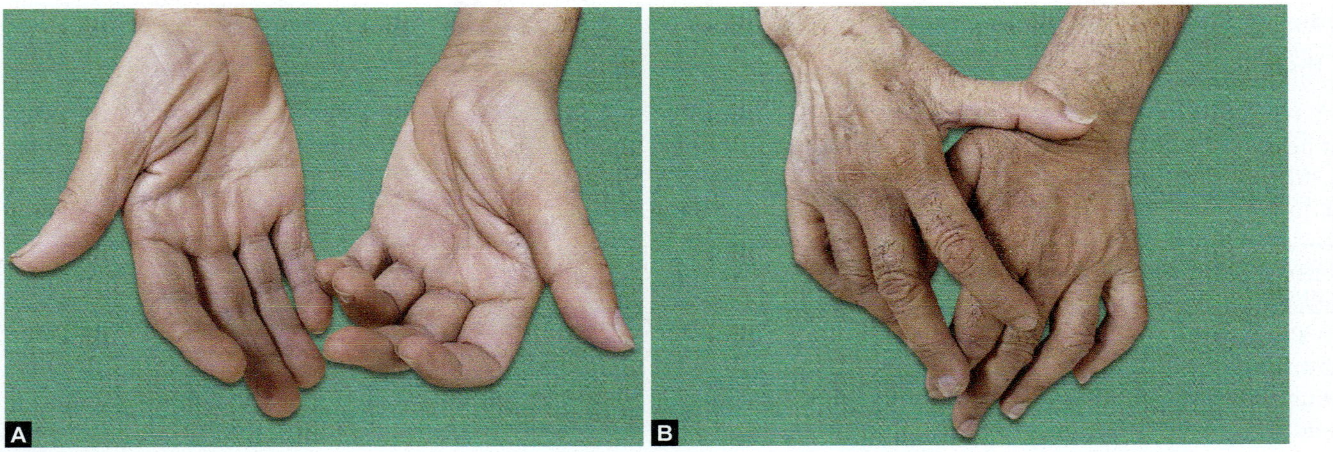

FIGS. 1A AND B: Split hand sign: (A) wasting of the thenar muscles, sparing muscle of hypothenar muscles (B) wasting of first dorsal interosseous.[1]

nontraumatic etiologies. The most common nontraumatic etiology is neuralgic amyotrophy (Parsonage–Turner syndrome) which is characterized by unilateral involvement, pain, and involvement of the upper or middle brachial plexus with scapular winging. Other nontraumatic causes of brachial plexus lesions are neoplastic, radiation-associated, hereditary, thoracic outlet syndrome, and associated with diabetes.

There is associated root involvement in >50% of those with LS plexopathy with a positive SLR test. The knee jerk is involved in the lumbar plexus and the ankle jerk in sacral plexopathy. Sensory abnormality in the anterior thigh, medial thigh, and medial leg indicates involvement of the lumbar plexus and in those with sacral plexus involvement, there is a sensory abnormality in the dorsum of the foot, posterior thigh, and the perianal area. LS plexopathy can be caused by various pathologies inflammation, idiopathic, direct trauma or stretch on the plexus (including pregnancy/during childbirth), diabetes, ischemia, malignancy (direct infiltration, metastasis, or compression by an abdomino-pelvic malignancy), and postradiotherapy. In those with malignancy-associated LS plexopathy, the L4-S1 segment is involved in >50% of cases, L1–L4 in 31%, and pan plexopathy in 10%.[4] Diabetic lumbar-radiculoplexus-neuropathy (diabetic amyotrophy or Bruns–Garland syndrome) occurs predominantly in those with type II diabetes in a unilateral distribution with severe dysesthetic pain, may become bilateral in some over 3 months, and is associated with constitutional symptoms like weight loss.

Peripheral Nerve

Most peripheral neuropathies are due to diseases involving the axon that present as a distal, symmetric, and sensory-motor (or motor-sensory) weakness. Both the weakness and sensory loss follow a distal to proximal gradient (due to the dying back phenomenon—the distal part is more affected than the proximal). This is associated with a glove and stocking pattern of sensory loss, distal reflex loss, and distal weakness with atrophy.

On the other hand, the demyelinating neuropathies (AIDP and CIDP) present with proximal weakness ≥ distal weakness, generalized areflexia without atrophy. Multifocal motor neuropathy with conduction block (MMNCB)[5] is a nodopathy that presents with a pure motor, distal > proximal, upper limbs > lower limb, asymmetric weakness mimicking a motor neuron disease (MND). MADSAM (multifocal acquired demyelinating sensory and motor neuropathy; Lewis–Sumner syndrome) presents as an asymmetric motor-sensory weakness, distal > proximal, involving upper limbs > lower limbs with multifocal or diffuse reflex loss.

Peripheral neuropathy can present as a mononeuropathy, mononeuritis multiplex (MM), or symmetric polyneuropathy. Mononeuropathies present with weakness (and sensory loss) in a single nerve distribution (caused by trauma, compression—carpal tunnel syndrome, ischemia, neoplastic infiltration, or as a part of generalized disorder such as diabetes, hypothyroidism, acromegaly, or in hereditary neuropathies like hereditary neuropathy with pressure palsies).

Mononeuritis multiplex neuropathies are asymmetric neuropathies due to nerve-by-nerve involvement that occurs over a variable period and eventually become symmetric like a polyneuropathy (hence, it is important to focus on early events to diagnose a MM neuropathy as its etiologic differential diagnosis is limited). Leprosy is the most common cause of painless MM; vasculitis causes a painful MM and MADSAM a demyelinating motor-sensory MM.

Polyneuropathies (axonal > demyelinating) are more common than MM. Common etiologies with motor weakness are immune [Guillain–Barré syndrome (GBS) and chronic inflammatory demyelinating polyneuropathy (CIDP)], metabolic (diabetes and renal dysfunction), drugs/toxins (lead, mercury, organophosphate poisoning, dapsone, and alcohol), critical illness neuropathy, paraprotein neuropathy, and inherited neuropathies. One should suspect an inherited neuropathy if the history is chronic and in those with skeletal deformities (pes cavus and hammertoes).

Polyradiculoneuropathies such as AIDP, CIDP, and porphyria neuropathy have both proximal and distal weakness (with associated weakness of the paraspinal muscles). Pain is an associated feature due to root involvement.

Weakness with autonomic features can be prominent in some neuropathies such as the GBS, neuropathy associated with porphyria, and toxins like vincristine.

Neuromuscular Junction

Lesions of the neuromuscular junction (NMJ) are usually asymmetric, pure motor, and can be distal or proximal. Cranial nerve involvement is common (especially asymmetric ptosis, involvement of the EOMs, and bifacial weakness). Neck drop due to involvement of the neck extensor muscles may be the presenting feature of NMJ pathologies.

Clinical differences in lesions involving the pre- and postsynaptic NMJ are given in **Table 2**.

The hallmark of postsynaptic NMJ weakness is the presence of fatigability. The presence of fatigable weakness can be demonstrated at the bedside: sustained up gaze (60–180 seconds) to demonstrate ptosis, sustained eye closure to demonstrate the fatigable weakness of orbicularis oculi resulting in the "peek sign", sustained lateral gaze for 60 seconds to demonstrate diplopia, abduction of the arm for 120 seconds, sustained leg elevation (90 seconds) while lying supine and counting aloud to 100 to demonstrate the fatigable change in voice. NMJ transmission improves with cooling. This is the basis of improvement in muscle weakness with the ice pack test (improvement in ptosis by > 2 mm after applying ice pack on the affected upper eyelid for 2–5 minutes) and iced drink test in those with suspected bulbar myasthenia.[6] The most common cause of NMJ abnormality is the acquired MG. In the majority, MG is due to antibodies against the postsynaptic acetylcholine receptor (AchR).

TABLE 2: Clinical differences in lesions involving the pre- and postsynaptic neuromuscular junction.

Clinical features	Presynaptic	Postsynaptic
Prototype	Lambert–Eaton myasthenic syndrome (LEMS)	Acetylcholine receptor (AchR) antibody myasthenia gravis (MG)
Fatigable weakness	Yes	Yes
The pattern of muscle weakness	Hip girdle	Face, extraocular muscle, upper limbs
Symmetric weakness	Yes	No
Postexercise improvement in weakness/deep tendon reflexes (DTR)	Yes	No
Autonomic abnormality	Yes	No
DTR	Absent	Present
Pain	Yes	No
Respiratory muscle involvement	Rare; late	Common; may be early

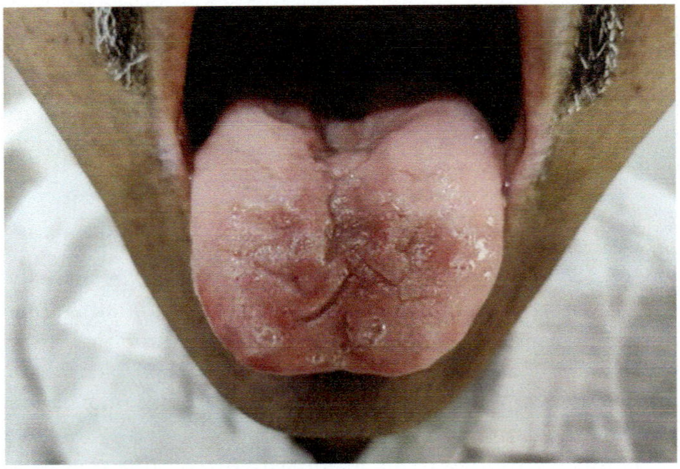

FIG. 2: Tongue atrophy in MuSK myasthenia.

Muscle-specific Kinase Antibody Myasthenia

As compared to AchR antibody myasthenia; weakness in muscle-specific kinase antibody myasthenia (MuSK) myasthenia tends to be more focal with severe involvement of the neck, shoulder, face, and bulbar muscles. If the extremities are involved, proximal muscle weakness is more common than distal muscle weakness. Ptosis tends to be mild and if present, symmetric. Many patients have prominent wasting of muscles including the tongue **(Fig. 2)**. Pyridostigmine is ineffective or even worsens MuSK myasthenia.[7]

Congenital Myasthenia Syndromes

These are inherited diseases caused by mutations in the genes that encode proteins that are important for the integrity of the NMJ. Clinical presentation may be variable with onset since birth or in the second or third decade. Most present with fatigable weakness of the face, eyes, and limbs; some may present with an isolated limb-girdle syndrome mimicking LGMD, respiratory insufficiency since birth, or skeletal abnormality (arthrogryposis multiplex congenita).

Muscle

Individuals with myopathies generally present with pure motor, symmetric, shoulder, or hip girdle weakness, with variable involvement of the cranial musculature. The weakness of the hip girdle muscles (especially of the gluteus medius muscle) results in the characteristic waddling gait. However, muscle disease can begin distally mimicking peripheral neuropathy (however, even in those with distal myopathies the extensor digitorum brevis muscle is usually spared or even hypertrophic; it is atrophic in those with peripheral neuropathy). Myopathies can be inherited or acquired.

Inherited myopathies can be due to dystrophies, myotonic disorders, congenital myopathy, channelopathy, storage disorders, and mitochondrial diseases. The clue to a specific diagnosis of inherited myopathies depends on the age of onset, the pattern of inheritance, and the pattern of muscle weakness. Dystrophies (the most common inherited myopathy) can present in all age groups [Duchenne muscular dystrophy (DMD) in the first decade, LGMDs in the first to third decade, and oculopharyngeal muscular dystrophy (OPMD) in the fifth decade] and can have variable inheritance (autosomal, X linked, or mitochondrial).

Clinical Pointers to the Etiology of Myopathy

- *Hypertrophy*: Most commonly seen in the calves in those with DMD, hypothyroidism, and some LGMD—sarcoglycanopathies, LGMD 2I and 1C. Tongue hypertrophy can be seen in DMD, LGMD 2I, amyloidosis, glycogen storage disorder, and hypothyroidism. Differential muscle weakness is another feature of dystrophies—muscle groups around a joint can be variably affected (e.g., in those with certain LGMDs; the hip adductors may be more involved than the hip abductors resulting in the "hip abduction sign"[8] on attempting to get up from a squatting position).
  In some dystrophies, atrophy and hypertrophy can be observed in the same muscle **(Fig. 3)**.
- *Prominent bifacial weakness*: Seen in myotonic dystrophy, facioscapulohumeral muscular dystrophy (FSHD), and congenital myopathies (central core, nemaline, myotubular, and fiber type disproportion).
- *Ocular paralysis (ptosis with/without EOM involvement) with/without limb weakness*: Seen in FSHD, myotonic dystrophy, OPMD, congenital myopathy (centronuclear, multicore/minicore), mitochondrial and dysthyroid ophthalmopathy.
- *Neck extensor weakness (dropped head syndrome)*: Commonly observed in polymyositis (PM), inclusion

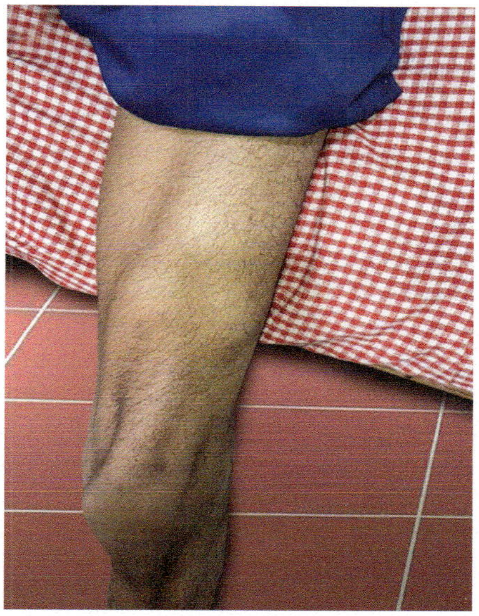

FIG. 3: Diamond on quadriceps sign: Atrophy and hypertrophy of the quadriceps muscle.[9]

body myositis (IBM), nemaline myopathy, mitochondrial, FSHD, myotonic dystrophy, and carnitine deficiency.

- *Prominent winging of the scapula*: Seen in those with calpainopathy (do not have facial weakness and have early tendoachilles contractures) and FSHD (have a prominent facial weakness).
- *Myopathies with prominent contractures*: Seen in Emery–Dreifuss muscular dystrophy (EDMD) (at the elbow), DMD (tendoachilles), congenital muscular dystrophy, collagen VI-related myopathies (spectrum ranging from the severe Ullrich muscular dystrophy to the milder Bethlem myopathy), juvenile dermatomyositis (DM), congenital myopathies (centronuclear, multicore/minicore), and calpainopathy.
- *Prominent myotonia (observed in both percussion and grip)*: Seen in myotonic dystrophy (also have distal weakness, ptosis, wasting of the facial musculature, baldness, and systemic features), myotonia congenita, paramyotonia congenita, and in some channelopathies (hyperkalemic paralysis).
- *Muscle diseases with cardiac involvement (cardiomyopathy or arrhythmia)*: Dystrophinopathy (DMD/Becker's muscular dystrophy), mitochondrial myopathy, EDMD, desminopathy, LGMD 1B, myotonic dystrophy, carnitine deficiency, and acid maltase deficiency.[10]
- *Muscle diseases with early respiratory muscle involvement*: LGMD 2I, titinopathy, OPMD, certain congenital myopathies, acid maltase deficiency, and debrancher enzyme deficiency.
- *Distal myopathies*: Those predominantly starting distally in the lower limbs include GNE myopathy, Miyoshi myopathy, myotonic dystrophy, telethioneinopathy, titinopathy (Udd's myopathy), Markesbery-Grigg's myopathy, and Laing myopathy. Some of the distal myopathies involving the upper limbs are IBM, desminopathy, myotonic dystrophy, and Welander's myopathy.
- *Storage disorder myopathy*: Most common presentation is exercise intolerance which when triggered by short, high-intensity exercises suggest a glycogen storage disorder[11] and when it occurs after sustained activity suggests a fatty acid oxidation defect. Improvement in muscle weakness with sustained muscle activity (the second wind phenomenon) is seen in McArdle disease. Another presentation of storage myopathies is with fixed muscle weakness which can mimic a dystrophic process. Most also have prominent cramps, myalgia, and early contractures.
- *Mitochondrial myopathies*: Most are associated with multisystem involvement (muscle weakness, neuropathy, cerebellar ataxia, hearing abnormality, retinal abnormality, cataracts, cardiac conduction defects, etc.), skeletal abnormality (short stature), and fatigue even with trivial exertion.
- *Episodic muscle weakness*: Many of these etiologies present with proximal (more than distal) muscle weakness and hence, in the acute setting (or if it is the first episode) can mimic GBS. These are the channelopathies (sodium, potassium, or calcium) that are either inherited in an autosomal dominant manner or can be acquired (associated with thyrotoxicosis, renal tubular acidosis, drugs, etc.). Thyrotoxic periodic paralysis is common in Asians and is associated with hypokalemia.
- *Endocrine myopathies*: Osteomalacic myopathy (due to hypovitaminosis D3) presents with painful hip girdle weakness with hyperreflexia. Steroid myopathy presents with painless hip girdle weakness. In those with dysthyroid myopathy, there is proximal muscle weakness with calf hypertrophy.
- *Inflammatory myopathies[12] [PM, DM, IBM, and necrotizing autoimmune myopathy (NAM)]*: Most present with symmetric; subacute, or acute (NAM); proximal (more than distal) limb weakness. An exception to this presentation is in those with IBM where asymmetric muscle involvement (involvement of the long finger flexors in the upper limb and quadriceps in the lower limbs) mimicking an MND or MMNCB is observed. Inflammatory myopathies may be associated with connective tissue disorders or be associated with an underlying malignancy (DM). Certain skin signs aid in the diagnosis of DM such as the characteristic heliotrope (violaceous) rash on the upper eyelid with or without edema, Gottron's papules (dorsal metacarpophalangeal and interphalangeal joints may show the presence of erythematous/violaceous rash with or without scaling and ulceration); and presence of the V sign or the shawl sign (depending on the distribution of the erythema: over the front of the chest or the posterior aspect of the neck and upper back respectively). The presence of mechanic's hands (hyperkeratotic eruption,

TABLE 3: Clinical features of neurogenic weakness and myogenic weakness.

Clinical features	Neurogenic weakness	Myogenic weakness
Pattern of limb weakness	Distal > proximal	Proximal > distal
Facial muscles	Usually spared	Can be involved
Extraocular muscles	Usually spared	Can be involved
Extensor digitorum brevis muscle	Atrophic	Preserved or hypertrophic
Fasciculations	Yes	No
Hypertrophy	No	Can be seen
Sensory abnormality	May be present	Absent
Autonomic abnormality	Can be seen	Absent
Tremors in the upper limbs	May be present	No
Electromyography (EMG)	Neurogenic	Myogenic

desquamation, and fissuring in the ulnar aspect of the thumb and radial aspect of the index finger) points to the diagnosis of antisynthetase (usually, anti-Jo-1) antibody inflammatory myopathy.

There are certain clinical and laboratory pointers which help differentiate neurogenic weakness from myogenic weakness **(Table 3)**.

INVESTIGATIONS TO AID/CONFIRM LOCALIZATION OF THE MOTOR WEAKNESS

A detailed history and a careful clinical examination of the pattern/site of weakness differentiate a UMN from an LMN lesion and help direct the investigations needed to confirm the diagnosis/etiology of the weakness.

- *Creatine phosphokinase (CPK)*: Elevated in those with muscle disease, especially in those with inflammatory myopathies (severe in those with NAM), muscular dystrophies (levels tend to decrease with worsening atrophy of the muscles), drug-induced myopathies (statins), hypothyroidism (sometimes, >50 times normal with mild weakness) and even in hypo/hyperkalemia. HyperCKemia can be seen not only in those with myogenic weakness but also in those with neurogenic weakness (mild-to-moderate elevation) like in ALS.
- *Serum lactate*: Elevated serum lactate and blood lactate/pyruvate ratio have high specificity for the diagnosis of mitochondrial myopathies.[13]
- *Autoantibody testing*: In those with neurogenic weakness, antiganglioside antibody testing may indicate certain subtypes like IgG anti-GM1 antibody in the AMAN (acute motor axonal neuropathy) variant of GBS and IgM anti-GM1 antibody in MMNCB.
- *Myositis-specific antibodies*: Myositis-specific antibodies can help characterize and prognosticate myositis. Presence of myositis with anti-TIF1γ or anti-NXP2 antibodies = high risk for malignancy in adults; anti-Jo-1 = antisynthetase syndrome [myositis, interstitial lung disease (ILD), mechanic hands, and Raynaud's phenomenon, polyarthritis]; anti-Mi-2 = typical DM with skin lesions and mild myositis; anti-signal recognition particle (SRP) = NAM; anti-MDA5 = amyopathic DM, rapidly progressive ILD, palmar papules (inverse Gottron papules), and arthritis.
- *Autoantibody in NMJ diseases*: Anti-AChR (seen in 85% of those with generalized MG), anti-MuSK (7–10%), and anti-lipoprotein receptor-related protein 4 (LRP4) (2%) antibodies are observed in those with acquired MG.
- *Nerve conduction study (NCS)*: Useful in those with suspected neuropathy to confirm the diagnosis and the type of neuropathy (axonal or demyelinating). Nonuniform slowing of the conduction velocity is seen in acquired demyelinating neuropathies and uniform slowing is seen in inherited demyelinating neuropathies. The presence of demyelinating conduction block in an asymmetric, motor predominant neuropathy indicates MMNCB. NCS can aid in the diagnosis of a nodopathy[14] [AMAN is the prototype nodopathy characterized by the presence of axonal conduction block (not associated with temporal dispersion or slowing of the conduction velocity) and improvement demonstrated with serial NCS]. In those with suspected NMJ disorders, the presence of a low CMAP amplitude and its facilitation after a brief period of exercise indicates a presynaptic NMJ abnormality.
- *Repetitive nerve stimulation study (RNS)*: RNS exploits the depletion of readily available ACh stores with low stimulation frequencies to unmask the reduced safety factor common to all NMJ disorders. This results in a reduced number of endplate potentials (EPP) and is reflected by a reduction of compound motor action potential (CMAP) amplitudes with successive stimulation or "decrement" in those with postsynaptic NMJ disorders. In presynaptic disorders, there is an augmentation of presynaptic calcium concentration with high stimulation frequencies or following brief exercise which increases EPP amplitudes and the CMAP amplitudes resulting in "facilitation".
- *Electromyography (EMG)*: Needle EMG is useful to confirm the presence of a myogenic (short/normal duration polyphasic) or neurogenic process (long-duration polyphasic) **(Figs. 4A to C)**.
  In those with inflammatory myositis, there will be an increase in spontaneous activity (also seen in MND) during EMG.
- *Magnetic resonance imaging (MRI)*: It is the best modality to demonstrate the cause of weakness due to a brain or spinal cord lesion. It is also being used increasingly in LMN disorders, especially in diseases involving the muscle and peripheral nerves. It is also the best noninvasive modality to demonstrate muscle involvement, especially to identify the group of muscles

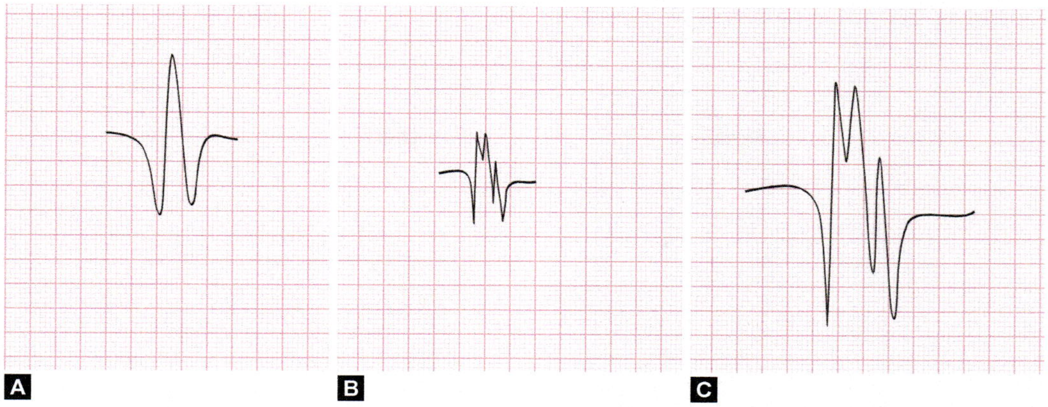

FIGS. 4A TO C: EMG in health and disease: (A) normal MUAP; (B) myopathic; and (C) neurogenic polyphasic.
(EMG: electromyography; MUAP: motor unit action potential)

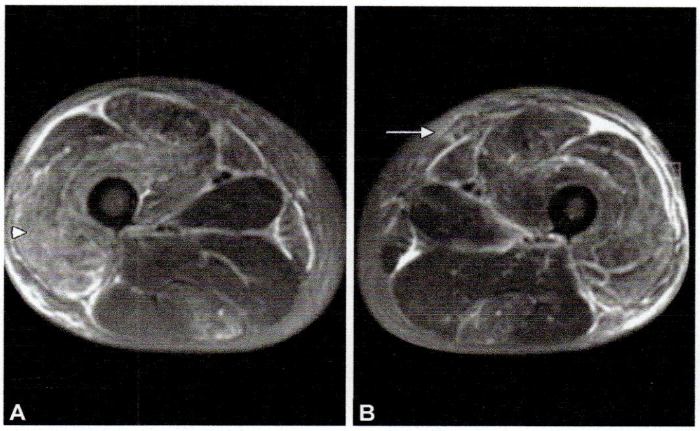

FIGS. 5A AND B: Dermatomyositis—diffuse hyperintensity in vastus lateralis muscle and increased signal in subcutaneous tissue septa with skin thickening.

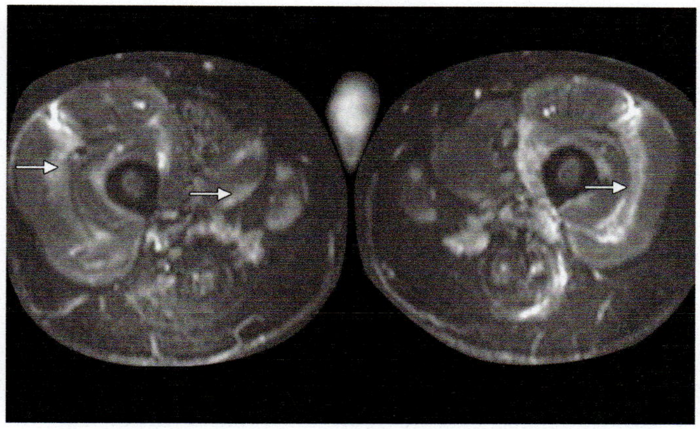

FIG. 6: Antisignal recognition particle myopathy—myofascial orientation of edema and inflammation.

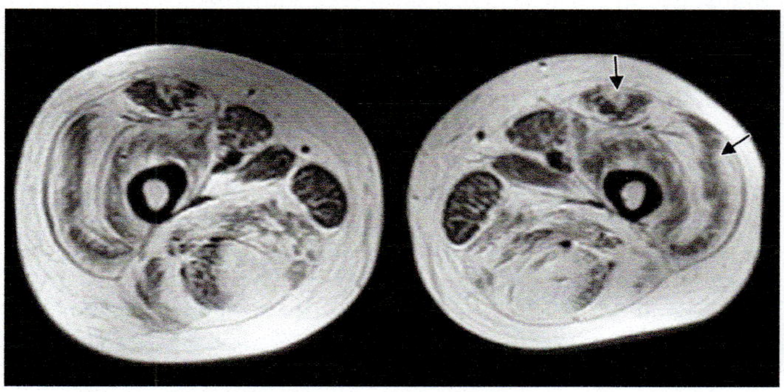

FIG. 7: Collagen VI myopathy—"target" sign in the rectus femoris and a "sandwich" sign in the vastus lateralis muscle.

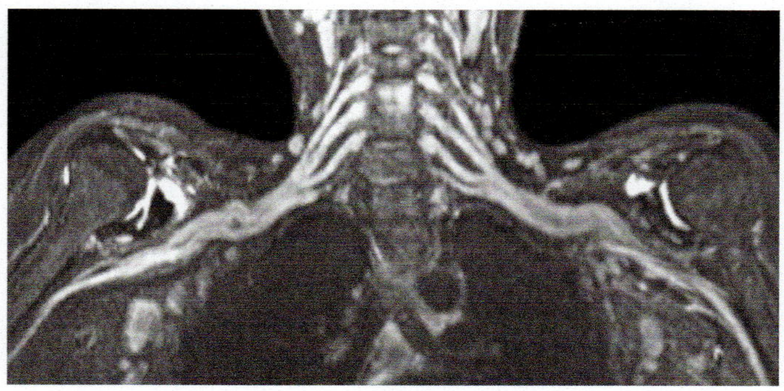

FIG. 8: Enlarged nerve roots and brachial plexus in chronic inflammatory demyelinating polyradiculoneuropathy.

involved, is best for focal muscle involvement and can be used to track changes during therapy. The pattern of muscle/subcutaneous involvement on MRI can point toward specific etiologies **(Figs. 5 to 7)**.

- *MR neurography*: Best noninvasive modality to demonstrate certain disorders of the roots, nerves, or plexus needs a higher resolution (3T) MRI scanner **(Fig. 8)**.

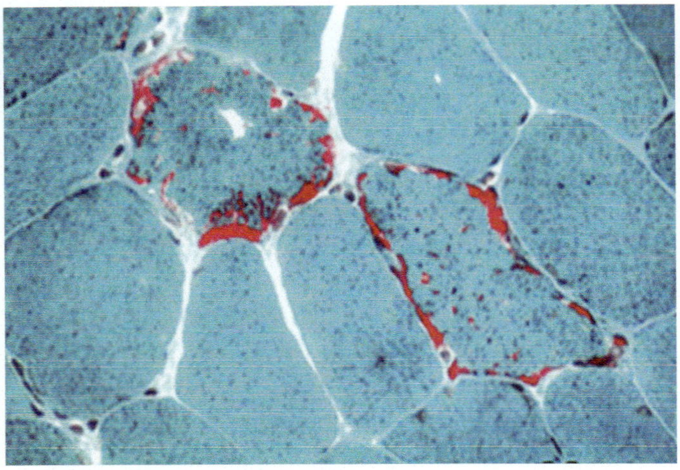

FIG. 9: Mitochondrial myopathy—ragged red fibers on Gomori trichrome stain.

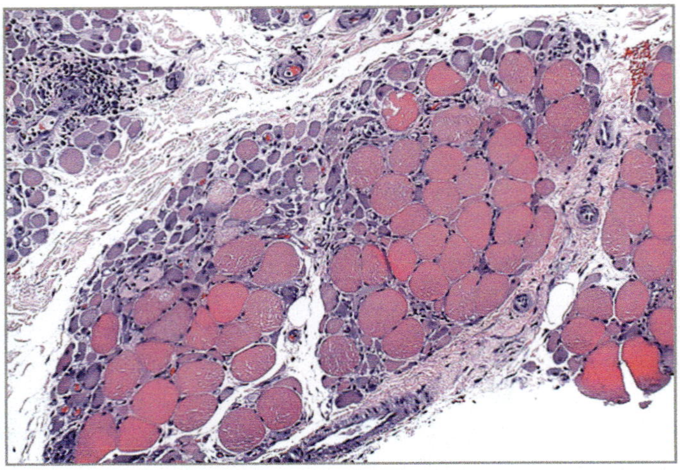

FIG. 10: Inflammatory myositis—dermatomyositis perifascicular atrophy with inflammation.

- *Nerve biopsy*: It is done when leprosy, vasculitis, sarcoidosis, or certain-inherited neuropathies like giant axonal neuropathy are suspected as a cause of the neuropathy.
- *Muscle biopsy*: It confirms the presence of muscle disease and also helps in specific etiologic diagnosis **(Figs. 9 and 10)**.
- *Genetic studies*: In those with suspected inherited causes for muscle weakness.

CONCLUSION

Motor weakness can be seen in diseases involving the entire neuroaxis; from the UMN (brain, spinal cord) to LMN pathologies (AHC, root, plexus, peripheral nerve, NMJ, and muscle). Motor weakness can be symmetric or asymmetric; proximal or distal; and with or without pain/atrophy or hypertrophy/sensory abnormality. Accurate localization of the site of weakness by history and clinical examination helps choose investigations to confirm the diagnosis and also, unearth the possible etiology of weakness. MRI is being increasingly used as a noninvasive modality to study diseases of the LMN (especially, diseases of the muscle and nerve).

ACKNOWLEDGMENT

I thank Bhagyadhan Patel for sharing image 2 and Pramod Dhonde for image 3.

REFERENCES

1. Benny R, Shetty K. The split hand sign. Ann Indian Acad Neurol. 2012;15(3):175-6.
2. Manzano R, Sorarú G, Grunseich C, Fratta P, Zuccaro E, Pennuto M, et al. Beyond motor neurons: expanding the clinical spectrum in Kennedy's disease. J Neurol Neurosurg Psychiatry. 2018;89:808-12.
3. Jones SJ, Miller JMM. Spurling Test. Treasure Island (FL): StatPearls Publishing; 2023.
4. Jaeckle KA, Young DF, Foley KM. The natural history of lumbosacral plexopathy in cancer. Neurology. 1985;35(1):8-15.
5. Lawson VH, Arnold WD. Multifocal motor neuropathy: a review of pathogenesis, diagnosis, and treatment. Neuropsychiatr Dis Treat. 2014;10:567-76.
6. Sawal N. The iced drink test—A bedside test for diagnosis of bulbar myasthenia. J Neurol Disord. 2007;5:333.
7. Engel AG. Why does acetylcholine exacerbate myasthenia caused by anti-MuSK antibodies? J Physiol. 2013;591(10):2377.
8. Khadilkar SV, Singh RK. Hip abduction sign: A new clinical sign in sarcoglycanopathies. J Clin Neuromusc Dis. 2001;3(1):13-5.
9. Pradhan S. Diamond on quadriceps: A frequent sign in dysferlinopathy. Neurology. 2008;70(4):322.
10. Verhaert D, Richards K, Rafael-Fortney JA, Raman SV. Cardiac involvement in patients with muscular dystrophies: magnetic resonance imaging phenotype and genotypic considerations. Circ Cardiovasc Imaging. 2011;4(1):67-76.
11. Tarnopolsky MA. Myopathies related to glycogen metabolism disorders. Neurotherapeutics. 2018;15(4):915-27.
12. Schmidt J. Current classification and management of inflammatory myopathies. J Neuromuscul Dis. 2018;5(2):109-29.
13. Parikh S, Goldstein A, Koenig MK, Scaglia F, Enns GM, Saneto R, et al. Diagnosis and management of mitochondrial disease: a consensus statement from the Mitochondrial Medicine Society. Genet Med. 2015;17(9):689-701.
14. Uncini A, Kuwabara S. Nodopathies of the peripheral nerve: an emerging concept. J Neurol Neurosurg Psychiatry. 2015;86(11):1186-95.

44

CHAPTER

Approach to Muscle Pain and Cramps

Swati H Shah

INTRODUCTION

Myalgia, defined as any pain perceived in muscle, is a very common complaint encountered in clinical practice. The incidence of myalgia in the general population is estimated to be about 10%.[1] Patients use various descriptive terms to describe pain such as aching, burning, soreness, tightness, stiffness, tenderness, or spasms. Myalgia is rarely due to primary muscle disease rather pain is frequently referred from ligaments, joints, bones, and the peripheral and central nervous system. The neurological examination in these patients is usually normal making a specific diagnosis difficult. However, myalgia can be successfully evaluated and treated in many instances with judicious use of history, clinical examination, and laboratory tests.

A muscle cramp is a sudden, involuntary, painful contraction of skeletal muscle or part of it and is often associated with a visible, palpable hardness of the muscle. It is clinically characterized by rapid or abrupt onset, acute pain triggered by trivial movement or forceful contraction, and relieved by passive stretching or counters contraction of agonist. There may be persistent soreness of affected muscle lasting 2–3 days and elevation in creatine kinase (CK). Postcramp pain and elevation in CK suggest that contraction of muscle during cramp was excessive and has caused some local injury to a muscle, or hypoxic/metabolic damage.[2] Commonly affected muscles are calf and foot muscles followed by hamstring and quadriceps. Contractures are clinically indistinguishable from cramps but are related to glucose or glycogen metabolism defects and can be differentiated from a cramp by electromyography (EMG). Cramps appear as irregular, high frequency, repetitive discharges of normal appearing motor units which increase and subside slowly on EMG. Contracture, on the other hand, is electrically silent. Cramps may occur in healthy individuals during sleep, pregnancy, with strenuous exercise or in subjects with nervous and metabolic disorders, inherited syndromes, or acute extracellular volume depletion. Dehydration and/or electrolyte imbalance is the presumed cause of cramps during or immediately after physical exertion. Data from animal studies have now shown that exercise-associated muscle cramps are caused by abnormal α motor neuron activity caused by aberrant control at the spinal level.[2,3] Increased excitatory and decreased inhibitory input to motor neurons during exercise, leading to sustained motoneuron activity, enhanced by supraspinal projections to motoneurons may trigger cramps in most exercised muscles. This mechanism also explains cramps associated with increased motoneuron excitability seen in pregnancy, hemodialysis, amyotrophic lateral sclerosis, post-polio syndrome, and certain metabolic disorders like hypothyroidism. The main risk factors for exercise-associated muscle cramps include a family history of cramping, previous occurrence of cramping with exercise, increased exercise intensity and duration, and inadequate conditioning for the exercise.[4] The lifetime prevalence of cramps in athletes and sedentary healthy subjects (aged 65 years or older) is as high as 30–50%.[4]

CHARACTERIZATION OF MYALGIA AND MUSCLE CRAMPS

Myalgia (Box 1)

Myalgia is classified in relation to activity and whether symptoms are focal or generalized. Myalgia at rest, especially in absence of weakness, is unlikely due to primary muscle disease. Acute exertion or strenuous exercise is the most common cause of muscle pain in healthy individuals. It is acute, localized, caused by muscle ischemia or accumulation of metabolites and resolves on completion of the activity. Postexertional pain results from eccentric contractions, caused by uneven muscle tension which can lead to microtears and edema.[5] Myalgia associated with primary myopathies is usually exertional. Muscle pain can also result from repetitive use of muscle most often related to occupation, referred to as overuse syndrome. This is

BOX 1 Causes of myalgia.

- Trauma
- Ischemia
- Muscle use/overuse
- Idiopathic
- *Inflammatory and immune disorders:*
  - Infection
    - Viral (influenza, CMV, HIV, coxsackie B virus, Epstein–Barr virus)
    - Bacterial (pyomyositis)
    - Fungal
    - Parasitic (trichinosis, toxoplasmosis, and cysticercosis)
  - Inflammatory/infiltrative myopathies associated with myalgia
    - Dermatomyositis/polymyositis/antisynthetase syndrome
    - Sarcoidosis
    - Eosinophilic myositis
    - Focal nodular myositis
  - Connective tissue disorders
    - Rheumatoid arthritis
    - Progressive system sclerosis
    - Systemic lupus erythematosus
    - Vasculitis
    - Sjögren's syndrome
  - Polymyalgia rheumatica
  - Primary fibromyalgia
  - Chronic myalgia/fatigue syndrome
  - Postviral
- *Metabolic and endocrine:*
  - Hypothyroid
  - Hypoparathyroidism
  - Hypoadrenalism
  - Osteomalacia
  - Liver failure
  - Uremia
  - Hemodialysis
  - Magnesium deficiency
  - Selenium deficiency
  - Thiamine deficiency
- *Neurologic:*
  - Myopathy
  - Neuropathy
  - Motor neuron disorder
  - Central nervous system
  - Psychiatric
- *Drugs and substances:*
  - Statins and fibrates
  - Cyclosporin
  - Zidovudine
  - Retinoids
  - Colchicine
  - D-penicillamine, gold
  - Interferon-α
  - Antimalarial drugs

Continued

Continued

  - Tumor necrosis factor α inhibitors
  - Labetalol
  - L-tryptophan
  - Captopril and enalapril
  - Lithium
  - Salbutamol
  - Cimetidine
  - Vincristine
  - Alcohol
  - Cocaine, heroin, amphetamine, and phencyclidine
  - Animal venom: tetanus toxoid, and strychnine
  - Related to hypokalemia: Diuretics, licorice (glycyrrhizinic acid), carbenoxolone, and amphotericin B

(CMV: cytomegalovirus; HIV: human immunodeficiency virus)

common in people playing a musical instrument, typing, thumb usage in mobile phone users, and so on. The chronic repetitive movement results in spasms of involved muscles which can be painful and sometimes associated with muscle weakness and swelling. These spasms are considered a form of focal dystonia and are of central origin.[5,6]

Idiopathic Leg Aches in Children

Approximately 20% of children experience recurrent leg pain, referred to as "growing pains".[4,7] These pains are benign, usually localized to the anterior thigh, posterior knee, and calves. They tend to occur in the late evening and night and disappear in the morning. There is no consistent relationship with activity. Neurological examination and blood investigations are typically normal.

Inflammatory and Immune Disorders

Muscle pain is a common manifestation of inflammatory or immune-mediated disorders. Most people have experienced myalgia in association with influenza or some other viral illness. This is usually benign but occasionally may be associated with severe muscle weakness as in cases of chikungunya, dengue, or West Nile virus.[5,8] Myalgia and/or myositis can also be seen with retroviral illness or as complications of the therapy (zidovudine). Human immunodeficiency virus (HIV)-associated myopathy is clinically and pathologically similar to autoimmune myositis seen in HIV-negative patients. It can occur at any stage of HIV disease, and is characterized by slowly progressive weakness symmetrically affecting the proximal muscles. Myalgias are often present. Myalgia is prominent in acute suppurative myositis usually secondary to staphylococcal or streptococcal or with disseminated fungal infection.[5,8] Parasitic infections such as toxoplasmosis, cysticercosis, and trichinosis are also commonly associated with myalgia.[5,8]

Muscle pain can be prominent in idiopathic inflammatory muscle disorders like polymyositis (PM), dermatomyositis (DM), and antisynthetase syndrome-overlap myositis in particular, due to the involvement of fascia.[5,8-10] Pain may be generalized or focal with muscle tenderness. It is present at rest and aggravated by movement and exercise. In these patients, myalgia is accompanied by objective muscle weakness, elevated serum CK, myopathic findings on EMG, and the presence of inflammatory infiltrates of T-cells, and macrophages primarily in the endomysial parenchyma on muscle biopsy. Patients with connective tissue disorder may have myalgia in absence of true PM/DM.

Polymyalgia rheumatica is a cause of myalgia in the elderly. Typically, elderly women present with bilateral aching and stiffness persisting for ≥1 month, involving two of the following: Neck or torso, shoulders or proximal regions of the arms, and hips or proximal areas of the thighs.[11] Systemic symptoms like anorexia, weight loss, and low-grade fever are common. ESR is invariably elevated but the muscle strength, CK, and EMG are normal; helping it differentiates from PM. The 50% of cases are associated with giant cell arteritis.

Primary fibromyalgia is now accepted as a distinct relatively common syndrome. Patients with fibromyalgia present with widespread musculoskeletal pain as well as a variety of symptoms including fatigue, cognitive dysfunction, sleep difficulties, irritable bowel, stiffness, anxiety, and depressed mood. A diagnosis of fibromyalgia requires widespread pain to be present for at least 3 months in absence of a disorder that would otherwise explain the pain.[5,12,13] Systemic and rheumatic diseases need to be ruled out by a detailed history, physical examination, and laboratory investigations. Fibromyalgia is more common in women <50 years of age with a chronic, nonprogressive course.

Psychogenic myalgia may be difficult to differentiate from fibromyalgia. Features supporting psychogenic myalgia are a bizarre description of symptoms, varying sites of discomfort, lack of modulating factors, lack of diurnal variation, overreaction to physical examination, and no response to medication or physical therapy.

Another similar entity is chronic myalgia/fatigue syndrome or postviral fatigue syndrome. A history of acute viral illness is often but not always present. The course may be constant or may have periodic remissions and exacerbations. Tender points typical of fibromyalgia are not seen. Although diffuse muscle tenderness may be present. Routine neurological examination, laboratory tests, EMG, and muscle biopsy are normal. In one patient with postvaricella myalgia/fatigue syndrome, excessive intracellular acidosis was documented on ^{31}P nuclear magnetic resonance spectroscopy.[5] Total 28 out of 40 patients with postviral myalgia/fatigue syndrome had increased jitter on single fiber EMG suggesting muscle membrane abnormality.[5]

Metabolic

Enzyme Defects

McArdle's disease (muscle phosphorylase deficiency) is the most well-known disorder of carbohydrate metabolism associated with exertional myalgia.[5,14] Typical history consists of childhood onset, exercise intolerance with exertional myalgia and cramps associated with high-intensity anaerobic exercise. The CK levels are elevated at rest (>1,000 U/I). About 50% of patients experience episodes of exertional muscle necrosis with myoglobinuria. Two key differentiating features are the development of contractures and the second wind phenomenon. Patients describe that they can continue the same level of exercise without the degree of fatigue that they noticed initially after 6–8 minutes of sustained low or moderate-intensity exercise. This happens due to the increased availability of extramuscular fuels, blood glucose, and free fatty acids. Inheritance is autosomal recessive. In the forearm exercise test, there is no rise in lactate and little or no phosphorylase activity in muscle biopsy studies. Muscle biopsy should be avoided within the month of rhabdomyolysis as regenerating fibers can express nonspecific isoforms of the enzyme leading to false-negative results. Other defects in carbohydrate metabolism such as phosphofructokinase, phosphoglycerate kinase, phosphoglycerate mutase, and lactate dehydrogenase are uncommon but may have a similar presentation. Diagnosis is based on biochemical demonstration of a specific enzyme defect.

Carnitine palmitoyltransferase II (CPT II) deficiency is autosomal recessive and the most common cause of recurrent myoglobinuria induced by intense or prolonged exertion, infection, fasting, cold weather, and rarely emotional stress.[5,14] There is associated exertional myalgia and muscle stiffness but no true cramps. Neurological examination and CK are usually normal between the attacks, and there is a normal rise in lactate on exercise testing. Routine muscle biopsy is usually normal and diagnosis is based on biochemical demonstration of decreased CPT activity or genetic testing of the *CPT2* gene (chromosome 1p32) with *p.S113L* mutant allele in 65–95% of cases. Other lipid metabolism disorders like primary or secondary carnitine deficiency may also be associated with exertional myalgia, myoglobinuria, and progressive muscle weakness. Muscle biopsy shows lipid accumulation.

Patients with myoadenylate deaminase deficiency (MAD) may also develop exertional myalgia and fatigue. It is the most common enzyme deficiency in muscle, noted in 1–2% of muscle biopsies.[5,14] The neurological examination is typically normal. CK might be mildly elevated and EMG may reveal minor nonspecific abnormalities. Patients with MAD deficiency show a lack of rise in ammonia on the forearm exercise test as MAD is involved in ammonia production through adenine monophosphate metabolism. The relationship between a MAD deficiency and exertional myalgia is controversial as many patients with MAD deficiency are asymptomatic.

Defects in the mitochondrial respiratory chain, especially NADH-coenzyme Q reductase (complex I) deficiency can also be associated with exertional myalgia and weakness. Mitochondrial disorders are heterogeneous with onset early in childhood and usually have associated features such as ataxia, ophthalmoparesis, dementia, and areflexia.

Endocrine Disorders

Muscle pain, stiffness, and cramps are commonly observed in hypothyroidism. Most patients with hypothyroidism have mild elevation in CK and myopathic features on needle EMG in proximal muscles. Occasionally, a more profound myopathy may be present. Myxedema, myoedema on percussion, delayed tendon reflexes, dry skin, constipation, weight gain, and bradycardia are some other features of hypothyroidism.[5,15] Myalgia can also be associated with thyrotoxic myopathy.

Cramps and muscle pain may also occur in 50% of patients with hypoadrenalism.[5,15] Weakness and pain, usually of bone origin are common in osteomalacia. Hypocalcemia associated with hypothyroidism leads to tetany and painful spasms.[5,15] Myalgia and muscle stiffness are also present in panhypopituitarism.

Mineral and Electrolyte Disorders

Chronic hypokalemia is associated with weakness, fatigability, myalgia, and cramps.[5,16] Conditions related to hypokalemia include metabolic acidosis, diuretic therapy, laxative abuse, diarrhea, hyperaldosteronism, and licorice ingestion. Acute severe hypokalemia is associated with more fulminant myopathy, myalgia, elevated CK, and rhabdomyolysis. Hypocalcemia results in tetany which is associated with painful muscle spasms. Alkalosis from any cause including hyperventilation leads to increased serum calcium binding and a decrease in serum ionized calcium with resultant hypocalcemia and tetany. Tetany and spasm are also associated with hypomagnesemia. Additional features of hypomagnesemia include weakness, tremor, myoclonus, exaggerated startle response, and hyperreflexia. Chronic hypophosphatemia can cause acute painful myopathy. Acute hyponatremia caused by free water replenishment after strenuous exertion or profuse sweating may cause cramps.

Drugs and Toxins

Many drugs and toxins produce muscle pain and are associated with myopathy.[5] The myopathy can be acute or subacute, proximal or generalized and may involve muscle necrosis. Chronic alcohol use can lead to painful, acute necrotizing, or chronic myopathy. These patients may develop myopathy in relation to hypokalemia and/or hypophosphatemia. Vincristine is associated with painful proximal myopathy; heroin and phencyclidine cause painful necrotizing myopathy and penicillamine, PM. Drug hypersensitivity reactions related to drugs like trazodone can have prominent myalgia with fever, rash, and elevated CK. Snake and spider venom can produce painful spams, cramps, and muscle pains. Tetanus toxin and strychnine poisoning may also result in cramps.

Neurologic Disorders

Myopathy

Muscle pain is not a common feature of muscular dystrophy with exception of limb girdle muscular dystrophy 2I (LGMD2I), LGMD 2B, LGMD 2L, and myotonic dystrophy 2.[5,17,18] Exertional and postexertional muscle pain and cramps have been described in young patients with Becker muscular dystrophy. Painful muscle contraction has also been reported in some individuals with myotonia congenita. Patients with chronic muscle pain and cramps and with no objective clinical or laboratory abnormalities have nonspecific abnormalities on muscle biopsy like tubular aggregates, internalized capillaries, and type 2 fiber predominance.

Two large retrospective muscle biopsy reviews have shown the presence of tubular aggregates in 1% of biopsy specimens.[5] Half of these patients with tubular aggregates had severe myalgia with a normal neurological examination. Patients were predominantly male with normal serum CK, EMG, ischemic exercise test, and responses to serum potassium manipulation. In addition, autosomal dominant families with the tubular aggregate-myalgia syndrome have been described.

Rippling muscle disease (RMD) is a myopathy characterized by transitory local muscle molding and involuntary rolling movements of the muscles after stretching or percussion.[19] EMG during these abnormal movements is "electrically silent" without any motor unit potentials or myotonic discharges suggesting hyperexcitability of the muscles. CKs are consistently elevated. Mutation in caveolin 3 (*CAV3*) gene has been implicated in pathophysiology of RMD. Persistent muscle cramps disturb the quality of life of these patients.

Neuropathy

Muscle pain is associated with neuropathies like brachial neuritis, diabetic amyotrophy, chronic inflammatory polyneuropathy, and acute intermittent porphyria.

Isaacs syndrome also referred to as acquired neuromyotonia is a peripheral nerve hyperexcitability syndrome characterized by involuntary, continuous motor overactivity.[20] Clinical features include muscle cramps, fasciculations, myokymia (undulating, wavelike movement visible on the muscle surface), and pseudomyotonia (slow relaxation after voluntary contraction). Nerve conduction studies demonstrate characteristic afterdischarges, and needle EMG shows various forms of abnormal spontaneous activity including fasciculation potentials, myokymic discharges, and neuromyotonic discharges. Classic Isaacs syndrome is an autoimmune disorder characterized by continuous muscle twitching, muscle hypertrophy, hyperhidrosis, and weight loss. Strength and tendon reflexes are usually normal. It is more common in men and the average age of onset is the mid-40s. Voltage-gated potassium channels (VGKCs) play an important role in the pathophysiology of Isaacs syndrome. In addition to the peripheral and autonomic nervous systems, VGKCs are present in the central nervous system as well. Neuronal hyperexcitability in the central nervous system results in related disorders, Morvan syndrome, and limbic encephalitis.

Autoantibodies to VGKCs are seen in 38–50% of patients with Isaacs syndrome. The antibodies are directed against leucine-rich glioma-inactivated protein 1 (LGI1) and contactin-associated protein-2 (CASPR2). LGI1 expression is very weak in peripheral nerves and antibodies to LGI1 are not seen in Isaacs syndrome. Isaacs syndrome is associated with various other autoimmune disorders such as myasthenia gravis, thymoma, Addison disease, Hashimoto thyroiditis, vitamin B12 deficiency, celiac disease, and connective tissue disorders. There is also an association with malignancies including thymoma, lung cancer, Hodgkin's lymphoma, plasmacytoma, lymphoblastic lymphoma, hemangioblastoma, and ovarian and bladder cancer. Tumor antigens trigger immune responses that generate antibodies that cross-react with neuronal voltage-gated ion channels. CASPR2 antibodies in particular have a strong paraneoplastic association.

Motor Neuron Disorders

Cramps are common in amyotrophic lateral sclerosis. Other clinical features include progressive muscle weakness, atrophy, fasciculations, signs of ongoing denervation, and chronic reinnervation on EMG and muscle biopsy. Although cramps are a feared symptom of motor neuron disorder; the majority of patients with chronic cramps and/or fasciculations do not have weakness and atrophy or evidence of denervation on EMG. The majority of these patients have benign cramp-fasciculation syndrome which is characterized by muscle twitching, muscle cramps, and exercise intolerance. Electrodiagnostic studies may show after discharges on repetitive nerve stimulation and fasciculations will be evident on needle EMG. One reported case of benign cramp and fasciculation did progress after many years and went on to develop severe motor neuron disorder with weakness, atrophy, and denervation.[5,21]

Central Nervous System

Some central nervous system disorders may also be associated with muscle pain and cramps. Patients with multiple sclerosis can develop paroxysmal, painful tonic muscle spasms, and dystonic posturing. Stiff-person syndrome is characterized by episodic axial rigidity and stiffness followed by generalized symmetric continuous muscular stiffness with superimposed stimulus triggered painful muscular spasms. The hyperexcitability is central in origin due to antibodies to GAD. EMG shows continuous firing of relatively normal motor unit potentials. Neuromyotonic discharges and myokymic discharges are not seen. Sleep and neuromuscular blocking agents abolish the stiffness and spasms.[5] Patients with Morvan syndrome have findings similar to Isaacs syndrome, but have encephalopathy, headache, drowsiness, and hallucinations in addition to peripheral nerve hyperexcitability.

Cramps (Box 2)

Nocturnal or Resting Cramps

Occasional nocturnal cramps are common in otherwise healthy individuals, especially the elderly. They may occur in association with pregnancy, electrolyte imbalance, or after strenuous exercise.

BOX 2 Classification of cramps.

- *Idiopathic*: Ordinary cramps; nocturnal/resting
- Exercise-induced cramps (mainly leg muscles)
- Pregnancy
- *Congenital*:
  - Metabolic myopathy:
    - McArdle's disease
    - Carnitine palmitoyltransferase II (CPT II) deficiency
    - Mitochondrial myopathy
  - Rippling muscle disease
  - Myotonic dystrophy type 2
  - Dystrophinopathies
  - Autosomal dominant cramping disease
- *Occupational (focal dystonias)*: Muscle cramps in writers, musicians, miners, and athletes
- *Neoplasms*: Neoplastic peripheral nerve invasion
- *Endocrine-metabolic diseases*:
  - Hypohyperthyroidism
  - Hypohyperparathyroidism
  - Hypoadrenalism
  - Diabetes mellitus
  - Uremia
  - Cirrhosis
- *Hydroelectrolyte disorders*: Fluid and electrolyte disturbance (including hemodialysis-induced cramps)
  - Hypoglycemia
  - Hypohypernatremia
  - Hypohypercalcemia (parathyroid disease)
  - Hypomagnesemia
  - Hypohyperkalemia
  - Hyperventilation, respiratory alkalosis (transient fall in free Ca^{+})
  - Dehydration and heat cramp
- *Toxicity or poisoning:*
  - Strychnine poisoning
  - Lead toxicity
  - Tetanus
  - Black widow (spider) bite
  - Snake
- *Vascular disease:*
  - Peripheral vascular disease (claudication)
  - Varicose leg veins

Continued

Continued

- *Central and peripheral nervous system diseases:*
  - Motor neuron disease
  - Post-polio syndrome
  - Kennedy disease
  - Cramp-fasciculation syndrome
  - Neuralgic amyotrophy
  - Radiculopathy
  - Peripheral neuropathy
  - Isaac's syndrome
  - Satoyoshi syndrome
  - Stiff person syndrome
  - Multiple sclerosis
  - Parkinson's disease
- *Drugs*:
  - Statins
  - Calcium channel blockers: Nifedipine
  - Antiarrhythmics
  - B-adrenergic agonists
  - Chemotherapeutic agents
  - Depolarizing muscle relaxants: Suxamethonium
  - Cyclosporin
  - Cimetidine
  - Lithium carbonate
  - Salbutamol
  - Gold therapy
  - Terbutaline
  - Ethanol
  - *Fibrates*: Clofibrate
  - D-penicillamine
  - Nicotinic acid
  - Diuretics
  - Morphine
  - Phenothiazines

Symptomatic Cramps

Symptomatic cramps can be seen in disorders of the central (e.g., Parkinson's disease) and peripheral (amyotrophic lateral sclerosis) nervous system. Cramps are common in patients with peripheral neuropathies, including uremia, diabetic, chemotherapy-induced, inherited polyneuropathies, and radiculopathy.[2,22] Exercise-induced cramps are the hallmark of metabolic myopathies. Cramps are also common in patients with arterial or venous insufficiency of the lower extremity. Electrolyte imbalance, in particular low ionizable serum magnesium and calcium levels, produces severe cramps (i.e., tetany) and involuntary contractions of hands and feet (carpopedal spasm). Tetany is a state of nervous system hypersensitivity and cramps are attributed to unstable axonal depolarization. Similarly, hypokalemia related to diuretic use or low sodium may also cause cramps. Patients requiring hemodialysis present with cramps from hypo-osmolarity or extracellular volume depletion. Heat cramps develop after prolonged exertion in hot and humid conditions. Etiology is likely sweating-induced hyponatremia or osmotic shift secondary to fluid replacement.[2,22]

Medical conditions such as liver cirrhosis, uremia and severe malnutrition, hypothyroidism, and diabetes mellitus can be associated with exercise intolerance and cramps. A wide spectrum of drugs are associated with cramps. One should always inquire about the use of lipid lower agents (statins, clofibrate, fenofibrate, and bezafibrate); antihypertensives (diuretics, β-blockers, calcium channel blockers, and angiotensin-converting enzyme inhibitors), β-agonists (terbutaline and salbutamol), insulin, oral contraceptives, alcohol, and creatine.[2,22] Statin-associated myotoxicity, with myalgia, cramp, or weakness has been reported in 7–29% of patients taking statin.[2]

EVALUATION OF MYALGIA AND CRAMPS (BOX 3)

A comprehensive history enlisting the nature of pain, frequency, distribution, severity, aggravating factors, and associated conditions is the single most cost-effective measure in the evaluation of myalgia. Routine blood investigations complete blood count, serum creatine, liver profile, CK, erythrocyte sedimentation rate (ESR), and other tests like electrolytes including plasma calcium, magnesium and phosphorus, rheumatoid factor, antinuclear factor, thyroxine, and fasting lipids are ordered where indicated. Several decades ago, one prospective study showed the usefulness of CPK level and ESR in deciding to proceed with EMG and muscle biopsy in patients with chronic muscle pain.[23] In this study, patients lacking specific abnormality of testing were more likely to have pain for >10 years, widespread in nature with elaborate or histrionic descriptions. Also, in this group of patients, associated swelling of painful muscles was common. The relationship between pain to exercise or lack of physical signs was not good predictors of the need for further investigation.

It is important to establish if there is associated muscle weakness with pain. Muscle strength can be quantified using the strain gauge method, isokinetic dynamometry, or hand-held dynamometer. For routine clinical practice, medical research council (MRC) scale for grading muscle strength can be used to establish the presence of weakness and follow the progression over time.

The nonischemic forearm exercise test is a sensitive and specific screening tool for disorders of carbohydrate carbohydrate metabolism and myoadenylate deaminase (MADA) deficiency. After securing venous access, the patient is asked to strenuously open and close the hand for 1 minute. Blood samples are drawn before exercise and at 1-, 2-, 4- and 6-minute postexercise to check ammonia, lactate, and pyruvate levels. In most glycogen storage disorders (GSDs), there is a rise in ammonia levels which serves as a control to ensure adequate exercise, but there is

BOX 3 Evaluation of myalgia.

- History
- Physical and neurological examination
- *Laboratory*:
  - *Serum*: ESR, CRP, CK, electrolytes, calcium, magnesium, phosphorus, urea, creatine, liver profile, complete blood count, RF, antinuclear antibody, thyroid function, parathyroid, cortisol, and myoglobin
  - *Urine*: Myoglobin and drug screen
  - Resting lactate (respiratory chain defect)
  - Dry blood spot or acid maltase in leukocytes for GSD II
  - Fasting acylcarnitine blood spot profile (fatty acid oxidation defects)
  - CPT II in leukocytes and cultured fibroblasts (CPT II deficiency)
  - Genetic screening for common mutations of suspected myopathy
- *Procedures*:
  - EMG, nerve conduction studies
  - Muscle strength and exercise tests
  - Nonischemic forearm exercise test (glycolytic enzyme defects)
  - Magnetic resonance imaging (local and diffuse inflammatory myopathies)
  - Muscle biopsy

(CK: creatine kinase; CRP: C-reactive protein; CPT: carnitine palmitoyltransferase; GSD: glycogen storage disorder; EMG: electromyography; ESR: erythrocyte sedimentation rate; RF: rheumatoid factor)

no or minimal rise in lactate and pyruvate levels. A rise in lactate but not ammonia is diagnostic of MADA deficiency. In a normal individual, all three parameters rise three to four times above the baseline value.

Electromyography and nerve conduction studies are an extension of history taking and clinical examination especially in patients with abnormalities on examination or elevated CKs. They help in evaluating for the presence of myopathy, neuropathy, or motor neuron disorder. Special investigative procedures like single fiber EMG can be considered for further evaluation of myopathic disorders.

Muscle biopsy is the definitive procedure in patients with chronic myalgia. The European Federation of Neurological Societies Task Force review on the role of muscle biopsy in the investigation of myalgia concluded that a muscle biopsy is more likely to be diagnostically useful if myalgia is exertional and if one or more of the following apply—(A) there is myoglobinuria, (2) there is second wind phenomenon, (3) there is muscle weakness, (4) there is muscle hypertrophy/atrophy, (5) there is hyperCKemia (>2–3 X normal), and (6) there is myopathic EMG.[18] In a prospective study, 180 consecutive patients ≥18 years of age with chronic isolated myalgia (chronic diffuse muscle pain lasting >1 year) were evaluated with EMG and muscle biopsy.[24] The notable result of this study was that EMG is an excellent screening tool for the diagnosis of muscle disease in clinically normal patients with chronic diffuse muscle pain. In this study, EMG was normal in 178 of the 180 patients who turned out to have no muscle disease and abnormal in two patients with the genetic myotonic disorder; myotonic dystrophy type 2 and SCN4A-related channelopathy. Patients with DM2 and muscle channelopathies may present with isolated myalgia with minimum or absent myotonic discharges on EMG and normal muscle pathology. In another study, DM2 screening was performed in 63 patients with chronic myalgia and was found to be positive in 2 (3.2%).[24] In a prospective study of 109 patients with muscle pain, 103 underwent quadriceps muscle needle biopsy. Tissue abnormalities were found in 49; 34 with specific diagnosis and 15 with nonspecific changes.[23] The investigators of this study found muscle biopsy to be very sensitive and specific in establishing a diagnosis. Complete evaluation of muscle biopsy in patients with myalgia involves a variety of frozen section stains, electron microscopy for ultrastructural changes, and tests of mitochondrial function.

In patients presenting with recurrent cramps, the role of the clinician is to establish if the subject has exercise-induced cramps or an associated medication condition. History should focus on triggering factors, family history of cramps, drug use, and presence of myoglobinuria. A complete physical examination including detailed orthopedic, and neurological assessments should be carried out. Particular attention should be paid to muscle atrophy and weakness which may suggest underlying motor neuron loss. Laboratory tests including complete blood count, serum electrolytes, CK, and thyroid-stimulating hormone should be checked and when needed, imaging studies like magnetic resonance imaging can be done to evaluate for degenerative disk disease.

TREATMENT

Irrespective of the specific diagnosis, patients with chronic myalgia require symptomatic relief. A variety of treatment options are available, most not based on controlled trials. Nonpharmacological treatments can also be useful.

Treatment of leg cramps can be difficult. For mild cramps, a trial of stretching exercises can be prescribed. Gentle motion, like standing or walking may relieve the shortened muscle position and relieve cramp.[2,5,22] Massage is extremely helpful. Another simple technique that can be beneficial is elevating the foot end of the bed by approximately 9 inches. This prevents venous stasis and accumulation of metabolites responsible for nocturnal cramps. The application of heat, ice, mechanical vibration, and transcutaneous electrical stimulation is also beneficial in the treatment of cramps and chronic muscle pain. Cold spray or ice reduces motor neuron activity by reflex inhibition. Acupuncture stimulates small afferent myelinated fibers to the spinal cord which releases opioids and other neurotransmitters such as serotonin, noradrenaline, and γ-aminobutyric acid, which in turn modifies the efferent motor neuron activity. Transcutaneous nerve stimulation over the dermatome, at a low frequency of 15–30 Hz stimulation can relieve the cramps.

Quinine is considered traditional therapy for the treatment of cramps. However, in 1987 a double-blind, placebo-controlled crossover trial of quinine bisulfate at a 300 mg dose in 22 patients with leg cramps failed to show any significant reduction in cramp frequency or severity.[22] Similarly, in 1986, Lim reported the ineffectiveness of quinine in relieving leg cramps in 25 patients.[22] A Cochrane review of quinine in patients with various causes of cramps found moderate evidence that quinine was safe and effective.[25] Quinine increases the muscle refractory period and reduces the excitability of the muscle end plate. Quinine may rarely cause cinchonism; presenting with nausea, vomiting, tinnitus, and blurred vision. It may progress to deafness, optic atrophy, severe gastrointestinal symptoms, renal failure, cardiac arrhythmias, and death. Quinine is contraindicated in pregnant women due to its abortifacient action and fetal damage. There is a risk of interaction with other drugs via CYP3A4 and CYP450-isoenzymes. As per American Academy of Neurology recommendations, quinine may be used as a last resort in the management of cramps.[26]

Roca and coworkers reported vitamin E to be effective in controlling leg cramps in dialysis patients based on a small, randomized, double-blind study.[22] Ayers and Mihan also found vitamin E to be helpful in 82% of their patients.[22]

Sodium channel blocking drugs, e.g., phenytoin, carbamazepine, or mexiletine are sometimes prescribed based on a few case reports. A small open-label pilot study of levetiracetam for cramps and spasticity in patients with amyotrophic lateral sclerosis (ALS) found a significant reduction in cramp severity and frequency, on initiation of levetiracetam.[27] In addition, there was a reduction in phasic but not tonic spasticity. Another small randomized, double-blind cross-over study of mexiletine 150 mg twice daily in 20 patients with ALS provided a weak beneficial effect of mexiletine.[28] Average cramp reduction, based on t tests, was 1.8 cramps per day (a reduction from 5.3 with placebo to 3.5 with mexiletine).

Resting or exertional myalgias can be treated with nonsteroidal anti-inflammatory agents. Calcium channel blockers like verapamil and nifedipine are a good choice for idiopathic exertional myalgias. In a double-blind, placebo-controlled, crossover study of eight patients with exertional myalgia, four patients had a partial response with 240 mg of verapamil daily after 6 weeks of therapy.[5]

Treatment of myalgia associated with specific disorders requires treatment of the underlying disease. For example, myalgia associated with PM responds to treatment with steroids. Occupational overuse syndromes respond to rest and avoidance of precipitating tasks. Treatment of fibromyalgia is more complicated and requires a holistic approach with reassurance, pain management, antidepressants, graded physical therapy, and intervention procedures like Botox or local anesthetic injection to painful spots. Alternative therapies like acupressure or acupuncture can also be beneficial in these patients. Special diets can be prescribed to patients with specific enzyme defects like myophosphorylase and CPT deficiency. Valproic acid, phenytoin, or carbamazepine can be beneficial in patients with continuous muscle fiber activity.

CONCLUSION

Muscle pain is a prominent symptom in a wide variety of conditions. A targeted approach for the investigation of these patients is needed. Despite exhaustive investigation in a large portion of these patients, no definite cause is found. Many of them may have a depressive state with myalgia as a prominent symptom. However, a significant number of these patients have abnormalities of muscle structure or function. Their muscles are likely sensitive to damage or they have a specific metabolic disorder that remains to be identified. Given the persistence of symptoms and credibility of patient's complaints, investigations with a high specificity like CK and EMG should be used as screening tests in the first place. If these initial tests are abnormal, then more sensitive tests like muscle biopsy or enzyme assays should be done.

REFERENCES

1. Wolfe F, Ross K, Anderson J, Russell IJ, Hebert L. The prevalence and characteristics of fibromyalgia in the general population. Arthritis Rheum. 1995;38:19-28.
2. Swash M, Czesnik D, de Carvalho M. Muscular cramp: causes and management. Eur J Neurol. 2019;26(2):214-21.
3. Maquirriain J, Merello M. The athlete with muscular cramps: clinical approach. J Am Acad Orthop Surg. 2007;15(7):425-31.
4. Minetto MA, Holobar A, Botter A, Farina D . Origin and development of muscle cramps. Exerc Sport Sci Rev. 2013;41(1):3-10.
5. Roy EP, Gutmann L. Myalgia. Neurol Clin. 1988;6(3):621-36.
6. Sheehy MP, Marsden CD. Writer's cramp-a focal dystonia. Brain. 1982;105(Pt 3):461-80.
7. Peterson HA. Leg aches. Pediatr Clin North Am. 1977;24(4):731-6.
8. Mastaglia FL, Ojeda VJ. Inflammatory myopathies: Part 1. Ann Neurol. 1985;17(3):215-27.
9. Mastaglia FL, Ojeda VJ. Inflammatory myopathies: Part 2. Ann Neurol. 1985;17(4):317-23.
10. Marco JL, Collins BF. Clinical manifestations and treatment of antisynthetase syndrome. Best Pract Res Clin Rheumatol. 2020;34(4):101503.
11. Salvarani C, Macchioni P, Boiardi L. Polymyalgia rheumatica. Lancet. 1997;350(9070):43-7.
12. Arnold LM, Gebke KB, Choy EH. Fibromyalgia: management strategies for primary care providers. Int J Clin Pract. 2016;70(2):99-112.
13. Wolfe F, Clauw DJ, Fitzcharles MA, Goldenberg DL, Katz RS, Mease P, et al. The American College of Rheumatology preliminary diagnostic criteria for fibromyalgia and measurement of symptom severity. Arthritis Care Res (Hoboken). 2010;62(5):600-10.

14. Adler M, Shieh PB. Metabolic myopathies. Semin Neurol. 2015;35(4): 385-97.
15. Ruff RL. Endocrine Myopathies (Hyper- and Hypofunction of Adrenal, Thyroid, Pituitary, and Parathyroid Glands and latrogenic Steroid Myopathy). In: Engel AG, Banker BQ (eds): Myology. New York: McGraw Hill; 1986. pp. 1871-906.
16. Corbett AJ. Electrolyte disorders affecting muscle. Sem Neurology. 1983;3:248-57.
17. Quinlivan R, Jungbluth H. Myopathic causes of exercise intolerance with rhabdomyolysis. Dev Med Child Neurol. 2012;54(10):886-91.
18. Kyriakides T, Angelini C, Schaefer J, Mongini T, Siciliano G, Sacconi S, et al. EFNS review on the role of muscle biopsy in the investigation of myalgia. Eur J Neurol. 2013;20(7):997-1005.
19. Arimura K. Rippling muscle syndrome. Intern Med. 2002;41(5): 325-6.
20. Ahmed A, Simmons Z. Isaacs syndrome: A review. Muscle Nerve. 2015;52(1):5-12.
21. Fleet WS, Watson RT. From benign fasciculations and cramps to motor neuron disease. Neurology. 1986;36(7):997-8.
22. Riley JD, Antony SJ. Leg cramps: Differential diagnosis and management. Am Fam Physician. 1995;52(6):1794-8.
23. Mills KR, Edwards RH. Investigative strategies for muscle pain. J Neurol Sci. 1983;58(1):73-8.
24. Echaniz-Laguna A, Chanson JB. Electromyography and muscle biopsy in chronic isolated Myalgia: A prospective study. Muscle Nerve. 2016;54(2):321-4.
25. El-Tawil S, Al Musa T, Valli H, Lunn MPT, Brassington R, El-Tawil T, et al. Quinine for muscle cramps. Cochrane Database Syst Rev. 2015;(4):CD005044.
26. Miller RG, Jackson CE, Kasarskis EJ, England JD, Forshew D, Johnston W, et al. Practice parameter update: The care of the patient with amyotrophic lateral sclerosis: Drug, nutritional, and respiratory therapies (an evidence-based review): report of the Quality Standards Subcommittee of the American Academy of Neurology. Neurology. 2009;73:1281-2134.
27. Bedlack RS, Pastula DM, Hawes J, Heydt D. Open-label pilot trial of levetiracetam for cramps and spasticity in patients with motor neuron disease. Amyotroph Lateral Scler. 2009;10(4):210-5.
28. Oskarsson B, Moore D, Mozaffar T, Ravits J, Wiedau-Pazos M, Parziale N, et al. Mexiletine for muscle cramps in amyotrophic lateral sclerosis: A randomized, double-blind crossover trial. Muscle Nerve. 2018;10.1002/mus.26117.

45

CHAPTER

Approach to Neck and Back Pain

Meenakshisundaram Umaiorubahan, Sreenivas U Meenakshisundaram

INTRODUCTION

Neck and back pain are among the most common complaints seen in the neurology outpatient clinic. A worldwide review estimated an age-standardized prevalence rate of 27.0 per 1,000 population[1] while a study in Brazil has shown that neck pain can have a prevalence of up to 20% in the population, with a tendency to be higher among those with poor socioeconomic conditions and people suffering from other chronic diseases.[2]

Lower back pain is one of the most common worldwide problems with a point prevalence or about 7.5% of the global population, or around 577.0 million people, estimated in 2019. The Global Burden of Diseases study group estimated that low back pain is the leading cause of years lived with disability worldwide since 1990,[3] while neck pain ranked fourth.[4]

In 20% of patients with acute neck pain, the pain evolves into chronic neck pain. The main predictor of these is traumatic causes, especially whiplash injury. [5]

The role of the neurologist in these situations is to determine the presence of neurological involvement and the possible etiology. This will help guide investigation and further management, leading to better long-term care of the patient.

Thorough knowledge of the anatomy of the nerve supply of the upper and lower limbs is essential to make sense of the type of neurological deficit which is elicited by a thorough and focused examination. Hence, good clinical acumen is essential to be able to assess neck and back pain.

REVISION OF CLINIC-ANATOMICAL CORRELATES

Before we look at the clinical approach to someone with neck pain or back pain, it would be prudent to revisit the neuroanatomical correlates in the limbs, which are essential for clinical correlation.

For ease of use and practicality, there are certain muscles and areas of sensory distribution, which can be pathognomonic of certain root involvements.

Upper Limb

Upper limb anatomy encompasses multiple cranial nerves from C2 to T2. The corresponding clinical correlates are listed in **Table 1**.

Lower Limb

Knowledge of these clinico-anatomical markers is necessary to be able to localize neck/back and limb pain and to decide on the course of the investigation **(Table 2)**.

TABLE 1: Clinico-anatomic correlates in upper limb.

Root	Sensory/pain distribution	Primary muscle affected	Reflex
C2	Occipital region	-	-
C3	The angle of mandible, upper neck	-	Trapezius reflex
C4	Lower neck, upper scapula	-	Trapezius reflex
C5	Over the deltoid, lateral neck	Deltoid, biceps brachii	Biceps jerk
C6	Thumb, dorsolateral upper limb	Brachioradialis, wrist extensors	Brachioradialis jerk
C7	Dorsal upper limb, middle finger	Triceps brachii	Triceps reflex
C8	Medial hand, little finger	Finger flexors	Finger flexor reflex (occasional)
T1	Medial forearm	Intrinsic muscle of the hand	-
T2	Axilla	-	-

TABLE 2: Clinico-anatomic correlates in lower limbs.

Root	Sensory/pain distribution	Primary muscle affected	Reflex
L1	Groin	-	Cremasteric reflex
L2	Anteromedial upper thigh	Iliopsoas	-
L3	Anterior thigh	Knee extension	Quadriceps reflex
L4	Lateral knee and medial leg	Tibialis anterior	Quadriceps reflex
L5	Lateral leg and dorsum of foot	Extensor hallucis longus	Medial hamstring reflex
S1	The plantar surface of the foot, posterior thigh and leg	Gastrocnemius and soleus	Achilles reflex, plantar
S2	Posterior thigh and leg	Knee flexors	-
S3	Groin, medial thigh to knee	-	-
S4	Perianal	-	-

CLINICAL APPROACH

The clinical approach, as with all conditions in neurology, starts with the history, followed by examination and creating a differential based on possible etiologies.

History

The main aspects of history, along with possible red flags for sinister causes of the pain are listed in **Tables 3 and 4**, for neck and back pain respectively.

While all these red flags are targeted to determine radicular involvement/spinal cord involvement as part of the process causing the neck/back pain, there are a few red flags that can help determine the etiology as well **(Table 5)**.

Apart from these, a specific history to ask for in people with neck pain, especially if they complain of unsteadiness or dizziness or difficulty walking, is any recent neck manipulation such as a massage or chiropractic adjustment, or a session of lifting heavy weights. This should point to a possibility of dissection.

Examination

The clinical examination starts with the assessment of the general condition as a whole.

The presence of a cast or bandage or a large bruise on the skin should raise a concern of a traumatic injury. If the patient is febrile, this raises the possibility of an epidural abscess or ongoing osteomyelitis as a cause for the pain.

The presence of rashes all over the body should make us think of possible meningitis, while a cachectic appearance should raise the possibility of an underlying malignancy or long-standing infection/inflammation, such as tuberculosis (TB) or ankylosing spondylitis.

Anemia on examination, with signs of renal failure such as asterixis and pedal edema, suggests a possibility of myeloma. Conversely, if a patient is dehydrated, one should think of hypercalcemia due to malignancy with bone metastasis or accelerated bone metabolism due

TABLE 3: Red flags in history for neck pain.

Aspects	Red flag
Onset	Acute/sudden
Duration	-
Progression of symptoms	Ellsberg phenomenon
Character	Sharp, shooting, burning
Radiation	Presence along any radicular distribution
Diurnal variation	Increased at night
Aggravating factors	Cough, sneezing, straining
Relieving factors	-
Sensory symptoms	If present
Limb weakness	If present
Postural variation	Worsening on sitting/standing up (or) bending forward

TABLE 4: Red flags in history for back pain.

Aspects	Red flag
Onset	Acute/sudden
Duration	-
Character	Sharp, shooting, burning
Radiation	Presence along any radicular distribution
Diurnal variation	Increased at night
Aggravating factors	Cough, sneezing, straining
Relieving factors	-
Sensory symptoms	If present
Limb weakness	If present
Bladder/bowel involvement	If present

TABLE 5: Red flags for emergency causes of neck and back pain.

Etiology	Red flags
Malignancy	Fever, night sweats, and loss of weight
Spinal TB	Fever, loss of weight, and evening rise in temperature
Myelopathy	Decreased dexterity, numbness/paresthesia in the feet, and urinary urgency
Spinal abscess	Fever, immunocompromised, and intravenous drug usage

to paraneoplastic parathyroid hormone-related protein (PTHrP) secretion.

The presence of jaundice can suggest multiple possibilities, such as liver metastasis, malabsorption syndrome, or chronic alcoholism, all of which can lead to pathological fractures in the form of osteoporosis or bone metastasis.

The presence of a distended bladder could suggest either acute urinary retention due to myelopathy, or a prostate carcinoma with metastasis to the spine.

The presence of multiple lymph node enlargements raises the possibility of lymphoma or malignancy, while matted noted suggest tuberculosis.

On examination of the back, start with observation, looking for signs of scoliosis or kyphosis. If there is obvious scoliosis, see if it improves on bending forward or on lying down. These help to differentiate muscular causes from skeletal causes.

A specific finding to look for in people with back pain, especially if they have difficulty walking, is exaggerated lumbar lordosis. This, coupled with difficulty in bending forward, suggests a possibility of stiff person syndrome.

Eliciting local tenderness over the spine is extremely useful to localize the site of pathology, as well as detecting bony abnormalities which might be contributing to the pain. You should also look for tenderness in the muscle pressure points and tenderness over the temporal artery, while evaluating neck pain. This can suggest fibromyalgia or polymyalgia rheumatica.

A stiff back or a stiff neck with restricted anteroposterior or rotational mobility could mean ankylosing spondylitis as the cause.

Neck pain with a stiff neck should lead to an assessment of Kernig's or Brudzinski's sign to rule out meningitis/subarachnoid hemorrhage (SAH) as a possibility.

Always observe the head and neck at rest before starting the examination for any evidence of cervical dystonia or dyskinesia. This is an often unrecognized cause of neck pain and has even been found to cause secondary disc changes over time. The best technique to recognize an abnormality is to look at the occiput and the chin and see if they align with the long axis of the neck and body. An elevated shoulder on one side might also point toward a dystonia. Occasionally, a hypertrophied sternocleidomastoid muscle may be the only clue to an underlying compensated dystonia.

Neurological examination should include examination of the cranial nerves, especially looking for Horner's syndrome and the lower cranial nerves. Horner's syndrome is seen in cervical dissection, while lower cranial nerves can be involved in craniovertebral junction pathologies.

Upper limb examination should include sensory, motor and reflex testing:

- The sensory testing should ideally be in a radicular pattern, looking predominantly for pinprick and touch
- Motor examination can be focused and testing for the cardinal muscle for each nerve root is usually adequate.
- The caveat is to remember to test multiple different muscles around the shoulder if the sensory loss is patchy, since this raises the possibility of a brachial plexopathy.
- Look for subtle differences in reflexes between both sides and for inversion of reflexes—highly localizing.

When doing reflex testing, it is important to hold the limb in the appropriate position, since this can lead to false positive inversion of reflexes, especially the triceps reflex, when the elbow is too flexed when tested.

In neck pain, it is useful to do a quick examination of the lower limbs as well, especially looking for signs of pyramidal involvement, such as upgoing plantars or brisk reflexes. This suggests spinal cord compression at the cervical level.

Examination of lower limbs needs targeted sensory, motor, and reflex testing:

- Sensory dermatomal testing is important, including perianal testing.
- Motor testing should target specific muscles for each root, with special attention to the difference in power between ankle dorsiflexion and big toe dorsiflexion—this helps to differentiate L4 and L5 radiculopathy.
- Examination of anal tone might not be practically possible in the outpatient setting but should be tested if the patient has complaints of bowel or bladder symptoms.
- Straight leg raising test is useful in detecting lumbar disc herniation. This is performed by raising the patient's leg, with the knee extended, to 30–70°. Pain at an elevation below 60° increases the likelihood of a lumbar disc herniation
- Stork test—ask the patient to stand on one leg and, with support, hyperextend the back. Repeat this on the other leg. If this produces pain, it indicates a pars interarticularis defect.

Remember to examine both sides, even if the pain is only on one side. The upper limbs and lower limbs, for neck pain and back pain, respectively, can show some evidence of radiculopathy, either in the form of sensory, motor, or reflex abnormalities. Sometimes these may be subtle and comparison with the normal side may be the only way to differentiate normal from abnormal.

It is worth remembering that there is usually no dissociation between sensory modalities in radiculopathy and if present, should suggest intra-axial spinal cord pathology. However, intra-axial pathologies are associated with long tract signs, and if absent, a functional sensory deficit should be thought of.

In back pain and associated leg pain, it is prudent to look for myokymia in the lower limbs, especially in the thigh and calf muscles, which might point toward neuromyotonia.

Etiological Approach

The knowledge of the various etiologies which can cause neck pain or back pain is essential before we start to clinically approach a patient. The clinical setting, history, and clinical findings all help to create a list of differentials, which determines the investigation and management plan.

Based on the tempo of the presentation, the differentials for neck pain are:

- *Hyperacute*:
  - Whiplash injury
  - Traumatic/nontraumatic fracture (pathological)
  - Arterial dissection
- *Acute*:
  - Meningitis—viral and bacterial
  - Herpes zoster—associated with skin eruptions
  - Osteomyelitis
  - Epidural abscess
  - *Subacute*: Polymyalgia rheumatic
- *Chronic*:
  - Osteoarthritis
  - Rheumatoid arthritis
  - Ankylosing spondylitis
  - Fibromyalgia
  - Cervical dystonia

The corresponding differentials for back pain are:

- *Hyperacute*:
  - Mechanical injury, especially due to lifting heavy loads or bending over (lumbago)
  - Traumatic/nontraumatic fracture (pathological)
- *Acute*:
  - Herpes zoster—associated with skin eruptions
  - Osteomyelitis
  - Epidural abscess
- *Subacute*:
  - Stiff person syndrome
  - Neuromyotonia
- *Chronic*:
  - Osteoarthritis
  - Rheumatoid arthritis
  - Ankylosing spondylitis
  - Fibromyalgia
  - Kyphoscoliosis

Investigations

The primary investigations in the evaluation of back and neck pain are imaging and neurophysiological studies. The choice of imaging is determined by the possible etiology.

If bony defects or prominent kyphoscoliosis are detected, an urgent X-ray of the lumbosacral spine with anteroposterior and lateral views should detect the anomaly. If a bony defect is detected in the background of acute onset back pain, the chances of a fracture are high and hence urgent computed tomography (CT) of the spine may be prudent.

Magnetic resonance imaging (MRI) spine is advised in the presence of any neurological deficit either in the form of radicular pain on history or sensory or motor deficits on examination. Selection of the appropriate site to request imaging is pertinent, since axial imaging is necessary to evaluate nerve root involvement or spinal canal compromise. The use of contrast imaging is limited, depending on the suspected etiology or the findings on plain imaging. Contrast imaging is useful to differentiate metastasis from other masses in the spine, as well as detecting significant spinal cord compression, i.e., the "pancake" sign.

Contrast imaging can be useful in rarer causes such as brachial/lumbosacral plexopathy or nerve root infiltrative diseases which can result in radicular pain.

Neurophysiological investigations are important to confirm the involvement of the nerve roots. The major tests are nerve conduction studies and needle electromyography (EMG).

Nerve conduction changes in radiculopathy:

- Prolongation of F wave latency in the nerve corresponding to the root involved
- Axonal changes in the corresponding compound muscle action potential (CMAP) if long-standing
- No changes in sensory nerve action potentials (SNAPs)
- Impaired H-reflex in S1 radiculopathy

Electromyography changes in radiculopathy:

- Neurogenic changes such as spontaneous discharges, high amplitude polyphasic motor unit action potentials (MUAPs), incomplete interference, and decreased recruitment in the muscles supplied by the implicated nerve root.
- Neurogenic changes in the paraspinal muscles supplied by the same root.

Paraspinal muscle involvement is the most specific neurophysiological sign to confirm a nerve root involvement.

Neurophysiology may occasionally pick up unexpected and rarer causes of pain:

- Patchy sensory involvement and multiple nerve involvement—suggesting plexopathies
- Continuous motor unit activity at rest, especially in the paraspinals—suggesting stiff person syndrome
- Multiple spontaneous discharges with complex repetitive discharges (CRDs) and myotonic discharges—suggesting neuromyotonia

Other neurophysiological testing which can be useful is somatosensory evoked potential (SSEP) and transcranial magnetic stimulation (TMS). The SSEP detects the intactness of the posterior columns in the spinal cord, as well as the proximal root and plexus, while the TMS can detect the integrity of the corticospinal tract. Both these tests are more useful when there is suspicion of long tract involvement in the spinal cord but the imaging is doubtful or noncontributory.

Other investigations are guided based on possible etiology as a result of imaging and neurophysiological studies. Some of the commonly useful tests are:

- Prostate-specific antigen (PSA) if metastasis detected
- X-ray chest and interferon-gamma if an epidural abscess is seen.
- Human immunodeficiency virus (HIV) and glycated hemoglobin (HbA1c) if osteomyelitis is detected.
- Serum protein electrophoresis if multiple punched-out lesions in vertebral column are seen.
- Serum calcium, dual-energy X-ray absorptiometry (DEXA) scan, PTH, and PTHrP levels if pathological fracture detected.
- Anti-GAD, Anti-CASPR2 Abs, if suspected clinically.

CONCLUSION

Neck and back pain are common complaints in the neurology outpatient setting. The causes can be varied and may range from local musculoskeletal pain to autoimmune or paraneoplastic processes. A detailed history, along with focused examination, is usually helpful in creating a possible list of differential diagnosis. The ability to recognize red flags is especially important in clinical practice to differentiate benign and malignant causes, which in turn will guide the investigation and management. A strong grasp of anatomy and the clinico-anatomical correlation is important tools in evaluation.

REFERENCES

1. Kazeminasab S, Nejadghaderi SA, Amiri P, Pourfathi H, Araj-Khodaei M, Sullman MJM, et al. Neck pain: global epidemiology, trends and risk factors. BMC Musculoskelet Disord. 2022;23:26.
2. Genebra CVDS, Maciel NM, Bento TPF, Simeão SFAP, Vitta A. Prevalence and factors associated with neck pain: a population-based study. Braz J Phys Ther. 2017;21(4):274-80.
3. Wu A, March L, Zheng X, Huang J, Wang X, Zhao J, et al. Global low back pain prevalence and years lived with disability from 1990 to 2017: estimates from the Global Burden of Disease Study 2017. Ann Trans Med. 2020;8(6):299-313.
4. Hoy D, March L, Woolf A, Blyth F, Brooks P, Smith E, et al. The global burden of neck pain: estimates from the global burden of disease 2010 study. Ann Rheum Dis. 2014;73(7):1309-15.
5. Sihawong R, Sitthipornvorakul E, Paksaichol A, Janwantanakul P, et al. Predictors for chronic neck and low back pain in office workers: a 1-year prospective cohort study. J Occup Health. 2016;58(1):16-24.

46

CHAPTER

Approach to Global Developmental Delay

Sonali Singh, Gautam Kamila, Sanjeeda, Sheffali Gulati

INTRODUCTION

Every child develops in a unique way. It depends on the child's innate abilities as well as the environmental stimuli that they are exposed to during their formative years. Although there are variations, age-based norms are available as a point of reference to help identify children who are beyond the physiological range and who need workup and care. The following areas of a child's development are assessed—motor (gross/fine), speech/language, cognition, social/personal, and activities of daily living.[1] Developmental delay can be global or in a single domain. A performance which is two or more standard deviations lower than the mean indicates a significant delay. The type of developmental delay offers a glimpse into the underlying disorder. A delay in the speech/language domain alone points toward a hearing impairment. A delay solely in the motor domain points toward a neuromuscular disorder. A child with delay in speech/language and social/personal domains is screened for autism spectrum disorder. A significant delay in two or more of the developmental domains is termed as global developmental delay (GDD). The affection of individual domains in a child with GDD may be differential. Cerebral palsy is a neurodevelopmental disorder where child presents with motor predominant GDD. The term GDD is reserved for children <5 years. The diagnosis of intellectual disability is possible in older children when they can undergo standardized IQ tests. Those below 5 years of age with GDD usually fulfil the criteria of intellectual disability later.[1,2]

CLINICAL APPROACH

The most important step in approaching a child who visits a pediatrician/pediatric neurologist with developmental concern is taking a detailed history. Various important aspects in history taking with respect to GDD are as follows:

- *Developmental history*: Identifies the domains in which a child is delayed. American Academy of Pediatrics (AAP) recommends developmental screening at every health supervision visit. Standardized screening should be done for children at 9, 18, and 30 months or at any time whenever developmental concern is raised.[3] Norm referenced standardized tests of development are administered by trained professionals to confirm the developmental delay. Differential involvement of different domains in a child with GDD is interpreted differently. Motor predominant GDD with increased tone and postural abnormalities point toward cerebral palsy. Similar pattern of GDD but in association with floppiness points toward congenital muscle disorders with central nervous system (CNS) involvement. Language/speech predominant GDD is usually found in syndromic causes of GDD such as trisomy 21, Fragile X syndrome, and other chromosomal and genetic causes of GDD.
- *Birth history*: It gives the etiological clue in most of the cases. Important points in the birth history for a clinician to take note are enumerated in **Table 1**.

TABLE 1: Important points on birth history.

Clinical cues	Etiology
Repeated early trimester abortions in the mother	Chromosomal disorders
Fever, lymphadenopathy, and rash in mother	Intrauterine infections
Fetal distress, meconium-stained liquor, difficult delivery, delayed cry at birth, and neonatal seizures within 24 hours of life	Perinatal asphyxia
Diabetes in the mother, poor feeding, and unresponsiveness in the baby, documented hypoglycemia in the baby	Hypoglycemic injury
Lethargy, vomiting, seizures, and breathing difficulties 48–72 hours after initiation of feeds	Metabolic disorders
History of neonatal hyperbilirubinemia, neonatal sepsis, meningitis, and intracranial bleed	Postnatal complications

- *Family history*: It is of paramount importance in evaluating a child with GDD.[4] Parental consanguinity is a strong clue to genetic causes of GDD. A three-generation detailed pedigree is mandatory in these patients. Once a positive family history is elicited, clinical details and clinical photographs help to identify syndromic causes of GDD. Pattern of inheritance shades light on the likely etiology. Prototype examples are enumerated below **(Table 2)**. The typical family history of males being severely affected and mildly affected females points toward X-linked GDD like Fragile X. A number of affected family members in one generation points toward an autosomal recessive pattern of inheritance. Vertical pattern of inheritance across generations points toward autosomal dominant pattern of inheritance.[5]
- *Psychosocial factors*: Emotional and sensory deprivation are important causes for children not being at par with their peers. This important aspect should always be looked into when evaluating a child with GDD.
- *Associated symptoms*: A child presenting with GDD may have various associated complaints. A child with history of neonatal or early infantile epileptic encephalopathies such as Ohtahara syndrome or west syndrome tends to have GDD. Developmental and epileptic encephalopathy is a recently termed entity. Epileptic encephalopathies have a causal relationship between epilepsy and developmental delay. Developmental encephalopathies are genetic etiologies which are responsible for developmental delay independent of the epilepsy **(Box 1)**.

After history taking, a detailed clinical examination is a must in evaluation of a child with GDD. Anthropometry usually reveals short stature and microcephaly. A head-to-toe examination is important to identify the facies, cleft lip and palate, neurocutaneous markers, and abnormalities of skull and spine, external genitalia, skin hyperpigmentation, hypertrichosis, umbilical, inguinal hernia, and anal opening. Other systemic examinations with special emphasis on cardiovascular system are crucial. Dysmorphism and multisystem involvement are found in children with syndromic GDD. Trisomy 21 is the most common cause of syndromic GDD. Presence of café-au-lait spots and other neurocutaneous markers in the child or the family members and early-onset seizures points toward tuberous sclerosis. Other classical syndromic causes of GDD and the clinical clues on history are enumerated in **Table 3**. Characteristic facial features, ocular, and skeletal abnormalities are also seen in large molecule storage disorders. Presence of organomegaly points toward storage disorders. Ocular examination may reveal ptosis, cataract, cherry red spot, and pigmentary changes in retina.[4]

TABLE 2: Etiological clues depending on the pattern of inheritance.

X-linked	Fragile X and Rett syndrome
Autosomal recessive (AR)	Metabolic disorders, creatine deficiency disorders, and homocystinuria
Autosomal dominant (AD)	ARID1B, SCN2A, ANKRD11, SATB2, SYNGAP1, DYRK1A, MED13L, STXBP1, CTNNB1, KCNQ2, KMT2A, and FOXP1

BOX 1 Common genes implicated in developmental and epileptic encephalopathies.

- Cyclin-dependent kinase-like-related epileptic encephalopathy [or CDKL5 deficiency disorder (CDD)]
- *SCN1A* gene (alpha subunit of voltage-gated sodium ion channel)
- KCNQ2/KCNQ3 (potassium channels Kv7.2 and Kv7.3, respectively)
- PCDH19-related disorder
- SCN2A/SCN8A (sodium channels Nav1.2 and Nav1.6, respectively)
- TSC1/TSC2 (tuberous sclerosis)

TABLE 3: Classical syndromic causes of global developmental delay (GDD).

Fragile X	Large head, long face, prominent chin, protruding ear, behavioral abnormalities in males, and behavioral abnormalities in females
Angelman syndrome	Severe GDD, gait imbalance, tremulousness of limbs, happy demeanor, small head, and seizures
Prader–Willi syndrome	Neonatal hypotonia and poor suck, GDD, hyperphagia, and obesity beyond the infancy
Rett syndrome	Female with normal early development followed by regression later, microcephaly, loss of purposeful hand movements, and ataxia
Velocardiofacial/DiGeorge syndrome	Congenital heart abnormalities (tetralogy of Fallot), cleft palate, characteristic facies, learning disabilities, immune deficiencies, and hypocalcemia
Williams–Beuren syndrome (WBS)	Cardiovascular disease (supravalvular aortic stenosis, pulmonary stenosis), typical facies (periorbital fullness, full lips), short stature, endocrine abnormalities (hypercalcemia, hypothyroidism), voice, and "cocktail personality"
Rubinstein–Taybi syndrome	Typical facies, broad angulated thumbs and great toes, short stature
Trisomy like Down syndrome (trisomy 21), Edward syndrome (trisomy 18), and Patau syndrome (trisomy 13)	Typical facies, characteristic musculoskeletal, ophthalmological, cardiovascular, and other systemic involvement

DEVELOPMENTAL SCREENING AND SURVEILLANCE

All children should be screened for developmental delay routinely till 2 years of age. Every visit for immunization should be utilized for screening a child's development. Besides the usual assessment, every child should be screened with standardized tools at 9–12 months, 18–24 months, and at school entry. A number of standardized screening tools **(Table 4)** as well as diagnostic tools are available **(Table 5)**.[6-16]

TABLE 4: Standardized screening tools.

Name	Age group	Administration time	Comments
Denver developmental screening test (DDST)	0–6 years	20 minutes	• Simple to administer • Best used to detect children who have a moderate-to-severe motor or cognitive deficit • High specificity
Cognitive adaptive test (CAT)/Clinical Linguistic Auditory Milestone Scales (CALMS)	1 month–3 years	20 minutes	• Quantitative development quotients for nonverbal visual motor (CAT DQ) and language (CLAMS DQ) abilities, as well as a cognitive function composite score • Assists in differentiating children with Intellectual disability from those with communication difficulties • Indian adaptation of the scales not available
Early Language Milestone Scale (ELMS)	6 months–3 years	15 minutes	• Two methods for scoring the scale: i. *Pass/fail grading*: Quick screening of low-risk people ii. *Point scoring*: Expresses linguistic level using percentile scores especially in high-risk settings (neurodevelopmental clinics, audiology clinics, and neonatal high-risk follow-up clinics) • Parental feedback can lead to a biased result
Ages and Stages Questionnaires, 3rd edition (ASQ-3)	1 month–5.5 years	10–15 minutes	• Available in Arabic, Chinese, English, French, Spanish, and Vietnamese • Emphasis on child's strengths and issues • Teach parents about their children's development and abilities • Easier to keep track of children at risk • Highlights findings falling into "monitoring zone" • Can be done at home, in a waiting room or during a phone or in-person interview
Developmental Profile-3 (DP3)	Birth–12 years 11 months	20–40 minutes	• Effectively used in variety of settings • Quickly assesses the likelihood of delay • Helps in planning interventions • Identifies neurotypical children, those with developmental delay and also children with different clinical impairments • Helpful in establishing eligibility for special education and planning IEPS • Can be used in multiple settings
Gesell Developmental Schedules (GDS)	1–72 months	30–40 minutes	• Standardized procedure to evaluate the course of development in child's daily life • Gives a quick and clear picture of child's behavioral level • Doesn't consider other problems that a child might have
Indian screening tools			
Developmental Screening Test (DST)	Birth–15 years	25 minutes	• Assess how appropriate a child's development is for his age • Diagnosis and planning of treatment program • Loaded with speech and language items • Must be interpreted cautiously in children with cerebral palsy, autism, and speech and hearing impairment
Test for Indian Children Trivandrum Development Screening Chart (TDSC)	0–3 years	5 minutes	• Developed in India • Requires very little equipment and training • Low sensitivity therefore not very useful in detecting developmental impairment

Continued

Continued

Name	Age group	Administration time	Comments
Baroda Development Screening Test for Infants	Birth–30 months	10 minutes	• Created for community workers • These tests are simple to do
Disability Screening Schedule	Birth–6 years	5 minutes	Simple to use, understandable, and quick to administer
Screening Test Battery for Assessment of Psychosocial Development (STBAPD)	Birth–6 years (rural)	No prescribed time limit	• Culturally relevant, straightforward, and simple to use by community health professionals • Community health professionals require at least 7 years of experience to use the test
Gesell's Drawing Test (GDT)	15 months–7 years	No prescribed time limit	• Reliable screening test of development • Not a valid test for the children who have not attended school or have no experience with a pencil or children with specific finger dexterity problem

TABLE 5: Diagnostic tools for developmental delay.

Name	Age group	Administration time	Comments
Bayley Scales of Infant and Toddler Development IV (BSID IV)	1–42 months	30–60 minutes	• Helps to design intervention measures • Cognitive and language scales • Internationally validated tool • Time-consuming and needs proper training • Scores represent mainly the population of US
Vineland Adaptive Behavior Scales III (VABS III)	3–21 years 11 months	20–90 minutes	• Helps in diagnosis and developing educational and treatment plans • Measures adaptive behavior of intellectual disability, autism spectrum disorder (ASD), attention deficit hyperactivity disorder (ADHD), hearing impairment, and posttraumatic brain injury • Graduate training is required in administration and interpretation
Indian tools			
Development Assessment Scales for Indian Infants (DASII)	0–30 months	40 minutes	• Gold standard scale • Most widely used scale in India • Needs proper training
Binet Kamat Test (BKT)	3–22 months	30–90 minutes	• Standardized in Indian vernacular languages (Marathi, Kannada, and Gujarati) • Cannot be used when the child's verbal ability is compromised • Cannot be used to rule out "subnormal intelligence" as it is required, in a child who is suspected of having specific learning disability (SLD) • Its use has decreased with the introduction of other tests, for example, Wechsler's tests with Indian norms
Stanford–Binet Intelligence Scale (Indian Adaptation by SK Kulshreshtha)	2–22 years	45–90 minutes	• More suitable for Hindi-speaking population • Did not include people with low intelligence in the sample
Seguin Form Board Test (SFBT) (Indian Adaptation by Bharatraj)	4–20 years old; all age groups for people with ID	10 minutes	• A quick measure of general intelligence • Easy to administer • Can be used as early as 3 years of age when most cognitive test cannot be performed • Not much valid for children aged above 11 years of age • Measure of visuo-motor speed rather than intelligence
Vineland Social Maturity Scale (Indian Adaptation Malin)	0–15 years	25 minutes	• Measures culturally appropriate adaptive behavior • Gives a comprehensive profile of adaptive behavior • Assesses social competence and intelligence too when child is not cooperative or having poor verbal skills • May need revision in tune with the changing concepts of adaptive behavior

Every child with GDD should be screened for autism spectrum disorder at 18–24 months and again at 3 years of age (if initial screening is negative).[2]

INVESTIGATIONS

Investigations, planned in the work up of GDD, are aimed to identify the etiology (especially the treatable ones) and the associated comorbidities. Another important aspect of investigating a child with GDD is also to identify the risk of recurrence in the future pregnancies.

The causes of GDD can be broadly divided into prenatal (intrinsic as well as extrinsic), perinatal, and postnatal causes.[2,17] The intrinsic/genetic causes of GDD are a large group comprising the chromosomal disorders (e.g., trisomy 21), monogenic disorders (e.g., Fragile X), metabolic disorders (such as phenylketonuria and homocystinuria) and cerebral malformations. The intrauterine infections, drug abuse, or medications like valproate in the mother are the prenatal extrinsic causes of GDD. Perinatal causes leading to GDD are hypoxic ischemic encephalopathy, birth trauma, prematurity, neonatal sepsis, neonatal meningitis, and other neonatal complications such as intracranial bleed and bilirubin encephalopathy. Postnatal causes are varied. Hypothyroidism, trauma, neurological disorders, nutritional deficiencies, toxins, and various social causes can lead to developmental delay.

A simple approach to investigating a child with GDD has been depicted in **Flowchart 1**.[1,2,17,18] After doing the initial history taking and clinical examination, children with GDD can be divided into two broad categories. The first group consists of children where a particular diagnosis is suspected. There is usually a history to suggest acquired cause of GDD as mentioned earlier. Neuroimaging in these cases helps to characterize the nature and extent of CNS insult. Magnetic resonance imaging (MRI) brain is preferred over computed tomography (CT) head. Another category in this group is children with distinct syndromic characteristics (e.g., trisomy 21, Fragile X, William syndrome, Turner syndrome, etc.) where a targeted test for the specific disorder can be done. Family history gives a clue in most of these disorders. In case of a similarly affected family member with proven genetic disorder, the specific test can be ordered. The common genetic tests are karyotype, chromosomal microarray analysis (CMA), fluorescence in situ hybridization (FISH), multiplex ligation-dependent probe amplification (MLPA), and next-generation sequencing (NGS). **Table 6** summarizes the common clinical scenarios when different genetic tests are used. The diagnostic yield of the genetic test varies in patients with GDD. The yield is higher in those with syndromic features. The diagnostic yield of microarray testing is approximately 7.8% (patients with GDD) and 10.6% (patients with syndromic features). Karyotype and FISH studies are abnormal in 4% and 3.5% of subjects with GDD. The yield of these two tests in syndromic GDD is 18.6% and 4.2%, respectively.

The second category comprises the children with unexplained GDD. These children have no typical syndromic characteristics. Hence, a tier system is followed to evaluate children. The stepwise evaluation helps to identify the treatable etiologies first. Children are screened for hypothyroidism, nutritional deficiencies such as vitamin B12, iron deficiency, toxin exposure like lead (when suspected), and biotinidase deficiency.

The yield of metabolic testing in children with isolated GDD is low. The yield can be increased by choosing the right candidates. Parental consanguinity, history of developmental regression, waxing, and waning course of disorder point toward small molecule disorder, whereas coarse facies, dysmorphism, and organomegaly point to complex molecule disorder. Diagnosis may require confirmation by molecular testing.

The role of neuroimaging in the workup of children with GDD is known. The diagnostic yield is higher in those with neurological signs (microcephaly, focal deficits, and disorders of tone and posture), than those with isolated GDD. MR spectroscopy helps in children with suspected mitochondrial cytopathy and treatable etiology like creatine deficiency. Neuroimaging may reveal cortical malformations, cortical atrophy, ischemic changes, hypomyelination and other white matter disorders, phacomatoses, and enlarged Virchow–Robin spaces.[1]

Epilepsy and behavioral issues are common comorbidities in children with GDD. Epileptic encephalopathies such as west syndrome, Lennox–Gastaut syndrome, and electrical status epilepticus in sleep (ESES) usually present with a developmental regression and significant cognitive and behavioral issues, unlike the relatively static to slowly

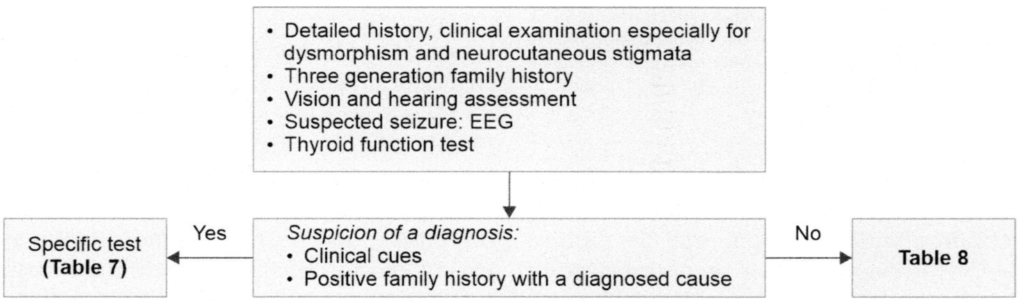

FLOWCHART 1: An approach to investigating a child with global developmental delay.

TABLE 6: Genetic testing in children with GDD.

Genetic test	Common disorders detected by the test	Remarks
Karyotype	• Trisomy 21, 18, and 13 • Ring chromosome 20	• Characteristic phenotype • Multiple congenital abnormalities • Detects abnormality >5–10 Mb in size
Triplet repeat primed-PCR (TP-PCR)	Fragile X	• Triplet repeats (CGG) are detected • Normal: ≤44; intermediate: 45–54; premutation: 55–200; full mutation: >200
FISH	Microdeletion syndromes (<5 Mb) such as Willian syndrome, 1p36 del, and DiGeorge syndrome	• Done when there is a strong suspicion of a specific syndrome (targeted FISH) • CMA is the next test to go for, if the suspected diagnosis is not confirmed by FISH
MLPA	Rett syndrome (MECP2), DMD other microdeletion/duplication syndromes as mentioned above	• Specific MLPA kits are available for GDD patients suspected to have microdeletions/duplications which include many known syndromes • Rapid turnaround time
CMA	Unexplained GDD ± ASD ± multiple congenital anomalies	• Microdeletions (<5 Mb), submicroscopic deletions (1–2 Mb) are detected by CMA • Also identifies regions of homozygosity, which can be assessed for autosomal recessive conditions and imprinting disorders • Does not detect balanced translocations
NGS	• Single gene disorders • Family history suggests Mendelian disorders	• Tests available are clinical exome sequencing (CES), whole-exome sequencing (WES), targeted gene panels • Does not detect the triplet repeats, large deletions and duplications, and intronic mutations • Intronic variations are detected by whole-genome sequencing (WGS)

(ASD: autism spectrum disorder; CMA: chromosomal microarray analysis; GDD: global developmental delay; DMD: Duchenne muscular dystrophy; FISH: fluorescence in situ hybridization; MLPA: multiplex ligation-dependent probe amplification; NGS: next-generation sequencing; PCR: polymerase chain reaction)

TABLE 7: Summary of the investigations for GDD.

Blood investigations	• Thyroid function tests • Complete blood count, vitamin B12, and iron study • Serum lead, biotinidase, and creatinine kinase
Metabolic tests	• *Screening*: Glucose, arterial lactate, ammonia, and ketones • *Small molecule disorders*: TMS/GCMS • *Large molecule disorders*: Enzyme assay • Molecular testing
Neuroimaging	• MRI brain is preferred over CT head • MR spectroscopy in selected cases
EEG	• EEG sleep and awake • Prolonged EEG when indicated
Genetic tests	• CMA/WES (unexplained GDD) • Karyotype/MLPA/FISH (syndromic GDD)

(CT: computed tomography; CMA: chromosomal microarray analysis; EEG: electroencephalogram; GCMS: gas chromatography–mass spectrometry; GDD: global developmental delay; FISH: fluorescence in situ hybridization; MLPA: multiplex ligation-dependent probe amplification; MRI: magnetic resonance imaging; TMS: tandem mass spectrometry; WES: whole-exome sequencing)

improving course in a child with developmental delay. There have been attempts to study the role of electroencephalogram (EEG) in children with developmental disabilities without epilepsy.[19] However, current recommendation supports use of EEG in selected children with history of seizure **(Table 7)**.

TREATMENT

Children with GDD require primary healthcare, routine immunizations, and management of usual childhood non-neurological illness, as any other neurotypical child. In addition, they require individualized management. The management of every child with GDD can be divided into three broad categories—(1) pharmacotherapy for the treatable causes, (2) multidisciplinary management to improve the functional capacity of the child, and (3) management of the comorbidities. **Table 8** enumerates the common treatable cause of GDD and their treatment options. Metabolic disorders comprise another large group of causes where treatment is available. Referral to specialists experienced with treating children with metabolic disorders, is recommended. While managing children with lead poisoning, the treatment modality depends on blood level, source of exposure, etc. So experts experienced in managing poisoning should be consulted.[20]

Hypothyroidism, nutritional deficiencies should be screened in all children, even when an alternative cause of GDD has already been identified.

Comorbidities are common in children with GDD **(Table 9)**. Identification and redressal of these issues help in overall improvement of the functional capacity of children. Some of the comorbidities such as recurrent infections, malnutrition, and cardiovascular diseases may become life threatening in absence of timely intervention. Once a syndrome has been identified, targeted surveillance should be done to look for all the

TABLE 8: Pharmacotherapy given in few selected cases of global developmental delay.[21-23]

Disorder	Drug preparation	Dosage	Remarks
Hypothyroidism	Oral thyroxine	• *Neonates*: 10–15 µg/kg/day • *1–3 years*: 4–6 µg/kg • *3–10 years*: 3–5 µg/kg/day • *10–16 years*: 2–4 µg/kg/day	Refer to pediatric endocrinologist for detailed workup
Vitamin B12 deficiency	Cyanocobalamin or methylcobalamin or hydroxycobalamin	• *Oral*: 500–1,000 µg/day daily for 4–6 weeks, then once a week • *Parenteral*: 1,000 µg/day intramuscular/intravenous for 2 weeks or thrice weekly for 2 weeks followed by weekly for another six doses till hematocrit returns to normal	• Refer to pediatric hematologist if refractory • In combined deficiency of vitamin B12 and folate, vitamin B12 should be initiated before folate
Iron deficiency anemia	Ferrous sulfate Alternatives: Ferrous fumarate, ascorbate, or gluconate	*Oral*: 3 mg/kg/day of elemental iron, once daily, in the morning, or between meals, administered with water or juice. To be continued for two additional months after Hb is normal	Refer to pediatric hematologist if refractory
Biotinidase deficiency	Biotin	10–20 mg/day	Requires life long

TABLE 9: Comorbidities in children with global developmental delay (GDD).[2]

Neurological	Non-neurological	Behavioral	Other systemic involvement (syndromic GDD)
• Visual deficits • Hearing impairment • Epilepsy • Cerebral palsy • Sleep issues	• Recurrent infections • Protein energy malnutrition • Drooling • Constipation • Nutritional anemia • Feeding difficulties • Frequent injury	• Attention deficit hyperactivity disorder • Autism spectrum disorder • Stereotypic movement disorders (with/without self-injurious behaviors) • Aggressive behavior • Mood disorder • Anxiety disorder	• Congenital heart disease, coarctation of aorta • Musculoskeletal deformities, dislocations • Hepatic and gastrointestinal (GI) abnormalities • Urogenital

known systemic conditions associated with the syndrome. Multidisciplinary management is important for the holistic care of the child.

Irrespective of the cause of GDD, the introduction of early developmental interventions in the management plan is crucial for the functional outcome of the child. Multiple modalities are used to improvise the functional skills. The team comprises developmental pediatrics/pediatric neurologist, special educator, clinical psychologist, occupational therapist/physiotherapist, and speech pathologist. Individualized intervention plan is charted. Child's current functional status as well as the target development is taken into account while making the plan. Parents are actively involved in the process. Age-appropriate positive parenting practices and developmental stimulations are explained to parents. Reading materials with self-explanatory graphics are available to help parents understand the concept of early intervention in high-risk neonates and infants.[24-26]

CONCLUSION

- Global developmental delay is multifactorial with variable outcome.
- Standardized culturally acceptable screening and diagnostic tools are available for evaluation of children with GDD.
- In every child with GDD, focus should be on identifying the treatable factors.
- Once diagnosis has been established, risk of recurrence and measures to reduce it should be discussed with the family.
- Genetic tests should be used judiciously. There is no single test which can be applied in all.
- Timely referral to experts is crucial.
- Early individualized developmental interventions is the cornerstone in the management of children with GDD.
- Prevention rather than the cure should be the mantra for GDD.

CASE VIGNETTES

Case 1

A 7-year-old boy was brought to the OPD with complaints of poor cognitive skills and behavioral issues in the form of autistic features, which were noticed in the child at 2.5 years of age. There was no history of seizures or focal neurological deficits. On examination, the child had high forehead, large protuberant ears, hyperextensible joints, soft and velvety palmar skin with redundancy on the dorsum of the hands, and large testes. Psychometric evaluation revealed that the child fulfilled the criteria for autism spectrum disorder and had moderate intellectual disability. Genetic testing was done considering the possibility of *Fragile X syndrome*. TP-PCR revealed > 200 CGG repeats in the *FMR1* gene, suggesting a full mutation.

Comment: The pathogenetic process is responsible for the entire spectrum of symptoms associated with the syndrome, is also responsible for the intellectual impairment in these children with *syndromic GDD/ID*. Younger children have subtle dysmorphism, which may be missed; therefore, Fragile X testing is recommended in all children especially males with idiopathic ID even in the absence of a family history.

Case 2

A 6-year-old boy presented with poor growth, speech, and learning difficulties. She had delayed milestones (GDD), poor growth, and reduced activity compared to her siblings. On examination, she had short stature, macroglossia, and coarse dry skin. Thyroid function test (TFT) revealed elevated TSH (85 μIU/mL), and very low T3 and T4 levels (0.02 and 0.1 ng/dL). Thyroid ultrasound scan revealed hypoplasia. X-rays were suggestive of delayed bone age and 2D-ECHO revealed mild pericardial effusion. A final diagnosis of *hypothyroidism* was made, and he was started on L-thyroxine therapy, following which there was remarkable improvement in overall performance as well as the TFT profile over the next 2 years.

Comment: Hypothyroidism is a *treatable cause of developmental delay* and intellectual disability. Hence, in all cases of GDD/ID, one should always rule out the possibility of hypothyroidism. An early diagnosis and prompt initiation of therapy can lead to a remarkable improvement in the symptoms.

Case 3

A 12-year-old girl was brought to the OPD with profound intellectual impairment. She had no history of epilepsy or focal neurological deficits. She had behavioral issues in the form of autistic features with aggressive and disruptive behavior. She was born to a third-degree consanguineous couple, at 34 weeks of gestation through vaginal delivery in view of premature rupture of membranes. Her birth weight was ~ 2 kg and she has an elder brother (16-year-old boy) with similar complaints of severe intellectual disability. All her milestones were delayed, with independent walking at 3 years, speaking one to two words at 5 years, indicating toilet needs at 8 years, and has very poor social interaction skills. On examination, no features of dysmorphism or neurocutaneous markers were observed. Apart from the higher mental functions, rest of the neurological examination was normal. Her social quotient on Vineland Social Maturity Scale (VSMS) was 10 at the age of 12 years. MRI brain and metabolic testing did not reveal any abnormality. WES of the family trioidentified a heterozygous variant in the *SYNGAP1* gene in the patient, which was confirmed using Sanger sequencing.

Comment: Over the last decade, many single gene causes of *nonsyndromic intellectual disability (NS-ID)* have been identified. Most of these genes are also associated with ASD and epilepsy, suggesting that other genetic modifiers or environmental factors may be involved in the disease process. Thus, a detailed genotype-phenotype comparison, which is often difficult to elucidate, is of paramount importance.

Case 4

A 3-year-old girl, presented with GDD noticed by parents since early infancy, with recurrent generalized tonic-clonic seizures, along with weakness of all the four limbs. The child also had intermittent episodes of dystonia. She had an adverse perinatal history. The child was born through emergency lower segment cesarean section (LSCS) at 36 weeks of gestation, in view of fetal distress. The child did not cry at birth requiring bag and mask ventilation, following which she was in neonatal intensive care unit (NICU) for a week. On examination, the child had poor visual fixation and following, poor response to sound stimulus, spastic quadriparesis, and brisk reflexes and extensor planta response. MRI brain revealed T2-weighted/fluid-attenuated inversion recovery (T2/FLAIR) hyperintensities of the bilateral basal ganglia, bilateral parieto-occipital regions along with cystic changes **(Figs. 1A to C)**. Child was diagnosed with *spastic quadriparetic cerebral palsy*, due to *hypoxic ischemic encephalopathy*.

Comment: The cause for GDD in this case is *structural*, due to the damage to various structures of the brain involved in cognitive processes, secondary to a hypoxic ischemic insult. So, GDD can be a part of overall structural damage to the brain.

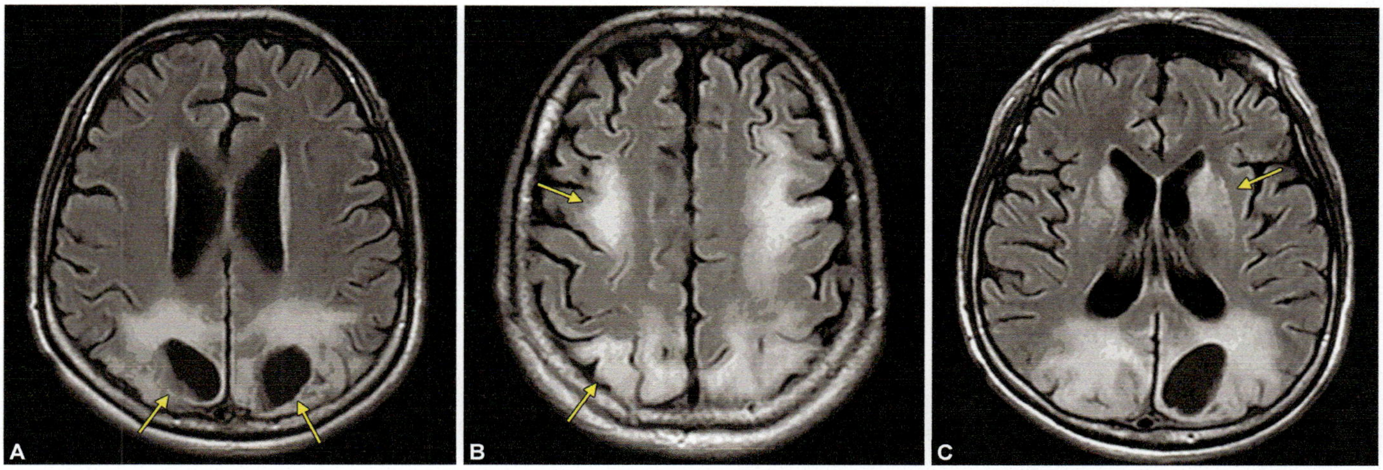

FIGS. 1A TO C: MRI brain (FLAIR) shows hyperintensities in the bilateral basal ganglia, parietooccipital region, and perirolandic areas with cystic changes in the bilateral occipital regions.

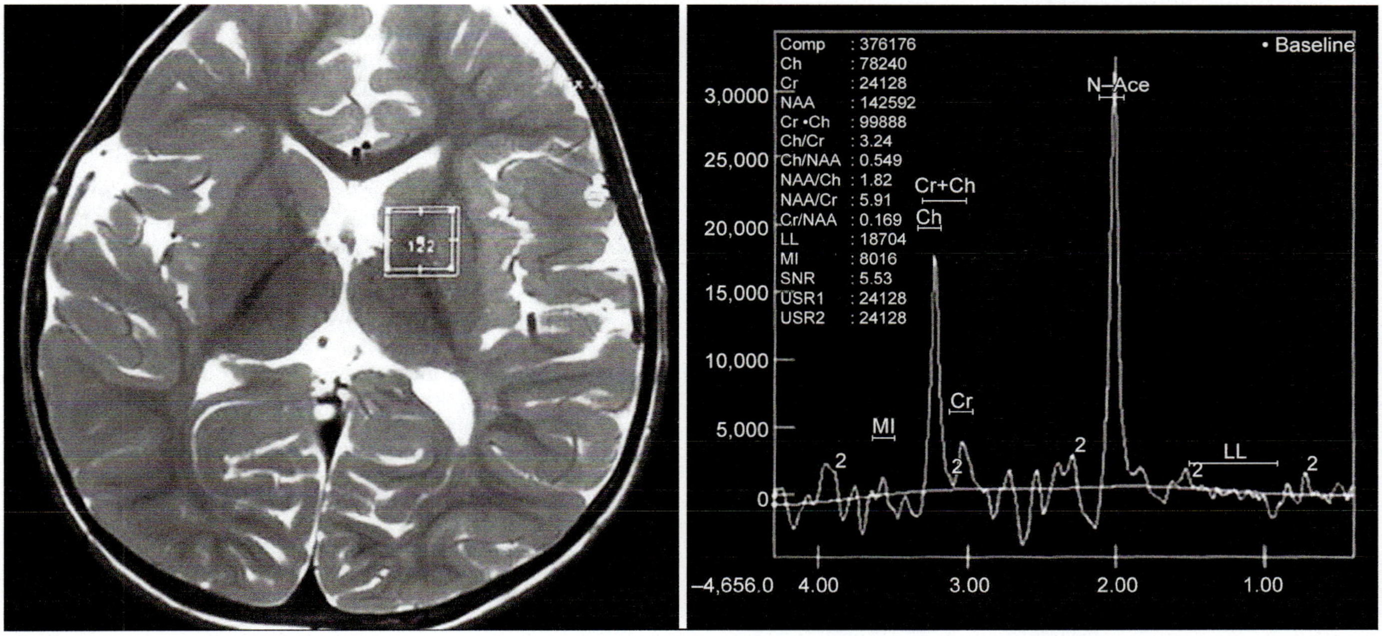

FIG. 2: Magnetic resonance spectroscopy brain of a 9-year-old male showing absence of creatine peak at 3 ppm.

Case 5

A curious case of two siblings (3-years-old male and 9-year-old male), both the siblings had an uneventful antenatal and perinatal period but were noted to have GDD since around 5–6 months of age, along with autistic features and behavioral issues in the form of aggressive and disruptive behavior. There was no history of any seizures or focal neurological deficits. Neither of them had any dysmorphism or neurocutaneous markers. Rest of the neurological examination was normal. MRI brain of the elder sibling was normal. However, the MRS showed absence of creatine peak at 3 ppm **(Fig. 2)**. NGS revealed a missense mutation in the *SLC6A8* gene of *Xq28* chromosome suggestive of *X-linked Creatine transporter defect.*

Comment: GDD in this case was associated with behavioral issues along with autistic features. And similar clinical features were seen in two siblings who were both boys along with similar family histories in maternal uncle. Thus, in this case, the cause of GDD was attributable to the *metabolic imbalance,* which led to a direct effect on the cognitive processes of the brain.

REFERENCES

1. Shevell M, Ashwal S, Donley D, Flint J, Gingold M, Hirtz D, et al. CME Practice parameter: Evaluation of the child with global developmental delay: Quality Standards Subcommittee of the American Academy of Neurology; Practice Committee of the Child Neurology Society. Neurology. 2003;60(3):367-80.
2. Juneja M, Gupta A, Sairam S, Jain R, Sharma M, Thadani A, et al. Diagnosis and Management of Global Development Delay: Consensus Guidelines of Growth, Development and Behavioral Pediatrics Chapter, Neurology Chapter and Neurodevelopment Pediatrics Chapter of the Indian Academy of Pediatrics. Indian Pediatr. 2022;59(5):401-15.
3. Lipkin PH, Macias MM, Council on Children with Disabilities, Section on Developmental and Behavioral Pediatrics. Promoting optimal development: Identifying infants and young children with developmental disorders through developmental surveillance and screening. Pediatrics. 2020;145(1):e20193449.
4. Vasudevan P, Suri M. A clinical approach to developmental delay and intellectual disability. Clin Med. 2017;17(6):558-61.
5. Wieczorek D. Autosomal dominant intellectual disability. Med Genet. 2018;30(3):318-22.
6. Specchio N, Curatolo P. Developmental and epileptic encephalopathies: what we do and do not know. Brain J Neurol. 2021;144(1): 32-43.
7. Kamat VV. A revision of the Binet scale for Indian children (Kanarese and Marathi Speaking). Br J Educ Psychol. 1934;4(3):296-309.
8. Indian Pediatrics. (2012). Ages and Stages Questionnaire as a Screening Tool for Developmental Delay in Indian Children. [online] Available from https://indianpediatrics.net/june2012/june-457-461.htm [Last accessed May, 2023].
9. Balasundaram P, Avulakunta ID. Bayley scales of infant and toddler development. Treasure Island (FL): StatPearls Publishing; 2021.
10. Department of Empowerment of Persons with Disabilities. (2023). Home—National Institute for the Empowerment of Persons with Intellectual Disabilities. . [online] Available from https://niepid.nic.in/public.php# [Last accessed May 2023].
11. Kulshreshtha SK. (1960). Indian Adaptation of Binet Simon Scale. [online]. Available from https://prasadpsycho.com/product/indian-adaptation-of-binet-simon-scale-1960/ [Last accessed May, 2023].
12. Niwlikar B. (2019). Malin's Intelligence Scale for Indian Children (MISIC) . [online] Available from: https://www.careershodh.com/malins-intelligence-scale-for-indian-children-misic/ [Last accessed May, 2023].
13. Goel SK, Sen AK. Mental retardation and learning. Agra, India: National Psychological Corp.; 1984.
14. Venkatesan S. Revalidation of Seguin Form Board Test for Indian children. Indian J Appl Psychol. 1998;35:38-42.
15. Roopesh B. Seguin Form Board Test: A proposal for appropriate norms. Indian J Appl Res. 2021;11:16-22.
16. Sparrow SS. Vineland Adaptive Behavior Scales. In: Kreutzer JS, DeLuca J, Caplan B (Eds). Encyclopedia of Clinical Neuropsychology. New York, NY: Springer; 2011.
17. Bélanger SA, Caron J. Evaluation of the child with global developmental delay and intellectual disability. Paediatr Child Health. 2018;23(6):403-10.
18. Shevell MI, Majnemer A, Rosenbaum P, Abrahamowicz M. Etiologic determination of childhood developmental delay. Brain Dev. 2001;23(4):228-35.
19. Asadi-Pooya AA. Yield of EEG monitoring in children with developmental disabilities is high. Epilepsy Behav. 2018;84:105-6.
20. American Academy of Pediatrics. (2023). Treatment of Lead Poisoning. [online]. Available from http://www.aap.org/en/patient-care/lead-exposure/treatment-of-lead-poisoning/ [Last accessed May, 2023].
21. Indian Academy of Pediatrics. (2022). Ch-012-Hypothyroidism. [online]. Available from https://iapindia.org/pdf/Ch-012-Hypothyroidism.pdf [Last accessed May, 2023].
22. Indian Academy of Pediatrics. (2022). Ch-044-Megaloblastic anemia. [online]. Available from https://iapindia.org/pdf/Ch-044-Megaloblastic-Anemia.pdf [Last accessed May, 2023].
23. Indian Academy of Pediatrics. (2022). Iron Deficiency Anemia. [online]. Available from https://iapindia.org/pdf/Ch-059-stg-Iron-Deficiency-Anemia.pdf [Last accessed May, 2023].
24. All India Institute of Medical Sciences. (2022). Developmental Stimulation. [online]. Available from: http://pedneuroaiims.org/pdf-2020/developmental-eng.pdf [Last accessed May, 2023].
25. All India Institute of Medical Sciences. (2022). Developmental Stimulation (Hindi). [online]. Available from: http://pedneuroaiims.org/pdf-2020/developmental-hindi.pdf [Last accessed May, 2023].
26. Ministry of Health and Family Welfare, Ministry of Women and Child Development. (2018). Guidebook for Mother-Child Protection Card 2018 for ANM, ASHA, AWW. Available from https://www.nhm.gov.in/New_Updates_2018/NHM_Components/Immunization/Guildelines_for_immunization/MCP_Guide_Book.pdf [Last accessed May, 2023].

47

CHAPTER

Approach to Developmental Regression

Vaishakh Anand, KP Vinayan

INTRODUCTION

Developmental regression denotes the loss of previously attained functional skills due to an underlying neurological or non-neurological disorder. However, a true neurological regression secondary to an ongoing pathological process is relatively rare, which is to be identified as early as possible to prevent or limit the irreversible damage wherever possible.

DEFINITION

Various terminologies are used in the literature for denoting neuroregression like "progressive encephalopathy", "neurodegenerative disorder", "degenerative brain disease (DBD)", and "progressive intellectual and neurological deterioration (PIND)." The study conducted by the British Paediatric Surveillance Unit (BPSU) defined PIND as progressive loss of already attained intellectual or developmental abilities with the development of abnormal neurological signs in any child <16 years old, with the deterioration lasting for 3 months or more.[1] Such a definition captures all the essential prerequisites for a neuroregressive syndrome. The only caveat is the exclusion of acute neurological worsening, which might occur in certain neurometabolic disorders like mitochondrial cytopathies. Children with sequelae of acute or hyperacute neurological insults like hypoxic-ischemic encephalopathy, meningoencephalitis, traumatic brain injuries, ischemic strokes or hemorrhages, and acute demyelination, are generally excluded according to this conceptual definition. In addition, developmental encephalopathies like Rett syndrome, where the natural course is initial regression followed by stabilization; epileptic encephalopathies like West syndrome and Landau-Kleffner syndrome (LKS) with the intellectual deterioration associated with the epileptic activity which might get better with the control of epileptic activity are usually considered as outside of the scope of PIND.

The few available studies on PIND noted a cumulative incidence of 0.1–0.6 per 1,000 live births.[1,2] The incidence decreases with age, and the highest incidence of PIND is seen in the neonatal period. The majority of cases of PIND are due to genetic causes barring a few acquired causes like human immunodeficiency virus (HIV) encephalopathy, subacute sclerosing panencephalitis (SSPE), or chronic lead poisoning. The identifiable genetic causes are either an inborn error of metabolism (IEM) or a neurodegenerative disorder.

Inborn errors of metabolism constitute the most common cause of PIND in all age groups[3] and many are potentially amenable to treatment including dietary modifications, supplementations, enzyme replacement therapy, or bone marrow transplantation. IEMs can be broadly grouped into three classes based on their pathophysiology.[4] The first group involves the disorders that give rise to intoxication due to the accumulation of toxic compounds proximal to the metabolic block. This group mainly involves aminoacidopathies, organic acidemias, and urea cycle disorders **(Table 1)**. The second group includes inborn errors involving energy metabolism. The symptoms are caused by the failure in energy production or utilization within the tissues like the liver, brain, heart, or muscle. It can either be due to mitochondrial cytopathies like Krebs cycle defects, pyruvate dehydrogenase deficiency, etc., or cytoplasmic energy defects like the disorders of glycolysis and glycogen metabolism, etc. Group three includes conditions involving complex molecules due to defective cellular organelles including the storage disorders like lysosomal storage disorders, mucopolysaccharidoses, and peroxisomal disorders.

TABLE 1: Inborn errors of metabolism associated with developmental regression.

Group I: Small molecule disorders leading to intoxication	• *Amino acidopathies:* ○ PKU ○ MSUD ○ Tyrosinemia ○ Homocystinuria • *Organic acidurias:* ○ MMA ○ PA ○ IVA • *Urea cycle disorders:* ○ OTC deficiency ○ CPS deficiency • *Carbohydrate intolerance:* ○ Galactosemia ○ HFI • *Metal intoxication:* ○ Wilson disease ○ NBIA ○ Menkes ○ Porphyrin metabolism
Group II: Disorders involving energy metabolism	• *Mitochondrial disorders:* ○ Congenital lactic acidemia ○ PDH ○ PC ○ Krebs cycle defects ○ Respiratory chain defects ○ Complex I, II, COX, CoQ deficiencies ○ FAOD • *Cytoplasmic energy defects:* ○ Disorders of glycolysis ○ Disorders of glycogen synthesis ○ Disorders of gluconeogenesis ○ Creatine metabolism defects
Group III: Disorders involving complex molecules	• LSD • MPS • Peroxisomal disorders • CDG • Inborn errors of cholesterol synthesis

(CDG: congenital disorders of glycosylation; CoQ: coenzyme Q; COX: cytochrome c oxidase; CPS: carbamoyl phosphate synthetase; FAOD: fatty acid oxidation disorders; HFI: hereditary fructose intolerance; LSD: lysosomal storage diseases; MMA: methylmalonic acidemia; MPS: mucopolysaccharidosis; MSUD: maple syrup urine disease; NBIA: neurodegeneration with brain iron accumulation; OTC: ornithine transcarbamylase; PA: propionic acidemia; PC: pyruvate carboxylase; PDH: pyruvate dehydrogenase; PKU: phenylketonuria)

Nonmetabolic causes of PIND are commonly called neurodegenerative disorders since there is neuronal loss at the cellular level, which can be identified as cerebral atrophy on neuroimaging. This group was traditionally classified as predominantly white matter disorders (leukodystrophies) or gray matter disorders (poliodystrophies). Although the clinical and radiological features help differentiate them initially, the late-stage presentations are usually indistinguishable without a genetic evaluation **(Table 2)**.

TABLE 2: Comparison of white matter disorders and gray matter disorders.

Feature	White matter disorders	Gray matter disorders
Seizures and cognitive decline	Late	Early
Spasticity and other pyramidal tract signs	Early	Late
Extrapyramidal signs and symptoms	Late	Early
Visual deficits	Late	Early
Fundus	Pigmentary changes, cherry red spot	Optic atrophy
Abnormal evoked potentials (VEP and BERA)	Early	Late
Examples	MLD, Canavan disease, Krabbe disease	NCL, GM1 gangliosidosis

(BERA: brainstem electric response audiometry; GM1: glutaric aciduria type 1; MLD: metachromatic leukodystrophy; NCL: neuronal ceroid lipofuscinosis; VEP: visual evoked potential)

APPROACH TO SUSPECTED DEVELOPMENTAL REGRESSION

Step 1: True Regression versus Pseudo Regression

The first step in approaching a child with developmental regression involves differentiating true regression from apparent regression of milestones or pseudo regression. In a child with static encephalopathy like cerebral palsy, multiple causes might contribute to the loss of previously attained milestones **(Box 1)**. Contrary to true regression, in such cases the lost milestones may be restored if the cause is correctly identified and treated **(Fig. 1)**.

Step 2: Age of Onset

As mentioned before, the incidence of PIND is highest in younger age groups. The age of onset of symptoms helps narrow down the differentials **(Table 3)**. A 1-year-old child with prominent extrapyramidal symptoms would suggest possibilities like glutaric aciduria type 1 (GA1) or mitochondrial cytopathy. At the same time, similar symptoms in a 10-year-old child should raise the first possibility of Wilson disease (WD).

Step 3: Neurological Involvement Pattern

Different PINDs involve different parts of the neuraxis giving rise to the characteristic pattern of signs and symptoms complex of that disease. A detailed history and examination should reach a syndromic diagnosis with possible anatomic localizations, which can help in planning further etiology-directed investigations. Though helpful in the initial part of the evaluation, the dichotomization into white matter DBD and gray matter DBD may not be possible in all cases **(Table 2)**.

BOX 1 **Causes of apparent developmental regression in static encephalopathy.**

- Increasing spasticity or contractures
- New onset movement disorders
- New onset seizures
- Progressive hydrocephalus
- Psychosocial causes
- Nutritional deficiencies

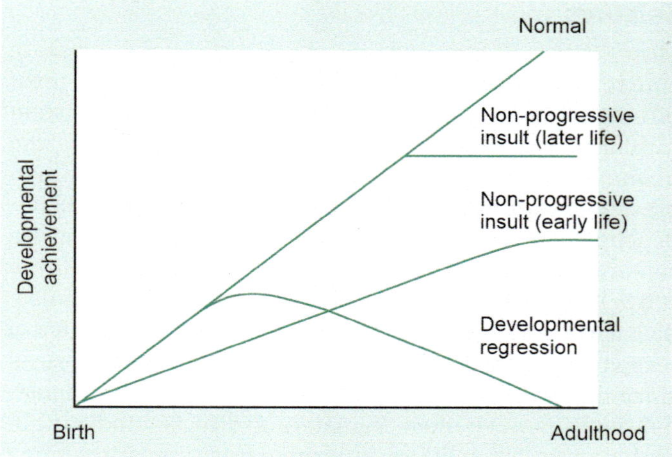

FIG. 1: Developmental trajectories in various conditions.

Source: Adapted from Holland J, Brown R. Developmental regression: Assessment and investigation. Paediatr Child Health. 2017;27(6):253-9.

TABLE 3: Classification of PINDs based on the age of onset of symptoms.

	Less than 2 years	2–5 years	5–15 years
IEM: Group 1	• *Amino acid metabolism*: PKU, homocystinuria, MSUD, GA1, and neurotransmitter deficiencies • *Organic acidemias*: MMA, PA, IVA • *Urea cycle defects*	• PKAN • Homocystinuria • GA1 • Lesch Nyhan • UCD	• Wilson disease • PKAN • Homocystinuria • UCD
Group 2	• *Carbohydrate metabolism defects*: Galactosemia and HFI • *Mitochondrial disorders*: Alexander, MELAS, Alpers, Leigh, Menkes • *FAOD*	Alpers, GAMT	
Group 3	• *Lysosomal*: GM1 and GM2 gangliosidosis, Gaucher 2, NPD A, Krabbe, MLD, Peroxisomal disorders, and GSD • *Mucopolysaccharidosis*: MPS I and MPS III • *Mucolipidosis*: I cell disease, ML4, and sialidosis 2	• *Lysosomal disorders*: Gaucher III, NPD C, Juvenile GM1 gangliosidosis, GM2 gangliosidosis • *Mucopolysaccharidosis and mucolipidosis*: MPS II, III and VII, Mannosidosis, Fucosidosis, ML4	MPS III, Gaucher III, NPD C, juvenile GM1 gangliosidosis , GM2 gangliosidosis
Gray matter disorders (Poliodystrophies)	NCL (CLN1), INAD, Lesch Nyhan, Biotinidase deficiency, Menkes disease	NCL (CLN2), MERRF, Xeroderma pigmentosum	• NCL (CLN3) • MERRF • ULD • Lafora • HD
White matter disorders (Leukodystrophies)	Canavan, MLC, Neonatal ALD, PMD, VWM	Late-onset Krabbe, late-onset MLD, ALD, Alexander, cerebrotendinous xanthomatosis, VWM	Juvenile MLD, juvenile Krabbe, ALD, juvenile Alexander, classical Refsum disease, and cerebrotendinous xanthomatosis
Basal ganglia disorders (Corencephalopathies)	• Mitochondrial • NBIA • OA	• NBIA • ATX	• HD • NBIA • WD

(ALD: adrenoleukodystrophy; ATX: ataxia-telangiectasia; FAOD: fatty acid oxidation disorder; GA1: glutaric aciduria type 1; GAMT: guanidinoacetate methyltransferase deficiency; GSD: glycogen storage disease; HD: Huntington's disease; HFI: hereditary fructose intolerance; IEM: inborn errors of metabolism; INAD: infantile neuroaxonal dystrophy; IVA: isovaleric acidemia; MELAS: mitochondrial encephalomyopathy, lactic acidosis and stroke-like episodes; MERRF: myoclonic epilepsy with ragged-red fibers; MLD: metachromatic leukodystrophy; MMA: Methylmalonic acidemia; MSUD: maple syrup urine disease; NBIA: neurodegeneration with brain iron accumulation; NCL: neuronal ceroid lipofuscinosis; NPD: Niemann–Pick disease; OA: organic acidemia; OTC: ornithine transcarbamylase deficiency; PA: propionic acidemia; PIND: progressive intellectual and neurological deterioration; PMD: Pelizaeus–Merzbacher disease; PKAN: pantothenate kinase-associated neurodegeneration; PKU: phenylketonuria; UCD: urea cycle disorder; ULD: Unverricht–Lundborg disease; VWM: vanishing white matter disease; WD: Wilson disease)

Seizures

Most PINDs will have seizures at some stage of the disease course. But in some cases, seizures may be the most prominent neurological complaint and are often resistant to pharmacotherapy. Drug refractory epilepsy since the neonatal or early infantile period is the most common presentation of vitamin-responsive IEMs like pyridoxine-dependent epilepsy (PDE), pyridoxal-phosphate responsive seizures due to pyridox(am)ine 5'-phosphate oxidase (PNPO) deficiency, biotinidase deficiency, cerebral folate deficiency, and serine synthesis defects. The importance of recognizing these disorders early cannot be overemphasized since the response to supplementation with the particular deficient vitamin is often dramatic and disease-modifying in the long term. Other IEMs with prominent seizures presenting in the first year include nonketotic hyperglycinemia (NKH), sulfite oxidase/molybdenum cofactor deficiency, phenylketonuria (PKU), Menkes disease, Alpers disease, and infantile NCL (neuronal ceroid lipofuscinosis).

The most common cause of neurodegeneration with prominent seizures presenting after 1–2 years of age includes different types of NCL, mostly preceded by progressive vision loss. Other differentials include mitochondrial cytopathies such as Alper's disease, MERRF (myoclonic epilepsy with ragged-red fibers), and Gaucher's type III.

Progressive myoclonic epilepsy (PME) is the term used when there is prominent myoclonic epilepsy associated with neurodegeneration. The most common cause of PME is different types of NCL. Other causes of PME presenting before 5 years include Sialidoses II, MERRF, Gaucher III, and Niemann–Pick disease type C (NPD-C). PMEs presenting after 5 years include juvenile variants of NCL, Unverricht–Lundborg disease (ULD), Lafora body disease, MERRF, dentatorubral-pallidoluysian atrophy (DRPLA), and sialidoses. SSPE, an acquired condition, should be considered a differential of PME-like presentation.

Psychiatric Symptoms

Occasionally, severe behavioral abnormalities and psychiatric symptoms may precede frank neurological deterioration. Early onset self-mutilation is a characteristic feature of Lesch–Nyhan syndrome. Extreme hyperactivity and autistic features may be associated with mucopolysaccharidosis (MPS) III, cerebral creatine deficiency, cerebral folate deficiency, succinic semialdehyde dehydrogenase deficiency (SSADH), Smith–Lemli–Opitz syndrome (SLOS), and PKU. Other examples include OTC (Ornithine transcarbamylase) deficiency, classic homocystinuria, methylenetetrahydrofolate reductase (MTHFR) mutation, cobalamin transporter defects, and Juvenile Huntington's disease (HD).

Pyramidal Tract Involvement

White matter DBD or leukodystrophies typically present with motor regression with prominent signs of pyramidal tract involvement. The common leukodystrophies presenting before the age of 2 years include Krabbe disease, Metachromatic leukodystrophy (MLD), vanishing white matter disease (VWM), megalencephalic leukoencephalopathy with subcortical cysts (MLC), Pelizaeus–Merzbacher disease (PMD), Alexander disease, Canavan disease, and mitochondrial cytopathies. Lysosomal storage diseases such as Gaucher type 2, GM1 gangliosidosis, and GM2 gangliosidosis also have pyramidal tract involvement with spasticity and long-tract signs. The conditions which present later with prominent pyramidal tract involvement are X-linked adrenoleukodystrophy (ALD), juvenile MLD, juvenile Krabbe, juvenile Alexander, and cerebrotendinous xanthomatosis (CTX).

Spastic paraparesis phenotype is associated with hereditary spastic paraparesis (HSP), arginase deficiency, hyperornithinemia-hyperammonemia-homocitrullinuria (HHH) syndrome, PKU, late-onset Krabbe, MLD and Alexander, CTX, and Sjögren–Larsson Syndrome (SLS).

Movement Disorders

Many PINDs have abnormal movements as the primary manifestation. Movement disorders may be brady/hypokinetic or hyperkinetic.

Bradykinesia implies reduced or slow movements often associated with rigidity, postural instability, and parkinsonian features. Hypokinetic rigid syndromes are relatively rare in children. Juvenile Parkinson's disease is a condition with bradykinesia with the most common gene associated being *Parkin* (PARK2). Other conditions with prominent bradykinesia are WD, HD, and neurodegeneration with brain iron accumulation (NBIA).

Hyperkinetic movement disorders have excess and abnormal involuntary movements. Dystonia, chorea, athetosis, ballismus, tremors, and myoclonus are the common hyperkinetic movements associated with various PINDs. Early-onset hyperkinetic movements in the form of dystonia, oculogyric crisis, and diurnal variation of symptoms should raise the suspicion of neurotransmitter deficiencies like tyrosine hydroxylase (TH) deficiency or aromatic L-amino acid decarboxylase (AADC) deficiency. Acute metabolic decompensation with dystonia in infancy is a common presentation of organic acidemias such as methylmalonic acidemia (MMA), isovaleric acidemia (IVA), and GA1. Mitochondrial cytopathies involving respiratory chain pathways can present similarly, commonly known as Leigh syndrome. Biotin-thiamine responsive basal ganglia disease (BTBGD) deserves special attention since it is a treatable condition presenting similarly.

Neurodegeneration with prominent extrapyramidal involvement after 2 years of age is associated with NBIA disorders like pantothenate kinase-associated neurodegeneration (PKAN) and PLA2G6-associated neurodegeneration (PLAN). Late presentation of organic acidurias, Lesch–Nyhan disease, Genetic (DYT) dystonias,

WD, and juvenile HD should be considered in cases presenting after 5 years of age.

Cerebellar Symptoms

Chronic progressive ataxia is the most common cerebellar phenotype associated with PINDs. Intermittent ataxias may be associated with certain IEMs, particularly during the acute decompensation phases. Early onset chronic progressive ataxia with recurrent infections and relatively preserved cognition is the typical presentation of ataxia-telangiectasia (ATX), the most common cause of progressive ataxia. Other causes of early-onset progressive ataxias include ataxia-telangiectasia-like disorder (ATLD), mitochondrial cytopathies, early-onset spinocerebellar ataxia (SCA), Marinesco-Sjögren disease, congenital disorders of glycosylation (CDG), and NPD-C. Progressive ataxias presenting after 5 years include Friedreich ataxia (FA), ATX, ataxia with oculomotor apraxia (AOA), ataxia with vitamin E deficiency (AVED), SCA, and Refsum disease.

Peripheral Neuropathy

Different types of neuropathies may be associated with PINDs. Peroxisomal disorders and mitochondrial cytopathies may be associated with axonal or demyelinating polyneuropathy. Krabbe disease and MLD are characteristically associated with demyelinating polyneuropathy. Mucopolysaccharidoses may be associated with compressive neuropathies.

Step 4: Extra Neurological Manifestations

General examination and other system examinations provide valuable etiological clues.

Head Size

Macrocephaly is defined as a head circumference >2 standard deviations above the mean for age and sex. Leukodystrophies associated with macrocephaly are MLC, Canavan, Alexander, and occasionally MLD. Other PINDs associated with macrocephaly are GM2 gangliosidosis, MPS, GA1, and L2 hydroxyglutaric aciduria.

Microcephaly is defined as a head circumference >2 standard deviations below the mean for age and sex. Krabbe and Aicardi–Goutieres syndrome (AGS) are the leukodystrophies typically associated with microcephaly. Many IEMs, including PKU, serine synthesis defects, sulfite oxidase deficiency, cerebral folate deficiency, etc., are also associated with microcephaly.

Facial Dysmorphism

Typical coarse facies associated with MPS is unmistakably identifiable and often serve as the initial clue toward the diagnosis. Similar coarse facies may be associated with other lysosomal storage disorders like GM1 gangliosidosis, mucolipidoses, sialic acid storage disorders, fucosidosis, and mannosidosis. Peroxisomal biogenesis defects like Zellweger syndrome also can have early facial dysmorphism. Other IEMs associated with facial dysmorphism are PDH deficiency, GA2, SLOS, and CDG. CDG may be associated with abnormal fat distribution with inverted nipples.

Skin and Hair

Flexural rashes and alopecia in an infant with drug-refractory seizures should raise the suspicion of biotinidase deficiency and warrant immediate biotin supplementation. Friable and brittle hair with elastic skin is a clue towards Menkes kinky hair disease. Excess body hair is noticed in certain mitochondrial cytopathies like SURF1 mutations. Excessive Mongolian spots are seen in GM1 gangliosidosis. Neuroichthyosis is a group of disorders with neurological involvement associated with ichthyotic skin lesions, the common ones being Refsum disease and SLS. Chilblain lesions strongly favor the AGS diagnosis and may even present in rheumatology clinics initially. New-onset skin hyperpigmentation and behavioral issues in a young boy can be the presentation of X-ALD. Photosensitivity is commonly seen in various porphyrias; disorders with defective nucleotide excision repair (NER) like xeroderma pigmentosum, Cockayne syndrome, and trichothiodystrophy and chromosomal instability disorders like Bloom syndrome.

Apart from Menkes disease, trichothiodystrophy also may be associated with brittle hair. Trichorrhexis nodosa, a hair shaft disorder, is associated with urea cycle defects like argininosuccinate lyase (ASL) deficiency.

Eyes

Ophthalmic examination is an inevitable part of PIND evaluation at any age. **Table 4** enumerates various ocular manifestations associated with PINDs presenting in <2 years and after 2 years.

Hearing Abnormalities

Impaired hearing is commonly associated with peroxisome biogenesis disorders (PBD) such as infantile Refsum disease, rhizomelic chondrodysplasia punctata (RCDP), and Zellweger syndrome. Mitochondrial disorders such as MELAS, MERRF, Kearns–Sayre Syndrome (KSS), MPS, Cockayne syndrome, and Alport syndrome are also associated with impaired hearing.

Excessive startle is associated characteristically with Tay–Sachs disease (TSD), Krabbe disease, SO deficiency, and asparagine synthetase deficiency.

Organomegaly

Organomegaly is an essential clue toward storage disorders. Hepatosplenomegaly associated with facial dysmorphism and dysostosis multiplex is present in MPS, GM1 gangliosidosis, I cell disease, sialidosis II, and

TABLE 4: Ophthalmological manifestations of various PINDs.

<2 years	>2 years
Cherry-red spot: NPD A, GM1 and GM2 gangliosidosis, sialidosis 2, MLD, Farber, and cytochrome C deficiency	*Cherry-red spot*: Sialidosis 1, delayed and late-onset NPD C
Optic atrophy: Canavan, Krabbe, MLD, NCL, GM2 gangliosidosis, PMD, INAD, and PEHO	
Retinitis pigmentosa: NCL, peroxisomal, PKAN, mitochondrial, abetalipoproteinemia, and CDG	*Retinitis pigmentosa*: NCL, peroxisomal, PKAN, mitochondrial, abetalipoproteinemia, and CDG
Cataract: Zellweger, galactosemia, Cockayne, Marinesco–Sjögren, serine deficiency, and Lowe	*Cataract*: CTX, Wilson
Lens dislocation: Sulfite oxidase deficiency, molybdenum cofactor deficiency	*Lens dislocation*: Homocystinuria
Corneal clouding: MPS, ML4	*Corneal clouding*: MPS
• *Oculogyric crisis*: Neurotransmitter deficiency (AAAD deficiency) • *Supranuclear gaze paralysis*: NPD-C, Gaucher • *Strabismus*: CDG 1a • *Pendular nystagmus*: PMD • *Ocular telangiectasias*: ATX	• *Progressive external ophthalmoplegia*: POLG, KSS, and CPEO • *Ocular telangiectasias*: ATX • *KF ring*: Wilson

(AAAD: aromatic L-amino acid decarboxylase; ATX: ataxia-telangiectasia; CDG: congenital disorders of glycosylation; CTX: cerebrotendinous xanthomatosis; GA1: glutaric aciduria type 1; INAD: infantile neuroaxonal dystrophy; IVA: isovaleric acidemia; KSS: Kearns–Sayre syndrome; ML: mucolipidoses; MLD: metachromatic leukodystrophy; NCL: neuronal ceroid lipofuscinosis; NPD: Niemann-Pick disease; PIND: progressive intellectual and neurological deterioration; PKAN: pantothenate kinase-associated neurodegeneration; PMD: Pelizaeus–Merzbacher disease; SO: sulfite oxidase)

Zellweger syndrome. HSM without dysmorphism is present in NPD, Gaucher, and Sandhoff. Hepatosplenomegaly with cardiomegaly is seen in GSDs.

Cardiac

Detection of cardiac abnormalities has diagnostic as well as prognostic implications. Cardiomyopathy with arrhythmias and conduction defects is associated with fatty acid oxidation disorder (FAOD) and D2 hydroxy glutaric acidemia. Cardiomyopathy is seen in respiratory chain defects, CDG, Pompe disease, Fabry disease, GM1 gangliosidosis, and MPS.

Step 5: Investigations

Hematological

A simple complete blood count (CBC) with a peripheral smear often provides important etiological clues. Different types of anemias are associated with abetalipoproteinemia, galactosemia, Wilson, porphyria, cobalamin, and folate metabolism defects. Bi/pancytopenia may be seen in OAs, Gaucher III, cobalamin, and folate metabolism defects. Vacuolated lymphocytes in PS are seen in MPS, I cell, sialidosis, GM1 gangliosidosis, NCL, Pompe, and NPD A. Acanthocytosis in PS is an important finding and is seen in abetalipoproteinemia, PKAN, and other neuro-acanthocytosis. Neuroacanthocytosis is a group of disorders of neurodegeneration associated with acanthocytes in PS. Typical examples include McLeod syndrome, chorea-acanthocytosis, and HD-like 2.

X-ray

The characteristic constellation of skeletal changes associated with MPS and other storage disorders like sialidoses 2 and GM1 gangliosidosis is called dysostosis multiplex and serves as an important diagnostic clue. Punctate calcification of the epiphyses is seen in PBD like Zellweger syndrome and RCDP. Osteopenia of long bones is present in homocystinuria, CDG, CTX, and GSD1. The presence of Wormian bones is associated with Menkes disease.

Neuroimaging

Though magnetic resonance imaging (MRI) brain is the imaging modality of choice in PIND, computed tomography (CT) brain can be utilized in some instances, especially to detect cerebral calcification. PINDs associated with calcification are AGS, Krabbe disease, Cockayne syndrome, MELAS, Leigh, KSS, GM2 gangliosidosis, CTX, and leukoencephalopthy, cerebral calcifications, and cysts (LCC)/Labrune syndrome.

Magnetic Resonance Imaging Brain

- *Central nervous system (CNS) malformations*: Many PINDs, especially IEMs, are associated with CNS malformations ranging from CC thinning to severe cortical malformations like polymicrogyria. The most common entities are CDG1a, GA1 and 2, Menkes disease, NKH, mitochondrial diseases; especially respiratory chain deficiencies, PBDs like Zellweger syndrome and infantile Refsum disease, congenital muscular dystrophy (CMD), and SLOS.
- *White matter dysmyelination*: The most important assessment in suspected leukoencephalopathies is the pattern recognition of brain lesions using MRI **(Flowchart 1)**.
- Early white matter involvement is seen in Alexander disease, MLD, and a frontal variant of ALD. Parieto-occipital predominance is seen in X-ALD, SLS, and Krabbe disease. Subcortical U fibers are early involved in L2OHGA, KSS, Canavan disease, and urea cycle defects. Periventricular white matter early involvement is seen in MLD, Krabbe disease, and SLS. Diffuse cerebral white matter involvement is seen in MLC, VWM, and merosin-negative CMD.
- *Hypomyelinating disorders*: Hypomyelinating disorders are a distinct group of conditions associated with failure to develop normal myelin. PMD is the prototype hypo-

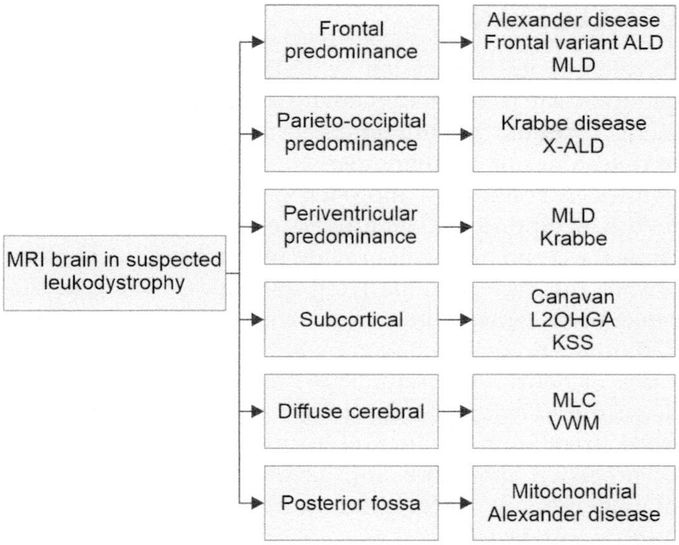

FLOWCHART 1: MRI-based approach in suspected leukodystrophy. (ALD: adrenoleukodystrophy; MLC: megalencephalic leukoencephalopathy with subcortical cysts; MLD: metachromatic leukodystrophy; MRI: magnetic resonance imaging; KSS: Kearns–Sayre syndrome; VWM: vanishing white matter disease)

myelinating disorder with characteristic clinical findings of nystagmus and spasticity. Other hypomyelinating disorders are Cockayne syndrome, 4H syndrome (hypomyelination, hypodontia, hypogonadotropic hypogonadism syndrome), trichothiodystrophy, 18q-syndrome, fucosidosis, hypomyelination with atrophy of basal ganglia, and cerebellum (HABC) and hypomyelination with congenital cataract (HCC).

Characteristic involvement of deep gray matter structures may be noted in certain PINDs:

- *Striatum*: Caudate nucleus and putamen constitute the striatum. Striatal involvement in the form of T2/FLAIR hyperintensity is seen in various PINDs, mainly Leigh syndrome, MELAS, WD, Alexander disease, OA, GA1, molybdenum cofactor deficiency, HD, biotinidase deficiency, BTBGD, and Cockayne syndrome.
- *Globus Pallidi (GP)*: NBIAs are a group of disorders with iron deposition mainly in the basal ganglia. The most common NBIA disorders are PLAN and PKAN, where the GP is T2 hypointense due to iron deposition. Iron-sensitive MRI sequences like susceptibility-weighted images (SWI) may be utilized to better detect iron deposition in suspected cases. Other mineral deposition diseases also involve GP and other BG components variably, like WD and manganese transporter defects. GP T2 hyperintensity is seen in GAMT deficiency, MMA, PDH deficiency, SSADH, and KSS. GP and thalami are involved in Canavan disease.
- *Thalamus*: Thalamus is characteristically and early involved in Krabbe disease along with corticospinal tract and cerebellar nuclei. GM1 and GM2 gangliosidosis, and WD also may affect thalami.
- *Cerebellum*: Brainstem and cerebellum involvement is typical of mitochondrial disorders. T2 hyperintensity of cerebellar nuclei is present in Leigh, OA, BTBGD, and GA1. Corresponding T2 hypointensity is present in CTX. Cerebellar atrophy is seen in many mitochondrial disorders as well as PLAN, ATX, and CDG.
- *Brainstem*: T2 hyperintensity in periaqueductal gray matter is seen with Leigh syndrome, WD, and Wernicke. Other PINDs with brainstem involvement are LBSL, MSUD, peroxisomal biogenesis disorders (PBD), Alexander, and Leigh syndrome.
- *Magnetic resonance spectroscopy (MRS)*: MRS can supplement the etiological workup in many cases of PINDs. N-acetylaspartate (NAA) peak is striking and characteristic of Canavan disease. An inverted lactate peak is associated with many mitochondrial diseases. Cerebral creatine deficiency disorders have a low creatine peak and can be restored with creatine supplementation in selected cases.
- *Genetic and metabolic testing*: Many IEMs like amino acidopathies, organic acidemias, and FAODs might present with acute metabolic decompensation. Tandem mass spectrometry (TMS) in blood and gas chromatography-mass spectrometry (GCMS) in urine are especially useful in such situations. Most of the PINDs including IEMs are due to single gene mutations and are inherited in an autosomal recessive fashion. Targeted gene sequencing or exome sequencing through next-generation sequencing (NGS) can detect causative pathogenic variations. However, chromosomal deletions and duplications are not detected by the NGS platform. Trinucleotide repeat disorders such as HD, FA, and many SCAs also are not detected by NGS.

DIFFERENTIAL DIAGNOSES

- *Static encephalopathies*: As mentioned before, pseudo-regression in the context of an acquired static brain injury must be excluded through history, clinical examination, and proper investigations. These conditions are not associated with neuronal loss at cellular levels, toxic metabolite accumulation, energy failure, or substrate deficiency.
- *Developmental/epileptic encephalopathies*: The term epileptic encephalopathy was previously used to denote any drug-resistant early-onset epilepsy associated with developmental delay. However, recent studies and new gene discoveries indicate that in most cases, developmental delay cannot be explained solely by epileptic activity and separate pathways exist for

developmental delay. Hence the term developmental and epileptic encephalopathy (DEE) is preferred now. In most of these disorders, development may be severely affected due to cortical dysfunction in the active progressive phase in infancy and early childhood. However, most of these children later enter a stable phase with residual static disabilities. There is no relentless progression of the deficits as in classical neurodegenerative disorders.

- *Cortical malformations*: Malformations of cortical development (MCD) usually have varied presentations from mild intellectual disability to severe encephalopathy. Many of these children might develop pharmacoresistant epilepsy with associated epileptic encephalopathies which might simulate a regressive disorder. Moreover, some of these conditions, like tubulinopathies are recently noted to have progressive neuronal loss similar to DBDs.

CONCLUSION

Developmental regression is a significant symptom in children which needs immediate attention and management. It should be differentiated from an apparent loss of milestones or a pseudoregression in static encephalopathies. A systematic approach giving proper attention to the evolution of symptoms followed by a focused clinical examination will provide important clinical clues toward the various underlying etiologies. Owing to the rapid advancements in genetics and imaging techniques, definitive etiological diagnoses are now possible in most cases of neuroregression. This has helped in providing disease-modifying therapies for some conditions which were thought to be incurable previously. These types of precision medicine approaches might help in the management of more and more degenerative brain disorders in the future.

REFERENCES

1. Verity C, Baker E, Maunder P, Pal S, Winstone AM. Differential diagnosis of progressive intellectual and neurological deterioration in children. Dev Med Child Neurol. 2021;63(3):287-94.
2. Stromme P, Kanavin OJ, Abdelnoor M, Woldseth B, Rootwelt T, Diderichsen J, et al. Incidence rates of progressive childhood encephalopathy in Oslo, Norway: A population based study. BMC Pediatr. 2007;7(1):1-8.
3. James Farrer M, Cooper-Knock J, Santorelli FM, G Warmerdam HA, Termeulen-Ferreira EA, Tseng LA, et al. A scoping review of inborn errors of metabolism causing progressive intellectual and neurologic deterioration (PIND). Front Neurol. 2020;10:1369.
4. Saudubray JM, Garcia-Cazorla A. Clinical approach to inborn errors of metabolism in pediatrics. Inborn Metab Dis. 2016;3:70.

48

CHAPTER

Approach to Hypotonia in Neonates and Infants

Viraj Sanghi

INTRODUCTION

Hypotonia (low muscle tone) is defined as decreased resistance to passive movement. This may or may not be accompanied with decreased muscle strength. It may also be defined as difficulty in sustaining postural control and movement against gravity. An infant with hypotonia appears floppy due to the lack of normal flexor tone observed in healthy newborns. The floppy infant presents with delayed motor development, poor control of movement, altered postural control, excessive joint mobility, and abnormal stability. In the most severe cases, the floppy infant has the appearance of a rag doll.

PHYSIOLOGY OF MUSCLE TONE

Muscle tone is influenced by neurological inputs from supraspinal or suprasegmental structures and motor unit or segmental structures.

Supraspinal influences include those that arise from discrete structures within the brain concerned with movement and motor control. The motor strip is a facilitator of tone and a discrete lesion in this will result in hypotonia in the corresponding group of muscles. The basal ganglia and red nucleus are inhibitors of tone and lesions in these result in pathologically increased tone in the extremities. The cerebellum facilitates tone and damage to the midline cerebellum results in axial hypotonia while lateral lesions in the cerebellar hemispheres result in appendicular hypotonia. Segmental or motor units are influenced by components of the reflex arc. Supraspinal inputs as well as diffuse cerebral states such as level of consciousness, anxiety, etc. control the resting state of discharge of the motor neuron. Lesions of the motor unit almost always result in hypotonia and loss of the stretch reflex.

ASSESSMENT OF TONE IN INFANTS

Evaluation of the floppy infant presents a significant challenge to many physicians. Assessment begins with observation of the infant's head size and shape, posture, and movement. There is often plagiocephaly and the infant lies with its limbs abducted and extended. Objective assessment of tone using scales such as the Ashworth scale are only moderately reliable and reproducible, even when performed by the same examiner.[1] There are some maneuvers that have been found to be particularly helpful in gauging low tone in neonates and infants. These include the following:

- *Traction*: The supine infant's hands are grasped and gently pulled to bring the infant to a sitting position. In neonates, there is a head lag. This progressively decreases as age advances and should be minimal or absent by 2 months of age. This is useful for assessing axial tone of the neck and back muscles and to some extent appendicular tone of the shoulders.
- *Scarf sign*: The supine infant's hand is grasped and pulled across the chest. In normal circumstances, the elbow can be brought up to the midline of the chin and chest. If hypotonic, the elbow can be pulled well beyond the midline. This test measures appendicular tone of the shoulders.
- *Ventral (horizontal) suspension*: The infant is suspended in the prone position with the examiner's palm under the chest. Usually, the infant flexes the arms and legs and briefly lifts its head above the horizontal line. The hypotonic infant hangs limply forming an inverted "U" posture.
- *Shoulder (vertical) suspension*: The infant is picked up holding the body under the shoulders in a vertical position. The hypotonic infant slips through the arms.

In addition to these maneuvers, additional signs of hypotonia may be seen including astasias, exaggerated hip abduction, "frog-legging", excessive ankle dorsiflexion, W-sitting, a wide-based gait, and hyperpronation of the feet.

LOCALIZATION OF HYPOTONIA

It is important to localize the pathological process within the nervous system. In a simplified approach, the first step is to ascertain if the hypotonia originates from a central or peripheral lesion. Within the central nervous system (CNS), it must further be determined if there is diffuse cerebral pathology or a focal lesion within the brain, brainstem, or spinal cord. Peripheral hypotonia arises from the anterior horn cell, peripheral nerve, neuromuscular junction, or muscle.

The first step toward this process is obtaining a detailed history followed by a thorough clinical examination which, apart from tone, must include the evaluation of dysmorphic features, muscle strength, and the myotatic (stretch) reflexes.

Typically, central hypotonia will be associated with preserved or exaggerated myotatic reflexes and peripheral hypotonia with absent reflexes. The myasthenic syndromes may have normal reflexes. Altered mental status, dysmorphic features, impaired visual tracking, seizures, relatively preserved muscle strength and the Babinski sign are indicative of a central cause. Presence of fasciculations, muscle wasting, and decreased muscle strength are features of peripheral hypotonia.

ETIOLOGY OF NEONATAL AND INFANTILE HYPOTONIA

Central hypotonia accounts for 60–80% of patients whereas peripheral hypotonia is identified in 15–30% of the cases.[1-3] The differential diagnosis of hypotonia is provided herewith **(Table 1)**.

The most frequently encountered cause of hypotonia in the newborn is systemic disease that diffusely affects the CNS. These include hypoxic-ischemic encephalopathy (HIE), sepsis, and congestive heart failure due to significant congenital heart disease.[1,4] The syndromic genetic disorders are another significant cause of hypotonia in infants. Of these, Down syndrome (DS) and Prader–Willi syndrome (PWS) are the most common. A careful search for dysmorphic features is thus essential in the evaluation **(Box 1)**.

The presence of muscle weakness and joint contractures are indicators of underlying neuromuscular disease. Poor fetal movements and polyhydramnios (suggesting prenatal weakness of swallowing musculature) are also important clues. Among the disorders that cause peripheral (motor unit) hypotonia, spinal muscular atrophy (SMA), and congenital myotonic dystrophy (CDM) are the most frequent. The congenital myopathies and congenital muscular dystrophies are less frequently encountered and the myasthenic syndromes are rare **(Flowchart 1)**.[3,4]

TABLE 1: Causes of neonatal and infantile hypotonia.

Central hypotonia	Systemic	Sepsis
		Congestive heart failure
	Brain and brainstem	Hypoxic-ischemic encephalopathy
		Syndromic genetic disorders
		CNS malformations
		Subtle cerebral dysgenesis
	Spinal cord	Spinal cord injury
	Metabolic	Hypothyroidism
		Peroxisomal disorders
		Respiratory chain disorders
Peripheral hypotonia	*Anterior horn cell*	Spinal muscular atrophy
	Peripheral nerve	Charcot–Marie–Tooth disease
	Muscle	Congenital myotonic dystrophy
		Congenital myopathies
		Congenital muscular dystrophies
	Neuromuscular junction	Congenital myasthenic syndromes
		Neonatal myasthenia gravis
Benign congenital hypotonia (primary/essential hypotonia)		
Indeterminate		Unknown

(CNS: central nervous system)

BOX 1 **Syndromic genetic disorders associated with hypotonia.**

- Down
- Prader–Willi
- Fragile X
- Trisomy 18
- Smith–Lemli–Opitz
- Sotos
- Angelman
- DiGeorge
- Williams
- Coffin–Lowry
- Trisomy 13
- Cri–du–chat

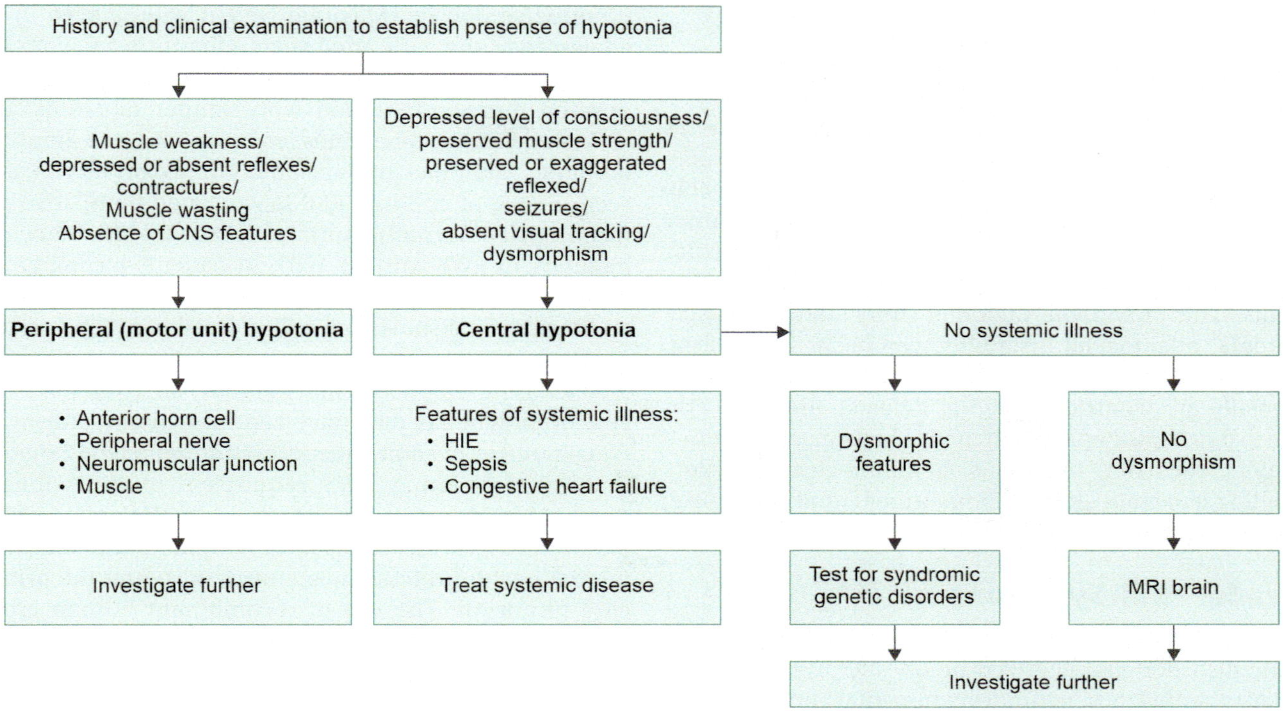

FLOWCHART 1: Clinical approach to hypotonia.
(CNS: central nervous system; HIE: hypoxic-ischemic encephalopathy)

SPECIFIC DISORDERS AND SYNDROMES

Some of the most frequent disorders that result in neonatal and infantile hypotonia will be discussed in further detail.

Hypoxic-ischemic Encephalopathy

Hypoxic-ischemic encephalopathy is a major cause of disability in the term neonate despite the widespread use of therapeutic hypothermia. The incidence of HIE ranges from approximately 1–8 per 1,000 live births in developed countries to 26 per 1,000 live births in developing countries.[5] Documented intrapartum sentinel events such as placental abruption, uterine rupture, shoulder dystocia, or cord prolapse are seen in only 15–30% of cases.[6] The resultant neonatal encephalopathy is characterized by depressed level of consciousness, hypotonia, variable muscle weakness, abnormal cranial nerve function, and seizures. Low Apgar scores and metabolic acidosis are essential for the diagnosis. Concomitant injury to other tissues such as the liver, the kidneys, and/or the heart provide further evidence of HIE. The extent of injury is classified into stage I (mild), stage II (moderate), and stage III (severe) as per the Sarnat staging system. Neurological examination, MRI, and EEG monitoring are the main tools to evaluate the extent of injury, prognosticate and assess the response to therapeutic interventions. MRI is the imaging modality of choice in neonates with HIE. In the first week of life, diffusion-weighted imaging with quantification of the apparent diffusion coefficient can be useful in assessing the extent of injury. Magnetic resonance spectroscopy can also detect early, acute injury. An elevated ratio of lactate to N-acetyl aspartate in the basal ganglia can be seen within the first 48 hours of hypoxic injury and can predict poor long-term neurological outcome.[7] Systemic supportive care is the cornerstone of management and includes care of respiratory, cardiac and renal function, fluid and electrolyte balance, and nutrition.[8] Therapeutic hypothermia (in the range of 33–35°C) is the standard of care for neonates with HIE and is both safe and efficacious. It has been shown to reduce both mortality as well as major adverse neurological outcomes in neonates with moderate and severe HIE.[9]

Ataxic-hypotonic Cerebral Palsy

Cerebral palsy (CP) is a heterogeneous group of disorders that impacts the early development of movement and posture secondary to a nonprogressive pathology of the developing brain. The ataxic-hypotonic variant is the rarest subtype of CP and accounts for <5% of all cases.[10] Some data suggests that patients with this subtype were more likely to be born at term and have significantly less perinatal adversity than the other subtypes. Intrauterine growth restriction (IUGR) and congenital malformations of the brain were more frequently encountered as risk factors in this variant.[10]

Down Syndrome

Down syndrome is the most common genetic condition responsible for intellectual disability and is caused by the presence of a supernumerary chromosome 21 (trisomy 21). Approximately 200–300 genes on chromosome 21 in addition to several epigenetic factors are responsible for the clinical features. DS is a multisystem disorder characterized by dysmorphic features and particular involvement of the nervous, musculoskeletal, and cardiac systems. The phenotype includes short stature, muscle hypotonia, atlantoaxial instability, cerebellar hypoplasia, intellectual disability, and congenital heart defects (especially atrioventricular septal defects). They are also prone to developing epilepsy, hypothyroidism, autoimmune disorders, recurrent infections, hematological disorders (including leukemia), hearing impairment, and early-onset Alzheimer's disease.[11,12]

Prader–Willi Syndrome

Prader–Willi syndrome is a rare and complex multisystem genetic disorder characterized by obesity, hypothalamic-pituitary insufficiency, neurodevelopmental and behavioral anomalies, and dysmorphism. PWS is caused by defective genomic imprinting by three different mechanisms. First, paternal deletion of the 15q11-q13 region results in a lack of expression of genes in this region. This is seen in about 60–70% of cases. Second, maternal uniparental disomy of chromosome 15 where both chromosome 15s are inherited from the mother is seen in 25–35% of patients. Genes on chromosome 15 inherited from the mother are normally silenced by epigenetic factors through methylation. In the remainder of patients, defects within the imprinting center of 15q11-q13 result in abnormal methylation or microdeletions.

Prader -Willi syndrome is most often a sporadic disorder. However, familial cases can occur rarely. This can happen when the father transmits a microdeletion of the imprinting center received from his mother. Recurrence of maternal uniparental disomy is also rare and occurs is <1% of cases. Imprinting center defects (which occur in <3% of PWS patients) are associated with a 50% risk of familial recurrence.[13,14] PWS occurs in 1 in 10,000–30,000 individuals.[14] Features of PWS are manifest at birth and affected newborns display profound hypotonia along with a poor suck and difficulty feeding. Patients have characteristic craniofacial features—dolichocephaly, almond-shaped eyes, thin upper lips, downturned mouth, and micrognathia. These problems persist into infancy along with muscle hypotonia and global developmental delay. Developmental milestones are typically achieved at double the age. Intellectual disability is common with an average IQ of 65–75 along with impaired communication and social skills. After the first year of life there is progressive weight gain due to decreased metabolic rate. After the age of 8 years, hyperphagia is severe with decreased satiety and progressive obesity. Maximal weight gain is seen in late adolescence and early adult years. Obesity is a major cause of morbidity and mortality in PWS. Behavioral problems develop during childhood with temper tantrums, food seeking behavior, repetitions, compulsions, and emotional outbursts. Skin picking (episodic skin excoriation) can be seen in 60% of children and is worsened by relative pain insensitivity. Hypothalamic-pituitary insufficiency is a hallmark of PWS with 40–100% of patients having growth hormone deficiency. Short stature along with hypogonadism and hypogenitalism is seen with a small penis and cryptorchidism in males and hypoplastic labia and clitoris in females. Delayed puberty and infertility are common. About 25% of individuals may have central hypothyroidism and equal number of adult patients may develop type 2 diabetes mellitus.[13] Treating PWS requires a multidisciplinary approach with a team that includes a clinical geneticist, endocrinologist, neurologist, developmental pediatrician, mental health professionals, nutritionist, and the primary care physician. The use of recombinant human growth hormone is increasingly important for promoting lean body mass and reducing fat mass. It should be started in early infancy soon after the diagnosis is made and may also have benefit in promoting development. Replacement of other deficient hormones is essential. Strict dietary control along with securing the food environment, regular exercise, and behavior therapy is important for controlling hyperphagia and obesity.

Spinal Muscular Atrophy

Spinal muscular atrophy is an inherited autosomal recessive neuromuscular disease with progressive weakness of skeletal and respiratory muscle weakness, atrophy, and significant disability. SMA occurs in approximately 1 in 6,000–11,000 live births and is one of the most common genetic causes of mortality in infants <2 years.[15-18]

There are two nearly identical forms of the *SMN* gene on chromosome 5q13: SMN1 (telomeric) which produces full length mRNA transcripts which encode for a fully functional SMN protein and SMN2 which mostly produces a truncated and nonfunctional SMN protein. Up to 15% of SMN2 mRNA transcripts contain exon 7 and can produce some functional protein. SMA is caused by homozygous deletion of exon 7 of the *SMN1* gene. In 5% of cases, there is a compound heterozygous deletion and point mutation. The clinical variability of SMA depends on the number of copies of SMN2 and the severity of the disease is inversely proportional to this. Certain variants within the *SMN2* gene itself can also increase full length SMN protein and thus also impact phenotypic variability.

Spinal muscular atrophy type 1 is the most common and severe phenotype, occurring in about 45-60% of all cases.[17,18] Patients typically have 1–2 copies of *SMN2* gene and develop symptoms in the neonatal or infantile period before the age of 6 months. These babies have severe hypotonia with a splayed-leg posture (frog-legging), poor feeding, and a weak cry. Tongue fasciculations are often present. Progressive limb and respiratory muscle weakness occur with respiratory distress and paradoxical breathing. Cognition is strikingly preserved. They never achieve sitting and death in untreated patients occurs before the age of 2 years. Some authors describe an even more severe phenotype, SMA type 0, with affected patients having only one copy of the *SMN2* gene and death in utero or manifesting in utero with decreased fetal movements and arthrogryposis. They have severe hypotonia and respiratory distress at birth and die within few weeks of delivery **(Table 2)**.[15,18,19]

There are now innovative SMN-dependent disease-modifying therapies available for SMA. These include two SMN2 splice modulators and gene therapy. Nusinersen, an antisense oligonucleotide acts on SMN2 exon 7 splicing and was approved for treatment of SMA in 2016. Onasemnogene abeparvovec is an adeno-associated virus serotype 9 (*AAV9*)-mediated gene therapy approved in 2019. Risdiplam, approved in 2020, is the first orally deliverable small molecule therapy that modifies SMN2 pre-mRNA splicing.[19-21] These are summarized here **(Table 3)**.

Patients must receive multidisciplinary care which includes specialist neurology, respiratory, and orthopedic care as well as rehabilitation, nutrition, and genetic counseling with active treatment of comorbidities.

Congenital Myotonic Dystrophy

Congenital myotonic dystrophy is an autosomal dominant, muscle disease with multisystem involvement. It is a subtype of myotonic dystrophy type 1 and is caused by expanded cytosine-thymine-guanine (CTG) trinucleotide in the myotonic dystrophy protein kinase (*DMPK*) gene on chromosome 19q13. In the majority of cases, CDM is transmitted from a maternal origin. Prenatal symptoms include polyhydramnios, decreased fetal movements, preterm delivery, and small for gestation size. In the neonatal period, there is profound hypotonia associated with limb muscle weakness (distal more than proximal). Neck flexors are also weak and typical facies (characterized by ptosis, facial diplegia, atrophy of temporalis muscles, and a tent-shaped mouth) may be seen. Newborns may have congenital talipes equinovarus, contractures, and

TABLE 2: Spinal muscular atrophy (SMA) classification.

SMA type	Age of onset	No of *SMN2* gene copies	Frequency	Motor function	Typical age of death (without invasive or disease modifying treatment)
0	Prenatal/birth	0–1	<5%	• Decreased movements in utero • Arthrogryposis • Severe neonatal weakness	Neonatal period
1	0–6 months	1–2	45–60%	• Werdnig–Hoffmann disease • Never sits independently (nonsitters)	<2 years
2	6–18 months	2–3	10–20%	• Dubowitz disease • Able to sit • Never walks (sitters)	>2 years (majority are alive at 25 years)
3	>18 months	3–4	5–10%	• Kugelberg–Welander disease • Variability in onset • Can stand and walk • Waddling gait (walkers)	Normal life expectancy
4	>21 years	4 or more	15–20%	Adult-onset mild proximal weaknes	Normal life expectancy

TABLE 3: Current disease-modifying therapies for spinal muscular atrophy (SMA).

Therapy	Indication	Administration
Nusinersen	• SMA types 1–3 • Initiated before 18 years age • Starting treatment before 6 weeks of age has dramatic results • Emerging data for efficacy and safety in adults	• Intrathecal • Four loading injections in first 2 months Then ongoing maintenance every 4 months
Onasemnogene abeparvovec	• SMA with 1–3 copies of *SMN2* gene • Treat before age 9 months	Single dose of virus vector given once intravenously
Risdiplam	• SMA types 1–3 • Initiate treatment between 2 months and 18 years	Daily oral medication

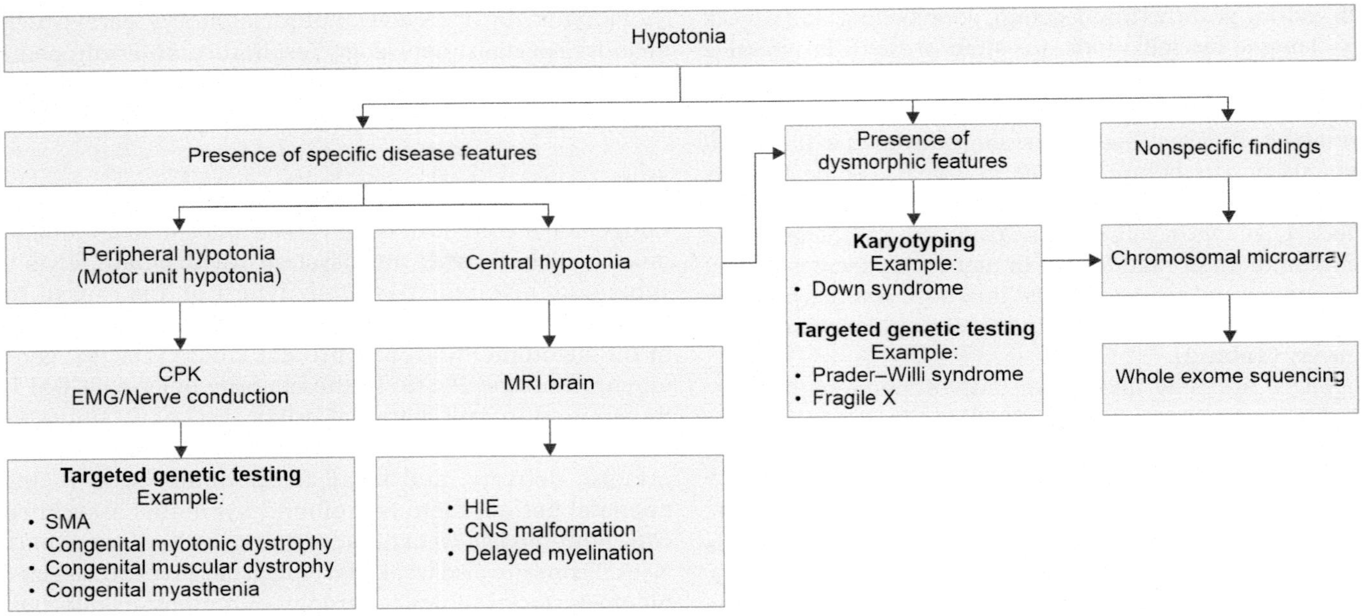

FLOWCHART 2: Algorithm for the diagnosis of neonatal and infantile hypotonia.
(CNS: central nervous system; CPK: creatine phosphokinase; EMG: electromyography; HIE: hypoxic-ischemic encephalopathy; SMA: spinal muscular atrophy)

arthrogryposis. Respiratory muscle weakness and distress is encountered in about half of neonates often requiring ventilatory support. In addition, poor sucking and feeding difficulties are seen along with gastroesophageal reflux disease. Some patients have gastroparesis and may even develop pseudo-obstruction. Clinical myotonia is not observed in newborns and infants with CDM. Cataracts are rare in this age group and only develop at a later age as do significant cardiac defects and diabetes mellitus. Cryptorchidism is common in males. Examination of the mother is an important aspect of clinical evaluation and must not be overlooked. Electromyography in the patient with CDM may show fibrillation potentials, positive sharp waves, and myopathic units in distal muscles. Classic myotonia with waxing and waning is rare in neonates and infants. Neonatal mortality is high (reported to be 16%) with respiratory failure as the primary cause.[22,23] Outside the neonatal period, most patients survive but only few become independent and most have significant intellectual disability **(Flowchart 2)**.

SUMMARY

Neonatal and infantile hypotonia may be caused by a wide range of disorders. Good clinical examination remains an essential step in determining the etiology despite the advances in available diagnostic procedures including genetics. Early recognition and diagnosis is essential to adequately counsel families regarding outcomes and to ensure timely intervention.

REFERENCES

1. Bodensteiner JB. The evaluation of the hypotonic infant. Semin Pediatr Neurol. 2008;15(1):10-20.
2. Sparks SE. Neonatal Hypotonia. Clin Perinatol. 2015;42(2):363-71.
3. Peredo DE, Hannibal MC. The floppy infant: evaluation of hypotonia. Pediatr Rev. 2009;30(9):e66-76.
4. Laugel V, Cossée M, Matis J, de Saint-Martin A, Echaniz-Laguna A, Mandel JL, et al. Diagnostic approach to neonatal hypotonia: retrospective study on 144 neonates. Eur J Pediatr. 2008;167(5): 517-23.
5. Kurinczuk JJ, White-Koning M, Badawi N. Epidemiology of neonatal encephalopathy and hypoxic-ischaemic encephalopathy. Early Hum Dev. 2010;86(6):329-38.
6. Nelson KB, Bingham P, Edwards EM, Horbar JD, Kenny MJ, Inder T, et al. Antecedents of neonatal encephalopathy in the Vermont Oxford Network Encephalopathy Registry. Pediatrics. 2012;130(5): 878-86.
7. Heinz ER, Provenzale JM. Imaging findings in neonatal hypoxia: a practical review. AJR Am J Roentgenol. 2009;192(1):41-7.
8. Douglas-Escobar M, Weiss MD. Hypoxic-ischemic encephalopathy: a review for the clinician. JAMA Pediatr. 2015;169(4): 397-403.
9. Tagin MA, Woolcott CG, Vincer MJ, Whyte RK, Stinson DA. Hypothermia for neonatal hypoxic ischemic encephalopathy: an updated systematic review and meta-analysis. Arch Pediatr Adolesc Med. 2012;166(6):558-66.
10. Levy JP, Oskoui M, Ng P, Andersen J, Buckley D, Fehlings D, et al. Ataxic-hypotonic cerebral palsy in a cerebral palsy registry: Insights into a distinct subtype. Neurol Clin Pract. 2020;10(2): 131-9.
11. Antonarakis SE, Skotko BG, Rafii MS, Strydom A, Pape SE, Bianchi DW, et al. Down syndrome. Nat Rev Dis Primers. 2020;6(1):9.
12. Bull MJ. Down Syndrome. N Engl J Med. 2020;382(24):2344-52.

13. Butler MG, Miller JL, Forster JL. Prader-Willi Syndrome—Clinical genetics, diagnosis and treatment approaches: An Update. Curr Pediatr Rev. 2019;15(4):207-44.
14. Passone CB, Pasqualucci PL, Franco RR, Ito SS, Mattar LBF, Koiffmann CP, et al. Prader-Willi syndrome: what is the general pediatrician supposed to do?—a review. Rev Paul Pediatr. 2018;36(3):345-52.
15. Waldrop MA, Kolb SJ. Current Treatment Options in Neurology—SMA Therapeutics. Curr Treat Options Neurol. 2019;21(6):25.
16. Ramdas S, Servais L. New treatments in spinal muscular atrophy: an overview of currently available data. Expert Opin Pharmacother. 2020;21(3):307-15.
17. Davidson JE, Farrar MA. The changing therapeutic landscape of spinal muscular atrophy. Aust J Gen Pract. 2022;51(1-2):38-42.
18. Arnold WD, Kassar D, Kissel JT. Spinal muscular atrophy: diagnosis and management in a new therapeutic era. Muscle Nerve. 2015;51(2):157-67.
19. Ross LF, Kwon JM. Spinal Muscular Atrophy: Past, Present, and Future. Neoreviews. 2019;20(8):e437-e451.
20. Messina S, Sframeli M. New Treatments in Spinal Muscular Atrophy: Positive results and new challenges. J Clin Med. 2020;9(7):2222.
21. Rossoll W, Singh RN. Commentary: Current status of gene therapy for spinal muscular atrophy. Front Cell Neurosci. 2022;16:916065.
22. Zapata-Aldana E, Ceballos-Sáenz D, Hicks R, Campbell C. Prenatal, neonatal, and early childhood features in congenital myotonic dystrophy. J Neuromuscul Dis. 2018;5(3):331-40.
23. Stokes M, Varughese N, Iannaccone S, Castro D. Clinical and genetic characteristics of childhood-onset myotonic dystrophy. Muscle Nerve. 2019;60(6):732-8.

4

SECTION

Diseases of the Nervous System

Part 4A: Vascular Diseases

49

CHAPTER

Ischemic Cerebrovascular Disease

MV Padma Srivastava, Ayush Agarwal

INTRODUCTION

Stroke is one of the leading causes of death and disability throughout the world. It can be broadly categorized into ischemic and hemorrhagic forms. Ischemic stroke is defined as infarction of the brain, retina, or spinal cord[1] and accounts for approximately 71% of all strokes.[2] Much of the initial neurological deficit in ischemic stroke is due to an electrically nonfunctional, hibernating, hypoperfused penumbra.[3] This penumbral brain can be salvaged and returned to normal function by reperfusion, barring which it progressively converts to an irreversibly damaged tissue (ischemic core). This tenet led to the elucidation of reperfusion therapies that have since transformed stroke outcomes and stroke care, worldwide.[4] Recent advances in neuroimaging have transformed the ischemic stroke definition from a largely clinical and time-based one to a tissue-based one [clinical transient ischemic attacks (TIAs) with an infarct on magnetic resonance imaging (MRI) are now classified as ischemic stroke].

Optimal stroke management should take place in stroke units, which comprise a team of neurologists, nursing staff, physiotherapists and best-evidence management guidelines, including thrombolysis and endovascular thrombectomy (EVT).[5] The latter although most beneficial are time-critical and therefore engineering the healthcare system and raising public stroke awareness in order to accelerate treatment is a key unmet challenge.[6]

EPIDEMIOLOGY

Stroke affects 13.7 million people and causes 5.5 million deaths per year globally.[7] 25% individuals will have a stroke in their lifetime and more than 80 million individuals are stroke survivors.[2,8] The global incidence, mortality, and disability related to ischemic stroke decreased between 1990 and 2013 with a concomitant increase in stroke prevalence. This is probably related to reduced stroke mortality, better diagnosis, and secondary prevention strategies.[9] However, this epidemiological trend is restricted to high-income countries and not lower- and middle-income countries.[10]

RISK FACTORS

These can be divided into nonmodifiable and modifiable factors. The former includes age, gender, and genetic factors. The stroke risk increases with age and is higher in men.[11] Although most cases of stroke are sporadic, the estimated heritability is approximately 38% by genome-wide analysis.[12] The most important modifiable risk factors include hypertension, sedentary lifestyle, diet, obesity, smoking, high alcohol consumption, depression, stress, cardiac disorders, diabetes mellitus, and high apolipoprotein B (apoB):apoA1 ratio. These account for over 90% of the population attributable risk, with hypertension being the strongest risk factor.[13] Other risk factors include chronic kidney disease, obstructive sleep apnea, periodontal disease, air pollution, and chronic inflammatory disorders.[14,15]

ETIOLOGY

Stroke etiology can be broadly categorized into atherosclerotic large vessel disease, small vessel disease, cardioembolic and other rarer causes **(Fig. 1)**. The latter includes arterial dissection, genetic monogenic stroke syndromes such as CADASIL (cerebral autosomal dominant arteriopathy with subcortical infarcts and leukoencephalopathy), hematological disorders, and vasculitis. Understanding etiology behind stroke is paramount as it guides investigations, treatment, and appropriate secondary prevention strategy.[8] **Table 1** lists the common causes of ischemic stroke along with corresponding managements strategies. Of particular emphasis is that intracranial atherosclerotic disease causes 30–50% of ischemic strokes in Asian patients, compared to 5–10% in the west.[16] Common causes of cardioembolic stroke include atrial fibrillation

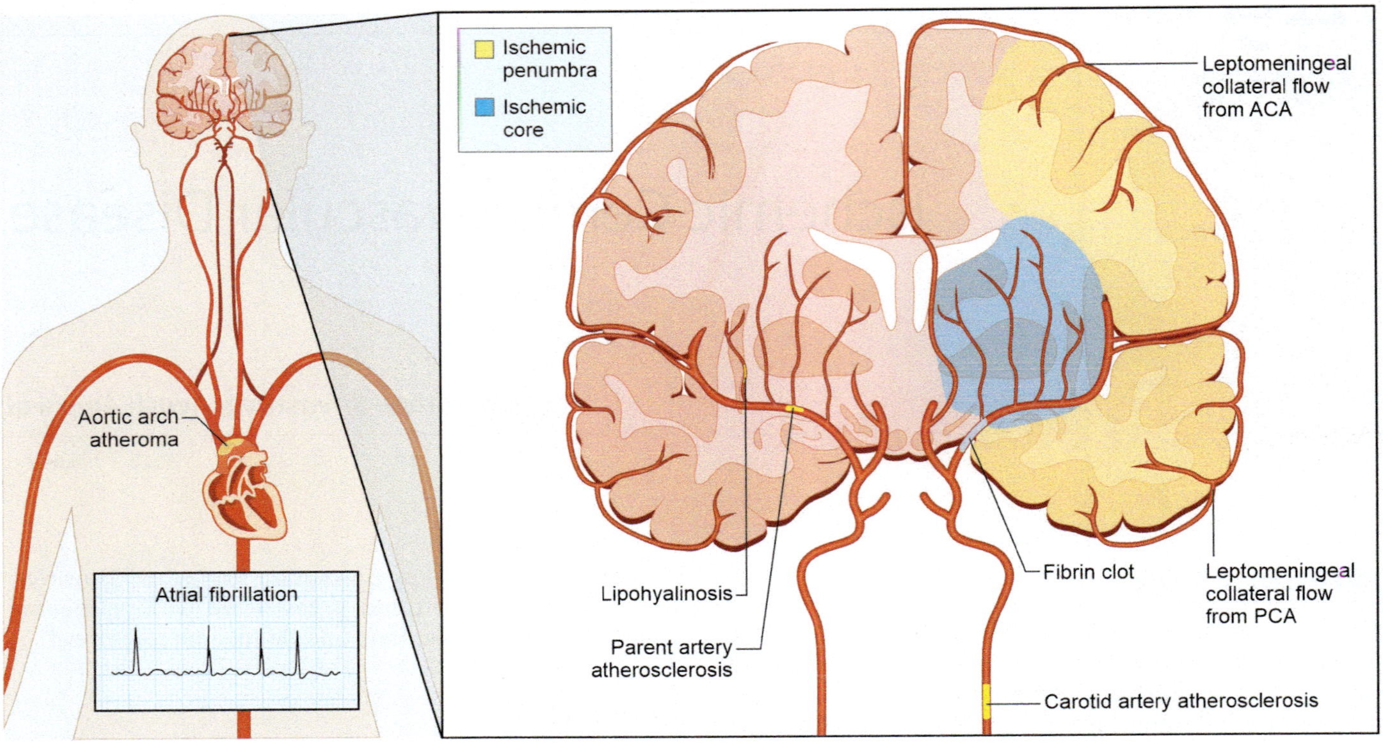

FIG. 1: Stroke pathophysiology.[8]
(ACA: anterior cerebral artery; PCA: posterior cerebral artery)

TABLE 1: Stroke pathophysiology guiding management.

Etiology	Investigations	Secondary prevention
Atherosclerosis	• CTA • MRA • Carotid doppler	• Antiplatelets • High-dose statins • Carotid artery stenting or endarterectomy if extracranial stenosis ≥70%
Cardioembolism	• Two-dimensional echocardiography • Holter/loop recorder	• Anticoagulants • Left atrial appendage occlusion • Percutaneous closure of PFO
Small vessel disease	MRI brain	Same as atherosclerotic disease
Vasculitis	• CTA/MRA • CSF examination • Digital subtraction angiography (DSA) • CSF analysis • Brain biopsy	• High-dose steroids • Cyclophosphamide/rituximab/intravenous immunoglobulin
Arterial dissection	CTA/MRA	Antiplatelets

(CSF: cerebrospinal fluid; CT: computed tomography angiography; MRA: magnetic resonance angiography; MRI: magnetic resonance imaging; PFO: patent foramen ovale)

(AF), rheumatic heart disease, patent foramen ovale (PFO), infective endocarditis, dilated cardiomyopathy, and post-acute myocardial infarction status.

PATHOPHYSIOLOGY

Occlusion of an artery supplying the brain leads to recruitment of alternative blood flow pathways ("collaterals") to sustain the penumbra. The extent of collateral flow varies between individuals and has both environmental and genetic determinants.[17] Collaterals are responsible for the amount of ischemic core and penumbral tissue and the circle of Willis is the most important collateral flow channel **(Fig. 2)**. They can be assessed by multiple imaging modalities but multiphasic computed tomography (CT) angiography (CTA) is most commonly used **(Fig. 2)**. If reperfusion is not undertaken, these collaterals eventually fail converting the penumbral tissue into more ischemic core.

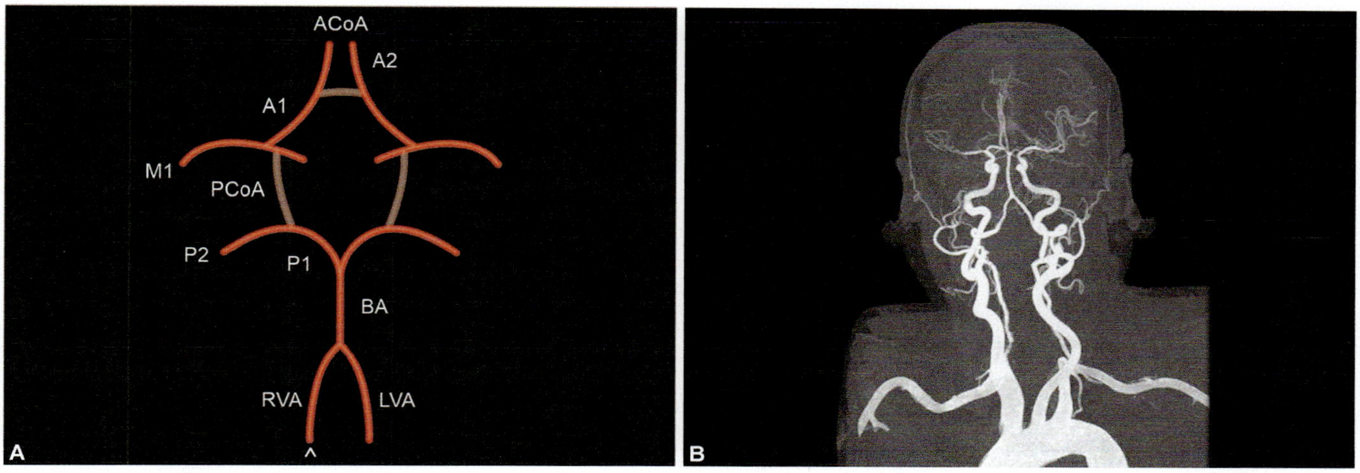

FIGS. 2A AND B: Circle of Willis.

(A1 and A2: anterior cerebral artery segments; ACoA: anterior communicating artery; BA: basilar artery; LVA: left vertebral artery; M1: middle cerebral artery segment; P1 and P2: posterior cerebral artery segments; PCoA: posterior communicating artery; RVA: right vertebral artery)

On a cellular level, ischemia leads to oxygen depletion and subsequent cellular and molecular changes culminating in apoptosis and cell death[18] **(Fig. 3)**. Post-ischemia recovery occurs because of *neuroplasticity*. This involves synaptogenesis, local sprouting, and strengthening transmission at the preexisting synapses. Early rehabilitative strategies promote neuroplasticity and should always be incorporated as a standard of care. However, patients can complain of increasing fatigue during this phase due to recruitment of larger networks leading to inability to deploy them for prolonged periods.[19,20]

DIAGNOSIS

The clinical presentation of sudden-onset focal neurological deficit conforming to a vascular territory is indicative of an ischemic stroke. The common presentations include hemiparesis, hemisensory loss, hemianopia, and aphasia. Stroke severity is gauged according to the National Institute of Health Stroke Severity (NIHSS) score[21] and disability on the modified Rankin Scale (mRS).[22]

Neuroimaging is done to confirm the diagnosis. MRI is more sensitive and provides better spatial resolution but its nonavailability in the emergency setting in most centers and increased time for imaging are drawbacks. Neuroimaging has now become even more important because certain sequences [diffusion-weighted imaging (DWI), fluid-attenuated inversion repeat (FLAIR), CT, and MR perfusion] allow for more sensitive estimation of ischemic core and penumbra and an increasing use of reperfusion therapies. At the same time, however, ruling out potential mimics such as seizures, migraine, metabolic derangements, and functional disorders is crucial.

Noncontrast Computed Tomography Head

- It is nearly 100% sensitive in diagnosing intraparenchymal hemorrhage.
- Early ischemic changes are graded based on ASPECTS (Alberta Stroke Program Early CT Score)[23] → noncontrast CT (NCCT) head is read at ganglionic and supraganglionic levels and one point each is subtracted for involvement of caudate, lentiform, internal capsule, insula, and M1–M6. A final score is attained out of 10 with higher scores indicative of a smaller infarct **(Fig. 4)**. Traditionally, score ≥6 can be taken up for reperfusion therapy.

Computed Tomography Angiography and Computed Tomography Perfusion

- CTA allows for detection of arterial stenosis, occlusion, or dissection and involves neuroimaging following intravenous contrast administration. Multiphase CTA should be acquired from the aortic arch to vertex in all acute ischemic stroke (AIS) patients as it helps provide insights into possible stroke etiology. It also helps in the assessment of the collaterals **(Fig. 5)** which is paramount when making an assessment for EVT.[24]
- Computed tomography perfusion (CTP) generates maps postcontrast delivery indicating cerebral blood flow (CBF) and the degree of delay, if any. Cerebral blood volume (CBV), CBF, mean transit time (MTT) and time-to-maximum (Tmax) are the main parameters calculated. Using these calculations, an automated software determines the volumes of the ischemic core and penumbra and helps in patient selection for reperfusion (thrombolysis or EVT) in the extended

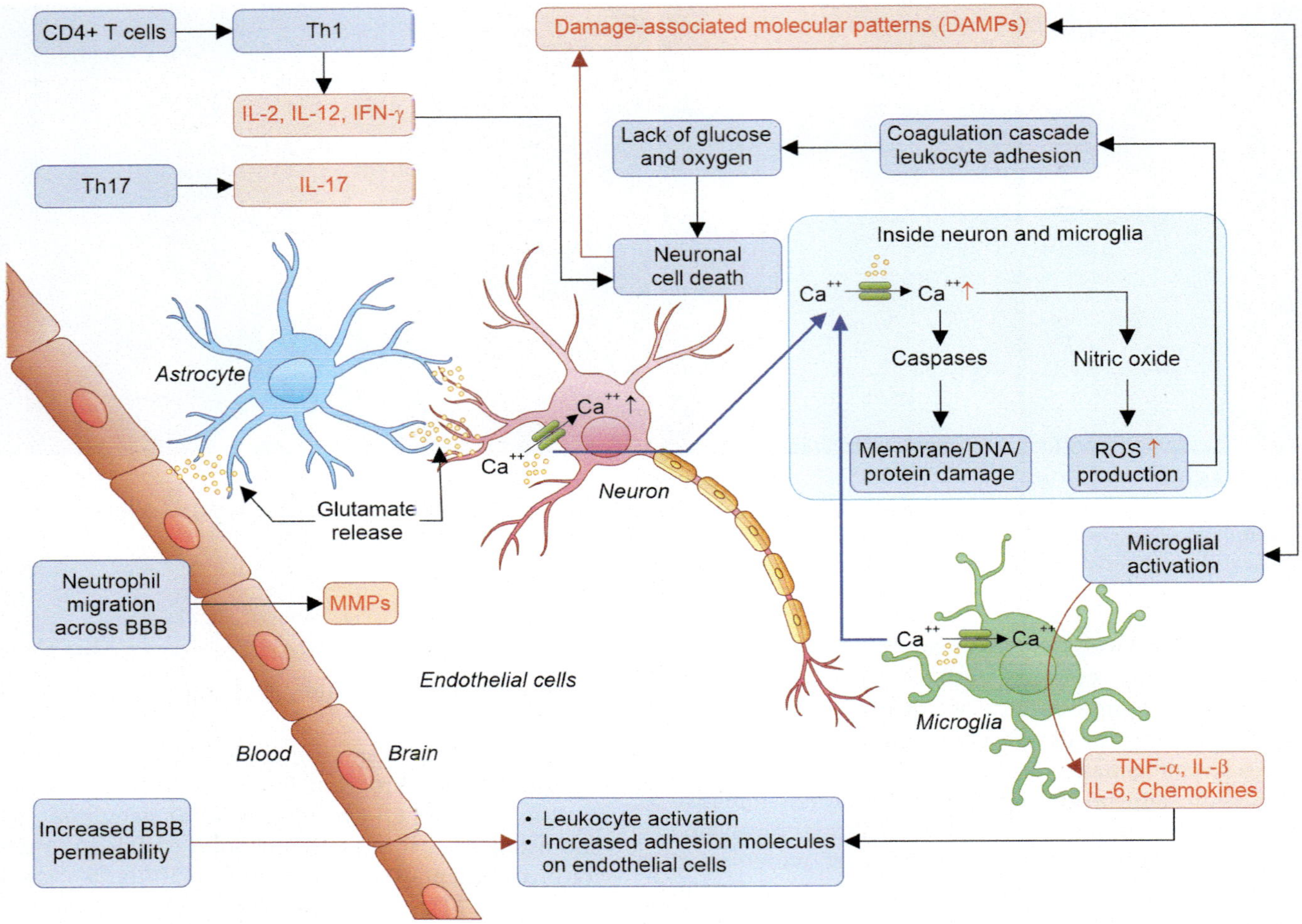

FIG. 3: Cellular effects of ischemia.[18]

(BBB: blood–brain barrier; CD4: cluster of differentiation 4; IFN-γ: interferon gamma; IL: interleukin; MMPs: matrix metalloproteinases; ROS: reactive oxygen species; Th: T helper cell; TNF-α: tumor necrosis factor alpha)

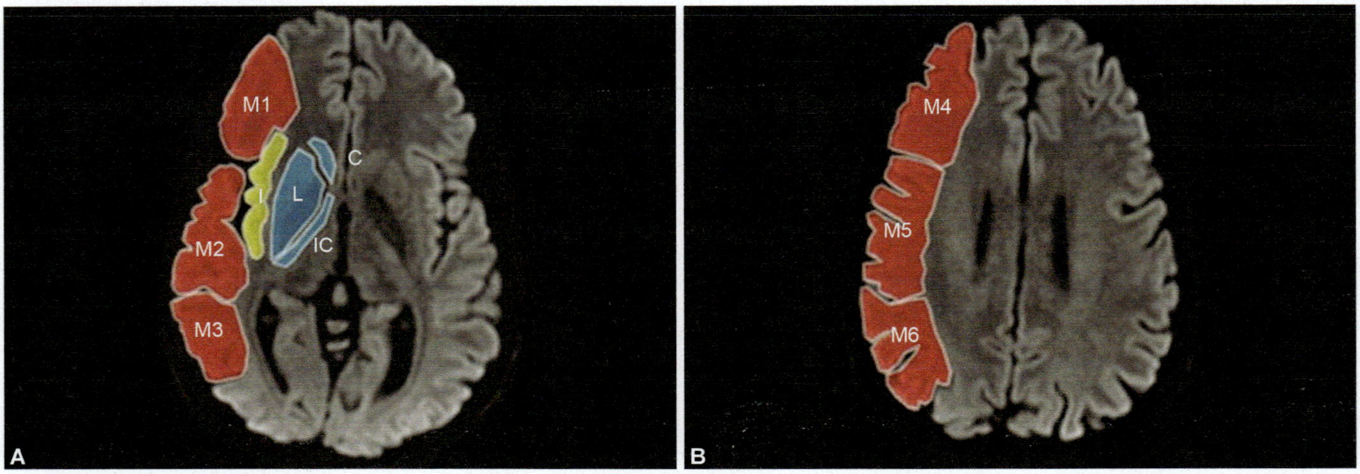

FIGS. 4A AND B: Alberta Stroke Program Early CT Score (ASPECTS) calculation on noncontrast computed tomography (NCCT) head.

(C: caudate; I: insula; IC: internal capsule; L: lentiform; M1 to M6: middle cerebral artery segments)

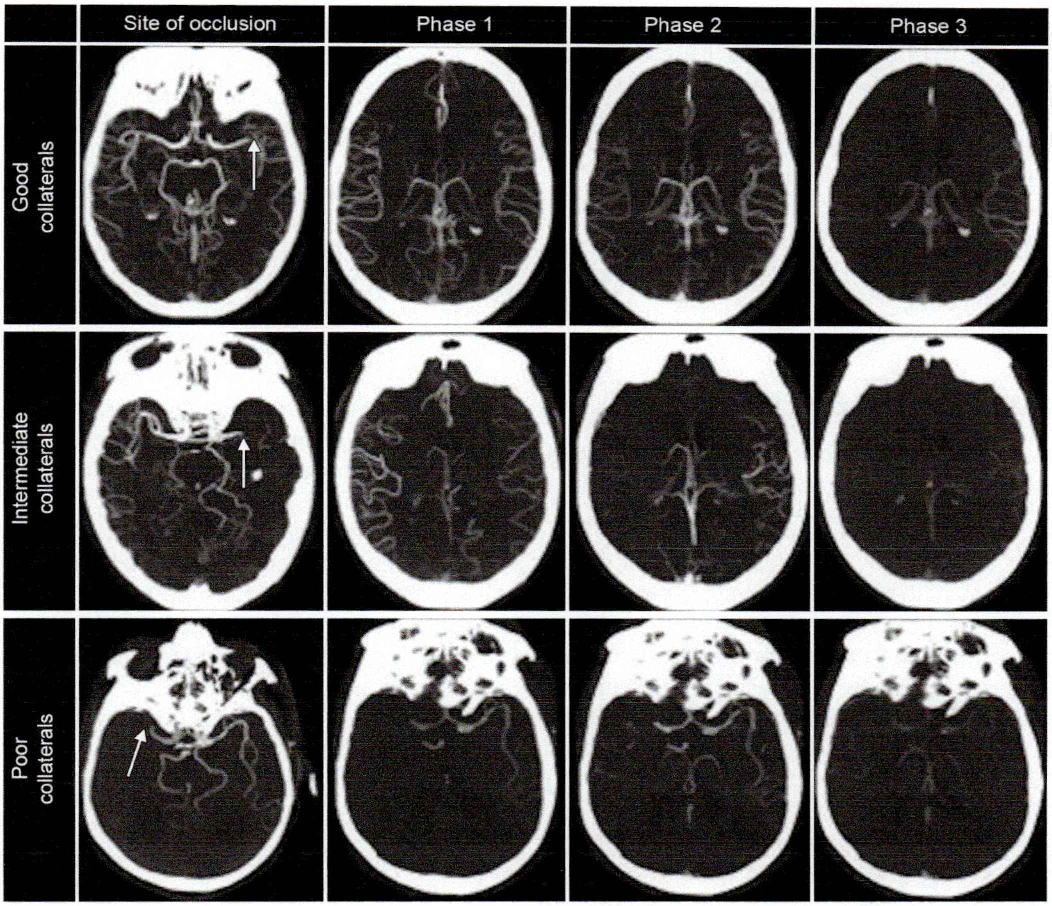

FIG. 5: Good, intermediate, and poor collaterals on multiphasic computed tomography (CT) angiography.

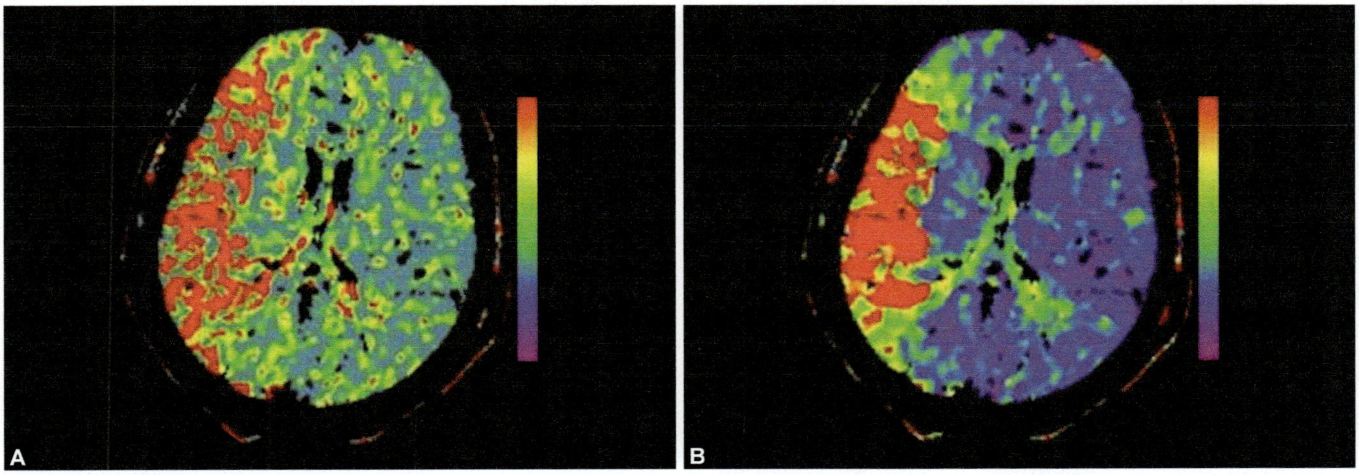

FIGS. 6A AND B: Computed tomography perfusion (CTP)-guided reperfusion

window. The typical criteria used is a penumbra/core ratio ≥1.2 with a minimum difference of 10 mL.[25] **Figure 6** illustrates this example.

Magnetic Resonance Imaging

- DWI sequences are the most sensitive in detecting brain ischemia and become abnormal within minutes of an ischemic stroke.[26] They detect the movement of water molecules and diffusion is restricted in infarcted regions (cytotoxic edema). Diffusion-restricted regions do not usually recover to baseline status (histologically or radiologically) despite reperfusion therapy.[27]
- T2-FLAIR sequences become abnormal after the development of vasogenic edema over the few hours.[28]

- Diffusion-FLAIR mismatch (infarct present on DWI but absent on FLAIR) has been used as a criteria for thrombolysis for patients presenting during the extended time window.[29]
- Time-of-Flight (ToF) sequences help in rough estimation of the intra- and extracranial vasculature, utilizing signals from endogenous blood flow.
- Susceptibility-weighted imaging (SWI) is extremely sensitive for detecting intraparenchymal bleeding (including microbleeds).
- MRI perfusion works on the same principles of CTP.

ACUTE STROKE MANAGEMENT

Thrombolysis and EVT form the cornerstone for acute stroke management and have revolutionized stroke care worldwide.

Thrombolysis

Two main drugs are available, namely: (i) alteplase and (ii) tenecteplase (TNK).

Alteplase is a recombinant tissue plasminogen activator (rTPA) which converts plasminogen to plasmin, which in turn degrades fibrin and causes thrombus lysis. Non-thrombus-bound thrombin is readily inactivated by antiplasmin leading to a short half-life, necessitating continuous infusion for an hour. Dose: 0.9 mg/kg body weight, with a maximum of 90 mg.

Previously, thrombolysis could only be performed up to 4.5 hours from symptom onset, with emphasis on it being performed as early as possible.[4] The numbers needed to treat (NNTs) for excellent outcome are approximately 4.5 within 90 minutes and approximately 15 between 3–4.5 hours. This is because the amount of salvageable penumbra and susceptibility of the thrombus to lysis decreases with time. EXTEND (Extending the Time for Thrombolysis in Emergency Neurological Deficits)[25] and WAKE UP[29] trials have now proven that thrombolysis can be performed till 9 hours, in select patient groups.

Tenecteplase is a genetically modified TPA with advantages of longer half time, greater selectivity for fibrin, and resistance to plasminogen activator inhibitors.[30] These properties allow for bolus infusion of its dose 0.25 mg/kg body weight, with a maximum dose of 25 mg.

Recent trials have proven TNK to at least be non-inferior and equally safe, with EXTEND IA TNK proving it to be superior in large-vessel occlusion (LVO) patients (22% patients achieved reperfusion more than 50% of the occluded territory in the TNK arm compared to 10% in the alteplase arm).[31]

All patients with AIS, presenting within 4.5 hours and ASPECTS ≥7 are eligible for thrombolysis by either alteplase or TNK. Selected patients fulfilling the criteria for thrombolysis in the extended window (EXTEND and WAKE UP trials) can be thrombolyzed by alteplase.

However, before thrombolysis, the contraindications should be sought for and ruled out to prevent complications **(Table 2)**.

Endovascular Thrombectomy

The publication of five landmark trials on EVT revolutionized stroke reperfusion therapy **(Table 3)**.[32-36] A meta-analysis of these trials[37] showed that EVT was superior to medical management alone of AIS associated with LVO [terminal internal carotid artery (ICA) or M1-middle cerebral artery (MCA)], if performed within 6 hours of symptom onset, with ASPECTS ≥6. The NNT to reduce disability by one level on the functional rating scale was 2.6.

The recently published DEFUSE-3 (Endovascular Therapy Following Imaging Evaluation for Ischemic Stroke 3)[38] and DAWN (DWI or CTP Assessment with Clinical Mismatch in the Triage of Wake-Up and Late Presenting Strokes Undergoing Neurointervention with Trevo)[39] trials have shown that some carefully selected patients can benefit from EVT treatment up to 16 and 24 hours of symptom onset respectively. The criteria for selection was by either perfusion–core mismatch[38] or clinical-radiological mismatch[39] and these trials recruited the patients with slow or medium infarct growth.

With improvement in patient selection and devices used for EVT, an increasing number of patients are becoming eligible for reperfusion therapies with better functional outcomes.

Cytoprotection

Many previous neuroprotection trials for AIS were found to be unsuccessful.[40,41] Enhanced understanding of stroke pathophysiology has shown that ischemic affects not only the neurons but also astrocytes, pericytes, microglia, and endothelial blood vessel lining in the ischemic zone: *Neurovascular unit*. Therapies targeting this neurovascular unit comprise cytoprotection and the ones targeting multiple components are more likely to be effective than the previous solely neuroprotective ones. These cytoprotective drugs should ideally be given prior to reperfusion therapies in order to reduce the infarct progression before perfusion is restored. Thereafter, they might even prevent post reperfusion injury.[18] Also, there should be no interaction between these agents and thrombolytics (e.g., nerinitide and rTPA interacted with the latter decreasing drug levels of the former possibly leading to the negative trial result).[42] Many cytoprotective trials are ongoing.

SECONDARY PREVENTION

An important part of stroke treatment is secondary prevention. This entails the use of "blood thinners" (either, antiplatelets or anticoagulants) apart from risk factor management. The blood thinner chosen depends upon the stroke severity and probable etiology. Antiplatelets are used in atherosclerotic disease whereas anticoagulants are used in cardioembolic ones.

CHANCE (Clopidogrel in High-risk Patients with Acute Nondisabling Cerebrovascular Events)[43] and POINT

TABLE 2: Contraindications to thrombolysis.

Definite exclusion criteria	Significant head trauma or prior stroke in the past 3 months	
	Subarachnoid hemorrhage	
	Arterial puncture at a noncompressible site in the past 1 week	
	History of intracranial hemorrhage	
	Intracranial neoplasm, arteriovenous malformation, or aneurysm	
	Recent intracranial or intraspinal surgery	
	Active internal bleeding	
	Elevated blood pressure (systolic >185 mm Hg, diastolic >110 mm Hg)	
	Acute bleeding diathesis, including but not limited to:	Platelet count <100,000/mm^3
		Heparin received in the past 48 hours resulting in abnormally elevated aPTT above the upper limit of normal
		Current use of anticoagulant with INR >1.7 or PT >15 seconds
		Current use of direct thrombin or direct factor Xa inhibitors within the past 48 hours
	Blood glucose <50 mg/dL	
	CT demonstrates multilobe infarction (hypodensity in >1/3 of cerebral hemisphere)	
Relative exclusion criteria	Minor or rapidly improving stroke symptoms	
	Pregnancy	
	Seizure at onset with postictal residual neurological impairments	
	Major surgery or serious trauma within the previous 2 weeks	
	Recent gastrointestinal or urinary tract hemorrhage in the past 3 weeks	
	Recent myocardial infarction in the past 3 months	
Relative criteria at 3–4.5 hours	Age >80 years	
	NIHSS >25	
	History of oral anticoagulant intake irrespective of INR	

(aPTT: activated partial thromboplastin time; CT: computed tomography; INR: international normalized ratio; NIHSS: National Institute of Health Stroke Severity; PT: prothrombin time)

TABLE 3: Important characteristics of landmark endovascular thrombectomy (EVT) trials.

	MR CLEAN	**EXTEND-IA**	**ESCAPE**	**SWIFT–PRIME**	**REVASCAT**
Occlusion site chosen	Distal ICA/M1/M2/ A1/A2	ICA/M1/M2	ICA/M1/M2	Intracranial ICA/M1	Intracranial ICA/M1
Intervention used	Choice of the interventionist	Solitaire stent retriever	Choice of the interventionist	Solitaire stent retriever	Solitaire stent retriever
Time from stroke onset allowed	6 hours	4.5 hours	10 hours	4.5 hours	8 hours
Number of patients	500	70	315	196	206
TICI score 2b–3	58.7%	86%	72.4%	88%	65.7%
NNT to achieve mRS 0–2	7.1	3.2	4.2	4.0	6.3

(A1 and A2: anterior cerebral artery segments; EXTEND: Extending the Time for Thrombolysis in Emergency Neurological Deficits; ICA: internal carotid artery; M1 and M2: middle cerebral artery segments; mRS: modified Rankin Scale; NNT: number needed to treat; SWIFT–PRIME: Solitaire with the Intention for Thrombectomy as Primary Endovascular Treatment; TICI: Thrombolysis in Cerebral Infarction)

(Platelet-Oriented Inhibition in New TIA and Minor Ischemic Stroke)[44] trials provided evidence for the use of short duration dual antiplatelets (21 days) in patients presenting with minor strokes and TIAs. This is followed by continuation of only single antiplatelet thereafter in the interest of safety and reducing side effects.

Cardioembolic strokes are treated with anticoagulants. The absence of need for repeated monitoring, easy dosing, and improved safety profile (decreased risk of intracranial bleeding) have led to increased use of direct-acting oral anticoagulants (dabigatran, apixaban, and rivaroxaban) in patients with nonvalvular AF associated strokes. The elucidation of reversal agents (idarucizumab for dabigatran, andexanet alfa for apixaban) has provided further confidence. Vitamin K antagonists (e.g., warfarin) continue to be the drug of choice in valvular AF.

Anticoagulation is not superior to antiplatelet use in patients with arterial dissection and is probably associated with increased bleeding risk.[45] Therefore, arterial dissection is often treated with single or dual antiplatelet therapy.

MOBILE STROKE UNITS—THE WAY FORWARD

Mobile stroke units (MSUs) represent a new approach to management where the stroke unit is brought to the patient. They are specially designed ambulances with CT scanners and medical/paramedical personnel that can triage AIS patients and perform thrombolysis. Through them, more patients are likely to get thrombolyzed within the golden hour (first 60 minutes after stroke onset) and therefore have better functional outcomes. A German study showed that thrombolysis occurred nearly half an hour earlier through MSU use.[46] LVO predictive scores for prehospital triage such as RACE (Rapid Arterial Occlusion Evaluation)[47] and LAMS (Los Angeles Motor Scale)[48] have been developed to facilitate direct transfer of patients with high likelihood of LVO to EVT equipped centers.

CONCLUSION

The management of acute ischemic stroke has evolved from time window to tissue window. Rapid recognition of symptoms and presentation to a stroke ready hospital are paramount to achieve thrombolysis/endovascular thrombectomy, leading to better functional outcomes.

Despite the advent of these acute management therapies, appropriate secondary prevention strategies along with correction of modifiable risk factors remain a very important cog in the wheel of stroke care.

REFERENCES

1. Sacco RL, Kasner SE, Broderick JP, Caplan LR, Connors JJ, Culebras A, et al; American Heart Association Stroke Council, Council on Cardiovascular Surgery and Anesthesia; Council on Cardiovascular Radiology and Intervention; Council on Cardiovascular and Stroke Nursing; Council on Epidemiology and Prevention; Council on Peripheral Vascular Disease; Council on Nutrition, Physical Activity and Metabolism. An Updated Definition of Stroke for the 21st Century: A Statement for Healthcare Professionals From the American Heart Association/American Stroke Association. Stroke. 2013;44(7):2064-89.
2. GBD 2016 Lifetime Risk of Stroke Collaborators; Feigin VL, Nguyen G, Cercy K, Johnson CO, Alam T, Parmar PG, et al. Global, Regional, and Country-Specific Lifetime Risks of Stroke, 1990 and 2016. N Engl J Med. 2018;379(25):2429-37.
3. Astrup J, Siesjö BK, Symon L. Thresholds in cerebral ischemia—the ischemic penumbra. Stroke. 1981;12:723-5.
4. National Institute of Neurological Disorders and Stroke rt-PA Stroke Study Group. Tissue Plasminogen Activator for Acute Ischemic Stroke. N Engl J Med. 1995;333:1581-8.
5. Collaborative systematic review of the randomised trials of organised inpatient (stroke unit) care after stroke. Stroke Unit Trialists' Collaboration. BMJ. 1997;314(7088):1151-9.
6. Emberson J, Lees KR, Lyden P, Blackwell L, Albers G, Bluhmki E, et al; Stroke Thrombolysis Trialists' Collaborative Group. Effect of treatment delay, age, and stroke severity on the effects of intravenous thrombolysis with alteplase for acute ischaemic stroke: a meta-analysis of individual patient data from randomised trials. Lancet. 2014;384(9958):1929-35.
7. GBD 2016 Stroke Collaborators. Global, regional, and national burden of stroke, 1990-2016: a systematic analysis for the Global Burden of Disease Study 2016. Lancet Neuro . 2019;18(5):439-58.
8. Campbell BCV, De Silva DA, Macleod MR, Coutts SB, Schwamm LH, Davis SM, et al. Ischaemic stroke. Nat Rev Dis Primers. 2019;5(1):70.
9. Feigin VL, Krishnamurthi RV, Parmar P, Norrving B, Mensah GA, Bennett DA, et al; GBD 2013 Writing Group; GBD 2013 Stroke Panel Experts Group. Update on the Global Burden of Ischemic and Hemorrhagic Stroke in 1990-2013: The GBD 2013 Study. Neuroepidemiology. 2015;45(3):161-76.
10. Krishnamurthi RV, Feigin VL, Forouzanfar MH, Mensah GA, Connor M, Bennett DA, et al; Global Burden of Diseases, Injuries, Risk Factors Study 2010 (GBD 2010); GBD Stroke Experts Group. Global and regional burden of first-ever ischaemic and haemorrhagic stroke during 1990-2010: findings from the Global Burden of Disease Study 2010. Lancet Glob Health. 2013;1(5):e259-81.
11. Feigin VL, Norrving B, Mensah GA. Global Burden of Stroke. Circ Res. 2017;120(3):439-48.
12. Bevan S, Traylor M, Adib-Samii P, Malik R, Paul NLM, Jackson C, et al. Genetic heritability of ischemic stroke and the contribution of previously reported candidate gene and genomewide associations. Stroke. 2012;43(12):3161-7.
13. O'Donnell MJ, Xavier D, Liu L, Zhang H, Chin SL, Rao-Melacini P, et al; INTERSTROKE investigators. Risk factors for ischaemic and intracerebral haemorrhagic stroke in 22 countries (the INTERSTROKE study): a case-control study. Lancet. 2010;376(9735):112-23.
14. Bang OY, Ovbiagele B, Kim JS. Nontraditional Risk Factors for Ischemic Stroke: An Update. Stroke. 2015;46(12):3571-8.
15. Shah AS, Lee KK, McAllister DA, Hunter A, Nair H, Whiteley W, et al. Short term exposure to air pollution and stroke: systematic review and meta-analysis. BMJ. 2015;350:h1295.
16. Holmstedt CA, Turan TN, Chimowitz MI. Atherosclerotic intracranial arterial stenosis: risk factors, diagnosis, and treatment. Lancet Neurol. 2013;12(11):1106-14.
17. Zhang H, Prabhakar P, Sealock R, Faber JE. Wide genetic variation in the native pial collateral circulation is a major determinant of variation in severity of stroke. J Cereb Blood Flow Metab. 2010;30(5):923-34.
18. Xiong Y, Wakhloo AK, Fisher M. Advances in Acute Ischemic Stroke Therapy. Circ Res. 2022;130(8):1230-51.
19. Wu S, Mead G, Macleod M, Chalder T. Model of Understanding Fatigue After Stroke. Stroke. 2015;46(3):893-8.
20. Desowska A, Turner DL. Dynamics of brain connectivity after stroke. Rev Neurosci. 2019;30(6):605-23.
21. Brott T, Adams HP Jr, Olinger CP, Marler JR, Barsan WG, Biller J, et al. Measurements of acute cerebral infarction: a clinical examination scale. Stroke. 1989;20(7):864-70.

22. van Swieten JC, Koudstaal PJ, Visser MC, Schouten HJ, van Gijn J. Interobserver agreement for the assessment of handicap in stroke patients. Stroke. 1988;19(5):604-7.
23. Pexman JHW, Barber PA, Hill MD, Sevick RJ, Demchuk AM, Hudon ME, et al. Use of the Alberta Stroke Program Early CT Score (ASPECTS) for Assessing CT Scans in Patients with Acute Stroke. AJNR Am J Neuroradiol. 2001;22(8):1534-42.
24. Román LS, Menon BK, Blasco J, Hernández-Pérez M, Dávalos A, Majoie CBLM, et al; HERMES collaborators. Imaging features and safety and efficacy of endovascular stroke treatment: a meta-analysis of individual patient-level data. Lancet Neurol. 2018;17(10):895-904.
25. Ma H, Campbell BCV, Parsons MW, Churilov L, Levi CR, Hsu C, et al; EXTEND Investigators. Thrombolysis Guided by Perfusion Imaging up to 9 Hours after Onset of Stroke. N Engl J Med. 2019;380(19):1795-803.
26. Hjort N, Christensen S, Sølling C, Ashkanian M, Wu O, Røhl L, et al. Ischemic injury detected by diffusion imaging 11 minutes after stroke. Ann Neurol. 2005;58(3):462-5.
27. Campbell BCV, Purushotham A, Christensen S, Desmond PM, Nagakane Y, Parsons MW, et al; EPITHET–DEFUSE Investigators. The infarct core is well represented by the acute diffusion lesion: sustained reversal is infrequent. J Cereb Blood Flow Metab. 2012;32(1):50-6.
28. Simard JM, Kent TA, Chen M, Tarasov KV, Gerzanich V. Brain oedema in focal ischaemia: molecular pathophysiology and theoretical implications. Lancet Neurol. 2007;6(3):258-68.
29. Thomalla G, Simonsen CZ, Boutitie F, Andersen G, Berthezene Y, Cheng B, et al; WAKE-UP Investigators. MRI-Guided Thrombolysis for Stroke with Unknown Time of Onset. N Engl J Med. 2018;379(7):611-22.
30. Tanswell P, Modi N, Combs D, Danays T. Pharmacokinetics and pharmacodynamics of tenecteplase in fibrinolytic therapy of acute myocardial infarction. Clin Pharmacokinet. 2002;41(15): 1229-45.
31. Campbell BCV, Mitchell PJ, Churilov L, Yassi N, Kleinig TJ, Dowling RJ, et al; EXTEND-IA TNK Investigators. Tenecteplase versus Alteplase before Thrombectomy for Ischemic Stroke. N Engl J Med. 2018;378(17):1573-82.
32. Saver JL, Goyal M, Bonafe A, Diener HC, Levy EI, Pereira VM, et al; SWIFT PRIME Investigators. Stent-Retriever Thrombectomy after Intravenous t-PA vs. t-PA Alone in Stroke. N Engl J Med. 2015;372(24):2285-95.
33. Goyal M, Demchuk AM, Menon BK, Eesa M, Rempel JL, Thornton J, et al; ESCAPE Trial Investigators. Randomized Assessment of Rapid Endovascular Treatment of Ischemic Stroke. N Engl J Med. 2015;372(11):1019-30.
34. Berkhemer OA, Fransen PSS, Beumer D, van den Berg LA, Lingsma HF, Yoo AJ, et al; MR CLEAN Investigators. A Randomized Trial of Intraarterial Treatment for Acute Ischemic Stroke. N Engl J Med. 2015;372(1):11-20.
35. Jovin TG, Chamorro A, Cobo E, de Miquel MA, Molina CA, Rovira A, et al; REVASCAT Trial Investigators. Thrombectomy within 8 Hours after Symptom Onset in Ischemic Stroke. N Engl J Med. 2015;372:2296-306.
36. Campbell BC, Mitchell PJ, Kleinig TJ, Dewey HM, Churilov L, Yassi N, et al; EXTEND-IA Investigators. Endovascular Therapy for Ischemic Stroke with Perfusion-Imaging Selection. N Engl J Med. 2015;372(11):1009-18.
37. Goyal M, Menon BK, van Zwam WH, Dippel DWJ, Mitchell PJ, Demchuk AM, et al; HERMES collaborators. Endovascular thrombectomy after large-vessel ischaemic stroke: a meta-analysis of individual patient data from five randomised trials. Lancet Lond Engl. 2016;387(10029):1723-31.
38. Albers GW, Marks MP, Kemp S, Christensen S, Tsai JP, Ortega-Gutierrez S, et al; DEFUSE 3 Investigators. Thrombectomy for Stroke at 6 to 16 Hours with Selection by Perfusion Imaging. N Engl J Med. 2018;378(8):708-18.
39. Nogueira RG, Jadhav AP, Haussen DC, Bonafe A, Budzik RF, Bhuva P, et al; DAWN Trial Investigators. Thrombectomy 6 to 24 Hours after Stroke with a Mismatch between Deficit and Infarct. N Engl J Med. 2018;378(1):11-21.
40. Hill MD, Goyal M, Menon BK, Nogueira RG, McTaggart RA, Demchuk AM, et al; ESCAPE-NA1 Investigators. Efficacy and safety of nerinetide for the treatment of acute ischaemic stroke (ESCAPE-NA1): a multicentre, double-blind, randomised controlled trial. Lancet. 2020;395(10227):878-87.
41. Dávalos A, Alvarez-Sabín J, Castillo J, Díez-Tejedor E, Ferro J, Martínez-Vila E, et al; International Citicoline Trial on acUte Stroke (ICTUS) trial investigators. Citicoline in the treatment of acute ischaemic stroke: an international, randomised, multicentre, placebo-controlled study (ICTUS trial). Lancet. 2012;380(9839):349-57.
42. Mayor-Nunez D, Ji Z, Sun X, Teves L, Garman JD, Tymianski M. Plasmin-resistant PSD-95 inhibitors resolve effect-modifying drug-drug interactions between alteplase and nerinetide in acute stroke. Sci Transl Med. 2021;13(588):eabb1498.
43. Wang Y, Wang Y, Zhao X, Liu L, Wang D, Wang C, et al; CHANCE Investigators. Clopidogrel with Aspirin in Acute Minor Stroke or Transient Ischemic Attack. N Engl J Med. 2013;369(1):11-9.
44. Johnston SC, Easton JD, Farrant M, Barsan W, Conwit RA, Elm JJ, et al; Clinical Research Collaboration, Neurological Emergencies Treatment Trials Network, and the POINT Investigators. Clopidogrel and Aspirin in Acute Ischemic Stroke and High-Risk TIA. N Engl J Med. 2018;379(3):215-25.
45. Markus HS, Levi C, King A, Madigan J, Norris J; Cervical Artery Dissection in Stroke Study (CADISS) Investigators. Antiplatelet Therapy vs Anticoagulation Therapy in Cervical Artery Dissection: The Cervical Artery Dissection in Stroke Study (CADISS) Randomized Clinical Trial Final Results. JAMA Neurol. 2019;76(6):657-64.
46. Ebinger M, Winter B, Wendt M, Weber JE, Waldschmidt C, Rozanski M, et al; STEMO Consortium. Effect of the use of ambulance-based thrombolysis on time to thrombolysis in acute ischemic stroke: a randomized clinical trial. JAMA. 2014;311(16):1622-31.
47. Pérez de la Ossa N, Carrera D, Gorchs M, Querol M, Millán M, Gomis M, et al. Design and validation of a prehospital stroke scale to predict large arterial occlusion: the rapid arterial occlusion evaluation scale. Stroke. 2014;45(1):87-91.
48. Llanes JN, Kidwell CS, Starkman S, Leary MC, Eckstein M, Saver JL. The Los Angeles Motor Scale (LAMS): a new measure to characterize stroke severity in the field. Prehosp Emerg Care. 2004;8(1):46-50.

50 CHAPTER

Intracerebral Hemorrhage

Radhika Nair, Jeyaraj Durai Pandian, Mahesh P Kate

INTRODUCTION

Spontaneous intracerebral hemorrhage (ICH) is defined as bleeding within the brain parenchyma **(Fig. 1)**. It is the most common type of nontraumatic intracranial bleed. ICH is associated with higher morbidity and mortality when compared to ischemic stroke. Globally, there were 12.2 million strokes in the year 2019 and ICH accounted for 3.14 million.[1] Unfortunately, the incidence of ICH is stable or increasing over the years, however, the outcome after ICH has not improved over the last few decades in comparison to ischemic stroke.[2-4]

EPIDEMIOLOGY

Intracerebral hemorrhage is the second most common cause of stroke **(Fig. 1)**. ICH accounts for about 10–15% of all strokes in the western population. According to the global burden of diseases 2019, the ischemic stroke incidence constituted 62.4% of all strokes, followed by ICH and subarachnoid hemorrhage which constituted 27.9% and 9.7%, respectively. When comparing low- to upper-middle-income countries to high-income countries, the proportion of ICH was about two-fold higher.[1] The African and Asian populations have a higher prevalence of ICH.[5] The prevalence of ICH in India ranged from 10.1% in Thiruvananthapuram to 35% in Kolkata. ICH rates are higher in the eastern part of India.[6-9] ICH becomes increasingly common as people get older, with people over 75 years being the most affected.[10,11] In comparison to the western population, where the mean age is 70–79 years, the incidence of ICH is predominantly in the younger population; nonetheless, the majority of Indian studies indicated mean ages of 50–59 years. In India, hypertensive ICH occurs 15–20 years earlier than in the west, and there is also a higher incidence among men.[12,13]

PATHOLOGY

Spontaneous ICH can be divided into primary and secondary. Primary ICH accounts for about 80–85% of all spontaneous ICH. Primary ICH results from spontaneous rupture of blood vessels due to hypertension or amyloid angiopathy.[14,15]

- *ICH associated with hypertension*: The untreated or poorly treated arterial hypertension increases the risk of stroke two- to four-fold. Deep perforator arteriopathy or small vessel disease is linked with hypertension and is a common cause of nonlobar or deep ICH **(Fig. 1)**. It is commonly seen in the putamen, caudate, thalamus, brain stem, and deep cerebellar nuclei; but may

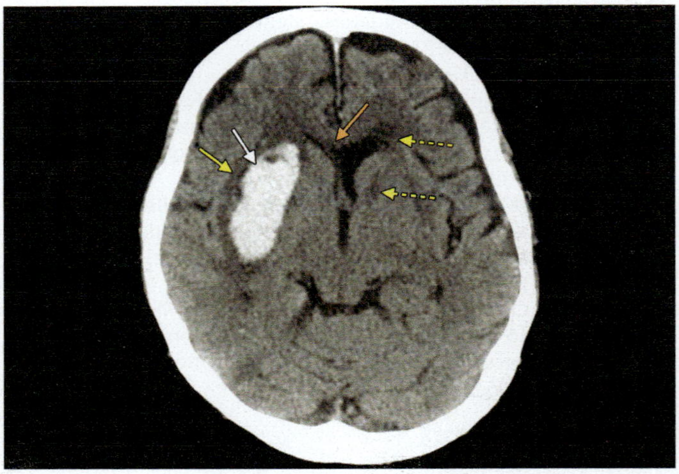

FIG. 1: Right basal ganglia intracerebral hemorrhage. White arrow: intracerebral hemorrhage hyperdensity, yellow arrow: surrounding the ICH is hypodensity that is perihematomal edema, orange arrow: mass effect of the intracerebral hemorrhage, dotted yellow arrow: small vessel disease periventricular hypodensity and deep white matter hypodensity.

also contribute to lobar hemorrhage. Long-standing hypertension leads to smooth muscle cell proliferation and necrosis; which subsequently results in the replacement of smooth muscles with collagen in arterioles. As a result, the arterioles become rigid, and brittle, which might dilate and form a Charcot–Bouchard aneurysm. These vessel microballoons can burst when subjected to high pressure or fluctuating pressure, as in deep thalamic, pontine, or striatal vessels because of their downstream proximity to relatively large pial arteries, they can burst to cause deep ICH.[16,17] The natural history of ICH is variable **(Fig. 2)**. Approximately, 15–25% of people have hematoma expansion, 60% of people have a stable hematoma, and 10–15% of people develop hematoma contraction.

- *ICH associated with cerebral amyloid angiopathy*: In CAA, there is a deposition of β-amyloid in the media and adventitia of cortical leptomeningeal blood vessels, causing weakening of arterial walls and rupture of vessels resulting in ICH. As the disease progresses, all layers of vessel walls including smooth muscle cells are replaced by Aβ. As a result, there is microaneurysm formation, fibrinoid necrosis, and perivascular leakage. Such weakened blood vessels are prone to vessel rupture resulting in cerebral microbleeds or lobar ICH **(Fig. 3)**.[17,18] The ICH related to cerebral amyloid angiopathy (CAA) occurs primarily in the lobar locations or in the subarachnoid spaces over the convexities. Studies have suggested that apolipoprotein E (ApoE) 2 or 4 alleles are at a greater risk of developing CAA and ICH.[19]

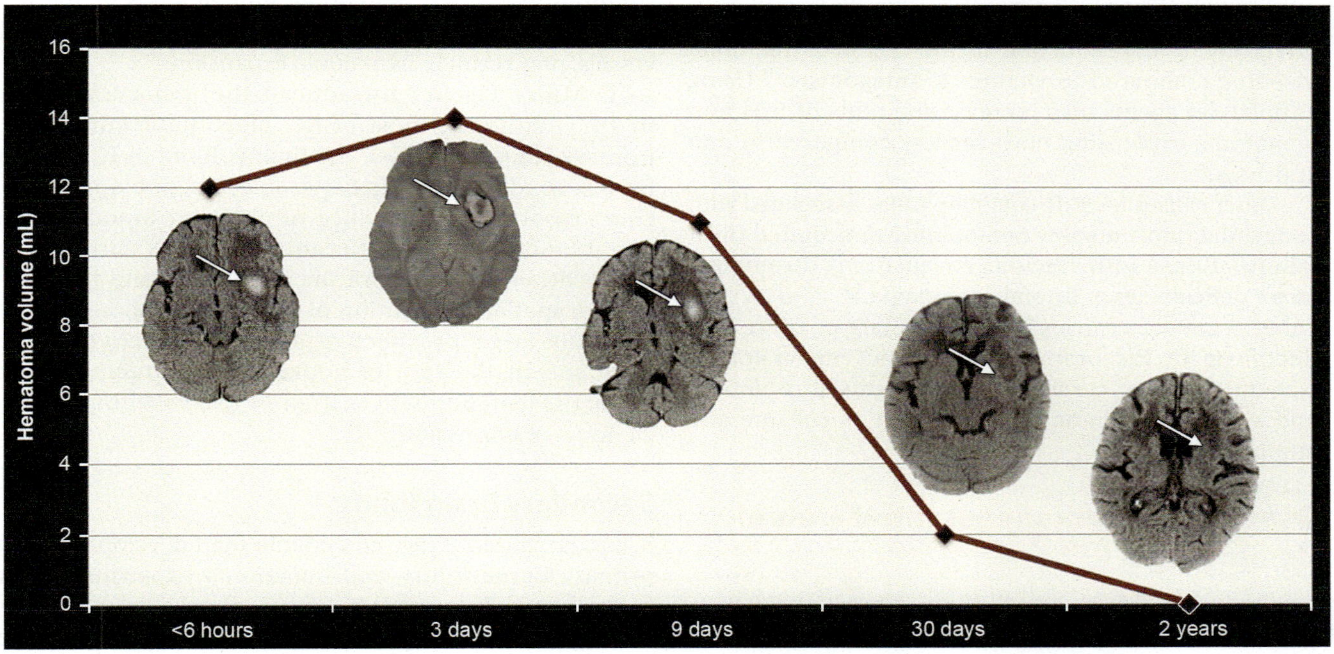

FIG. 2: Natural history of intracerebral hemorrhage over a period. Initial hematoma expansion followed by hematoma contraction.

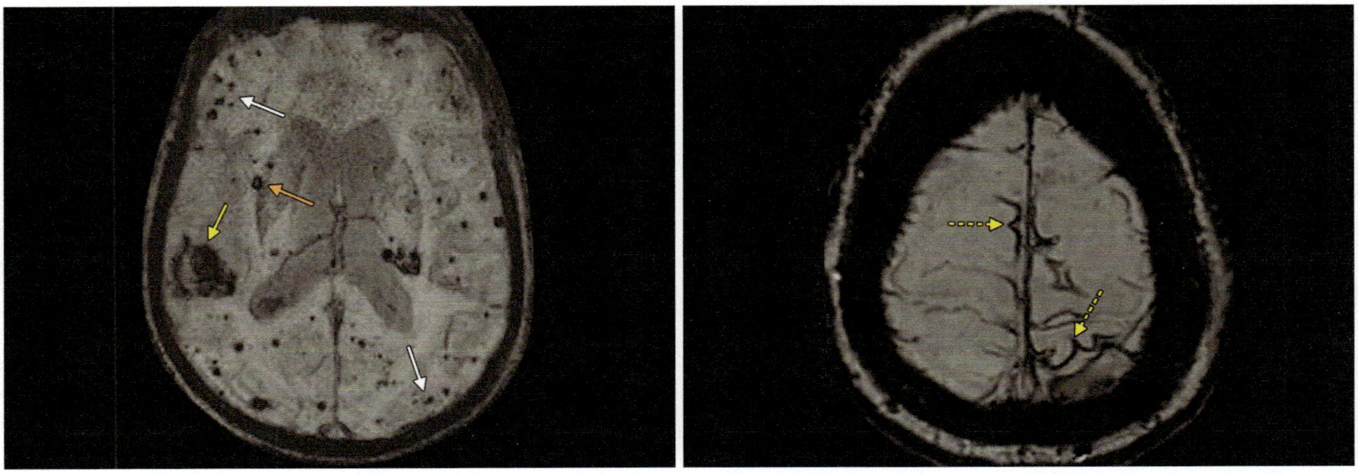

FIG. 3: Susceptibility-weighted imaging in magnetic resonance imaging shows the left temporal lobe, cortical intracerebral hemorrhage (yellow arrow), cortical microbleeds (white arrows), and deep microbleeds (orange arrow). Cortical superficial siderosis (dotted yellow arrow).

Secondary ICH can be caused by:

- Structural abnormalities of underlying blood vessels like cavernous angiomas, aneurysms, arteriovenous, fistula, etc. These are more often encountered in young and individuals without vascular risk factors like hypertension.
- *Coagulopathies*: The most common acquired causes are due to the use of anticoagulants, antithrombotic, and thrombolytic agents. A proportion of patients use anticoagulants or antiplatelet medicines for secondary prevention of cardiovascular disorders. The highest risk of ICH is with the use of vitamin K antagonists like warfarin. The absolute annual risk of ICH in person on oral anticoagulants ranges from 0.25 to 1.1%, which is 7–10 times higher than the incidence in the general population. Direct oral anticoagulants (DOACs) are also associated with a higher risk of ICH compared to aspirin, the overall favorable safety profile of DOACs is indeed driven by a 50% reduction in the risk of intracranial bleeding compared to vitamin K antagonists.[20] Using antiplatelet agents also increase the odds of ICH and hematoma expansion, however less compared to oral anticoagulants.

  Other causes include coagulopathies associated with congenital (most notably hemophilia) or acquired (liver failure, diffuse intravascular coagulation) thrombotic factor deficiencies or thrombocytopenia.[19]
- Other secondary causes include primary or metastatic neoplasm of the brain, hemorrhagic conversion of ischemic stroke, cerebral venous sinus thrombosis, and sympathomimetic drug use such as cocaine and amphetamines.[14,15]

Genetics of Spontaneous Intracerebral Hemorrhage

A population-based case-control study reported that having a first-degree relative with ICH leads to a six-fold increase in the risk of ICH.[21] Genome-wide association studies have identified epsilon variants within ApoE, the rs4311 variant of the angiotensin-converting enzyme (*ACE*) gene, rs9588151 of the collagen type IV alpha 2 (*COL4A2*) gene are associated with increased risk for ICH. 1q22 is identified as a susceptibility locus for nonlobar ICH, a locus potentially relevant to small vessel diseases. Familial amyloid angiopathy where there are mutations in APP—the beta-amyloid precursor protein gene also has a higher incidence of ICH.[22]

Pathophysiology of Intracerebral Hemorrhage

Direct Neuronal Injury

An acute hemorrhage in the brain parenchyma causes immediate tissue injury from hematoma due to compression and disorganization of neurons. This leads to disruption of signaling pathways and may cause focal neurological deficits. If the hemorrhage is within the brainstem, the manifestations may be altered sensorium with or without cardiorespiratory distress.[23]

Secondary Hematoma Growth

Secondary stationary growth or secondary hematoma growth usually follows the initial hematoma growth and the prognosis is largely determined by this. The initial hematoma expansion exerts pressure on the surrounding tissues and blood vessels. In response to the pressure, the surrounding tissues exert counter pressure. The pressure increases in proportion to the hematoma growth. If this counter pressure can overcome the force of the jet of blood from a primary ruptured vessel, the hematoma growth stops or reduces. If the pressure is high enough to rupture the surrounding vessels, may result in hematoma expansion.[16]

C Miller Fischer introduced the *avalanche* model in 1971, although most of the bleeding occurs from a primary ruptured vessel, the final volume in ICH results from secondary shearing between adjacent blood vessels. One vessel triggers rupture of adjacent blood vessels, and blood flows in different directions, influencing the location and shape of the hematoma and forming a unique spatial distribution of intracranial hemorrhage.[24] Previous large prospective and retrospective studies have shown the rate of hematoma enlargement after initial presentation ranges from 14 to 38% within the first 24 hours of admission.[25,26]

Secondary Brain Injury

Secondary brain injury and edema then develop following primary tissue injury and hematoma expansion. There is a release of neutrophils, macrophages, and activated microglia that secrete cytotoxic enzymes, oxygen-free radicals, and nitric oxide resulting in secondary neuronal injury and death.[27]

A decrease in blood flow to the perihematomal region may result in ischemia. Perihematomal edema during the hyperacute phase is caused by changes in intracellular osmotic pressure, cytotoxicity, and clot retracement, and occurs within 1–2 hours. There is the activation of the coagulation cascade and thrombin in the acute phase, which results in vasogenic edema. After 72 hours, there is hemoglobin-induced cytotoxicity. The progression of edema lasts for more than 24 hours is stable for up to 4 days and gradually reduces after a few days to weeks.[28,29] The expanding edema causes increased intracranial pressure (ICP), movement of adjacent tissues, and mass effect, which can result in herniation syndromes. It may also result in decreased perfusion pressure, further accelerating secondary brain injury.[23]

CLINICAL PRESENTATION

The classic presentation is a sudden onset of focal neurological deficits, which may rapidly worsen over a few hours. The type of neurological deficits will depend on the location of ICH. ICH in the supratentorial region may cause contralateral weakness, hemisensory deficits, aphasia, hemineglect, hemianopia, or gaze paresis. An infratentorial ICH may present with altered sensorium, cranial nerve defects, and ataxia **(Fig. 4)**.

- ICH patients often experience headaches, nausea, and vomiting
- Examination often reveals elevated blood pressure
- If there is hematoma extension to subarachnoid space, the patient may have neck stiffness.
- Seizures are less common and may be seen in up to 10% of patients.[30]
- Rarely, bleeding can rupture into ventricles [intraventricular hemorrhage (IVH)] causing hydrocephalus, a large hemorrhage may cause a sudden increase in ICP leading to mass effect, brain herniation, and death due to compression of the brainstem.
- At the bedside, it is difficult to distinguish an ischemic stroke from a hemorrhagic stroke. Certain features such as rapidly progressive neurodeficits, headache, vomiting, seizures, and alerted level of consciousness may suggest ICH is more likely.

DIAGNOSIS

Acute Evaluation

Intracerebral hemorrhage is a life-threatening neuro-emergency that necessitates prompt diagnosis; because brain imaging is necessary to reliably distinguish ICH from ischemic stroke, the emergency workflow for patients suspected of either ICH or ischemic stroke should be the same, which includes routine application of a neurological baseline severity score. The National Institute of Health Stroke scale (NIHSS) score is feasible and useful. NIHSS is 11 items with 42 points assessment scale that includes the level of consciousness, consciousness questions, consciousness commands, best gaze, visual field loss, facial palsy, motor weakness in the arms and in the legs, limb ataxia, sensory loss, language assessment, dysarthria assessment, extinction, and inattention. The Glasgow Coma Scale (GCS) is a widely used, quick, and reproducible tool for assessing consciousness. In all patients focused history should be taken, including any trauma, past medical history of bleeding diathesis, use of antiplatelet or anticoagulant drugs, and drug abuse. General medical assessments including airways, blood pressure, and circulation should be carried out on all the patients.[31] The ICH score **(Table 1)** is a reliable and validated scale for the rapid assessment of ICH severity.[32]

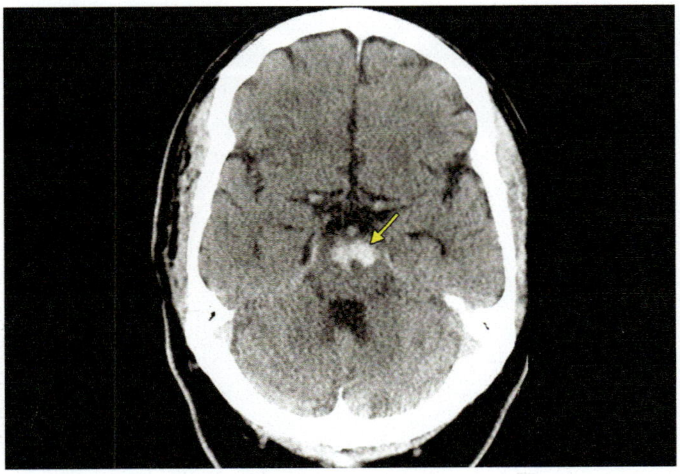

FIG. 4: Infratentorial hemorrhage, acute ventral pontine hemorrhage.

Mortality rate based on ICH score: ICH scores with corresponding mortality risk are as follows: 0 points: 0%, 1 point: 13%, 2 points: 26%, 3 points: 72%, 4 points: 97%, 5 points: 100%, and 6 points: 100% (estimated).

Imaging

Noncontrast Computed Tomography Brain

- It is a rapid, highly specific, and sensitive test for diagnosing all forms of ICH. It is considered the gold standard test for diagnosis of ICH.[31]

TABLE 1: ICH score components.

Component	ICH score points
Glasgow Coma Scale score at presentation	
3–4	2
5–12	1
13–15	0
ICH volume (mL)	
≥30	1
<30	0
Intraventricular extension	
Yes	1
No	0
Infratentorial origin	
Yes	1
No	0
Age, years	
≥80	1
<80	0
Total ICH score	

(ICH: intracerebral hemorrhage)

- A CT scan of the brain can be used to assess the location of hemorrhage, intraventricular extension, hydrocephalus, cerebral edema, mass effect, midline shift, and brain herniation.
- CT head can help detect small vessel ischemic changes and leukoaraiosis **(Fig. 1)**.
- Certain CT head signs increase the possibility of hematoma expansion island sign, swirl sign, or meniscus sign **(Fig. 5)**.
- Using noncontrast computed tomography (NCCT) head we can calculate hematoma volume. It can be estimated using the formula ABC/2 and it is a strong predictor of ICH outcome **(Fig. 6)**. Patients with a parenchymal hemorrhage volume of 60 cm^3 or more on their initial CT and a GCS of eight or less had a 30-day death rate of 91%. Patients with a volume smaller than 30 cm^3 and a GCS of 9 or higher had a predicted 30-day death rate of 19%.[33]

Computed Tomography Angiography

- Computed tomography angiography (CTA) is a noninvasive technique for the diagnosis of vascular malformation resulting in secondary ICH.
- CTA should be ordered when there is a high suspicion of vascular malformation or other causes of secondary ICH like the presence of lobar ICH, younger age at

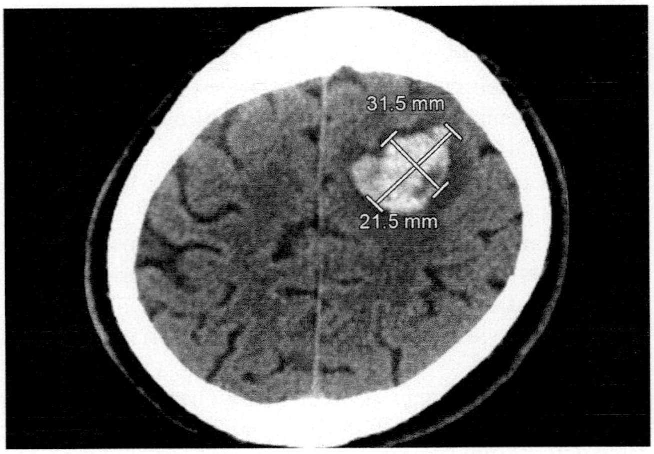

FIG. 6: Hematoma volume calculation, ABC/2 (mL). Measure the (A) longest diameter, (B) widest diameter, and (C) longest height. The height is measured by counting the slices of the CT scan where the ICH hyperdensity is first noted and continues to measure last seen. We must know the interslice distance typically it is 5 mm.

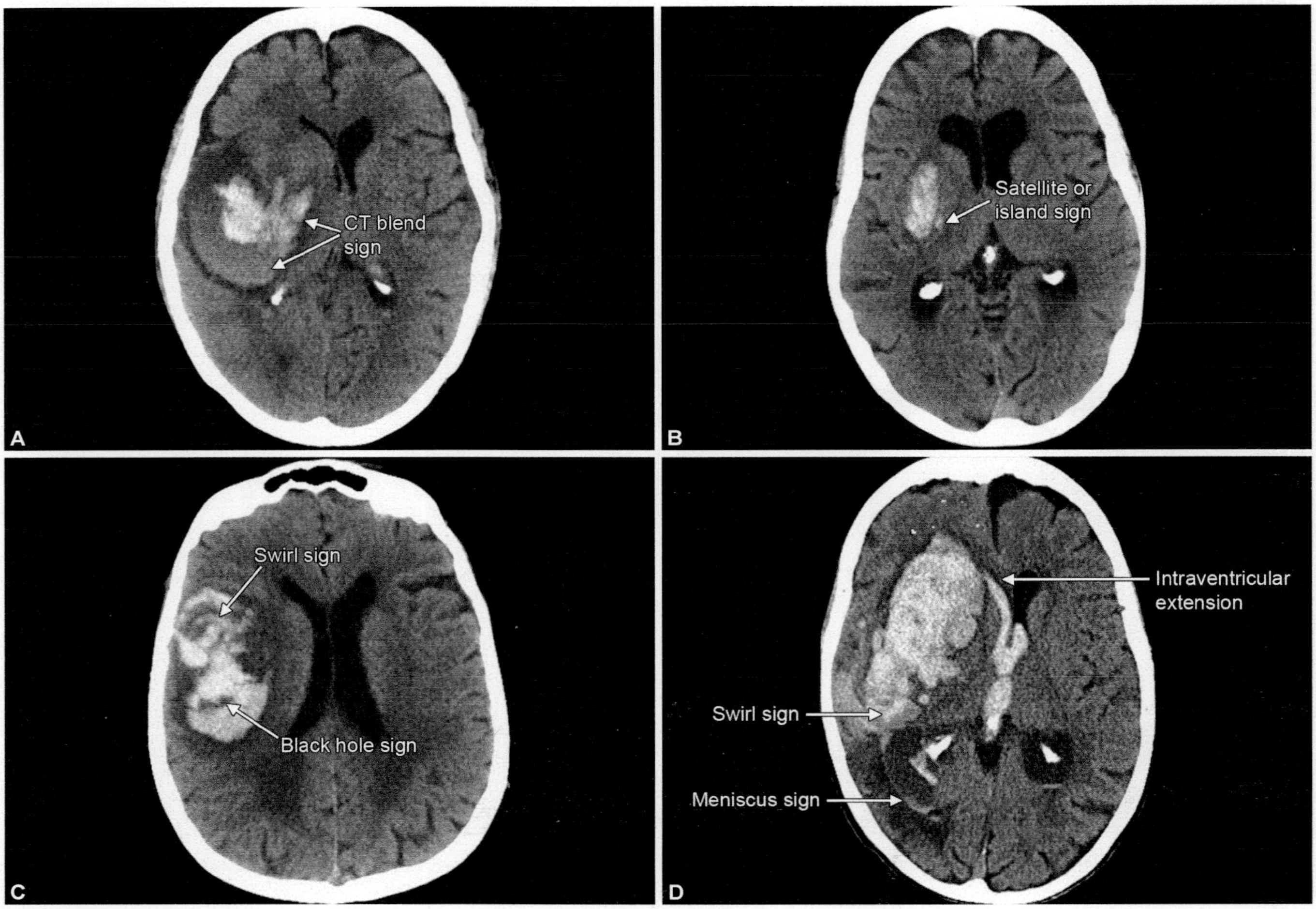

FIGS. 5A TO D: Intracerebral hemorrhage features on computed tomography (CT) head associated with the risk of hematoma expansion.

presentation, significant intraventricular expansion, and absence of traditional cerebrovascular risk factors.[31]

- Prompt diagnosis of vascular malformations is important for management.
- *Spot sign*: CTA sign in acute ICH that represents the focal accumulation or extravasation of contrast-containing blood within the hematomas **(Fig. 7)**. It is an independent predictor of hematoma expansion and the presence of spot signs indicates poor outcomes in patients with supratentorial ICH.[34]
- Drawbacks of CTA are radiation exposure, contrast allergy, and contrast-induced nephropathy.

Magnetic Resonance Imaging Brain

- Sensitivity is equivalent to NCCT head in diagnosing ICH. Magnetic resonance imaging (MRI) is more accurate than CT in revealing chronic bleeding in the brain, particularly microbleeds.[35]
- MRI also aids in the etiological diagnosis of amyloid angiopathy (cortical microhemorrhages in susceptibility imaging), neoplastic lesions, and hemorrhagic transformation of ischemic stroke.[36]
- MRI is sensitive to flow abnormalities in vascular structures. This property makes MRI an ideal tool for the detection of vascular malformations. MRI can sometimes pick up lesions that are not detected by angiography.[36,37]

Cerebral Angiography

- For the diagnosis of vascular anomalies in ICH, conventional cerebral angiography remains the gold standard.[38]
- Conventional angiography is needed to completely exclude a vascular lesion even if a CT angiogram, MR image, and MR angiogram are negative.
- A conventional angiogram is also used to confirm a vascular malformation diagnosis as it is a dynamic study that provides additional information about the active filling/emptying phases of the veins and arteries.[14]
- Although the risk of angiography is low, the diagnostic yield must be weighed against the procedural risk at each institution.[15]

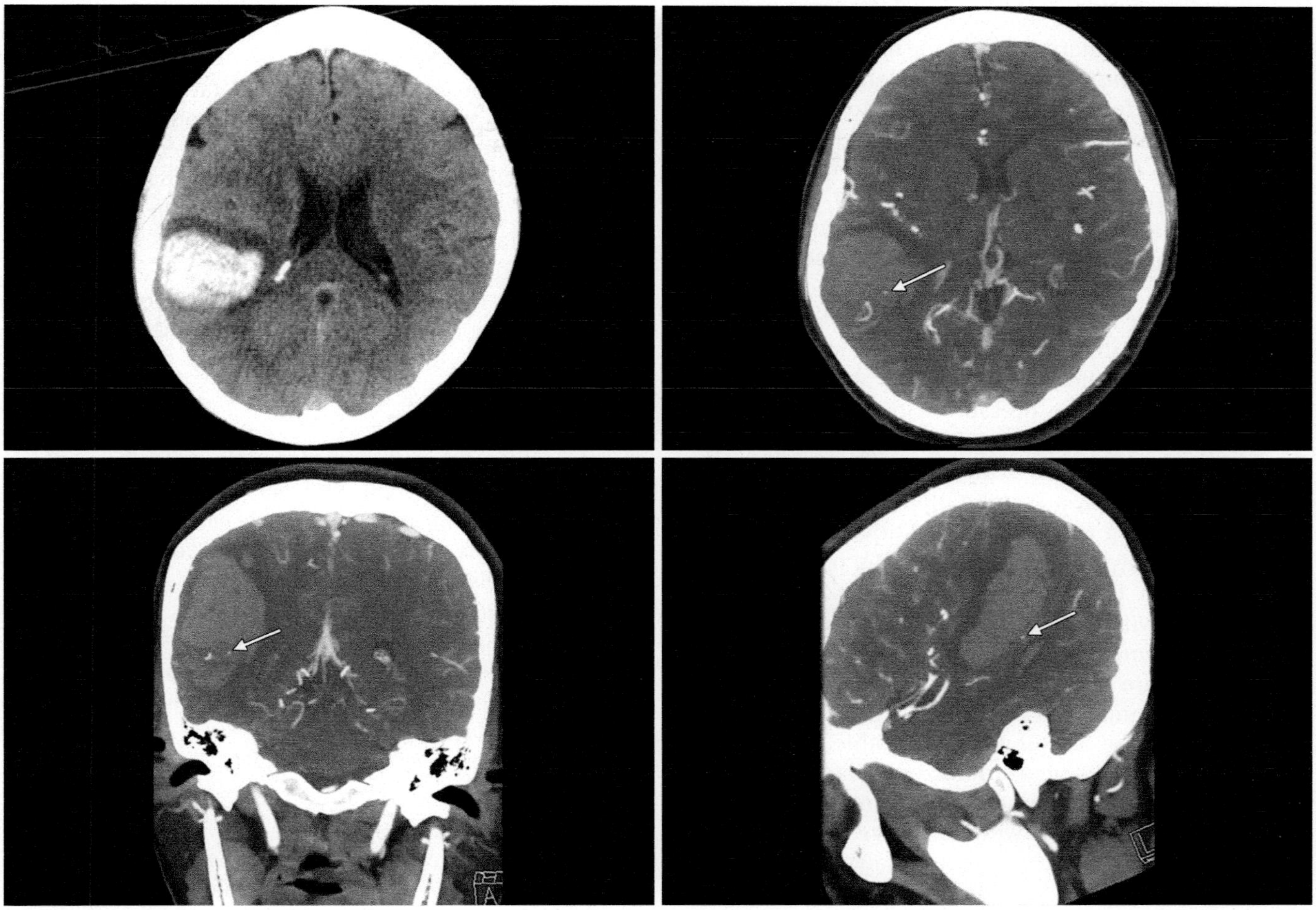

FIG. 7: Right frontal hemorrhage with computed tomography (CT) angiogram showing spot sign in axial, coronal, and sagittal images (white arrows).

Laboratory Test

Complete blood count, coagulation studies, serum creatinine, electrolytes, and blood glucose should be obtained.

MANAGEMENT

Acute Medical Management

Intracerebral hemorrhage is a neurological emergency like an acute ischemic stroke. The concept of time is brain holds good for ICH too. One of the independent predictors of outcome is hematoma expansion which usually occurs early in the course of the disease.[39,40] The expanding hematoma and edema can lead to an increase in ICP and may result in brain herniation. Timely treatment for optimal blood pressure management, reversal of anticoagulation, and neurosurgical care is the key to the treatment of ICH.[25]

Stroke Unit Management

A meta-analysis reported a reduction in death and dependence rates in ICH patients admitted to a stroke unit. All ICH patients should be admitted to an acute or hyperacute stroke unit as soon as feasible and those at high risk of neurological deterioration to the intensive care unit.[41]

- *Airway maintenance*: Patients with large ICH or ICH in the posterior fossa may have respiratory distress and difficulty maintaining the airway. Patients with declining GCS or GCS of ≤8 should be evaluated for respiratory distress and may require endotracheal intubation.[42] Pretreatment with lidocaine before intubation may be helpful as it may blunt a rise in ICP associated with intubation.[43,44]
- *Blood pressure management*: Very high blood pressure is associated with hematoma expansion in patients with ICH. Previously, there were concerns about a reduction in cerebral perfusion pressure with rapid lowering of blood pressure in patients with ICH. Recent research, on the other hand, has disproved the concern.[45,46] For patients with ICH, a systolic blood pressure target of 140–160 mm Hg for the first 24–48 hours is ideal, and a more intensive reduction of systolic blood pressure of <140 mm Hg should be considered in patients presenting within 6 hours of the onset of symptoms, patient on anticoagulant therapy, presenting systolic blood pressure not >220 mm Hg and the neuroimaging suggesting hematoma expansion.[42] The BP reduction should be done as quickly as possible. ATACH and INTERACT 2, two large, randomized trials on rapid blood pressure reduction, found no substantial reduction in mortality or disability with intensive blood pressure reduction.[47,48] However, a meta-analysis of these and other smaller trials has found that individuals with lower target blood pressure within 24 hours of symptom onset had better functional outcomes.[49] For acute blood pressure reduction, parenteral labetalol, hydralazine, nicardipine, and/or enalaprilat (oral or intravenous) may be recommended.[42]
- *Management of anticoagulant-associated ICH*: The annual rate of ICH ranges from 0.3 to 0.6% in patients taking vitamin K antagonists and 0.1 to 0.2% in those taking DOACs. DOACs are associated with an overall 50% reduction in the rate of ICH.[50] Oral anticoagulants are thought to exacerbate the spontaneous ICH, and sustain and cause expansion. Studies report around 35–50% of hematoma expansion in patients taking anticoagulants.[51] The goal is to stop the anticoagulant and reverse it as quickly as possible.

For vitamin K antagonist (warfarin):

- Stop warfarin immediately
- Patients with international normalized ratio (INR) of ≥1.4 at the time of admission should be considered for reversal.
- The goal of the reversal treatment is to reduce the INR to under 1.4 as quickly as possible.
- *Treatment includes*:
  - Vitamin K 10 mg administered IV over 20–30 minutes
  - It may take up to 12 hours for vitamin K to reduce INR level and therefore 4-factor prothrombin complex concentrate (PCC) should be given with vitamin K. Dosage for INR 2–3.9: >25 units/kg, INR of 4–6: >35 units/kg, INR of >6: >50 units/kg.
  - If PCC is not available, consider fresh frozen plasma. However, large volume of plasma is required.
- For the first 24 hours, INR should be monitored every 3–6-hour intervals to detect rebound coagulopathy and other complications.[40]

For direct oral anticoagulants:

- *Dabigatran*:
  - Stop dabigatran immediately
  - Drug levels can be tested using thrombin time, dilute thrombin time, and ecarin clot time.
  - Reversal should be considered for dabigatran levels >30 ng/dL
  - *Treatment*:
    - *Specific reversal agent*: Idarucizumab. The recommended dose is 5 g, provided as two separate vials each containing 2.5 g/50 mL idarucizumab.
    - *Other agents*: 4-factor PCC.[40]

Factor Xa inhibitors:

- Stop the dug immediately
- Drug levels can be tested using Factor Xa assay
- *Specific reversal agent*: Andexanet alpha.
- *Other agents*: 4-factor PCC.[40]

Heparin:

- Stop heparin infusion/low molecular weight heparin (LMWH)
- Protamine sulfate slow infusion: 1 mg/100 units of heparin if activated partial thromboplastin time is prolonged or if heparin is infused within 2 hours. The maximum dose is 50 mg.
- Protamine sulfate partially neutralizes the effect of LMWH. The same dosing strategy can be used.[40]

  Patients with coagulopathies should receive an appropriate replacement of deficient factors. For patients using antiplatelet agents, there is no specific therapy. Platelet transfusion has not shown benefit in these patients.

- *Seizure management*: Several studies investigated the efficacy and safety of using prophylactic antiepileptic medicines for ICH with no studies finding a benefit for prophylactic treatment. Several studies concluded worse cognitive or neurological outcomes in patients treated with antiepileptic drugs. Given these findings, antiepileptic drugs are no longer indicated for seizure prophylaxis.[52,53]
- *Intracranial pressure management*: Patients with ICH associated with mass effect, cerebral edema, and hydrocephalus with ventricular outflow obstruction have been associated with increased ICP. The role of osmotic therapy is limited. Hypertonic or mannitol can be used to reduce raised ICP but this is not associated with improved outcomes.
- *Neurosurgical management*: ICH in supratentorial fossa is generally managed conservatively. The standard surgical intervention is open craniotomy. One of the largest RCTs in ICH, STICH I trial found no meaningful difference between the surgical and medical groups at 6 months in terms of mortality or outcome.[54,55] However, a meta-analysis of trials has shown early surgery may be beneficial.

  When there is the development of malignant edema or mass effect due to hemorrhage, hemicraniectomy may be necessary to prevent the mass effect and midline shift. This should be offered to the younger patient and the family should be informed about the enhanced probability of survival with long-term disability.

  The extension of hematoma into ventricles may result in obstruction of the outflow tract resulting in hydrocephalus. This is an indication of emergency external ventricular drain placement for cerebrospinal fluid (CSF) diversion and helps to monitor intracerebral pressure.[56] The CLEAR trial, aimed to test whether attempts to remove IVH with alteplase versus saline irrigation improved the outcome at 3 months, however, the trial showed no significant difference between the group.[57]

  In recent years, the potential for minimally invasive surgery to evacuate intracerebral bleed has been investigated. These trials have failed to show a significant difference between medical management and surgical evacuation group.[58,59] The MISTIE trial, which investigated minimally invasive catheter evacuation followed by thrombolysis with alteplase in ICH, showed alteplase to be safe in patients with intracerebral bleed, although there was an increase in asymptomatic hemorrhage.[59] The STICH II trial in which the patients were randomly assigned to surgical hematoma evacuation plus medical treatment with medical treatment only, showed early surgery did not increase the rate of death or disability at 6 months. The study concluded that the surgical group might have a small but clinically relevant advantage in spontaneous superficial ICH without intraventricular extension.[60]

  Because of the confined space, even a small volume hemorrhage in the infratentorial fossa can result in life-threatening complications such as compression of the brainstem and hydrocephalus. For cerebellar ICH of >3 cm or those with lesser bleeds that result in hydrocephalus or compression of the brainstem, surgical therapy with posterior decompressive evacuation, and/or ventricular catheter placement should be explored.[61]
- *Deep venous thrombosis prophylaxis*: Initiate sequential compression stockings device from admission if there is even minor immobility. After 48 hours if the CT head shows stable hematoma volume, we can consider initiation of LMWH prophylaxis.

ABC Care Bundle Approach for Management of ICH

Anticoagulation reversal, intensive blood pressure control, neurosurgery, and access to critical care in patients with ICH were associated with lower 30 days case fatality rates when compared to standard treatment which included the following:

- Rapid anticoagulant reversal, within 90 minutes of arrival in patients who are on anticoagulants with 4-factor PCC for vitamin K antagonists and anti-Xa antagonists or idarucizumab for dabigatran.
- Intensive BP lowering to a systolic target of 130–140 mm Hg for patients arriving within 6 hours of onset with a systolic blood pressure of >150 mm Hg within 60 minutes of arrival to the hospital.

Immediate neurosurgical referral of all patients with good premorbid function [modified Rankin scale (mRS) score ≤2] and any of the following: GCS <9, posterior fossa ICH, an obstructed third/fourth ventricle, or hematoma volume >30 mL.[62]

Chronic Management

Long-term blood pressure is important with a systolic BP target of <130 mm Hg. The usual BP treatment agents are ACE inhibitors including perindopril, angiotensin receptor blocker, calcium channel blocker, and β-blocker. This is to prevent recurrent hemorrhage **(Fig. 8)**.

CONCLUSION

The concept of "time is brain" holds good in ICH, timely treatment to reduce hematoma expansion, perihematomal edema, and inflammation. This includes treating high blood pressure, and reversal of anticoagulation should be addressed immediately. To diagnose the ICH, complications such as hydrocephalus and mass effects, brain, and vascular imaging should be performed as soon as possible for timely intervention.

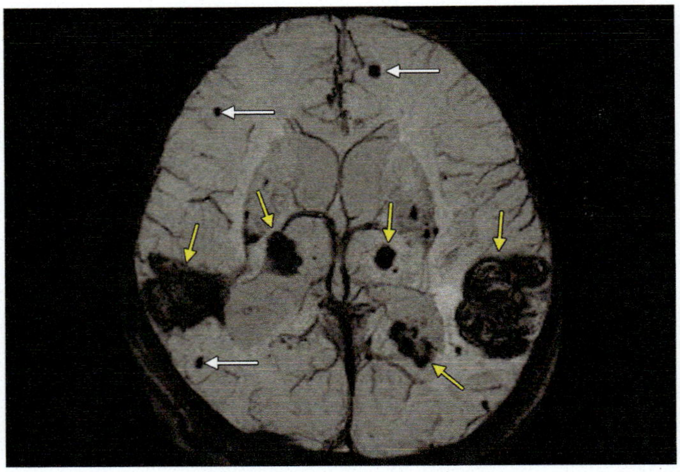

FIG. 8: Multiple intracerebral hemorrhages both deep and cortical (yellow arrows). Evidence of microbleeds (white arrow).

REFERENCES

1. GBD 2019 Stroke Collaborators. Global, regional, and national burden of stroke and its risk factors, 1990-2019: a systematic analysis for the Global Burden of Disease Study 2019. Lancet Neurol. 2021;20(10):795-820.
2. Van Asch CJ, Luitse MJ, Rinkel GJ, van der Tweel I, Algra A, Klijn CJ. Incidence, case fatality, and functional outcome of intracerebral haemorrhage over time, according to age, sex, and ethnic origin: a systematic review and meta-analysis. Lancet Neurol. 2010;9(2):167-76.
3. Bejot Y, Cordonnier C, Durier J, Aboa-Eboulé C, Rouaud O, Giroud M. Intracerebral haemorrhage profiles are changing: results from the Dijon population-based study. Brain. 2013;136(Pt 2):658-64.
4. Hostettler IC, Seiffge DJ, Werring DJ. Intracerebral hemorrhage: an update on diagnosis and treatment. Expert Rev Neurother. 2019;19(7):679-94.
5. Rymer MM. Hemorrhagic stroke: intracerebral hemorrhage. Mo Med. 2011;108(1):50-4.
6. Sridharan SE, Unnikrishnan JP, Sukumaran S, Nayak SD, Sarma PS, Radhakrishnan K. Incidence, types, risk factors, and outcome of stroke in a developing country: the Trivandrum Stroke Registry. Stroke. 2009;40(4):1212-8.
7. Das SK, Banerjee TK, Biswas A, Raut DK, Mukherjee CS, Chaudhuri A, et al. A prospective community-based study of stroke in Kolkata, India. Stroke. 2007;38:906-10.
8. Pandian JD, Singh G, Kaur P, Bansal R, Paul BS, Singla M, et al. Incidence, short-term outcome, and spatial distribution of stroke patients in Ludhiana, India. Neurology. 2016;86:425-33.
9. India State-Level Disease Burden Initiative CVD Collaborators. The changing patterns of cardiovascular diseases and their risk factors in the states of India: the Global Burden of Disease Study 1990-2016. Lancet Glob Health. 2018;6(12):e1339-51.
10. Broderick J, Brott T, Tomsick T, Miller R, Huster G. Intracerebral hemorrhage more than twice as common as subarachnoid hemorrhage. J Neurosurg. 1993;78:188-91.
11. Lovelock CE, Molyneux AJ, Rothwell PM, Oxford Vascular Study. Change in incidence and aetiology of intracerebral haemorrhage in Oxfordshire, UK, between 1981 and 2006: a population-based study. Lancet Neurol. 2007;6(6):487-93.
12. Giroud M, Delpont B, Daubail B, Blanc C, Durier J, Giroud M, et al. Temporal trends in sex differences with regard to stroke incidence: the Dijon Stroke Registry (1987-2012). Stroke. 2017;48(4):846-9.
13. Hegde A, Menon G. Modifying the intracerebral hemorrhage score to suit the needs of the developing world. Ann Indian Acad Neurol. 2018;21(4):270-4.
14. Rajashekar D, Liang JW. Intracerebral Hemorrhage. In: StatPearls [Internet]. Treasure Island (FL): StatPearls Publishing; 2022.
15. Fewel ME, Thompson BG Jr, Hoff JT. Spontanoeus intracerebral hemorrhage: a review. Neurosurg Focus. 2003:15(4):E1.
16. Schlunk F, Greenberg SM. The Pathophysiology of Intracerebral Hemorrhage Formation and Expansion. Transl Stroke Res. 2015;6:257-63.
17. Ziai WC, Carhuapoma JR. Intracerebral Hemorrhage. Continuum (Minneap Minn). 2018;24(6):1603-22.
18. Revesz T, Holton JL, Lashley T, Plant G, Rostagno A, Ghiso J, et al. Sporadic and familial cerebral amyloid angiopathies. Brain Pathol. 2002;12:343-57.
19. Bernstein JM, Girard R, Polster S, Srinath A, Romanos S, Awad IA, et al. Cerebral Hemorrhage: Pathophysiology, Treatment, and Future Directions. Circ Res. 2022;130:1204-29.
20. Morotti A, Goldstein JN. Anticoagulant-associated intracerebral hemorrhage. Brain Hemorrhages. 2020;1(1):89-94.
21. Woo D, Sauerbeck LR, Kissela BM, Khoury JC, Szaflarski JP, Gebel J, et al. Genetic and environmental risk factors for intracerebral hemorrhage: preliminary results of a population-based study. Stroke. 2002;33(5):1190-5.
22. Falcone GJ, Woo D. Genetics of spontaneous intracerebral hemorrhage. Stroke. 2017;48(12):3420-4.
23. Aiyagari V. The clinical management of acute intracerebral hemorrhage. Expert Rev Neurother. 2015;15(12):1421-32.
24. Fisher CM. Pathological observations in hypertensive cerebral hemorrhage. J Neuropathol Exp Neurol. 1971;30:536-50.
25. Brott T, Broderick J, Kothari R, Barsan W, Tomsick T, Sauerbeck L, et al. Early hemorrhage growth in patients with intracerebral hemorrhage. Stroke. 1997;28:1-5.
26. Fujii Y, Takeuchi S, Sasaki O, Minakawa T, Tanaka R. Multivariate analysis of predictors of hematoma enlargement in spontaneous intracerebral hemorrhage. Stroke. 1998;29:1160-6.
27. Yang GY, Betz AL, Chenevert TL, Brunberg JA, Hoff JT. Experimental intracerebral hemorrhage: relationship between brain edema, blood flow, and blood-brain barrier permeability in rats. J Neurosurg. 1994;81:93-102.

28. Lim-Hing K, Rincon F. Secondary hematoma expansion and perihemorrhagic edema after intracerebral hemorrhage: from bench work to practical aspects. Front Neurol. 2017;8:74.
29. Xie H, Qin Z, Yin X. Classification mechanism and clinical analysis of perihematomal edema in intracerebral hemorrhage. Brain Hemorrhages. 2020;1:141-5.
30. Bladin CF, Alexandrov AV, Bellavance A, Bornstein N, Chambers B, Cote R, et al. Seizures after stroke: a prospective multicenter study. Arch Neurol. 2000;57:1617-22.
31. Cordonnier C, Demchuk A, Ziai W, Anderson CS. Intracerebral haemorrhage: current approaches to acute management. Lancet. 2018;392:1257-68.
32. Hemphill JC 3rd, Greenberg SM, Anderson CS, Becker K, Bendok BR, Cushman M, et al. Guidelines for the management of spontaneous intracerebral hemorrhage: a guideline for healthcare professionals from the American Heart Association/American Stroke Association. Stroke. 2015;46:2032-60.
33. Hemphill JC, Bonovich DC, Besmertis L, Manley GT, Johnston SC. The ICH score: a simple, reliable grading scale for intracerebral hemorrhage. Stroke. 2001;32(4):891-7.
34. Broderick JP, Brott TG, Duldner JE, Tomsick T, Huster G. Volume of intracerebral hemorrhage. A powerful and easy-to-use predictor of 30-day mortality. Stroke. 1993;24(7):987-93.
35. Demchuk A, Dowlatshahi D, Rodriguez-Luna D, Molina CA, Blas YS, Dzialowski I, et al. Prediction of haematoma growth and outcome in patients with intracerebral haemorrhage using the CT-angiography spot sign (PREDICT): A prospective observational study. Lancet Neurol. 2012;11(4):307-14.
36. Kidwell CS, Chalela JA, Saver JL, Starkman S, Hill MD, Demchuk AM, et al. Comparison of MRI and CT for detection of acute intracerebral hemorrhage. JAMA. 2004;292:1823-30.
37. Macellari F, Paciaroni M, Agnelli G, Caso V. Neuroimaging in intracerebral hemorrhage. Stroke. 2014;45(3):903-8.
38. Siddiqui FM, Bekker SV, Qureshi AI. Neuroimaging of hemorrhage and vascular defects. Neurotherapeutics. 2011;8(1):28-38.
39. Balami JS, Buchan AM. Complications of intracerebral haemorrhage. Lancet Neurol. 2012;11:101-18.
40. McGurgan IJ, Ziai WC, Werring DJ, Al-Shahi Salman R, Parry-Jones AR. Acute intracerebral haemorrhage: diagnosis and management. Pract Neurol. 2021;21:128-36.
41. Langhorne P, Fearon P, Ronning OM, Kaste M, Palomaki H, Vemmos K, et al. Stroke unit care benefits patients with intracerebral hemorrhage: systematic review and meta-analysis. Stroke. 2013;44(11): 3044-9.
42. Shoamanesh A, Lindsay PM, Castellucci LA, Cayley A, Crowther M, de Wit K, et al. Canadian stroke best practice recommendations: Management of Spontaneous Intracerebral Hemorrhage, 7th Edition Update 2020. Int J Stroke. 2021;16(3):321-41.
43. Morotti A, Goldstein JN. Diagnosis and Management of Acute Intracerebral Hemorrhage. Emerg Med Clin North Am. 2016;34(4):883-99.
44. Salhi B, Stettner E. In defense of the use of lidocaine in rapid sequence intubation. Ann Emerg Med. 2007;49(1):84-6.
45. Butcher KS, Jeerakathil T, Hill M, Demchuk AM, Dowlatshahi, Coutts SB et al. The intracerebral hemorrhage acutely decreasing arterial pressure trial. Stroke. 2013;44:620-6.
46. Gould B, McCourt R, Asdaghi N, Dowlatshahi D, Jeerakathil T, Kate M, et al. Autoregulation of cerebral blood flow is preserved in primary intracerebral hemorrhage. Stroke. 2013;44:1726-8.
47. Anderson CS, Heeley E, Huang Y, Wang J, Stapf C, Delcourt C, et al. Rapid blood-pressure lowering in patients with acute intracerebral hemorrhage. N Engl J Med. 2013;368:2355-65.
48. Qureshi AI, Palesch YY, Barsan WG, Barsan WG, Hanley DF, Hsu CY, et al. Intensive blood-pressure lowering in patients with acute cerebral hemorrhage. N Engl J Med. 2016;375:1033-43.
49. Moullaali TJ, Wang X, Martin RH, Shipes VB, Robinson. TG, Chalmers J, et al. Blood pressure control and clinical outcomes in acute intracerebral haemorrhage: a preplanned pooled analysis of individual participant data. Lancet Neurol. 2019;18:857-64.
50. Hart RG, Diener HC, Yang S, Wallentin L, Reilly PA, Ezekowitz MD, et al. Intracranial hemorrhage in atrial fibrillation patients during anticoagulation with warfarin or dabigatran: the RE-LY trial. Stroke. 2012;43:1511-7.
51. Flibotte JJ, Hagan N, O'Donnell J, Greenberg SM, Rosand J. Warfarin, hematoma expansion, and outcome of intracerebral hemorrhage. Neurology. 2004;63:1059-64.
52. Sheth KN, Martini SR, Moomaw CJ, Koch S, Elkind MS, Sung G, et al. Prophylactic Antiepileptic Drug Use and Outcome in the Ethnic/ Racial Variations of Intracerebral Hemorrhage Study. Stroke. 2015;46:3532-5.
53. Mackey J, Blatsioris AD, Moser EAS, Carter RJL, Saha C, Stevenson A, et al. Prophylactic Anticonvulsants in Intracerebral Hemorrhage. Neurocrit Care. 2017;27:220-8.
54. Mendelow AD, Gregson BA, Fernandes HM, Murray GD, Teasdale GM, Hope DT, et al. Early surgery versus initial conservative treatment in patients with spontaneous supratentorial intracerebral haematomas in the international surgical trial in intracerebral haemorrhage (STICH): a randomised trial. Lancet. 2005;365(9457):387-97.
55. Esquenazi Y, Savitz.SI, El Khoury R, McIntosh MA, Grotta JC, Tandon N. Decompressive hemicraniectomy with or without clot evacuation for large spontaneous supratentorial intracerebral hemorrhages. Clin Neurol Neurosurg. 2015;128:117-22.
56. Bhattathiri PS, Gregson B, Prasad KS, Mendelow AD; STICH Investigators. Intraventricular hemorrhage and hydrocephalus after spontaneous intracerebral hemorrhage: results from the STICH trials. Acta Neurochir Suppl. 2006;96:65-8.
57. Hanley DF, Lane K, McBee N, Ziai W, Tuhrim S, Lees KR, et al. Thrombolytic removal of intraventricular haemorrhage in treatment of severe stroke: results of the randomised, multicentre, multiregion, placebo-controlled CLEAR III trial. Lancet. 2017;389(10069):603-11.
58. Kellner CP, Chartrain AG, Nistal DA, Scaggiante J, Hom D, Ghatan S, et al. The stereotactic intracerebral hemorrhage underwater blood aspiration (SCUBA) technique for minimally invasive endoscopic intracerebral hemorrhage evacuation. J Neurointerv Surg. 2018;10(8):771-6.
59. Hanley DF, Thompson RE, Muschelli J, Rosenblum M, McBee N, Bistran-Hall AJ, et al. Safety and efficacy of minimally invasive surgery plus alteplase in intracerebral haemorrhage evacuation (MISTIE): a randomised, controlled, open-label, phase 2 trial. Lancet Neurol. 2016;15(12):1228-37.
60. Mendelow AD, Gregson BA, Rowan EN, Murray GD, Gholkar A, Mitchell PM, et al. Early surgery versus initial conservative treatment in patients with spontaneous supratentorial lobar intracerebral haematomas (STICH II): a randomised trial. Lancet. 2013;382(9890):397-408.
61. Kirollos RW, Tyagi AK, Ross SA, van Hille PT, Marks PV. Management of spontaneous cerebellar hematomas: a prospective treatment protocol. Neurosurgery. 2001;49(6):1378-86. discussion 1386-77.
62. Parry-Jones AR, Sammut-Powell C, Paroutoglou K, Birleson E, Rowland J, Lee S, et al. An Intracerebral Hemorrhage Care Bundle Is Associated with Lower Case Fatality. Ann Neurol. 2019;86(4): 495-503.

51

CHAPTER

Subarachnoid Hemorrhage

Jagarlapudi MK Murthy

INTRODUCTION

Spontaneous subarachnoid hemorrhage (SAH) accounts for 2–7% of all strokes. Ruptured intracranial aneurysm [aneurysmal SAH (aSAH)] is the most common cause and accounts for 85% of cases. The reported annual incidence of aSAH in high-income countries is 6 per 100,000 individuals, and there is a declining trend in the incidence. Survival from aSAH has increased in the past two decades. However, the functional outcome is still suboptimal. This is partly due to serious complications, particularly delayed cerebral ischemia (DCI).

CLINICAL FEATURES

The striking symptom of aSAH is an abrupt onset of severe headache classically described as the "worst headache of my life." Headache may be accompanied by a brief loss of consciousness, nausea or vomiting, and seizures. Neurologic examination may show meningeal signs and focal deficits. Intraocular hemorrhages of different types have been documented in aSAH. Terson syndrome refers to subhyaloid and/or vitreous hemorrhage. About 10–40% of patients with aSAH experience sentinel headaches, a severe headache occurring days to weeks before aneurysmal rupture. Important risk factors for aneurysmal rupture are uncontrolled hypertension, cigarette smoking, alcohol abuse, female sex, and older age.

DIAGNOSIS

Noncontrast computed tomography (CT) is the first imaging modality, and it will show blood in the subarachnoid space, typically in the basal cisterns, around the circle of Willis, major fissures ("star sign"), and within the ventricles **(Figs. 1A and B)**. In patients with aSAH, the sensitivity of CT approaches 100% in the first 24 hours and is only 60% at 1 week. Subarachnoid blood along the cerebral convexity is often due to nonaneurysmal causes. Perimesencephalic hemorrhage is of venous origin and is associated with good outcomes **(Figs. 2A and B)**. If the initial CT is non-diagnostic, the traditional next step is a lumbar puncture to evaluate for xanthochromia. However, recent studies suggest that if the initial CT is obtained on a third-generation or higher machine within 6 hours of headache onset in a neurologically intact patient and is interpreted as normal by a neuroradiologist, then SAH is ruled out, and no further investigations are necessary.

Digital subtraction angiography (DSA) is the gold standard diagnostic modality for detecting the source of bleeding, and with three-dimensional reconstruction, even a small aneurysm can be identified. However, CT angiography (CTA) is a widely used modality as it obviates DSA-attended risks **(Fig. 3)**. A meta-analysis of studies of CTA reported a pooled sensitivity of 97% and specificity of 91% for detecting an intracranial aneurysm. Aneurysms <3 mm in size may escape detection with CTA and this threshold may be less with most CT scanners. Magnetic resonance angiography (MRA) is inferior to DSA and CTA for aneurysm detection. A meta-analysis of MRA studies reported a sensitivity of 95% and specificity of 89%. In patients with an aneurysmal pattern of SAH and no etiology identified, DSA is a preferred diagnostic modality and should be repeated days to weeks later, and the yield is 10%.

MANAGEMENT

The first step in the management of patients with aSAH is to assign the disease severity grade using the World Federation of Neurosurgical Societies (WFNS) or the Hunt and Hess scale and modified Fisher's radiologic (CT scan) grading scales **(Tables 1 and 2)**. The amount of subarachnoid blood and the presence of intracerebral hemorrhage (ICH) or intraventricular hemorrhage (IVH) are associated with

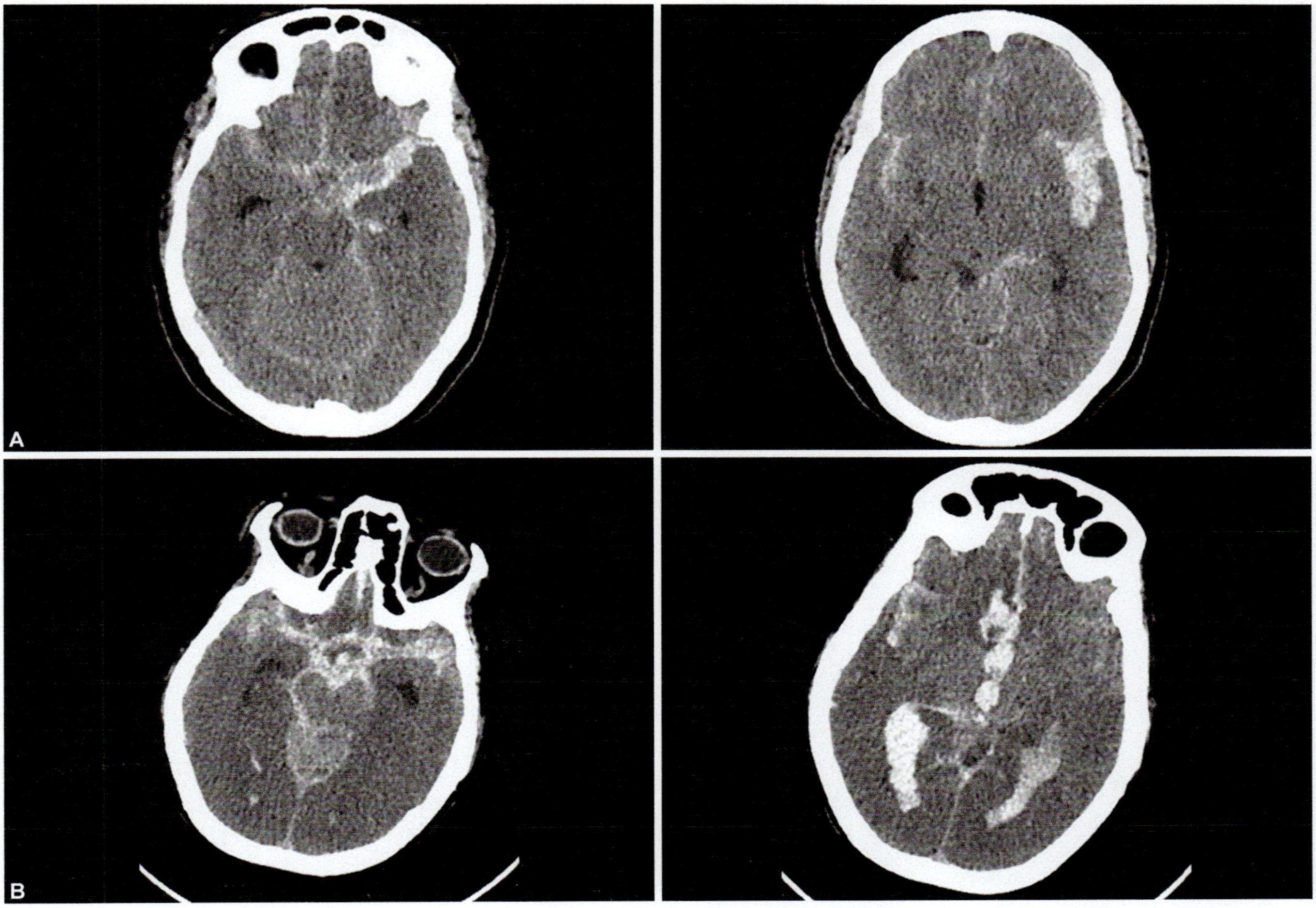

FIGS. 1A AND B: Noncontrast computed tomography (CT) scan showing (A) Blood in the subarachnoid spaces—modified Fisher's grade 3; and (B) Blood in the subarachnoid spaces and the ventricles—modified Fisher's grade 4.

subsequent vasospasm and neurological deficits. Initial Fisher's scale was modified and has been shown to predict vasospasm more accurately.

The admission grade of aSAH determines the outcome and directs treatment strategies. The rupture of the aneurysm triggers a cascade of events that are all interlinked. The course of the illness can be divided into three phases: acute phase (0–24 hours), subacute phase (≤72 hours), and delayed or chronic phase (>7 days) **(Box 1)**.

Acute Phase

The acute phase encompasses what happens in the first 24 hours and sets the stage for the later events. During this time, complications that may occur include rebleeding, cardiopulmonary complications, hydrocephalus, and seizures.

Cardiopulmonary Complication

Increasing sympathetic activity and excessive catecholamine release occur in the immediate phase of aSAH. Acute catecholamine surge results in cardiopulmonary complications such as neurogenic-stunned myocardium and neurogenic pulmonary edema.

Of the cardiac abnormalities, electrocardiogram (ECG) changes are the most common, occurring in 25–75% and life-threatening arrhythmias in 8% of patients. Cardiac troponin I (cTI) elevations are common (20–30%), but are generally below the threshold for myocardial infarction. Troponin I elevation >2 μ/L is strongly associated with depression of ejection fraction, vasospasm, cerebral infarction, and death. The presence of ejection fraction <40% and cT1 < 2–8 ng/mL is consistent with stunned myocardium. The clinical syndrome is characterized by T-wave inversions with prolonged QT interval, reversible regional wall motion abnormality (RWMA) beyond a single vascular territory (Takotsubo cardiomyopathy), cardiogenic shock, pulmonary edema, and transient metabolic acidosis. Treatment is supportive, and has the potential for improvement with time.

Aneurysmal SAH leads to pulmonary dysfunction at the capillary level, leading to neurogenic pulmonary edema.

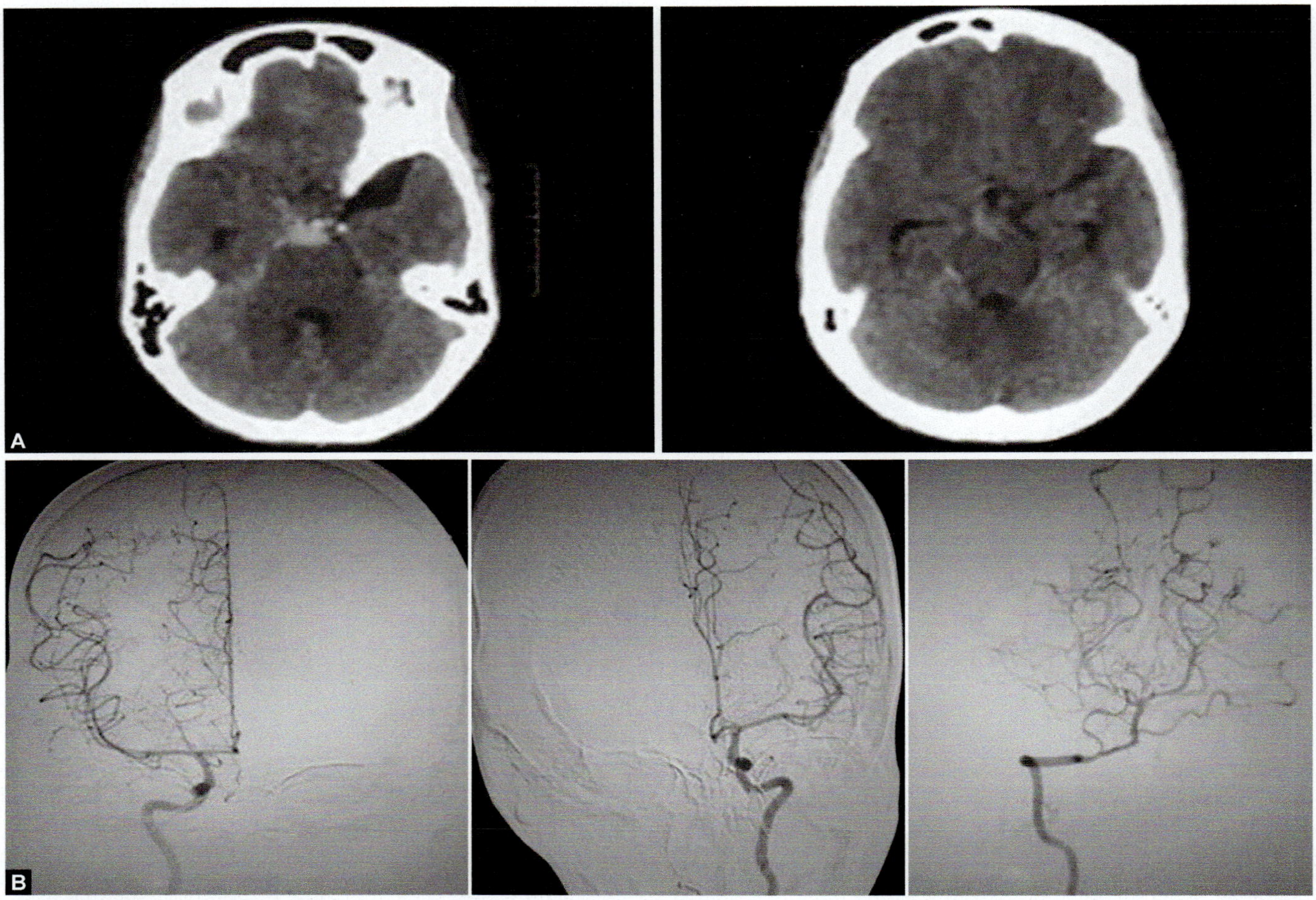

FIGS. 2A AND B: Computed tomography (CT) angiography in a patient with subarachnoid hemorrhage showing right side middle cerebral artery.

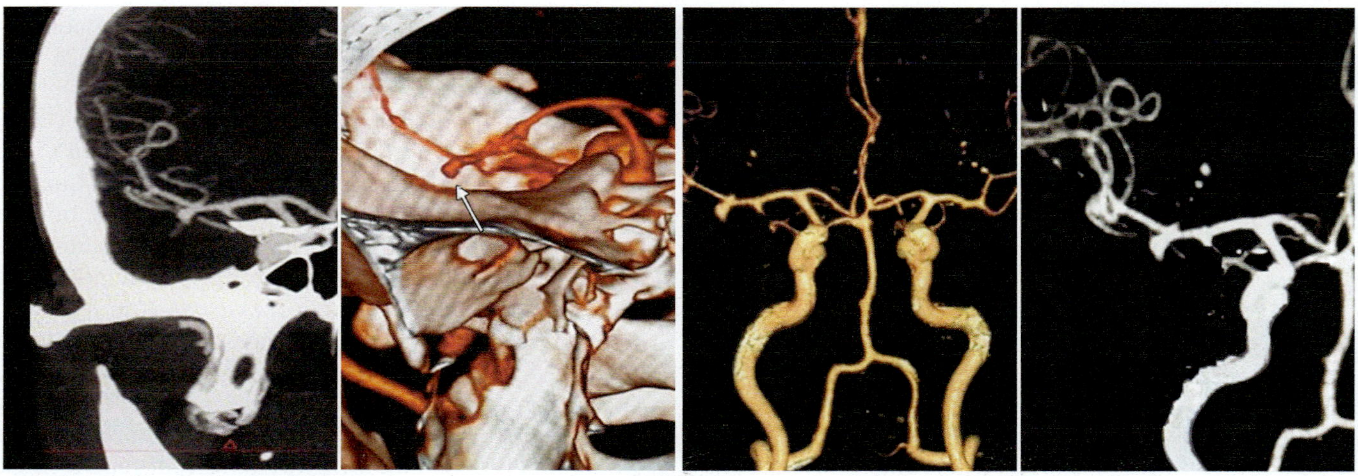

FIG. 3: Noncontrast computed tomography (CT) showing perimesencephalic hemorrhage and normal digital subtraction angiogram.

Pulmonary edema may occur with normal echocardiographic left ventricular function in the absence of volume overload. This may lead to impaired oxygen exchange, and increased work of breathing, and may require mechanical ventilation. In such a scenario, increased positive end-expiratory pressure may be necessary.

TABLE 1: The aSAH severity grading scales.

		World Federation of Neurological Societies scale	
	Hunt and Hess scale		
Grade	Symptoms	GCS	Motor symptoms
I	Asymptotic or mild headache	15	Absent
II	Moderate-to-severe headache, nuchal rigidity, with or without cranial nerve deficits	14–13	Absent
III	Confusion, lethargy, or mild focal symptoms	14–13	Present
IV	Stupor and/or hemiparesis	12–7	Present or absent
V	Comatose and/or extensor posturing	6–3	Present or absent

(aSAH: aneurysmal subarachnoid hemorrhage; GCS: Glasgow Coma Scale)

TABLE 2: Aneurysmal SAH: Modified Fisher's CT severity rating scale.

Grade	CT criteria
0	No SAH or IVH
1	Minimal thin SAH, no IVH in both lateral ventricles
2	Minimal thin SAH, with IVH in both lateral ventricles
3	Thick SAH,* no IVH in both lateral ventricles
4	Thick SAH,* with IVH in both lateral ventricles

*Complete filling ≥ one cistern or fissure.

(CT: computed tomography; IVH: intraventricular hemorrhage; SAH: subarachnoid hemorrhage)

BOX 1 Aneurysmal SAH: Disease phases and complications.

Acute phase (0–24 hours):

- Rebleeding
- Cardiopulmonary complications
- Hyponatremia
- Hydrocephalus
- Acute seizures

Subacute phase (≤72 hours):

- Early brain injury

Chronic phase (>7 days):

- Arterial vasospasm and DCI

(DCI: delayed cerebral ischemia; SAH: subarachnoid hemorrhage)

Hyponatremia

Hyponatremia is the most common electrolyte abnormality occurring in 30–50% of patients with aSAH. Hypovolemia occurs in 17–30% of patients. Both hypovolemia and hyponatremia are associated with negative outcomes. Hyponatremia is associated with a risk of vasospasm. Hyponatremia is either due to a syndrome of inappropriate antidiuretic hormone secretion (SIADH, euvolemic) or due to cerebral salt wasting syndrome (CSWS, hypovolemic). CSWS is caused by excessive secretion of natriuretic peptides, which provoke not only hyponatremia but also volume contraction. Treatment includes aggressive volume resuscitation by using crystalloids or colloids and also hypertonic saline to correct hyponatremia. Randomized control studies show that fludrocortisone is effective for correcting the negative balance and reduces the need for fluids in this setting. Fluid restriction should be avoided in treating hyponatremia due to the risk of developing DCI. SIADH is best treated by fluid restriction while maintaining a euvolemic state. Alternatively, vasopressin receptor antagonists have been proposed and trailed in small studies.

Acute Seizures

Fewer than 26% of patients with aSAH have acute seizures, most frequently at the ictus of aneurysmal rupture. Seizures occurring after this time are rare and occur in about 2–8% of patients. Nonconvulsive status epilepticus (NCSE) is common in patients with high-grade aSAH in up to 20%, and patients with altered mental status should have continuous electroencephalogram (EEG) monitoring to detect NCSE. Acute seizures should be treated with nonsedative intravenous antiseizure medications (ASMs) as seizures can contribute to elevated intracranial pressure (ICP) and cerebral hypoperfusion. However, routine use of seizure prophylaxis is not recommended. Several observational studies found that routine ASM prophylaxis is associated with poor cognitive outcomes as well as increased hospital complications. A recent randomized, double-blind, placebo-controlled, phase 3 trial showed that levetiracetam might be effective in preventing acute seizures in ICH. However, larger studies are needed to determine whether seizure prophylaxis improves functional outcomes in patients with ICH.

Hydrocephalus

Acute hydrocephalus occurs in about 30% of patients with severe grades of aSAH within 3 days of ictus **(Fig. 4)**. Symptomatic hydrocephalus may be associated with elevated ICP. It can be treated with external ventricular drainage (EVD). Placement of EVD will also provide a means of monitoring ICP. There is a theoretical risk that cerebrospinal fluid (CSF) diversion will lead to increased transmural pressure and rerupture of the aneurysm. A recent systematic review and meta-analysis suggested that a causal relationship between EVD and aneurysm rebleeding could be a plausible hypothesis, at least in certain cases. In patients with a high risk for rebleeding, aggressive drainage is often avoided until the aneurysm is secured. Some patients may develop chronic hydrocephalus requiring a permanent CSF diversion procedure. A recent meta-analysis found that high Fisher grade, acute hydrocephalus, IVH, high Hunt and Hess grade, rebleeding, posterior circulation aneurysm, and age ≥60 years are among the risk factors for permanent CSF diversion requirements.

Rebleeding

The most threatening early complication and predictor of poor outcome after aSAH is a rebleed. A recent meta-analysis reported rebleeding in 7–26% of patients with aSAH. Most of the rebleeds occurred within 24 hours with a median time interval between initial hemorrhage and rebleed of 180 minutes. Factors associated with rebleeding risk were in proximity to the first hemorrhage, higher blood pressure (BP), worse neurological grade, IVH or ICH, and larger aneurysm.

The possible strategies to prevent rebleeding are treating acute hypertension, securing the aneurysm (clipping or coiling) early, and short-term antifibrinolytic treatment. The current recommended guideline is the early definitive treatment of the aneurysm, clipping, or coiling to prevent rebleeding. Multiple factors affect the approach utilized to treat a cerebral aneurysm: aneurysm location, size, and neck size. Endovascular treatment is the preferred option in the elderly and for posterior circulation aneurysms **(Fig. 5)**. Surgery is the option for the aneurysms in the middle cerebral artery and ruptured aneurysms with large ICH **(Fig. 6)**. In the International Subarachnoid Aneurysm Trial (ISAT), 1-year outcomes demonstrated a reduction in

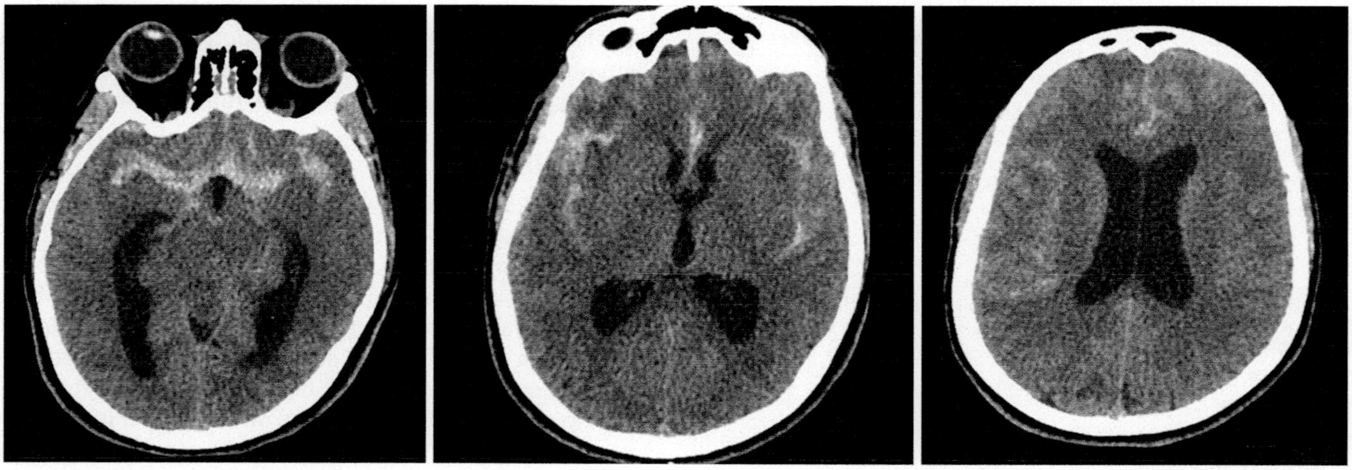

FIG. 4: Noncontrast computed tomography (CT) in a patient with subarachnoid hemorrhage due to bilobed middle cerebral artery aneurysm showing acute communicating hydrocephalus.

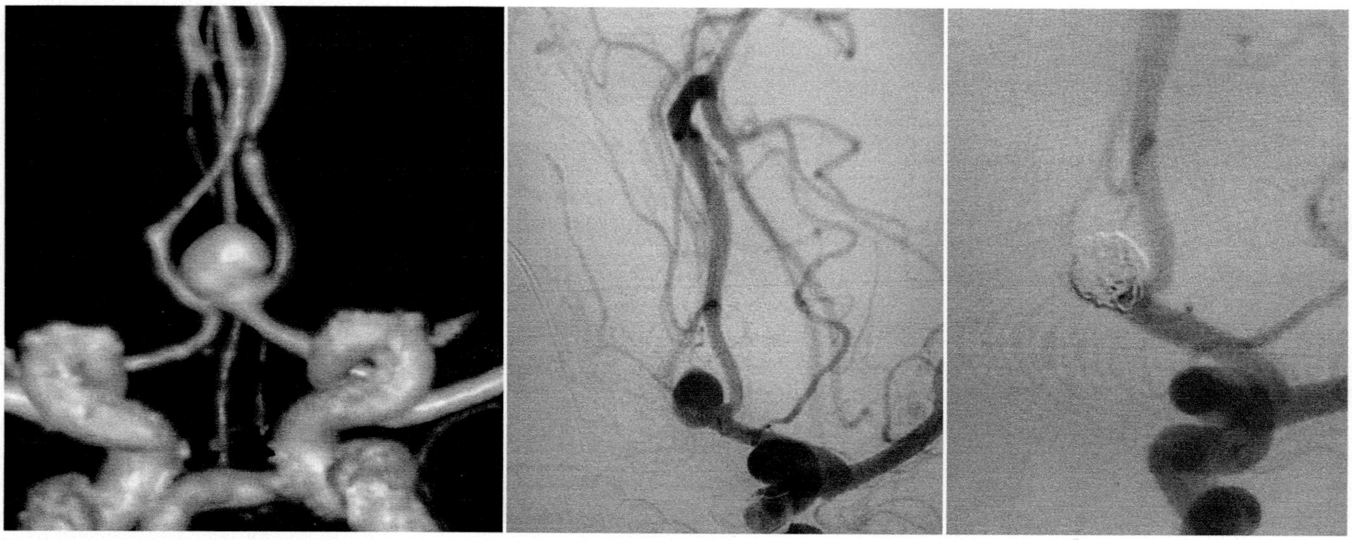

FIG. 5: Reconstructed computed tomography (CT) angiogram image showing an anterior communicating aneurysm; the same aneurysm was coiled, precoiled, and postcoiled images.

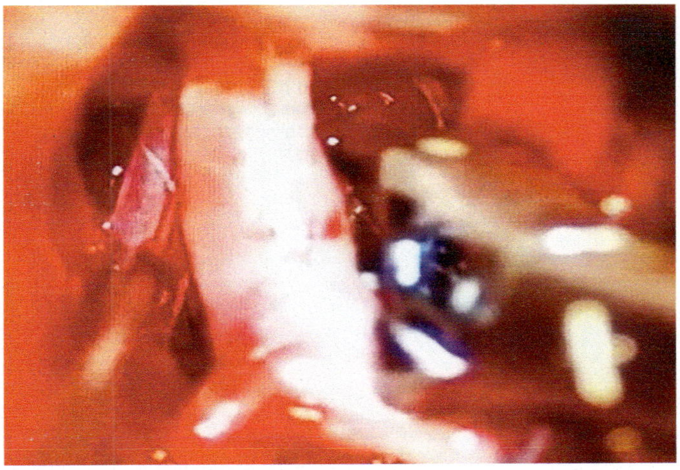

FIG. 6: Intraoperative photograph showing clipped middle cerebral artery aneurysm.

death and disability from 31% in the microsurgery group to 24% in the endovascular group. Rebleeding occurred more commonly in the endovascular group (2.9% vs. 0.9%). The rate of complete aneurysm occlusion was lower with coiling (58% vs. 81%). It is prudent to evaluate both options on a case-to-case basis.

Observational studies on large cohorts suggest that acute hypertension, particularly systolic BP > 160 mm Hg, is associated with a risk of rebleed. Current guidelines suggest treating severe hypertension in patients with an unsecured ruptured aneurysm; a decrease in systolic BP to <160 mm Hg is reasonable. The American Heart Association/American Stroke Association (AHA/ASA) and Neurocritical Care Society guidelines acknowledge the lack of quality data about BP control in aSAH patients and suggest only that BP should be monitored and controlled to "balance the risk of stroke, hypertension-associated rebleeding, and maintenance of the cerebral perfusion pressure (CPP)."[1] Modest hypertension (mean arterial pressure or MAP < 110 mm Hg) may not require treatment.[2]

Preoperative short-term antifibrinolytic treatment with either epsilon aminocaproic acid or tranexamic acid is another option. The evidence for such an approach is not robust, and the strategy remains investigational. Because of its procoagulant properties, antifibrinolytic treatment is associated with the risk of venous and arterial thrombosis. Patients with severe-grade aSAH are also at a higher risk of vasospasm and DCI.

Subacute Phase

Early brain injury (EBI) is a new concept and refers to the immediate brain injury during the first 72 hours after the aneurysm rupture.[3] EBI is caused by initial physiological changes after aneurysm rupture, such as elevated ICP, transient global cerebral ischemia, mechanical brain injuries caused by ICH, and acute hydrocephalus. The clinical correlate would be the neurological state of the patient. EBI is a precursor to DCI and microcirculatory disturbances **(Flowchart 1)** and also increases the vulnerability of the brain to secondary brain injury.

There is currently no therapeutic intervention to target prevention or treatment for EBI. Secondary brain injury may be prevented by providing adequate oxygen delivery to meet cerebral metabolic demands. Recognition and treating the complications that occur during the acute phase might mitigate brain damage related to EBI. Maintaining CPP above 70 mm Hg early on may improve brain tissue oxygenation and brain perfusion. Multimodality monitoring may assist in individualizing treatment strategies. Recent studies indicate that not only large artery vasospasm but also disturbances in cerebral microcirculation contribute to the development of DCI.

Chronic Phase

The chronic phase is marked by the development of intracranial large artery vasospasm and microvascular disturbances, which contribute to DCI **(Flowchart 1)**. DCI is defined as any neurological deterioration, focal deficit, or decline in the Glasgow Coma Scale (GCS) by 2 or more points, lasting for more than 1 hour and not attributable to any other cause. It is the leading cause of morbidity in survivors.

VASOSPASM AND DELAYED CEREBRAL INFARCT

Cerebral vasospasm after aSAH is defined as the narrowing of the large and medium-sized intracranial arteries. The risk typically begins around day 3, peaks around days 4–10, and typically resolves 21 days after the aneurysmal rupture. Angiographic vasospasm is seen in 30–70% of patients with aSAH, and clinical or symptomatic vasospasm is seen in 20–30% of patients. Cerebral vasospasm is a clinical diagnosis, and radiographic studies support the diagnosis. Multiple signaling pathways have been implicated in the pathogenesis of arterial spasm. The principle initiating factors blood degradation products in the subarachnoid space. They act as triggers for the development of endothelial dysfunction and intramural inflammatory response. In addition to large artery vasospasm, disturbed microcirculation due to microvasospasm, microthrombosis, impaired autoregulation, cortical spreading ischemia, and blood–brain barrier disruption may contribute to the development of DCI **(Flowchart 1)**. **Table 3** gives various techniques to monitor vasospasm.

Treatment of Vasospasm and Delayed Cerebral Infarct

Management of cerebral vasospasm should focus on the reduction of ischemic neuronal damage by improving

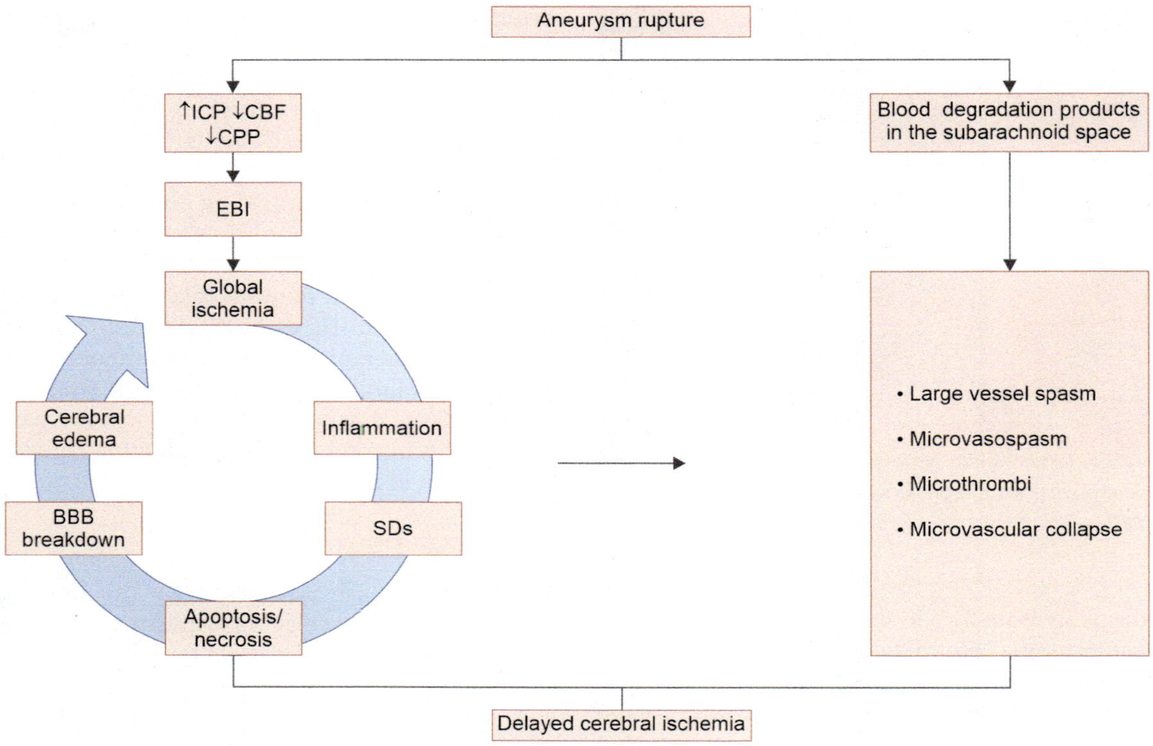

FLOWCHART 1: Postulated mechanism of EBI and delayed cerebral ischemia.

(BBB: blood–brain barrier; CBF: cerebral blood flow; CPP: cerebral perfusion pressure; EBI: early brain injury; ICP: intracranial pressure; SDs: spreading depolarizations)

Source: Modified from the figure in reference 3.

TABLE 3: Monitoring for vasospasm.

Modality	Ischemic findings	Advantages
Transcranial doppler	Mean velocity >140 or Lindegaard ratio >3.0	Noninvasive, good NPV
CTA/perfusion	Proximal spasm or hypoperfusion of vascular tertiary	Good correlation with proximal angiographic spasm
MRA/perfusion	Hypoperfusion of vascular tertiary	Perfusion images without contrast
Cerebral angiography	Proximal vessel spasm or poor distal flow	Gold standard for vasospasm
Continuous EEG	Increased alpha–delta ratio	Noninvasive
$PbtO_2$	<20 mm Hg	Direct measure of brain metabolism
Brain glucose	<20 mg/dL	Direct measure of brain metabolism
Lactate/pyruvate ratio	> 40 or rising	Direct measure of brain metabolism

(CTA: computed tomography angiography; EEG: electroencephalogram; MRA: magnetic resonance angiography; NPV: negative predictive value; $PbtO_2$: partial brain tissue oxygen)

cerebral blood flow (CBF) and brain oxygen delivery. General measures include preventing and treating the possible risk factors associated with vasospasm and DCI. Physiological variables such as body temperature, body fluid volumes, glucose levels, hemoglobin levels, and electrolytes should be maintained within normal ranges. An insufficient supply of oxygen to the brain should be avoided **(Box 2)**. Studies failed to show the benefit of prophylactic "triple-H" treatment.

BOX 2 Initial treatment of aSAH.

- *Respiratory system*: Airway protection and ventilation
- *Fluid management*: Goal—euvolemia, avoid hypotonic fluids, no role for prophylactic triple-H therapy
- *Blood pressure management*: Target systolic blood pressure <160 mm Hg until the aneurysm is secured; avoid fluctuation
- *Antifibrinolytic treatment*: Tranexamic acid 1 g every 6 hours × 72 hours or until the aneurysm is secured or aminocaproic acid 4 g × 1 hour then 1 g/h until 4 hours before angiography or 72 hours
- *Seizure treatment*: Acute treatment—IV benzodiazepine; short-term ASM prophylaxis—levetiracetam/lacosamide
- *Glycemic control*: To maintain the blood glucose level of about 140 mg/dL, and the control should be smooth
- *Temperature*: Target normothermia ≤38°C; treatment-refractory fever: TTM cooling devices

(aSAH: aneurysmal subarachnoid hemorrhage; ASM: antiseizure medication; IV: intravenous; TTM: target temperature management)

Pharmacologic Agents

Nimodipine and fasudil have been shown to improve DCI, neurological outcomes, and mortality after aSAH. There has been no convincing evidence for the use of nicardipine, cilostazol, statins, clazosentan, magnesium, and heparin in patients with aSAH.

Nimodipine, an L-type dihydropyridine calcium channel blocker, currently remains the only pharmacologic agent approved. A meta-analysis has shown that nimodipine reduces the risk of poor outcomes [risk ratio (RR) of 0.70]. The beneficial effect of nimodipine on clinical outcomes after aSAH has been achieved without angiographic evidence of cerebral vasodilation. The precise mechanisms of the action of nimodipine are unknown. Experimental studies suggest that the beneficial effect of nimodipine is probably by preventing cortical spreading ischemia. The current regimen recommended by the AHA/ASA (class I, level of evidence A) is oral nimodipine 60 mg given every 4 hours for 21 days.

Fasudil exerts its vasodilatory action by inhibiting Rho-associated kinase (ROCK) activity and decreasing Ca^{2+} sensitivity. A systematic meta-analysis has shown that fasudil treatment significantly reduces angiographic vasospasm and cerebral infarction and improves the clinical outcome in patients with aSAH. The drug has been approved for its use in patients with aSAH in Japan and China. Fasudil is administered intravenously (3 mg for dose 3 doses in a day) from the time of presentation until 14 days after the onset of SAH in Japan.

"Triple-H" Therapy

The "triple-H" therapy includes inducing hypertension, hypervolemia, and hemodilution and is thought to increase the MAP and cerebral perfusion. Hypervolemia and hemodilution have fallen out of favor as current treatment modalities for vasospasm. Hypervolemia may increase the risk of pulmonary edema, myocardial ischemia, and cerebral edema. Hemodilution may result in reduced oxygen delivery capacity and may not increase the overall CBF oxygen delivery. The induced hypertension component of "triple-H" therapy is more effective in increasing CBF. The AHA/ASA guidelines for the management of aSAH have noted that hyperdynamic therapy is a class IIa, level of evidence B modality for the treatment of symptomatic cerebral vasospasm. Current guidelines recommend euvolemia instead of hypervolemia using isotonic crystalloid fluid resuscitation. Hemodynamic augmentation using pressors to augment BP and inotropes to augment cardiac output (CO) continues to remain an important component of first-line treatment. Vasopressors norepinephrine, dopamine, and phenylephrine are effective in improving CBF and neurological outcomes. The consensus goal of systolic BP is 140–240 mm Hg, with an associated MAP of 70–210 mm Hg. Hypertension can be adjusted in a stepwise fashion depending on the clinical response of the patient and titrated as needed for an optimal response. The preferred ionotropic agent is dobutamine or milrinone to induce a hyperdynamic state and the target CO > 4.0 L/min **(Box 3)**.

BOX 3 Treatment approaches for vasospasm.

First-line therapy:
- Nimodipine: Oral 60 mg q4h for 21 days
- Fasudil: Intravenous from the time of presentation until 14 days from the onset of aSAH
- Blood pressure augmentation: SBP 140–240 mm Hg by 20 mm Hg increments with MAP
- Vasopressors: Norepinephrine, dopamine, phenylephrine
- Euvolemia: Isotonic crystalloids

Medically refractory vasospasm—Rescue therapy:
- Hemodynamic augmentation: Target cardiac output >4.0 L/min
- Ionotropic agents: Dobutamine, milrinone
- Endovascular, both mechanical and chemical
- Pharmacological agents: Verapamil, nicardipine, milrinone
- Intraventricular nicardipine

(aSAH: aneurysmal subarachnoid hemorrhage; MAP: mean arterial pressure; SBP: systolic blood pressure)

Rescue Therapy for Medically Refractory Vasospasm

Endovascular Therapies

Endovascular therapies are options in patients with medically refractory vasospasm. Endovascular options are included as a class IIb, level of evidence B modality in current AHA/ASA guidelines. Mechanical dilatation and percutaneous transluminal balloon angioplasty (PTCA) have become the treatment option for symptomatic focal vasospasm of the larger cerebral arteries refractory to medical treatment. Angioplasty has high success rates in proximal arteries including the internal carotid and vertebral arteries. Complications can occur in about 5% of patients and include thrombosis, vessel rupture, and dissection. The risk of complication increases in more distal branches.

Chemical angioplasty, intra-arterial administration of vasodilators, is generally used for diffuse vasospasm involving smaller arterial branches. The agents that have shown vasodilatation are milrinone (2.5–15 mg), nicardipine (0.5–22 mg), and verapamil (3 mg). These patients should be monitored during the drug administration as these agents have the potential to increase ICP by increasing the cerebral blood volume (CBV). Currently, papaverine use is limited in aSAH. A recent meta-analysis of 55 studies on intra-arterial therapy reported 89% angiographic improvement, 57% neurological improvement, 66% good clinical outcome, and 9% deaths **(Box 3)**.

In small case series, intraventricular nicardipine is associated with moderate-to-good outcomes. The NEWTON (Nimodipine Microparticles to Enhance Recovery While

Reducing TOxicity After SubarachNoid Hemorrhage) trial defined 800 mg as a safe and tolerable intraventricular dose, and NEWTON 2, a phase III randomized clinical trial, is currently underway.

PROGNOSIS

The 30-day mortality rate after aSAH ranges from 33 to 50%. Poor-grade aSAH is associated with high morbidity and mortality. A recent multivariate analysis revealed that older age, lower GCS score, the absence of pupillary reactivity, higher modified Fisher grade, and conservative treatment were independent predictors of poor outcomes. Based on these observations an outcome risk score, WFNS grade-age-pupillary reactivity (WAP), was developed to assess the outcomes in patients with aSAH. The score ranges from 0 to 4, and the predicted risk of poor outcome ranged from 25.5% for a WAP score of 0 to 96.2% for a WAP score of 4. The WAP risk score had good discrimination **(Table 4)**.

TABLE 4: WAP score components and weightings.

Variable	Score
WFNS grade	
WFNS IV	0
WFNS V	1
Age (years)	
<60	0
60–64	1
≥65	2
Pupillary reactivity	
Nonreactive	1
Reactive	0

(WAP: World Federation Neurosurgical Societies grade, age, and pupillary reactivity; WFNS: World Federation of Neurological Societies)

CONCLUSION

Aneurysmal SAH is a serious neurological emergency associated with high mortality and significant morbidity despite the medical advances made in the last three decades. Recent data shifts the focus onto EBI as the precursor to DCI. Nimodipine currently remains the only pharmacologic agent approved, and all patients with aSAH should receive nimodipine for 21 days. There are no evidence-based guidelines for the treatment of DCI. The recommended therapies include induced hypertension and endovascular treatment. BP augmentation remains the only component of "triple-H" therapy that effectively increases cerebral perfusion and brain oxygenation. BP should be titrated in a stepwise manner until clinical improvement. When neurologic deficits persist, endovascular therapies are indicated. Further clinical studies of the mechanisms underlying DCI and the development of effective therapeutic strategies for DCI are necessary to further improve the functional outcome and mortality in patients with aSAH.[4]

REFERENCES

1. Connolly ES Jr, Rabinstein AA, Carhuapoma JR, Derdeyn CP, Dion J, Higashida RT, et al. Guidelines for the management of aneurysmal subarachnoid hemorrhage: a guideline for healthcare professionals from the American Heart Association/American Stroke Association. Stroke. 2012;43:1711-37.
2. Maher M, Schweizer TA, Macdonald RL. Treatment of spontaneous subarachnoid hemorrhage guidelines and gaps. Stroke. 2020;51: 1326-32.
3. Osgood ML. Aneurysmal subarachnoid hemorrhage: review of the pathophysiology and management strategies. Curr Neurol Neurosci Rep. 2021;21(9):50.
4. Zheng K, Zhong M, Zhao B, Chen SY, Tan XX, Li ZQ, et al. Poor-grade aneurysmal subarachnoid hemorrhage: risk factors affecting clinical outcomes in intracranial aneurysm patients in a multicenter study. Front Neurol. 2019;10:123.

52 CHAPTER

Stroke Syndromes

Debasish Hota, Arvind Sharma, Stuti Shah, Shlok Patel

INTRODUCTION

A stroke is defined as a sudden-onset, focal, neurological deficit that is attributable to a vascular cause. It is a clinical event, and brain imaging is used to confirm the diagnosis. The clinical presentation of cerebrovascular events is highly variable due to the complex anatomy of the brain and its vascular supply.

Stroke is broadly classified into ischemic and hemorrhagic strokes. An ischemic stroke usually manifests as a group of clinical features ascribable to certain areas of the brain supplied by a single vascular region. Intracranial hemorrhage produces signs and symptoms due to mass effect or intracranial pressure, which may not be confined to a vascular territory.

EPIDEMIOLOGY[1,2]

Stroke is one of the leading causes of morbidity and mortality in India. The estimated incidence is 105–152 per lakh population, and prevalence ranged from 45 to 559 per lakh. In the last decade there has been an increase in the incidence of stroke in the younger population and even more in post-COVID-19 era attributed to the prothrombotic state after COVID-19 infection and vaccination. Out of all strokes, 85% are ischemic and 15% are hemorrhagic.

Out of all ischemic strokes, 17% are attributed to atrial fibrillation, 4% are due to carotid disease, and the rest 64% are due to other specific causes. In the case of hemorrhagic strokes, 7% are hypertensive bleeds, 4% are aneurysmal subarachnoid bleeds, and the rest are due to unknown causes.

PATHOPHYSIOLOGY OF STROKE[3]

Stroke syndrome includes a constellation of signs and symptoms imputable to an arterial territory. Mechanisms of stroke whether atherothrombosis or embolization from a proximal artery or heart are very vital for the management and prevention of stroke.

Before we confirm the diagnosis of stroke, we need to be familiar with various terminologies closely mimicking stroke.

Cerebral ischemia is due to a reduction in blood flow that sustains longer than few seconds. Transient ischemic attack (TIA) refers to a condition wherein all neurological signs and symptoms resolve within 24 hours without evidence of brain infarction on imaging. Syncope is the generalized reduction in cerebral blood flow due to systemic hypotension of any cause. If low cerebral blood persists longer, then that will lead to border zone infarction and even more severe hypoxic ischemic encephalopathy.

Grossly, brain is supplied by four major vessels originating from the arch of the aorta: two pairs of internal carotid arteries (ICAs) constituting anterior circulation and two pairs of vertebral arteries joining each other, forming basilar artery that constitutes posterior circulation. All these major vessels form the circle of Willis at ventral side of the brain. Normal cardiac output is 5 L/min and the brain constitutes 20% of it. Total blood flow to the brain is approximately 1 L/min, out of which each carotid artery carries 400 mL each, and each vertebral artery carries 100 mL blood each minute.

Stroke is a vascular disease, and brain vasculature is quite like a systemic vascular bed. The distribution of oxygen and glucose and removal of byproducts are very essential for the optimal function of neurons. Acute occlusion of an intracranial vessel causes a reduction in blood flow to the brain area. The magnitude of flow reduction depends upon collateral blood flow, individual vascular anatomy, site of occlusion, and systemic blood pressure. A decrease in cerebral blood flow to near zero causes death of tissue within 4–10 minutes. Normal cerebral flow is 50 mL/100 g/min. Reduction of flow <16–18 mL/min will cause infarction within an hour, and value <20 mL/min will cause ischemia if prolonged for a few hours. The threshold for membrane failure is <8 mL/min. If blood flow is restored to ischemic tissue before infarction develops, it will present like a TIA. Another terminology includes ischemic penumbra, which is defined as ischemic but reversibly abnormal tissue surrounding the core area of infarction. The penumbra can be identified by computed tomography (CT) or magnetic resonance imaging (MRI) perfusion. This ischemic penumbra will eventually progress to infarction if blood flow does not restore.

PATHOLOGY OF STROKE[4]

The pathological characteristic mechanism of ischemic stroke depends upon stroke mechanism, size of artery occluded, and collateral flow availability. The brain surface in the area of infarction is pale. When ischemia is caused by hypotension or hemodynamic changes, the watershed zone is vulnerable. A wedge-shaped infarct area is seen when one main artery is occluded with good collaterals, but the whole area is infarcted if there are poor collaterals. If the large artery is occluded like ICA, then there will be multilobar infarct with flattening of gyri and sulci and cerebral edema. In the case of a lacunar infarct (size 1.5 cm or less), cerebral edema is less and barely seen. Reperfusion of infarct areas will lead to hemorrhagic transformation.

The microscopic changes seen after infarction occur due to either a necrotic pathway (cellular cytoskeleton is broken down) or an apoptotic pathway (programmed cell death). Ischemia leads to necrosis by cutting off glucose and oxygen, which in turn results in mitochondrial shutdown. Without adenosine triphosphate (ATP), cell metabolism fails with intracellular calcium accumulation, glutamate release, and free radical production. This array of metabolites will cause permanent neuron destruction with neuronal swelling. Subsequently, there will be neutrophils followed by foamy macrophage infiltration, which will engulf necrotic materials with a cavity consisting of glial and fibrovascular elements, but areas of ischemic penumbra will show lesser damage due to favoring apoptotic cellular death if not reversed. Fever and hypoglycemia worsen brain injury during ischemia.

CLINICAL PRESENTATION OF STROKE AND ITS DIAGNOSIS[5-8]

Carotid Syndrome

Right common carotid artery (CCA) arises from the brachiocephalic trunk, but left CCA arises directly from the arch of aorta. Many variations do exist for the origin of CCA, but common variations are depicted in the following pictures. Both CCAs divide into internal and external carotid arteries at the level of C4 vertebrae posteriorly and base of thyroid cartilage anteriorly. The carotid vessel is more prone to narrowing, atherothrombotic occlusion, arterial dissection, and rarely vasculitis **(Fig. 1)**.

Common carotid occlusion is very rare but can be occluded by plaque or years after radiation exposure. Manifestation of ICA occlusion largely depends upon the patency of the circle of Willis. If there is no communication from the other side or from posterior circulation, then that will result in massive infarction of the anterior two-third cerebral hemisphere. If both anterior cerebral arteries (ACAs) originate from a single ICA, then it will result in bilateral ACA territory infarction. If posterior cerebral artery (PCA) is fetal type, then that will lead to posterior circulation manifestation. The high variability of symptoms is because ICA is not an end artery and no part of the brain is completely dependent on its supply. Therefore, occlusion in the proximal part of ICA after bifurcation is many times clinically silent. If one side of the ICA is stenotic then occlusion of the other side causes bilateral infarction, leading to coma with quadriparesis and metronomic horizontal eye movements. Occlusion of distal ICA will present like a combination of middle cerebral artery (MCA) and ACA occlusion in the form of contralateral hemiplegia, hemianesthesia, and aphasia along with leg paralysis. Additional features include mild headache above the eyebrow, but when one of the ICA is already compromised then there will be two zones of maximum ischemia in the border region of MCA and ACA, one of them cortical watershed and the other a deep watershed. The site of infarction is the high parietal and frontal cortex manifesting as weakness of the hip and shoulder regions more than the hand and leg **(Figs. 2 to 4)**.

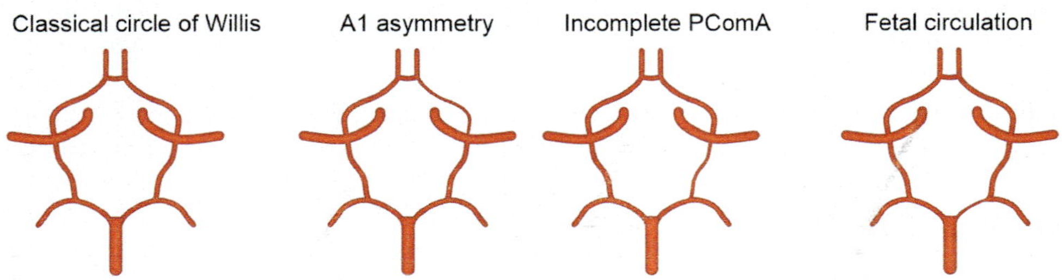

FIG. 1: Variants of circle of Willis.
(PComA: posterior communicating artery)

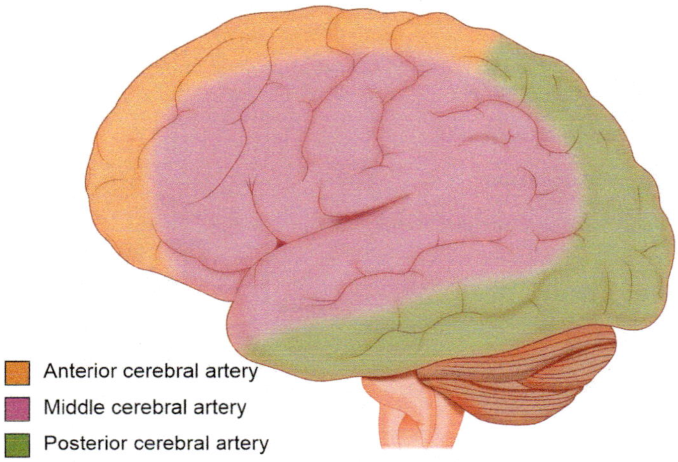

FIG. 2: Blood supply of superolateral surface of cortex.

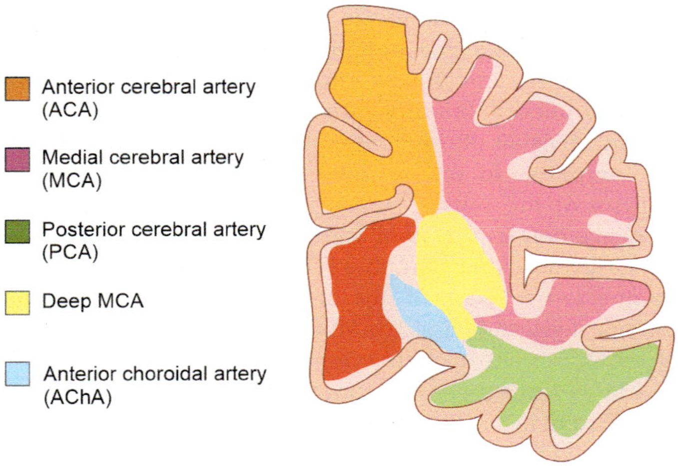

FIG. 3: Blood supply of coronal section cortex.

Longer standing ICA occlusion will shift areas of oligemia to downward, presenting as facial weakness or nonfluent aphasia, whereas deep watershed area will involve subfrontal and subparietal regions. In a nutshell, signs of carotid occlusion include transient monocular blindness or dimness of vision with exercise or on exposure to bright light. Common carotid occlusion will lead to claudication of jaw muscles.

Middle Cerebral Artery Syndrome[9]

Middle cerebral artery originates from bifurcation of ICA. Occlusion of MCA is mostly due to embolus (artery to artery, cardiac, or unknown) or atherosclerosis. Cortical branches of MCA supply the lateral surface of the hemisphere except for the frontal pole and a strip along the superomedial border of frontal and parietal lobes. Proximal MCA (M1 segment) gives rise to lenticulostriate arteries that supply putamen, globus pallidus, posterior limb of internal capsule (IC), and caudate nucleus. In the Sylvian fissure MCA divides into superior and inferior divisions (M2 segments) supplying frontal and superior parietal cortex via superior division and temporal cortex and inferior parietal via inferior division **(Fig. 5 and Table 1)**.

If MCA stem is occluded at its origin (penetrating and cortical branches are occluded), the clinical finding will be contralateral hemiplegia (involving face, arm, and leg proportionately due to infarction of posterior limb of IC), hemianesthesia, homonymous hemianopia [infarction of lateral geniculate body (LGB)], and gaze shifted to the ipsilateral side. Dysarthria is common because of facial weakness. When a dominant hemisphere is involved then global aphasia is seen, and when a nondominant hemisphere is affected anosognosia, constructional apraxia, and neglect are seen. If distal M1 is occluded, then there are unaffected, deep, penetrating branches.

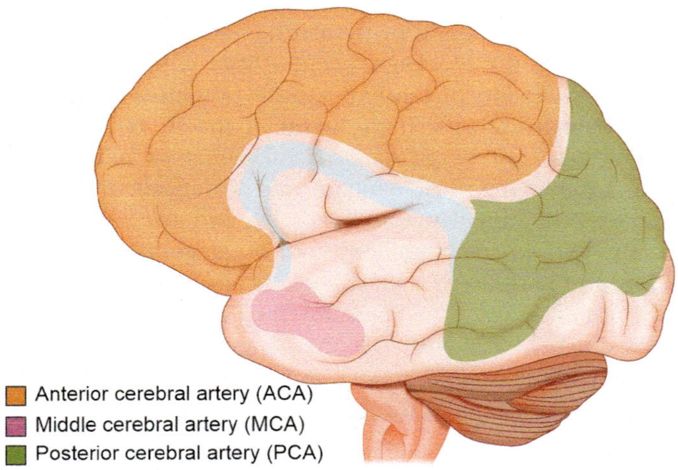

FIG. 4: Blood supply of medical surface of cortex.

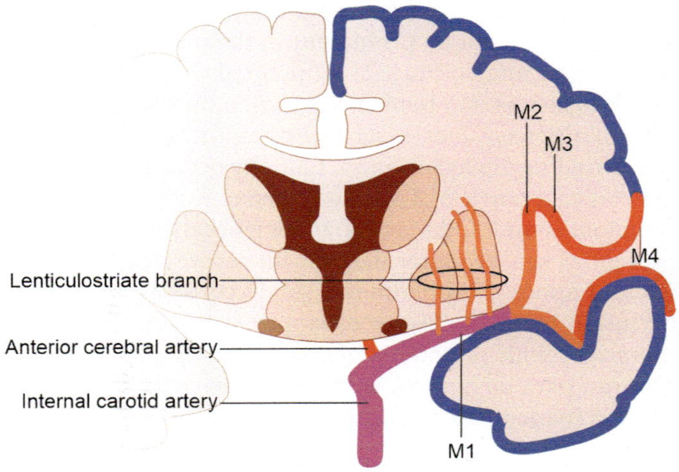

FIG. 5: Left middle cerebral artery (MCA) division.

TABLE 1: Summary of middle cerebral artery (MCA) territory and its symptoms.

Areas of brain	Function	Deficit
Primary motor area (except superomedial part)	Motor movement of arm, face > leg	Contralateral face and arm weakness > leg
Broca area	Fluency	Nonfluent aphasia
Parietal operculum	Speech coordination	Conduction aphasia
Perisylvian area (dominant side)	Comprehension	Fluent aphasia
Nondominant parietal lobe	Visuospatial function	• Constructional apraxia • Dressing apraxia • Hemineglect
Frontal eye field	Voluntary eye movement to the opposite side	Gaze palsy toward the lesion
Optic radiation	Visual information transfer	Homonymous hemianopia
Primary sensory area	All modalities of sensation + cortical sensation (face, arm > leg)	Sensory impairment over face, arm

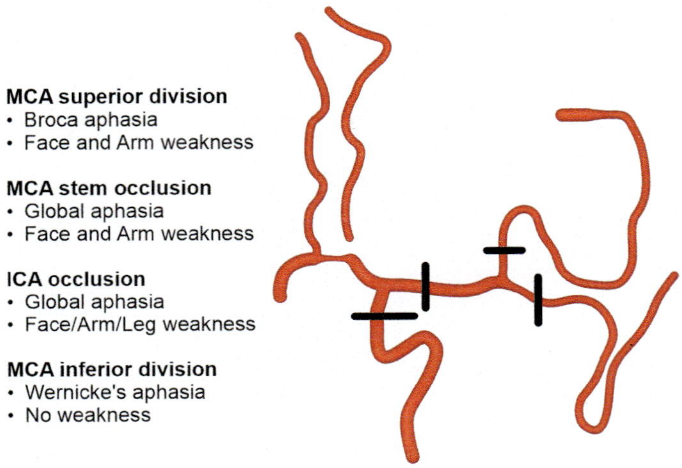

FIG. 6: Left ICA branches with clinical pictures.
(ICA: internal carotid artery; MCA: middle cerebral artery)

Superior Division Syndrome[10]

Frequently partial syndromes are seen depending on the strength of the collaterals and degree of occlusion of the stem. If the collateral system is robust over the surface, then components of deep structure occlusion will be evident. Combination of hemianesthesia (contralateral face and arm), nonfluent aphasia, hemiparesis (faciobrachial predominant), and ipsilateral deviation of head and eye will be due to occlusion of dominant superior division, but faciobrachial weakness without significant nonfluent aphasia will be due to localization to nondominant superior division. MCA M2 superior occlusion differs from MCA stem occlusion in the form of relative sparing of leg weakness. The sensory deficit will be prominent in the contralateral side like thalamic infarcts but in M2 superior division, the sensory deficit is less severe than motor deficit and mostly in the form of stereoanesthesia, agraphesthesia, impaired position sense, and tactile localization. Embolic occlusion of one of the cortical branches of MCA will lead to further fractionate symptom complex like central branch occlusion, which will present as sensorimotor deficit with severe dysarthria but without aphasia. Sometimes a single cortical end branch occlusion may manifest as monoplegia or hand weakness that may mimic peripheral neuropathy. Nevertheless, only superior parietal branch occlusion presents as conduction aphasia (parietal operculum infarct) or ideomotor apraxia.

Inferior Division Syndrome

Inferior division occlusion is less frequent than superior division and nearly always results from embolism. If fluent aphasia, jargon speech, and inability to comprehend written and spoken language with homonymous superior quadrantanopia are seen, then dominant inferior division is the culprit. In other words, visual hemineglect with superior quadrantanopia without weakness is seen if the inferior division of nondominant hemisphere is involved. As compared to the superior division where there is mutism at the outset, here there is a severe receptive language deficit. Tetrad of finger agnosia, acalculia, right–left confusion, and agraphia (Gerstmann syndrome) will be due to occlusion of one of the terminal branches of inferior division (angular branch) supplying angular gyrus of the dominant hemisphere, though rarely occlusion of end branches supplying supramarginal gyrus will present as difficulty in receptive language processing with limited empathy **(Fig. 6)**.

Lenticulostriate Syndrome[11]

Occlusion of lenticulostriate branches produces stroke within IC, presenting as pure motor or sensory motor stroke or clumsy hand or dysarthria variant contralateral to the site of the blockage. Lacunar infarct results mostly due to occlusion of lenticulostriate branches by means of atherothrombosis. If the genu of the IC is involved, presentation will be primarily facial weakness followed by arm and then leg as ischemia moves posteriorly. If there is proportionate involvement of the leg and arm along with components of hemianopia without language affection, gaze palsy, and visual hemineglect, then localization of the lesion is confined to the IC, suggesting deep penetrating branch occlusion not the superficial cortex. Lacunar infarct affecting globus pallidus and putamen may present as hemiballismus and parkinsonism very rarely.

Anterior Cerebral Artery Syndrome

Anterior cerebral artery supplies anterior three-fourth of medial surface of frontal lobe with the frontal pole,

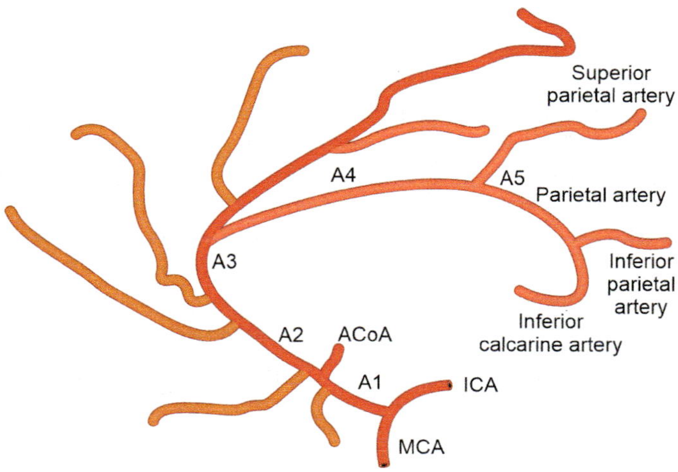

FIG. 7: ACA segment and branches.
(ACA: anterior cerebral artery; ACoA: anterior communicating artery; ICA: internal carotid artery; MCA: middle cerebral artery)

TABLE 2: Summary of anterior cerebral artery (ACA) territory and its syndromes.

Area of brain	Function	Deficit
Primary motor area (leg)	Motor movement of lower limb	Contralateral weakness of leg > arm and face
Primary sensory area (lower limb)	Sensation over lower limb + cortical sensation	Cortical sensory loss over toe, foot, leg
Paracentral lobule	Continence of bladder	Urinary incontinence
Supplementary motor area	Control of frontal reflex	Contralateral grasp reflex, sucking reflex, and paratonic rigidity
Cingulate gyrus	Emotion and behavior	Abulia, lack of spontaneity, distractibility
Cortex near leg motor area	Gait and stance	Gait apraxia

anterior four-fifth of the corpus callosum, and a strip of the superolateral surface. Deep branches arising from anterior communicating and A1 segment supply the anterior limb of IC, head of caudate nucleus, and globus pallidus. The largest deep branch is called the recurrent artery of Heubner, which supplies the anterior part of IC and caudate nucleus through lenticulostriate branches. Symptoms of ACA occlusion will depend upon the site of the lesion [either precommunicating or distal to anterior communicating artery (ACom) origin] and patency of the circle of Willis **(Fig. 7 and Table 2)**.

A1 (Precommunicating) Syndrome

A1 occlusion is usually well tolerated if ACom is patent as flow from the other side of ACA will supply distribution of A2 segment. Significant symptoms appear when both A2 segments originate from single ACA stem; in such a case, presentation will be paraplegia, incontinence, abulia, and frontal personality changes.

A2 (Postcommunicating Syndrome)

A2 occlusion will manifest as sensorimotor deficit in contralateral foot and leg with a lesser degree of weakness of the arm, with sparing of face and hand. Sometimes additional symptoms in the form of deviation of the head and eye to the side of lesion, urinary incontinence, contralateral grasp reflex, and paratonia rigidity are evident. Language deficits like transcortical aphasia will occur along with behavioral disturbances in the form of abulia, lack of spontaneity in reaction, muteness, and distractibility. Terminal end branch occlusion further fragments the syndrome, like spastic weakness of the opposite leg and foot only.

Penetrating Branch Syndrome

Occlusion of the medial lenticulostriate branch will disturb blood supply to the IC and caudate, presenting with dysarthria, abulia, and transient hemiparesis. With the dominant side lesion, stuttering and language difficulty are seen, and nondominant side lesion manifests with visuospatial neglect. Occlusion of the artery of Heubner will present as contralateral hemiparesis (predominant in leg) with grasping and groping responses, buccofacial apraxia, and transcortical motor aphasia (inability to name objects with preservation of repetition). Bilateral lenticulostriate occlusion supply caudate lobe will produce inattentiveness, abulia, agitation, and psychosis with transient choreoathetosis.

Anterior Choroidal Artery Syndrome

Anterior choroidal artery (AChA) is a branch of the ICA just distal to the origin of the posterior communicating artery (PCom). It supplies the globus pallidus, posterior limb of the IC, optic tract, and choroid plexus. Being a slender artery, the common mode of occlusion is due to atherosclerosis. Specifically, AChA supplies medial and lateral portions of the LGB.

Occlusion of the AChA will manifest in the form of contralateral hemiplegia (lesion of posterior IC), hemihypesthesia, and homonymous sectoral hemianopia (optic tract and LGB). Usually, a lesion involving the LGB supplied by AChA will present as sectoral quadrantanopia sparing a sector along the equator. In contrast, occlusion of the posterior choroidal artery will cause sectoral quadrantanopia involving the equatorial sector. Contralateral motor, sensory, and visual deficits with preserved language and cognition will distinguish this from MCA cortical infarct. Only contralateral sensorimotor deficit without visual deficit like homonymous hemianopia or any other features will localize the lesion to lenticulostriate penetrating branches of MCA. While considering totality most of time presentation of occlusion of AChA artery will be minimal and recovers substantially as there is an overlapping supply of this area by PCom, posterior choroidal, and penetrating arteries from the MCA.

Posterior Cerebral Artery Syndrome[12]

In 75% of cases PCA will arise from the bifurcation of basilar artery. In 20% of cases, it will arise from one of the ipsilateral ICAs (fetal PCA), and in 5% of cases each PCA arises from respective ipsilateral ICA. Most of the strokes in PCA are embolic in nature. For convenience of discussion PCA syndrome is categorized into (1) proximal/central (P1) syndrome, (2) cortical/peripheral (P2) syndrome, and (3) bilateral syndrome **(Fig. 8)**.

P1 Syndrome

Posterior cerebral artery is grossly divided into proximal (P1) and distal (P2) segments. P1 segment (from the bifurcation of the basilar artery to the ostium of the PCom) gives rise to the interpeduncular branch, which supplies red nuclei, substantia nigra, cerebral peduncles, III and IV cranial nerve nuclei reticular activating system, medial longitudinal fasciculus, and medial lemnisci.

In most of the cases two mesencephalic arteries arise symmetrically but, in some cases, a single artery arises from the proximal PCA stem, which supplies both side of midbrain and medial thalamic region known as the artery of Percheron. Occlusion of artery of Percheron will cause butterfly-shaped lesion in the bilateral thalamus, leading to vertical gaze palsy, confusion to coma, and memory loss.

P1 segment also give rise to thalamoperforating branches and thalamogeniculate branches. Thalamoperforating branches arise slightly distal to stem nearer to PCom junction, which supply anterior, medial, and inferior thalamus. Thalamogeniculate branches arise more distally,

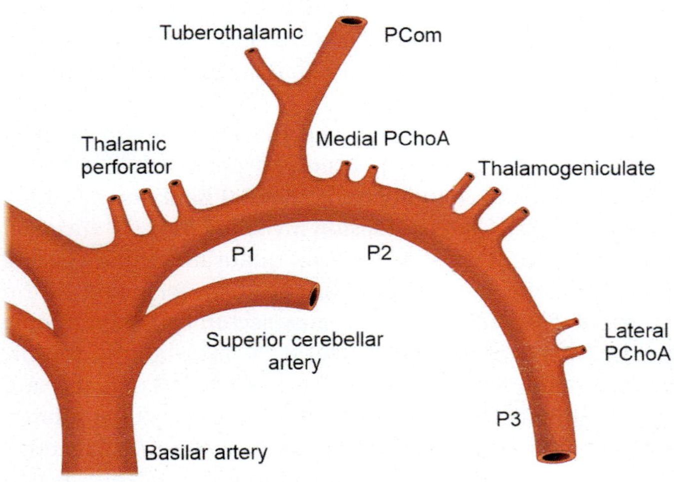

FIG. 8: PCA segments and branches.
(PCA: posterior cerebral artery; PChoA: posterior choroidal artery; PComA: posterior communicating artery)

which supply the LGB and central and posterior thalamus. Dejerine-Roussy syndrome is due to infarction of the sensory relay nuclei of the thalamus imputable to occlusion of thalamogeniculate branches, which manifest as deep and cutaneous sensory loss in severe degrees of the contralateral side including face and trunk. Sometimes homonymous hemianopia may be associated. The characteristic feature is always sensory loss involving entire hemi side, but infrequently there is dissociated sensory loss in the form of pain and temperature being more affected. After a few days, the patient will complain of pain and hyperpathia in affected parts.

Thalamoperforating branch occlusion will cause anteromedial thalamic syndrome, which manifests as extrapyramidal involvement (hemiballismus and hemichoreoathetosis) and memory loss, deep sensory loss, hemiataxia, or tremor. Hemiballismus is the result of occlusion of a small branch supplying subthalamic nucleus. Specifically, occlusion of paramedian branches/thalamoperforate supplying mediodorsal nucleus is manifested as an amnestic syndrome (Korsakoff syndrome). This may mimic infarction of hippocampi due to cortical branch occlusion but later occurs more frequently.

Occlusion of interpeduncular branches will manifest depending upon the region of the midbrain affected. One of common occlusion is ipsilateral III nerve palsy in case of the tegmental lesion. We have enlisted a table below for different midbrain syndromes as per the part of the midbrain affected, which is divided into base, tegmentum, and tectum **(Table 3 and Fig. 9)**.

Cortical Syndrome of PCA

After supplying brainstem structure, PCA moves posteriorly for supplying the medial and inferior temporal lobes and occipital cortex. Occlusion of the calcarine branch supplying the primary visual cortex (striate cortex) will cause homonymous hemianopia, but it may be incomplete and involve upper quadrants of the visual field more commonly. Macular sparing is an important feature due to collateral supply from the MCA. Other infrequent features include visual hallucinations (peduncular hallucinosis), metamorphopsia, and palinopsia. Dominant occipital lobe lesion will manifest as alexia without agraphia (splenium of corpus callosum involvement), visual agnosia for objects and mathematical symbols, color anomia, and anomic aphasia/amnestic aphasia with paraphasia. Occlusion of an artery supplying the medial temporal lobe and hippocampus will cause disturbances in memory, but it lasts shorter as memory has bilateral representation **(Fig. 10 and Table 4)**.

Bilateral PCA Syndrome

Occlusion of upper basilar artery or global circulation failure will lead to infarction of bilateral occipital territory. Extensive bilateral damage will cause cortical blindness (blindness with preserved pupillary reflex and normal optic disc) and unformed hallucination. Sometimes the

TABLE 3: Different types of midbrain syndromes (based on location).

Eponym	Site	CN involved	Tract affected	Signs
Weber syndrome	Base of midbrain	III nerve	Corticospinal	III nerve palsy (ipsilateral) + contralateral hemiplegia (crossed)
Claude syndrome	Tegmentum of midbrain	III nerve	Red nucleus + superior cerebellar peduncles	III nerve palsy (ipsilateral) + contralateral cerebellar ataxia and tremor
Benedikt syndrome	Base + tegmentum	III nerve	Red nucleus + SCP + CST	Ipsilateral III nerve palsy with contralateral hemiparesis + ataxia
Nothnagel syndrome	Tectum of midbrain	III and IV nerves	Superior cerebellar peduncles	Gaze palsy + nystagmus + ataxia
Parinaud syndrome	Dorsal midbrain		Supranuclear gaze mechanism + periaqueductal gray	Vertical gaze palsy + accommodation defect

(CN: cranial nerve; CST: corticospinal tract; SCP: superior cerebellar peduncle)

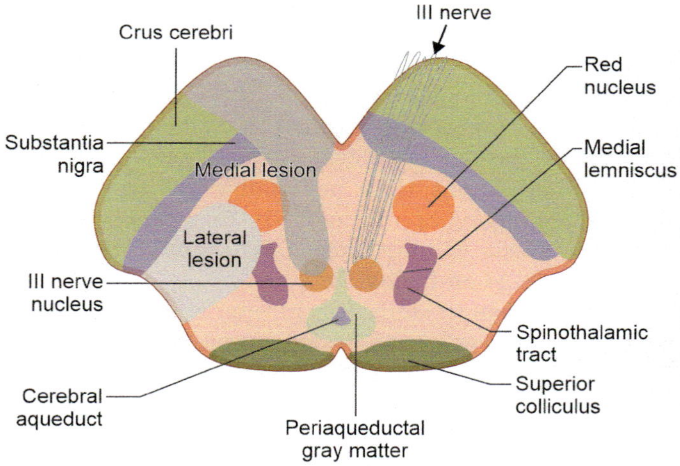

FIG. 9: Midbrain cross-section with its lesion.

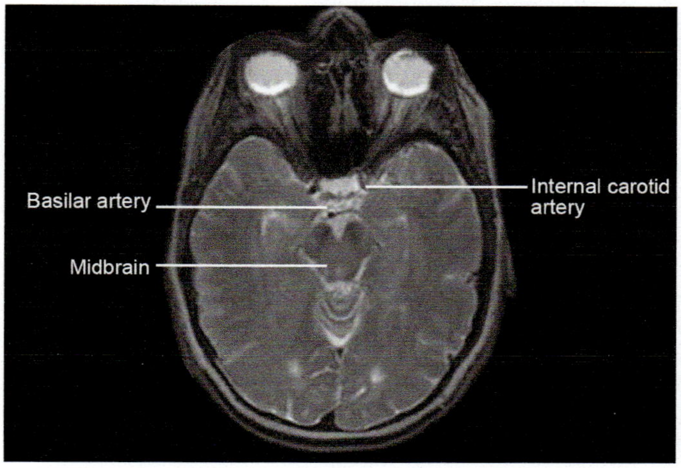

TABLE 4: Summary of posterior circulation areas and their functions.

Area of brain	Function	Deficit
Visual cortex (striate cortex)	Primary visual construct	Cortical blindness, complex hallucination
Visual processing area (extrastriate cortex)	Visual recognition and processing	Visual agnosia
Splenium of corpus callosum	Connecting reading area to writing area	Alexia without agraphia
Hippocampus	Memory processing	Short-term memory loss
Lingual gyrus	Face recognition	Prosopagnosia
Calcarine cortex (nondominant side)	Posterior visual pathway	Homonymous hemianopia and topographic disorientation
Calcarine cortex (dominant side)	Complex visual processing	Simultanagnosia

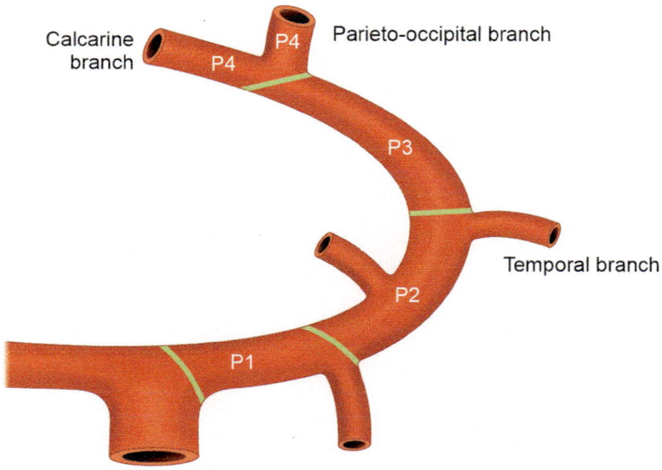

FIG. 10: Posterior cerebral artery (PCA) segments and branches.

patient is unaware of his/her blindness and denies the existence of the problem, which is called Anton syndrome. Usually, in most cases, cortical blindness is incomplete, which will cause sectoral visual remnants compelling the patient to excessive movements to capture the totality of scene. Only occipital pole lesions bilaterally will cause homonymous central scotoma. Altitudinal field defects are due to the involvement of upper or lower banks of calcarine sulci. Lesion of bilateral occipitoparietal border zone infarcts will cause Balint syndrome (optic ataxia, oculomotor apraxia, and dorsal simultanagnosia) due to posterior circulatory collapse. Likewise, bilateral inferomedial temporal lobe lesions will cause impairment of memory or severe Korsakoff amnestic state. Bilateral occipitotemporal lesions will cause a lack of recognition of faces (prosopagnosia).

Vertebral Artery Stroke Syndrome

Vertebral artery originates from posterior superior surface of the first part of the subclavian artery. It is divided into four parts:

1. *V1*: From origin to entry into cervical transverse foramen
2. *V2*: From C6 transverse foramen to C2 foramen
3. *V3*: From exit of C2 foramen to dural penetration at foramen magnum
4. *V4*: It is an intradural portion. V4 segments are joined from the contralateral side to form the basilar artery.

The vertebral artery supplies major part of the medulla (medial and lateral parts), medial lemniscus, and posterior-inferior part of the cerebellum. In 10% cases, one of the vertebral arteries is nonfunctional. The dominant vertebral artery is identified by the convexity of the basilar artery, which swings in a direction opposite to the dominant vertebral artery. Without collateral flow from the ICA, single functional vertebral artery occlusion is equivalent to basilar artery occlusion. The most common mode of occlusion is due to atherothrombosis of the intracranial portion. Infrequently, vertebral artery dissection will present with brainstem deficit.

Extracranial occlusion of the vertebral artery is usually asymptomatic due to contralateral flow from the other side. Intracranial occlusion proximal to the posterior inferior cerebellar artery (PICA) with intact second vertebral artery will be symptomless because of contralateral retrograde flow from another vertebral artery. If the blockage occurs at the level of PICA origin, then characteristic lateral medullary syndrome occurs. If the subclavian artery is blocked at the origin, then the exercise of the ipsilateral hand will cause retrograde flow in the vertebral artery, leading to the symptoms of basilar insufficiency.

Lateral Medullary Syndrome

Lateral medullary syndrome is due to occlusion of either the vertebral artery or more specifically the PICA, which is a branch of the vertebral artery. It supplies the lateral surface of the medulla lying posterior to the olivary nucleus along with the inferior surface of the cerebellum. The PICA has one proximal caudal loop and distal cranial loop. The highest point on the cranial loop is called as the choroidal point. Occlusion of the PICA distal to the choroidal point will spare brainstem symptoms as the penetrating branch supplying the medulla originates proximal to it. There will be vertigo, vomiting, ataxia without Horner syndrome, and palatal paralysis **(Fig. 11 and Table 5)**.

Partial lateral medullary syndrome is more frequent. Vertigo is the most common symptom followed by ipsilateral ataxia and dysphagia. Nystagmus is always direction changing associated with skew deviation and hypometria saccades toward the side of the lesion.

Medial Medullary Syndrome

Occlusion of penetrating branches directly originating from the vertebral artery will lead to the medial medullary

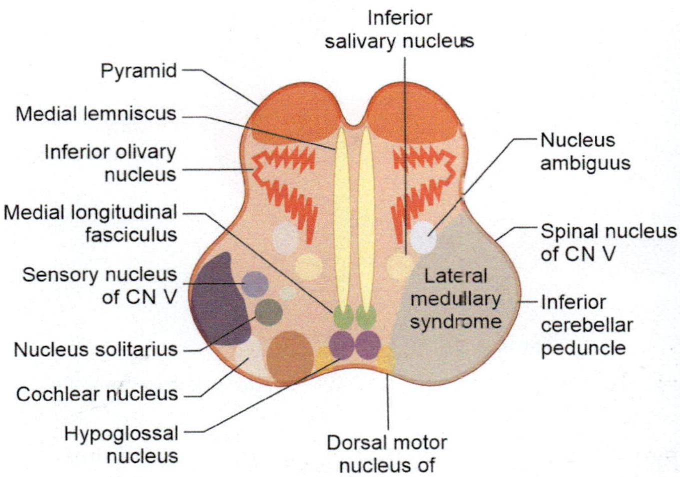

FIG. 11: Medullary cross-section with lateral medullary syndrome.
(CN V: cranial nerve V)

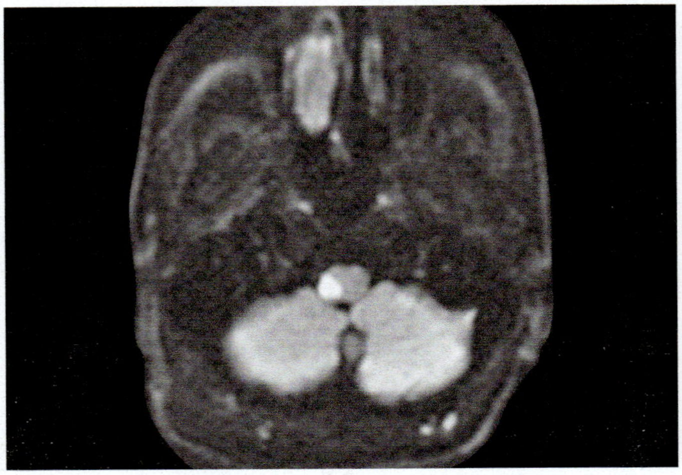

TABLE 5: Lateral medullary syndrome (occlusion of vertebral artery or posterior inferior cerebellar artery).

On the side of lesion (ipsilateral)		Opposite to the side of lesion (contralateral)	
Structure involved	**Features**	**Structure involved**	**Features**
Spinal nucleus of V nerve	Pain, numbness, impaired sensation	Spinothalamic tract	Impaired pain and thermal sensation over half of the body
Cerebellar hemisphere	Ataxia of limbs, fall toward the side of lesion		
Vestibular nerve	Vertigo, nausea and vomiting, nystagmus, diplopia, oscillopsia		
Descending sympathetic tract	Horner syndrome		
IX and X nerve nuclei	Dysphasia, hoarseness, palatal paralysis		

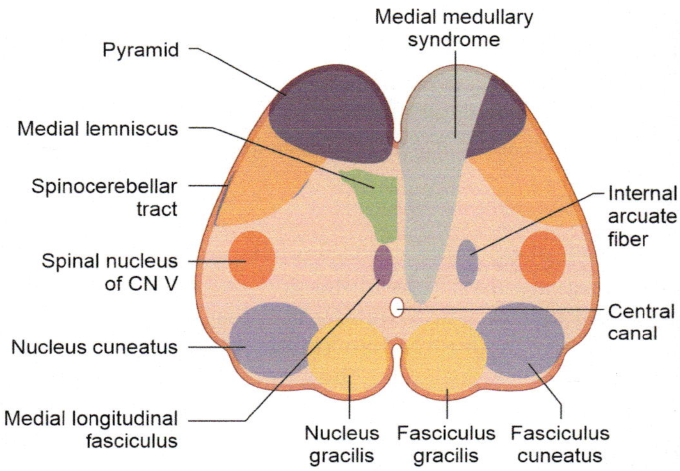

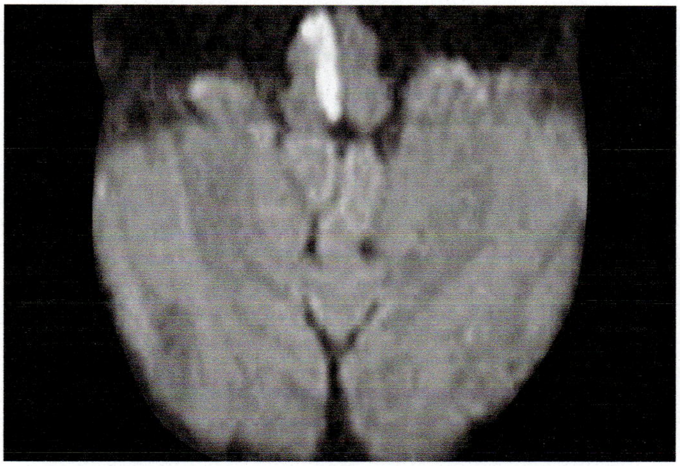

FIG. 12: Medullary cross-section with medial medullary syndrome.
(CN V: cranial nerve V)

TABLE 6: Medial medullary syndrome (occlusion of vertebra artery or branch of vertebral or proximal basilar).

On the side of lesion (ipsilateral)		Opposite side of lesion (contralateral)	
Structure involved	**Features**	**Structure involved**	**Clinical features**
XII nerve palsy	Paralysis and atrophy of ipsilateral tongue	Pyramidal tract	Paralysis of arm and leg, sparing face
		Medial lemniscus	Impaired tactile and proprioceptive sensation

syndrome. Areas supplied by penetrating branches include the medullary pyramid, medial lemniscus, and emerging hypoglossal nerve. Clinical features of the medial medullary syndrome are mentioned below **(Fig. 12 and Table 6)**.

Anterior Spinal Artery Syndrome

Anterior spinal artery originates from stem joining from both sides of vertebral artery. It supplies anterior two-third of the spinal cord. Occlusion of one vertebral artery or one stem of the anterior spinal artery will go unnoticed as their flow on the other side will prevent infarction of the cervical cord. Occlusion of the anterior spinal artery after fusion will cause dissociated sensory loss with paraplegia. The anterior two-third of spinal cord contains lateral spinothalamic tracts with the corticospinal tract on both sides. The sensory deficit will exclusively involve pain and temperature sensation with sparing joint position sense and vibration.

On summary, vertebral artery occlusion or posterior circulation stroke involving the cerebellum can lead to respiratory arrest due to a high chance of brainstem herniation attributed to swelling within the closed compartment and hydrocephalus by blockage of the aqueduct of Sylvius. Clinicians should have a high index of suspicion for impending hemodynamic instability in such a situation.

Basilar Artery Syndrome

Basilar artery is formed by joining of vertebral arteries at pontomedullary junction. Usually, there are four types of branches of basilar artery:

1. *Paramedian branches*: Seven-to-ten pairs directly originating from basilar artery supplying wedge-shaped areas of pons in the midline
2. *Short circumferential branches*: Five-to-seven pairs supplying lateral two-third of pons and middle cerebellar peduncles

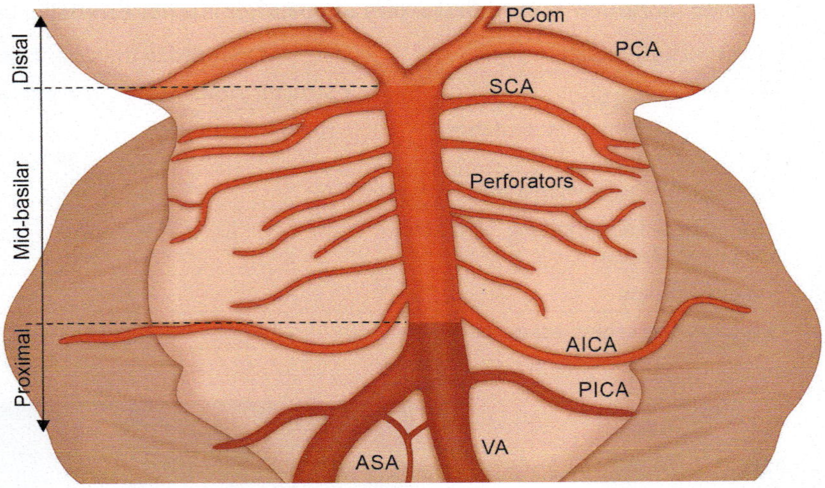

FIG. 13: Basilar artery segments and its branches.
(AICA: anteroinferior cerebellar artery; ASA: anterior spinal artery; PCA: posterior cerebral artery; PCom: posterior communicating artery; PICA: posterior inferior cerebellar artery; SCA: superior cerebellar artery; VA: vertebral artery)

3. *Long circumferential branches*: They include a pair of superior cerebellar artery and anterior inferior cerebellar artery supplying lateral and superior surface of the cerebellum.
4. *Interpeduncular and terminal branches*: Several paramedian branches supply the midbrain, and two PCAs supply the occipital and temporal lobes.

The most common mode of occlusion is thrombotic over the preexisting atherothrombotic plaque. Embolization usually occurs in the distal portion of the basilar artery as the clot, which passes the vertebral artery, can easily traverse the basilar artery, which is larger in diameter. The full syndrome of complete basilar artery occlusion is coma, quadriparesis, and ophthalmoplegia. Infrequently, there may be spontaneous posturing with jerky components resembling seizure activity. In many instances, clinical picture varies widely depending upon retrograde flow from the PCom **(Fig. 13)**.

Proximal Basilar Occlusion Syndrome

Proximal basilar occlusion syndrome is usually associated with V4 occlusion before the origin of paramedian branches supplying pons. The presentation will be contralateral hemiparesis of the arm and leg (due to corticospinal tract involvement), ipsilateral facial palsy, and diplopia (VI nerve involvement). Associated occlusion of V4 region will manifest as a vertebral artery or PICA syndrome described earlier **(Fig. 14 and Tables 7 and 8)**.

Mid-basilar Occlusion Syndrome

Mid-basilar occlusion syndrome is mainly due to the involvement of paramedian branches supplying both sides of pons along the midline. There is involvement of bilateral corticospinal tract and corticobulbar tract manifesting as quadriparesis, anarthria/mute, and dysphagia, respectively, and diplopia/horizontal gaze palsy due to VI nerve involvement or paramedian reticular formation (PPRF) involvement, respectively. The pupil becomes extremely narrow with some reactivity. There is a sparing of vertical gaze and ability to elevate eyelids along with intact consciousness called locked-in syndrome. Ataxia (due to cerebellar tract lesion) and Horner syndrome (descending sympathetic tract) may be associated. Infrequently, there may be hearing loss associated due to cochlear nuclei affection **(Fig. 15 and Tables 9 and 10)**.

Top of the Basilar Syndrome

Occlusion of basilar artery at its distal end will involve midbrain, thalamus, and distribution of PCA. This will manifest as transient loss of consciousness to coma (reticular activating system involvement), oculomotor disturbances (upward gaze defect with eye moving inward and downward), hemianopia (optic radiation involvement), bilateral ptosis, and skew deviation (midbrain lesion containing III nerve). There is also contralateral hemiplegia and peduncular hallucinosis depending upon the patency of the circle of Willis via the PCom **(Fig. 16 and Tables 11 and 12)**.

Basilar Artery Branch Occlusion Syndrome

Occlusion at terminal bifurcation branches will present such as thalamic, subthalamic, and midbrain occlusions. Most of the times, basilar branch occlusion features are rather unilateral in nature as compared to basilar occlusion where it affects both sides.

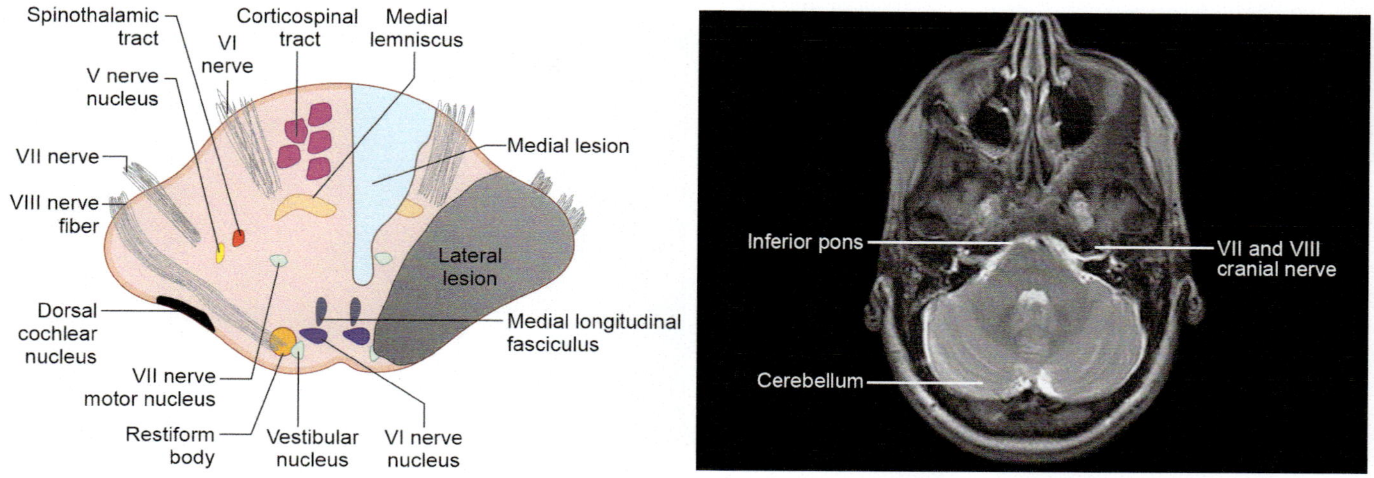

FIG. 14: Inferior pontine cross-section and its lesion.

TABLE 7: Medial inferior pontine syndrome (occlusion of paramedian branch of basilar artery).

On the side of lesion (ipsilateral)		Opposite to side of lesion (contralateral)	
Structure involved	**Features**	**Structure involved**	**Features**
Parapontine reticular formation (PPRF)	Paralysis of conjugate gaze to the side of lesion	Corticospinal tract	Paralysis of arm and leg
Vestibular nucleus	Vertigo, nystagmus	Corticobulbar tract	Paralysis of face
Middle cerebellar peduncles	Ataxia of limb and gait	Medical lemniscus	Impaired tactile and proprioception of the half of the body
Abducens nerve	Diplopia		

TABLE 8: Lateral inferior pontine syndrome (occlusion of anterior inferior cerebellar artery).

On the side of lesion (ipsilateral)		Opposite to the side of lesion (contralateral)	
Structure involved	**Features**	**Structure involved**	**Features**
Vestibular nuclei	Vertigo, nystagmus, nausea, and vomiting	Spinothalamic tract	Impaired pain and thermal sensation over one half of the body
VII nerve	UMN facial palsy		
PPRF	Paralysis of gaze to side of lesion		
Cochlear nuclei	Deafness and tinnitus		
Middle cerebellar peduncles	Ataxia of limbs and gait		
V nerve	Impaired sensation over face		

(PPRF: parapontine reticular formation; UMN: upper motor neuron)

TABLE 9: Medial midpontine syndrome (paramedian branch occlusion).

On side of lesion (ipsilateral)		Opposite to the side of lesion (contralateral)	
Structure involved	**Features**	**Structure involved**	**Features**
Pontine nuclei	Ataxia to limbs and gait	Medial lemniscus	Impaired joint position sense and touch
		Corticospinal tract	Paralysis of face, leg, and arm

TABLE 10: Lateral midpontine syndrome (occlusion of small circumferential artery).

On the side of lesion (ipsilateral)		Opposite to side of the lesion (contralateral)	
Structure involved	**Features**	**Structure involved**	**Features**
Middle cerebellar peduncles	Ataxia of limbs	Lateral spinothalamic tract	Impaired pain and thermal sensation of half of the body
Motor nuclei of V nerve	Paralysis of muscle of mastication		
Principal sensory nuclei of V nerve	Impaired sensation over face		

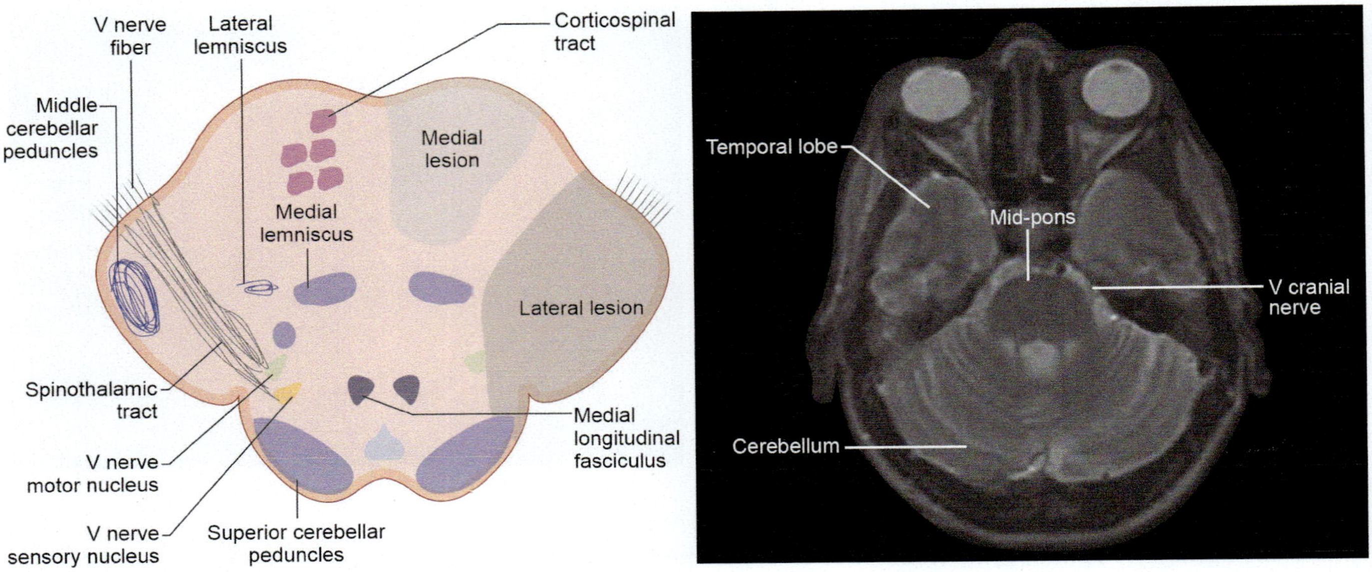

FIG. 15: Midpontine cross-section and its lesion.

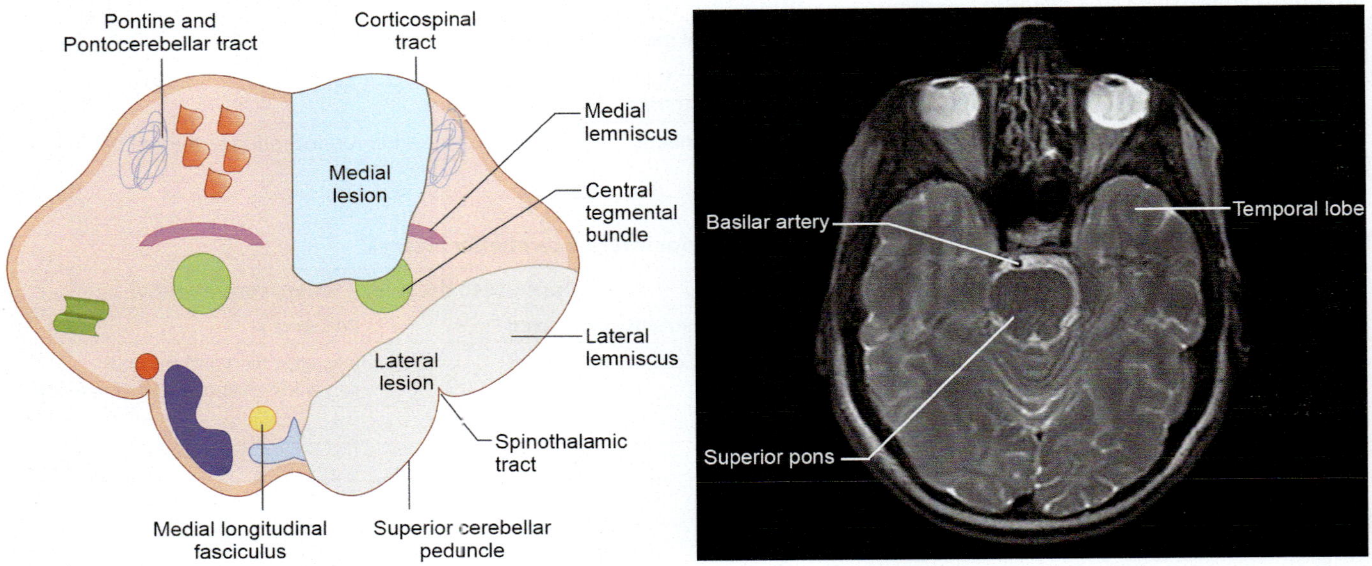

FIG. 16: Superior pontine cross-section and its lesion.

TABLE 11: Medial superior pontine syndrome (paramedian branch of upper basilar artery).

On the side of lesion (ipsilateral)		On the opposite side of lesion (contralateral)	
Structure involved	**Features**	**Structure involved**	**Features**
Superior cerebellar peduncles	Ataxia of limbs	Medial lemniscus	Impaired touch and proprioception
Medial longitudinal fasciculus	Intranuclear ophthalmoplegia	Corticospinal	Paralysis of arm and leg
Central tegmental bundle	Palatal myoclonus	Corticobulbar	Paralysis of face

Penetrating Branch Occlusion

Small infarct usually occurs due to occlusion of small penetrating vessels, which manifests heterogeneously in various combinations such as contralateral hemiparesis, ipsilateral facial numbness, or tingling sensation. The mechanism of stroke can be embolic or atherosclerotic depending upon the patient's comorbidity or risk factor. The presence of atrial fibrillation will favor embolization whereas long-standing diabetes and hypertension shift our preference to another side.

Superior Cerebellar Artery Occlusion

Superior cerebellar artery is the most rostral branch of the basilar artery. Occlusion of this artery will manifest as

TABLE 12: Lateral superior pontine syndrome (occlusion of superior cerebellar artery).

On the side of lesion (ipsilateral)		Opposite to the side of lesion (contralateral)	
Structure involved	**Features**	**Structure involved**	**Features**
Superior cerebellar peduncles	Ataxia of limb and gait	Lateral spinothalamic tract	Loss of pain and temperature of hemibody
Vestibular nuclei	Dizziness, nausea, and vomiting		
Descending sympathetic fiber	Horner syndrome		
Dentatorubrothalamic pathway	Tremor		

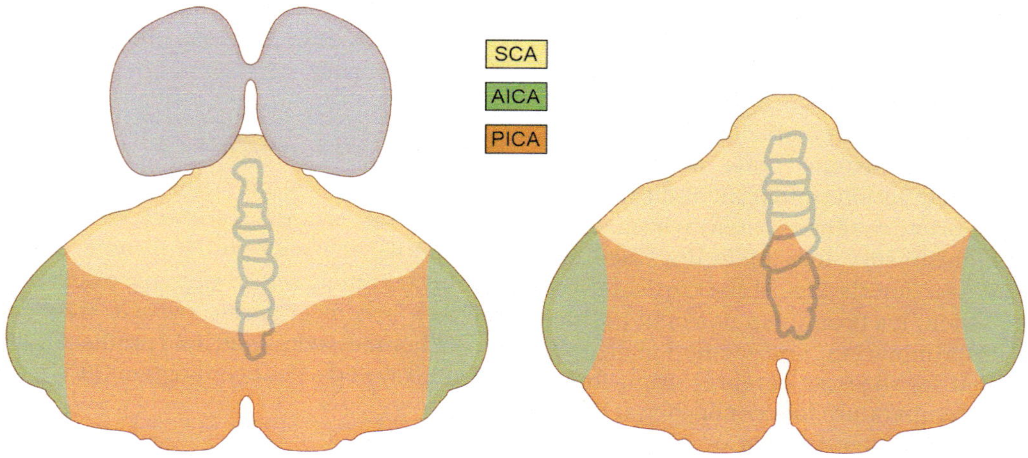

FIG. 17: Blood supply of cerebellum.
(AICA: anteroinferior cerebellar artery; PICA: posterior inferior cerebellar artery; SCA: superior cerebellar artery)

ipsilateral cerebellar ataxia of limbs (middle and superior cerebellar peduncle involvement) with an ataxic tremor of ipsilateral upper limb, nausea and vomiting (vestibular nuclei), slurred speech, loss of pain and thermal sensation over the contralateral side, ipsilateral Horner syndrome, and palatal myoclonus rarely **(Fig. 17)**.

Anterior Inferior Cerebellar Artery Occlusion

Anterior inferior cerebellar artery is a branch of basilar artery, but sometimes it originates combinedly from basilar and vertebral artery junction as single stem then divided into anterior inferior cerebellar artery and PICA. It is a small, slender artery, but often its size and distribution complement with PICA. The clinical picture of its occlusion manifests as following:

- *Nausea and vomiting, vertigo, and nystagmus*: Vestibular nuclei defect
- *Unilateral deafness*: Cochlear nuclei lesion
- *Facial weakness*: VII nerve lesion
- *Ipsilateral cerebellar ataxia*: Inferior and middle cerebral peduncle lesion
- *Ipsilateral Horner syndrome*: Descending sympathetic tract defect
- *Paresis of conjugate lateral gaze*: Paramedian pontine reticular formation
- *Contralateral loss of pain and thermal sensation of arm, trunk, and leg*: Lateral spinothalamic tract involvement

Sometimes occlusion at the origin causes contralateral hemiplegia, and end distal occlusion will present as isolated unilateral deafness.

The most characteristic features of basilar branch occlusion are crossed long tract sensory or motor deficit and cranial nerve involvement, which represents unilateral infarction of the brainstem.

SUMMARY AND LOCALIZATION OF ANTERIOR AND POSTERIOR CIRCULATION STROKE SYNDROME

Anterior circulation strokes (75%) are more common than posterior circulation (25%). Anterior circulation typically presents with unilateral symptoms, but posterior circulation is either unilateral or bilateral. Posterior circulation has high chance of affecting consciousness and autonomic disturbances (fever, respiratory alteration).

Contralateral motor deficit including face, arm, hand, leg, and foot is affected in brainstem infarction, posterior limb of IC lesion, and cortical infarction in primary motor areas. In brainstem lesions, there is associated cranial involvement depending upon the level of lesion in the brainstem such as III and IV cranial nerve involvement in midbrain infarction; VI, VII, and VIII cranial nerve involvement in pontine infarct; and IX, X, and XII cranial nerve involvement in the medullary lesion. Ipsilateral trigeminal nerve involvement can be seen in pontine and medullary infarcts. The presence of ipsilateral ataxia is usually seen in brainstem lesions as compared to the capsular or cortical lesion. In hemiplegia of pontine origin, eye will be deviated to contralateral side due to affection of paramedian pontine reticular formation, whereas ipsilateral eye deviation is seen in supratentorial lesions/ MCA territory lesion (M2 superior division) but no eye deviation seen in isolated posterior IC lesion. Another important feature includes crossed sensory deficit (ipsilateral face and contralateral half of body), which usually indicates a lesion of the lower brainstem (pons and medulla), whereas upper brainstem lesion (midbrain and thalamus) and parietal lesion (primary sensory area) will manifest as contralateral hemisensory loss including face and involving all modalities. For distinguishing cortical lesion from the thalamic lesion, if a prominent defect in position sense, two-point discrimination, and tactile localization are observed, then it localizes to cerebral origin but if prominent pain and temperature loss occur then it points toward thalamic origin. Bilateral motor or sensory signs will conclude to be a brainstem lesion. Additional features that favor brainstem lesions include vertigo, diplopia, ataxia, and Horner syndrome. Coexistence of hemiparesis with hemisensory loss (all modalities) will point toward supratentorial lesion, but the capsular lesion is most of the time either pure sensory or motor or sensorimotor (still it can be differentiated from cortical lesion based on the absence of language, cognition, and hemianopia).

DIFFERENTIAL DIAGNOSIS OF STROKE[13]

Any acute focal neurological deficit should be considered as stroke unless proven otherwise. Stroke is basically a clinical diagnosis. The list of stroke mimics is mentioned below:

- Brain tumor
- Subdural hematoma
- Seizures/postictal Todd's palsy
- Hypoglycemia
- Hyperglycemic chorea
- Migraine/familial hemiplegic migraine
- Mononeuritis
- Encephalopathy
- Bell's palsy
- Conversion disorder

These mimics should be identified at the earliest to save brain tissue and prevent a catastrophic outcome.

INVESTIGATIONS[14,15]

Any abrupt-onset focal neurological deficit should be addressed at the earliest. On presentation to emergency department there should be brief neurological examination along with detailed assessment as per the National Institutes of Health Stroke Scale (NIHSS). The exact time of onset should be noted either by the patient or by the bystander if the patient is aphasic or confused or has a loss of consciousness. Once clinical examination is complete the patient should be sent to an imaging study for confirming clinical diagnosis. Before proceeding with imaging, it should be made dictum to do blood glucose estimation for ruling out hypoglycemia.

Essential Laboratory Investigation[15]

The important blood investigations include complete blood count, prothrombin time, international normalized ratio (INR), activated partial thromboplastin time (aPTT), serum creatinine, serum glutamic oxaloacetic transaminase (SGOT), serum glutamic pyruvic transaminase (SGPT), serum homocysteine, and lipid profile. Another test includes chest X-ray and electrocardiogram (ECG).

CT Scans

Computed tomography is the first imaging of choice for stroke diagnosis. It is extremely important to differentiate ischemic stroke from hemorrhagic stroke. It is also helpful to identify extra-axial hemorrhage, neoplasm, and ring-enhancing lesion that masquerade as stroke. The most important advantage of this imaging is very minimal time consumption. The disadvantage of CT scan is that it won't pick up any infarct properly in the early hour of a stroke and usually takes minimum 24–48-hour time to reliably identify a stroke. It is also ineffective for small ischemic stroke and posterior fossa stroke.

For the identification of anterior circulation stroke, there is a standardized ASPECT (Alberta Stroke Program Early CT) score, which is helpful in deciding stroke severity and plan for appropriate management. For identification of early signs of ischemic stroke, it is vital to look for loss of gray/ white differentiation, sulcal effacement, and obscuration of the lentiform nucleus. The large vessel occlusion has a typical dense MCA sign, Sylvian fissure dot sign, and dense basilar sign before infarction becomes visible.

Computed tomography angiography (CTA) is one of the most accurate noninvasive investigations to delineate site of occlusion of large vessel causing stroke. CT perfusion is one of the advanced investigations to detect tissue at risk of death or salvageable brain areas.

MRI Study

Magnetic resonance imaging is also highly sensitive for identifying stroke. It is better than CT scan in terms of higher resolution, can pick up very early stroke, and is best for identification for posterior circulation stroke. The sequences required for stroke identification are diffusion-weighted image (DWI) which can pick up as early as 30 minutes from the onset, apparent diffusion coefficient (ADC) which is a constructed image for assuring true diffusion restriction, susceptibility-weighted angiography (SWAN) for identification of microbleed/hemorrhages, and fluid-attenuated inversion recovery (FLAIR), which is very informative to know the age of infarction. Another study like magnetic resonance angiography (MRA) is also helpful to identify large vessel occlusion but has less sensitivity than CTA as it is flow dependent. MR perfusion is very informative to identify the ischemic core and penumbra.

Cerebral Angiography

Cerebral angiography is the gold standard investigation for detecting vascular pathology. It accurately determines the size and localization of vascular pathology. It is very much required in stroke for mechanical removal of the clot. It is also helpful in detecting specific causes such as cervico-cephalic arterial dissection, vasculitis, moyamoya disease, aneurysm, and differentiating between atherosclerosis and nonatherosclerotic vasculopathy.

Echo and Holter Study

Echo and Holter study are complementary tests to be done for distinguishing cardiovascular source of embolization.

MANAGEMENT OF STROKE[15,16]

The first goal of stroke treatment is to prevent or reverse brain injury. It is our high priority to save salvageable tissue. Before starting treatment, secure the patient airway, breathing, and circulation and treat hypo- or hyperglycemia. Treatment protocol involves six categories:
1. Intravenous thrombolysis
2. Endovascular revascularization
3. Medical support
4. Antithrombotic treatment
5. Neuroprotection
6. Rehabilitation

Intravenous Thrombolysis and Endovascular Treatment[17-20]

Whenever a patient with suspected stroke reaches emergency, detailed neurological assessment is done with the NIHSS score. Urgently shift to CT room to rule out any hemorrhage. Based on the NIHSS score if 0–5 (minor stroke), conventional supportive treatment is preferred.

TABLE 13: Mechanical thrombectomy trial.

Inclusion criteria	DEFUSE-3	DAWN
Time window	6–16 hours since time last known well	6–24 hours since time last known well
Age	18–90 years	≥18 years
mRS score before qualifying stroke	≤2; life expectancy ≥ 6 months	≤1; life expectancy ≥ 6 months
NIHSS score	≥6	≥10 (see below)
Arterial occlusion	ICA and/or M1	ICA and/or M1
Mismatch definition	*Target mismatch profile on CT or MR perfusion imaging, as determined by an automated image postprocessing system*: Infarct core volume <70 mL, mismatch volume >15 mL (T_{max} >6 seconds), and mismatch ratio (penumbra/core) >1.8	Clinical imaging mismatch age <80 years, NIHSS score >10, and infarct core volume 0–30 mL or age <80 years, NIHSS score >20, and infarct core volume 31–51 mL or age ≥80 years, NIHSS score >10, and infarct core volume 0–20 mL

(CT: computed tomography; DAWN: Diffusion-weighted imaging or computerized tomography perfusion assessment with clinical mismatch in the triage of wake-up and late presenting strokes undergoing neurointervention with Trevo; DEFUSE-3: endovascular therapy following imaging evaluation for ischemic stroke 3; ICA: internal carotid artery; MR: magnetic resonance; mRS: modified Rankin scale; NIHSS: National Institutes of Health Stroke Scale)

Now guidelines suggest in favor of thrombolysis if a minor stroke is disabling. If the NIHSS > 6, ASPECT score (CT score for MCA territory) <6, and symptom onset is <4.5 hours, then the patient should be thermolyzed with intravenous tissue-type plasminogen activator (tPA). In the Indian context, tenecteplase (TNK) is also approved for this with time limit of within 3 hours from onset. As per the new Canadian trail, TNK is a very effective choice with ease of administration for acute ischemic stroke up to 4.5 hours from the onset. Endovascular treatment is very much effective for large vessel occlusion. The time window is extended till 24 hours, but earlier intervention will give a good outcome **(Table 13, Box 1, and Flowchart 1)**.

CONCLUSION

Stroke is a devastating disease with high mortality and morbidity if left untreated timely. It is a clinical diagnosis, and imaging studies only support clinical suspicion. Protocol for stroke management is time dependent and keeps evolving on a yearly basis. For the clinician, to address stroke there should be high index of intuition and to prioritize thought on the mechanism and territory of stroke rather than name eponyms. Revascularization in a timely manner is the cornerstone of treatment. For better outcomes comprehensive stroke care includes a team of healthcare professionals and nursing caregivers.

BOX 1 **Inclusion and exclusion criteria for IVT.**

Inclusion criteria

- Clinical diagnosis of ischemic stroke causing measurable neurological deficit
- Onset of symptoms <4.5 hours before treatment; if the exact time of onset of stroke is unknown, it is defined as the last time the patient was known to be normal or at neurological disease
- Age > 18 years

Exclusion criteria

Patient history:

- Ischemic stroke or severe head trauma in the previous 3 months
- Previous intracranial hemorrhage
- Intra-axial intracranial neoplasm
- Gastrointestinal malignancy
- Gastrointestinal hemorrhage in the previous 21 days
- Intracranial or intraspinal surgery within the prior 3 months

Clinical:

- Symptoms suggestive of subarachnoid hemorrhage
- Persistent blood pressure elevation (systolic ≥185 mm Hg or diastolic ≥110 mm Hg)
- Active intracranial bleeding
- Presentation consistent with infective endocarditis
- Stroke known or suspected to be associated with aortic arch dissection
- Acute bleeding diathesis, including but not limited to conditions defined under "hematologic"

Hematologic:

- Platelet count <100,000/mm^3
- Current anticoagulant use with INR >1.7 or PT >15 seconds or aPTT >40 seconds
- Therapeutic doses of low-molecular-weight heparin received within 24 hours (e.g., to treat VTE and ACS); this exclusion does not apply to prophylactic doses (e.g., to prevent VTE)

Current use (last dose within 48 hours in a patient with normal renal function) of a direct thrombin inhibitor or direct factor Xa inhibitor with evidence of anticoagulant effect by laboratory tests such as aPTT, INR, ECT, TT, or appropriate factor Xa assays

Head CT:

- Evidence of hemorrhage
- Extensive regions of obvious hypodensity consistent with irreversible injury

Warnings:

- Only miner and isolated neurological signed or rapidly improving symptoms
- Serum glucose < 50 mg/dL (2.8 mmol/L)
- Serious trauma in the previous 14 days
- Major surgery in the previous 14 days
- History of gastrointestinal bleeding (remote) or genitourinary bleeding
- Pregnancy
- Arterial puncture at a noncompressible site in the previous 7 days
- Large (>10 mm), untreated, unruptured intracranial aneurysm
- Untreated intracranial vascular malformation

Additional warnings for treatment from 3 to 4.5 hours from symptom onset:

- Age > 80 years
- Oral anticoagulant use regardless of INR
- Severe stroke (NIHSS score > 25)
- Combination of both previous ischemic stroke and diabetes mellitus

(ACS: acute coronary syndrome; aPTT: activated partial thromboplastin time; CT: computed tomography; ECT: electroconvulsive therapy; INR: international normalized ratio; IVT: intravenous thrombolysis; NIHSS: National Institutes of Health Stroke Scale; PT: prothrombin time; PTT: partial thromboplastin time; TT: thrombin time; VTE: venous thromboembolism)

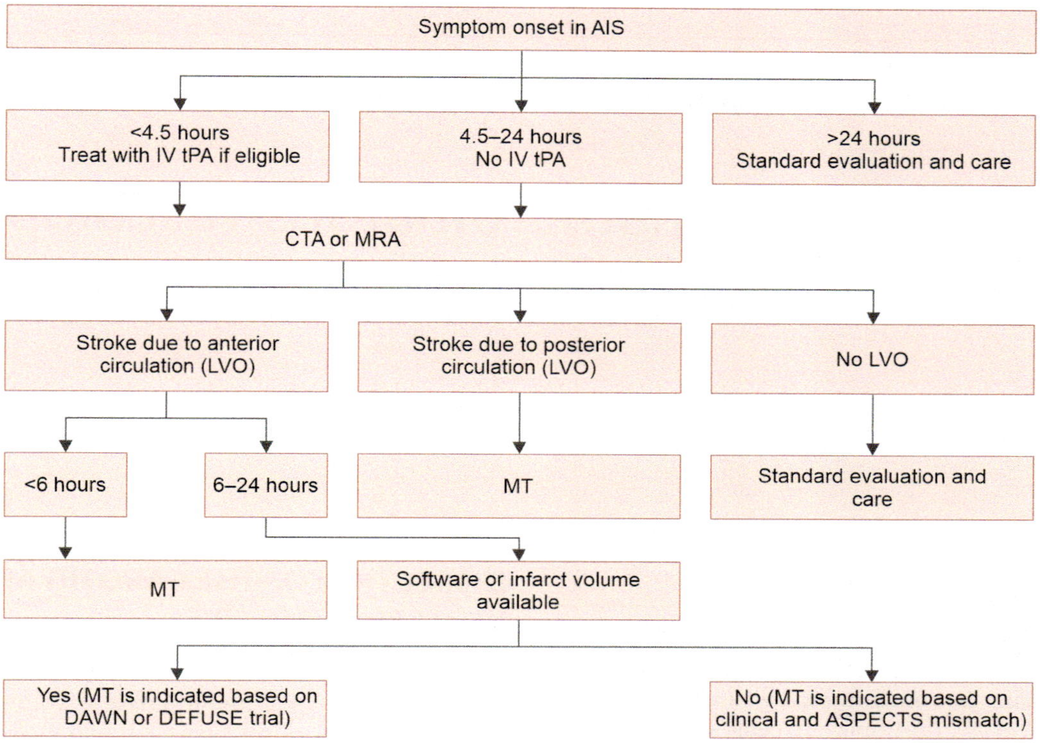

FLOWCHART 1: Treatment algorithm of AIS.

(AIS: acute ischemic stroke; ASPECTS: Alberta Stroke Program Early CT score; CTA: computed tomography angiography; DAWN: diffusion-weighted imaging or computerized tomography perfusion assessment with clinical mismatch in the triage of wake-up and late presenting strokes undergoing neurointervention with Trevo; DEFUSE: endovascular therapy following imaging evaluation for ischemic stroke 3; IV: intravenous; LVO: large vessel occlusion; MRA: magnetic resonance angiography; MT: mechanical thrombectomy; tPA: tissue-type plasminogen activator)

REFERENCES

1. Benjamin EJ, Blaha MJ, Chiuve SE, Cushman M, Das SR, Deo R, et al. Heart disease and stroke statistics—2017 update: a report from the American Heart Association. Circulation. 2017;135(10):e146-603.
2. Pandian JD, Sudhan P. Stroke epidemiology and stroke care services in India. J Stroke. 2013;15(3):128.
3. Bell R, Severson MA, Armonda RA. Neurovascular anatomy: a practical guide. Neurosurg Clin N Am. 2009;20(3):265-78.
4. Kuriakose D, Xiao Z. Pathophysiology and treatment of stroke: present status and future perspectives. Int J Mol Sci. 2020;21(20):7609.
5. Murphy SJ, Werring DJ. Stroke: causes and clinical features. Medicine. 2020;48(9):561-6.
6. Allen CM. Clinical diagnosis of the acute stroke syndrome. Q J Med. 1983;52(4):515-23.
7. Caplan LR (Ed). Caplan's Stroke. Cambridge: Cambridge University Press; 2016.
8. Koroshetz WJ, Ropper AH. Artery-to-artery embolism causing stroke in the posterior circulation. Neurology. 1987;37(2):292-5.
9. Smith WS, Lev MH, English JD, Camargo EC, Chou M, Johnston SC, et al. Significance of large vessel intracranial occlusion causing acute ischemic stroke and TIA. Stroke. 2009;40(12):3834-40.
10. Adams Jr HP, Bendixen BH, Kappelle LJ, Biller J, Love BB, Gordon DL, et al. Classification of subtype of acute ischemic stroke. Definitions for use in a multicenter clinical trial. TOAST. Trial of Org 10172 in acute stroke treatment. Stroke. 1993;24(1):35-41.
11. Hui C, Tadi P, Patti L. Ischemic Stroke. In: StatPearls [Internet]. Florida: StatPearls Publishing; 2022.
12. Banerjee G, Stone SP, Werring DJ. Posterior circulation ischemic stroke. BMJ. 2018;361:k1185.
13. Vilela P. Acute stroke differential diagnosis: stroke mimics. Eur J Radiol. 2017;96:133-44.
14. Vo KD, Yoo AJ, Gupta A, Qiao Y, Vagal AS, Hirsch JA, et al. Multimodal diagnostic imaging for hyperacute stroke. Am J Neuroradiol. 2015;36(12):2206-13.
15. Cassella CR, Jagoda A. Ischemic stroke: advances in diagnosis and management. Emerg Med Clin North Am. 2017;35(4):911-30.
16. Bhalla A, Patel M, Birns J. An update on hyperacute management of ischemic stroke. Clin Med (Lond). 2021;21(3):215.
17. Demaerschalk BM, Kleindorfer DO, Adeoye OM, Demchuk AM, Fugate JE, Grotta JC, et al. Scientific rationale for the inclusion and exclusion criteria for intravenous alteplase in acute ischemic stroke: a statement for healthcare professionals from the American Heart Association/American Stroke Association. Stroke. 2016;47(2):581-641.
18. Nogueira RG, Jadhav AP, Haussen DC, Bonafe A, Budzik RF, Bhuva P, et al. Thrombectomy 6 to 24 hours after stroke with a mismatch between deficit and infarct. N Engl J Med. 2018;378(1):11-21.
19. Albers GW, Marks MP, Kemp S, Christensen S, Tsai JP, Ortega-Gutierrez S, et al. Thrombectomy for stroke at 6 to 16 hours with selection by perfusion imaging. N Engl J Med. 2018;378(8):708-18.
20. Cho YH, Choi JH. Outcomes of mechanical thrombectomy in patients with large diffusion-weighted imaging lesions. J Korean Neurosurg Soc. 2022;65(1):22-9.

53

CHAPTER

Nonatheromatous Vasculopathies

Soumya Sundaram, Sapna Erat Sreedharan, PN Sylaja

INTRODUCTION

Atherosclerotic disease of cerebral vasculature is one of the most common causes of ischemic stroke.[1,2] A proportion of ischemic stroke is contributed by nonatheromatous vasculopathies (NAVs). The important causes of NAV leading on to stroke include dissection, central nervous system (CNS) vasculitis, moyamoya disease (MMD), Takayasu arteritis (TA), fibromuscular dysplasia (FMD), and carotid web (CaW).[3,4] They are an important cause of stroke in children and young adults.[3] Magnetic resonance imaging (MRI) helps establish the nature of lesion and the extent of brain involvement. Luminal imaging with either MR angiography (MRA) or computed tomography angiography (CTA) plays a key role in the diagnosis of NAV and identification of the underlying cause. The MR vessel wall imaging has emerged as an additional tool in delineating the abnormality in arterial walls by direct visualization. Conventional angiography (CA) and meningo-cortical biopsy are considered when above investigations fail to identify the underlying cause.[5] The list of NAV is exhaustive **(Box 1)**, and addressing each of these conditions in this chapter is not possible. Hence, we will be discussing the most common causes of NAV, namely dissection, CNS vasculitis, FMD, CaW, and MMD.

BOX 1 Causes of nonatheromatous vasculopathy.

- Central nervous system vasculitis
- Reversible cerebral vasoconstriction syndrome
- Dissection
- Fibromuscular dysplasia
- Radiation-induced vasculopathy
- Moyamoya disease
- Cerebral amyloid angiopathy
- Cerebral autosomal dominant arteriopathy with subcortical infarcts and leukoencephalopathy
- Sickle cell disease
- Drug-induced vasculopathy

DISSECTION OF THE CAROTID AND VERTEBRAL ARTERIES

Dissection of the carotid and vertebral arteries (VAs) is an important cause of ischemic stroke in young and accounts for around 2.5% of all first ever ischemic strokes.[6,7] The clinical presentation depends on the vessel involved and also whether the dissection is intracranial or extracranial.[7]

Pathophysiology

Arterial dissection results from an intimal tear or vasa vasorum rupture with bleeding into tunica media, which produces separation of vessel wall layers and false lumen formation. In subintimal dissection, the hematoma will expand toward the lumen-causing luminal narrowing or occlusion of the vessel, but in subadventitial dissection it expands outside toward the adventitia, causing pseudoaneurysm.[8] The subintimal dissection usually presents with ischemic symptoms due to artery-to-artery embolism or hemodynamic compromise or both. The subadventitial dissection can present with subarachnoid hemorrhage (SAH). The arterial wall weakness can be due to genetic causes with contribution from environmental factors such as infection and minor trauma. Genetic conditions such as FMD, Ehlers–Danlos syndrome (EDS), Marfan's syndrome, and osteogenesis imperfecta can predispose to dissection. These conditions can also lead to recurrent or multivessel dissection. Certain risk factors such as hypertension, migraine, hyperhomocysteinemia, and recent infections have been associated with dissection.[9,10] Our study showed that cervical carotid artery dissection has also been associated with long styloid process, suggesting that mechanical injury from styloid process can predispose to dissection.[11]

Clinical Features

The arterial dissection presents with either local, ischemic, or hemorrhagic symptoms. Local symptoms alone may be present in 23–33% of patients, when the diagnosis can be missed.[12] Carotid dissection can present with local symptoms such as ipsilateral neck pain and/or headache (25–66%), Horner's syndrome (up to 50%), and lower cranial nerve palsies (12%) with or without retinal and cerebral ischemic symptoms (50–90%). About 3–8% of the patients present with SAH. In adults, 1–10% of all nontraumatic SAH is due to dissection. The SAH presentation is more common in posterior circulation compared to anterior circulation since intradural VA has a thin media with fewer elastic fibers.[13]

Imaging

Early and accurate diagnosis of arterial dissection is important for initiating immediate treatment. CT scan and MRI of brain may show single **(Figs. 1A and B)** or multiple infarcts in embolic, hemodynamic, or mixed pattern. It can rarely show SAH. With advances in noninvasive vascular imaging (CTA and MRA) **(Figs. 1C and D)**, the gold standard CA is required only in very few situations. CTA is the preferred diagnostic modality as it is fast, can screen from aortic arch to vertex, and can be used in unstable patients. The classical findings in arterial dissection are irregular/asymmetric wall intramural hematoma, intimal flap, flame-shaped occlusion **(Figs. 1E and F)**, and dissecting aneurysm.[14] The diagnostic accuracy of CTA compared with gold standard CA has a sensitivity and specificity ranging from 60 to 100%.[15] CTA is preferred over MRA in suspected VA dissection, due to smaller luminal caliber of the affected vessel and due to its proximity to bony structures. In patients with intracranial dissection and dissecting aneurysms, CA is preferred over CTA. MRA with MRI T1-weighted fat-suppressed sequences is optimal for imaging in suspected dissection **(Figs. 1G and H)**, where even small intramural hematomas can be visualized. The dissection is seen as region of crescentic hyperintensity on T1 fat-saturated images, suggesting intramural hematoma. In addition, there may be luminal narrowing and enlargement of the vessel wall diameter. Compared to CA, MRA has 50–100% sensitivity and 30–100% specificity for detecting cervical arterial dissection (CAD).[16] As a screening tool, Doppler ultrasound (DUS) is useful in excluding extracranial carotid dissection in patients presenting with cerebral ischemia. The ultrasound (US) features reported in dissection are hypoechogenic increase

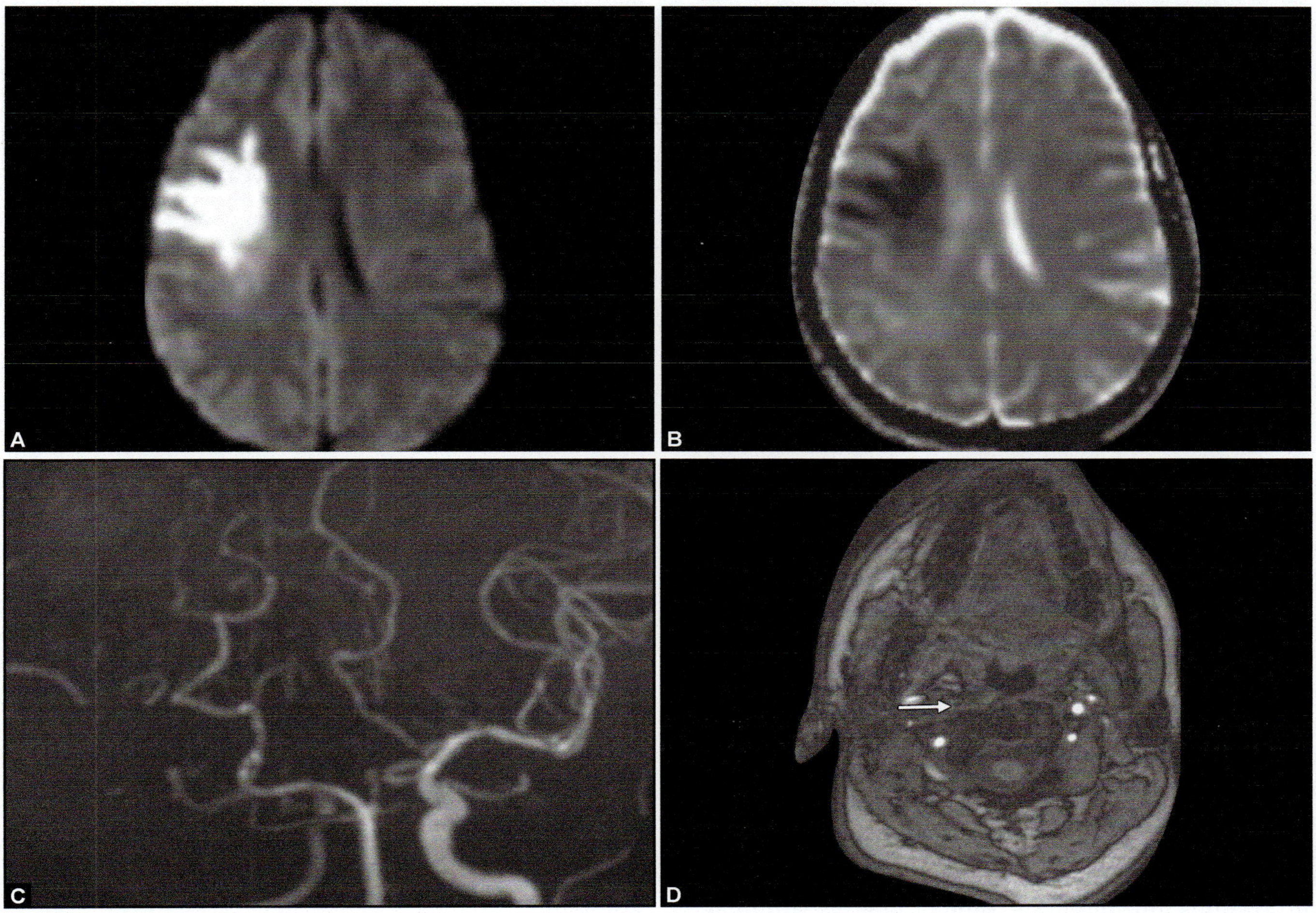

FIGS. 1A TO H: *Continued*

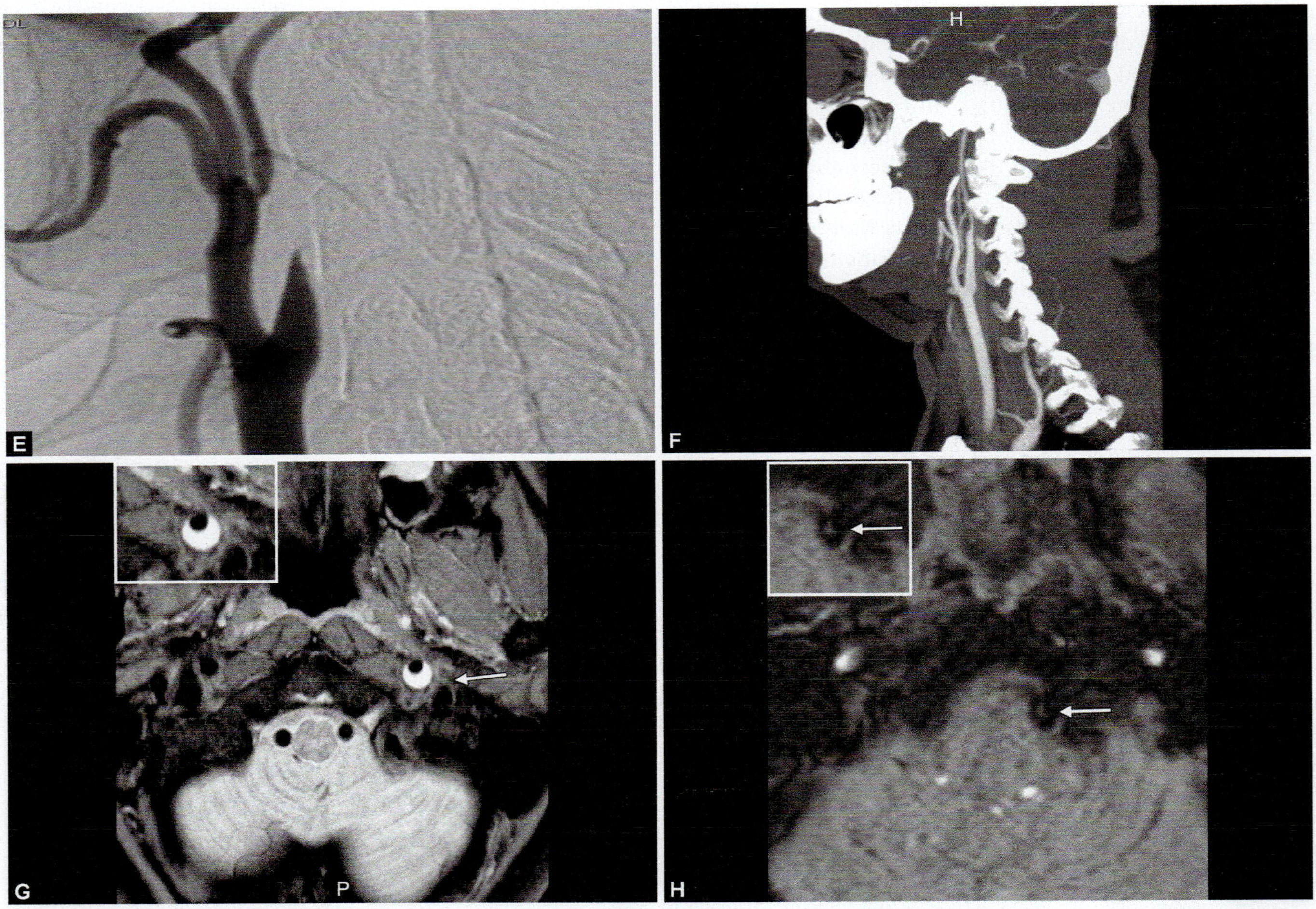

FIGS. 1A TO H: Neuroimaging findings in dissection. Top panel shows the imaging features of a 34-year-old male patient who presented with sudden-onset headache and left hemiplegia. (A and B) MR imaging showed acute infarct; (C) Time-of-flight MR angiogram revealed attenuation of right ICA with poor distal flow; (D) Source image showed narrow caliber of right ICA. Bottom panel represents the imaging features seen in dissection. (E) Conventional cerebral angiogram showing left ICA flame-shaped tapering and occlusion; (F) CT angiogram showing right ICA long-segment tapering and occlusion; (G) Axial fat suppressed T1W image showing left ICA crescent sign; (H) Susceptibility-weighted image showing left V4 thrombus with dissection flap.

(CT: computed tomography; ICA: internal carotid artery; MR: magnetic resonance; T1W: T1-weighted)

in wall thickness, false lumen, and hyperechogenic flap. Currently the role of CA is only when the noninvasive imaging modalities are inconclusive, when patient presents with SAH, and when interventional management is planned.[14]

Management

The management of ischemic stroke due to CAD involves hyperacute treatment and secondary prevention. Studies have investigated the safety and efficacy of intravenous thrombolysis in hyperacute ischemic stroke due to CAD. The rate of favorable outcome and safety profile was similar to patients thrombolyzed for other etiologies.[17,18] Though there is a theoretical risk of intramural hematoma expansion, intravenous thrombolysis should not be withheld in ischemic stroke due to dissection. After acute treatment, the patient can be started on antithrombotic therapy to prevent stroke recurrences. There is no superiority for anticoagulation over antiplatelets in preventing stroke recurrence, except in situations where there are ischemic events in spite of antiplatelets or if there is a thrombus on vascular imaging.[19,20] The management remains same for intracranial dissection when the patient presents with ischemic symptoms alone. The duration of antiplatelet therapy in patients with dissection is still unknown. The recurrence risk after dissection is very low. In patients with ischemic stroke presentation, the role for endovascular treatment is limited.[20,21]

Mechanical thrombectomy is the preferred treatment in patients with acute ischemic stroke with cervical dissection presenting with intracranial large vessel occlusion and when they present within 24 hours from stroke onset.[21]

Endovascular/surgical management may be required in patients who present with SAH or pressure effects secondary to dissecting aneurysm, especially intracranially.[13]

CENTRAL NERVOUS SYSTEM VASCULITIS

Inflammation of the blood vessels of CNS is termed as CNS vasculitis and is a heterogenous group of disorders. CNS vasculitis occurring secondary to systemic infections, autoimmune disorders, connective tissue diseases, and malignancy is termed secondary CNS vasculitis. But when it occurs in isolation without any systemic features then the condition is labelled as primary CNS vasculitis (PCNSV) or primary angiitis of CNS (PACNS).[22] The clinical features are nonspecific and protean, which include headache, encephalopathy, focal neurological deficits, seizures, neuropsychiatric manifestations, and dementia. Cranial nerve palsies and myelopathy can occur. In secondary vasculitis, systemic features and constitutional symptoms comprising fever, loss of appetite, and weight loss are seen. In CNS vasculitis, the clinical, imaging, and pathological features are almost similar except for certain distinguishing features in each of the individual conditions.[23]

Primary Angiitis of Central Nervous System

Primary angiitis of CNS is a rare vasculitis that exclusively affects the blood vessels of brain, meninges, and spinal cord.[24] The prevalence from North America is estimated to be 2.4 per 1,000,000 person-years.[25] It can affect both children and adults, and the median age of onset is 50 years. The diagnosis of PACNS is arrived at only when all the secondary causes of cerebral vasculitis and the vasculitis mimics are excluded.[26]

Clinical Features

The clinical features of PACNS are similar to any other forms of cerebral vasculitis, which includes stroke and rapidly progressive dementia as the predominant clinical syndrome. Headache is a common accompanying symptom, the character of which is different from that of the thunderclap headache in reversible cerebral vasoconstriction syndrome (RCVS).[27] In the largest series from India, the clinical features reported were ischemic stroke (33%), headache (25%), seizures (18%), cognitive decline (11%), and intracranial hemorrhage (9%). The other rare manifestations include tumor-like mass lesions and myelopathy.[28] In PACNS, fever, anorexia, weight loss, and arthralgia are infrequent.[29] Some patients can progress rapidly with fatal outcome.[30] In PACNS, any size of cerebral vessel can get involved. Large-medium-sized vessel involvement can manifest as stroke or transient ischemic attack (TIA), whereas small-vessel involvement can present as encephalopathy, dementia, and seizures.[29,31]

Imaging and Other Investigations

Normal MRI brain excludes PACNS. MRI brain findings reflect the type of vessels involved. Infarcts are the most common findings **(Figs. 2A and B)**. Acute, subacute, and chronic infarcts can coexist in a single patient. The infarcts span over multiple arterial territories bilaterally and mostly over supratentorial location. Subcortical and deep white matter, deep gray matter, and cerebral cortex are also involved.[32] Small-vessel involvement can lead to lacunar infarcts and ischemic demyelination of the periventricular white matter, which is often graded as per Fazekas grading.[32,33] Intracranial hemorrhage can be due to either hemorrhagic conversion of the infarct or direct bleed from rupture of inflamed vessel with necrosis.[32,34] Intraventricular hemorrhage (IVH) is very rare in PACNS.[35] Cortical and subcortical microbleeds **(Fig. 2C)** can point toward the diagnosis of CNS vasculitis. Gadolinium enhancement of the parenchyma **(Fig. 2D)**, especially of the noninfarct region, and leptomeninges is also observed. Rather than a single finding, a constellation of the above imaging features helps in the diagnosis.[32] Time-of-flight MRA (TOF-MRA) at 3T can detect the typical angiographic features of vasculitis. However, the distal vessels are less appreciated.[36] CA is obviously the first choice of investigation in the evaluation of CNS vasculitis due to its better spatial and temporal resolution. However, the specificity is very low. Angiography shows stenosis and dilatations, giving rise to a "string of beads" appearance, microaneurysms, and vessel occlusions **(Figs. 2E and F)**. Apart from secondary vasculitis, intracranial atherosclerotic disease and RCVS can also mimic the angiographic findings of CNS vasculitis **(Box 2)**.[37] Some of these conditions can be differentiated from PACNS by proper clinical history and investigations. Cerebral vessels <500 μm cannot be appreciated in the CA.[26] High-resolution MR vessel wall imaging (HRVWI) is a promising tool to differentiate various vasculopathies such as intracranial atherosclerosis, RCVS, and MMD from CNS vasculitis.[38] In PACNS, concentric thickening of vessel wall accompanied by concentric enhancement is the classical feature **(Figs. 2G and H)**.[39]

Meningo-cortical biopsy is the gold standard investigation for the diagnosis of PACNS. The histopathological findings in PACNS are classified into granulomatous, necrotizing, lymphocytic, and mixed patterns. Targeted biopsy from radiologically abnormal area is preferred to blind biopsy from nondominant temporal or frontal pole due to low yield from blind biopsy. Biopsy can also be negative due to patchy inflammatory process. Predominant large-vessel vasculitis can also be missed in biopsy as large vessels are not included in the biopsy.[40,41]

Calabrese and Malek diagnostic criteria **(Table 1)** is usually followed in PACNS; however, Birnbaum and Hellmann proposed a definite and probable subcategorization according to the evidence of vasculitis from histopathology and angiogram, respectively.[42,43]

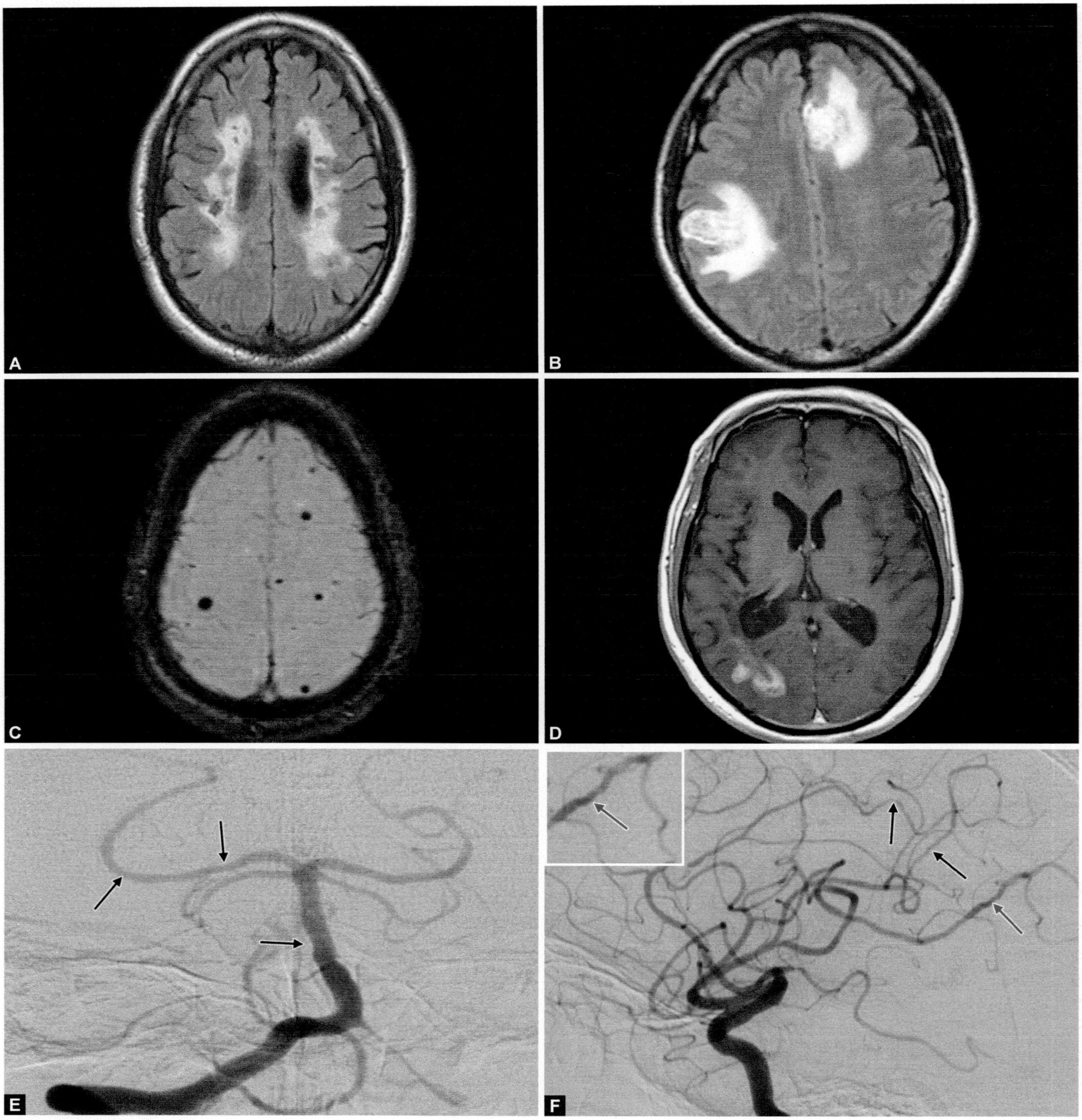

FIGS. 2A TO H: *Continued*

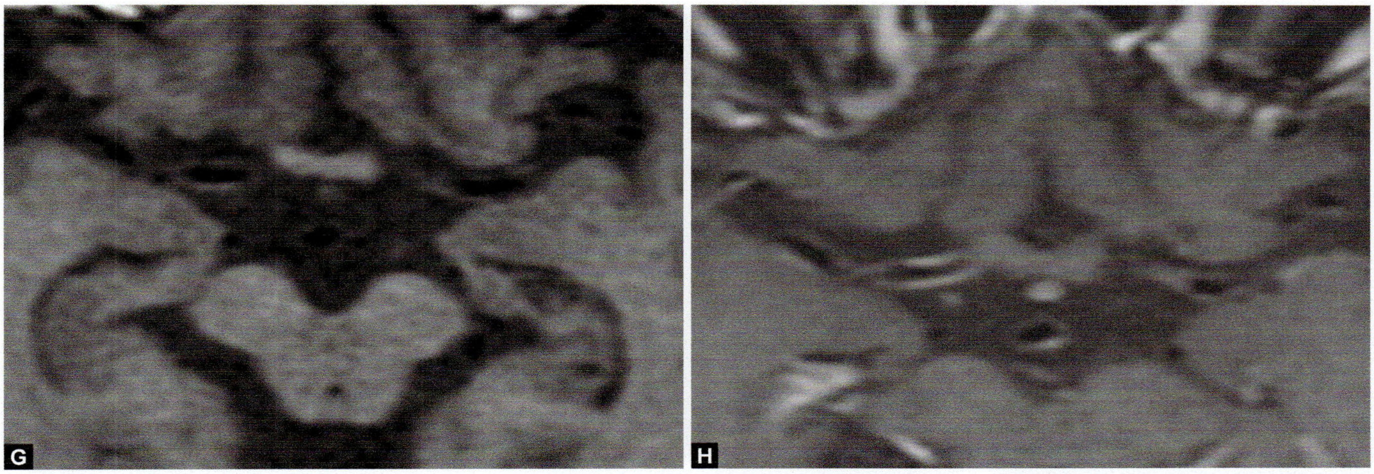

FIGS. 2A TO H: Neuroimaging features in patients with primary angiitis of central nervous system. Fluid attenuation inversion recovery images shows (A) Grade 3 Fazekas small-vessel ischemic changes and (B) tumor-like mass lesions; (C) Susceptibility-weighted image shows multiple microbleeds; (D) T1W image shows postcontrast parenchymal enhancement; (E and F) Conventional angiogram shows stenosis (black arrows) and string of bead appearance (blue arrows) of multiple arteries; (G) High-resolution MR vessel wall T1W sequences showing concentric thickening; (H) Concentric vessel wall enhancement of right middle cerebral artery and basilar artery after gadolinium injection.
(MR: magnetic resonance; T1W: T1-weighted)

BOX 2 Angiographic mimics of vasculitis.

- Reversible cerebral vasoconstriction syndrome
- Radiation-induced vasculopathy
- Fibromuscular dysplasia
- Intracranial atherosclerotic disease
- Drug-induced vasoconstriction (cocaine, ephedrine, and amphetamines)
- Intravascular lymphoma
- Marfan's syndrome
- Ehlers–Danlos syndromes

Management

Induction therapy with glucocorticoids and cyclophosphamide followed by maintenance therapy with azathioprine, mycophenolate mofetil (MMF), or methotrexate is the current practice.[44,45] In refractory cases, rituximab, an anti-CD20 monoclonal antibody, and tumor necrosis factor (TNF)-α inhibitors (infliximab and etanercept) can be tried.[45,46]

Secondary Central Nervous System Vasculitis

Cerebral vasculature can get involved in systemic inflammatory disorders and infections during their natural course and in them the diagnosis is easier as the neurological illness is presumed to be due the same condition.[22] Sometimes, CNS involvement may be the first sign or only manifestation of a systemic disorder, making the diagnosis challenging.[47]

TABLE 1: Diagnostic criteria for PACNS.

Calabrese and Mallek criteria	
1	Clinical history and findings suggestive of an acquired neurological deficit, which remains unexplained after an appropriate initial evaluation comprising blood counts, blood biochemistry, CSF analysis, neuroimaging, and serological tests
2	Evidence of vasculitis in the central nervous system by angiogram or biopsy
3	No evidence of systemic vasculitis or any other condition to which the angiography or histopathology is attributed
All the three criteria should be satisfied for the diagnosis of PACNS	
Birnbaum and Hellmann criteria	
Definite diagnosis	Confirmation of vasculitis in brain tissue biopsy specimen
Probable diagnosis	In the absence of tissue confirmation, if there are high-probability findings of vasculitis on an angiogram with abnormal findings on MRI and a CSF profile consistent with PACNS

(CSF: cerebrospinal fluid; MRI: magnetic resonance imaging; PACNS: primary angiitis of central nervous system)

Infections due to varicella zoster virus **(Figs. 3A to D)**, *Mycobacterium tuberculosis, Treponema pallidum, Borrelia burgdorferi*, and various fungal organisms cause CNS vasculitis **(Box 3)**.[48] Primary systemic vasculitis is classified into large-, medium-, and small-vessel vasculitides **(Table 2)** based on the size of the involved vessel.[49] Among the systemic vasculitides, Behcet's disease, polyarteritis nodosa (PAN), microscopic polyangiitis, Wegener's

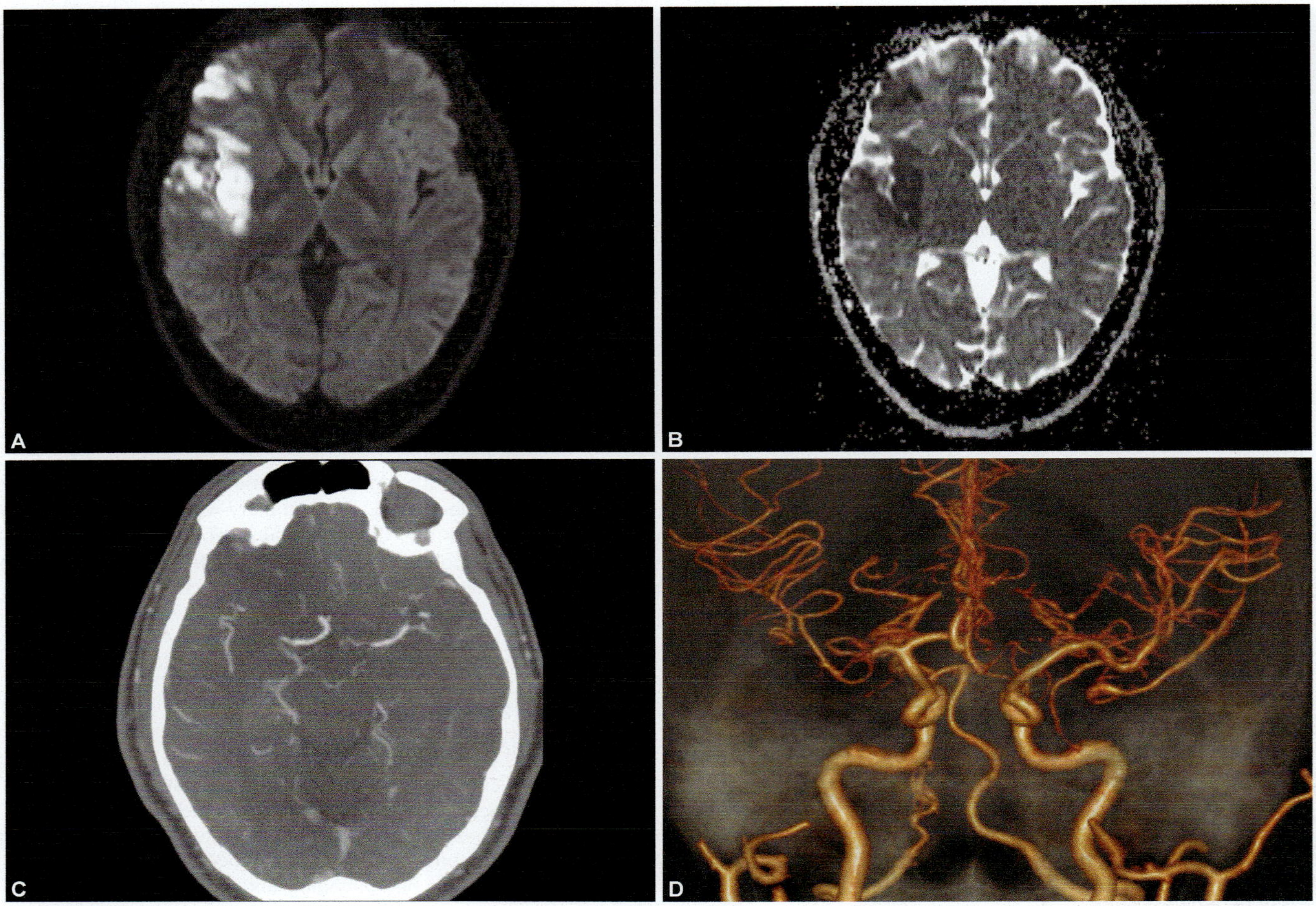

FIGS. 3A TO D: Neuroimaging in varicella zoster associated vasculitis. A 31-year-old male had one episode of transient left-sided weakness followed by acute-onset left hemiplegia 3 weeks later. He had varicella zoster infection 1 month prior to the neurological illness. (C and D) MR imaging showed acute infarct in the right MCA territory (A and B) with CT angiogram showing right right MCA occlusion (C and D).
(CT: computed tomography; MCA: middle cerebral artery; MR: magnetic resonance)

granulomatosis, and Churg–Strauss syndrome can cause CNS vasculitis. Connective tissue disorders such as systemic lupus erythematosus **(Figs. 4A to D)**, Sjögren's syndrome, rheumatoid arthritis, mixed connective tissue disorders, and dermatomyositis can also cause CNS vasculitis. Vasculitis can also occur with lymphoproliferative disorders such as Hodgkin's and non-Hodgkin's lymphoma. These disorders can arise within or outside CNS.[22]

Magnetic resonance imaging findings are nonspecific and reveal multiple infarcts, small-vessel ischemic changes, hemorrhage, microbleeds, and parenchymal and leptomeningeal enhancements. They can reveal basilar exudates (tuberculosis), sinus involvement (fungal infection), skull base lesions (bacterial or fungal infection), and space-occupying lesions (lymphoma), which can give clue regarding the underlying cause.[47] The presence of vasculitis is usually established by luminal imaging techniques; however, biopsy may be required if angiography is negative. **Table 3** shows the detailed investigations to be performed in suspected cases of CNS vasculitis. Once the diagnosis is established, the treatment of secondary CNS vasculitis is directed at the underlying cause.[22]

BOX 3 Infectious causes of CNS vasculitis.

- *Bacteria*: *Staphylococcus aureus, Streptococcus pneumonia, Streptococcus viridans, Haemophilus influenza, Neisseria meningitides, Pseudomonas aeruginosa, Mycobacterium tuberculosis, Treponema pallidum, Brucella, Borrelia, Listeria monocytogenes, Nocardia*
- *Virus*: Herpes simplex virus, varicella zoster virus, Epstein–Barr virus, cytomegalovirus, influenza, HIV
- *Fungi*: *Aspergillus*, Mucormycosis, *Cryptococcus neoformans, Histoplasma capsulatum, Coccidioides immitis*
- *Parasites*: *Toxoplasma gondii, Plasmodium* species, *Acanthamoeba*

(CNS: central nervous system; HIV: human immunodeficiency virus)

TABLE 2: Chapel Hill Consensus Conference (CHCC): The primary systemic vasculitides

Type of vasculitis	Condition
Large-vessel vasculitis	• Giant cell arteritis • Takayasu arteritis
Medium-vessel vasculitis	• Polyarteritis nodosa • Kawasaki disease
Small-vessel vasculitis	• Systemic lupus erythematosus • Rheumatoid arthritis • Cryoglobulinemia • Henoch–Schönlein purpura • Churg–Strauss syndrome • Wegener's granulomatosis • Microscopic polyangiitis

Takayasu Arteritis

Takayasu arteritis is a rare form of large-vessel vasculitis observed most frequently in young females of Asian descent. The prevalence of this disorder is estimated to be 1–2 per million, and the incidence rate is 1.1 per million person-years.[50,51]

Pathophysiology

The inflammatory process preferentially affects the aorta and its large branches. The exact mechanism behind the immune-mediated phenomenon in TA is unclear and as in any immune-mediated disorders, a pathogen-driven inflammatory cascade in genetically predisposed individuals

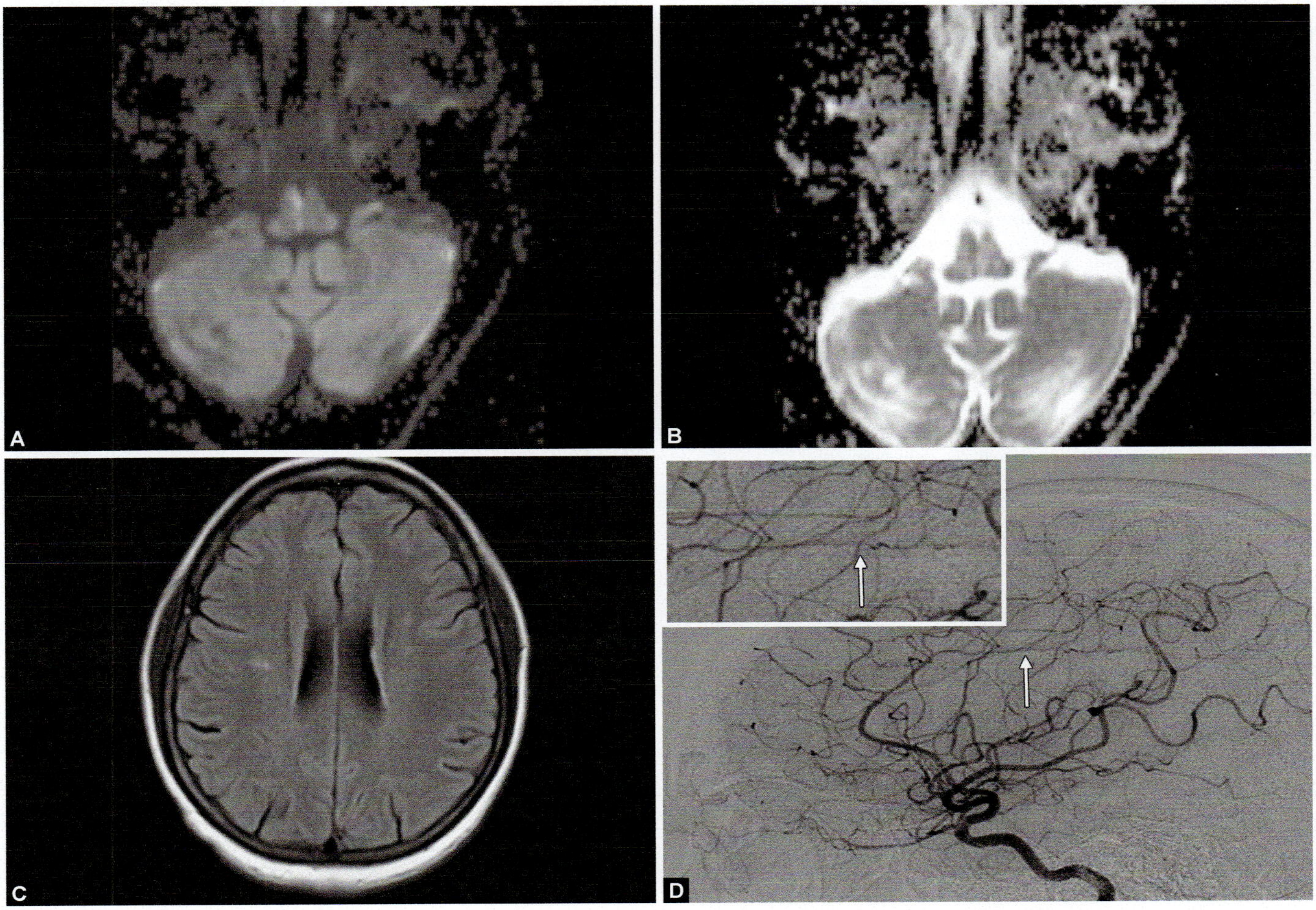

FIGS. 4A TO D: Neuroimaging in CNS vasculitis due to systemic lupus erythematosus. (A and B) MR image of a 39-year-old female patient with systemic lupus erythematosus shows acute infarct in the right medial pontomedullary junction; (C) A small hyperintensity in the right corona radiata in fluid attenuation inversion recovery image; (D) Conventional cerebral angiogram lateral view of internal carotid artery injection demonstrating significant long-segment narrowing of pericallosal segment of anterior cerebral artery with nonvisualization of cortical branches arising from the corresponding segment.

(CNS: central nervous system; MR: magnetic resonance)

TABLE 3: Investigations in suspected CNS vasculitis.

Parameters	Investigations
Routine hemogram	Hemoglobin, total and differential leukocyte count, platelet counts, peripheral smear
Acute phase reactants	Erythrocyte sedimentation rate, C-reactive protein
Metabolic parameters	Renal function test, liver function tests, blood sugars, serum ammonia and lactate levels, urine routine
Electrolytes	Serum sodium, potassium, calcium, and magnesium levels
Endocrine	Thyroid function tests, serum cortisol
Serological testing	Varicella zoster virus, *Treponema pallidum* hemagglutination, hepatitis B and C, HIV, Lyme disease
Immunological tests	Antinuclear antibody, anti-double-stranded DNA, anti-Smith (Sm) antibodies, antineutrophil cytoplasmic antibodies (PR3 and MPO), antihistone antibodies, antibodies to Ro (SSA) and La (SSB), cryoglobulins, rheumatoid factor, antithyroid antibodies
CSF analysis	Protein, cell count, glucose, Gram-stain, ZN, fungal stain, Indian ink stain, PCR for virus, bacteria and *Mycobacterium tuberculosis*, cultures, flow cytometry
Imaging	MRI brain with gadolinium contrast, CT chest, abdomen, and pelvis

(CNS: central nervous system; CSF: cerebrospinal fluid; CT: computed tomography; DNA: deoxyribonucleic acid; HIV: human immunodeficiency virus; MPO: myeloperoxidase; MRI: magnetic resonance imaging; PCR: polymerase chain reaction; PR3: proteinase 3; SSA: Sjögren's-syndrome-related antigen A; SSB: Sjögren's-syndrome-related antigen B; ZN: Ziehl–Neelsen)

is hypothesized. HLAB*52 has been strongly associated with this entity. Vessel walls are infiltrated by T lymphocytes and macrophages, which can elicit a granulomatous inflammation in the early stages of active disease. The chronic stage is marked by adventitial fibrosis and intimal smooth muscle proliferation, leading to stenosis of the affected vessels.[52]

Clinical Features

The clinical features are nonspecific in the early stages wherein constitutional symptoms such as myalgia, arthralgia, weight loss, and anorexia predominate. Once the stenosis occurs, ischemic symptoms and signs start appearing depending on the vessel involved. This includes claudication pain, discrepancy in the pulse volume and blood pressure in the limbs, arterial bruit, amaurosis fugax, TIA, and stroke. Visual loss is a dreadful complication of TA, which occurs due to central retinal hypoperfusion secondary to carotid artery occlusion. Other complications include aortic regurgitation secondary to aortic root dilatation, coronary vessel stenosis, pulmonary artery hypertension,

TABLE 4: Diagnostic criteria for Takayasu arteritis by the American College of Rheumatology.

Criteria	Definition
Age at disease onset <40 years	Onset of symptoms or signs related to Takayasu arteritis ≤40 years of age
Claudication of extremities	Development and worsening of fatigue and discomfort in muscles of one or more extremities while in use, especially the upper extremities
Decreased brachial artery pulse	Decreased pulsation of one or both brachial arteries
Blood pressure (BP) difference >10 mm Hg	Difference of >10 mm Hg in systolic BP between arms
Bruit over subclavian arteries or aorta	Bruit audible on auscultation over one or both subclavian arteries or abdominal aorta
Angiographic abnormality	Narrowing or occlusion of the entire aorta, its primary branches, or large arteries in the proximal upper or lower extremities. These findings should not be recorded due to atherosclerosis, fibromuscular dysplasia, or similar causes. The changes observed are usually focal or segmental

and renovascular hypertension.[50,53] Supradiaphragmatic vessels are mainly involved in females, whereas abdominal aorta and its branches are typically involved in males. Dermatological manifestations include erythema nodosum, erythema induratum, pyoderma gangrenosum, and ulcerative skin lesions.[50]

Imaging and Other Investigations

Investigations reveal elevated acute phase reactants along with thrombocytosis, leukocytosis, and anemia. CA of aorta and its branches is considered as gold standard investigation; however, since it is an invasive procedure with lack of vessel wall information, MRA and CTA are preferred. Both are noninvasive and can give information on the vessel wall pathology and the lumen. High-resolution US imaging can also be used to detect the active inflammation of TA; however, only carotid, subclavian, and axillary arteries are accessible for meaningful interpretation.[50,54]

Management

Once the diagnosis of TA is confirmed **(Table 4)**, the treatment with glucocorticoids (oral prednisolone at 1 mg/kg/day) for 3–6 months followed by low-dose maintenance therapy after achieving remission is carried out.[55] Azathioprine, MMF, methotrexate, leflunomide, and cyclophosphamide can also be used for maintenance therapy. If refractory biological agents like TNF-α inhibitors can be added to the treatment regimen. Other agents that can be considered are rituximab, tocilizumab, and abatacept.[56,57] Antiplatelet therapy is indicated in carotid or vertebrobasilar involvement. In chronic stages of TA, endovascular procedures such as angioplasty and stenting for short-segment stenosis or surgical bypass for long-segment involvement are required.[50] Acute phase reactants and noninvasive imaging techniques can be utilized for assessing the treatment response.[57]

FIBROMUSCULAR DYSPLASIA

Fibromuscular dysplasia is a rare idiopathic nonatheromatous and noninflammatory disease of the arterial walls predominantly affecting the renal and carotid arteries.[58] The prevalence of renal FMD is 4 per 1,000 persons and that of cerebrovascular FMD is probably half.[59] This condition is more commonly seen in young adults and females.[60] The mean age of diagnosis of cervical FMD is around 50 years.

Pathophysiology

The exact etiology of FMD is unknown; genetic, mechanical, environmental (tobacco smoking), and hormonal factors (estrogen) are attributed. About 10% of FMD is familial.[58,60] FMD results from proliferation of smooth muscle cells and fibrosis, which can cause stenosis and aneurysm of the affected arteries, leading to various clinical manifestations.[59] Aorta, subclavian, brachial, iliac, popliteal, tibial, splanchnic, hepatic, and coronary arteries can also get involved.[61] Carotid arteries and VAs are affected in cerebrovascular FMD and can be asymptomatic. Extracranial carotid is more frequently involved, especially in the mid and distal portions at the level of C1 and C2 vertebrae. The affection can be bilateral. The usual site of VA involvement is V3 and V4 segments, which can also be seen along with carotid artery FMD. Intracranial arteries are rarely affected.[58,60]

Clinical Features

The most common symptoms reported were headache, dizziness, and tinnitus, which are nonspecific. The headache is often similar to migraine, and the tinnitus may be pulsatile or nonpulsatile.[58] Dissection of the extracranial or intracranial arteries can occur in FMD, which causes headache, neck pain, Horner's syndrome, and stroke.[60] The critical stenosis or occlusion of the arteries or embolism from proximal arterial thrombi can lead to TIA, amaurosis fugax, or stroke. Other manifestations include vertigo and syncope. Aneurysm rupture can cause intracerebral hemorrhage or SAH. Examination may reveal cervical bruit.[61] In suspected case of craniocervical FMD, renal artery involvement should be screened and when present can aid in the diagnosis. Intervention for renal artery stenosis needs to be contemplated if critical stenosis is present. Renovascular hypertension is the most common presentation of renal FMD, and US may reveal atrophic kidney.[59] Renal artery dissection can cause renal ischemia and symptoms include flank pain, hematuria, and accelerated hypertension.[60]

Imaging

Arterial doppler can detect the carotid artery involvement at the cervical region; however, the preferred noninvasive diagnostic modalities for FMD are MRA and CTA as they can delineate the intracranial vessels, aneurysms, and dissection.[59] Angiographic pattern is classified into two types—multifocal and focal.[58] Multifocal type is characterized by the classical "string of beads" appearance due to multiple stenosis alternating with dilatation of the involved vessel, which is often associated with medial type of FMD **(Figs. 5A to D)**. Other abnormalities that can be seen include focal stenosis and aneurysms.[60] Focal type can be unifocal (<1 cm) or tubular (>1 cm) stenosis on angiography and is seen typically in intimal FMD and rarely in adventitial type. The close differential diagnosis includes atherosclerotic arterial disease, vascular EDS, Marfan's syndrome, Loeys–Dietz syndrome, and *ACTA2* gene mutations.[58] The vessel wall abnormalities are mostly seen in the mid or distal segments of the arteries as compared to the proximal segments near to ostium as often seen in atherosclerotic disease.[60]

Management

There are no randomized controlled trials in cerebrovascular FMD, and management relies upon cohort studies and expert opinion.[62] The risk of recurrence is very low and in a mean follow-up of 3 years, only 2% had new dissection and 0.7% had new stroke and none of them had a new aneurysm. Therefore, only symptomatic cerebrovascular FMD is considered for any intervention, and the decision for revascularization should be individualized.[58] The current guidelines for management of acute ischemic stroke and aneurysm should also be followed in patients with FMD. For secondary prevention of ischemic stroke, aspirin is recommended. Statins are only indicated if there is concomitant atherosclerotic process. In asymptomatic FMD, low-dose aspirin (75–100 mg/day) can be advised, but bleeding from unruptured aneurysm is a concern.[62] Endovascular therapy such as carotid angioplasty with or without stenting is recommended in patients with recurrent events despite optimal medical management.[58,62] The neurological manifestations, the type and extent of lesions, patient preferences, and experience of each center are the factors to be taken into consideration for any treatment decisions.[59] On initial diagnosis of FMD, head-to-toe angiography should be performed for assessing the extent of vascular involvement, and surveillance is usually by arterial doppler for carotid FMD. The patient should be encouraged to stop smoking and avoid chiropractic spinal manipulation and activities causing extreme neck movements as in contact sports.[58]

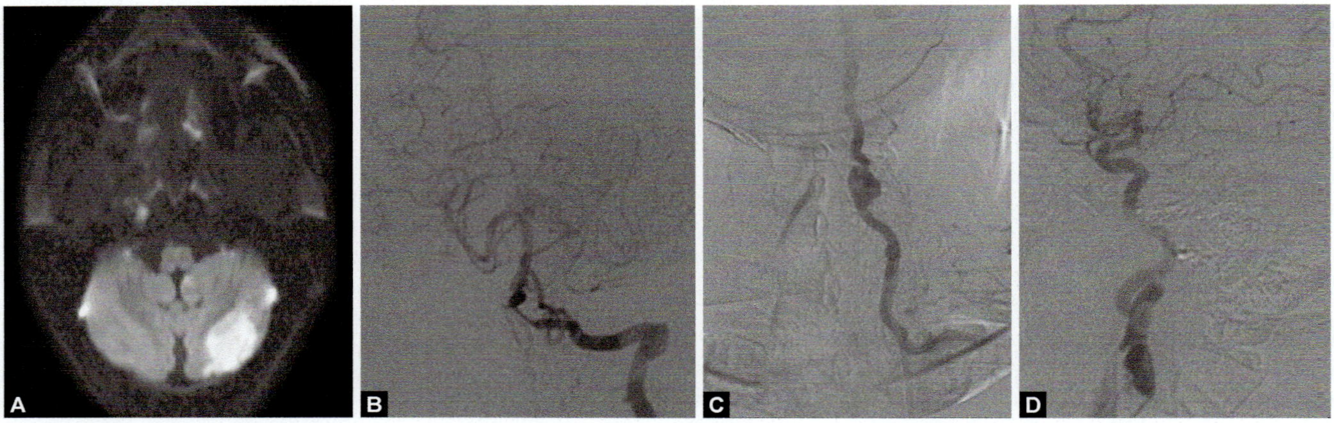

FIGS. 5A TO D: Neuroimaging in fibromuscular dysplasia. A 26-year-old male presented with acute-onset headache, vomiting, and dysarthria and his MR brain image (A) showed acute infarct in the left cerebellum; Conventional CA with left vertebral artery injection showed (B) V3 and V4 aneurysms and beading and (C) V1 aneurysm and beading, and left ICA injection (D) showed left cervical ICA aneurysm and beading.
(CA: cerebral angiography; ICA: internal carotid artery; MR: magnetic resonance)

CAROTID WEB

Carotid webs have been recently identified to be an important cause among patients with cryptogenic ischemic stroke.[63] This condition is often overlooked in the evaluation of stroke, and lack of awareness in the medical community is largely attributed.[64] This rare entity has to be suspected in any patient presenting with embolic stroke of undetermined source (ESUS). In a single-center study of 466 patients with anterior circulation stroke referred for mechanical thrombectomy, the prevalence of ipsilateral CaW was 1.9%, 12.5 times more common in patients with ESUS than in other causes of ischemic stroke.[65] The population prevalence of CaW is unknown, but in case control studies the prevalence ranged from 9% to 37% in cryptogenic stroke and two-thirds were females.[63,64,66] The median age of the pathologically confirmed cases was 40.5 years.[67]

Pathophysiology

Pathological studies have shown that CaW is an intimal type of FMD, fibrosis affecting the innermost layer of the arterial wall. It has a shelf-like (web-like/ridge-like) endoluminal protrusion due to focal fibrous dysplasia situated at the origin of internal carotid artery (ICA) in the carotid bulb.[67] This shelf-like lesion causes a local hemodynamic disturbance as it creates a pocket wherein it acts as a nidus for local thrombosis. Once formed, thrombus can fragment and embolize, leading to stroke.[66]

Imaging

In order to diagnose the CaW accurately, luminal and vessel wall imaging is required. US can give an idea about the vessel wall, lumen, and blood flow, but the sensitivity in detecting the CaW is poor. The CaW appears as a shelf-like outgrowth or as a protrusion into the lumen and is hyperechoic. However, this finding can often get misinterpreted as atherosclerotic plaque. Overestimation of the degree of stenosis is another drawback in US. CTA is the preferred investigation for CaW as it has much better spatial resolution, and the multiplanar reconstruction in axial, sagittal, and coronal projections allow the detection of CaW efficiently. The superimposed thrombus can also be identified in CTA. The lesion composition and flow dynamics cannot be assessed using this technique. The CA, although invasive, has high spatial and temporal resolution and is the confirmatory investigation (gold standard).[68] The three-dimensional (3D) rotational angiography can create a multiplanar reconstruction, which is needed to detect CaW as the standard posteroanterior or lateral projection may miss the posteriorly located CaW. The dynamic assessment can also reveal the stagnation of contrast in the area (pocket) just above the web and is able to detect the superimposed thrombus.[66] The interpretation of CaW in digital subtraction angiography (DSA) and CTA is comparable and much better than US.[69] The close differentials based on the imaging are atherosclerotic plaque and dissection. The presence of vascular risk factors and older age of stroke are historical clues toward the possibility of atherosclerotic cause. The surface of atherosclerotic plaque is irregular as compared to the smooth contour of the web. The most common sites of atherosclerotic plaque are distal part of common carotid and distal portions of the carotid bulb as opposed to the carotid bulb for CaW. The presence of vessel wall thickening and calcification is the other pointer for atherosclerotic plaque.[66] CaW can be mistaken for a dissection flap in the CTA/MRA; however, the presence of dilation of arterial wall due to false lumen and history of neck pain can favor dissection.[66,69]

Management

There are no randomized controlled trials for forming guidelines for the treatment of symptomatic CaW. Antiplatelets, anticoagulants, surgical resection, and carotid stenting are the various treatment options.[67,70] Secondary prevention of stroke by antiplatelet therapy in symptomatic

CaW might be insufficient in further prevention of stroke as there were recurrences with single and dual antiplatelet therapies. Since thrombosis and clot fragmentation are the pathological basis for the stroke in CaW, anticoagulation has been proposed as an alternative treatment option; however, lifelong therapy with anticoagulation poses risk for hemorrhagic complications.[66] A recent study had demonstrated that one in six symptomatic patients with CaW had recurrent stroke despite receiving antiplatelet agents or anticoagulants. Hence, in selected patients with recurrence, carotid endarterectomy or stenting may be considered.[71]

MOYAMOYA DISEASE AND SYNDROMES

Moyamoya disease is a neurovascular syndrome characterized by progressive stenosis and obliteration of intracranial ICA and its proximal branches with reduction in blood flow in the major vessels of anterior circulation with compensatory collateral development.[72,73] While most of our understanding about the disease is from Japan and other East Asian countries, now the disease, albeit in low numbers, is being reported from all across the world.[74] The highest number of cases are reported from East Asia, with incidence ranging from 0.94–2.3/100,000 population in Japan and South Korea to <0.09/100,000 in North America. 10–15% of patients can have a family history, more so in Asian ancestry, implicating a possible genetic link. The condition shows a bimodal age of distribution with early peak around 5 years of age and second peak in the third decade, with presentation differing between pediatric and adult-onset MMD. While ischemic presentation is more often reported in pediatric age group, both ischemic and hemorrhagic presentations are reported in adult-onset MMD.[73,74]

TABLE 5: Associations with moyamoya vasculopathy.

Conditions	Prevalence
Idiopathic moyamoya disease	80–90%
Less common moyamoya syndromes: • Down syndrome • Neurofibromatosis type 1 • Sickle cell disease • Other hemoglobinopathies • Cranial irradiation	10–20%
Very rare associations: • Congenital cyanotic heart disease—tetralogy of Fallot/Ebstein's anomaly • Hereditary spherocytosis • Renal artery stenosis • Giant hemangiomas • Hyperthyroidism	<1%—case reports/series only

TABLE 6: Clinical presentation and their frequencies in pediatric and adult MMD.

Clinical presentation	Pediatric	Adults
Common:		
• Ischemic stroke	68–87%	50–98%
• TIAs	50–65%	50%
• Hemorrhage	2.8%	20–42%
• Headaches	20–63%	22–41%
Less common:		
• Seizures	5%	
• Chorea/involuntary movements	<4%	
• Cognitive/psychiatric presentation		

(MMD: moyamoya disease; TIAs: transient ischemic attacks)

Pathophysiology

In 80–90% of patients, no underlying cause is identified where it is referred to as MMD. Around 10–20% of patients can have the condition secondary to or in association with other syndromes/conditions, which is given in **Table 5**, and is often referred to as moyamoya syndrome.[73] The high prevalence in East Asian population of this rare syndrome points to a plausible genetic link, which has been proved with genome-wide association studies (GWAS). A whole GWAS identified a novel susceptibility gene, ring finger protein 213 (*RNF213*) in a cohort of MMD, which was subsequently confirmed in eight MMD families as well.[75,76] A low-frequency variation of *RNF213* (c.14576G>A, p.R4810K) has been reported to significantly increase the risk of MMD in East Asian populations, suggesting a possible founder effect, as this mutation has not been reported from studies on Caucasian population. While MMD patients with homozygous *RNF213* p.R4810K mutation showed more severe disease, onset before 5 years of age, and more cognitive deficits at onset, long-term surgical outcome was not inferior to those without mutation in Japanese, Korean, and Chinese cohorts.[77,78]

Clinical Features

The clinical presentations in this condition are given in **Table 6**. Ischemic symptoms are the most common across all age groups, and transient cerebral hypoperfusion can be precipitated by crying, playing wind instruments like flute, and after exertion in children. Anterior circulation symptoms are more common than posterior circulation, and patients can present with weakness, aphasia, sensory symptoms, or seizures. Seizures as a presentation are more reported in pediatric age group. Recurrent ischemic events can lead to global developmental delay or regression as well.[79,80] Headache is another common presentation in MMD and can remain even after successful revascularization, though 80% reports complete benefit in 1 year after surgery. Hemorrhagic presentation of MMD is more often reported in adult-onset MMD in Asian population, and bleeding can occur in anterior circulation-dependent territories. Fundus finding of "morning glory disk," an enlargement of the optic disk, with concomitant retinovascular anomalies in a stroke patient should alert the physician to investigate for MMD.[81]

Imaging

Though CA is the gold standard for diagnosis of MMD and differentiates it from other stroke syndromes, noninvasive investigations such as MRI with angiogram and vessel wall imaging are also being widely used for diagnosis of this rare entity. Parenchymal imaging may show infarcts of different ages, predominantly in the anterior circulation **(Figs. 6A to F)**. The infarct topography may not be corresponding to classical vascular territories because of the altered vascular supply secondary to long-standing major vessel occlusion and subsequent collateral development. Infarct patterns reported in MR-based studies are more often atypical (gyral 44%, atypical territorial 13%, and honeycomb 11%) in MMD. Watershed and gyral patterns of infarcts are more often seen in children, whereas a honeycomb pattern is more common in adult patients with advanced vascular stages. Although posterior circulation stroke has been considered uncommon, recent reports suggest that angiographically posterior cerebral artery (PCA) may be involved in around 29% of patients, with 17% developing strokes as well.[82] Other nonspecific signs such as "ivy sign," on fluid-attenuated inversion recovery (FLAIR) sequence, diffuse leptomeningeal enhancement in contrast-enhanced MRI, and "brush sign," increased visibility of deep medullary veins seen best on susceptibility-weighted MR, are also reported. MRA will show narrowing of supraclinoid ICA extending to anterior cerebral artery (ACA) and middle cerebral artery (MCA) with/without basal collaterals, which often needs CA for confirmation. Approximately 30% of adult MMD patients present with parenchymal hemorrhage secondary to rupture of friable collaterals/microaneurysms. The common locations of hemorrhage in MMD are intraventricular (37.6%) followed by lobar (23.7%) and putaminal (22.6%).[83] Susceptibility-weighted MRI may identify cerebral microbleeds (CMBs) in 28–46% of MMD patients. CMBs often occur in deep and periventricular areas and are associated with dilated anterior choroidal or posterior communicating arteries and have an association with future risk for IVH.[84]

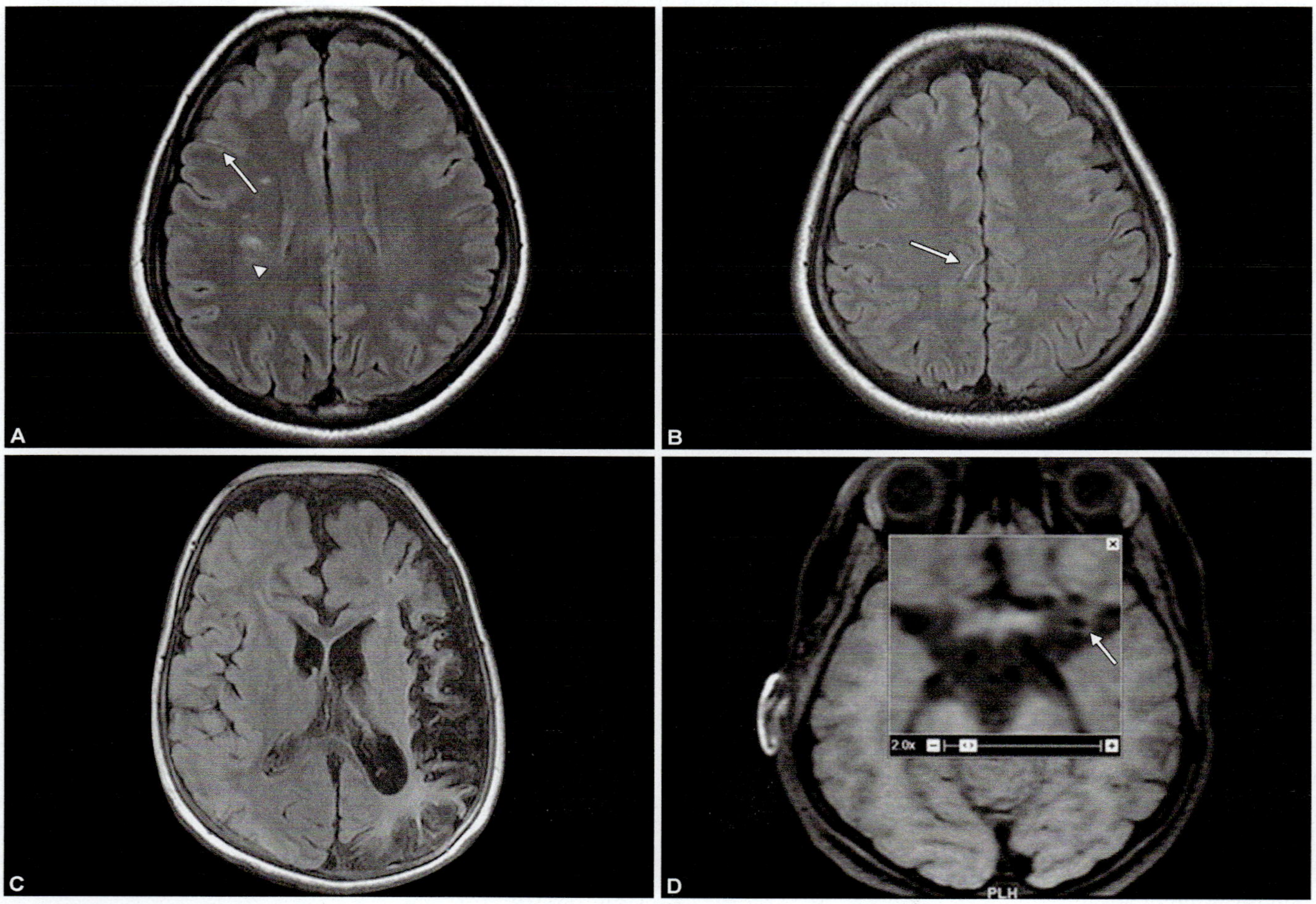

FIGS. 6A TO F: *Continued*

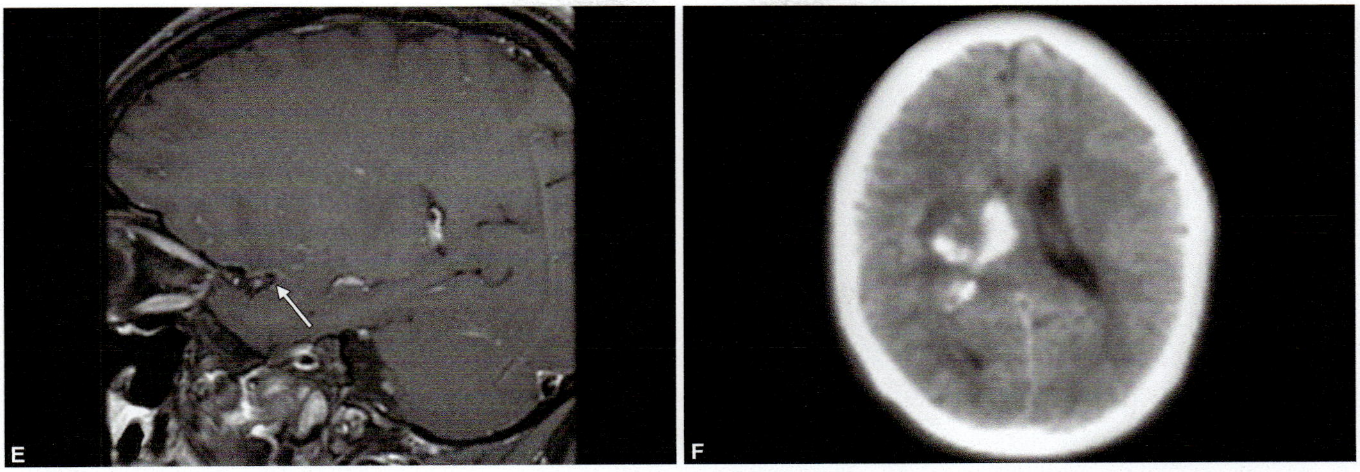

FIGS. 6A TO F: Brain parenchymal imaging in MMD. MRI and CT images of patients with MMD. (A and B) FLAIR images with small subcortical chronic infarcts (arrow head) and ivy sign (arrow) in the sulcus representing collaterals (arrow); (C) MRI FLAIR of a patient with bihemispheric strokes—chronic infarct in the left MCA and PCA territories and acute infarct right MCA territory; vessel wall imaging-T1 axial fat suppressed sequences (D) shows left intracranial ICA wall thickening (arrow) with (E) faint uniform contrast enhancement of MCA-M1(arrow); (F) CT plain images of a patient with no vascular risk factors presenting with right corona radiata hemorrhage extending to ventricle whose angiogram showed MMD Suzuki grade III on the right side and IV on the left side.

(CT: computed tomography; FLAIR: fluid-attenuated inversion recovery; ICA: internal carotid artery; MCA: middle cerebral artery; MMD: moyamoya disease; MRI: magnetic resonance imaging; PCA: posterior cerebral artery)

High-resolution MR vessel wall imaging is emerging as a useful tool for supporting diagnosis of MMD in the early stages and differentiating it from other intracranial vasculopathies, especially where angiographic abnormalities may be subtle or unilateral. Outer diameter narrowing of the affected intracranial vessels as demonstrated by 3D constructive interference in steady state (CISS) imaging called negative remodeling is reported as an early characteristic change of MMD.[85,86] Besides outer diameter narrowing, concentric enhancement of symptomatic segments also has been reported, which has been associated with future recurrent events as well.[87,88] The definitive diagnosis is based on CA showing stenosis of the distal intracranial ICA, extending to the proximal ACA and MCA. Disease severity is classified using Suzuki's grading system into five grades depending on the severity of stenosis and extent of collateralization **(Figs. 7A to F)**. When performing angiogram, injection of external carotid arteries (ECAs) is essential to identify any preexisting collateral vessels before planning for surgical bypass procedures. Aneurysms and rare arteriovenous malformation are often found in MMD with hemorrhagic presentation, which needs angiogram for confirmation.[79] The diagnostic criteria for definitive MMD is given in **Box 4**. As per the recent guidelines, MRA findings of stenosis and abnormal vascular networks are enough for a definitive diagnosis of MMD. Quasi-MMD or moyamoya syndrome is a vasculopathy similar to MMD, which is secondary to an underlying cause. The cause may differ in adult and pediatric age groups, with atherosclerosis and thyroid disorders more often reported in adults.[89]

Management

There are only very few natural history studies on MMD, which shows that the condition is progressive. Asymptomatic MMD not treated surgically has an annual incidence of cerebrovascular events, including TIA, of 2.4–5.7%, while symptomatic subjects have reported a progression rate of 20% over 6 years.[90] Though none of the medications have been proven to be beneficial in preventing the progression of stenosis or reversing the occlusion and improving perfusion, antithrombotics are given in patients presenting with ischemic symptoms with some studies showing a favorable functional status.[91] But there is lack of evidence in favor of preventing recurrent ischemic events and an added hemorrhagic risk, especially in adult MMD, with long-term use of antiplatelets. Seizures and headache can be managed symptomatically, with some surgical series reporting relief of headache in majority of subjects after a successful revascularization procedure. Surgical revascularization is recommended for all patients with MMD with impaired hemodynamics with an aim to improve cerebral perfusion. Even in patients with asymptomatic disease or those with stable hemodynamics, annual stroke risk is not negligible, ranging from 3.2 to 4.5%, with female gender, hypertension, and posterior circulation involvement increasing the ischemic stroke risk. Pediatric patients are more likely to have a progressive course and revascularization should be pursued in them carefully, considering the perioperative risk and surgical expertise of the center.

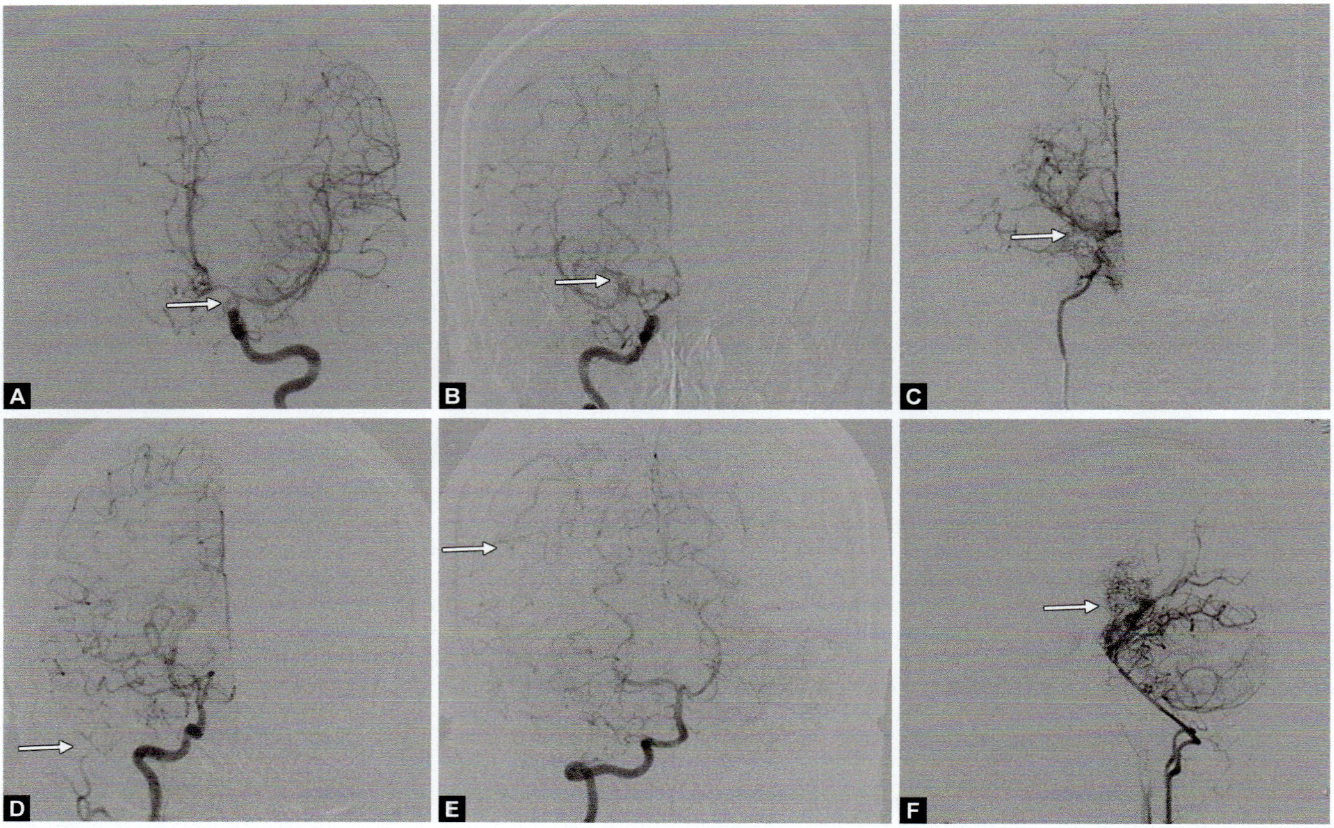

FIGS. 7A TO F: Suzuki grading system of angiographic findings in moyamoya disease (by Suzuki and Takaku). (A) Grade I-left ICA injection showing narrowing of ICA apex, indicated by arrow. (B) Right ICA AP view showing narrowing of terminal ICA and MCA and ACA with initiation of moyamoya collaterals depicted by arrow. (C) Grade III-Right ICA AP view showing intensification of basal collaterals (arrow) with progressive stenosis of ICA and occlusion of ACA. ECA does not show collateralization. (D) Grade IV development of ECA collaterals, ICA occlusion beyond ophthalmic segment, and reduction in moyamoya blush. This is followed by Grade V with intensification of ECA collaterals and finally Grade VI with total occlusion of ICA and its branches with ECA being the sole supply to brain. (E) Right VA injection in a patient with Suzuki Grade III showing VB system supplying right MCA territory (arrow). (F) Right VA lateral view of a patient with Suzuki Grade IV disease showing extensive collaterals (arrow) from both PCA.

(ACA: anterior cerebral artery; AP: anteroposterior; ECA: external carotid artery; ICA: internal carotid artery; MCA: middle cerebral artery; PCA: posterior cerebral artery; VA: vertebral artery; VB: vertebrobasilar)

BOX 4 Diagnostic criteria for moyamoya disease.

The diagnostic criteria for definitive moyamoya disease include all of the following items based on the conventional angiographic findings:

- Stenosis or occlusion of the terminal portion of the intracranial ICA or proximal portions of the ACA and/or the MCA
- Development of abnormal vascular networks near the occlusive or stenotic lesions in the arterial phase
- Bilateral lesion

(ACA: anterior cerebral artery; ICA: internal carotid artery; MCA: middle cerebral artery)

The arteriopathy of moyamoya spares the ECA and its branches, enabling the surgeon to use the vessel for intracranial revascularization. Two general methods of revascularization used are direct and indirect anastomoses. In direct anastomosis, a branch of the ECA (usually the superficial temporal artery) is directly anastomosed to a cortical artery, usually MCA. Indirect anastomoses involve the placement of vascularized tissues supplied by the ECA (e.g., dura, temporalis muscle, or the superficial temporal artery itself termed encephalo-duro-myo-arterio-synangiosis) in direct contact with the brain, leading to new vessel developing and supplying the underlying cerebral cortex. While a direct anastomosis establishes cerebral perfusion immediately, indirect anastomosis takes time for its benefit to establish. However, in children where a direct approach is often difficult due to small caliber of vessels, indirect bypass is preferred in majority of surgical centers. There are recent reports of a combined approach being superior to either of the procedures in achieving good cerebral perfusion, with minimal complications.[92]

Though efficacy of surgery in preventing ischemic events is well established, its utility in hemorrhagic disease is less certain. Though earlier reports showed unsatisfactory results with surgery in hemorrhagic subgroup, recent studies have shown that recurrent hemorrhagic stroke risk falls from 11.5% in the conservative group to 1.6% annually following revascularization procedures. Perioperative complications include ischemic events leading to permanent disability (1.6–16%), hemorrhagic complications (0.6–7%), hyperperfusion syndrome, and local scalp ischemia. Maintaining euvolemia, adequate blood pressure, and hemoglobin level during surgery and early perioperative period can help in preventing ischemic and hemorrhagic complications.

Conservatively managed patients with MMD experienced stroke at a rate ranging between 3.2% and 15.0% annually. Following direct anastomosis, the stroke risk falls to 0–1.6% annually, when patients are followed up for >3 years. Indirect anastomosis in pediatric patients is also effective in reducing stroke risk on long-term follow-up. Recent studies have also shown that hemorrhagic moyamoya also benefits from revascularization by reducing both ischemic and hemorrhagic stroke risks.

Indian Perspective

Earliest report on moyamoya syndrome from India dates back to 1995 from Kolkata where an association with beta thalassemia was found.[93] Subsequently there have been multiple case reports and case series on MMD and moyamoya syndrome from across the country, mostly from East India, suggesting a possible genetic link, which needs to be explored further. Genetic studies on South Indian cohort have shown a homozygous allele of RNF variant to be associated with more severe phenotypes.[94] While there are some reports suggesting that the disease may be less aggressive in Indian patients even without surgery,[95] surgical series from South India have shown good outcome with indirect anastomosis in children.[96]

CONCLUSION

Dissection, CNS vasculitis, MMD, and FMD are important NAVs causing stroke in young individuals and need to be evaluated by various luminal and vessel wall imaging techniques. Advances in noninvasive imaging by MRA and CTA have obviated the need for CA for the diagnosis of most of these conditions. CA is still the preferred investigation in CNS vasculitis and in situations of discordance between noninvasive imaging. MR vessel wall imaging is a recent addition to the vast array of investigations, which has proven to be useful in the diagnosis of intracranial atherosclerotic disease, CNS vasculitis, and MMD.

The treatment depends on the underlying etiology. Antiplatelets are the cornerstone in the management of dissection and FMD, whereas corticosteroids and other immunomodulatory agents are used in CNS vasculitis. Endovascular/surgical treatments are pursued in dissection in patients who present with SAH and if they have recurrent ischemic events despite medical management. MMD is primarily treated by direct or indirect surgical revascularization. Carotid endarterectomy or stenting needs consideration if there is recurrence of stroke while on antiplatelets in patients with CaW.

REFERENCES

1. Radu RA, Terecoasă EO, Băjenaru OA, Tiu C. Etiologic classification of ischemic stroke: where do we stand? Clin Neurol Neurosurg. 2017;159:93-106.
2. Sylaja PN, Pandian JD, Kaul S, Srivastava MVP, Khurana D, Schwamm LH, et al. Ischemic stroke profile, risk factors, and outcomes in India: the Indo-US Collaborative Stroke Project. Stroke. 2018;49(1): 219-22.
3. Camilo O, Goldstein LB. Nonatherosclerotic vascular disease in the young. J Thromb Thrombolysis. 2005;20(2):93-103.
4. Osehobo EM, Nogueira RG, Koneru S, Al-Bayati AR, de Camara CP, Nahab F, et al. Carotid web: an under-recognized and misdiagnosed ischemic stroke etiology. J Neurointerv Surg. 2022;14(2):138-42.
5. Agarwal A, Bathla G, Kanekar S. Imaging of nonatherosclerotic vasculopathies. J Clin Imaging Sci. 2020;10:62.
6. Lee VH, Brown RD Jr, Mandrekar JN, Mokri B. Incidence and outcome of cervical artery dissection: a population-based study. Neurology. 2006;67(10):1809-12.
7. Thanvi B, Munshi SK, Dawson SL, Robinson TG. Carotid and vertebral artery dissection syndromes. Postgrad Med J. 2005;81:383-8.
8. Volker W, Dittrich R, Grewe S, Nassenstein I, Csiba L, Herczeg L, et al. The outer arterial wall layers are primarily affected in spontaneous cervical artery dissection. Neurology. 2011;76:1463-71.
9. Dittrich R, Heidbreder A, Rohsbach D, Schmalhorst J, Nassenstein I, Maintz D, et al. Connective tissue and vascular phenotype in patients with cervical artery dissection. Neurology. 2007;68:2120-4.
10. Engelter ST, Grond-Ginsbach C, Metso TM, Metso AJ, Kloss M, Debette S, et al. Cervical artery dissection: trauma and other potential mechanical trigger events. Neurology. 2013;80:1950-7.
11. Muthusami P, Kesavadas C, Sylaja PN, Thomas B, Harsha KJ, Kapilamoorthy TR. Implicating the long styloid process in cervical carotid artery dissection. Neuroradiology. 2013;55:861-7.
12. Debette S, Leys D. Cervical-artery dissections: predisposing factors, diagnosis, and outcome. Lancet Neurol. 2009;8(7):668-78.
13. Schievink WI. Spontaneous dissection of the carotid and vertebral arteries. N Engl J Med. 2001;344:898-906.
14. Hakimi R, Sivakumar S. Imaging of carotid dissection. Curr Pain Headache Rep. 2019;23(1):2.
15. Vertinsky AT, Schwartz NE, Fischbein NJ, Rosenberg J, Albers GW, Zaharchuk G. Comparison of multidetector CT angiography and MR imaging of cervical artery dissection. Am J Neuroradiol. 2008;29:1753-60.
16. JM Provenzale, B Sarikaya. Comparison of test performance characteristics of MRI, MR angiography, and CT angiography in the diagnosis of carotid and vertebral artery dissection: a review of literature. AJR Am J Roentgenol. 2009;193(4):1167-74.
17. Engelter ST, Dallongeville J, Kloss M, Metso TM, Leys D, Brandt T, et al. Thrombolysis in cervical artery dissection—data from the Cervical Artery Dissection and Ischemic Stroke Patients (CADISP) database. Eur J Neurol. 2012;19:1199-206.

18. Engelter ST, Rutgers MP, Hatz F, Georgiadis D, Fluri F, Sekoranja L, et al. Intravenous thrombolysis in stroke attributable to cervical artery dissection. Stroke 2009;40:3772-6.
19. Markus HS, Levi C, King A, Madigan J, Norris J; Cervical Artery Dissection in Stroke Study (CADISS) investigators. Antiplatelet therapy vs. anticoagulation therapy in cervical artery dissection: the Cervical Artery Dissection in Stroke Study (CADISS) randomized clinical trial final results. JAMA Neurol. 2019;76(6):657-64.
20. Vineetha VS, Sreedharan SE, Sarma S, Sylaja PN. Antiplatelets versus anticoagulants in the treatment of extracranial carotid and vertebral artery dissection. Neurol India. 2019;67:1056-9.
21. Haussen DC, Jadhav A, Jovin T, Grossberg JA, Grigoryan M, Nahab F, et al. Endovascular management versus intravenous thrombolysis for acute stroke secondary to carotid artery dissection: local experience and systematic review. Neurosurgery. 2016;78:709-16.
22. Hajj-Ali RA, Calabrese LH. Central nervous system vasculitis. Curr Opin Rheumatol. 2009;21(1):10-8.
23. Berlit P. Diagnosis and treatment of cerebral vasculitis. Ther Adv Neurol Disord. 2010;3(1):29-42.
24. Godasi R, Pang G, Chauhan S, Bollu PC. Primary Central Nervous System Vasculitis. In: StatPearls [Internet]. Treasure Island (FL): StatPearls Publishing; 2022.
25. Salvarani C, Brown RD Jr, Calamia KT, Christianson TJ, Weigand SD, Miller DV, et al. Primary central nervous system vasculitis: analysis of 101 patients. Ann Neurol. 2007;62(5):442-51.
26. Salvarani C, Brown RD Jr, Hunder GG. Adult primary central nervous system vasculitis. Lancet. 2012;380(9843):767-77.
27. de Boysson H, Parienti JJ, Mawet J, Arquizan C, Boulouis G, Burcin C, et al. Primary angiitis of the CNS and reversible cerebral vasoconstriction syndrome: a comparative study. Neurology. 2018;91(16):e1468-78.
28. Sundaram S, Menon D, Khatri P, Sreedharan SE, Jayadevan ER, Sarma P, et al. Primary angiitis of the central nervous system: clinical profiles and outcomes of 45 patients. Neurol India. 2019;67(1):105-12.
29. Salvarani C, Brown RD Jr, Christianson TJ, Huston J 3rd, Giannini C, Miller DV, et al. Adult primary central nervous system vasculitis treatment and course: analysis of one hundred sixty-three patients. Arthritis Rheumatol. 2015;67(6):1637-45.
30. Salvarani C, Brown RD Jr, Calamia KT, Christianson TJ, Huston J 3rd, Meschia JF, et al. Rapidly progressive primary central nervous system vasculitis. Rheumatology (Oxford). 2011;50(2):349-58.
31. de Boysson H, Zuber M, Naggara O, Neau JP, Gray F, Bousser MG, et al; French Vasculitis Study Group and the French NeuroVascular Society. Primary angiitis of the central nervous system: description of the first fifty-two adults enrolled in the French cohort of patients with primary vasculitis of the central nervous system. Arthritis Rheumatol. 2014;66(5):1315-26.
32. Boulouis G, de Boysson H, Zuber M, Guillevin L, Meary E, Costalat V, et al. Primary angiitis of the central nervous system: magnetic resonance imaging spectrum of parenchymal, meningeal, and vascular lesions at baseline. Stroke. 2017;48(5):1248-55.
33. Fazekas F, Chawluk JB, Alavi A, Hurtig HI, Zimmerman RA. MR signal abnormalities at 1.5 T in Alzheimer's dementia and normal aging. AJR Am J Roentgenol. 1987;149:351-6.
34. Giannini C, Salvarani C, Hunder G, Brown RD. Primary central nervous system vasculitis: pathology and mechanisms. Acta Neuropathol. 2012;123(6):759-72.
35. Pillai SH, Sreedharan SE, Menon G, Kannoth S, Pn S. Primary CNS vasculitis presenting as intraventricular bleeding. Ann Indian Acad Neurol. 2016;19(3):406-8.
36. Aviv RI, Benseler SM, DeVeber G, Silverman ED, Tyrrell PN, Tsang LM, et al. Angiography of primary central nervous system angiitis of childhood: conventional angiography versus magnetic resonance angiography at presentation. Am J Neuroradiol. 2007;28(1):9-15.
37. Duna GF, Calabrese LH. Limitations of invasive modalities in the diagnosis of primary angiitis of the central nervous system. J Rheumatol. 1995;22:662-7.
38. Kesav P, Krishnavadana B, Kesavadas C, Sreedharan SE, Rajendran A, Sukumaran S, et al. Utility of intracranial high-resolution vessel wall magnetic resonance imaging in differentiating intracranial vasculopathic diseases causing ischemic stroke. Neuroradiology. 2019;61:389-96.
39. Sundaram S, Kumar PN, Sharma DP, Kesavadas C, Sreedharan SE, Prasad BA, et al. High-resolution vessel wall imaging in primary angiitis of central nervous system. Ann Indian Acad Neurol. 2021;24(4):524-30.
40. Suri V, Kakkar A, Sharma MC, Padma MV, Garg A, Sarkar C. Primary angiitis of the central nervous system: a study of histopathological patterns and review of the literature. Folia Neuropathol. 2014;52(2):187-96.
41. Miller DV, Salvarani C, Hunder GG, Brown RD, Parisi JE, Christianson TJ, et al. Biopsy findings in primary angiitis of the central nervous system. Am J Surg Pathol. 2009;33(1):35-43.
42. Calabrese LH, Mallek JA. Primary angiitis of the central nervous system. Report of 8 new cases, review of the literature, and proposal for diagnostic criteria. Medicine (Baltimore). 1988;67(1):20-39.
43. Birnbaum J, Hellmann DB. Primary angiitis of the central nervous system. Arch Neurol. 2009;66(6):704-9.
44. de Boysson H, Arquizan C, Touzé E, Zuber M, Boulouis G, Naggara O, et al. Treatment and long-term outcomes of primary central nervous system vasculitis. Stroke. 2018;49(8):1946-52.
45. Beuker C, Strunk D, Rawal R, Schmidt-Pogoda A, Werring N, Milles L, et al. Primary angiitis of the CNS: a systematic review and meta-analysis. Neurol Neuroimmunol Neuroinflamm. 2021;8(6):e1093.
46. Paramasivan NK, Sundaram S, Sharma DP, Sreedharan SE, Sylaja PN. Rituximab for refractory primary angiitis of the central nervous system: experience in two patients. Mult Scler Relat Disord. 2021;51:102907.
47. Abdel Razek AA, Alvarez H, Bagg S, Refaat S, Castillo M. Imaging spectrum of CNS vasculitis. Radiographics. 2014;34(4):873-94.
48. Carod Artal FJ. Clinical management of infectious cerebral vasculitides. Expert Rev Neurother. 2016;16(2):205-21.
49. Jennette JC, Falk RJ. Nosology of primary vasculitis. Curr Opin Rheumatol. 2007;19(1):10-6.
50. Zaldivar Villon MLF, de la Rocha JAL, Espinoza LR. Takayasu arteritis: recent developments. Curr Rheumatol Rep. 2019;21(9):45.
51. Rutter M, Bowley J, Lanyon PC, Grainge MJ, Pearce FA. A systematic review and meta-analysis of the incidence rate of Takayasu arteritis. Rheumatology (Oxford). 2021;60(11):4982-90.
52. Watanabe R, Berry GJ, Liang DH, Goronzy JJ, Weyand CM. Pathogenesis of giant cell arteritis and Takayasu arteritis: similarities and differences. Curr Rheumatol Rep. 2020;22(10):68.
53. Comarmond C, Biard L, Lambert M, Mekinian A, Ferfar Y, Kahn JE, et al; French Takayasu Network. Long-term outcomes and prognostic factors of complications in Takayasu arteritis: a multicenter study of 318 patients. Circulation. 2017;136(12):1114-22.
54. de Souza AW, de Carvalho JF. Diagnostic and classification criteria of Takayasu arteritis. J Autoimmun. 2014;48-49:79-83.
55. Arend WP, Michel BA, Bloch DA, Hunder GG, Calabrese LH, Edworthy SM, et al. The American College of Rheumatology 1990 criteria for the classification of Takayasu arteritis. Arthritis Rheum. 1990;33(8):1129-34.
56. Misra DP, Rathore U, Patro P, Agarwal V, Sharma A. Disease-modifying antirheumatic drugs for the management of Takayasu arteritis: a systematic review and meta-analysis. Clin Rheumatol. 2021;40(11):4391-416.
57. Águeda AF, Monti S, Luqmani RA, Buttgereit F, Cid M, Dasgupta B, et al. Management of Takayasu arteritis: a systematic literature review informing the 2018 update of the EULAR recommendation

for the management of large vessel vasculitis. RMD Open. 2019;5(2):e001020.

58. Harriott AM, Zimmerman E, Singhal AB, Jaff MR, Lindsay ME, Rordorf GA. Cerebrovascular fibromuscular dysplasia: the MGH cohort and literature review. Neurol Clin Pract. 2017;7(3):225-36.
59. Persu A, Touzé E, Mousseaux E, Barral X, Joffre F, Plouin PF. Diagnosis and management of fibromuscular dysplasia: an expert consensus. Eur J Clin Invest. 2012;42(3):338-47.
60. Plouin PF, Perdu J, La Batide-Alanore A, Boutouyrie P, Gimenez-Roqueplo AP, Jeunemaitre X. Fibromuscular dysplasia. Orphanet J Rare Dis. 2007;2:28.
61. Slovut DP, Olin JW. Fibromuscular dysplasia. N Engl J Med. 2004;350(18):1862-71.
62. Touzé E, Southerland AM, Boulanger M, Labeyrie PE, Azizi M, Bouatia-Naji N, et al. Fibromuscular dysplasia and its neurologic manifestations: a systematic review. JAMA Neurol. 2019;76(2): 217-26.
63. Compagne KCJ, van Es ACGM, Berkhemer OA, Borst J, Roos YBWEM, van Oostenbrugge RJ, et al. Prevalence of carotid web in patients with acute intracranial stroke due to intracranial large vessel occlusion. Radiology. 2018;286:1000-7.
64. Coutinho JM, Derkatch S, Potvin ARJ, Tomlinson G, Casaubon LK, Silver FL, et al. Carotid artery web and ischemic stroke: a case-control study. Neurology. 2017;88:65-9.
65. Labeyrie MA, Serrano F, Civelli V, Jourdaine C, Reiner P, Saint-Maurice JP, et al. Carotid artery webs in embolic stroke of undetermined source with large intracranial vessel occlusion. Int J Stroke. 2021;16(4):392-5.
66. Kim SJ, Allen JW, Bouslama M, Nahab F, Frankel MR, Nogueira RG, et al. Carotid webs in cryptogenic ischemic strokes: a matched case-control study. J Stroke Cerebrovasc Dis. 2019;28:104402.
67. Zhang AJ, Dhruv P, Choi P, Bakker C, Koffel J, Anderson D, et al. A systematic literature review of patients with carotid web and acute ischemic stroke. Stroke. 2018;49:2872-6.
68. Pereira BJ, Batista UC, Tosello RT, Ströher IN, Baeta AM, Piske RL. Web vessels: literature review and neurointerventional management. World Neurosurg. 2017;110:e907-16.
69. Madaelil TP, Grossberg JA, Nogueira RG, Anderson A, Barreira C, Frankel M, et al. Multimodality imaging in carotid web. Front Neurol. 2019;10:220.
70. Haussen DC, Grossberg JA, Bouslama M, Pradilla G, Belagaje S, Bianchi N, et al. Carotid web (intimal fibromuscular dysplasia) has high stroke recurrence risk and is amenable to stenting. Stroke. 2017;48(11):3134-7.
71. Guglielmi V, Compagne KCJ, Sarrami AH, Sluis WM, van den Berg LA, van der Sluijs PM, et al.; MR CLEAN trial and MR CLEAN Registry Investigators. Assessment of recurrent stroke risk in patients with a carotid web. JAMA Neurol. 2021;78(7):826-33.
72. Takeuchi K, Shimizu K. Hypoplasia of the bilateral internal carotid arteries. Brain Nerve. 1957;9:37-43.
73. Scott RM, Smith ER. Moyamoya disease and moyamoya syndrome progress review. N Engl J Med. 2009;360:1226-3.
74. Zhang H, Zheng L, Feng L. Epidemiology, diagnosis and treatment of moyamoya disease. Exp Ther Med. 2019;17(3):1977-84.
75. Kamada F, Aoki Y, Narisawa A, Abe Y, Komatsuzaki S, Kikuchi A, et al. A genome-wide association study identifies *RNF213* as the first moyamoya disease gene. J Hum Genet. 2011;56:34-40.
76. Liu W, Morito D, Takashima S, Mineharu Y, Kobayashi H, Hitomi T, et al. Identification of *RNF213* as a susceptibility gene for moyamoya disease and its possible role in vascular development. PLoS One. 2011;6(7):e22542.
77. Kim EH, Yum MS, Ra YS, Park JB, Ahn JS, Kim GH, et al. Importance of RNF213 polymorphism on clinical features and long-term outcome in moyamoya disease. J Neurosurg. 2016;124:1221-7.
78. Mertens R, Graupera M, Gerhardt H, Bersano A, Tournier-Lasserve E, Mensah MA, et al. The genetic basis of moyamoya disease. Transl Stroke Res. 2022;13(1):25-45.
79. Kim JS. Moyamoya disease: epidemiology, clinical features, and diagnosis. J Stroke. 2016;18(1):2-11.
80. Starke RM, Komotar RJ, Hickman ZL, Paz YE, Pugliese AG, Otten ML, et al. Clinical features, surgical treatment, and long-term outcome of adult moyamoya patients. J Neurosurg. 2009;111(5):936-42.
81. Hirano Y, Miyawaki S, Imai H, Hongo H, Teranishi Y, Dofuku S, et al. Differences in clinical features among different onset patterns in moyamoya disease. J Clin Med. 2021;10(13):2815.
82. Cho HJ, Jung YH, Kim YD, Nam HS, Kim DS, Heo JH. The different infarct patterns between adulthood-onset and childhood-onset moyamoya disease. J Neurol Neurosurg Psychiatry. 2011;82:38-40
83. Nah HW, Kwon SU, Kang DW, Ahn JS, Kwun BD, Kim JS. Moyamoya disease-related versus primary intracerebral hemorrhage: location and outcomes are different. Stroke. 2012;43:1947-50.
84. Kikuta K, Takagi Y, Nozaki K, Sawamoto N, Fukuyama H, Hashimoto N. The presence of multiple microbleeds as a predictor of subsequent cerebral hemorrhage in patients with moyamoya disease. Neurosurgery. 2008;62:104-11.
85. Kaku Y, Morioka M, Ohmori Y, Kawano T, Kai Y, Fukuoka H, et al. Outer-diameter narrowing of the internal carotid and middle cerebral arteries in moyamoya disease detected on 3D constructive interference in steady-state MR image: is arterial constrictive remodeling a major pathogenesis? Acta Neurochir (Wien). 2012;154:2151-7.
86. Yuan M, Liu ZQ, Wang ZQ, Li B, Xu LJ, Xiao XL. High-resolution MR imaging of the arterial wall in moyamoya disease. Neurosci Lett. 2015;584:77-82.
87. Ryoo S, Cha J, Kim SJ, Choi JW, Ki CS, Kim KH, et al. High-resolution magnetic resonance wall imaging findings of moyamoya disease. Stroke. 2014;45:2457-60.
88. Kathuveetil A, Sylaja PN, Senthilvelan S, Kesavadas C, Banerjee M, Jayanand Sudhir B. Vessel wall thickening and enhancement in high-resolution intracranial vessel wall imaging: a predictor of future ischemic events in moyamoya disease. AJNR Am J Neuroradiol. 2020;41(1):100-5.
89. Fujimura M, Tominaga T. Diagnosis of moyamoya disease: international standard and regional differences. Neurol Med Chir (Tokyo). 2015;55(3):189-93.
90. Kuroda S, Ishikawa T, Houkin K, Nanba R, Hokari M, Iwasaki Y. Incidence and clinical features of disease progression in adult moyamoya disease. Stroke. 2005;36:2148-53.
91. Onozuka D, Hagihara A, Nishimura K, Kada A, Nakagawara J, Ogasawara K, et al. Prehospital antiplatelet use and functional status on admission of patients with nonhemorrhagic moyamoya disease: a nationwide retrospective cohort study (J-ASPECT study). BMJ Open. 2016;6:e009942.
92. Kim T, Oh CW, Bang JS, Kim JE, Cho WS. Moyamoya Disease: Treatment and Outcomes. J Stroke. 2016;18(1):21-30.
93. Mukherjee A. Moyamoya disease and beta-thalassemia. J Assoc Physicians India. 1995;43(10):710-1.
94. K A, Shafeeque CM, Sudhir JB, Banerjee M, P N S. Ethnic variation and the relevance of homozygous RNF213 p.R4810.K variant in the phenotype of Indian moyamoya disease. PLoS One. 2020;15(12):e0243925.
95. Sundaram S, Sylaja PN, Menon G, Sudhir J, Jayadevan ER, Sukumaran S, et al. Moyamoya disease: a comparison of long-term outcome of conservative and surgical treatment in India. J Neurol Sci. 2014;336(1-2):99-102.
96. Furtado SV, Basu E, Mehta A, Vala K, Mohan D. Surgical outcome of encephaloduroarteriomyosynangiosis for moyamoya disease. Neurol India. 2021;69(5):1259-64.

54

CHAPTER

Central Nervous System Vasculitis

Raviteja Kakarla, Rajsrinivas Parthasarathy, Imtiyaz Khan, Karan Sharma, Sajad Ahmad Tak, Vipul Gupta

INTRODUCTION

Vasculitis is considered to be a group of heterogenous clinical entities characterized by inflammatory infiltration of the blood vessels of different sizes, resulting in reactive damage both to the vessel integrity (leading to rupture and bleeding) and to the diameter of the vessel (leading to downstream ischemia, necrosis, and subsequent tissue damage).[1] Blood vessels of different sizes ranging from large arteries to small arterioles and venules will be affected.

CLASSIFICATION

The revised Chapel Hill Consensus Conference helps us to have a better approach to understanding vasculitis by classifying it into different types of primary and secondary vasculitis based on the vessel caliber and also on primary or secondary affection.[1] Primary vasculitis is classified into large-vessel, medium-vessel, and small-vessel vasculitis based on the size of the vessel. In small-vessel vasculitis, intraparenchymal arteries, arterioles, veins, and venules are affected. There is also a variable vessel vasculitis that is classified without a predominant vessel size and caliber. It involves arteries, veins, and capillaries. Secondary vasculitis is termed when it occurs secondary to any systemic diseases more commonly like connective tissue diseases or when it is associated with a specific cause such as substance abuse or infection. Single-organ vasculitis is when the disease process is confined to a single organ such as the central nervous system (CNS) or peripheral nervous system (PNS). It involves both arteries or veins of any size without features of systemic vasculitis and includes primary angiitis of the CNS (PACNS) (adult or childhood). The other similar terms are adult (or childhood) primary CNS vasculitis, granulomatous angiitis of the brain **(Table 1)**.

TABLE 1: Classification of vasculitis and their subtypes, adapted from the revised 2012 Chapel Hill Consensus Conference (CHCC).[1]

Type of vessel/ localization	Vascular disease
Large vessels	• Giant cell arteritis • Takayasu arteritis
Medium vessels	• Polyarteritis nodosa • Kawasaki disease
Small vessels	• Antineutrophil cytoplasmic antibody associated vasculitis—ANCA • Microscopic polyangiitis granulomatosis with polyangiitis—Wegener's • Eosinophilic granulomatosis with polyangiitis—Churg–Strauss • Immune complex vasculitis • Cryoglobulinemia • Immunoglobulin (IgA) vasculitis—Henoch–Schönlein purpura • Hypocomplementemic urticarial vasculitis—anti-C1q
Variable vessel sizes	• Behçet's disease • Cogan syndrome
Single-organ vasculitis	• Primary angiitis of central nervous system (PACNS) • Nonsystemic peripheral nerve vasculitis • Idiopathic aortitis
Vasculitis associated with systemic connective disease	• Rheumatoid arthritis vasculitis • Systemic lupus erythematous vasculitis
Vasculitis associated with infection	• Acute bacterial meningitis vasculitis • Mycobacterial tuberculous vasculitis • Atypical mycobacteriosis vasculitis • Varicella zoster virus vasculitis • Human immunodeficiency virus vasculitis

Continued

Continued

Type of vessel/ localization	Vascular disease
	• COVID-19 vasculitis • Syphilis • Mycoses • Parasites • Fungal • Others
Other types	Vasculitis due to drugs and illicit substance abuse (amphetamines, cocaine, and opioids)

EPIDEMIOLOGY AND DEMOGRAPHY

Epidemiological studies are very rare. Available data shows an annual incidence rate of PACNS as 2.4 cases per 1 million person years.[2] CNS vasculitis can occur at any age and can affect both men and women. In adults PACNS usually occurs between the age of 40 and 60 years.[3] In adults more females are reported to have angiography-positive vasculitis whereas in angiography-negative vasculitis both sexes are equally affected.[4,5] Ethnic variation and predomination have not yet been reported.

PATHOGENESIS OF CENTRAL NERVOUS SYSTEM VASCULITIS

The integrity of blood–brain barrier (BBB) is of utmost importance as its disturbance leads to a number of primary and secondary neurological diseases including vasculitis.[6] There also has been a genetic predisposition for vasculitis where very highly polymorphic loci like human leukocyte antigen B (HLA-B), which is involved in the binding of the antigen to the CD8 cells and natural killer (NK) cells, has been found to be associated with vasculitis.[7] Another example for genetic predisposition is that the proteinase 3-antineutrophil cytoplasmic antibody (PR3-ANCA) vasculitis is associated with genes such as *SERPINA 1* (encoding alpha-1 antitrypsin) and *PRTN* (encoding PR3).[8] The complex genetic risk is usually because of the role of hundreds of loci, which have a very low independent effect, and hence genetic heritability can only be seen only in rare cases. The immune system and inflammatory responses play an important role in the pathogenesis of vasculitis, but some aspects are not yet clear.

Mechanisms include immune-mediated, cell-mediated, ANCA-mediated (cytoplasmic, perinuclear, and atypical ANCA), or direct spread to the brain from the blood through the BBB.[9] The immune-mediated damage is through complement activation, neutrophil-mediated phagocytosis, and granular secretion, resulting in vascular damage. Cell-mediated damage is through interferon (IFN) released by the cytotoxic CD8+ T cells, which recruit and activate macrophages.[10,11] All these mechanisms eventually cause ischemic or hemorrhagic strokes. These can affect both intraparenchymal and subependymal areas, resulting in significant disability. There will be degeneration, necrosis, demyelination, and reactive gliosis in the parenchyma.[12] In contrast to CNS vasculitis occurring secondarily as a part of diffuse disease, PACNS is much less frequent but fatal without any clear etiopathogenesis and typically involves the CNS without any systemic involvement.[13]

CLINICAL FEATURES

Central nervous system vasculitis may be primary or secondary.[14] In primary CNS vasculitis, the inflammation is restricted only to the brain and spinal cord with no identifiable cause being found, whereas in secondary CNS vasculitis, there is associated involvement of skin, lungs, sinuses, kidneys, cardiovascular system, or joints, and also there will be an underlying cause such as malignancy, drugs, substance abuse, and infection.

Usually, neurological symptoms are nonspecific, and they present with a wide range of neurologic and psychiatric symptoms as well. The multifocal characteristics of the lesions due to segmental or diffuse vessel involvement are responsible for the nonspecific symptomatology of different patients. The onset also varies widely, ranging from acute stroke symptoms to chronic progressive cognitive decline, even though most of them have an insidious onset with slow progression. Symptoms also depend on the affected vascular territory and the duration of the disease.[15] Headache is one of the most common symptoms, which is initially gradual and mild in nature in patients with PACNS. In addition, patients also complain of seizures, and focal deficits (because of stroke or hemorrhage), which are more common in children than adults who complain of diffuse progressive deficits **(Boxes 1 and 2)**.[16] CNS vasculitis presenting as encephalopathy, isolated myelopathy, and rarely as glioma is also described.[17,18]

BOX 1 Symptoms and signs of vasculitis—findings.

- Headache
- Cognitive dysfunction
- Stroke
- Transient ischemic attack
- Aphasia
- Weight loss, fever
- Seizure
- Ataxia
- Intracranial bleeding
- Amnestic syndrome
- Visual (visual field deficits, blurred vision, diplopia, papilledema)

BOX 2	**When to suspect vasculitis?**

- When recurrent strokes occur in young patients without unidentifiable cardiovascular or hypercoagulable risk factors
- Development of cognitive dysfunction with or without headaches
- Recurrent or focal neurological symptoms
- Abnormal cerebrovascular imaging in the setting of unexplained neurological deficit
- Unexplained spinal cord dysfunction not associated with systemic disease

DIAGNOSIS

Diagnosis is usually many times challenging, and many patients are either underdiagnosed or overdiagnosed. No test is sensitive or specific for diagnosing and confirming CNS vasculitis. Unlike secondary or systemic vasculitis, primary CNS vasculitis shows normal blood tests or nonspecific findings such as anemia, leukocytosis, and normal or mildly elevated routine inflammatory markers. However, in childhood PACNS Von Willebrand factor is a potential biomarker for childhood PACNS.[9]

Cerebrospinal fluid (CSF) analysis helps in ruling out differential diagnosis of vasculitis. Most infections can be ruled out after thorough microbiological testing. It is abnormal in 80–90% of biopsy-confirmed vasculitis. It can also be mild mimicking aseptic meningitis including modest pleocytosis and elevated protein levels in more than 90% of patients.[20] It has been found in angiographic-positive PACNS patients that they infrequently demonstrate CSF abnormalities.[4] Hence, a normal CSF analysis does not rule out CNS vasculitis. CSF analysis in suspicion of vasculitis requires a search for systemic inflammation including specific antibodies. It has been found that rarely autoantibodies (antinuclear, antineutrophil cytoplasmic, and anticardiolipin antibodies) are positive in vasculitis patients with PACNS.[16] Hence, they must be interpreted in the context of clinical and laboratory settings.

Neuroimaging

Neuroimaging helps to identify different types of lesions at one time point. Lesions can be ischemic, hemorrhagic, or inflammatory. Computed tomography (CT) scan can detect only 30% of lesions, and hence the preferred modality is contrast-enhanced magnetic resonance imaging (MRI) brain studies [include T1- and T2-weighted imaging, fluid-attenuated inversion recovery (FLAIR), gradient echo (GRE), diffusion-weighted imaging (DWI), apparent diffusion coefficient (ADC), high-resolution T1-weighted imaging after contrast injection with fat suppression and fat compensation to look for vessel wall enhancement] and MRI spinal cord studies (with T1- and T2-weighted imaging of the entire spinal cord as well as T1- and T2-weighted axial imaging as well as gadolinium-enhanced imaging of cord lesions) with vascular imaging [conventional digital subtraction angiography (DSA), CT angiography (CTA), and magnetic resonance angiography (MRA)], which was found to be abnormal in 97% of adults with CNS vasculitis.[21] Characteristic multiple and bilateral cortical and subcortical infarctions are seen.[4] In addition, ischemic and hemorrhagic lesions at different ages with focal or diffuse inflammation findings are also observed. It was also found that there was an increase in the ADC in patients with normal MRI scans.[22] Vessel wall contrast enhancement was found in 82% and wall thickening in 92% of patients with PACNS **(Figs. 1A and B)**.[23]

Vessel wall imaging (VWI) using black-blood T1 pre- and postcontrast sequences depicts wall enhancement in vasculitis involving CNS vessels. VWI has superior sensitivity over MRI/MRA and DSA in diagnosing CNS vasculitis, especially involving smaller vessels. Recently, three-dimensional VWI has added the advantage of isotropic spatial resolution and whole brain coverage with decreased period. VWI, unlike DSA, can detect and differentiate vasculitic lesions from nonvasculitic pathologies such as atherosclerotic plaques and reversible cerebral vasoconstriction syndrome (RCVS) **(Figs. 2A and B)**.

Conventional invasive angiography should be performed in every patient with suspicion of inflammatory brain disease and is considered the gold standard. However, stroke is the major complication of invasive angiography with its incidence being 0.25%.[24] MRA can also be considered as a reasonable alternative as few studies that compared MRA and conventional angiography did not show any difference in the ability to detect and characterize vascular abnormalities.[25] Typical features that are indicative of primary CNS vasculitis include multiple areas of narrowing and dilatation or multilocular occlusions of intracranial vessels (vessel beading appearance).[26] Vessel beading appearance is not specific and is also seen in noninflammatory vasculopathies and nonvasculitis conditions such as atherosclerosis, atrial myxoma, neurofibromatosis, infections, and vasospasm.[27] Sometimes fusiform dilatations, delayed contrast enhancement, and development of collateral circulation are also seen, but long-segment stenosis and complete occlusions are unlikely in PACNS.[28,29] When the inflammatory changes are limited to <500-μm-sized arteries, angiography will be normal and they must be guided to brain biopsy in such angiography-negative patients.[17]

Salvarni et al. from the Mayo clinic cohort in 2007 defined CNS vasculitis as a large-vessel and small-vessel CNS vasculitis. Large vessel was considered as the involvement of intracranial segment of internal carotid artery, proximal anterior cerebral, middle cerebral, and posterior cerebral artery, and it presents with focal deficits and acute lesions on MRI.[30] Small-vessel involvement was considered where there is the involvement of all vascular segments beyond the second branching. Small-vessel PACNS (SV-PACNS) is associated with more severe encephalopathic presentation

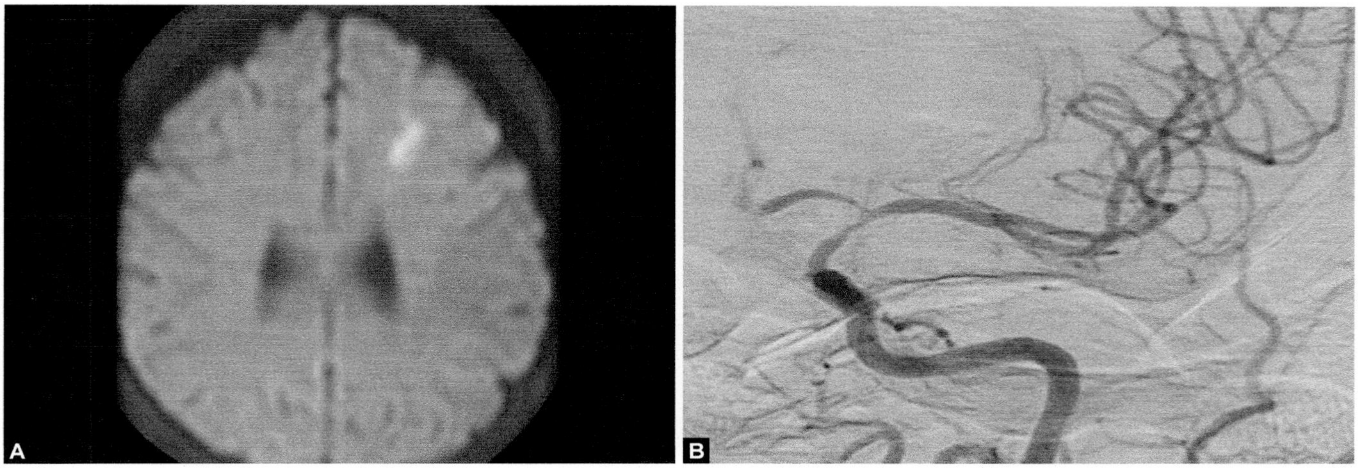

FIGS. 1A AND B: (A) DWI MRI shows acute diffusion restriction in left frontal subcortical white matter; (B) DSA image shows significant luminal narrowing in left supraclinoid ICA and A1-ACA.

(A1-ACA: A1 segment of the anterior cerebral artery; DWI: diffusion-weighted imaging; ICA: internal carotid artery; MRI: magnetic resonance imaging)

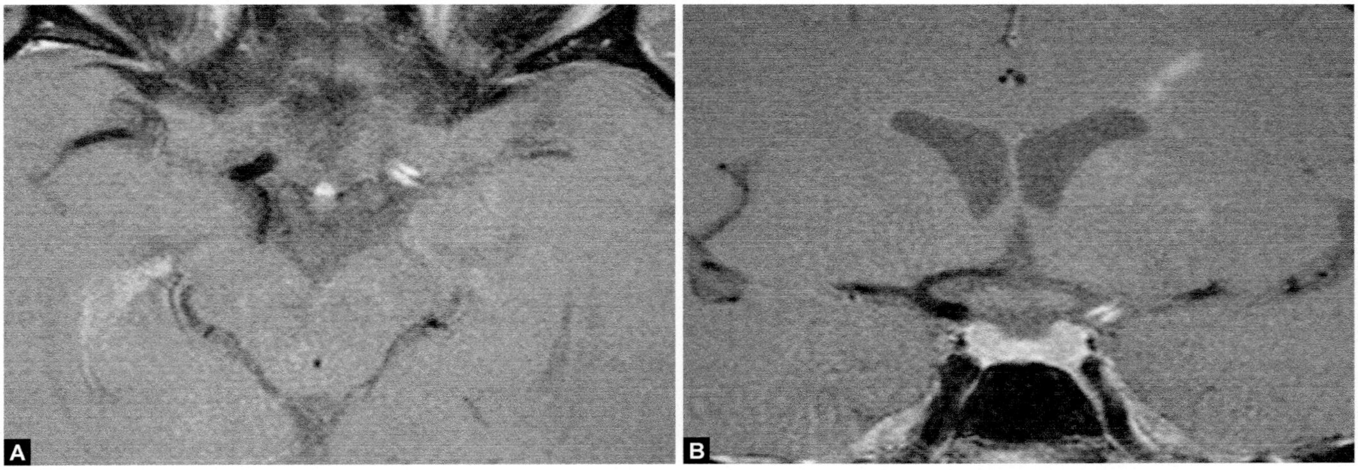

FIGS. 2A AND B: Vessel wall MRI (A) axial and (B) coronal show smooth concentric wall enhancement in left supraclinoid ICA.

(ICA: internal carotid artery; MRI: magnetic resonance imaging)

with cognitive impairment and seizures, more abnormal CSF analysis, and more diffuse gadolinium-enhanced lesions on MRI.[4,31]

Brain biopsy: The role of brain biopsy is initially well established in neoplastic lesions of the brain. Its role is also increasing in diagnosing vasculitis of the brain nowadays and is included in the algorithm for diagnosing inflammatory brain diseases. The overall diagnostic yield is considered to be 53–74%, but the yield can be increased to 80% by targeting areas of imaging abnormality.[32] Biopsy from the right dominant frontal lobe with its overlying leptomeninges is recommended if affected lesions are not surgically accessible. Even when performed by trained operators in specialized centers, brain biopsy can be complicated by intracranial hemorrhage, seizures, and altered mental status. The sensitivity or specificity of biopsy may be effected by prolonged time to biopsy, nonlesioned biopsy, prior steroid treatment, and inadequate sampling. A negative biopsy does not rule out a diagnosis of vasculitis.

A biopsy is important in not only diagnosing CNS vasculitis but also excluding other diseases such as malignancies, demyelination, infection, and Rasmussen encephalitis.[33] Primary CNS vasculitis involves small vessels, arterioles, and capillaries. Hence, transmural and segmental signs of inflammation are the main diagnostic findings. There occurs a transmural vasculocentric inflammation with vascular wall damage with or without fibrinoid necrosis.[34] The characteristic features in adults include necrotizing, granulomatous, or lymphocytic infiltration, whereas children exclusively demonstrated lymphocytic infiltration.[16] In addition, adults also showed amyloid deposition with no such deposition in the children. The most common pattern is granulomatous vasculitis, which includes T-cell and macrophage vessel wall infiltration resulting in the formation of granulomas with giant cells

TABLE 2: Findings in diagnostic workup in suspected vasculitis.

Diagnostic workup	Findings
Clinical features	• Headache • Seizures • Strokes • Encephalopathy • Altered cognition
Laboratory tests	Absence of systemic vasculitis-associated antibodies
Cerebrospinal fluid (CSF)	• Mild lymphomonocytic pleocytosis • Protein elevation • Presence of oligoclonal bands
Magnetic resonance imaging (MRI)	• Ischemic infarction • Microangiopathy • Hemorrhage • Contrast enhancement • Tumor-like lesions
Digital subtraction angiography (DSA)	• Vessel beading • Arterial wall narrowing with poststenotic dilatation
Biopsy	• Granulomatous lymphocytic • Acute necrotizing patterns • Lymphocytic pattern

and is also associated with amyloid deposition. Sarcoidosis is considered a differential diagnosis for granulomatous vasculitis. In lymphocytic vasculitis, there is predominant CD3+ and CD20+ lymphocytic infiltration with a small amount of plasma cells affecting the entire vessel wall.[12] Leukodystrophy is a differential diagnosis for this subtype. The less common necrotizing vasculitis shows transmural fibrinoid necrosis affecting small muscular arteries with rupture of the internal elastic lamina and may be associated with inflammatory lymphomonocyte infiltrate. These histological findings are often associated with ischemic stroke due to stenosis or total occlusion of a damaged vessel or with intraparenchymal hemorrhage due to damaged vessel rupture **(Table 2)**.

Table 3 gives the investigative workup needed before considering vasculitis.

SPECTRUM OF THE DISEASE AND VASCULITIS MIMICS

Central nervous system vasculitis has wide differential diagnosis including PACNS, secondary CNS vasculitis, nonvasculitis inflammatory brain diseases, and noninflammatory vasculopathies of the brain.

TABLE 3: Investigative workup needed before considering vasculitis.

Tests	Investigative workup
Routine blood tests	• Complete blood count (CBC) • Liver function tests • Kidney function tests • Erythrocyte sedimentation rate (ESR) • C-reactive protein (CRP) • Coagulation profile • Serum electrophoresis • Lipid profile • Ferritin • Lactate dehydrogenase (LDH) • Serum B12 • Serum folate • Serum homocysteine
Autoimmune screening	• Antineutrophil cytoplasmic antibodies (ANCAs) • Anti-double stranded DNA (anti-dsDNA) antibodies • Extractable nuclear antigen (ENA) antibodies • Antinuclear antibody (ANA) • Anti-thyroglobulin (TG) antibodies • Anti-thyroid peroxidase (TPO) antibody • Antimitochondrial antibody (AMA) • Gastric parietal cell antibodies (APCAs) • Anti-smooth muscle antibodies (ASMAs) • Anti-citrullinated peptide antibody (ACPA) • Rheumatoid factor (RF) • Anti-transglutaminase antibodies • *Complement*: C3, C4, CH50 • Angiotensin-converting enzyme (ACE) • Immunoglobulin (IgA, IgG, IgM) • Cryoglobulins • Lymphocyte subsets IgG4 • Ab anti-NMDAr, AMPA 1 e 2, GABAb1, LGI1 e CASPR2, Ab anti-GluR3
Nongenetic thrombophilic screening	• Anti-beta 2 glycoprotein I autoantibodies (IgG and IgM) • Anticardiolipin antibodies (IgG and IgM) • LAC (lupus anticoagulant) • C protein, S protein • Factor V G1691A and FII G20210A mutation
Neoplastic and paraneoplastic screening	• Prostate-specific antigen (PSA) • Cancer antigen (CA)-125 antibodies against neuronal antigens (Hu, Yo, Ri, amphiphysin ant - Ma1, anti-Ma2, anti-CV2 antibodies) • β2 microglobulin • Alpha-fetoprotein • CA 19–9 • Carcinoembryonic antigen (CEA)

Continued

Continued

Tests	Investigative workup
Viral and bacterial screening	• Anti-hepatitis C virus (HCV) antibodies • Anti-human immunodeficiency virus (HIV) antibodies • Venereal diseases research laboratories (VDRL) • Anti-herpes simplex virus (HSV) 1/2 antibodies (IgG and IgM) • Anti-varicella zoster virus (VZV) antibodies (IgG and IgM) • Anti-cytomegalovirus (CMV) antibodies (IgG and IgM) • Anti-Epstein–Barr virus (EBV) antibodies [IgG and IgM; including anti-EBV nuclear antigen 1 (EBNA1) antibodies] • Hepatitis B surface antigen (HbsAg), anti-HBsAg (aHBs), hepatitis B core antibody (HBcAb), and anti-hepatitis B e antibody (HbeAb) antibodies • Anti-severe acute respiratory syndrome coronavirus 2 (SARS-CoV-2) • Antibodies polymerase chain reaction (PCR) against neurotropic virus QuantiFERON • Anti-treponema antibodies [fluorescent treponemal antibody absorption test (FTA-ABS)/ treponema pallidum hemagglutination test (TPHA)]
Urinalysis	• Routine and microscopy • Urine electrophoresis • Drug tests (when clinically indicated)

Secondary Central Nervous System Vasculitis

The most common etiology for secondary CNS vasculitis is infection. It is identified by doing cultures and polymerase chain reactions (PCRs) of serum and CSF. Varicella zoster virus (VZV) is one such common infection which affects CNS and PNS. VZV reactivation commonly causes postvaricella angiopathy, which results in inflammatory stenosis of proximal large vessels.[35] Human immunodeficiency virus (HIV) infection can also sometimes mimic CNS vasculitis. Among fungal infections, *Candida* and aspergillosis can cause vasculitis.[36]

Central nervous system involvement in the form of strokes, transient ischemic attacks (TIAs), and hemorrhages also occurs in large-, medium-, and small-vessel vasculitis, which is differentiated from PACNS by their associated systemic symptoms and signs. Most often CNS involvement is seen in Behçet's disease, Wegener's granulomatosis, and Churg-Strauss syndrome.[17] In systemic diseases like systemic lupus erythematosus (SLE), CNS vasculitis is also known to occur and is characterized by fever, severe headaches, confusion episodes with rapid progression to psychiatric symptoms, seizures, and coma with the most common microscopic brain finding being microvasculopathy being described as healed vasculitis.[37] It also has been reported in postmortem findings of patients with rheumatoid arthritis. CNS vasculitis is also seen in Sjögren's syndrome, mixed connective tissue disease, and dermatomyositis.[17]

Occurrence of PACNS in association with Hodgkin's lymphoma, non-Hodgkin's lymphoma has been reported.[38] More importantly intravascular lymphoma, an extranodal diffuse large B-cell lymphoma subtype, has a predilection for CNS and hence is an important differential diagnosis for PACNS.[39]

Central Nervous System Vasculitis Mimics

Important disease entities that are considered as mimics are demyelinating diseases such as acute disseminated encephalomyelitis and multiple sclerosis; antibody-mediated diseases such as anti-N-methyl-d-aspartate receptor (NMDAR) encephalitis, limbic encephalitis, and neuromyelitis optica; Hashimoto's encephalitis; and celiac disease-mediated encephalitis. Sometimes noninflammatory vasculopathies can also mimic vasculitis. Hence, arteriosclerosis is an important disease entity that needs to be excluded before confirming vasculitis. Cerebral autosomal dominant arteriopathy with subcortical infarcts and leukoencephalopathy (CADASIL); mitochondrial myopathy, encephalopathy, lactic acidosis, and stroke-like episodes (MELAS); moyamoya angiopathy; and radiation vasculopathy are other noninflammatory vasculopathy entities. Likewise, conditions such as reversible vasoconstriction syndrome, migraine, and drugs, which can cause transient vasoconstriction, might also mimic CNS vasculitis. Drugs such as cocaine and amphetamines are known as mimics as well as the drugs causing secondary vasculitis **(Table 4)**.

DIAGNOSTIC CRITERIA

In 1988, Calabrese and Mallek suggested a diagnostic criterion, and a diagnosis is made if all three criteria were met. These include the presence of unexplained acquired neurological deficit after extensive investigation of other causes, the presence of evidence of inflammatory arteritic process within the CNS by either angiography or histopathological examination or both, and no other evidence of systemic vasculitis or any other disorders to which the angiographic or histopathological findings are secondary.[40] In 2009, to avoid misdiagnosis, Birnbaum and colleagues modified the criteria: Definite when there is histopathological confirmation of vasculitis by brain biopsy and probable when there is lacking brain biopsy but the evidence is supported by DSA and/or MRI/intracranial MRA and/or intracranial CTA in the form of alternating areas of stenosis, ectasia, or both in more than one vascular territory, which is unexplained by intracranial atherosclerosis or any other disease that may mimic PACNS and/or CSF analysis, which may reveal lymphocytic pleocytosis and elevated protein.[41]

TABLE 4: Differential diagnosis for central nervous system (CNS) vasculitis.[12]

Etiological entities	Diseases
Demyelinating diseases	• Multiple sclerosis • Optic neuritis
Antibody-mediated inflammatory brain diseases	• Anti-N-methyl-d-aspartate receptor (NMDAR) encephalitis • Antibody-mediated limbic encephalitis • Neuromyelitis optica • Hashimoto encephalitis • Postmycoplasma encephalitis, celiac disease-associated encephalitis • Hashimoto encephalopathy • Acute posterior multifocal placoid pigment epitheliopathy (APMPPE)
T cell-mediated inflammatory brain diseases	Rasmussen encephalitis (frequent and severe seizures, loss of motor skills and speech, hemiparesis, encephalitis, and dementia)
Granulomatous inflammatory brain diseases	• Neurosarcoidosis • Antineutrophil cytoplasmic antibody (ANCA)-associated vasculitis
Infections	• Tuberculosis • John Cunningham (JC) virus • Syphilis
Autoinflammatory syndromes	Familial Mediterranean fever
Tumors	Predominantly, glioma and lymphoma (although the latter is rare lesions)
Vasospastic diseases	• Reversible cerebral vasoconstriction syndrome • Migraines, vasospasms secondary to hypertension, drug exposure • Subarachnoid hemorrhage • Eclampsia • Pheochromocytoma • Hashimoto encephalopathy
Thromboembolic disease, bacterial endocarditis	
Hemoglobin disorders	
Antiphospholipid antibody syndrome	
Fibromuscular dysplasia	
Genetic diseases associated with obliterating cerebral vasculopathy	Degos disease [Kohlmeier–Degos disease or malignant atrophic papulosis (MAP)], retinocerebral vasculopathy with cerebral leukodystrophy (RVCL)
Other syndromes with associated cerebral vasculopathy	Cogan syndrome [vasculopathy plus inflammatory eye disease (interstitial keratitis) and vestibular auditory dysfunction], Susac syndrome (noninflammatory vasculopathy, retinopathy, hearing loss, and encephalopathy), Sneddon syndrome (progressive noninflammatory cerebral arteriopathy and livedo)

TREATMENT OF CENTRAL NERVOUS SYSTEM VASCULITIS

Flowchart 1 shows the treatment of CNS vasculitis.

Treatment of Primary Angiitis of Central Nervous System

Current treatment recommendations are based on observational studies or are derived from the management of systemic vasculitis.[42] PACNS treatment is divided into induction and maintenance therapies.[43]

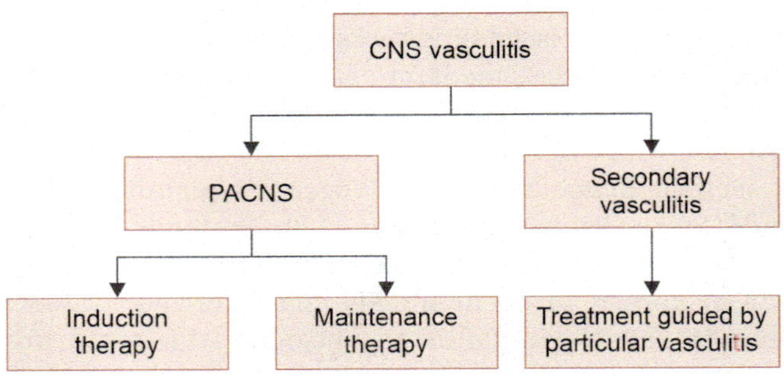

FLOWCHART 1: Treatment of CNS vasculitis.
(CNS: central nervous system; PACNS: primary angiitis of the CNS)

Induction Therapy[44]

Common regimens used include:

- Glucocorticoids plus cyclophosphamide
- Glucocorticoids plus rituximab
- Glucocorticoids only

Glucocorticoids

Oral prednisolone @ 1 mg/kg/day is started. Continue this dose for at least 6 weeks.

In severe cases, intravenous (IV) methylprednisolone @ 1 g/day for 3–5 days can be used. It is followed by oral prednisolone @ 1 mg/kg/day.[45]

Tapering Protocol of Steroids

After 6 weeks, prednisolone should be tapered by 10 mg each week until a dose of 40 mg/day is reached. After 1 week of 40 mg/day, the prednisolone dose should be tapered by 5 mg each week until the patient reaches 20 mg/day. After 1 week of 20 mg/day, the prednisolone dose should be tapered by 2.5 mg each week until the patient reaches 10 mg/day. After 1 week of 10 mg/day, the prednisolone dose should be tapered by 1 mg every 2 weeks until the patient reaches the maintenance dose of 5 mg/day.[46]

Cyclophosphamide

Intravenous cyclophosphamide pulses @ 1 g/month for at least 6 months are recommended. Oral cyclophosphamide with a median starting dose of 150 mg/day can also be used.[47]

Rituximab

It can be used in place of cyclophosphamide for induction therapy. Dosage @ 1 g IV infusion to be repeated after 2 weeks or weekly rituximab infusion @ 375 mg/m^2, with the maintenance dosage of 1 g every sixth month.[48]

Maintenance Therapy

A combination of immunosuppressants with oral glucocorticoids being gradually tapered is frequently used.[48] Common immunosuppressive agents are azathioprine (1.5 or 2 mg/kg/day), mycophenolate mofetil (2–3 g/day), and methotrexate (0.3–0.5 mg/kg/week or 7.5–20 mg/week).[2]

The best functional outcome is achieved by patients being treated with a combination of glucocorticoids and other immunosuppressive drugs followed by maintenance therapy. According to the data of de Boisson, maintenance drugs were started at the median time of 4 months after initiation of induction therapy for a median duration of 24 months.

Monitoring Treatment

Treatment is monitored by a periodic reassessment of symptoms, neurological findings, and neuroimaging abnormalities. A follow-up MRI should be obtained 4–6 weeks after starting treatment followed by every 3–6 months.

During the treatment patients require close clinical follow-up and laboratory monitoring to avoid preventable adverse effects of immunosuppressive therapy.

CONCLUSION

Central nervous system vasculitis forms an important group of modifiable diseases of the nervous system. Early recognition and prompt appropriate therapy go a long way in total outcome and prognosis.

REFERENCES

1. Jennette JC, Falk RJ, Bacon PA, Basu N, Cid MC, Ferrario F, et al. 2012 revised International Chapel Hill Consensus Conference nomenclature of vasculitides. Arthritis Rheum. 2013;65(1):1-11.
2. Salvarani C, Brown RD Jr, Christianson T, Miller DV, Giannini C, Huston J 3rd, et al. An update of the Mayo clinic cohort of patients with adult primary central nervous system vasculitis: description of 163 patients. Medicine (Baltimore). 2015;94(21):1-15.
3. Néel A, Pagnoux C. Primary angiitis of the central nervous system. Clin Exp Rheumatol. 2009;27(1):S95.
4. Salvarani C, Brown Jr RD, Calamia KT, Christianson TJH, Weigand SD, Miller DV, et al. Primary central nervous system vasculitis: analysis of 101 patients. Ann Neurol. 2007;62(5):442-51.
5. MacLaren K, Gillespie J, Shrestha S, Neary D, Ballardie FW. Primary angiitis of the central nervous system: emerging variants. QJM. 2005;98(9):643-54.
6. Younger DS. The blood–brain barrier: implications for vasculitis. Neurol Clin. 2019;37(2):235-48.
7. Carmona FD, López-Mejías R, Márquez A, Martín J, González-Gay MA. Genetic basis of vasculitides with neurologic involvement. Neurol Clin. 2019;37(2):219-34.
8. Rahmattulla C, Mooyaart AL, van Hooven D, Schoones JW, Bruijn JA, Dekkers OM, et al. Genetic variants in ANCA-associated vasculitis: a meta-analysis. Ann Rheum Dis. 2016;75(9):1687-92.
9. Shavit E, Alavi A, Sibbald RG. Vasculitis—what do we have to know? A review of literature. Int J Low Extrem Wounds. 2018;17(4):218-26.
10. Ozen S, Batu ED. Vasculitis pathogenesis: can we talk about precision medicine? Front Immunol. 2018;9:1892.
11. Yates M, Watts R. ANCA-associated vasculitis. Clin Med (Northfield Il). 2017;17(1):60.
12. Mansueto G, Lanza G, Fisicaro F, Alaouieh D, Hong E, Girolami S, et al. Central and peripheral nervous system complications of vasculitis syndromes from pathology to bedside: part 1—central nervous system. Curr Neurol Neurosci Rep. 2022;1-23.
13. Giannini C, Salvarani C, Hunder G, Brown RD. Primary central nervous system vasculitis: pathology and mechanisms. Acta Neuropathol. 2012;123(6):759-72.
14. Younger DS. Eleven themes in the history of systemic and nervous system vasculitides. Neurol Clin. 2019;37(2):149-70.
15. Smitka M, Bruck N, Engellandt K, Hahn G, Knoefler R, Von der Hagen M. Clinical perspective on primary angiitis of the central nervous system in childhood (cPACNS). Front Pediatr. 2020;8:281.
16. Twilt M, Benseler SM. The spectrum of CNS vasculitis in children and adults. Nat Rev Rheumatol. 2012;8(2):97-107.
17. Beuker C, Schmidt A, Strunk D, Sporns PB, Wiendl H, Meuth SG, et al. Primary angiitis of the central nervous system: diagnosis and treatment. Ther Adv Neurol Disord. 2018;11:1756286418785071.

18. Mullah M, More N, Devani K, Diyora BD. Primary CNS vasculitis mimicking glioma: A case report and literature review. Int J Neurooncol. 2021;4:56-60.
19. Cellucci T, Tyrrell PN, Pullenayegum E, Benseler SM. Von Willebrand factor antigen—a possible biomarker of disease activity in childhood central nervous system vasculitis? Rheumatology. 2012;51(10):1838-45.
20. Salvarani C, Brown Jr RD, Hunder GG. Adult primary central nervous system vasculitis. Lancet. 2012;380(9843):767-77.
21. Aviv RI, Benseler SM, Silverman ED, Tyrrell PN, Deveber G, Tsang LM, et al. MR imaging and angiography of primary CNS vasculitis of childhood. Am J Neuroradiol. 2006;27(1):192-9.
22. White ML, Zhang Y. Primary angiitis of the central nervous system: apparent diffusion coefficient lesion analysis. Clin Imaging. 2010;34(1):1-6.
23. Küker W, Gaertner S, Nägele T, Dopfer C, Schöning M, Fiehler J, et al. Vessel wall contrast enhancement: a diagnostic sign of cerebral vasculitis. Cerebrovasc Dis. 2008;26(1):23-9.
24. Willinsky RA, Taylor SM, TerBrugge K, Farb RI, Tomlinson G, Montanera W. Neurologic complications of cerebral angiography: prospective analysis of 2,899 procedures and review of the literature. Radiology. 2003;227(2):522-8.
25. Aviv RI, Benseler SM, DeVeber G, Silverman ED, Tyrrell PN, Tsang LM, et al. Angiography of primary central nervous system angiitis of childhood: conventional angiography versus magnetic resonance angiography at presentation. Am J Neuroradiol. 2007;28(1): 9-15.
26. Berlit P. Primary angiitis of the CNS—an enigma that needs worldwide efforts to be solved. Eur J Neurol. 2009;16(1):10-1.
27. Duna GF, Calabrese L. Limitations of invasive modalities in the diagnosis of primary angiitis of the central nervous system. J Rheumatol. 1995;22(4):662-7.
28. Hajj-Ali RA, Singhal AB, Benseler S, Molloy E, Calabrese LH. Primary angiitis of the CNS. Lancet Neurol. 2011;10(6):561-72.
29. Zuccoli G, Pipitone N, Haldipur A, Brown Jr RD, Hunder G, Salvarani C. Imaging findings in primary central nervous system vasculitis. Clin Exp Rheumatol Suppl. 2011;29(1):S104.
30. Salvarani C, Brown Jr RD, Christianson TJH, Huston III J, Giannini C, Miller DV, et al. Adult primary central nervous system vasculitis treatment and course: analysis of one hundred sixty-three patients. Arthritis Rheumatol. 2015;67(6):1637-45.
31. Salvarani C, Brown Jr RD, Calamia KT, Christianson TJH, Huston III J, Meschia JF, et al. Angiography-negative primary central nervous system vasculitis: a syndrome involving small cerebral vessels. Medicine (Baltimore). 2008;87(5):264-71.
32. Calabrese LH, Furlan AJ, Gragg LA, Ropos T. Primary angiitis of the central nervous system: diagnostic criteria and clinical approach. Cleve Clin J Med. 1992;59(3):293-306.
33. Alrawi A, Trobe JD, Blaivas M, Musch DC. Brain biopsy in primary angiitis of the central nervous system. Neurology. 1999;53(4): 858.
34. Suthiphosuwan S, Bharatha A, Hsu C-T, Lin AW, Maloney JA, Munoz DG, et al. Tumefactive primary central nervous system vasculitis: imaging findings of a rare and underrecognized neuroinflammatory disease. Am J Neuroradiol. 2020;41(11):2075-81.
35. Kleinschmidt-DeMasters BK, Gilden DH. Varicella-zoster virus infections of the nervous system: clinical and pathologic correlates. Arch Pathol Lab Med. 2001;125(6):770-80.
36. Nogueras C, Sala M, Sasal M, Vinas J, Garcia N, Bella M-R, et al. Recurrent stroke as a manifestation of primary angiitis of the central nervous system in a patient infected with human immunodeficiency virus. Arch Neurol. 2002;59(3):468-73.
37. Younger DS. Overview of the vasculitides. Neurol Clin. 2019;37(2): 171-200.
38. Calabrese LH, Duna GF, Lie JT. Vasculitis in the central nervous system. Arthritis Rheum. 1997;40(7):1189-201.
39. Dutra LA, de Souza AWS, Grinberg-Dias G, Barsottini OGP, Appenzeller S. Central nervous system vasculitis in adults: an update. Autoimmun Rev. 2017;16(2):123-31.
40. Calabrese LH, Mallek JA. Primary angiitis of the central nervous system. Report of 8 new cases, review of the literature, and proposal for diagnostic criteria. Medicine (Baltimore). 1988;67(1):20-39.
41. Birnbaum J, Hellmann DB. Primary angiitis of the central nervous system. Arch Neurol. 2009;66(6):704-9.
42. Mukhtyar C, Guillevin L, Cid MC, Dasgupta B, De Groot K, Gross W, et al. EULAR recommendations for the management of primary small and medium vessel vasculitis. Ann Rheum Dis. 2009;68(3): 310-7.
43. De Boysson H, Arquizan C, Touzé E, Zuber M, Boulouis G, Naggara O, et al. Treatment and long-term outcomes of primary central nervous system vasculitis: updated results from the French registry. Stroke. 2018;49(8):1946-52.
44. Beuker C, Strunk D, Rawal R, Schmidt-Pogoda A, Werring N, Milles L, et al. Primary angiitis of the CNS: a systematic review and meta-analysis. Neurol Neuroimmunol Neuroinflamm. 2021;8(6):1-11.
45. Salvarani C, Brown RD, Christianson TJH, Huston J, Giannini C, Hunder GG. Long-term remission, relapses, and maintenance therapy in adult primary central nervous system vasculitis: a single-center 35-year experience. Autoimmun Rev. 2020;19(4):102497.
46. Ribi C, Cohen P, Pagnoux C, Mahr A, Arène JP, Puéchal X, et al. Treatment of polyarteritis nodosa and microscopic polyangiitis without poor-prognosis factors: a prospective randomized study of one hundred twenty-four patients. Arthritis Rheum. 2010;62(4):1186-97.
47. Coronel-Restrepo N, Bonilla-Abadía F, Cortes OA, Izquierdo JH, Shinchi AM, Bravo JC, et al. Primary angiitis of the central nervous system: a report of three cases from a single colombian center. Case Rep Neurol Med. 2013;2013(Figure 1):1-4.
48. Schuster S, Ozga AK, Stellmann JP, Deb-Chatterji M, Häußler V, Matschke J, et al. Relapse rates and long-term outcome in primary angiitis of the central nervous system. J Neurol. 2019;266(6): 1481-9.

55

CHAPTER

Cerebral Venous Thrombosis

Pawan Ojha, Aditya Aundhakar, Arjun Shah, Aamna Maniyar

INTRODUCTION

Even though it is rarer than arterial strokes, cerebral venous thrombosis (CVT) is frequently encountered in developing countries like India, and most often affects younger people, especially women. It commonly presents with a combination of symptoms such as headache, seizures, focal neurological deficits, or coma. The list of underlying etiologies is ever expanding with better access to neuroimaging tools and an efficient evaluation of the hypercoagulable state. Recognizing these is essential, as timely initiation of anti-coagulation can considerably reduce morbidity and mortality.

EPIDEMIOLOGY

Cerebral venous thrombosis affects approximately 5 people per million annually worldwide and accounts for 0.5–1% of all strokes.[1] Most of the studies from India being hospital-based studies, the exact incidence is not known. A study from Portugal reported an incidence of 0.22/100,000/year[2] and another from Netherlands showed an incidence of 1.32/100,000/year.[3]

International Study on Cerebral Vein and Dural Sinus Thrombosis (ISCVT) trial evaluated 624 patients in 24 countries, affected at a median age of 37 years and 74% being females.[4] Similarly, in a large hospital-based cohort published by Narayan et al., the mean age of the patients was also found to be 31.3 years.[5]

According to older data, a higher proportion of women developed CVT as compared to men, female:male ratio being 3:1.[3] This gender bias was presumably due to well-recognized risk factors such as pregnancy, puerperium, usage of oral contraceptives (OCs), and hormone replacement therapy.[6,7] Some later Indian case series did not show the female preponderance.[5,8] In a large prospective study of 612 patients with CVT treated at various hospitals in Mumbai, the male to female ratio was 3:2. This new trend could be due to improved obstetric care.[8]

Seasonal variations in the incidence of CVT are a topic of interest. A Portuguese study showed peak incidence of CVT symptoms in the autumn and winter.[9] In a German study, there was a biphasic distribution with peaks both in summer and winter months.[10] In 2019, a study by Aaron et al. from India found a correlation between a rise in ambient temperature and an increase in the incidence of CVT cases.[11] The risk of CVT was more in women across all seasons. The puerperal period is high-risk period for CVT, but there was no correlation between hot seasons and the occurrence of postpartum CVT. They also found a weak positive correlation with rainfall. However, humidity and cloud cover did not seem to influence the occurrence of CVT.

Recently, an increased incidence of CVT was observed during the coronavirus disease 2019 (COVID-19) pandemic. CVT was also observed more frequently in association with thrombocytopenia with or without antibodies to antigenic complexes platelet factor-4 (PF4) in serum. This was termed vaccine-induced immune thrombotic thrombocytopenia (VITT), and was observed to occur in persons who had recently received the Oxford–AstraZeneca COVID-19 vaccine (ChAdOx1 nCoV-19).[12]

PATHOPHYSIOLOGY

The cerebral venous system can be divided into a superficial and a deep system. The superficial system comprises superior sagittal sinus, inferior sagittal sinus, and cortical veins (including the veins of Trolard and Labbe), which drain the superficial surfaces of both cerebral hemispheres. The deep system consists of the transverse sinus, straight sinus, and sigmoid sinus along with draining deeper cortical veins ultimately returning blood to the heart via the internal jugular veins. **Figure 1** depicts the anatomy of cerebral venous systems.

The risk factors for venous thrombosis can be easily understood about Virchow triad, i.e., stasis of blood, changes in the vessel wall, and changes in the composition

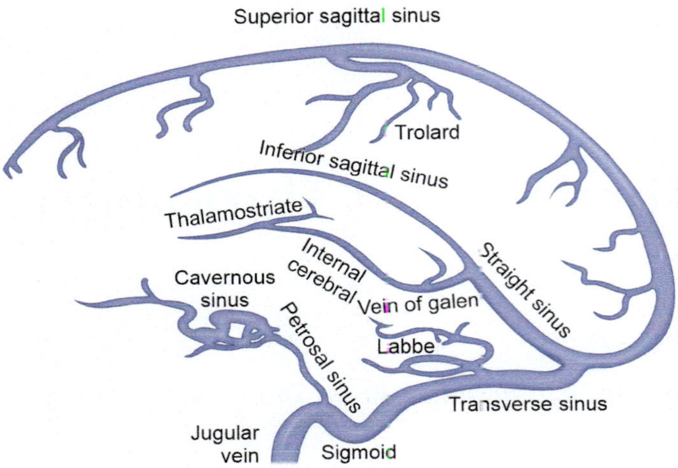

FIG. 1: Anatomy of cerebral venous systems.

of blood. An imbalance between prothrombotic and fibrinolytic processes usually predisposes to progressive venous thrombosis and its sequelae.

Two main pathophysiological mechanisms contribute to CVT:

1. Obstruction of veins causes increased venous pressure, reduced capillary perfusion, and locally increased cerebral blood volume. Initially, this is compensated by dilatation of cerebral veins and the recruitment of collateral vessels; however, continued elevation of venous pressure causes decreased cerebral perfusion pressure and cerebral blood flow resulting in ischemic injury and cytotoxic edema. Disruption of the blood–brain barrier leads to vasogenic edema, and venous and capillary rupture culminates in parenchymal hemorrhage. Thus, both cytotoxic and vasogenic edema can occur.[13]
2. CVT also hampers cerebrospinal fluid absorption through the arachnoid villi, which then leads to raised intracranial pressure (ICP) typically seen in association with superior sagittal sinus obstruction.

ETIOLOGY

The International Study on Cerebral Vein and Dural Sinus Thrombosis found that at least one risk factor can be identified in >85% of patients with CVT. The most common was use of OCs, followed by any prothrombotic condition in 34% of patients. A genetic prothrombotic condition was found in 22% of all patients.[4] Detailed classification and frequency of etiology have been described in **Table 1**.

They commonly included factor V Leiden, G20210A prothrombin gene mutation,[12] as well as antithrombin, protein C and S deficiency. Homozygosity for the C655T MTHFR polymorphism has been reported in approximately 10% of the population. It may predispose to hyperhomocysteinemia, which can lead to thrombosis.[14]

TABLE 1: Risk factor for cerebral venous thrombosis.[4]

Risk factor	%
Gender-specific risk factors:	
• Oral contraceptives use	54.3%
• Pregnancy	13.8%
• Puerperium	6.3%
• Hormonal replacement therapy	4.3%
Systemic conditions:	
• Iron deficiency anemia	9.2%
• Malignancy	7.4%
• Myeloproliferative diseases	2.9%
• Dehydration	1.9%
• Inflammatory bowel disease	1.6%
• Systemic lupus erythematosus	1%
• Behçet's disease	1%
• Thyroid disease	1.7%
• Neurosarcoidosis	0.2%
• Obesity	–
Genetic/acquired prothrombotic condition (thrombophilia):	22.4%/15.7%
• Antiphospholipid antibody syndrome	5.9%
• *MTHFR* gene mutation	4.5%
• Factor V Leiden mutation	–
• Prothrombin gene mutation	–
• Protein S/C deficiency	–
• Antithrombin deficiency	–
• Nephrotic syndrome	0.6%
• Polycythemia/thrombocythemia	–
Infections:	
• *Local*: Otitis, sinusitis, orbital cellulitis, tonsillitis, dental infection, stomatitis, cutaneous cellulitis, abscess, and subdural empyema	8.2%
• *Others*	4.3%
• *Central nervous system*: Meningitis, encephalitis	2.1%
Mechanical factors:	
• Surgery/neurosurgery	2.7%/0.6%
• Lumbar puncture	1.9%
• Head trauma	1.1%
Drugs:	
Cytotoxic	0.8%
Vascular abnormalities:	
• Dural arteriovenous fistulae	1.6%
• Arteriovenous malformations	0.2%
• Other venous abnormalities	0.2%

(MTHFR: methylenetetrahydrofolate reductase)

Pai et al. studied 612 patients from various hospitals of Mumbai for the common thrombophilia markers over a period of 9 years.[8] 18% of patients were positive with protein C deficiency being the most common thrombophilia marker followed by protein S deficiency, Factor V Leiden mutation, and antithrombin III deficiency. In this study, the proportion of genetic prothrombotic state was similar to that reported from developed countries.

The most common acquired prothrombotic states are pregnancy, puerperium, and use of OCs,[15] which explain the increased risk among childbearing women.[16] Antiphospholipid antibody syndrome is also an important treatable cause of CVT.[17] Dehydration increases the risk of CVT. In patients over 55 years of age, CVT is equally prevalent in both sexes,[18] and malignancy is a frequent cause seen in about 25% of patients.

Coronavirus disease 2019 was recently identified to be a risk factor for CVT by causing endothelial injury and prothrombotic state mediated by viral affinity to angiotensin-converting enzyme 2 (ACE2) receptor and various mechanisms. Asymptomatic severe acute respiratory syndrome coronavirus 2 (SARS-CoV-2) infection can be seen in patients with CVT and could be the trigger, especially in the absence of traditional prothrombotic factors.[19]

Other less common causes of CVT include:

- Local infection of ears, sinuses, mouth, face, or neck
- Head injury with trauma to the venous sinuses
- Iron deficiency anemia
- Inflammatory diseases [systemic lupus erythematosus (SLE), Behçet's disease, granulomatosis with polyangiitis, inflammatory bowel disease, and sarcoidosis]
- Hematological disorders (myeloproliferative diseases associated with *JAK2 V617F* mutations, paroxysmal nocturnal hemoglobinuria, and hemoglobinopathies).[20]

CLINICAL FEATURES OF CEREBRAL VENOUS SINUS THROMBOSIS

The clinical presentations of CVT are diverse, ranging from asymptomatic to comatose.[1] A common heuristic is to divide common presentations into three categories:

1. *Intracranial hypertension (IH) syndrome*: It presents with headache, vomiting, and papilledema.
2. *Focal syndrome*: Neurodeficits, seizures, or a mixture of the two
3. *Encephalopathy*: Multifocal signs, altered sensorium, stupor, or even coma. An encephalopathic presentation might be suggestive of deep venous thrombosis.

The pathophysiologic mechanism for the common neurological symptoms is described in **Flowchart 1**, and the symptoms are described in detail here.

Headache

Headache is the most common clinical symptom. According to the ISCVT, 89% of patients had headaches.[4] It can range from a dull, diffuse headache to a severe thunderclap headache that often represents an underlying bleed.

It is usually acute and progresses over hours to days, and can adopt a variety of distributions, including unilateral (in a third), holocranial, bifrontal, or at the vertex, the latter being rarer, but more specific. Raised intracranial pressure (ICP) can cause severe headache, that classically worsens

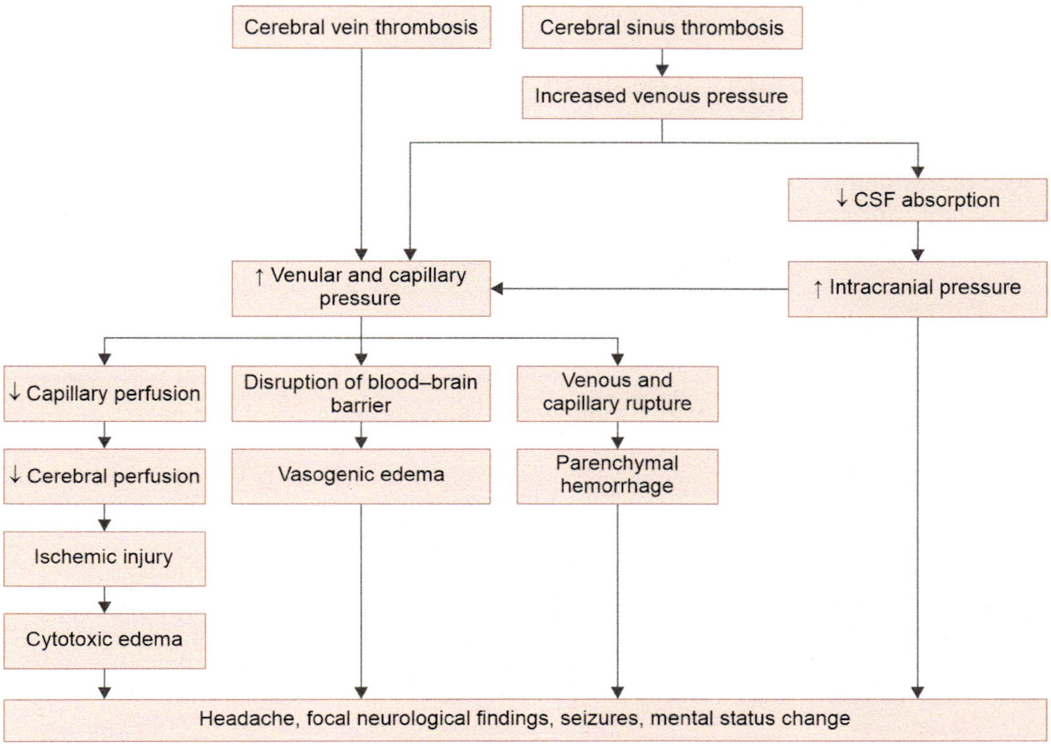

FLOWCHART 1: Pathophysiology of cerebral venous thrombosis.

with Valsalva and lying down.[21] Rarely, the headaches may be more chronic and can be confused with a migraine or tension-type headache.

Raised Intracranial Pressure

Several patients with idiopathic intracranial hypertension (IIH) are eventually diagnosed to have CVT. The clinical features in these patients are headaches and transient visual obscurations.[22] Fundoscopic finding of papilledema is often useful.

Seizures

The presence of seizures is commonplace in CVT. According to the ISCVT study, 39% of patients had seizures at onset and 7% after the diagnosis was made.[2] The seizures can be focal or generalized. Seizures are more likely to occur in supratentorial CVST sagittal sinus thrombosis, cortical vein thrombosis, and secondary bleeds.

New onset of seizures, in the presence of focal deficits, should prompt one to evaluate for the possibility of cerebral venous sinus thrombosis (CVST).

Focal Syndrome

This can be in the form of monoparesis, hemiparesis, or even quadriparesis. In the ISCVT study, 37% of patients had focal motor weakness. An aphasia may also be present, especially with left lateral sinus thrombosis. Although rare, sensory and visual deficits are also known to occur.

Encephalopathy

When severe, CVT can lead to loss of consciousness, altered sensorium, delirium, stupor, or even coma. Dysexecutive syndromes with seizures can also be seen. Multiple sinus thrombosis and deep vein thrombosis (DVT) can present this way. Drowsiness or stupor can arise from bilateral thalamic involvement or obstructive hydrocephalus.

Special Syndromes

- *Sagittal sinus syndrome* can present with bilateral motor deficits, or also as an isolated IIH.
- *Lateral sinus thrombosis* can present with isolated headaches, seizures, and, if the involvement of the dominant hemisphere, an aphasia.[23]
- Isolated cortical vein thrombosis can present with motor or sensory deficits or even seizures.[24]
- Deep cerebral vein thrombosis might be asymptomatic or even present with mental alterations. Occlusion of the *vein of Galen* can produce a most bizarre syndrome of inattention, spatial neglect, and amnesias, sometimes severe enough to cause an apathetic state. It can present as a bi-thalamic infarct.
- Since there is considerable variation in the anatomy of the deep cerebral veins, the presenting features are highly variable. However, one must note the possibilities of language disorders and aphasia in the *vein of Labbe* thrombosis. *Vein of Trolard* may also present with deficits attributed to the frontoparietal region including limb weakness or temporal lobe, including behavioral changes.[25]
- Jugular vein thrombosis can have pulsatile tinnitus or even present with multiple cranial nerve palsies, in concert with lateral sinus and the posterior fossa veins.

When the brain lesions or deficits do not respect arterial territories, it should alert one to the possibility of CVT.

DIAGNOSIS

Whenever the above-mentioned symptoms are seen to occur suddenly either singly or in combination, a diagnosis of CVT should be considered. The diagnosis of CVT can be confirmed by urgent neuroimaging.[26] The imaging findings can be categorized as:

- Direct visualization of cortical or dural sinus thrombus
- Indirect ischemic changes related to the venous outflow disturbance.

Cranial computed tomography (CT) is usually the first investigation in the emergency department, and it can at times reveal cerebral venous hyperdensity in patients with CVT. It could be normal in about 30% of patients and, even if abnormal, is not specific.[1,27] All patients with suspected CVT need to be confirmed with further imaging. The European Stroke Organization (ESO) guidelines suggest magnetic resonance venography (MRV) or CT venography (CTV) for confirming the diagnosis.[26] CT venography is done with an intravenous contrast agent and shows absent flow in thrombosed veins or sinuses and partial circumferential enhancement of thrombosed venous sinuses.

Certain specific signs seen on CT scans in CVT patients are enumerated below and in **Table 2**:

- *Dense triangle sign*: Noncontrast head CT shows a fresh thrombus in the posterior part of the sagittal sinus in a triangle shape.[28]
- *Cord sign*: Head CT with contrast shows hyperdense thrombosed cortical vein.[29]
- *Empty triangle or empty delta sign*: It is seen as nonfilling of the confluence of sinuses after contrast injection.[30]

  Contrast-enhanced CT scan also reveals indirect signs such as:
  - Local or generalized brain swelling
  - Enhancement of the falx and tentorium
  - Localized hypodense or hyperdense areas reflecting hemorrhagic transformation

Magnetic resonance imaging (MRI) is the most sensitive technique for demonstrating the presence of the thrombus. MR time-of-flight (TOF) venography is performed with TOF sequences which allow to assess the absence of flow in thrombosed sinuses, without the need for contrast medium[33] **(Figs. 5A to D)**. Contrast-enhanced MR venography is done using gadolinium-contrast agent.

Magnetic resonance imaging sequences can be used to date the likely onset of CVT because the appearance of the clot varies depending on its age as follows:

- *<1 week*: Isointense on T1 and hypointense in T2W images
- *1–2 weeks*: Hyperintense on T1 and T2W images
- *>2 weeks*: Variable on T1 and T2, hypointense in gradient-echo (GRE) and susceptibility-weighted imaging (SWI)

Magnetic resonance imaging is also the best technique to assess parenchymal involvement such as ischemia, hemorrhage, edema, or swelling **(Figs. 6A to C)**. Diffusion-weighted imaging (DWI)-hyperintense thrombosed sinuses have a reduced rate of recanalization.[34] According to the Indian guidelines for stroke management, MRI/MRV/CTV should only be done if the plain CT scan is negative in a patient with suspected CVT.[35] The venography was also recommended to define the extent of CVT, if the plain CT or MRI suggests the presence of a CVT.[36]

Cerebral catheter angiography is a technique rarely used to confirm CVT only when CT or MR venography is not diagnostic. It is also done in suspicious cases of dural arteriovenous fistula (dAVF).[26,36] A dAVF can rarely complicate CVT, which is presumed due to the opening of arteriovenous pathways in the wall of the sinus during occlusion or recanalization.

TABLE 2: Radiological (CT) signs in CVT.

Signs	CT brain
Cord sign **(Fig. 2)**	Curvilinear or linear hyperdensity from a thrombosed cortical vein typically found over the cerebral cortex
Dense clot sign Or Dense vessel sign Or Dense vein sign **(Fig. 3)**	Direct visualization of a clot in the cerebral veins on a non-enhanced CT scan
Empty delta sign[30,31] **(Fig. 4)**	Triangular pattern of contrast enhancement surrounding a central region without enhancement found in the posterior part of superior sagittal sinus
Dense triangle sign[32]	Triangular or round hyperdensity reflecting a thrombosed sinus on a cross-sectional view

(CT: computed tomography)

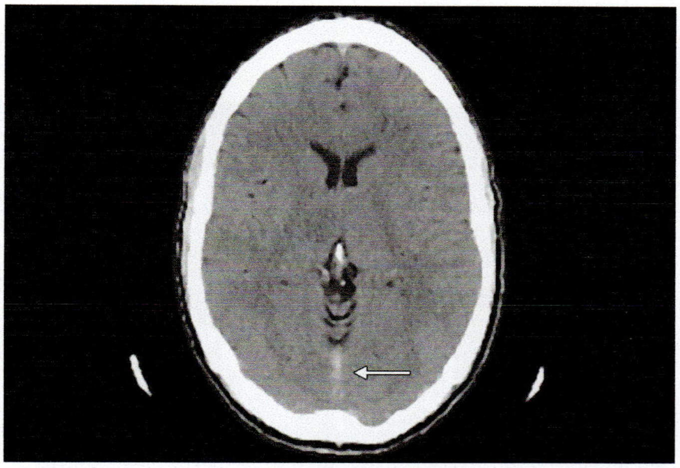

FIG. 2: A plain CT showing a hyperdense acute thrombus (arrow) in the occluded straight sinus: cord sign or dense sign.

(CT: computed tomography)

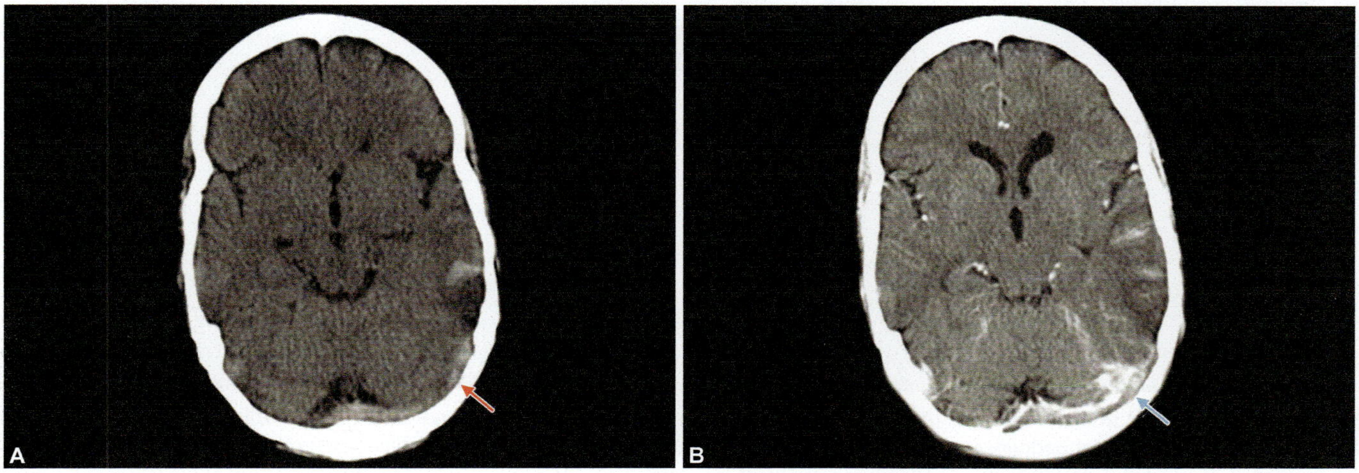

FIGS. 3A AND B: The image on the left is a nonenhanced CT brain image showing a dense thrombus within the transverse sinus. On the enhanced CT brain image on the right, there is a filling defect that can be seen in the transverse sinus.

(CT: computed tomography)

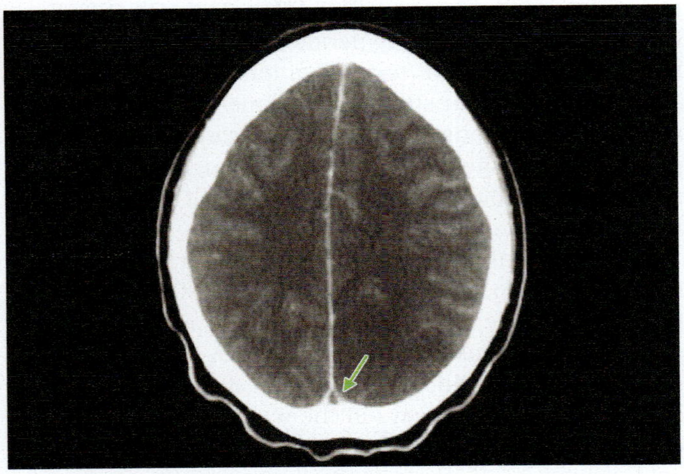

FIG. 4: Head CT with contrast, showing filling defect—empty delta sign.
(CT: computed tomography)

There is no laboratory test that can comprehensively rule in or rule out acute CVT. D-dimer level measurement could be used as a screening tool for the assessment of patients with possible CVT. It has a high negative predictive value (NPV) for excluding CVT in patients with isolated headache.[37] Therefore, it has been suggested as a component of a preimaging probability score, along with a normal neurological examination and CT scan of the head, to avoid unnecessary neuroimaging.[38] However, a normal D-dimer cannot rule out CVT especially in mild or chronic cases.[37,39] Misra et al. studied 26 patients with CVT proven by MRV. The sensitivity and specificity of D dimer in the diagnosis were 77% each, respectively.[40]

Routine blood studies including erythrocyte sedimentation rate, blood count, chemistry panel, prothrombin time, and activated partial thromboplastin time are recommended, ideally to be done before starting anticoagulation treatment.

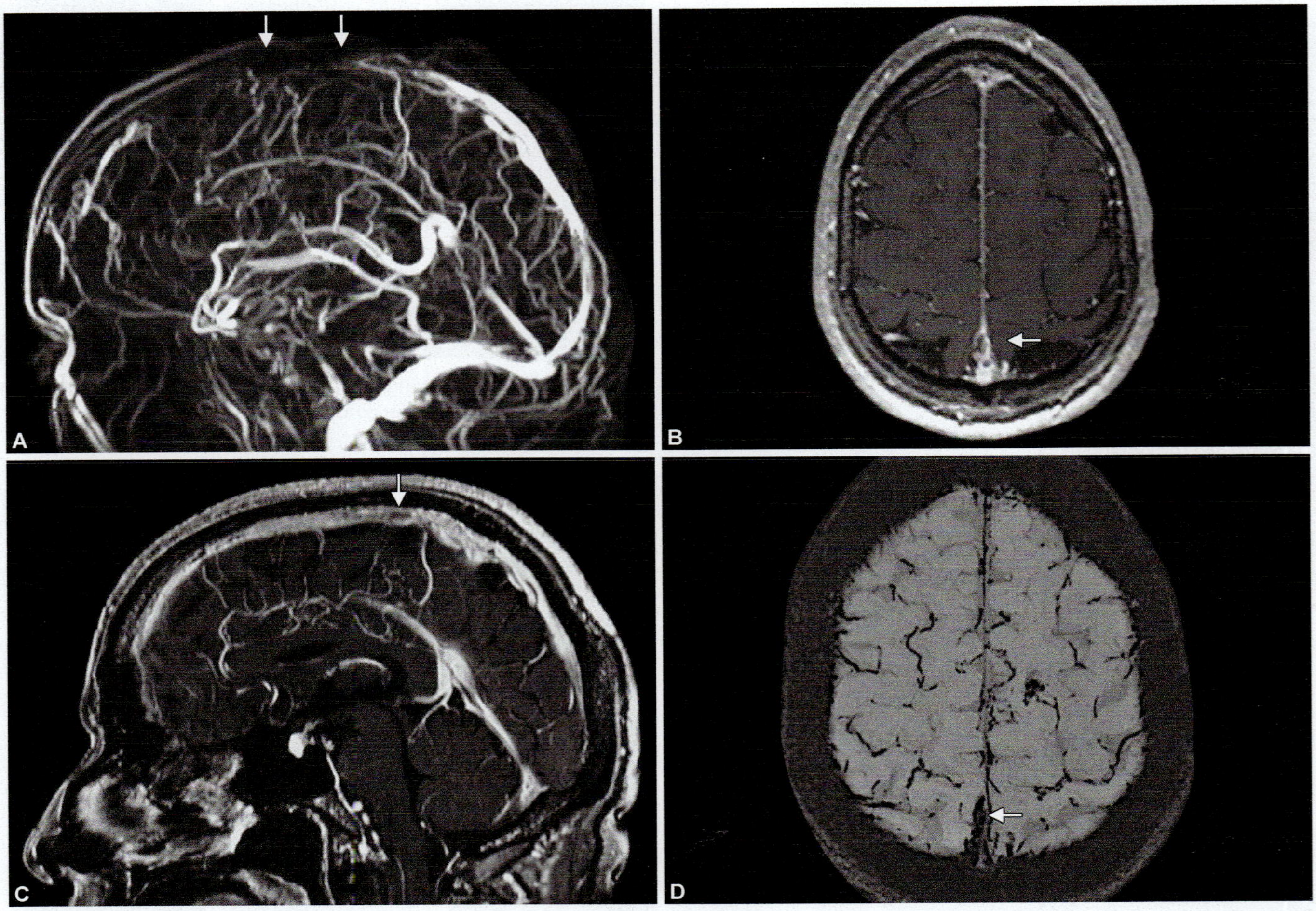

FIGS. 5A TO D: Sagittal sinus thrombosis. (A) MR venogram showing absent venous flow signal in the middle third of the superior sagittal sinus (white arrows); (B) Axial gadolinium-enhanced T1-weighted MR scan showing an irregular filling defect of the superior sagittal sinus (white arrow); (C) Sagittal gadolinium-enhanced T1-weighted MR scan also showing a focal filling defect indicating thrombus (white arrow); (D) Axial susceptibility-weighted imaging showing low signal indicating blood products (thrombus) in the superior sagittal sinus (white arrow).
(MR: magnetic resonance)

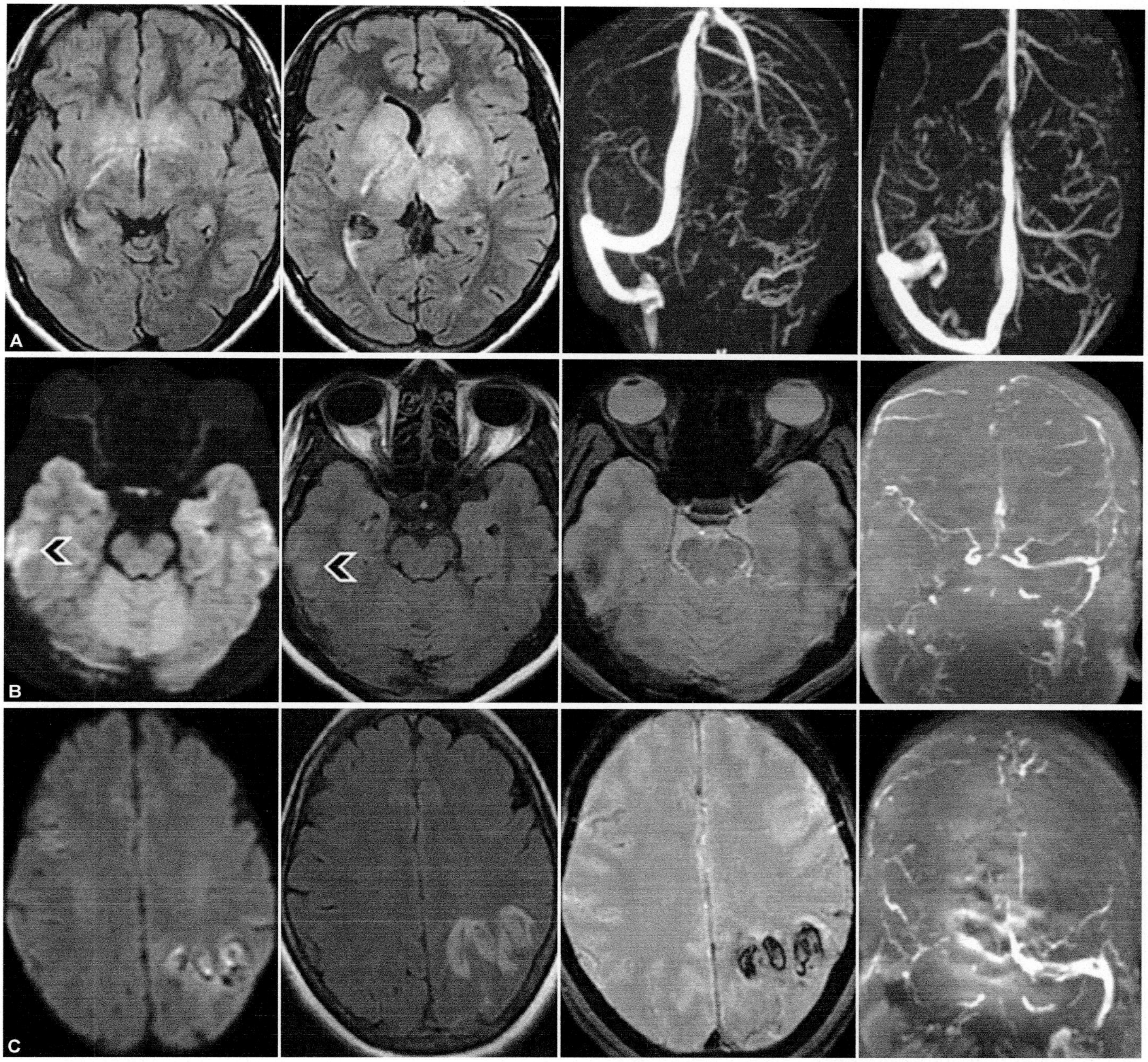

FIGS. 6A TO C: (A) FLAIR Axial and Venogram: Infarcts in the Deep Nuclei and Deep Vein and Left Sigmoid Sinus Thrombosis. (B) DWI, FLAIR, and GRE Axial Brain and Venogram: Right Lateral Temporal Infarct with Superior Sagittal and Right Transverse Sinus Thrombosis. (C) DWI, FLAIR, and GRE Axial Brain and Venogram: Left Frontoparietal Hemorrhagic Infarct with Superior Sagittal Sinus Thrombosis.
(DWI: diffusion-weighted image; FLAIR: fluid-attenuation inversion recovery; GRE: gradient echo)

Evaluation for a thrombophilic state should be done in CVT patients with a high probability of thrombophilia. This includes patients with:

- Personal and/or family history of venous thrombosis
- CVT at a young age
- CVT in the absence of a risk factor

Acute thrombosis transiently decreases the levels of antithrombin, protein C and S, so the utility of these tests in the acute phase of CVT is limited. Hence, it is recommended to conduct screening tests for inherited thrombophilia at least 2 weeks after oral anticoagulation has been discontinued. This is because warfarin reduces the protein C and protein S levels and may increase plasma antithrombin levels in patients with hereditary antithrombin deficiency. One can test for acquired thrombophilia, i.e., antiphospholipid antibodies in the acute phase of CVT, but it requires reconfirmation in later stages.

A practical approach to diagnosis is given in **Flowchart 2.**

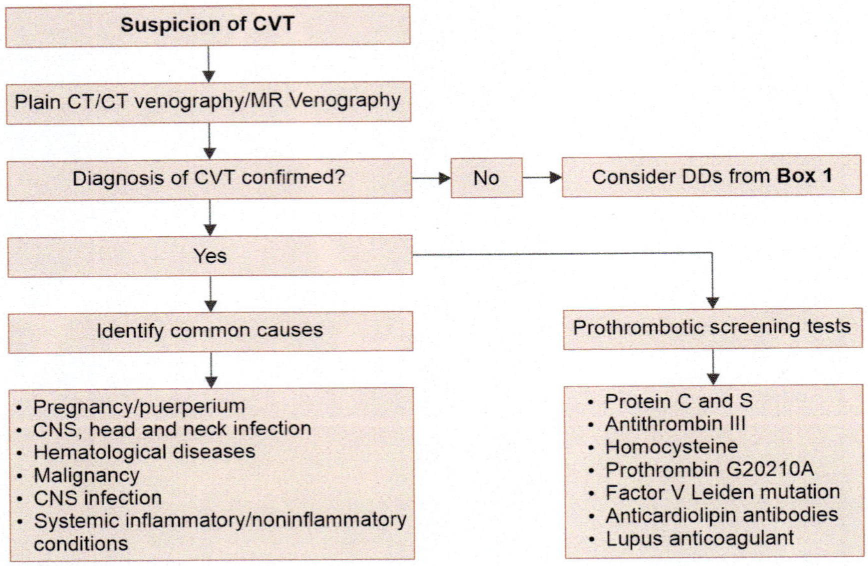

FLOWCHART 2: Approach to diagnosis of CVT.
(CNS: central nervous system; CT: computed tomography; CVT: cerebral venous thrombosis; MR: magnetic resonance)

DIFFERENTIAL DIAGNOSIS

The diagnosis of CVT can be challenging at times as the symptoms and signs often overlap with conditions that could range from migraine and meningitis to brain tumor. It could be worthwhile to use a prediction score to help arrive at the diagnosis. One such score is based on a prospective, multicenter study (2020)[41] that included consecutive patients with possible CVT. This clinical score is as follows:

1. Any (focal and/or generalized) seizure(s) at presentation (4 points)
2. Known thrombophilia (including hematological disease) (4 points)
3. Oral contraception (2 points)
4. Duration of symptoms >6 days (2 points)
5. Worst headache ever (patient reported) (1 point)
6. Focal neurological deficit at presentation (1 point)

The CVT was confirmed in 25.8% of patients. A low CVT probability score was defined as 0–2 points and had an NPV of 94.1%. The frequency of CVT increased with a higher clinical probability score. The best CVT prediction score was achieved by also adding D-dimer levels (>500 ng/mL fibrinogen equivalent units) to the clinical score: sensitivity—89.4% and specificity—66.4%.[41]

An approach to the differential diagnosis of CVT is suggested in **Box 1**.

MANAGEMENT OF CVST

Standard Therapy

Low-molecular-weight heparin (LMWH) or unfractionated heparin (UFH) is typically used during the initial phase for a few days, followed by the use of oral anticoagulants as continuation therapy. The European guidelines recommend treating acute CVT with heparin (LMWH being preferred to UFH) at therapeutic dosage, even in patients with an intracerebral hemorrhage at baseline, followed by vitamin K antagonists (VKAs) for a period of 3–12 months.[36,26]

Low-molecular-weight Heparin and Unfractionated Heparin

Research conducted in the 1990s showed that heparin treatment was effective, as proven by three small randomized trials.[42-44] Both types of heparins, LMWH and UFH, can be used to treat CVT, but some experts suggest that LMWH is generally more effective. However, if the patient requires surgical intervention, then UFH is better, as it can be easily halted and reversed.[45,46] In 2012, Misra et al. conducted a study comparing the effectiveness and safety of LMWH and UFH in CVT. The group that received UFH had a higher death rate ($p = 0.01$).[47]

A large multicenter study involving different countries found that patients treated with LMWH had a better outcome after 6 months. Those treated with LMWH were less likely to experience new intracranial bleeding, better appreciated in patients with intracranial lesions at baseline (adjusted odds ratio 0.19; CI 0.04–0.99).[45]

Vitamin K Antagonists

Vitamin K antagonists were used as the default oral anticoagulation of choice since their introduction in the 1960s.[48] There was never any controlled study for their efficacy, but these are consensus guideline-approved therapies.[49]

BOX 1 Approach to differential diagnosis of CVST.

A. **Syndrome of presentation with severe headaches:**
1. *Headache associated with vascular disorders:*
   - RCVS
   - Subarachnoid hemorrhage
   - Acute ischemic cerebrovascular disorder
   - Unruptured vascular malformation
   - Arteritis (e.g., temporal arteritis)
   - Carotid or vertebral artery pain
   - Arterial hypertension
2. *Headache associated with nonvascular intracranial disorder:*
   - Benign intracranial hypertension (pseudotumor cerebri)
   - Intracranial infection
   - Low cerebrospinal fluid pressure (e.g., headache subsequent to lumbar puncture)

B. **Syndrome of presentation with altered mental status (AMS):**
1. *AMS with CNS neoplasms:*
   - Primary CNS neoplasm
   - CNS metastasis
2. *AMS with CNS infections:*
   - Meningitis
   - Encephalitis
3. *AMS with cerebrovascular disease:*
   - Intracranial hemorrhage
   - Ischemic stroke
   - Hypertensive encephalopathy
4. *AMS with seizures:*
   - Seizures may be idiopathic (epilepsy)
   - Secondary to structural abnormalities, metabolic alterations, or drug intoxication/withdrawal
5. *AMS with metabolic abnormalities:*
   - Electrolyte abnormalities:
     - Hyponatremia
     - Hypernatremia
     - Hypercalcemia
   - Endocrine abnormalities:
     - Hypoglycemia
     - Hyperglycemia
     - Hypothyroidism
     - Hyperthyroidism
   - Hepatic or renal failure
   - Alcohol withdrawal

C. **Syndrome of presentation with focal neurological deficit:**
1. *Hemorrhage:*
   - Intracranial hemorrhage
   - Subarachnoid hemorrhage
   - Subdural hemorrhage
2. *Ischemic stroke*

(CNS: central nervous system; CVST: cerebral venous sinus thrombosis; RCVS: reversible cerebral vasoconstriction syndrome)

VKAs have a very narrow therapeutic range and significant interactions with food and drugs, this leads to difficulties with drug compliance. The duration of treatment continuation has been addressed below under the heading of Duration of continuing oral anticoagulation.

Vitamin K Antagonists versus Direct Oral Anticoagulants

Direct oral anticoagulants (DOACs) were introduced into practice in 2010 and have been compared in detail to the established standard of care, i.e., VKAs. Bose G et al. (2020) conducted a systematic review of 33 studies that met the inclusion criteria for evaluating the use of DOACs for CVT. The observational cohorts showed no significant difference in the risk of death between the DOAC and standard therapy groups (RR 2.12; 95% CI 0.29–15.59). A favorable modified Rankin Scale (mRS) between 0 and 2 was reported in 94% of DOAC-treated patients, which was more likely than standard therapy in observational cohorts (RR 1.13; 95% CI 1.02–1.25). The study suggests that DOACs are safe and effective for treating CVT, despite some variability in the timing and dose of treatment used across different studies.[50]

Another meta-analysis of 17 studies, that include those studies with or without a control group using VKAs, found that the occurrence of complete recanalization was more likely in the group of patients treated with DOACs compared to the group treated with VKAs. DOACs are preferable as they have a better safety profile and predictable pharmacokinetics than VKA. DOACs do not require regular monitoring of the INR, and they have a lower rate of intracranial hemorrhage. They have fewer interactions with other drugs and food.[51]

The ACTION-CVT study was a multicenter retrospective analysis of patients with CVT treated with oral anticoagulation between January 2015 and December 2020. The study aimed to compare DOACs to warfarin in a real-world CVT cohort.[52] They included 845 patients, among them, 33.0% received DOAC only, 51.8% received warfarin only, and 15.1% received both treatments at different times. The median follow-up was 345 days. The study found that DOAC treatment was associated with a similar risk of recurrent venous thrombosis [aHR 0.94 (95% CI 0.51–1.73); $p = 0.84$], death [aHR 0.78 (95% CI 0.22–2.76); $p = 0.70$], and rate of partial/complete recanalization [aOR 0.92 (95% CI 0.48–1.73); $p = 0.79$], but a lower risk of major hemorrhage [aHR 0.35 (95% CI 0.15–0.82); $p = 0.02$] when compared to warfarin. DOACs had similar clinic-radiographic outcomes but a more favorable safety profile when compared to warfarin.[52]

In RESPECT-CVT trial, which randomized 120 patients with CVT to dabigatran versus warfarin for 24 weeks, the patients did not show significant differences in efficacy and safety outcomes between the two treatment groups. There were no recurrent thromboembolic events, there was one case of major bleeding with dabigatran, and two cases of subdural hemorrhages with warfarin.[53] The DOAC-CVT study is ongoing to compare the safety and efficacy of DOACs compared to VKAs.[54]

Which DOAC is better: Head-to-head trials of different DOACs are missing in the treatment of CVT. However, comparative data on DOACs can also be partially inferred from previous trials on DVT, pulmonary embolism (PE), and atrial fibrillation (AF), as well as from the known characteristics of each DOAC. For patients with a history of gastrointestinal bleeding, apixaban or low-dose edoxaban may be preferred as they have been shown to have a similar or lower incidence of gastrointestinal bleeding compared to warfarin.[55] Rivaroxaban or edoxaban may be prescribed for patients who prefer once-daily dosing.[56] Dabigatran should be avoided for patients with a history of myocardial infarction.[57] A European Union-wide review has suggested that DOACs should be avoided in patients with the antiphospholipid syndrome (APS) as there might be an increased risk of recurrence of thrombotic events as compared to treatment with VKAs.[58]

Anticoagulation in the background of parenchymal hemorrhage: According to the findings from ISCVT, where 83% of patients were treated with heparin, the risk of new or increasing cerebral hemorrhages is low, but cannot be dismissed. However, the risk of not using anticoagulants is an enlarging thrombus, which could cause more venous infarcts.[59]

Ideal timing for initiating DOACs: The ideal timing for initiating DOACs is uncertain. Most studies have used LMWH or UFH before starting DOACs, with only a few studies using DOACs directly. However, the optimal timing and duration of DOAC therapy for CVT are still unclear and further research is needed to establish the best practice.

Duration of continuing oral anticoagulation: In the meta-analysis by Nepal G et al., the duration of DOAC anti-coagulation ranged from 3 months to indefinite, with the majority of studies reporting anticoagulation duration of 6–12 months. Due to the nonuniformity of the data, the optimal duration of anticoagulation in CVT remains inconclusive.[51] According to literature on DVT and PE caused by known temporary risk factors (provoked), a short course of anticoagulation (3–6 months) is typically recommended. Whereas, for patients with DVT and/or PE caused by chronic risk factors or unprovoked DVT and/or PE, anticoagulation therapy should be continued indefinitely. However, for a select group of patients who have chronic risk factors that are expected to improve over time, a longer course of anticoagulation (6–12 months) is prescribed.[60,61] It is assumed that these principles may potentially apply to CVT.

An ongoing prospective study, Benefit of EXtending oral antiCOAgulant treatment after Cerebral Vein and Dural Sinus Thrombosis (EXCOA-CVT), is comparing the effectiveness of short-term (3–6 months) versus long-term (12 months) oral anticoagulation therapy in preventing VTE (venous thromboembolism) after an episode of CVT. This study is part of the larger ISCVT2 project, which is a multinational collaboration aimed at improving the diagnosis, treatment, and prevention of CVT.[62]

Hence, the question regarding the duration of anti-coagulation remains unanswered till now, with the author suggesting a case-by-case approach to the duration of DOACs.

Neurointervention in CVST

Most patients have a positive outcome after being treated with anticoagulation. However, a clinical worsening despite anticoagulants can occur in one-fourth of CVT patients and may warrant additional treatments, such as intravascular thrombolysis or thrombectomy. **Box 2** enumerates indications for neurointervention. Intravascular thrombolysis treatment can be achieved by a combination of chemical and mechanical methods.

In a study by Li et al. (2013), 52 patients with severe CVT were treated using a combination of mechanical thrombectomy (MT) and injecting urokinase into the cerebral venous sinus. The results showed that 87% of the patients had complete recanalization, 6% had partial recanalization, and 7% had no recanalization. Six patients died, but the remaining patients had a good functional outcome at discharge, 3-month, and 6-month follow-up. The authors concluded that this treatment method is safe and effective for severe CVT that does not respond to anticoagulation therapy.[63]

Siddiqui et al. (2015) conducted a systematic analysis of 185 CVT patients in 42 different studies, where all patients underwent MT. These studies have shown that a combination of MT and chemical thrombolysis can lead to high recanalization rates and good functional outcomes. However, it is important to note that this treatment option requires clinical expertise and specialized equipment and may not be widely available in resource-limited settings. Additionally, there is a small risk of complications such as new bleeding during the perioperative period.[64]

BOX 2 Indications for neurointervention.

1. *Clinical worsening (one or more of the following):*
   - GCS <8 or decline in GCS from that at admission
   - The development or worsening of focal neurological deficits
   - New or recurrent seizures
2. *Worsening intracranial hypertension (IH) (one or more of the following):*
   - *Persistent symptoms of IH*: Severe headache, prolonged vomiting, slow heart rate, and high blood pressure
   - Repeat imaging showing increasing cerebral edema or venous infarct-related mass effect
3. Deep venous system thrombosis (straight sinus, vein of Galen, and internal cerebral veins)
4. Any contraindication to systemic anticoagulation such as severe thrombocytopenia, active systemic bleeding, or bleeding tendencies

(GCS: Glasgow Coma Scale)

A recent prospective study by Alwan A et al. (2023) from CMC, Vellore found that among 546 patients treated at their center for CVT during the study period, 10% (57 patients) required MT. Hemorrhagic venous infarction was seen in 50% of patients who received MT. The average time between starting medical treatment and receiving MT was 43 hours, and the most common indication for MT was clinical deterioration. A small number of patients (9%) required decompressive hemicraniectomy. The mortality rate at discharge was 5% and at the last follow-up visit was 7%. This study found that younger patients without hemorrhagic venous infarction and those whose frontoparietal lobes were not affected had the best outcomes. At discharge, 65% of patients had a favorable functional outcome as measured by the mRS, which improved to 77% at 1-year follow-up. They conclude that in a subset of patients with severe CVT who have clinical deterioration despite optimal medical management, the use of a technique called balloon-assisted MT is safe and effective.[65]

Role of Lumbar Puncture for Therapeutic Reduction of Raised Intracranial Pressure

The 75% of CVT patients who received therapeutic lumbar puncture (LP) had favorable outcomes in a prospective study.[22] However, in another study, there was no difference in outcomes (worsening, death or dependency at 6 months, or complete recovery) between patients with or without therapeutic LP.[4] Hence, available data is not enough to make a specific recommendation regarding the use of therapeutic LP as a treatment for improving outcomes in patients with CVT and signs of IH.

Role of Glucocorticoids

One prospective nonrandomized study showed that steroids were associated with worse outcomes and not recommended in general. However, they may be used in rare conditions such as SLE or Behçet's disease to treat the underlying disorder.[66]

Role of Acetazolamide and Diuretics

There is very limited nonrandomized data in the form of case series, hence is not recommended, but in isolated IH with severe headache or threatening vision, acetazolamide may be considered if the safety profile is acceptable.[36]

Role of Decompressive Surgery in the Management of Cerebral Edema

Cerebral edema can occur as a complication of CVT, either at presentation or after treatment with anticoagulation and can lead to a transtentorial herniation, which can be fatal if not treated promptly. This is often referred to as malignant CVT. In this clinical scenario, along with other standard therapies for raised ICT, such as head elevation, hypertonic saline, hyperventilation, and ICP monitoring, decompressive surgery may be lifesaving. Théaudin et al. (2010) conducted a study of 12 patients with malignant CVT. They found that all 4 patients who did not undergo decompressive surgery died. Of the remaining 8 patients, 6 had a good prognosis (mRS: 0–1) and one had an mRS of 3. One patient died of a PE after surgery. The study suggests that even in patients with bilateral pupil dilation, decompressive surgery may provide a meaningful benefit. The authors recommend that decompressive surgery should be considered in patients with malignant CVT who exhibit continuous and progressive symptoms, despite the presence of bilateral dilated pupils.[67]

In a retrospective case analysis conducted by Mahale et al. (2017), 30 patients with malignant CVT underwent decompressive craniectomy. They found that more than two-thirds of the patients had a good prognosis after the surgery. Factors associated with poor prognosis include patients >50 years old, those with a midline shift >10 mm, and those in which the basilar cistern had disappeared. These factors should be taken into consideration when deciding whether to perform decompressive craniectomy in patients with malignant CVT.[68]

The DECOMPRESS2 study was a large prospective study of decompressive surgery for CVT patients. The results revealed that two-thirds patients survived and one-third were independent at a follow-up of 1 year after decompressive surgery. The conclusion was that patients who have malignant CVT and large hemispheric lesions should undergo decompression surgery as soon as possible.[69]

An overview of the treatment algorithm is given in **Flowchart 3**.

Role of Antiepileptic Drugs for Preventing Seizures

There is currently a lack of well-designed randomized controlled trials regarding the primary or secondary prevention of seizures in CVST. Treatment decisions, including timing, type, dosage, and duration, are often individualized and based on expert opinion. A study by Coutinho et al. found large variations in the use of prophylactic antiepileptic drugs (AEDs) among experts, with 8% initiating prophylactic AED in all patients, 21% prescribing prophylactic therapy only in patients with focal cerebral lesions, and the remaining 71% not recommending prophylaxis.[70]

Based on current data, prophylactic treatment with AEDs is not recommended for patients without focal neurologic deficits or supratentorial lesions, as it may be harmful in these cases, as stated in the European Stroke Organization/European Academy of Neurology (ESO/EAN) and American Heart Association/American

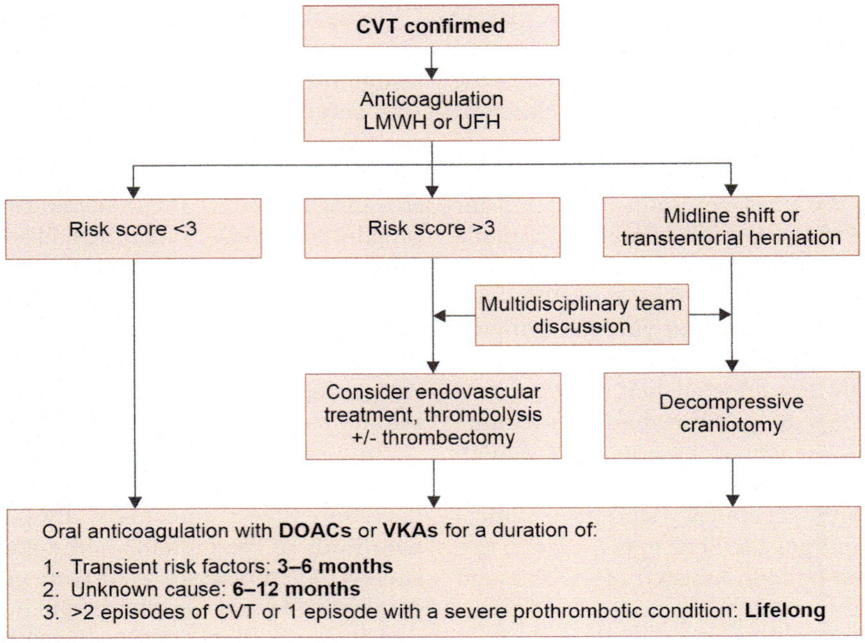

*Note: Risk score is as per Ferro JM et al.[71] outlined in **Table 3** of the text.*

FLOWCHART 3: Treatment algorithm for CVT.

(CVT: cerebral venous thrombosis; DOAC: direct oral anticoagulants; LMWH: low-molecular-weight heparin; UFH: unfractionated heparin; VKA: vitamin K antagonist)

Stroke Association (AHA/ASA) guidelines. The AHA/ASA guidelines also suggest that in patients with CVST and no supratentorial lesion or focal neurological deficits who experience a seizure, early initiation of AEDs for a defined period is probably recommended to prevent further seizures, but ESO/EAN guidelines do not provide recommendations for these subsets of patient.[26,36]

There is no consensus about the duration of treatment for post- CVST epilepsy (PCE). PCE commonly occurs within the first 6–12 months after the acute stage, treatment with AEDs for 1 year is recommended for patients with CVST and previously indicated risk factors. However, in patients without these risk factors who have received AED therapy, a gradual taper of AEDs after the acute stage seems reasonable with an approximate duration of 3 months. If seizures recur during or after drug tapering, a continuation of antiepileptic treatment for another 1–2 years or more is recommended. It should be noted that treatment with AEDs in the acute phase has no role in the prevention of PCE and, therefore, according to ESO/EAN guidelines, no recommendations can be made for the prevention of PCE at this time.[26]

There is no consensus on the most appropriate type and dosage of AEDs for PCE seizures. It is reasonable to select an AED with fewer drug interactions, similar to the treatment approach for seizures accompanying comorbidity. Injectable forms of levetiracetam, lacosamide, and probably sodium valproate should be considered for preventing further seizures in the acute phase.

PROGNOSIS OF CVST

In the acute situation, CVT has a good complete functional recovery in about 75% of patients.[4] The risk factors for a poor outcome, i.e., death or being dependent are the presence of malignancy, altered mental status, involvement of deeper veins, male gender, and intracranial hemorrhage. **Table 3** enumerates a risk score given by Ferro JM et al.[71] There may be some long-term sequelae in the form of depression, anxiety, headaches, or cognitive impairments as enumerated previously.

Long-term sequelae of CVT:

- *Headache, fatigue, depression, and concentration impairment*: In a long-term study (63 months follow-up), 75% of CVT patients reported impairment of mental concentration, 43% had headache, 30% were depressive, and 30% experienced fatigue, more frequently reported by patients than control subjects.[72] Up to 21% of previously employed patients were unable to work, and 34% found it difficult to work.
- *Late-onset seizures*: About 34% have early symptomatic seizures. Factors predicting early symptomatic seizures were sensory deficits and a parenchymal lesion on admission in neuroimaging. Up to 9.5% of patients had late seizures, which were more frequent in patients with early symptomatic seizures and who had a hemorrhage on admission. Pharmacological prevention should be limited to patients with early symptomatic seizures and cerebral lesions on admission in neuroimaging.[73]

TABLE 3: Risk score for CVT.[72]

Prognostic variable	Risk points
Malignancy	2
Coma	2
Deep venous thrombosis	2
Mental status disturbances	2
Male sex	1
Intracranial hemorrhage	1
<3: Low risk of poor outcome	
≥3: High risk of poor outcome	

(CVT: cerebral venous thrombosis)

- *Intracranial hypertension*: IH occurs in around 10% of patients after CVST and that patients with visual disturbances seem to be at higher risk for developing IH. Patients with IH after CVST were less likely to have recanalization of the occluded vessel on follow-up MRI.[74]
- *Dural arteriovenous fistula*: dAVF can be seen as complication of CVT on follow-up and requires a catheter angiogram for confirmation and it requires treatment with endovascular embolization. The formation of dAVF is postulated to be linked to CVT and may be related to changes in intracranial pressure and venous drainage pattern. The development of dAVF after 6 months of acute CVT is rare.[75,76]

SPECIAL POPULATIONS

Treatment of CVST in Pregnancy and Lactation

The standard treatment in the hyperacute phase is anticoagulation using LMWH in subcutaneous form or intravenous UFH. Both LMWH and UFH are considered safe during pregnancy, but UFH has been associated with increased risk of fetal bleeding and teratogenicity. After the hyperacute phase, oral anticoagulation is generally indicated, but VKAs and DOACs are contraindicated during pregnancy due to their potential to cross the placenta and cause neurodevelopmental disorders and fetal bleeding. Therefore, LMWH is continued in pregnant CVT patients after the hyperacute phase. There are no studies assessing the optimal duration of anticoagulation in pregnant CVT patients, but therapeutic LMWH is typically continued for at least 6 weeks postpartum. LMWH is the gold standard during breastfeeding as it does not transfer easily into breastmilk. UFH and warfarin are also acceptable during lactation, while DOACs should be avoided as no clinical data is available about their safety during lactation. Patients with recurrent VTEs or an associated prothrombotic condition with high thrombotic risk may need lifelong oral anticoagulation with VKAs. It is important to note that a medical history of CVT alone is not considered a contraindication for future pregnancies.[77] In a subsequent pregnancy, the risk of recurrent CVT is 80-fold higher and that of other VTE is 16-fold higher as compared to the general population.[78] Prophylaxis with LMWH during future pregnancies and 8 weeks post-partum is recommended.[66]

Treatment of CVT in Children

Cerebral venous thrombosis in children is treated on similar lines as that of adults. In 2022, the EINSTEIN-Jr trial study evaluated the safety and efficacy of rivaroxaban and standard anticoagulants in a subgroup of 114 children with CVT. They were randomized 2:1 to treatment with rivaroxaban or standard anticoagulants for 3 months. The primary efficacy outcome was recurrent VTE and the principal safety outcome was major or clinically relevant nonmajor bleeding. The study found that none of the 73 rivaroxaban recipients and 1 of the 41 standard anticoagulant recipients had symptomatic, recurrent VTE after 3 months, and clinically relevant bleeding occurred in 5 rivaroxaban recipients and 1 standard anticoagulant recipient. Sinus recanalization was a secondary outcome of the study, and the study found that among the rivaroxaban group, 25% had complete or partial sinus recanalization, while 53% had complete or partial sinus recanalization among the standard anticoagulant group. The difference was not statistically significant. The study concluded that in this sub-study, children with CVT treated with rivaroxaban or standard anticoagulation had a low risk of recurrent VTE and clinically relevant bleeding.[79]

Treatment of CVT in Antiphospholipid Syndrome

The medical treatment of CVT in patients with APS is mainly focused on the secondary prevention of thromboembolism events by the use of VKAs. However, patients with triple-positive laboratory tests (lupus anticoagulant, anticardiolipin antibodies, and anti-B2-glycoprotein I antibodies) have a high risk for recurrence of thromboembolism events, even while in the therapeutic INR range. The use of DOACs such as rivaroxaban is not recommended for triple-positive patients with APS, based on the results of the TRAPS trials, which was terminated prematurely due to an excess of arterial thromboembolism events in the rivaroxaban treatment arm. The possible explanation for this may be the interindividual variability of rivaroxaban plasma levels and the different mechanism of action between warfarin and rivaroxaban.[80]

In patients with recurrent thrombosis while receiving standard-intensity VKA treatment with a target INR range of 2.0–3.0, the current management approach is to increase the VKA treatment to a high-intensity regimen with a target INR of 3.5 (range 3.0–4.0), following an interim bridging with supplementary LMWH. It is recommended that these patients should be on indefinite warfarin treatment with a target INR of 3.0–4.0 and close INR monitoring. Some physicians add aspirin with a moderate warfarin goal of a target INR of 2.0–3.0, but this practice is not used at all centers due to the increased risk of bleeding. Fondaparinux, a synthetic pentasaccharide with anti-Xa activity, may have a beneficial role in patients with recurrent thrombotic events while receiving other anticoagulation. Adjunctive therapy such as hydroxychloroquine (HCQ) and statins may also be considered in refractory APS.[81]

CONCLUSION

Cerebral venous thrombosis can present with a variety of clinical manifestations ranging from asymptomatic to coma. Hence, it must be a consideration on the differential diagnosis for common neurological ailments such as unexplained headaches, encephalopathy, and focal deficits, especially considering the potential for reversal with prompt treatment. The list of underlying causes and differential diagnoses is large. A diligent search for an underlying cause is crucial and anticoagulation is the cornerstone of therapy. Those patients who progress despite anticoagulation might derive benefit from chemical or mechanical thrombolysis and or decompression surgery. Thus, although CVT is rare, it is also an important neurologic condition to be aware of and be armed with the knowledge of the different therapeutic management strategies available.

REFERENCES

1. Bousser MG, Ferro JM. Cerebral venous thrombosis: an update. Lancet Neurol. 2007;6:162-70.
2. Ferro JM, Correia M, Pontes C, Baptista MV, Pita F, Cerebral Venous Thrombosis Portuguese Collaborative Study Group (Venoport). Cerebral vein and dural sinus thrombosis in Portugal: 1980-1998. Cerebrovasc Dis. 2001;11:177-82.
3. Coutinho JM, Zuurbier SM, Aramideh M, Stam J. The incidence of cerebral venous thrombosis: A cross-sectional study. Stroke. 2012;43:3375-7.
4. Ferro JM, Canhão P, Stam J, Bousser MG, Barinagarrementeria F; ISCVT Investigators. Prognosis of cerebral vein and dural sinus thrombosis: results of the International Study on Cerebral Vein and Dural Sinus Thrombosis (ISCVT). Stroke. 2004;35(3):664-70
5. Narayan D, Kaul S, Ravishankar K, Suryaprabha T, Bandaru VC, Mridula KR, et al. Risk factors, clinical profile, and long-term outcome of 428 patients of cerebral sinus venous thrombosis: Insights from Nizam's Institute Venous Stroke Registry, Hyderabad (India). Neurol India. 2012;60:154-9.
6. Padmavati S, Gupta S, Singh B. A clinical study of 44 cases of hemiplegia in adult women. Neurol India. 1957;5:59-65.
7. Bansal BC, Gupta RR, Prakash C. Stroke during pregnancy and puerperium in young females below the age of 40 years as a result of cerebral venous/venous sinus thrombosis. Jpn Heart J. 1980;21:171-3.
8. Pai N, Ghosh K, Shetty S. Hereditary thrombophilia in cerebral venous thrombosis: a study from India. Blood Coagul Fibrinolysis. 2013;24(5):540-3.
9. Ferro JM, Lopes GC, Rosas MJ, Araújo C, Henriques I; Venoport Investigators. Chronobiology of cerebral vein and dural sinus thrombosis. Cerebrovasc Dis. 2002;14:265.
10. Stolz E, Klötzsch C, Rahimi A, Schlachetzki F, Kaps M. Seasonal variations in the incidence of cerebral venous thrombosis. Cerebrovasc Dis. 2003;16(4):455-6; author reply 456.
11. Aaron S, Lakshmanan J, Sunrsanam TD, Benjamin K, Durairaj J, Matew V, et al. Cerebral Venous Sinus Thrombosis, Seasonal Trends, and Climatic Influence: A Region-Specific Study. Ann Indian Acad Neurol. 2020;23(4):522-7.
12. Schultz NH, Sørvoll IH, Michelsen AE, Munthe LA, Lund-Johansen F, Ahlen MT, et al. Thrombosis and thrombocytopenia after ChAdOx1 nCoV-19 vaccination. N Engl J Med. 2021;384:2124-30.
13. Biousse V, Conard J, Brouzes C, Horellou MH, Ameri A, Bousser MG, et al. Frequency of the 20210 G-->A mutation in the 3'-untranslated region of the prothrombin gene in 35 cases of cerebral venous thrombosis. Stroke. 1998;29:1398-400.
14. Marjot T, Yadav S, Hasan N, Bentley P, Sharma P. Genes associated with adult cerebral venous thrombosis. Stroke. 2011;42:913-8.
15. Duman T, Uluduz D, Midi I, Bektas H, Kablan Y, Goksel BK, et al. A multicenter study of 1144 patients with cerebral venous thrombosis: the VENOST study. J Stroke Cerebrovasc Dis. 2017; 26:1848-57.
16. Stam J. Thrombosis of the cerebral veins and sinuses. N Engl J Med. 2005;352:1791-8.
17. Pengo V, Tripodi A, Reber G, Rand JH, Ortel TL, Galli M, et al. Update of the guidelines for lupus anticoagulant detection. Subcommittee on Lupus Anticoagulant/antiphospholipid Antibody of the Scientific and Standardisation Committee of the International Society on Thrombosis and Haemostasis. J Thromb Haemost. 2009;7:1737-40.
18. Ferro JM, Canhão P, Bousser MG, Stam J, Barinagarrementeria F; ISCVT Investigators. Cerebral vein and dural sinus thrombosis in elderly patients. Stroke. 2005;36:1927-32.
19. Pujari SS, Ojha PK, Kulkarni RV, Kharat S, Gupta D, Lalla R, et al. Cerebral Venous Sinus Thrombosis (CVST) as a Complication of SARS-CoV-2 Infection. J Stroke Med. 2022;5(1):32-9.
20. Passamonti SM, Biguzzi E, Cazzola M, Franchi F, Gianniello F, Bucciarelli P, et al. The JAK2V617F mutation in patients with cerebral venous thrombosis. J Thromb Haemost. 2012;10:998-1003.
21. Agostoni E. Headache in cerebral venous thrombosis. Neurol Sci. 2004;25 (Suppl 3):S206-10.
22. Biousse V, Ameri A, Bousser MG. Isolated intracranial hypertension as the only sign of cerebral venous thrombosis. Neurology. 1999;53(7):1537-42.
23. Jacobs K, Moulin T, Bogousslavsky J, Woimant F, Dehaene I, Tatu L, et al. The stroke syndrome of cortical vein thrombosis. Neurology. 1996;47(2):376-82.
24. Damak M, Crassard I, Wolff V, Bousser MG. Isolated lateral sinus thrombosis: a series of 62 patients. Stroke. 2009;40(2):476-81.
25. Ropper AH, Klein JP. Cerebral Venous Thrombosis. N Engl J Med. 2021;385(1):59-64.
26. Ferro JM, Bousser MG, Canhão P, Coutinho JM, Crassard I, Dentali F, et al. European Stroke Organization guideline for the diagnosis and treatment of cerebral venous thrombosis - endorsed by the European Academy of Neurology. Eur J Neurol. 2017;24(10): 1203-13.
27. Chiras J, Bousser MG, Meder JF, Koussa A, Bories J. CT in cerebral thrombophlebitis. Neuroradiology. 1985;27:145-54.

28. Sonoo T, Gunshin M, Son D, Nakajima S, Kitamura K, Yahagi N, et al. Cerebral venous thrombosis and "dense triangle sign" on unenhanced head computed tomographic scan. Am J Emerg Med. 2016;6:192e3-4.
29. Vijay RKP. The cord sign. Radiology. 2006;240:299-300.
30. Lee EJ. The empty delta sign. Radiology. 2002;224:788-9.
31. Virapongse C, Cazenave C, Quisling R, Sarwar M, Hunter S. The empty delta sign: frequency and significance in 76 cases of dural sinus thrombosis. Radiology. 1987;162(3):779.
32. Boukobza M, Crassard I, Bousser MG. when the 'dense triangle' in dural sinus thrombosis is round. Neurology. 2007;69(8):808.
33. Isensee C, Reul J, Thron A. Magnetic resonance imaging of thrombosed dural sinuses. Stroke. 1994;25:29-34.
34. Favrole P, Guichard JP, Crassard I, Bousser MG, Chabriat H. Diffusion-weighted imaging of intravascular clots in cerebral venous thrombosis. Stroke. 2004;35:99-103.
35. Prasad K, Kaul S, Padma MV, Gorthi SP, Khurana D, Bakshi A. Stroke management. Ann Indian Acad Neurol. 2011;14:S82-96.
36. Saposnik G, Barinagarrementeria F, Brown RD Jr, Bushnell CD, Cucchiara B, Cushman M, et al. Diagnosis and management of cerebral venous thrombosis: a statement for healthcare professionals from the American Heart Association/American Stroke Association. Stroke. 2011;42(4):1158-92.
37. Alons IME, Jellema K, Wermer MJH, Algra A. D-dimer for the exclusion of cerebral venous thrombosis: a meta-analysis of low risk patients with isolated headache. BMC Neurol. 2015;15:118.
38. Smith E, Kumar KV. BET 1: does a normal D-dimer rule out cerebral venous sinus thrombosis (CVST)? Emerg Med J. 2018;35:396-7.
39. Dentali F, Squizzato A, Marchesi C, Bonzini M, Ferro JM, Ageno W. D-dimer testing in the diagnosis of cerebral vein thrombosis: a systematic review and a meta-analysis of the literature. J Thromb Haemost. 2012;10:582-9.
40. Misra UK, Kalita J, Bansal V. D-dimer is useful in the diagnosis of cortical venous sinus thrombosis. Neurol India. 2009;57:50-4.
41. Heldner MR, Zuurbier SM, Li B, Von Martial R, Meijers JCM, Zimmermann R, et al. Prediction of cerebral venous thrombosis with a new clinical score and D-dimer levels. Neurology. 2020;95(7):e898-e909.
42. Einhaupl KM, Villringer A, Meister W, Mehraein S, Garner C, Pellkofer M, et al. Heparin treatment in sinus venous thrombosis. Lancet. 1991;338:597-600.
43. Nagaraja D, Rao BSS, Taly AB. Randomized controlled trial of heparin in puerperal cerebral venous/sinus thrombosis. Nimhans J. 1995;2:111-5.
44. de Bruijn SF, Stam J. Randomized, placebo-controlled trial of anticoagulant treatment with low-molecular-weight heparin for cerebral sinus thrombosis. Stroke. 1999;30:484-8.
45. Coutinho JM, Ferro JM, Canhao P, Barinagarrementeria F, Bousser MG, Stam J. Unfractionated or low-molecular weight heparin for the treatment of cerebral venous thrombosis. Stroke. 2010;41: 2575-80.
46. Einhäupl K, Stam J, Bousser MG, De Bruijn SF, Ferro JM, Martinelli I, et al. EFNS guideline on the treatment of cerebral venous and sinus thrombosis in adult patients. Eur J Neurol. 2010;17:1229-35.
47. Misra UK, Kalita J, Chandra S, Kumar B, Bansal V. Low molecular weight heparin versus unfractionated heparin in cerebral venous sinus thrombosis: a randomized controlled trial. Eur J Neurol. 2012;19:1030-6.
48. Heestermans M, Poenou G, Hamzeh-Cognasse H, Cognasse F, Bertoletti L. Anticoagulants: A Short History, Their Mechanism of Action, Pharmacology, and Indications. Cells. 2022;11:3214.
49. Einhäupl K, Bousser MG, de Bruijn SF, Ferro JM, Martinelli I, Masuhr F, et al. EFNS guideline on the treatment of cerebral venous and sinus thrombosis. Eur J Neurol. 2006;13(6):553-9.
50. Bose G, Graveline J, Yogendrakumar V, Shorr R, Fergusson DA, Le Gal G, et al. Direct oral anticoagulants in treatment of cerebral venous thrombosis: a systematic review. BMJ Open. 2021;11: e040212.
51. Nepal G, Kharel S, Bhagat R, Ka Shing Y, Ariel Coghlan M, Poudyal P, et al. Safety and efficacy of Direct Oral Anticoagulants in cerebral venous thrombosis: A meta-analysis. Acta Neurol Scand. 2022;145(1):10-23.
52. Yaghi S, Shu L, Bakradze E, Salehi Omran S, Giles JA, Amar JY, et al. Direct Oral Anticoagulants Versus Warfarin in the Treatment of Cerebral Venous Thrombosis (ACTION-CVT): A Multicenter International Study. Stroke. 2022;53(3):728-38.
53. Ferro JM, Coutinho JM, Dentali F, Kobayashi A, Alasheev A, Canhão P, et al.; RE-SPECT CVT Study Group. Safety and Efficacy of Dabigatran Etexilate vs Dose-Adjusted Warfarin in Patients With Cerebral Venous Thrombosis: A Randomized Clinical Trial. JAMA Neurol. 2019;76(12):1457-65.
54. CVT Consortium. DOAC–CVT: Direct oral anticoagulants. [online] Available from https://cerebralvenousthrombosis.com/professionals/doac-cvt/. [Last accessed March, 2023].
55. Abraham NS, Noseworthy PA, Yao X, Sangaralingham LR, Shah ND. Gastrointestinal safety of direct oral anticoagulants: a large population-based study. Gastroenterology. 2017;152(5):1014-22.e1.
56. Schaefer JK, McBane RD, Wysokinski WE. How to choose appropriate direct oral anticoagulant for patient with nonvalvular atrial fibrillation. Ann Hematol. 2016;95(3):437-49.
57. Jonathan D, Fanny B, François M, Minet V, Rabenda V, Reginster JY, et al. Dabigatran etexilate and risk of myocardial infarction, other cardiovascular events, major bleeding, and all-cause mortality: a systematic review and meta-analysis of randomized controlled trials. J Am Heart Assoc. 2021;3(3):e000515.
58. BMJ Publishing Group Limited. DOACs not recommended for people with antiphospholipid syndrome. Drug Ther Bull. 2019;57:182.
59. Coutinho JM, Stam J. How to treat cerebral venous and sinus thrombosis. J Thromb Haemost. 2010;8:877-83.
60. Ortel TL, Neumann I, Ageno W, Beyth R, Clark NP, Cuker A, et al. American Society of Hematology 2020 guidelines for management of venous thromboembolism: treatment of deep vein thrombosis and pulmonary embolism. Blood Adv. 2020;4(19):4693-738.
61. Burnett AE, Mahan CE, Vazquez SR, Oertel LB, Garcia DA, Ansell J. Guidance for the practical management of the direct oral anticoagulants (DOACs) in VTE treatment. J Thromb Thrombolysis. 2016;41(1):206-32.
62. Ferro, José M., et al. "Benefit of EXtending Oral anti-COAgulant Treatment after Cerebral Vein and Dural Sinus Thrombosis (EXCOA-CVT)." Welcome to the EXCOA-CVT Study Website, 1 Mar. 2014, [online] Available from https: www.excoa-cvt.com/Homepage.html.
63. Li G, Zeng X, Hussain M, Meng R, Liu Y, Yuan K, et al. Safety and validity of mechanical thrombectomy and thrombolysis on severe cerebral venous sinus thrombosis. Neurosurgery. 2013;72(5):730-8; discussion:730.
64. Siddiqui FM, Dandapat S, Banerjee C, Zuurbier SM, Johnson M, Stam J, et al. Mechanical thrombectomy in cerebral venous thrombosis: systematic review of 185 cases. Stroke. 2015;46: 1263-8.
65. Alwan A. Management of Severe Cerebral Venous Sinus Thrombosis Using Mechanical Balloon Assisted Thrombectomy. Stroke. 2023;3(1):e000574.
66. Canhão P, Cortesão A, Cabral M, Ferro JM, Stam J, Bousser MG, et al. Are steroids useful to treat cerebral venous thrombosis? Stroke. 2008;39(1):105-10.
67. Théaudin M, Crassard I, Bresson D, Saliou G, Favrole P, Vahedi K, et al. Should decompressive surgery be performed in malignant cerebral venous thrombosis? A series of 12 patients. Stroke. 2010;41:727-31.
68. Mahale R, Mehta A, Varma RG, Hegde AS, Acharya PT, Srinivasa R. Decompressive surgery in malignant cerebral venous sinus thrombosis: what predicts its outcome? J Thromb Thrombolysis. 2017;43:530-9.

69. Hughes S. (2021). Decompressive Surgery Saves Lives in Severe Cerebral Vein Thrombosis. [online] Available from https://www.medscape.com/viewarticle/958798. [Last accessed March, 2023].
70. Coutinho JM, Seelig R, Bousser MG, Canhão P, Ferro JM, Stam J. Treatment variations in cerebral venous thrombosis: an international survey. Cerebrovasc Dis. 2011;32:298-300.
71. Ferro JM, Bacelar-Nicolau H, Rodrigues T, Bacelar-Nicolau L, Canhão P, Crassard I, et al. Risk score to predict the outcome of patients with cerebral vein and dural sinus thrombosis. Cerebrovasc Dis. 2009;28:39-44.
72. Koopman K, Uyttenboogaart M, Vroomen PC, van der Meer J, De Keyser J, Luijckx GJ. Long-term sequelae after cerebral venous thrombosis in functionally independent patients. J Stroke Cerebrovasc Dis. 2009;18(3):198-202.
73. Ferro JM, Correia M, Rosas MJ, Pinto AN, Neves G; Cerebral Venous Thrombosis Portuguese Collaborative Study Group [Venoport]. Seizures in cerebral vein and dural sinus thrombosis. Cerebrovasc Dis. 2003;15(1-2):78-83.
74. Geisbüsch C, Herweh C, Gumbinger C, Ringleb PA, Möhlenbruch MA, Nagel S. Chronic intracranial hypertension after cerebral venous and sinus thrombosis - frequency and risk factors. Neurol Res Pract. 2021;3(1):28.
75. Ferro JM, Coutinho JM, Jansen O, Bendszus M, Dentali F, Kobayashi A, et al.; RE-SPECT CVT Study Group. Dural Arteriovenous Fistulae After Cerebral Venous Thrombosis. Stroke. 2020;51(11):3344-7.
76. Kang MK, Cho YD, Kang HS, Jung KH. Development of a dural arteriovenous fistula subsequent to cerebral venous thrombosis by venous hypertension. eNeurologicalSci. 2018;14:24-7.
77. Durmuş B, Yperzeele L, Zuurbier SM. Cerebral venous thrombosis in women of childbearing age: diagnosis, treatment, and prophylaxis during a future pregnancy. Ther Adv Neurol Disord. 2020;13:1756286420945169.
78. Bates SM, Middeldorp S, Rodger M, James AH, Greer I. Guidance for the treatment and prevention of obstetric-associated venous thromboembolism. J Thromb Thrombolysis. 2016;41(1):92-128.
79. Connor P, Sánchez van Kammen M, Lensing AWA, Chalmers E, Kállay K, Hege K, et al. Safety and efficacy of rivaroxaban in pediatric cerebral venous thrombosis (EINSTEIN-Jr CVT). Blood Adv. 2020;4(24):6250-8.
80. Pengo V, Denas G, Zoppellaro G, Jose SP, Hoxha A, Ruffatti A, et al. Rivaroxaban vs warfarin in high-risk patients with antiphospholipid syndrome. Blood. 2018;132:1365-71.
81. Tumian NR, Hunt BJ. Clinical Management of Thrombotic Antiphospholipid Syndrome. J Clin Med. 2022;11(3):735.

56

CHAPTER

Vascular Diseases of the Spinal Cord

Rakesh Singh, Narayan Deshmukh, Jagadish Annapureddy

INTRODUCTION

Vascular diseases of spinal cord are potentially treatable myelopathies. It is important to recognize them early in the course as treatment and long-term outcome are time dependent. They are often missed during evaluation of longitudinally extensive myelopathies.[1] The presentation could vary from acute, subacute, to chronic myelopathy with symptoms related to long tract functions, motor–sensory deficits, and bowel–bladder dysfunction, which may evolve over a period of time.[2] Neuroimaging techniques [magnetic resonance imaging (MRI) and/or computed tomography (CT) scan] supplemented with digital subtraction angiography (DSA) are important tools in diagnosing and planning management.

In this chapter, we review the common diseases causing arterial ischemia and spinal vascular malformations with varied manifestations.

VASCULAR ANATOMY OF SPINAL CORD

Brief introduction of the spinal cord vascular supply will be helpful for further understanding vascular myelopathies. Gross vascular anatomy of spinal cord is shown in **Figure 1**.[3-5]

- *Anterior spinal artery (ASA)*: Single ASA runs down in the anterior sulcus supplying anterior two-third of the spinal cord. It is formed by the fusion of two descending branches from the bilateral intracranial vertebral artery (VA) (V4 segment). It usually starts at C2–C4 and ends at conus. It is thinnest in the thoracic cord region and thickest at conus. It is not a continuous artery, but has multiple reinforcements and vascular anastomoses at different segments.
- *Posterior spinal artery (PSA)*: Paired PSAs arise either from the VA or from the posterior inferior cerebellar artery (PICA) on either side at foramen magnum. They supply the posterior one-third of the cord, i.e., mainly the posterior columns. The interarterial anastomosis and reinforcements from radiculomedullary arteries may look like ladders with crossover from either side.
- *Segmental arteries*: They are named by the segment they supply rather than from the site of origin. It has three branches: (1) dorsal branch supplying the dorsal skin and muscles, (2) ventral branch which continues as an intercostal nerve anteriorly, and (3) middle or spinal trunk dividing into spinal canal branch and radicular branches. They supply the vertebral bone, muscle, ligament, joints, dura, nerve root, and cord. Segmental arteries reinforce ASA and PSA. **Figure 2** shows segmental supply of cord and vertebra.

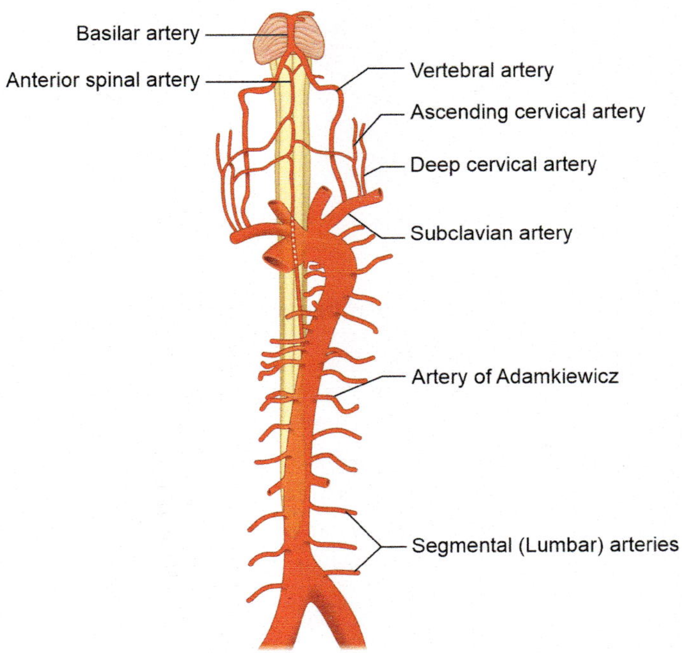

FIG. 1: Vascular anatomy of spinal cord.

Segmental arteries at different levels derive additional supply from various arteries as shown in **Table 1**.[6]

- *Radiculomedullary arteries*: In the fetal life, there are 31 pairs supplying each and every spinal segment; however, in the adult life only few radiculomedullary arteries are left supplying the cord. They are variable in number, on an average 6–10. There is a single large radiculomedullary artery arising between T9 and L2 , also known as artery of Adamkiewicz, on left side in 75% of the cases. It has a characteristic "hair pin" loop. It travels cranially from radicular branch, with sudden caudal turn before joining ASA. **Figure 3** shows artery of Adamkiewicz. Another enlarged cervical radiculomedullary artery is seen at C3, called artery of cervical enlargement. Radicular arteries along with ASA and PSA form a pial network over the surface of the cord called vasa corona. Penetrating branches from the ASA and vasa corona travel centripetally and supply the cord.
- *Intrinsic/intramedullary arterial system*: It can be divided into (1) central system (centrifugal) and (2) peripheral system (centripetal). Central system is constituted by sulcocommissural artery arising from the ASA in anterior central sulcus. Perforating radial arteries arise from the vasa corona and travel centripetally, supplying the periphery of the cord.[7] **Figure 4** shows intrinsic arterial system.

Venous drainage: Venous drainage of spinal cord is variable but follows more or less the arteries. The vertebral venous system is divided into three components: (1) internal vertebral venous plexus (IVVP), (2) external vertebral venous plexus (EVVP), and (3) basivertebral veins. The intramedullary veins, radially oriented and superficial pial veins, join on the surface of cord forming anterior and posterior spinal veins in subarachnoid space. They drain into internal vertebral plexus in epidural space via radiculomedullary veins. **Figure 5** shows venous drainage of spinal cord.

Internal vertebral venous plexus is an interconnected network of venous channels that lies within the epidural space of the spinal canal. It surrounds the thecal sac, running longitudinally from the cranium to the sacrum, and

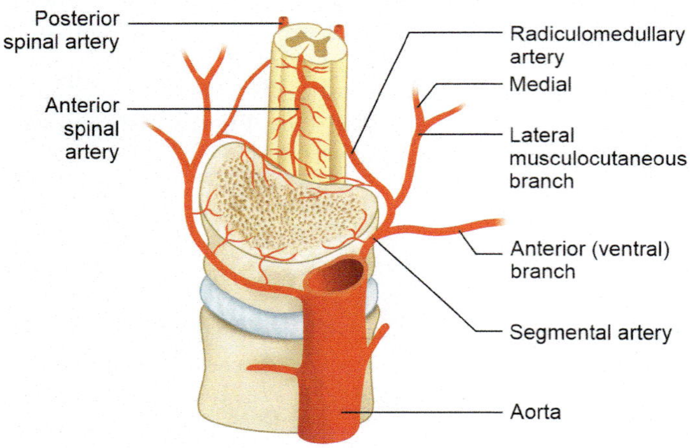

FIG. 2: Segmental arterial supply of vertebrae and the spinal cord.

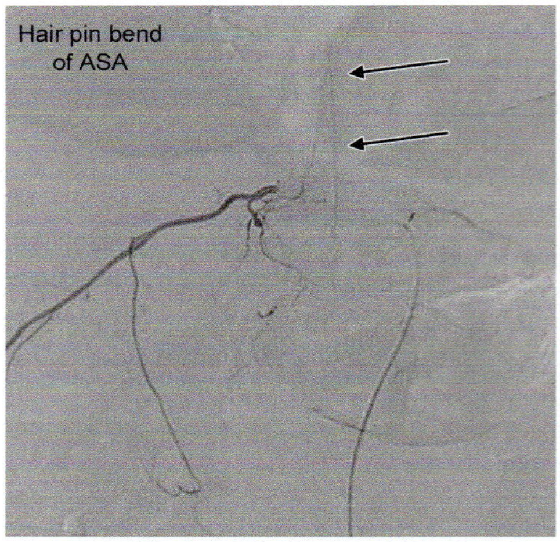

FIG. 3: DSA image of segmental artery supplying cord via radiculomedullary branches to ASA, i.e., artery of Adamkiewicz. Black arrows show hairpin bend of ASA.
(ASA: anterior spinal artery; DSA: digital subtraction angiography)

TABLE 1: Feeding arteries of different vertebral levels.

Vertebral level	Feeding artery
C1–C2	Ascending pharyngeal, occipital, vertebral, ascending cervical, deep cervical
C3–C7	Vertebral, ascending cervical, deep cervical
T1–T3	Supreme intercostal
T3–T4	T4 ("superior") intercostal
T5–T12	T5–T12 intercostal
L1–L4	Lumbar arteries
L5	Median sacral, iliolumbar
Sacrum	Median sacral, lateral sacral

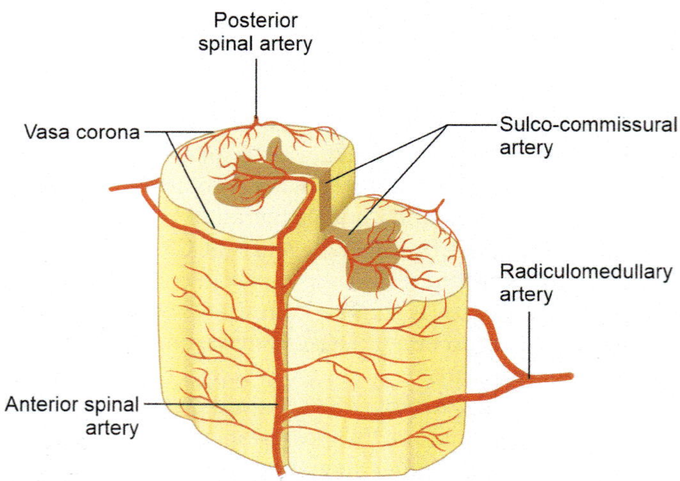

FIG. 4: Intrinsic arterial supply of the spinal cord.

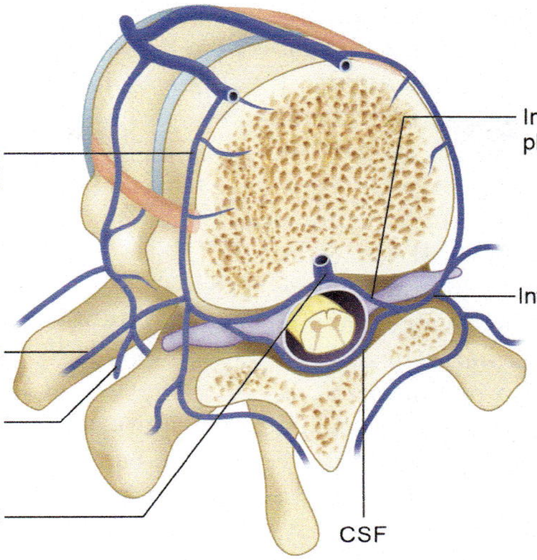

FIG. 5: Anatomy: Image of segmental venous drainage of vertebrae and spinal cord.
(CSF: cerebrospinal fluid)

receives drainage from the intrinsic venous system of the spinal cord.

External vertebral venous plexus lies outside of the spinal canal, surrounding the bony vertebral column anteriorly and the posterior spinal elements posteriorly. The EVVP communicates with the IVVP through veins that traverse the neural foramen, known as intervertebral veins. Muscular branches and lateral branches from the paraspinal muscles and intercostal spaces, respectively, also drain into the EVVP. Segmental spinal veins are part of the EVVP and run alongside the midportion of vertebral bodies to anastomose anteriorly with the azygous and hemiazygos venous systems, as well as with longitudinal lumbar veins. It finally drains into superior and inferior vena cava.

Basivertebral veins run through the vertebral bodies themselves, connecting the portion of the IVVP in the anterior epidural space with the EVVP along the anterior surfaces of the vertebral body.[8]

Epidural venous plexus is a valve-less structure, which communicates freely from skull base to sacrum, transmitting venous pressure in case of venous hypertension.

SPINAL CORD INFARCTION

Introduction: Spinal cord infarction (SCI) is uncommon compared to cerebral infarction. Aortic surgeries, especially repair of ruptured aortic aneurysm, are common procedures presenting with SCI. Hypotension, atherosclerotic aortic disease, vessel dissection (aorta, VA dissection), embolic events from fibrocartilaginous embolism, aortic atheroma, cardioembolic events, vasculitis, and infections such as syphilis, varicella zoster, tuberculosis, and substance abuse (cocaine, cannabis, etc.) are other etiologies for SCI. Most periprocedural SCI present with maximum deficit acute flaccid paraplegia with minimal pain in perioperative period. Spontaneous SCI usually has underlying vascular risk factors and may present with pain as predominant symptom at onset. Surfer's myelopathy is a characteristic syndrome due to infarction in thoracic cord during spine hyperextension in surfers. Various hypercoagulable states including lupus anticoagulant, malignancy, sickle cell disease, disseminated intravascular coagulation (DIC) may also cause SCI.[2]

Anatomical correlation: Each radiculomedullary artery has to supply multiple spinal segments and hence either has to ascend or descend from the site of the origin. Because of the ascending and descending branches, there creates an overlap or watershed zone which can be susceptible to ischemic insults. Involvement of single radiculomedullary artery can cause long-segment infarct in the cord. Proximal nerve roots also receive vascular supply from branches of the ASA and radiculomedullary arteries, highlighting root involvement in many patients with SCI.

Due to this varied blood supply, there are horizontal and vertical watershed zones, which can be prone to ischemia during insults like hypotension or hypovolemia. Horizontal watershed region lies at the junction of anterior two-third and posterior one-third of the cord. Vertical watershed lies at around T2–T3 region, which is more vulnerable. The entire thoracic cord is dependent on one or two radiculomedullary arteries, hence at high risk of ischemia.

Clinical features: Most patients have abrupt onset, with back or neck pain, with radicular symptoms. Vascular territory of ASA is often involved with acute flaccid paraplegia due to both corticospinal tracts, affecting pain and temperature sensation (lateral column) with sparing of posterior column sensations. Variable presentations including unilateral involvement, hemicord involvement, complete transverse myelopathy, only spinothalamic sensory deficits without motor deficits, or involvement of posterior cord due to PSA have been documented.

Investigation: Neuroimaging forms mainstay in diagnosis, and MRI is imaging modality of choice. High-resolution MRI with diffusion weighted imaging (DWI) and apparent diffusion coefficient (ADC) sequences help in identifying SCI. DWI hyperintensity with drop in signal in ADC is 50–70% sensitive for diagnosis of SCI and helps in early cord ischemia. In acute stage, MRI T2 sequence shows hyperintense signal. **Figures 6A to D** show MRI features of acute SCI. Involvement of adjacent vertebral body is a more specific sign of SCI. Vascular dissection can be seen on T1 fat-saturated sequence as meniscus sign or flap in the vessel. Thrombus in ASA can be visualized as T2-hyperintense signal. In subacute stage, signal intensity on T1 and T2 sequences can be variable with patchy contrast enhancement. In chronic stage, myelomalacia is usual imaging feature with T1 hypointensity, T2 hyperintensity, and volume loss. Magnetic resonance angiography (MRA) is of limited value in detecting SCI. Other adjuvant tests helpful for diagnosis of SCI are described in **Table 2**.[2]

Treatment: Goal of treatment is to improve perfusion through collaterals. Cerebrospinal fluid (CSF) drainage reduces spinal canal pressure, thereby decreasing resistance to blood flow. CSF drainage up to 10 mL every 2–4 hours, maintaining CSF pressure to 10 mm Hg, is desirable. Longer drainage can be achieved using lumbar drains. Increasing mean arterial pressure (MAP) to maintain perfusion can be also be useful. Target MAP is above 90 mm Hg. Limited data and conflicting results have been noted for using

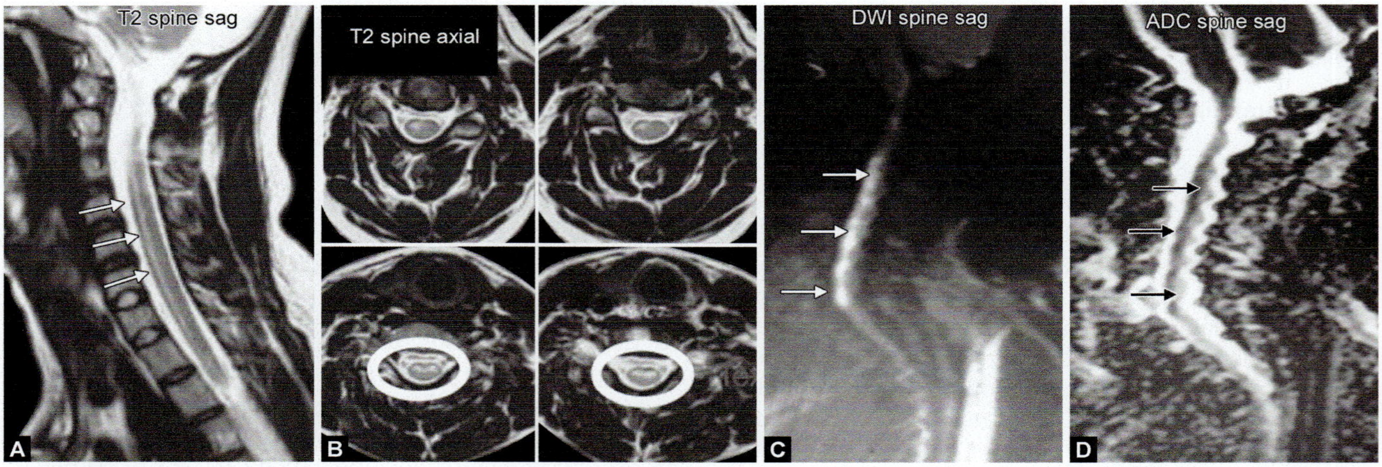

FIGS. 6A TO D: Acute spinal cord infarct presenting as quadriparesis. (A) MRI of cervical cord, T2 sagittal section showing long-segment hyperintense signal changes from C2 to C8 level (white arrows); (B) T2 axial spine showing classical "owl eye" sign with hyperintense signal changes in the anterior horn cells (white circle); (C and D) Sagittal DWI sequence showing hyperintense signal with corresponding ADC hypointense signal (white and black arrows).

(ADC: apparent diffusion coefficient; DWI: diffusion weighted imaging; MRI: magnetic resonance imaging)

Image courtesy: Dr Pramod Dhonde, Consultant Neurologist, Dhonde Hospital, Nanded, Maharashtra, India.

TABLE 2: Adjuvant tests for spinal cord infarction (SCI).

Test	
Vascular risk factors, routine blood tests	Complete blood count, fasting and post-lunch blood sugars, HbA1c, fasting lipids, prothrombin time/activated partial thromboplastin time, sedimentation rate, C-reactive protein
Cerebrospinal fluid (CSF)	Cell count, glucose, protein, IgG index, oligoclonal bands, varicella zoster-PCR, VDRL for syphilis, *Cryptococcus* antigen
CT chest/abdomen/pelvis; PET-CT	Malignancy
Serology	Aquaporin-4 IgG, MOG-IgG, syphilis serology (TPHA), ANA, ANCA, APLA, dsDNA
Cardiac workup	Echo, TEE, Holter
EMG/NCS	Guillain–Barré syndrome
Temporal artery biopsy	Giant cell arteritis

(ANA: antinuclear antibody; ANCA: antineutrophil cytoplasmic antibody; APLA: antiphospholipid antibody; CT: computed tomography; dsDNA: double-stranded deoxyribonucleic acid; EMG: electromyography; HbA1c: glycated hemoglobin; IgG: immunoglobulin G; MOG: myelin oligodendrocyte glycoprotein; NCS: nerve conduction studies; PCR: polymerase chain reaction; PET: positron emission tomography; TEE: transesophageal echocardiography; TPHA: treponema pallidum hemagglutination; VDRL: venereal disease research laboratory) prophylactic lumbar drain in patients undergoing aortic aneurysm repair. Established ischemia usually is difficult to treat. There is no beneficial role of steroids for acute ischemia.

Spontaneous spinal cord ischemia is relatively rare, so limited data is available on using alteplase [recombinant tissue plasminogen activator (rtPA)] for thrombolysis. If promptly suspected and confirmed on MRI, it is reasonable to discuss with family about risks and benefits of rtPA and consider for thrombolysis. Secondary prevention depends on underlying etiology, but antiplatelets with statins can be considered in the presence of atherosclerotic risk factors.[9]

SPINAL VASCULAR MALFORMATIONS

Introduction: Spinal vascular malformations are complex and rare disorders. There could be a single lesion or associated with multiple other lesions. They could be associated with genetic disorders [e.g., Cobb syndrome and hereditary hemorrhagic telangiectasia (HHT)]. The spinal dural arteriovenous fistula (dAVF) usually presents with congestive myelopathy, whereas spinal arteriovenous malformations (AVMs) have varied presentation. Principally, as compared to AVM, the AVF does not have intervening nidus between feeding artery and draining vein.

Clinical features: The spinal AVM can present with hematomyelia, venous hypertension, compression on spinal cord and nerve roots, subarachnoid hemorrhage (SAH) due to ruptured aneurysm, syringomyelia, steal phenomenon, thrombosis of draining vein, arachnoiditis, and necrosis of spinal cord. Infrequently spinal AVM can present with extradural hemorrhage. Patients presenting with acute-onset severe headache and backache with subarachnoid hemorrhage on imaging must be screened with spinal angiography to rule out spinal vascular malformation.

Classification: Over years multiple classification systems for spinal vascular malformations.[10-12] These classification systems use site and size of fistula, presence of intervening nidus, feeding arteries, draining vein location, involvement of vertebra and paravertebral structures, and associated syndromes as classifying features. A simplified five-point system describes spinal vascular malformations as follows:[13]

1. *Type I*: dAVF
2. *Type II*: Intramedullary AVM
3. *Type III*: Juvenile AVM
4. *Type IV*: Intradural perimedullary AVF
5. *Type V*: Extradural AVF

Brief anatomical details and clinical presentation are presented in **Table 3**.

Spinal Dural Arteriovenous Fistula

Introduction: Spinal dAVFs are the most common vascular malformations forming up to 70%. There is a direct connection between feeding radiculomedullary artery and spinal medullary vein. The etiology of spinal dAVF is poorly understood. In contrast to cranial dAVF, spinal dAVFs usually do not have preceding venous thrombosis. They can occur spontaneously, postinfection, trauma, or surgery as well. They usually present as insidious onset, gradually progressive myelopathy with bladder involvement and sensory level. Congestive myelopathy is due to arterialization of veins, causing significant increase in back pressure on intramedullary veins. It causes delayed venous outflow, stasis, and spinal cord edema. It is extremely important to recognize these as lack of specific treatment has worse prognosis. It is often missed and treated as idiopathic transverse myelitis.

Pathology: Pathophysiologically, the important factor is arterialization of spinal veins. Normally, the pial venous plexus of the spinal cord is protected against reflux from the epidural venous plexus. Fistula usually occurs at radicular branch of segmental artery in the nerve root sleeve as it enters dura. Often, these fistulas occur on dorsal aspect of nerve root sleeve. Due to fistula, arterial pressure is transmitted to radicular vein. This increases the pressure in perimedullary and intramedullary veins. This impairs the microcirculation in spinal cord and nerve root. The passive increase in venous pressure increases size of veins, and they appear turgid and red to naked eye and as serpiginous flow voids on MRI. The resistance to drainage of medullar veins which follows causes congestive myelopathy.[14]

TABLE 3: Arterial feeder, venous drainage, and presentation of spinal vascular malformations.

Type of AVF	Arterial feeder	Venous drainage	Predominant clinical presentation
Dural AVF	Radicular artery, within nerve root sleeve	Intradural venous plexus	Venous hypertension, congestive myelopathy
Intramedullary AVM	Anterior/posterolateral spinal artery	Medullary vein	Hemorrhage
Juvenile AVM	Intradural/extradural VA, radicular artery, or cervical artery	Medullary vein	Involvement of cord, vertebra, paraspinal muscles. Cobb syndrome
Intradural perimedullary AVF	Anterior/posterolateral spinal artery	Coronal plexus/segmental veins with varix at transition site	Progressive myeloradiculopathy
Extradural AVF	Extradural artery	Epidural venous plexus/Batson plexus	Compressive myelopathy

(AVF: arteriovenous fistula; AVM: arteriovenous malformation; VA: vertebral artery)

Clinical features: Spinal dAVF is more common in males (M:F—5:1), with mean age of onset 60 years (range: 28–83 years). Mean delay in diagnosis of spinal dAVF is 23 months from onset of symptoms. Most are located in lower thoracic or lumbar region, at or around T7–T9 level. The venous outflow may reach cranially up to high thoracic or cervical region. Gait abnormality is usually the first symptom. Gradually, they develop spastic paraparesis, less often as flaccid paraparesis, with sensory symptoms involving both lateral and posterior column. Both upper motor neuron and lower motor neuron signs could be present. Bladder and bowel dysfunction is frequently reported. Pain could be additional feature seen in more than 50% patients. There is peculiar worsening due to exertion or Valsalva maneuver. These patients often receive steroids for treatment as idiopathic transverse myelitis, and there is worsening in symptoms due to venous hypertension. If the dAVF is located further down the spine, patients may present with cauda-conus syndrome. Hemorrhage in fistula is relatively rare, but can cause acute deterioration.[15]

Investigation: MRI is sensitive but can miss the diagnosis early in course of disease. T2-hyperintense signal, patchy enhancement with longitudinally extending transverse myelitis, in thoracolumbar spine is typical. The abnormal T2 signal can extend sometimes up to conus. There could be multiple flow voids on dorsal surface of spinal cord. MRI with absent T2-hyperintense signal or flow voids could reliably exclude diagnosis. Contrast enhancement patterns are not disease specific, appear more often as patchy heterogenous enhancement.

Digital subtraction angiography remains the gold standard for diagnosis as well as planning treatment for dAVF. Thorough spine DSA cannulating both vertebral arteries, subclavian arteries, common carotid arteries, intercostal arteries, and internal iliac arteries is a must before ruling out dAVF. Site of fistula, number of feeding arteries, ASA, and origin artery of Adamkiewicz are noted during DSA. Draining vein and extent of drainage are important in planning embolization. **Figures 7A to E** show MRI and DSA features of dAVF, with resolution following treatment.

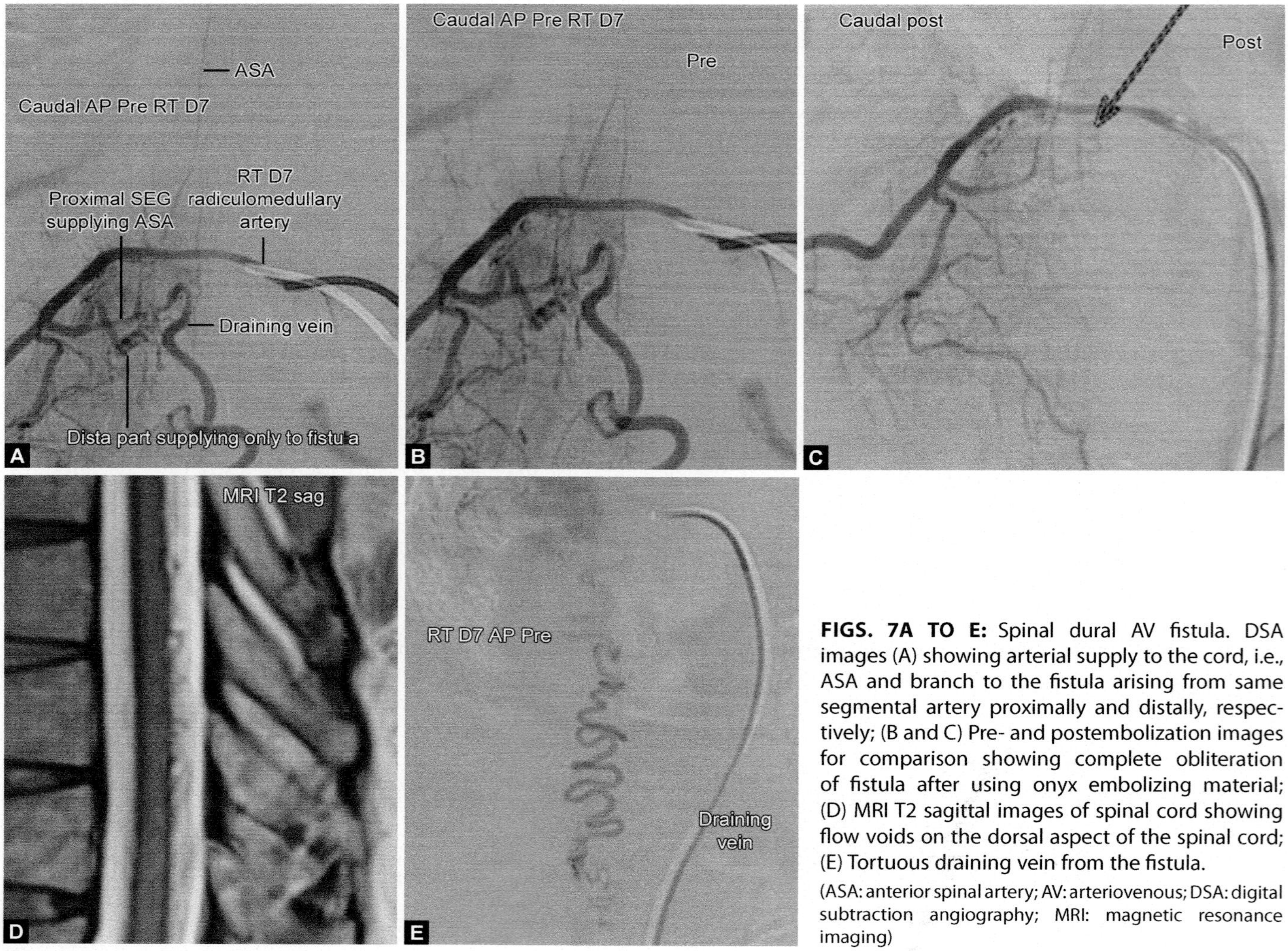

FIGS. 7A TO E: Spinal dural AV fistula. DSA images (A) showing arterial supply to the cord, i.e., ASA and branch to the fistula arising from same segmental artery proximally and distally, respectively; (B and C) Pre- and postembolization images for comparison showing complete obliteration of fistula after using onyx embolizing material; (D) MRI T2 sagittal images of spinal cord showing flow voids on the dorsal aspect of the spinal cord; (E) Tortuous draining vein from the fistula.

(ASA: anterior spinal artery; AV: arteriovenous; DSA: digital subtraction angiography; MRI: magnetic resonance imaging)

Treatment: Treatment options for spinal dAVF include surgical ligation of draining vein or embolization of fistula. Efficacy of surgical ligation is higher (95%), but correct identification and ligation of site of fistula are important. Endovascular embolization aims at curing dAVF by occluding foot of vein (site of fistula) using liquid embolic agents such as n-Butyl cyanoacrylate (NBCA—glue) or onyx (ethylene vinyl alcohol copolymer) dissolved in dimethyl sulfoxide (DMSO). Care should be taken to avoid embolization of ASA or artery of Adamkiewicz.[15]

Uncommon fistulous malformations include spinal epidural and pial AVFs, which have paraspinal and paravertebral arteries draining into epidural venous plexus. They present with congestive myelopathy, infrequently as compressive symptoms on nerve roots.

Spinal Arteriovenous Malformations

Introduction: Spinal AVMs are lesions with intervening nidus between feeding arteries and draining veins. These are more complex and may present with variety of manifestations. The most common presentation is hematomyelia, intraparenchymal spinal cord hemorrhage. The spinal cord malformations types 2–5 (type II: intramedullary AVM, type III: juvenile AVM, type IV: intradural perimedullary AVF, type V: extradural AVM) are clubbed together as spinal AVMs. They can be associated with spinal cord aneurysms in 30–40% cases. They can be associated with genetic syndromes such as HHT, Cobb syndrome, Klippel-Trenaunay-Weber syndrome, congenital lipomatous overgrowth, and epidermal nevi syndrome.[16]

Clinical features: They present with acute myelopathy due to hematomyelia, acute pain, or compressive symptoms. Some of the patients may recover spontaneously. Annual risk of rupture is around 4%, whereas risk after rupture may increase to 10%.

Investigation: MRI is the first modality of investigation, which may show blood products as hypointense signal on gradient-recalled echo (GRE). T1-hyperintense, T2-hypointense, and hypointense signals of GRE are characteristic of acute bleed. DSA remains gold standard for diagnosis and management.

Treatment: Treatment modalities include surgery for acute bleed, large lesions, endovascular embolization for surgically inoperable lesions, targeted embolization of aneurysms, palliative care, or radiotherapy. Combination strategy individualized for each case is better.

Intramedullary Arteriovenous Malformations: Type 2

These are second most common spinal vascular lesions. They present in the third or fourth decade, more common in males. They appear in thoracic (70%) or cervical (30%) cord. Genetic syndromes such as neurofibromatosis, Osler-Weber-Rendu disease, and Klippel-Trenaunay-Weber syndrome may be associated. These are common in thoracolumbar region followed by cervical cord. They can have multiple feeders. Aneurysms associated with AVMs usually present with hematomyelia. Recurrent hemorrhage in AVM occurs frequently. These lesions can also present with congestive myelopathy, or compressive symptoms on roots.

Magnetic resonance imaging can detect AVMs, and findings include multiple flow voids, T1-T2 sequence suggestive of hemosiderin deposition. T2-hyperintense lesions of spinal cord may suggest cord edema. DSA can detect feeding arteries, draining veins, and aneurysms. **Figures 8A to F** show spinal AVM type 2 with aneurysm on feeding artery.

Treatment options include surgery, endovascular embolization, and stereotactic radiosurgery. Natural improvement post hemorrhage is known, and emergency surgery is rarely needed. Surgical treatment is reserved for patients with recurrent hemorrhage and peripherally located compact nidus. Embolization may help in curing if all niduses are embolized, or palliative in case of multiple feeders with diffuse nidus. Embolization can be considered for targeted therapy for aneurysms. Combination of all three modalities may sometimes be needed.[2]

Juvenile AVMs: Type 3 Lesions (aka Juvenile, Metameric, or Extradural–Intradural AVMs)

These are complex AVMs; they have intradural and extradural components. They involve complete segment of the spinal cord, vertebra, and paraspinal muscles. They are usually high-flow AVMs with multiple feeders. This makes complete delineation by DSA difficult. Most cases may need staged embolization and surgical approach.

Cobb syndrome (cutaneomeningospinal angiomatosis) is a rare congenital disorder that has a combination of vascular skin naevi and a spinal vascular lesion involving within the same metameric segment. It has a somatic mutation of neural crest or mesodermal cells. The syndrome presents with characteristic dermal lesions—port wine stains and neurodeficits in corresponding dermatome.[16]

Intradural Perimedullary AVF: Type 4 Lesions (aka Perimedullary, or Ventral Intradural AVFs)

These are located on the pial surface of the spinal cord. The fistula is between a spinal cord artery or arteries (ASA or PSA) and the coronal venous plexus.

Figures 9A to H show intramural perimedullary congenital AVF.

Spinal Extradural AVF: Type 5 Lesions (aka Epidural AVFs, Extradural AVMs, or Perivertebral AVMs)

These are extremely rare. The fistula is located extradurally, with draining vein going in Batson plexus or piercing dural and draining in intradural plexus. The symptoms

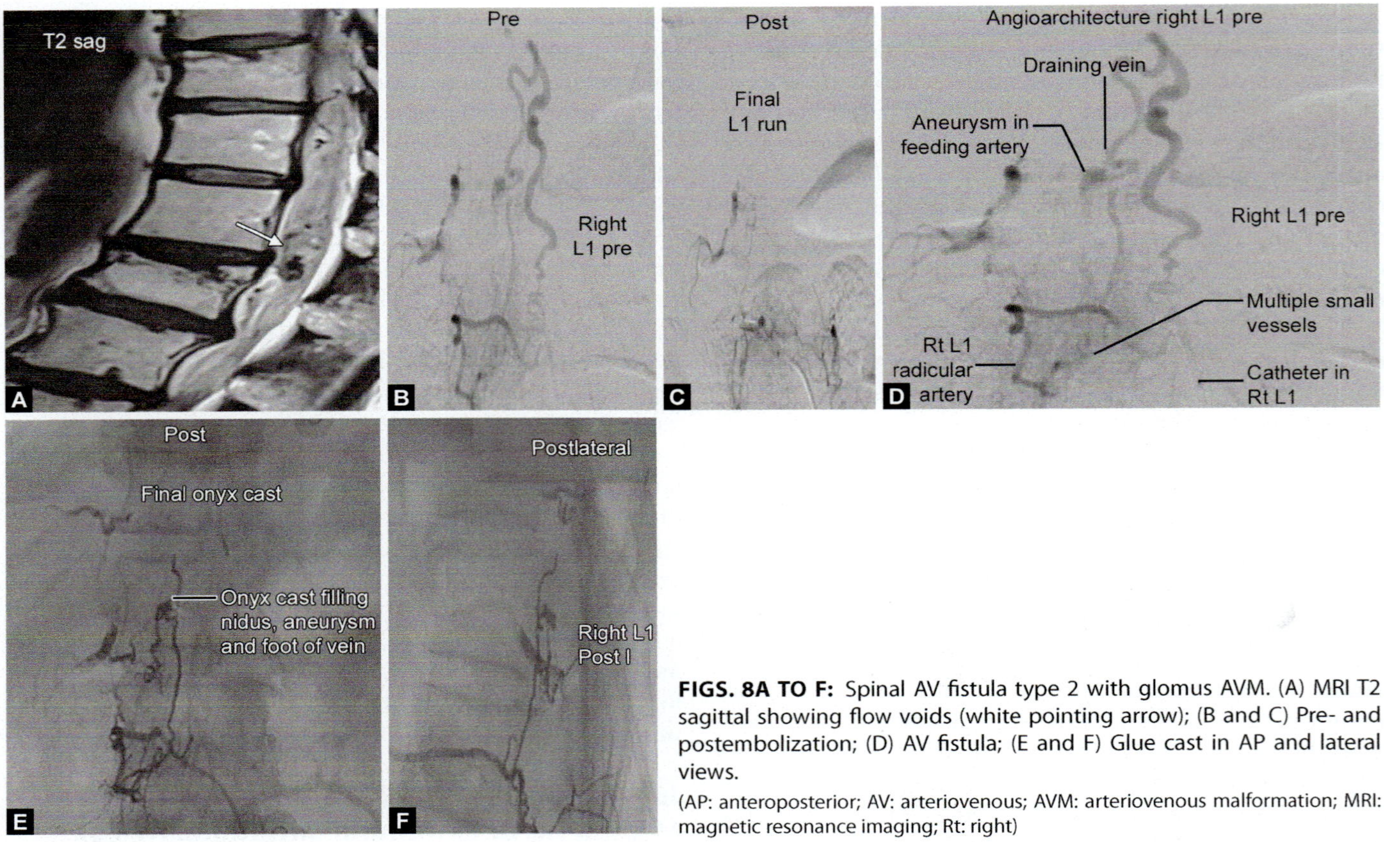

FIGS. 8A TO F: Spinal AV fistula type 2 with glomus AVM. (A) MRI T2 sagittal showing flow voids (white pointing arrow); (B and C) Pre- and postembolization; (D) AV fistula; (E and F) Glue cast in AP and lateral views.

(AP: anteroposterior; AV: arteriovenous; AVM: arteriovenous malformation; MRI: magnetic resonance imaging; Rt: right)

are mainly due to thecal sac compression with or without congestive myelopathy. The difference between type 5 lesions and spinal dAVF (type 1) lesions is the draining vein in dAVF is intradural in origin.

Intramedullary Cavernous Malformations

Spinal cavernous malformations are 5% of all central nervous system (CNS) cavernomas; around 25% spinal cavernomas have intracranial cavernomas. Cavernomas are pathologically a cluster of tightly packed sinusoidal veins, without intervening parenchyma, without any feeding artery or draining veins. Some cavernomas may have associated developmental venous anomaly.

Cavernomas have slightly male predominance, usually present in the fourth decade. Some patients may have familial predisposition. They present as acute hematomyelia. Annual risk of hemorrhage is 1–5%. Cavernomas of size more than 1 cm have higher risk of bleed. Pregnancy and puerperal periods are known to worsen cavernomas. MRI appearance of cavernoma is typical, lobulated mass lesion, heterogenous T1 and T2 signals with hypointense T2 signal. There is usually no contrast enhancement. Typical popcorn appearance on GRE sequence is often described. Surgery is reserved for large lesions (>1 cm), recurrent hemorrhage, and progressive neurological deficit, while expectant management is done for asymptomatic small cavernomas.[2]

Figures 10A and B show MRI of cervical cord cavernoma pre- and postsurgery of the patient who presented with recurrent hematomyelia.

Miscellaneous Lesions Presenting as Hematomyelia

Many other conditions may present with hematomyelia. These include vascular spinal tumors including hemangioma, hemangioblastoma, metastatic tumors, aneurysmal bone cyst, hemangiopericytoma, angiofibroma; anticoagulant-induced bleed, hemorrhage in SCI; and post-infections such as postinfluenza, varicella zoster virus, and herpes simplex virus 2 (HSV-2).

Hemangioma can present with hematomyelia or more often as cord compression. It is a highly vascular tumor, and embolization can be done presurgery to reduce the vascularity or with curative intent. **Figures 11A and B** show vertebral hemangioma with focal cord compression. It was embolized using glue **(Figs. 12A to D)**.

Vertebral metastasis of tumors or primary tumors like myeloma can be vascular and may present with cord hemorrhage or compressive myelopathy. **Figures 13A to D** show highly vascular myeloma presenting as compressive myelopathy, which was embolized with polyvinyl alcohol (PVA) particles prior to chemotherapy.

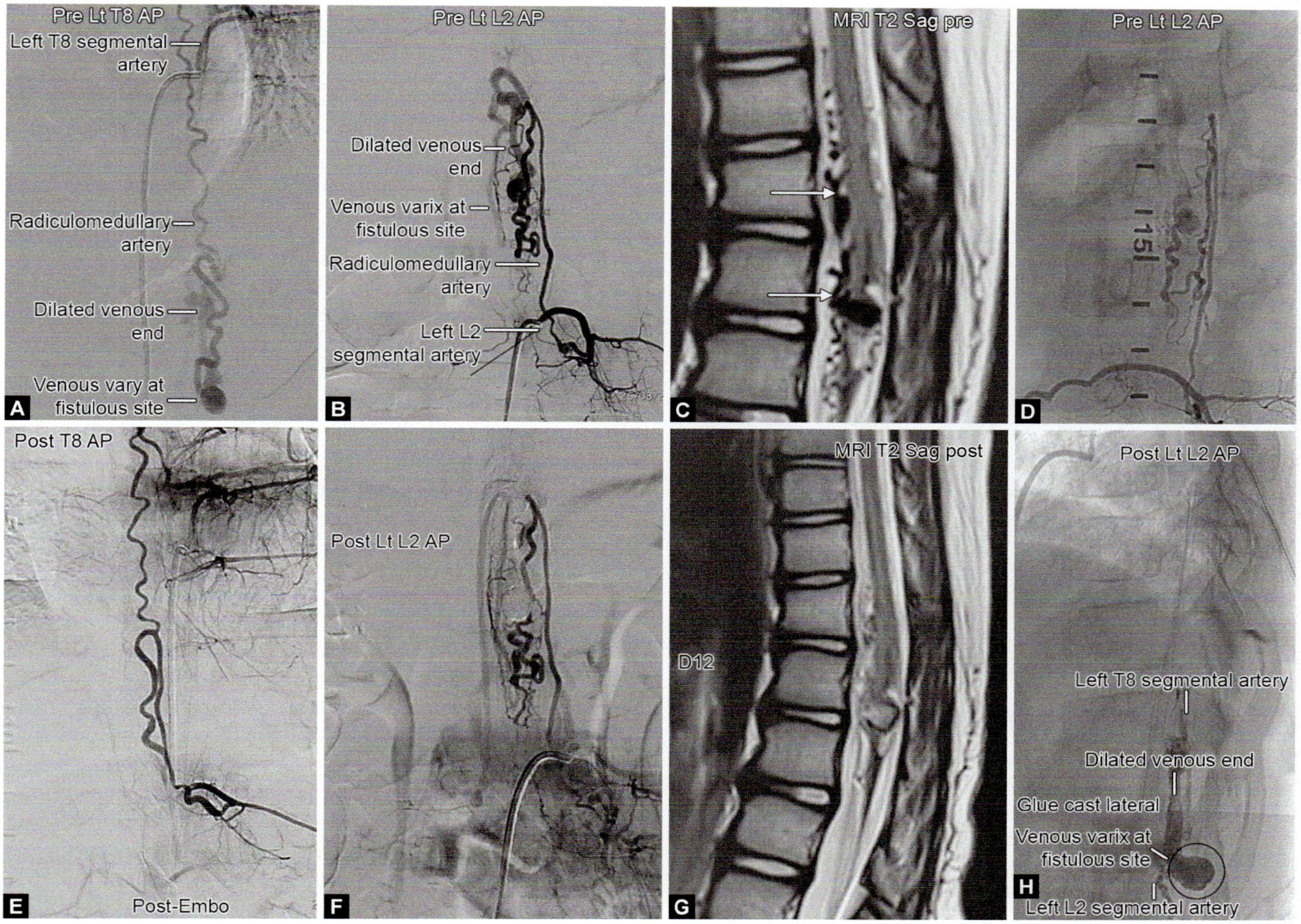

FIGS. 9A TO H: Congenital spinal AV fistula: Patient presented with acute paraplegia and loss of sensation from below T10 with urinary urgency. (A and B) Pial AV fistula at T10 supplied from left T8 arterial feeder flowing caudally and L2 feeder flowing cranially; (C and G) Pre- and postembolization MRI T2 sagittal images; (E and F) Postembolization showing no residual fistula; (H) Glue cast in the arterial feeder, fistulous site, and venous varix.

(AV: arteriovenous; MRI: magnetic resonance imaging)

Epidural Hematoma

Amongst the extraparenchymal spinal hemorrhage, epidural hepatoma is the most common presentation. It is caused by trauma, surgery, epidural catheterization, lumbar puncture, and coagulopathies (liver disorders). In post-spine surgery patients who present with intractable pain with or without new motor deficits, imaging of spine should be considered to rule out epidural hepatoma. It can be seen asymptomatically in many post-spinal surgery patients on radiological evaluation done with in the first week. Postsurgical is the common condition and to be suspected in patients with intractable pain with or without new motor deficits. MRI shows T2 hyperintensities in acute condition. Surgery may be required for emergency situation. **Figures 14A and B** show acute cervical epidural hematoma with cord compression with gradual resolution after 1 week.

Subdural Hematoma

Subdural hematoma (SDH) may present with acute back pain with radicular symptoms, and myelopathy. Nontraumatic causes commonly include iatrogenic procedures with history of antiplatelets and anticoagulant usage. Following spinal surgery, spinal SDH is not unusual. Treatment of underlying condition forms the mainstay.

Subarachnoid Hemorrhage

Spontaneous spinal SAH is rare in comparison to cerebral SAH. Patients may have intense neck or back pain, occasional headache, meningismus, and electrolyte disturbances. Underlying etiologies apart from trauma include:

- Medical conditions such as hypertension, blood dyscrasias, collagen vascular diseases, coarctation of aorta, aortic dissection, and anticoagulant usage

- Vascular pathologies such as type 1 dAVF, AVM, aneurysm, cavernoma, tumors like hemangioblastoma, and vasculitis

Management includes symptomatic treatment of SAH, its complications, and specific treatment of the underlying condition.[2]

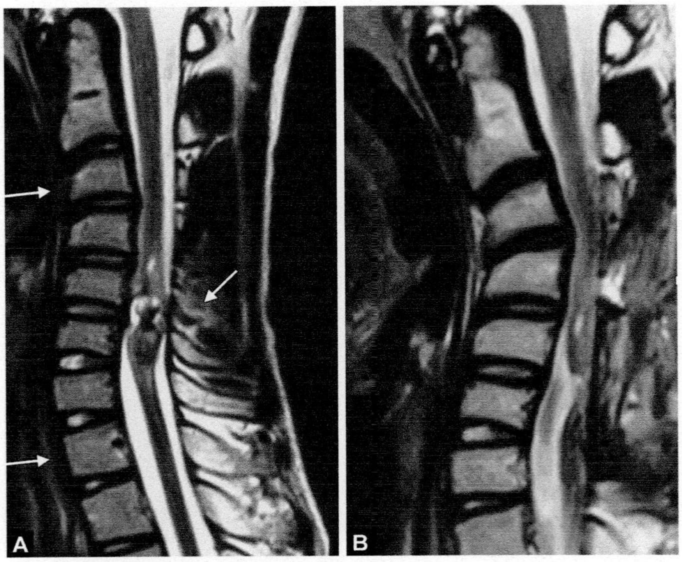

FIGS. 10A AND B: Cavernoma: Patient presented with recurrent quadriparesis secondary to bleed. Excision biopsy confirmed to have cavernoma. (A) Magnetic resonance imaging (MRI) T2 sagittal view showing lesion with central hypointensity (bleed) and patchy hyperintensities suggestive of calcification; (B) Post-cavernoma resection surgery, T2 showing normal cord without posterior elements.

CEREBROSPINAL FLUID–VENOUS FISTULAS

Introduction: This is an important cause of spontaneous intracranial hypotension (SIH). CSF–venous fistulas (CVFs) can be challenging to detect on conventional anatomic imaging because, unlike other types of spinal CSF leak, they do not typically result in pooling of fluid in the epidural space, and imaging signs of CVF may be subtle. They are abnormal connections between the spinal subarachnoid space and adjacent paraspinal veins that allow unregulated egress of CSF into the venous system. Resultant CSF depletion causes intracranial hypotension.

Cerebrospinal fluid–venous fistulas appear to be unidirectional, and CSF flows into the venous system because of high CSF pressure compared to venous pressure. They are often anatomically associated with fistulous connection from diverticulum of nerve sleeve. Overinterpretation of diverticula is to be avoided as they are commonly seen in patients without SIH. Two most common causes of CVF are transdural osteophytes and ruptured meningeal diverticula.

Pathogenesis: Spinal arachnoid granulations are in close relation with paraspinal vertebral plexus, mainly at thoracic spine. Hence, rupture of such granulation may be an inciting event in forming CVF. Alternatively, it is understood that CVF arises between the subarachnoid space of thecal sac, connecting the subarachnoid space to the extrinsic venous system that drains spinal cord parenchyma, with CSF flowing into radicular veins and ultimately into epidural venous plexuses. This alternative theory is supported by the fact that surgical ligation is the effective treatment option for CVF.

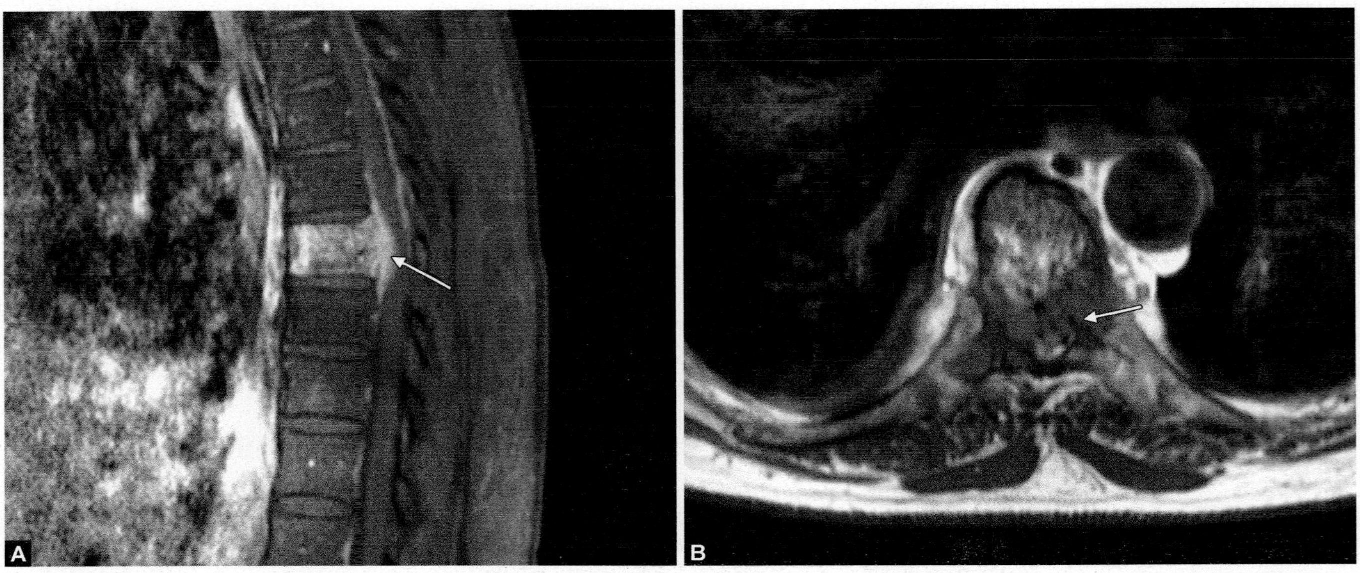

FIGS. 11A AND B: Magnetic resonance imaging (MRI) spine of vertebral hemangioma. (A) T1 postcontrast sagittal section showing enhancement of vertebral body with focal cord compression (arrow). (B) T1 axial section at the same level showed effacement of vertebra with compression of the spinal cord.

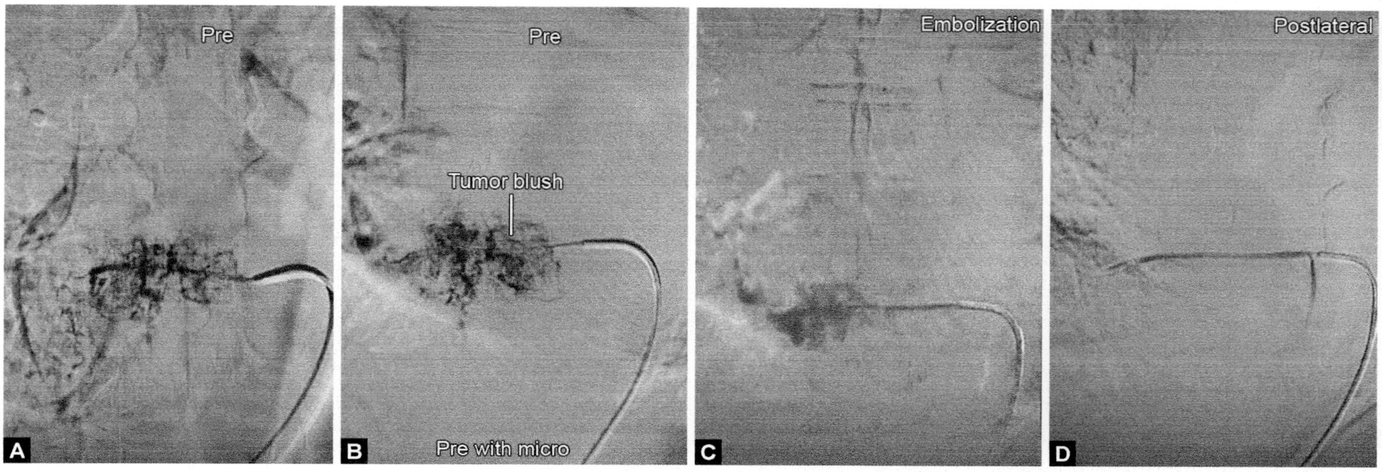

FIGS. 12A TO D: Vertebral hemangioma. (A and B) DSA images showed tumor blush at T10 level; (C) Embolization done with glue showed embolic agent at tumor site. (D) Postembolization angiogram showed no tumor blush, suggesting complete obliteration of the hemangioma.

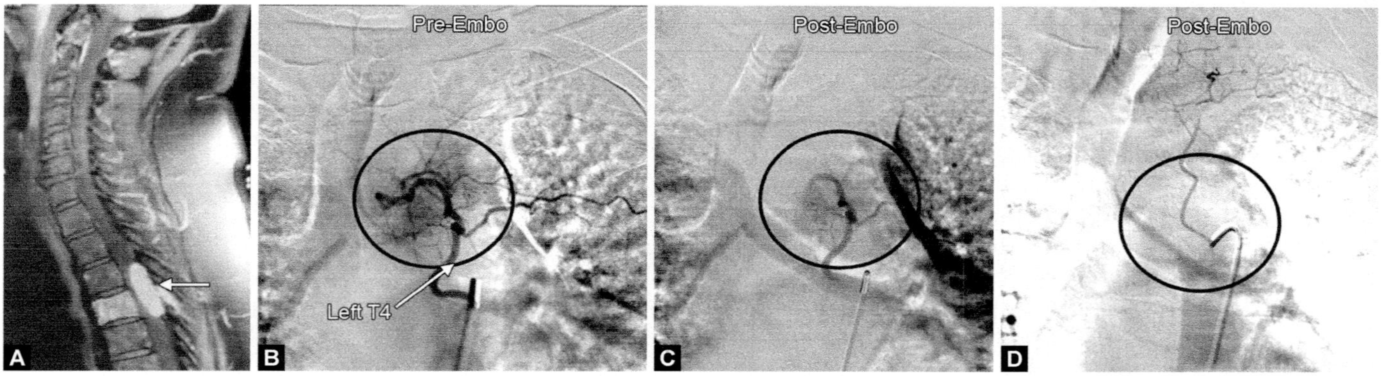

FIGS. 13A TO D: (A) Solitary myeloma, MRI T1 postcontrast sagittal section showing bright enhancing lesion of T4 vertebra and spinal cord (black arrow); (B to D) DSA images of the same patient showing tumor blush as marked by arrow in (B), embolized with PVA particles; (C and D) Postembolization images have not revealed tumor blush.

(DSA: digital subtraction angiography; MRI: magnetic resonance imaging; PVA: polyvinyl alcohol)

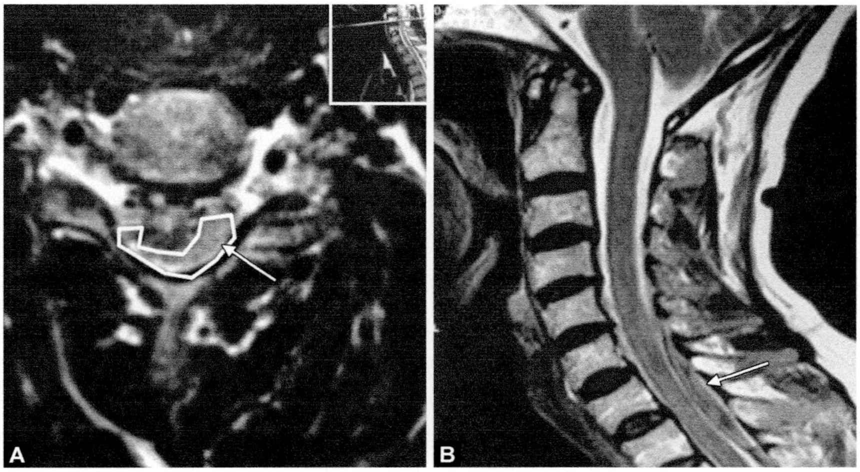

FIGS. 14A AND B: EDH MRI spine. (A) T1 axial of C-spine showing epidural hematoma compressing the cord (white arrow); (B) T2 sagittal cervical spine showing hypo- and isointense signal change dorsal to the cord suggestive of acute bleed (white arrow).

(EDH: epidural hematoma; MRI magnetic resonance imaging)

Clinical feature: Postural headache increases in severity in sitting/standing posture and subsides on lying down in recumbent position within few minutes. Headache is usually diffuse and dragging in nature, which can be more in the back of the head.

Investigations: MRI brain is done to identify features of intracranial hypotension such as pachymeningeal thickening, enhancement, engorged venous sinuses, tonsillar herniation, and subdural collection. These features may not be present, and quantitative findings such as reduced mamillopontine distance <5.5 mm, pontomesencephalic angle < 50°, and interpeduncular angle < 45° help in diagnosis. Identifying myelographic contrast opacifying the vein is the key for diagnosis and can be achieved by CT myelography or digital subtraction myelography. CSF pressure <6 cm H_2O in recumbent position helps in diagnosis of intracranial hypotension, but may not be seen in few cases.

Computed tomography myelography: It is performed in decubitus position after injecting contrast into the intrathecal space under fluoroscopy diagnosis. Hyperdense paraspinal vein (>70 HU) represents intrathecal contrast leaking into the circulation, and diagnosis relies on its identification.

Digital subtraction myelography: Contrast is injected into the intrathecal space of the patient in lying-down position on tilt table. Gradual tilting of the table helps in running along the suspected fistula region. Visualizing the passage of contrast directly from subarachnoid space into the paraspinal vein is diagnostic of CVF.

Management: Percutaneous epidural blood patch has been tried with limited success. Obliteration of fistulous communication by open surgical ligation is the standard treatment of CVF. Hemilaminectomy and laminectomy surgical techniques to reach the CVF then followed by coagulation/sectioning/ligation of enlarged paraspinal veins with coagulation/ligation of associated nerve are used. As this open surgical technique involves preprocedure general anesthesia, prolonged postoperative recovery and costs and endovascular selective embolization of the fistula site using liquid embolic agents are evolving. There are case reports of CT-guided percutaneous fibrin glue deposition to occlude the CVF.[17] Rebound headache due to intracranial hypertension after occlusion of CVF can occur and resolves usually after symptomatic management.[8]

CONCLUSION

Vascular myelopathies are uncommon and underrecognized neurologic disorders. Unless there is a high index of clinical suspicion in appropriate cases for a possible vascular etiology, the correct diagnosis will often be missed or delayed because of the overlapping clinical and imaging features that may mimic other causes of myelopathy. Prompt identification helps in optimal medical/surgical management at the right time and helps in avoiding unnecessary or harmful treatment.

ACKNOWLEDGMENTS

We would like to thank Dr Anil Karapurkar, Dr SV Khadilkar, and Dr Riddhi Patel.

REFERENCES

1. Brinjikji W, Nasr DM, Morris JM, Rabinstein AA, Lanzino G. Clinical outcomes of patients with delayed diagnosis of spinal dural arteriovenous fistulas. AJNR Am J Neuroradiol. 2016;37(2):380-6.
2. Zalewski NL. Vascular myelopathies. Continuum Minneap Minn. 2020;27(1, spinal cord disorders):30-61.
3. Caplan L, Massaro A. Spinal cord vascular disease. In: Caplan LR (Ed). Caplan's Stroke: A Clinical Approach. Cambridge: Cambridge University Press; 2016. pp. 534-43.
4. Colman MW, Hornicek FJ, Schwab JH. Spinal cord blood supply and its surgical implications. J Am Acad Orthop Surg. 2015;23(10):581-91.
5. Martirosyan NL, Feuerstein JS, Theodore N, Cavalcanti DD, Spetzler RF, Preul MC. Blood supply and vascular reactivity of the spinal cord under normal and pathological conditions. J Neurosurg Spine. 2011;15(3):238-51.
6. Harrigan MR, Deveikis JP. Essential Neurovascular anatomy. In: Handbook of Cerebrovascular Disease and Neurointerventional Technique, 2nd edition. New York: Springer; 2013. pp. 86-7.
7. Santillan A, Nacarino V, Greenberg E, Riina HA, Gobin YP, Patsalides A. Vascular anatomy of the spinal cord. J Neuro Intervent Surg. 2011;4:67-74.
8. Kranz PG, Gray L, Malinzak MD, Houk JL, Kim DK, Amrhein TJ. CSF-venous fistulas: anatomy and diagnostic imaging. AJR Am J Roentgenol. 2021;217(6):1418-29.
9. Harrigan MR, Deveikis JP. Spinal vascular lesions. In: Handbook of Cerebrovascular Disease and Neurointerventional Technique, 2nd edition. New York: Springer; 2013. pp. 814-7.
10. Borden JA, Wu JK, Shucart WA. A proposed classification for spinal and cranial dural arteriovenous fistulous malformations and implications for treatment. J Neurosurg. 1995;82:166-79.
11. Spetzler RF, Detwiler PW, Riina HA, Porter RW. Modified classification of spinal cord vascular lesions. J Neurosurg. 2002;96:145-56.
12. Bao YH, Ling F. Classification and therapeutic modalities of spinal vascular malformations in 80 patients. Neurosurgery. 1997;40:75-81.
13. Harrigan MR, Deveikis JP. Spinal vascular lesions. In: Handbook of Cerebrovascular Disease and Neurointerventional Technique, 2nd edition. New York: Springer; 2013. p. 803.
14. Morris P. Vascular malformations of the spine. In: Practical Neuroangiography, 3rd edition. Philadelphia: Lippincott Williams & Wilkins; 2013. pp. 359-65.
15. Harrigan MR, Deveikis JP. Spinal vascular lesions. In: Handbook of Cerebrovascular Disease and Neurointerventional Technique, 2nd edition. New York: Springer; 2013. pp. 803-6.
16. Harrigan MR, Deveikis JP. Spinal vascular lesions. In: Handbook of Cerebrovascular Disease and Neurointerventional Technique, 2nd edition. New York: Springer; 2013. pp. 806-12.
17. Mamlouk MD, Shen PY, Sedrak MF, Dillon WP. CT-guided fibrin glue occlusion of cerebrospinal fluid-venous fistulas. Radiology. 2021;299(2):409-18.

Part 4B: Infections

57 CHAPTER

Tuberculous Meningitis

Tanish Modi, Chamanjot Kaur, Manish Modi

INTRODUCTION

Tuberculosis (TB), caused by bacillus *Mycobacterium tuberculosis (MTB),* was the leading cause of death from a single infectious agent, ranking above human immunodeficiency virus/acquired immunodeficiency syndrome (HIV/AIDS) until the coronavirus disease 2019 (COVID-19) pandemic. Now, it is the second leading infectious killer after COVID-19.[1]

Amongst all the forms of TB, central nervous system (CNS) TB has the worst prognosis, resulting in death in approximately 20–50% of patients, and permanent neurological sequelae in 20–30% of the survivors. Of all presentations, tuberculous meningitis (TBM) has the most devastating course and constitutes about 10% of TB cases and 40% of deaths in developing countries.[2] Complications occur in about 78% of the patients with TBM, which include hydrocephalus, stroke, cranial nerve palsies, epileptic seizures, tuberculomas, myeloradiculopathy secondary to arachnoiditis, cortical blindness, syringomyelia, and hypothalamic syndrome to name a few. Stroke accounts for about 15–57% of all complications.[3]

Tubercular meningitis can be recognized by its subacute to chronic presentation and diagnosed with the help of cerebrospinal fluid (CSF) analysis (for biochemistry, Ziehl–Neelsen staining, various culture methods, and the newer nucleic acid amplification techniques) and neuroimaging. All these modalities of diagnosis have varied sensitivity and specificity. The diagnostic and treatment delay account for a high rate of morbidity and mortality in TBM. Moreover, the current treatment regimens are directly derived from pulmonary regimes, which have remained largely unchanged for the past 40 years, and do not take into account the varied ability of the first-line anti-TB drugs to penetrate the brain. These issues, together with coinfection with HIV and the increasing frequency of drug resistant bacteria, have made the management of TBM even more difficult. Many therapeutic trials are being conducted to address these issues, however, the delay in diagnosis and treatment needs to be addressed at the primary healthcare level in developing countries to improve outcomes from this deadly disease. In this chapter, we will discuss the basic pathogenesis of TBM, clinical manifestations, complications, and updates in diagnostic modalities and treatment.

EPIDEMIOLOGY

Due to the COVID-19 pandemic, there has been a large global drop in the number of newly diagnosed and reported TB patients. In 2019, 7.1 million TB cases were notified, which fell to 5.8 million in 2020. India was similarly affected by the COVID-19 pandemic. Due to this unprecedented infection, there was a decline of 38% in TB notifications after the initial 2 months of the pandemic. However, the count rose by 11% by the end of 2020, such that there was an 11% increase since April 2020. Up to 50% of the total notifications were contributed by five states—(1) Uttar Pradesh, (2) Maharashtra, (3) Madhya Pradesh, (4) Rajasthan, and (5) Gujarat.[4]

Despite the large drop in the number of people newly diagnosed with TB, there has been an increase in the number of people who died from TB at all levels—global, regional, and country level.[1] Worldwide, there were an estimated 1.3 million deaths among HIV-negative people in 2020, up from 1.2 million in 2019, and an additional 214,000 deaths among HIV-positive people, a small increase from 209,000 in 2019. The COVID-19 pandemic had reversed years of global progress in reducing the number of people who die from TB.

An estimated 9.9 million people were affected with TB in 2020, which showed a small decline as compared to 2019 data. Geographically, the largest number of new TB cases occurred in the World Health Organization (WHO) South-East Asian Region accounting for 43% of new cases. Eight countries accounted for two-thirds of the global total—(1) India (26%), (2) China (8.5%), (3) Indonesia (8.4%), (4) Philippines (6.0%), (5) Pakistan (5.8%), (6) Nigeria (4.6%), (7) Bangladesh (3.6%), and (8) South Africa (3.3%).[1]

Human immunodeficiency virus and TB form a lethal combination. People living with HIV are 18 times more likely to develop active TB. The risk of active TB is also greater in persons with undernutrition who are at three times more risk. Alcohol use disorder and tobacco smoking also increase the risk of TB disease by a factor of 3.3 and 1.6, respectively. In 2020, 0.74 million new TB cases worldwide were attributable to alcohol use disorder and 0.73 million were attributable to smoking.[1]

PATHOLOGY AND PATHOPHYSIOLOGY

Tubercular meningitis is the most common cause of subacute or chronic meningitis, especially in developing countries. It was first described in 1836 as a distinct clinical entity and in 1882, Robert Koch demonstrated the causative organism for TB as *MTB*.[5,6] *MTB* is an aerobic gram-positive rod that stains poorly with routine stains due to its thick cell wall containing lipids, peptidoglycans, and arabinomannans. Hence, Ziehl–Neelsen stain is used that prevents decolorization by acid or alcohol.[7]

Our understanding of the pathogenesis of CNS TB is from the original study of Arnold Rich and Howard Mc Cordock. It is always secondary to a TB focus elsewhere in the body, which may be latent or active. *MTB* bacilli enter the host through droplet inhalation and settle in alveolar macrophages. This escalates into a primary localized infection in the lungs which, along with dissemination to the regional lymph nodes, forms a primary complex. During this stage, there is significant bacteremia with seeding of tubercle bacilli to other organs. In the CNS, there is seeding to the meninges or the brain parenchyma that results in the formation of Rich's foci, which are small subpial or subependymal foci of metastatic caseous lesions. CNS involvement is more likely in the presence of miliary TB. Rupture of Rich's foci causes delivery of infectious material into the subarachnoid space (SAS) leading to dense inflammation and meningitis[8] **(Flowchart 1)**. The clinical manifestations of TBM are due to this inflammatory response.

The complications of TBM mainly occur by the following processes:[9]

- Leptomeningeal reaction and a*dhesion formation* from dense basal meningeal exudate resulting in CSF flow obstruction and hydrocephalus.
- *Obliterative vasculitis* of both small and large vessels resulting in infarction and strokes.
- Encephalitis or myelitis.

Studies have found elevated levels of interferon (IFN)-gamma and tumor necrosis factor-alpha (TNF-α) in TBM patients.[10] TNF-α plays very important role in the pathogenesis of TBM. Activated macrophages produce

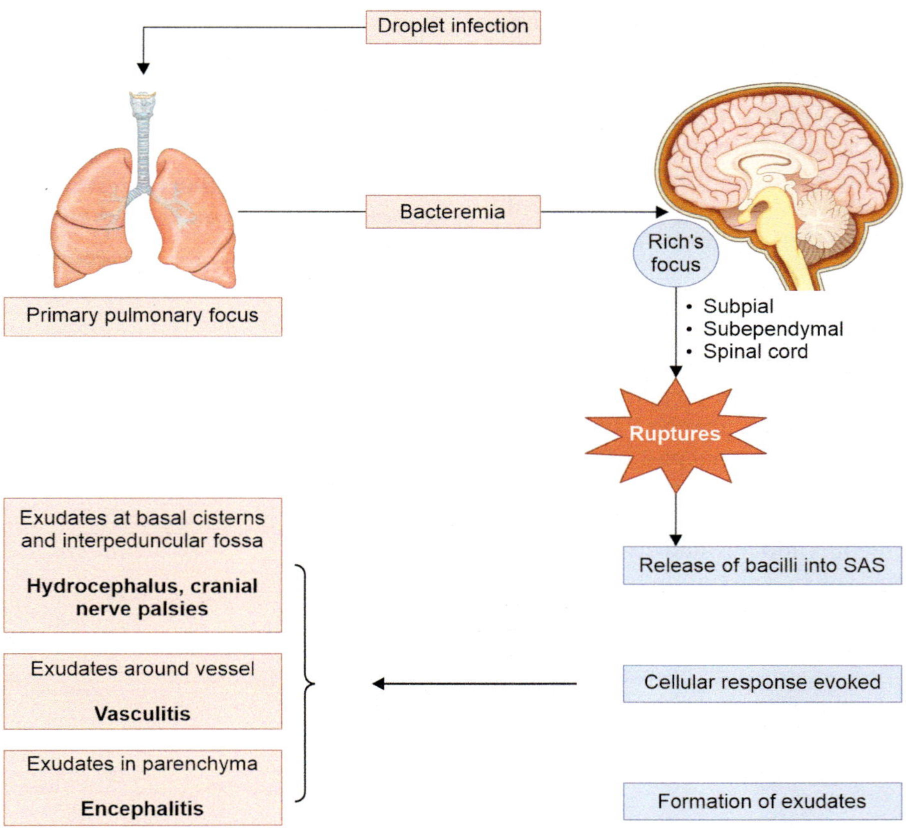

FLOWCHART 1: Pathogenesis of central nervous system (CNS) tuberculosis.

interleukin-1 beta (IL-1β) and TNF-α which are needed for granuloma formation and containment of mycobacterial infections. Local production of TNF-α leads to altered blood–brain barrier (BBB) permeability and CSF leukocytosis. CSF concentrations of TNF-α correlate with clinical progression of the disease as demonstrated in rabbit models. Further, intervention with the anti-TNF-α agents has been shown to have resulted in significant improvement and neurological outcome in these patients.[11] In a study by Sinha et al., it was found that levels of TNF-α in serum, and of IL-1β in serum, and CSF correlate significantly with the severity of the disease and also predicted the mortality in the patients.[12]

The brain parenchyma resides in a unique "immunologically privileged" environment. Not only is it protected by BBB, the immune reactivity in brain parenchyma to a foreign antigen is selective.[13] Antigen presentation is severely limited, dendritic cells are few and show lowered levels of major histocompatibility complex (MHC) class II molecules. Microglia (resident macrophages in the brain) have poor antigen-presenting capability and usually induce apoptosis of effector cells instead of proliferation. Also, T cells are converted into Fox-P3+ T regulatory cells which suppress inflammation by a neuron dependent process.[14] The main purpose of this limitation of immune reactivity is to limit inflammatory damage to the brain which has limited regenerative capacity. This explains why inflammatory meningitis does not occur immediately after disseminated TB.

The leptomeningeal reaction in TBM consists of serofibrinous exudate which lies between pia mater and arachnoid intermixed with areas of caseous necrosis. It may also occur in the form of proliferative arachnoiditis which is most prominent at the base of the brain and may involve optic chiasma resulting in optochiasmatic arachnoiditis. The exudates may also encircle the brainstem and disrupt functioning of other cranial nerves.[15] Ventriculitis resulting from involvement of the ependymal lining by this inflammatory process is seen consistently in TBM. The choroid plexus may show different degrees of inflammation.

Vasculitis—the vessels traversing the SAS are commonly involved in an inflammatory process resulting in vasculitis, resulting in spasm, constriction, and thrombosis of blood vessels. Vasculitis most frequently involves the proximal middle cerebral artery and the terminal part of the internal carotid artery in the Sylvian fissure. Therefore, most of the infarcts occur in the middle cerebral artery territory. The veins may also show phlebitis and thrombosis.[16]

Hydrocephalus develops in most of the cases symptomatic for >2 or 3 weeks, owing to blockage of CSF pathways.[17] In most cases, it occurs as communicating hydrocephalus due to blockage of CSF absorption by arachnoid villi. However, it can be of obstructive type due to narrowing and obstruction of the 3rd or 4th ventricle, cerebral aqueduct, or other CSF flow pathways by exudates or mass lesions such as tuberculomas.

Tubercular brain abscess is a unique presentation of CNS TB. It is an encapsulated pus collection with viable bacilli. It must be seen differently from tuberculoma with central caseation and liquefaction which may mimic pus. A tubercular brain abscess has a thicker abscess wall compared to a pyogenic abscess.[18]

CLINICAL PRESENTATION

Tubercular meningitis usually has subacute to chronic presentation, however, acute presentation is not unknown. TBM is mostly preceded by a variable period of nonspecific symptoms such as malaise, anorexia, fatigue, weight loss, myalgia, and headache. The most common presenting symptoms include fever, headache, nausea, vomiting, and altered sensorium.[19] Atypical clinical features are common in the elderly which often lead to a wrong diagnosis. In elderly patients, meningeal signs are less frequently present. In advanced stages, cranial nerve palsies, focal neurological deficits, and signs of raised intracranial pressure are present. The various clinical features of TBM are shown in the **Table 1**.

The presence of altered sensorium, old age, higher stage of disease, focal neurological deficit, cranial nerve deficits, and prolonged duration of illness at presentation is associated with poor outcome.[20-25]

Cranial nerve palsies are reported in up to 66% of cases. 6th nerve is most commonly involved.

Visual Abnormalities in TBM

The spectrum of visual disturbances ranges from mild blurring to complete vision loss. Optochiasmatic arachnoiditis accounts of a major chunk of patients with visual

TABLE 1: The presenting clinical features of tuberculous meningitis (TBM) in older children and adults.[23,24]

Symptoms	Percentage of patients with TBM
Fever	60–95%
Headache	50–80%
Anorexia/weight loss	60–80%
Photophobia	5–10%
Vomiting	30–60%
Clinical signs	
Neck stiffness	40–80%
Confusion	10–30%
Coma	30–60%
Cranial nerve palsy	30–50%
VI nerve palsy	30–40%
III nerve palsy	5–15%
VII nerve palsy	10–20%
Hemiparesis	10–20%
Paraparesis	5–10%
Seizures	*Children*: 50%; *Adults*: 5%

TABLE 2: Clinical staging of patients with tuberculous meningitis (TBM).[25]

Stage	Features
Stage I (early)	Nonspecific symptoms and signs
	No clouding of consciousness
	No neurologic deficits
Stage II (intermediate)	Lethargy or behavioral changes
	Meningeal irritation
	Minor neurologic deficits such as cranial nerves
Stage III (late)	Stupor or coma, abnormal movements
	Seizures
	Severe neurologic deficits such as paresis

loss. Optic nerve tuberculoma, optic neuritis, ethambutol toxicity, and hydrocephalus (ventricular dilatation leading of chiasma compression) are the main causes responsible for vision loss in TBM patients. Fundus abnormalities (papilledema/primary optic atrophy) are seen in 38.4%cases.[20]

Stroke

Cerebral infarctions are due to panarteritis with secondary thrombosis and occlusion of vessels. Hemiparesis at the time presentation is seen in about 17–26% of the patients. Involvement of anterior circulation is more common than that of posterior circulation.[20] The vascular involvement per se, apart from other neurological involvement is associated with higher risk of poor outcome, longer hospital stay, and recurrent hospital admissions as depicted in an Indian study.[22]

A staging system was introduced in 1947, which has since been widely adopted in the initial assessments of these patients and can be used to estimate prognosis **(Table 2)**.[25]

DIAGNOSIS

Cerebrospinal Fluid Analysis

Cerebrospinal fluid analysis usually reveals pleocytosis of >20 cells/mm^3 with lymphocytic predominance (>60%); proteins are usually >100 mg% and sugar <60% of the corresponding blood sugar.[26] The other tests performed on CSF to confirm the diagnosis of TBM include here.

Cerebrospinal Fluid Smear

Here, approximately 10 mL of CSF is collected. It is then centrifuged and stained with Ziehl–Neelsen and fluorescence staining. It is very cost-effective and is one of the definitive tests for the diagnosis of TBM. The major drawback of this test lies in its low sensitivity.[27]

Cerebrospinal Fluid Culture

Cerebrospinal fluid is inoculated in liquid culture media automated systems such as BACTEC MGIT 960 (Becton Dickinson, Sparks, MD, USA), radiometric BACTEC 460 (Becton Dickinson, Heidelberg, Germany), and ESP II (Difco Laboratories, Detroit, MI, USA). In a study of 5,162 positive cultures by any medium, 97% of cultures were positive by BACTEC method compared to 72% by LJ medium. The major advantage of BACTEC is shortening of time required for testing. It gives results of culture and antimycobacterial drug sensitivity [drug susceptibility testing (DST)] within 10–14 days. In this system, growth of *MTB* is detected by measuring $^{14}CO_2$ which is produced by metabolism of radiolabeled substrate in the medium. Recently, a nonradiometric version of BACTEC called BACTEC MGIT 960 TB system has been introduced.[28] Culture positivity, however, was found in only about 18.6% patients in a study.[19]

Cerebrospinal Fluid Adenosine Deaminase

Adenosine deaminase (ADA) is an enzyme involved in purine metabolism that catalyzes the conversion of deoxyadenosine to inosine and deoxyinosine. It is present mainly in active T lymphocytes. A cut off value of >10 IU/L was found to have a sensitivity of 82.14% and specificity of 90.91% for diagnosis of TBM.[29]

Techniques Based on Nucleic Acid Amplification

Nucleic Acid Amplification Test (NAAT) and Polymerase Chain Reaction (PCR)

NAAT is a molecular technique used to detect a virus or bacterium by its DNA which was first described nearly two decades ago. An advantage is that *MTB* DNA remains detectable for up to a month after starting therapy when culture and microscopic examination may become negative. NAATs are based on PCR, ligase chain reaction, and branched DNA (quantiplex bDNA) tests which use a molecule that links to specific genetic material.[30]

Many *MTB*-specific DNA sequences such as IS6110 insertion sequence, MPB64, protein antigen B, and 65kDa protein sequence have been used in NAATs. Overall sensitivity and specificity of IS6110-based assay for diagnosis of TBM range from 32 to 100% and 38 to 100%, respectively. *MPB64* gene is considered the most specific sequence for PCR assay for detection of *MTB* with sensitivity of 53–100% and specificity of 85–100% in various studies. Earlier PCR-based studies used a single gene target for amplification. Presently, multiplex PCR techniques are used which target and amplify several genes at once. For confirmed TBM cases, the sensitivity and specificity of multiplex PCR using protein B, MPB64, and IS6110 primers are 94.4% and 100%, respectively.[30]

When large volumes of CSF are processed, the diagnostic yield of NAAT increases. One disadvantage of PCR-based tests is that they are unable to differentiate been live and dead bacilli. The main reason for false positive PCR results is laboratory-induced contamination.

Loop-mediated Isothermal Amplification (LAMP)

It is a form of NAAT which is simple, rapid, and cost-effective. It operates in isothermal conditions and does not need sophisticated equipment or skilled personnel. Thus, it is an attractive and feasible option in resource limited settings.[31]

A small study on LAMP for diagnosis of TBM showed good performance with sensitivity of 88% and specificity of 90% with better sensitivity than nested PCR.[32] However, LAMP cannot be multiplexed, unlike PCR, so simultaneous drug resistance detection is only possible with selected isothermal amplification methods.

Nested PCR

It is a modified version of PCR that increases the efficiency of amplification and reduces the level of nonspecific PCR products. It has a higher sensitivity and specificity than conventional PCR.[33,34] According to studies, its sensitivity and specificity has been reported as 90–100% and this method was able to detect very low amounts of purified *MTB* DNA (1–10 copies/2 μL).[35]

GeneXpert System (Cepheid)

It is a novel point of care test that has been developed to address the issues of feasibility and sensitivity. The Cepheid GeneXpert *MTB*/rifampin (RIF) assay uses heminested reverse transcription (RT)-PCR to amplify *MTB*-specific sequence of *rpoB* gene. To determine RIF resistance, the rpoB gene is probed with molecular beacons within the rifampicin resistance-determining region (RRDR) region. This is a nearly fully automated assay, including bacterial lysis, nucleic acid extraction, amplification, and amplicon detection. The test is run on the GeneXpert platform using a disposable plastic cartridge with all required reagents. The major edge over other tests lies in the fact that this system detects mycobacterial DNA in approximately 2 hours. The assay detected *MTB* in all of the smear positive samples (29 of 29) (100%; 95% CI 85.4–100%) and in 38 of 53 smear-negative samples detected by culture.[35] This method is now widely used and endorsed by WHO for detection of pulmonary TB but its role in diagnosis of TBM is still not clear.[34,35] Xpert Ultra, its successor, has proven diagnostic accuracy over Xpert *MTB*/RIF assay in diagnosing TBM. In 2017, WHO released guidelines for using GeneXpert Ultra as the first-line diagnostic test for TBM.[36]

Truenat

Truenat (Molbio Diagnostics, Goa, India) is a chip-based NAAT platform developed indigenously to meet the requirements of Indian primary health centers. It functions on a portable, battery-operated Truelab device that can operate even at environmental temperature of 40°C, making it ideal for peripheral healthcare settings of this tropical country. It is another *MTB* DNA identification method. The preliminary data suggested similar diagnostic accuracy as GeneXpert system. Its role in TBM diagnosis was first published in 2021, according to which it had sensitivity for TBM as 79–86%.[36]

Newer Techniques

Lipoarabinomannan Assay

The first-generation lipoarabinomannan test has poor sensitivity of 24% but a high specificity of 95%.[37] The next-generation TB lipoarabinomannan assay (FujiLAM, Fujifilm, Tokyo, Japan) detects concentrations 30 times lower than the conventional lipoarabinomannan assay and is 35% more sensitive in detecting TB in adults with HIV.[38]

Metagenomic Next-generation Sequencing

It is a novel diagnostic test for the detection of untargeted pathogen in CSF. It has sensitivity of 84% and specificity of 100% as reported in a study by Yan et al.[39]

Serum Protein Biomarkers

Three serum biomarkers—(1) adipsin, (2) amyloid β42, and (3) IL-10 were implicated in a South African study of 47 children who were diagnosed with tuberculous meningitis. The combination of these markers had 83% diagnostic sensitivity and 75% specificity.[40]

Neuroimaging

Computed tomography (CT) and magnetic resonance imaging (MRI) are integral to the diagnosis of TBM. In a study on 67 patients of TBM, MRI brain was abnormal in 61 (91%) patients.[41]

Exudates

The most consistent feature of TBM on plain CT head is hyperdense signal changes in basal cisterns along with their obliteration, which is due to exudates. They display diffuse enhancement after contrast administration on MRI. These are seen in about 32–81% of cases. The most common site for exudates is basal cisterns, followed by cerebral convexities.[2,42-45] Dense exudates are found in about 14.8% cases, which are typically described as having a "spider-leg" appearance **(Fig. 1)**. These dense exudates can lead to

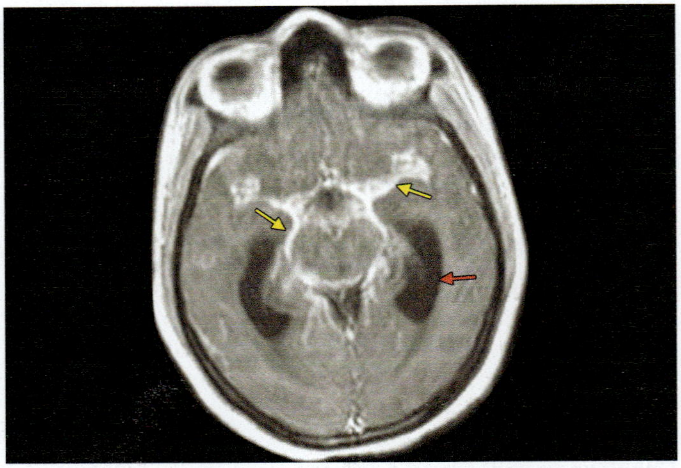

FIG. 1: Gadolinium-enhanced magnetic resonance imaging (MRI) brain of a 20-year-old female with definite tuberculous meningitis. T1-contrast axial section showing contrast enhancement in ambient, crural, perimesencephalic cisterns, depicting grade 3 exudates (yellow arrows). Note the enlargement of occipital horns of lateral ventricle (red arrow).

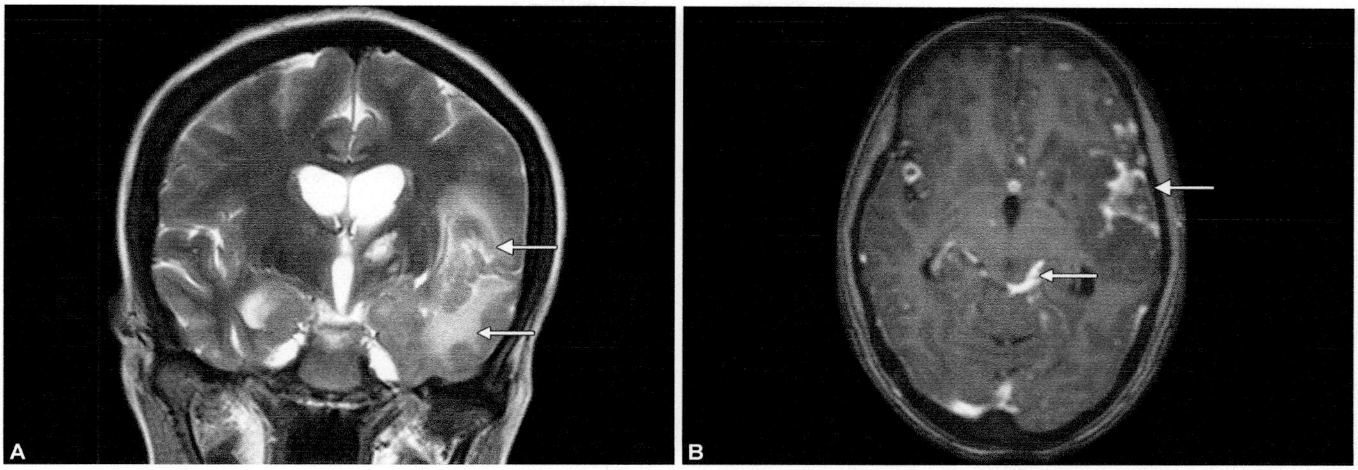

FIGS. 2A AND B: Border-zone encephalitis (BZE) affecting left perisylvian region in tubercular meningitis (TBM). (A) Intensive hyperintense signal changes (white arrows) T2W MR (T2-weighted magnetic resonance) images involving left temporoparietal region (white arrows); (B) Gadolinium-enhanced magnetic resonance (MR) images of brain showing thick enhancing exudates in left sylvian fissure and basal cisterns (white arrows).

edema and a perivascular reaction, that is known as border-zone reaction, and this reaction leads to encephalitis, known as border zone encephalitis **(Figs. 2A and B)**.

Hydrocephalus

Obstructive (extraventricular or intraventricular obstruction) or nonobstructive hydrocephalus is found in up to 56% of cases.[42]

Tuberculomas

Among the various forms of parenchymal TB, tuberculoma is the most common form. They have been noted in up to 77% of cases of TBM as reported in a study by Dian et al.[42] Their presence has been found to be as high as in 77% cases as reported in a study by Dian et al.[42] Radiological presentation varies depending upon whether the granuloma is noncaseating or caseating. Imaging characteristics of tuberculomas are often nonspecific. Differentials include other granulomatous processes such as sarcoidosis or fungal lesions, parasitic diseases like cysticercosis and toxoplasmosis, multicentric primary neoplasms as well as metastatic neoplasms.

Infarcts

Infarction patterns in TBM could be unilateral as well as bilateral. Involvement of anterior circulation is more common than that of posterior circulation. Venous system is usually spared.[44]

The subcortical area is divided into two zones—tubercular zone and ischemic zone, depending on the blood supply.[43] The tubercular zone is supplied by medial lenticulostriate, thalamotuberal, and thalamoperforating branches. This area consists of head of caudate nucleus, anterior limb, genu of internal capsule, and anteromedial thalamus. The ischemic zone is supplied by lateral lenticulostriate arteries, anterior choroidal, and thalamogeniculate arteries. Infarcts are more common in tubercular zone as compared to ischemic zone **(Figs. 3 and 4)**. Stroke occurrence is significantly related to stage of meningitis, presence of hydrocephalus, exudates, and hypertension. However, there was no difference in clinical or laboratory parameters in early and late strokes.[46,47] **Table 3** demonstrates the spectrum of infarcts in two major studies. MRA abnormalities were associated with poor outcome. They had found a significant correlation of disseminated irregular calibers of intracranial arteries with duration of the disease, presence of hydrocephalus, and age at presentation. The localized stenosis at the base of the brain was related to the stage of the disease, basal exudates, and infarction.[48]

DIAGNOSTIC CRITERIA FOR TUBERCULAR MENINGITIS

The diagnosis of TBM in early stages is very difficult, and a high index of suspicion is required when any patient of febrile encephalopathy is worked up for a definite etiology. It is primarily because of the paucibacillary nature of this disease that most of the available tests are lacking sensitivity to diagnose all cases of TBM. A positive test may confirm the diagnosis in a given clinical setting, but a negative test does not rule out TBM. So, for labeling a patient as TBM, the composite reference standard (CRS), [i.e., aggregate of clinical, radiological imaging, CSF analysis, and microbiological features (smear, NAAT and culture)] are used. Ahuja et al. proposed diagnostic

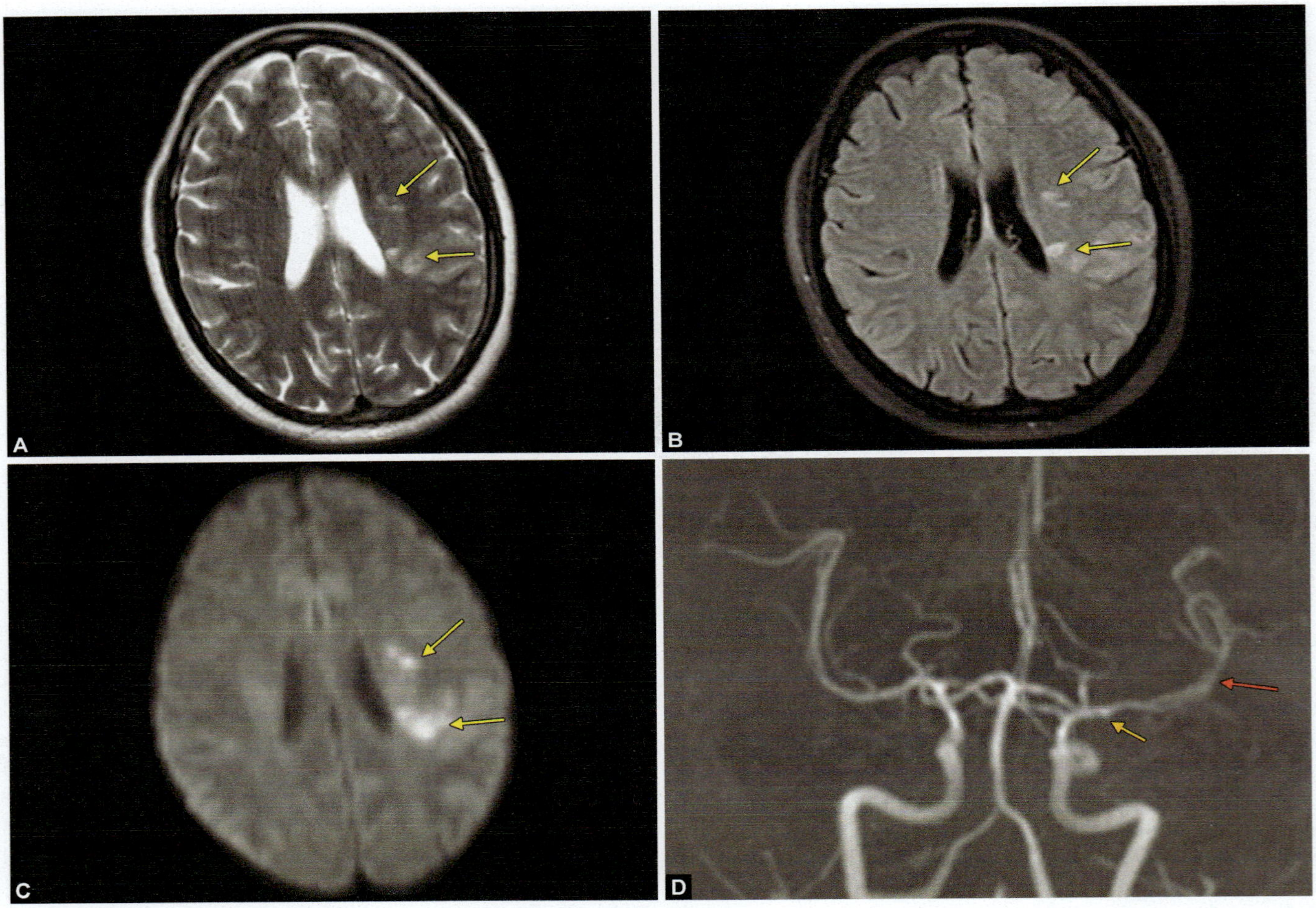

FIGS. 3A TO D: A 36-year-old female with definite TBM. Axial section of T2-weighted image (A) and FLAIR (B) image and diffusion-weighted image (C) showing acute multiple infarcts (yellow arrows) in left periventricular white matter corresponding to left MCA territory. MR angiography (D) showing left M1 MCA narrowing (orange arrow) with severe attenuation of left M2 MCA (red arrow).
(FLAIR: fluid-attenuated inversion recovery; MCA: middle cerebral artery; MR: magnetic resonance; TBM: tubercular meningitis)

criteria for TBM based on various clinical features in a patient presenting with fever and headaches, supported by radiological and CSF parameters and categorized them into definite, highly probable and probable groups.[49] Patients suspected of TBM were classified as definite when the organism was identified in CSF either by Ziehl–Neelsen stain or culture. However, at that time NAATs were not readily available for clinical use. To label a patient as a case of "definite TBM", isolation of the organism from the CSF is required. It was in the year 2010 that Marais et al.[50] included NAAT confirmation of presence of organism in CSF for "definite TBM" and proposed a uniform case definition that patients with suspected tuberculous meningitis be allocated to one of four diagnostic categories depending on the strength of clinical, laboratory, and radiological findings. The proposed categories are definite, probable, possible, and not tuberculous meningitis.

DIFFERENTIAL DIAGNOSIS

The differential diagnosis for a subacute to chronic meningitis with a CSF picture of raised protein, low glucose, and lymphocytic pleocytosis includes:

- *Fungal meningitis*: It shares a similar clinical picture of subacute presentation, which may be associated with cranial neuropathies. Common disorders include cryptococcosis, histoplasmosis, blastomycosis, and coccidiomycosis. The risk is increased in immunosuppressed states, and cryptococcosis is particularly associated with HIV with low CD4 counts. Definitive diagnosis is made by CSF culture, although other tests such as India Ink preparation may be utilized.
- *Bacterial meningitis*: Although, it typically presents acutely, the differentiation may not always be so straightforward, such as in cases of partially treated meningitis. Typically, neutrophilic predominance is seen rather than monocytic predominance.

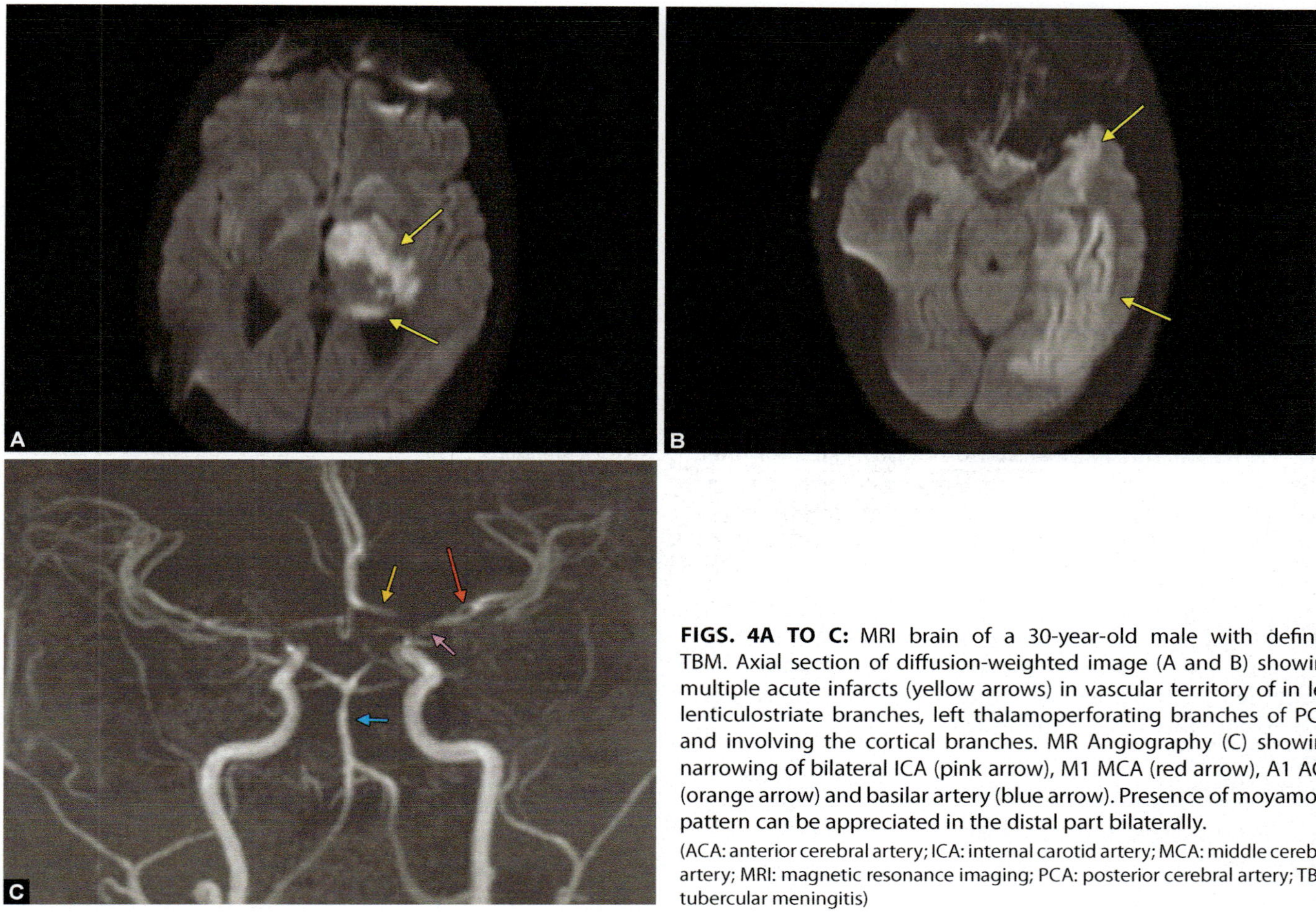

FIGS. 4A TO C: MRI brain of a 30-year-old male with definite TBM. Axial section of diffusion-weighted image (A and B) showing multiple acute infarcts (yellow arrows) in vascular territory of in left lenticulostriate branches, left thalamoperforating branches of PCA, and involving the cortical branches. MR Angiography (C) showing narrowing of bilateral ICA (pink arrow), M1 MCA (red arrow), A1 ACA (orange arrow) and basilar artery (blue arrow). Presence of moyamoya pattern can be appreciated in the distal part bilaterally.

(ACA: anterior cerebral artery; ICA: internal carotid artery; MCA: middle cerebral artery; MRI: magnetic resonance imaging; PCA: posterior cerebral artery; TBM: tubercular meningitis)

TABLE 3: Spectrum of infarcts in recent studies.

Parameter	Tai et al.[19] (*n* = 51)	Soni et al.[46] (*n* = 90)
Infarcts	34 (66.67%)	52 (57.7%)
Lateral lenticulostriate	25 (73%)	26 (50%)
Medial lenticulostriate	14 (41%)	12 (23%)
Cortical branches MCA/ACA/PCA	10 (29%)	5 (15.4%)
Thalamoperforating and thalamogeniculate	13 (38%)	26 (50%)
Perforating branches BA	4 (12%)	
Superior cerebellar	1 (3%)	1(2%)
AICA	2 (6%)	

(ACA: anterior cerebral artery; MCA: middle cerebral artery; PCA: posterior cerebral artery)

- *Viral meningitis*: It typically presents acutely. It is commonly caused by herpesviruses and enteroviruses. Glucose levels are usually normal. Diagnosis is established by CSF Pan viral test (PVT).
- *Neurosyphilis*: Neurosyphilis may manifest as syphilitic meningitis, with symptoms including headache, nausea, vomiting, nuchal rigidity, and confusion. Another form of neurosyphilis is meningovascular syphilis, which includes infectious arteritis affecting vessels in the SAS. This may result in ischemic events involving the CNS, which are also seen in TBM. Concomitant-ophthalmic disease commonly occurs in the form of uveitis, retinitis, or optic neuropathy. Diagnosis is established by serum treponemal and nontreponemal tests, and CSF venereal disease research laboratory test.
- *Neurobrucellosis*: Brucellosis typically presents with insidious onset of fever, malaise, night sweats, and arthralgias. It may be complicated by neurobrucellosis; manifestations include meningitis, encephalitis, brain abscess, myelitis, radiculitis, and/or neuritis (with involvement of cranial or peripheral nerves). CSF findings are similar to TBM and include a mononuclear pleocytosis (10–200 white blood cells), mild-to-moderately elevated protein levels, and reduced sugars. The diagnosis may be established via antibody or agglutination testing of spinal fluid.
- *Neoplastic meningitis*: Leptomeningeal metastases (LM), also known as carcinomatous meningitis, refer to the metastatic spread of primary tumors, most commonly breast, lung, and melanoma to the leptomeninges. Clinical manifestations include headache, nausea and

vomiting, limb weakness, altered mental status, diplopia, and cranial neuropathies. Typical MRI findings include linear and nodular leptomeningeal enhancement, thickening and enhancement of cranial nerves or nerve roots, and hydrocephalus. CSF findings include elevated opening pressure, mild pleocytosis, elevated protein, and decreased glucose concentrations. The diagnosis of LM is definitively established via demonstration of malignant cells in the CSF.

MANAGEMENT

Treatment of patients with TBM is complex and can be divided into four major areas. First, the core is formed by anti-TB treatment. Early initiation of anti-TB treatment, before the onset of coma, greatly increases chances of survival. Secondly, adjunctive immunomodulatory treatment is currently recommended for all grades and ages. Thirdly, supportive therapy consists of intracranial pressure control and management of other secondary complications, such as hyponatremia. Finally, for HIV-positive patients, antiretroviral treatment (ART) should be initiated or continued, with particular care for drug-drug interactions and the immune reconstitution syndrome (IRIS).

Antituberculosis Treatment in Drug Susceptible Tubercular Meningitis

The first-line TB agents recommended in global guidelines for the treatment of TBM are rifampicin (R), isoniazid (H), pyrazinamide (Z), ethambutol (E), and streptomycin (S). Currently, WHO recommends 2 months treatment with four first-line drugs in the intensive phase, followed by a continuation phase with at least rifampicin and isoniazid for 4–10 months.[51] The regimens recommended for TBM are derived from short-course treatment for pulmonary TB. However, optimal drug doses and duration of treatment for TBM have not been established by large clinical trials and the principles of tuberculous meningitis treatment are still derived from observational studies and clinical practice. They include the importance of starting antitubercular drugs early; the recognition that isoniazid and rifampicin are the key components of the regimen; the potentially fatal consequences of interrupting treatment, more so during the first 2 months; and the perceived need for long-term treatment (9–12 months) to prevent disease relapse.

The ability of the BBB to limit intracerebral concentrations of anti-TB drugs is an important consideration in the treatment of tuberculous meningitis. **Table 4** shows the recommended first-line and second-line drugs for management of tuberculous meningitis along with their estimated CSF penetration.[52,53]

TABLE 4: Daily dose of first- and second-line ant-tubercular drugs with their cerebrospinal fluid (CSF) to plasma concentration.

Drug	Dose	CSF to plasma concentration
First-line drugs		
Isoniazid	300 mg	80–90%
Rifampicin	450 mg (weight < 50 kg) or 600 mg (weight ≥ 50 kg)	10–20%
Pyrazinamide	1.5 g (weight < 50 kg) or 2.0 g (weight ≥ 50 kg)	90–100%
Ethambutol	15 mg/kg	20–30%
Streptomycin	15 mg/kg (1 g maximum)	10–20%
Second-line drugs		
Kanamycin	15 mg/kg	10–20%
Amikacin	15–20 mg/kg	10–20%
Moxifloxacin	400 mg	70–80%
Levofloxacin	1,000 mg	70–80%
p-aminosalicylic acid	10–12 g	No data
Ethionamide or protionamide	15–20 mg/kg (1 g maximum)	80–90%
Cycloserine	10–15 mg/kg	80–90%
Linezolid	1,200 mg	40–70%
Capreomycin	15–20 mg/kg	No data

Most of the regimens recommend either streptomycin or ethambutol as the fourth drug in standard treatment, although neither penetrates the CSF well in the absence of inflammation,[53] and both can produce serious adverse reactions. Streptomycin should not be given to patients who are pregnant or who have renal impairment, and streptomycin resistance is fairly common worldwide. Ethambutol-induced optic neuritis is a concern, especially in the treatment of comatose patients, although at the standard dose of 15–20 mg/kg the incidence is <3%.[54] Some centers in South Africa advocate ethionamide, which can penetrate healthy and inflamed BBBs and is safer than ethambutol and streptomycin.[55]

Investigators in Indonesia have tested the hypothesis that treatment intensification, through use of high-dose intravenous rifampicin and the addition of moxifloxacin, would enhance bacterial killing and improve outcome. About 60 adults with tuberculous meningitis were randomly allocated to treatment with daily rifampicin at either standard dose (450 mg, about 10 mg/kg) orally or high dose (600 mg, about 13 mg/kg) intravenously, and either 400 mg or 800 mg oral moxifloxacin or 750 mg ethambutol for the first 14 days of treatment. High-dose intravenous rifampicin led to a three-times increase in the plasma and CSF area under the concentration-time curve compared with the standard oral dose and was associated with a substantial drop in mortality (65% vs. 35%), which could not be accounted for by HIV status or baseline disease severity.[56]

This finding provides compelling evidence that the chemotherapeutic regimen for tuberculous meningitis needs to be optimized and that the recommended doses of rifampicin might be too low because of its poor CSF penetration.

Managing Drug-resistant Tubercular Meningitis

Drug-resistant TB is a growing problem globally. Globally, approximately 20% of isolates in TB are resistant to one drug, and 7% are resistant to at least H.[57] Isolated resistance to H with or without resistance to S may be more frequently found in high-burden settings.

Multidrug-resistant (MDR)-TBM (resistance to at least R and H) is highly lethal. Most patients die within 2 months after treatment initiation.[58] Timely drug-resistance detection is limited by the lack of rapid diagnostics. The timing of an adjusted treatment schedule for drug resistant TBM based on culture DST results is often too late to prevent neurological disability or death. There are no studies evaluating the optimal regimen for drug-resistant TBM. The advent of Xpert *MTB*/RIF may reveal resistance to R in an early stage and open the field for intervention trials of second-line treatment for drug resistant TBM.

Some commonly described patterns of drug resistance are:

- *Isoniazid-resistant (HR)-TB* refers to MTB strains that are resistant to isoniazid and susceptible to rifampicin, confirmed invitro.
- *Rifampicin-resistant (RR)-TB* is resistant to rifampicin on basis of DST and, is eligible for treatment with MDR-TB regimens.
- *Poly-resistance-TB* refers to resistance of more than one first line anti-TB drug, other than isoniazid and rifampicin together.
- *MDR-TB* refers to MTB strains that resistant to both isoniazid and rifampicin, the two most potent tuberculocidal drugs.
- *XDR-TB (extensively)* refers to the form of tb in which MTB strains have resistant to isoniazid, rifampicin, any of the fluoroquinolone and to at least one of the three injectable second-line drugs (amikacin, capreomycin, and kanamycin).
- *XXDR-TB (extremely drug-resistant TB)* refers to TB in which MTB strains are resistant to all first line as well as second-line drugs.

In pulmonary MDR-TB the WHO guidelines recommend the addition of an injectable drug (amikacin, kanamycin, or capreomycin) and a fluoroquinolone (moxifloxacin or levofloxacin) and at least two other agents to which the mycobacterium is susceptible.[55,57] There are no guidelines that specify treatment for MDR-TBM. Of the second-line agents, ethionamide, prothionamide, and cycloserine are able to penetrate the CSF and may be effective in TBM.[55,57] In patients with MDR/RR-TB who have not been exposed to treatment with second-line TB medicines, a shorter, all-oral, bedaquiline-containing regimen of 9–12 months' duration is recommended.[57]

Paradoxical responses—deterioration despite appropriate anti-TB treatment are frequently reported. This can be observed in all tissues, but most often in the lungs, lymph nodes, and the brain.[59] In the brain, tuberculoma may develop or enlarge during treatment for pulmonary TB or during TBM treatment. It may be accompanied by worsening symptoms or signs of a space occupying lesion, generally occurring within 1–4 months of treatment after initial improvement. If other causes of deterioration (such as drug resistance or infarcts) are ruled out, anti-TB therapy should be continued, and the addition of systemic corticosteroids or other immune-modulatory drugs may be considered.

Adjunctive Immune-modulatory Treatment

Corticosteroids

The rationale of adjunctive anti-inflammatory therapy is based on the hypothesis that a substantial part of the pathological morbidity in TBM is caused by an inappropriate inflammatory response to *MTB*. The use of corticosteroids in TBM has been the subject of numerous clinical trials in the past decades. These have been systematically reviewed by the Cochrane collaboration, whose meta-analysis concluded that corticosteroids improved outcome in HIV-negative adults and children with TBM.[60] However, the benefit in HIV-positive patients remains to be established.

Aspirin

There is a potential role of aspirin in reducing the brain infarcts and mortality due to TBM, in HIV-negative patients when used in high doses (1,000 mg/day). This beneficial effect is due to dose-dependent inhibition of prostanoids and upregulation of specialized proresolving mediators in CSF. Various phase 3 trials are ongoing in adults (NCT04145258 and NCT03927313) and in children to define the role of aspirin in patients with tuberculous meningitis.[61,62]

Thalidomide

In the earlier animal models of TBM, it was found that thalidomide reduced inflammation and improved survival. But when used in children with TBM, it was associated with increased mortality. Subsequently, there are only case series and reports to define the benefit of this drug. Further studies and clinical trials are required to define the role of adjuvant thalidomide in the treatment of tuberculous meningitis.[62]

Tumor Necrosis Factor-alpha Inhibitors

Infliximab has been used in adults and children with tuberculous meningitis as a rescue adjuvant therapy for refractory paradoxical reactions, or tuberculous meningitis-associated vasculopathy.[62]

Interleukin-1 Inhibitor

Anakinra has also been used at various centers to control tuberculous meningitis-associated paradoxical reactions.[62]

Antiretroviral Therapy

The main challenge in dealing with HIV and TBM coinfection is the drug interactions and the timing to start ART. The main risk of early ART initiation is IRIS, which occurs in up to 50% of those with tuberculous meningitis and results in substantial morbidity and mortality.[63] A trial indicated that prednisone given with ART could prevent TB-associated IRIS, although people with tuberculous meningitis were excluded. Whether corticosteroids prevent and treat tuberculous meningitis-associated IRIS is an important unanswered question.[64] Starting ART after 2 months of ATT was associated with lesser grade 4 adverse events as compared to when started immediately.[65]

Managing Hyponatremia

Hyponatremia in TBM is associated with worse outcomes. In resource-limited settings, it is difficult to discriminate between the different causes of low sodium, however, mostly implicated are the syndrome of inappropriate antidiuretic hormone secretion (SIADH) or cerebral salt wasting (CSW) syndrome, of which CSW is probably underdiagnosed in TBM. A pragmatic approach is to avoid both hypoosmolality and hypovolemia. Fluid restriction in CSW can be detrimental and is not recommended. General advice is to correct hyponatremia cautiously with hypertonic saline combined with fludrocortisone if indicated.[66] Pontine myelinolysis should be prevented by gradual correction.

Managing Hydrocephalus

Hydrocephalus is one of the most common complications of TBM, more so in children than in adults. It may develop both in the early and late stage of the disease. It occurs at an earlier stage and in more severe form in children. This may be acute in onset due to the presence of thick gelatinous exudates in the basal cisterns, especially interpeduncular (IPC) and peripontine cisterns, causing blockage of the SAS. In the later stage of the disease, these exudates cause blockage of arachnoid granulations thus preventing absorption of CSF. Overproduction of CSF due to the inflammation of the ependymal lining and choroid plexus also contributes to the hydrocephalus. A plain CT scan is the ideal imaging in acute setting as it is faster, easily available, and gives adequate information regarding size of the ventricles, periventricular lucency, basal exudates, and presence of infarcts.

Medical Management with Antitubercular Treatment

Steroids and diuretics such as frusemide and acetazolamide may be tried in acute stage of communicating hydrocephalous.

Surgical Management

Mainstay of management of TBM with hydrocephalus is CSF diversion. Early surgery may improve outcome and early discharge from hospital as prolonged monitoring on medical management may not be cost-effective. Ventriculoperitoneal (VP) shunt is the procedure of choice for management of hydrocephalus. Complications of VP shunt are higher in TBM than performed for hydrocephalus secondary to other causes due to higher cell counts and protein content in CSF. Various complications include frequent shunt blockage requiring multiple revisions, shunt infection, skin erosion, peritoneal pseudocyst formation, and adhesive peritonitis.[67] These complications, especially infection and shunt blockage, can be prevented to a large extent by taking strict measures in the operating room with respect to asepsis, using powder-free gloves and minimal touch technique to the shunt system. It is found that shorter the procedure lesser is the infection.

Role of Endoscopy

More and more interest in endoscopic CSF diversion has emerged to avoid foreign body insertion and accompanying complications. *Endoscopic third ventriculostomy (ETV)* theoretically is not a favored procedure in hydrocephalous due to TBM as mostly it is of communicating type. The success rate of ETV has been reported in 68–77% patients in different studies. Experience of surgeon in endoscopic procedures determines the success rate as TBM exudates and scarring cause difficulty in recognizing the anatomical landmarks at the floor of third ventricle to perform ventriculostomy. Patients with longer duration of symptoms and those who have received at least 4 weeks of ATT are more likely to benefit from ETV.[68,69]

CONCLUSION

- Early diagnosis and treatment of TBM save lives. A high index of suspicion in patients presenting with a meningitic syndrome lasting longer than few days to weeks is fundamental to diagnosis.
- TBM is a paucibacillary disease; hence, all available diagnostic modalities lack sensitivity. Treatment should be initiated based on a presumptive diagnosis even in the absence of microbiological confirmation. Clinical indicators suggestive of TBM are longstanding illness, cranial nerve palsy of the 4th, 3rd, or 2nd nerve, chest X-ray (pulmonary TB and military TB), brain imaging (hydrocephalus, nasal meningeal enhancement, and tuberculoma) and radiological or microbiological confirmation of extraneural TB.
- Xpert *MTB*/RIF ultra may have improved sensitivity over smear in most high-burden settings. It gives early results and if *MTB* is detected, gives additional information on rifampicin resistance within 2 hours. Early treatment adjustment is warranted for those patients in whom

MDR-TBM is detected. A negative Xpert *MTB*/RIF does not rule out TBM.

- Treatment should be started early, preferably before neurological deterioration. Isoniazid and rifampicin are key constituents of the treatment regimen and should be used whenever possible. Treatment interruption in the intensive phase of therapy is a risk factor for death.
- There is a great need for shorter, less toxic treatment regimens, new drugs, and better and shorter ways of evaluating new TB drugs and drug regimens.
- Early CSF diversion by shunt surgery provides better outcome in patients of TBM who develop hydrocephalus. ETV has its role in a particular subset of patients who show features of obstruction.

REFERENCES

1. World Health Organization. (2021). Global tuberculosis report 2021. [online] Available from https://www.who.int/publications/i/item/9789240037021 [Last accessed May, 2023].
2. Wasay M, Farooq S, Khowaja ZA, Bawa ZA, Ali SM, Awan S, et al. Cerebral infarction and tuberculoma in central nervous system tuberculosis: frequency and prognostic implications. J Neurol Neurosurg Psychiatry. 2014;85(11):1260-4.
3. Misra UK, Kalita J, Maurya PK. Stroke in tuberculous meningitis. J Neurol Sci. 2011;303(1-2):22-30.
4. National Tuberculosis Elimination Programme Annual report. (2021). India TB Report 2021. [online] Available from https://tbcindia.gov.in/showfile.php?lid=3587 [Last accessed May, 2023].
5. Green PH. Tubercular meningitis. Lancet. 1836;26(663):232-5.
6. Koch R. The etiology of tuberculosis. Berliner Kliniscben Wocbenschift. 1882;15:221-30.
7. Chen P, Shi M, Feng GD, Liu JY, Wang BJ, Shi XD, et al. A highly efficient Ziehl–Neelsen stain: Identifying de novo intracellular mycobacterium tuberculosis and improving detection of extracellular M. tuberculosis in cerebrospinal fluid. J Clin Microbiol. 2012;50(4):1166-70.
8. Rich AR, McCordock HA. The pathogenesis of tuberculous meningitis. Bull John Hopkins Hosp. 1933;52:5.
9. Dastur DK, Manghani DK, Udani PM. Pathology and pathogenetic mechanisms in neurotuberculosis. Radiol Clin North Am. 1995;33(4):733-52.
10. Mastroianni CM, Paoletti F, Lichtner M, D'Agostino C, Vullo V, Delia S. Cerebrospinal fluid cytokines in patients with tuberculous meningitis. Clin Immunol Immunopathol.1997;84(2):171-6.
11. Ramilo O, Sáez-Llorens X, Mertsola J, Jafari H, Olsen KD, Hansen EJ, et al. Tumor necrosis factor alpha/cachectin and interleukin 1 beta initiate meningeal inflammation. J Exp Med. 1990;172(2):497-507.
12. Sinha HP, Modi M, Prabhakar S, Singh P. Do cytokines correlate with disease activity in tuberculous meningitis? Neurol Asia. 2015;20(3):243-50.
13. Galea I, Bechmann I, Perry VH. What is immune privilege (not)? Trends Immunol. 2007;28(1):12-8.
14. Liu Y, Teige I, Birnir B, Issazadeh-Navikas S. Neuron-mediated generation of regulatory T cells from encephalitogenic T cells suppresses EAE. Nat Med. 2006;12(5):518-25.
15. Sharma SK, Mohan A. Tuberculosis. New Delhi: Jaypee Brothers Medical Publishers (P) Ltd;. 2009. pp.304-30.
16. Lammie GA, Hewlett RH, Schoeman JF, Donald PR. Tuberculous cerebrovascular disease: a review. J Infect. 2009;59(3):156-66.
17. Davis AG, Rohlwink UK, Proust A, Figaji AA, Wilkinson RJ. The pathogenesis of tuberculous meningitis. J Leukoc Biol. 2019;105(2):267-80.
18. Kumar R, Pandey CK, Bose N, Sahay S. Tuberculous brain abscess: clinical presentation, pathophysiology and treatment (in children). J Int Soc Pediatr Neurosurg. 2002;18(3-4):118-23.
19. Tai MLS, Viswanathan S, Rahmat K, Nor HM, Kadir KAA, Goh KJ, et al. Cerebral infarction pattern in tuberculous meningitis. Sci Rep. 2016;6(1):38802.
20. Sharma S, Goyal MK, Sharma K, Modi M, Sharma M, Khandelwal N, et al. Cytokines do play a role in pathogenesis of tuberculous meningitis: A prospective study from a tertiary care center in India. J Neurol Sci. 2017;379:131-6.
21. Misra UK, Kalita J, Srivastava M, Mandal SK. Prognosis of tuberculous meningitis: a multivariate analysis. J Neurol Sci. 1996;137(1):57-61.
22. Selvaraj JU, Sujalini BB, Rohitson MS, George AA, Arvind VH, Mishra AK. Identification of predictors of cerebrovascular infarcts in patients with tuberculous meningitis. Int J Mycobacteriol. 2020;9(3):303-8.
23. Farinha NJ, Razali KA, Holzel H, Morgan G, Novelli VM. Tuberculosis of the central nervous system in children: a 20-year survey. J Infect. 2000;41(1):61-8.
24. Hinman AR. Tuberculous meningitis in Cleveland Metropoliton General Hospital 1959 to 1963. Am Rev Resp Dis.1967;95:670-3.
25. Ahuja GK, Mohan KK, Prasad K, Behari M. Diagnostic criteria for tuberculous meningitis and their validation. Tuber Lung Dis. 1994;75(2):149-52.
26. Garg RK. Tuberculosis of the central nervous system. Postgrad Med J. 1999;75:133-40.
27. Koch ML, Cote RA. Comparison of fluorescence microscopy with ziehl-neelsen stain for demonstration of acid-fast bacilli in smear preparations and tissue sections. Am Rev Respir Dis. 1965;91:283-4.
28. Rodrigues CS, Shenai SV, Almeida D, Sadani MA, Goyal N, Vadher C, et al. Use of BACTEC 460 TB system in the diagnosis of tuberculosis. Indian J Med Microbiol. 2007;25(1):32-6.
29. Chander A, Shrestha CD. Cerebrospinal fluid adenosine deaminase levels as a diagnostic marker in tuberculous meningitis in adult Nepalese patients. Asian Pac J Trop Dis. 2013;3(1):16-9.
30. Sharma K, Sharma A, Ray P, Kumar SS, Modi M, Prabhakar S, et al. Multiplex PCR for rapid diagnosis of tuberculous meningitis. J Neurol. 2011;258(10):1781-7.
31. Boehme CC, Nabeta P, Hillemann D, Nicol MP, Shenai S, Krapp F, et al. Rapid molecular detection of tuberculosis and rifampin resistance. N Engl J Med. 2010;363(11):1005-15.
32. Nagdev KJ, Kashyap RS, Parida MM, Kapgate RC, Purohit HJ, Taori GM, et al. Loop-mediated isothermal amplification for rapid and reliable diagnosis of tuberculous meningitis. J Clin Microbiol. 2011;49(5):1861-5.
33. Takahashi T, Nakayama T, Tamura M, Ogawa K, Tsuda H, Morita A, et al. Nested polymerase chain reaction for assessing the clinical course of tuberculous meningitis. Neurology. 2005;64(10):1789-93.
34. Thwaites G, Chau TT, Mai NT, Drobniewski F, McAdam K, Farrar J. Tuberculous meningitis. J Neurol Neurosurg Psychiatry. 2000;68(3):289-99.
35. Philip N, William T, John DV. Diagnosis of tuberculous meningitis: Challenges and promises. Malays J Pathol. 2015;37(1):1-9.
36. Sharma K, Sharma M, Modi M, Singla N, Sharma A, Sharma S, et al. Comparative analysis of Truenat MTB Plus and Xpert Ultra in diagnosing tuberculous meningitis. Int J Tuberc Lung Dis. 2021;25:626-31.

37. Kwizera R, Cresswell FV, Mugumya G, Okirwoth M, Kagimu E, Bangdiwala AS, et al. Performance of lipoarabinomannan assay using cerebrospinal fluid for the diagnosis of tuberculous meningitis among HIV patients. Wellcome Open Res. 2019;4:123.
38. Sigal GB, Pinter A, Lowary TL, Kawasaki M, Li A, Mathew A, et al. A novel sensitive immunoassay targeting the 5-methylthio-d-xylofuranoselipoarabinomannan epitope meets the WHO's performance target for tuberculosis diagnosis. J Clin Microbiol. 2018;56:e01338-18.
39. Yan L, Sun W, Lu Z, Fan L. Metagenomic next-generation sequencing (mNGS) in cerebrospinal fluid for rapid diagnosis of tuberculosis meningitis in HIV-negative population. Int J Infect Dis. 2020;96:270-5.
40. Manyelo CM, Solomons RS, Snyders CI, Mutavhatsindi H, Manngo PM, Stanley K, et al. Potential of host serum protein biomarkers in the diagnosis of tuberculous meningitis in children. Front Pediatr. 2019;7:376.
41. Kalita J, Prasad S, Maurya PK, Kumar S, Misra UK. MR angiography in tuberculous meningitis. Acta Radiol Stockh Swed. 2012;53(3):324-9.
42. Dian S, Hermawan R, van Laarhoven A, Immaculata S, Achmad TH, Ruslami R, et al. Brain MRI findings in relation to clinical characteristics and outcome of tuberculous meningitis. PLoS One. 2020;15(11):e0241974.
43. Hsieh FY, Chia LG, Shen WC. Locations of cerebral infarctions in tuberculous meningitis. Neuroradiology. 1992;34(3):197-9.
44. Kalita J, Singh RK, Misra UK, Kumar S. Evaluation of cerebral arterial and venous system in tuberculous meningitis. J Neuroradiol. 2018;45(2):130-5.
45. Yaşar K, PehliVanoğlu F, Şengöz A, Şengöz G. Evaluation of radiological findings in 160 adult patients with tuberculous meningitis. Turk J Med Sci. 2012;42(2):259-67.
46. Soni N, Kumar S, Shimle A, Ora M, Bathla G, Mishra P. Cerebrovascular complications in tuberculous meningitis-A magnetic resonance imaging study in 90 patients from a tertiary care hospital. Neuroradiol J. 2020;33(1):3-16.
47. Kalita J, Misra UK, Nair PP. Predictors of stroke and its significance in the outcome of tuberculous meningitis. J Stroke Cerebrovasc Dis. 2009;18(4):251-8.
48. Lu TT, Lin XQ, Zhang L, Cai W, Dai YQ, Lu ZZ, et al. Magnetic resonance angiography manifestations and prognostic significance in HIV-negative tuberculosis meningitis. Int J Tuberc Lung Dis. 2015;19(12):1448-54.
49. Modi M, Sharma K, Prabhakar S, Goyal MK, Takkar A, Sharma N, et al. Clinical and radiological predictors of outcome in tubercular meningitis: A prospective study of 209 patients. Clin Neurol Neurosurg. 2017;161:29-34.
50. Marais S, Thwaites G, Schoeman JF, Török ME, Misra UK, Prasad K, et al. Tuberculous meningitis: a uniform case definition for use in clinical research. Lancet Infect Dis. 2010;10(11):803-12.
51. WHO. (2017). Guidelines for treatment of drug-susceptible tuberculosis and patient care, 2017 update. [online] Available from https://apps.who.int/iris/handle/10665/255052 [Last accessed May, 2023].
52. Thwaites G, Fisher M, Hemingway C, Scott G, Solomon T, Innes J. British Infection Society guidelines for the diagnosis and treatment of tuberculosis of the central nervous system in adults and children. J Infect. 2009;59:167-87.
53. Ellard GA, Humphries MJ, Allen BW. Cerebrospinal fluid drug concentrations and the treatment of tuberculous meningitis. Am Rev Respir Dis. 1993;148:650-5.
54. Donald PR, Maher D, Maritz JS, Qazi S. Ethambutol dosage for the treatment of children: literature review and recommendations. Int J Tuberc Lung Dis. 2006;10:1318-30.
55. Donald PR, Seifart HI. Cerebrospinal fluid concentrations of ethionamide in children with tuberculous meningitis. J Pediatr. 1989;115:483-86.
56. Ruslami R, Ganiem AR, Dian S, Apriani L, Achmad TH, van der Ven AJ, et al. Intensified regimen containing rifampicin and moxifloxacin for tuberculous meningitis: an open-label, randomised controlled phase 2 trial. Lancet Infect Dis. 2013;13:27-35.
57. WHO. Multidrug and extensively drug-resistant TB (M/XDR-TB) 2010 global report on surveillance and response. report. Geneva, Switzerland: World Health Organization 2010.
58. Thwaites GE, Lan NT, Dung NH, Quy HT, Oanh DTT, Thoa NTC, et al. Effect of antituberculosis drug resistance on response to treatment and outcome in adults with tuberculous meningitis. J Infect Dis. 2005;192(1):79-88.
59. Smith H. Paradoxical responses during the chemotherapy of tuberculosis. J Infect. 1987;15(1):1-3.
60. Prasad K, Singh MB. Corticosteroids for managing tuberculous meningitis. Cochrane Database Syst Rev. 2008(1):CD002244.
61. WHO. (2021) Rapid communication on updated guidance on the management of tuberculosis in children and adolescents. [online] Available from https://www.who.int/publications/i/item/9789240033450 [Last accessed May, 2023].
62. Huynh J, Donovan J, Phu N, Nghia HDT, Thuong NTT, Thwaites GE. Tuberculous meningitis: progress and remaining questions. Lancet Neurol. 2022;21(5):450-64.
63. Marais S, Meintjes G, Pepper DJ, Dodd LE, Schutz C, Ismail Z, et al. Frequency, severity, and prediction of tuberculous meningitis immune reconstitution inflammatory syndrome. Clin Infect Dis. 2013;56:450-6.
64. Meintjes G, Stek C, Blumenthal L, Thienemann F, Schutz C, Buyze J, et al. Prednisone for the prevention of paradoxical tuberculosis-associated IRIS. N Engl J Med. 2018;379:1915-25.
65. Török ME, Yen NT, Chau TT, et al. Timing of initiation of antiretroviral therapy in human immunodeficiency virus (HIV)-associated tuberculous meningitis. Clin Infect Dis. 2011;52:1374-83.
66. Figaji AA, Fieggen AG. The neurosurgical and acute care management of tuberculous meningitis: Evidence and current practice. Tuberculosis (Edinb). 2010;90(6):393-400.
67. Agrawal D, Gupta A, Mehta VS. Role of shunt surgery in pediatric tubercular meningitis with hydrocephalus. Indian Pediatr. 2005;42:245-50.
68. Singh D, Sachdev V, Singh AK, Sinha S. Endoscopic third ventriculostomy in post-tubercular meningitic hydrocephalus: A preliminary report. Minim Invasive Neurosurg. 2005;48:47-52.
69. Husain M, Jha DK, Rastogi M, Husain N, Gupta RK. Role of neuroendoscopy in the management of patients with tuberculous meningitis hydrocephalus. Neurosurg Rev. 2005;28:278-83.

58
CHAPTER

Neurocysticercosis

Gagandeep Singh

INTRODUCTION

Neurocysticercosis (NCC) refers to brain infestation with the larval stage of helminth, *Taenia solium*. It is considered the single major cause of acquired epilepsy in the world[1-4] and thus an important public health problem. The infection and resulting disease are highly endemic in all parts of the developing world where pigs are raised as a food source.[5] Cysticercosis is endemic throughout Latin America, most of Asia including India, and sub-Saharan Africa. NCC is now also increasingly diagnosed in high-income countries resulting from the immigration of tapeworm carriers from and travel to endemic regions of the world.[6,7]

Clinical manifestations reflect the compromise of the affected organs. Outside the nervous system, cysticercosis causes few symptoms and parasitic cysts are destroyed by the host's immune response. Symptoms or signs usually result from parasites located in the eye or the nervous system. Clinical manifestations of NCC are varied and nonspecific, related to individual differences in the number, size, and topography of lesions, and in the severity of the host's immune response to the parasites.[8]

LIFE CYCLE

Taenia solium has a complex two-host life cycle. Humans are the only definitive host and harbor the adult tapeworm, whereas both humans and pigs may act as intermediate hosts and harbor the larvae or cysticerci **(Fig. 1)**. Humans are infected by accidental ingestion of *Taenia* eggs by fecal–oral infection. The embryos contained in the eggs cross the intestinal mucosa and are then transported by the circulatory system and distributed throughout the body.[9] Once they reach a small terminal vessel, the embryos establish and encyst to form the larval vesicles or cysticerci, reaching their definitive size of 1–2 cm in 2–3 months. The cysts can lodge anywhere in the body, but encystment of the nervous system, subcutaneous tissue, muscle, and eyes are common. It is the infestation of the brain and eye, which produced serious clinical manifestations. Infestation of other organ systems is mostly asymptomatic.

EVOLUTIONARY STAGES

In the human central nervous system (CNS), cysticercosis may be located in the parenchyma, ventricles, and meninges, or in mixed distribution. Here, the cysts evolve through a series of well-defined pathological stages. Initially, the cysts are uniformly rounded or oval vesicles, varying in size from a few millimeters to 1–2 cm and rarely, these may grow to reach several centimeters in diameter. They have a translucent membrane through which the scolex is visible as a small 2-mm nodule. Its most frequent location in clinical cases is in the brain parenchyma, where cysts can be found in the cerebral hemispheres, mainly at the gray-white matter junction. This is the vesicular stage. On histology, it is characterized by a well-defined and intricate canalicular network, an intact cyst wall, and inflammation in the surrounding brain parenchyma. Vesicles vary in contents according to their evolutionary stage. After an undetermined length of time, degeneration begins and the vesicular fluid becomes opaque, dense, and the cyst's edges become irregular and shrink. The scolex may still be identified, while its canalicular network becomes degenerative. There is surrounding inflammation in the brain parenchyma. This is known as the colloidal stage of the cysticercus. Later, the scolex is no longer discernable, either macroscopically or histologically. The appearance is one of a granuloma; hence the name, granular nodular stage. Eventually, calcification starts, usually in the cephalic portion of the parasite and progresses to the vesicular wall. This leaves a round, hard, whitish, and calcareous nodule with fibrosis and little surrounding inflammation; hence the name, fibro-calcified stage.[10] These stages are adequately discernible on modern neuroimaging, particularly magnetic resonance imaging (MRI) **(Figs. 2A to I)**. The vesicular stage

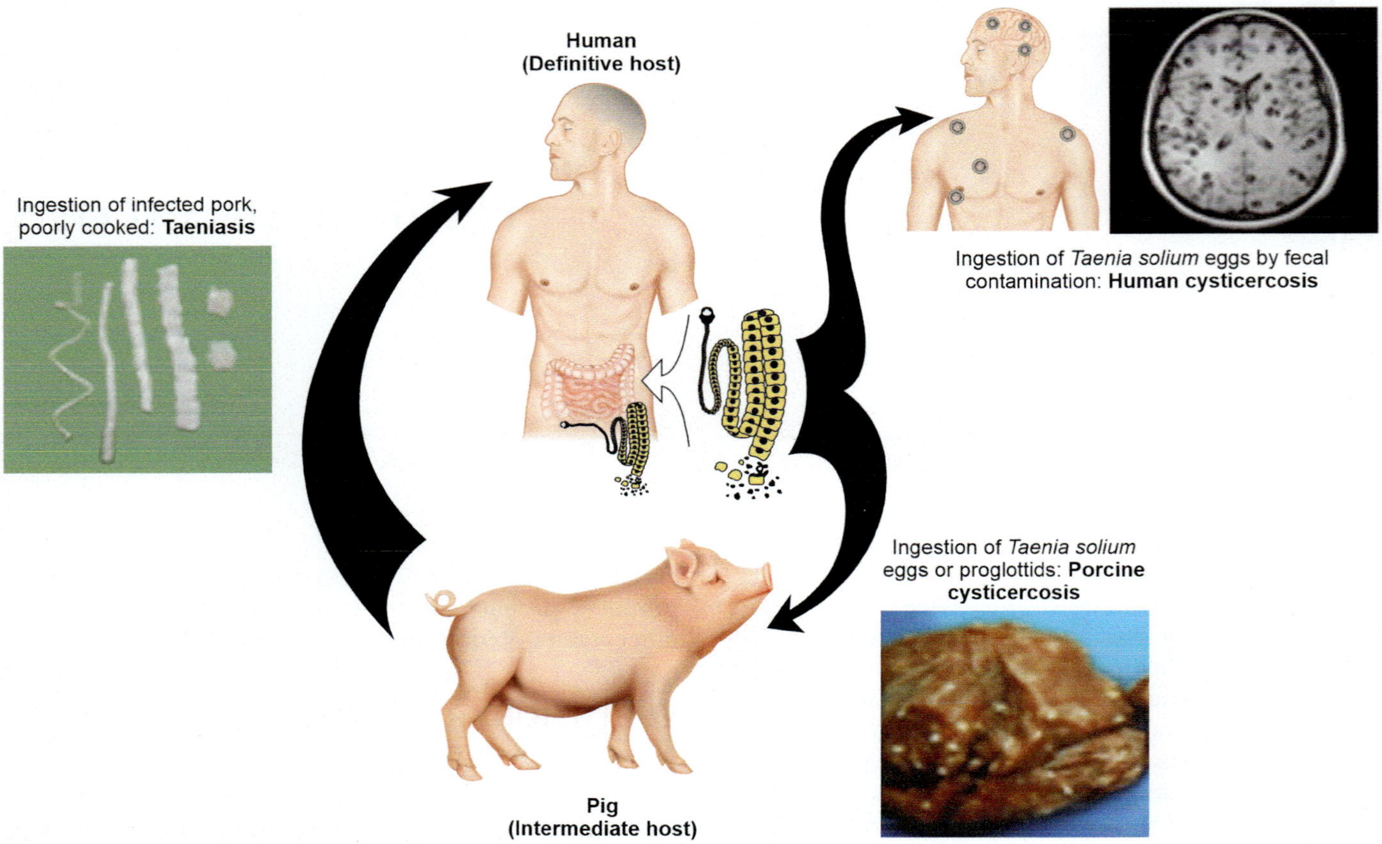

FIG. 1: Life cycle of *Taenia solium* emphasizing how humans get infested with cysticercosis.

is characterized as a clear cystic structure with an eccentric scolex. There is no surrounding edema around the cyst indicating the absence of inflammation and breakdown of the blood-brain barrier. As the cyst begins to degenerate, its fluid contents become proteinaceous and hence of different intensities in comparison to the cerebrospinal fluid (CSF). The scolex is still mostly discernible. There is surrounding edema outside of the cyst wall. This represents the vesicular stage. Later, the scolex completely degenerates and hence a granuloma with a thick ring enhancement, representing the inflamed wall of the cyst and considerable surrounding edema is visible; this is referred to as the granular nodular stage of the cysticercus. Lastly, the cyst completely involutes, leaving behind a small fibro-calcified nodule, known as the fibro-calcified stage.

The vesicular and colloidal stages denote the active or live stage of the cysticercus. The live or active stage can be recognized by the presence of an identifiable eccentric scolex. The granular nodular stage, seen as simply a ring-enhancing lesion devoid of the scolex, is considered as the transitional stage. This is an intermediate stage between the live and inactive or dead stages of the cysticercosis. The inactive or dead stage is essentially the fibro-calcified nodule. From the treatment standpoint, the live or active stage to a considerable extent and the granular nodular or transitional stage to a somewhat lesser extent but not the inactive, fibro-calcified stage are amenable to treatment with antihelminthic agents.

The fibro-calcified stage is typically associated with little inflammatory infiltrate in the surrounding brain parenchyma and hence, the absence of breakdown of the blood-brain barrier and the absence of surrounding edema on MRI. An elegant follow-up study of focal calcified lesions on brain imaging showed that roughly 35% of people with these lesions continue to have seizures over a period of 5 years. In roughly half of those who had seizures and brain MRI performed soon after the seizures, revealed surrounding edema and contrast enhancement. These findings were, however, absent in MRI studies in people who did not have seizures and who acted as controls in the study. Hence, perhaps some residual cyst contents are released from the fibro-calcified stage intermittently, leading to surrounding inflammation and hence, also perinodular edema **(Fig. 3)**. From a clinical standpoint, these phenomena are typically linked to the occurrence of seizures in people with calcified lesions.

Where community- or population-based epidemiological surveys have been conducted in highly cysticercosis-endemic regions of the world, imaging [mostly computed tomography (CT)] shows a large proportion of the

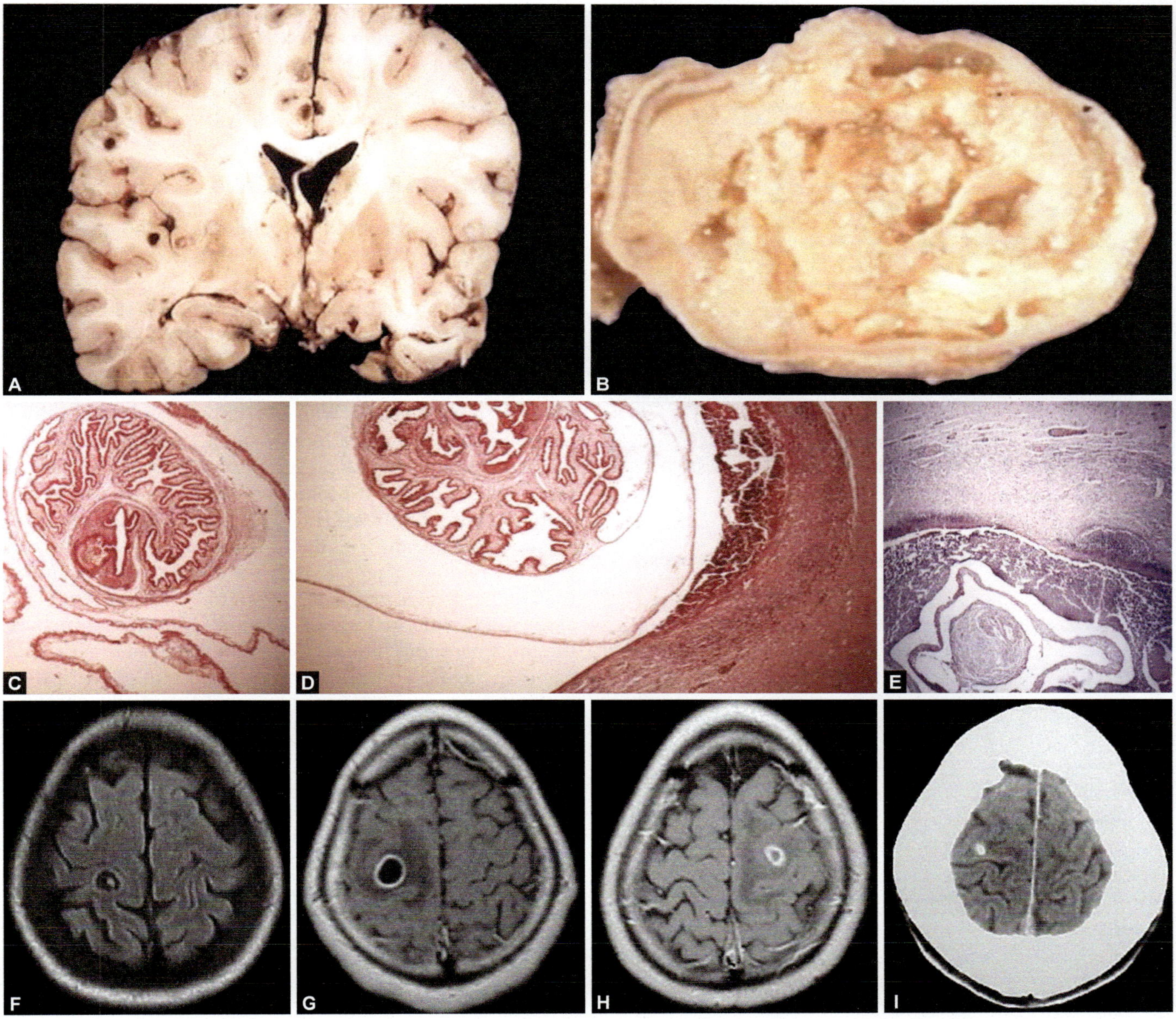

FIGS. 2A TO I: Evolutionary stages of cysticercosis—pathological (A and B), histological (C to E) and radiological (F to I) appearances. (A) Live active cysticercosis in cut section of human brain; (B) Gross appearance of a degenerating cysticercus; (C) Histological appearance of live active cysticercus in the vesicular stage (note the well preserved canalicular network within the cyst and the absence of inflammation in the surrounding parenchyma); (D) Colloidal stage with intense inflammation in the surrounding parenchyma; (E) Fibrocalcified nodule with little inflammation in the surrounding parenchyma; (F) Live active, vesicular cyst on MRI with well-defined eccentric scolex, clear cyst fluid and the absence of surrounding edema; (G) Colloidal, also known as degenerating or transitional stage with disappearing scolex and surrounding edema; (H) Granular-nodular stage with thick enhancing wall and surrounding edema; and (I) Calcified nodule on CT scan.

populations studied with mostly single and rarely, multiple calcified lesions, representing the inactive stage of cysticercosis. Many of these people are asymptomatic and have never had seizures in their life. Consistent with this, NCC has often been diagnosed on autopsy of people who never had symptoms in life in Latin America. At the same time, however, in community-based epidemiological studies, calcified lesions are more commonly encountered in people with a history of seizures in the past. It is rather rare to find active or granular nodular stages in images performed on a community scale. This contrasts to the frequent finding of active or granular nodular transitional stages in people who are scanned soon after their seizures in hospital facilities in endemic regions of the world. This implies, possibly that

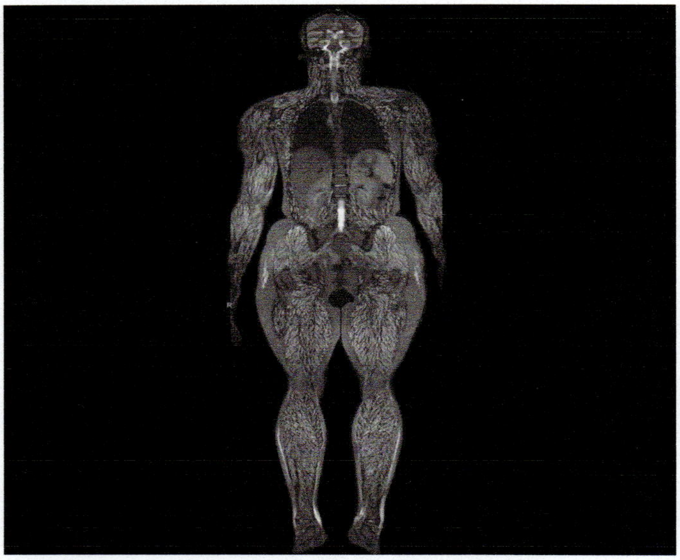

FIG. 3: MRI appearances of disseminated cysticercosis.

TABLE 1: Anatomical classification of neurocysticercosis.

Location	Clinical conditions
Parenchymal cysticercosis	• Solitary cysticercus granuloma • Multiple parenchymal cysticercosis • Cysticercotic encephalitis • Disseminated cysticercosis
Extraparenchymal cysticercosis	
Ventricular cysticercosis	• Free cysts • Inflamed and obstructing cysts
Meningeal–racemose cysticercosis	
Spinal cysticercosis	
Spinal intramedullary cysticercosis	
Spinal subarachnoid cysticercosis	

the cysticercus frequently lodges in the brain and passes through its series of evolutionary stages without producing any symptoms.

ANATOMICAL CLASSIFICATION OF NEUROCYSTICERCOSIS

Encystment of the brain parenchyma is most common **(Table 1)**. However, cysts can also be found in the ventricles as well as in the subarachnoid spaces including the basal cisterns and the spine (extraparenchymal NCC). This type of NCC is less frequent and presents mostly with mass effects and intracranial hypertension. In the subarachnoid space cysts tend to grow and large translucent vesicles, frequently lobulated, without a scolex, preferentially occur in the basis of the brain or in the ventricles.[11] As vesicles grow in number and adherence, they take over the chiasmatic, interpeduncular, and pontine and magna cisterns, appearing to be an infiltrating malignancy. Rarely, the cysts may lodge in the vertebral canal, including the subarachnoid space and the spinal cord itself.

CLINICAL MANIFESTATIONS

The clinical manifestations depend on: (1) the anatomical location, (2) number, and (3) evolutionary stage of the cysticerci.

The most common location is in the brain parenchyma, typically at the junction on the cortex and subcortex. In this location, the cyst predisposes to the occurrence of epileptic seizures. These seizures are typically focal with or without awareness impaired or with evolution to bilateral tonic–clonic seizures. However, many a time, the focal component may be eluding and the presentation is thus with bilateral tonic–clonic seizures. Moreover, the seizures can occur with all evolutionary stages of cysticerci. These, however, occur, most typically with the transitional, i.e., colloidal and granular nodular stages. Seizures are also common during the calcified stage and nearly one-half of them might be associated with perilesional edema. Overall, seizures are the most common neurological manifestation of NCC and occur in nearly 80% in hospital-based clinical series. In endemic regions of the world, one-third of all epilepsies might be attributed to NCC.

When the cysticerci are multiple instead of one, the manifestations include raised intracranial tension besides seizures and focal neurological deficits. There are two situations in which raised intracranial tension might be encountered in the setting of multiple parenchymal NCC. One is with the presence of hundreds of cysts in the brain, manifesting as raised intracranial tension, papilledema, and dementia or other cognitive impairments. When there is widespread distribution across the entire body, the condition is known as disseminated NCC **(Flowchart 1)**. The other condition is known as cysticercotic encephalitis. In this condition, there are multiple parenchymal cysticerci, all in degenerating stages and consequently massive cerebral edema. The latter can lead to rapid rise in intracranial tension and can be fatal as well.

Ventricular cysts can be stuck either in the foramen of Monro, the cerebral aqueduct, or the fourth ventricle outlet and lead to acute hydrocephalus. Besides, ventricular cysts can degenerate and lead to ependymitis and consequent hydrocephalus. When cysts are located in the subarachnoid cysts, they may behave as extra-axial space-occupying lesions. When these cysts degenerate, they induce a profound inflammatory arachnoiditis, which can involve the basal cranial nerves as well as the vessels of the brain. The latter leads to stroke associated with NCC. The inflammatory arachnoiditis can also lead to occlusion of the cerebrospinal outflow through the cisterns and hence, communicating hydrocephalus.

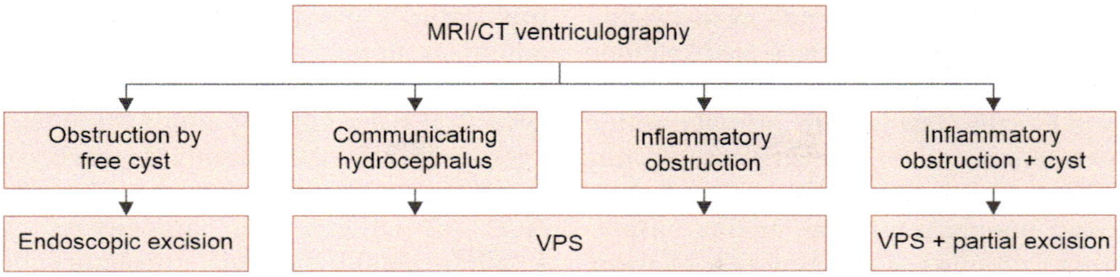

FLOWCHART 1: Management of interventricular cysticercosis.

(CT: computed tomography; MRI: magnetic resonance imaging; VPS: ventriculoperitoneal shunt)

Spinal cysticercosis is rare. The cysticerci may involve the intramedullary compartment via the hematogenous route. Alternatively, subarachnoid cysticercosis can lead to myelopathy after dropping down from the intracranial compartment. Regardless, the presentation is one of a myelopathy or myeloradiculopathy.

DIAGNOSIS

Neurocysticercosis is primarily diagnosed by neuroimaging studies, either CT or MRI.[12,13] In the past, when CT and MRI were not available, a presumptive diagnosis was often based on ventriculography or pneumoencephalography with histopathological conformation by biopsy of extraneural cysticercosis, mostly subcutaneous. Diagnostic sensitivity of CT is good for intraparenchymal NCC, but is lower for ventricular or subarachnoid disease. MRI is superior to CT for imaging cysticercosis and provides the best evaluation of the evolutionary stage of the parasite. It most accurately differentiates between vesicular, colloidal, and granular nodular stages of the cysticercus. MRI is more sensitive than CT scan for the diagnosis of NCC in brainstem as well as sellar locations. It is also more sensitive in recognizing small cysts or those located in the ventricles, brainstem, cerebellum, or intraocularly and the racemose vesicles at the level of the posterior fossae and basal cisterns. CT scan, however, is more sensitive for detecting calcifications. Modern MRI techniques such as the T2* imaging are promising for the detection of calcifications, but CT remains the gold standard.

Imaging not only provides valuable inputs for the diagnosis of NCC, but it is also immensely useful in follow-up studies. These studies might demonstrate involution or not of the cysticercus from various stages to eventually a fibro-calcified nodule. Follow-up studies might also demonstrate migration of ventricular cysts.

Extraparenchymal cysticercosis may take the form of either ventricular or meningeal-racemose cysticercosis. Ventricular cysts often present with free cysts in the ventricular pathways. These may then become stuck in the ventricular system and often degenerate in that location, leading on to inflammation in the surrounding edema. The presence of a stuck cyst with surrounding ependymitis is characteristic and has important therapeutic implications. When this happens in the fourth ventricle, it requires differentiation from a trapped fourth ventricle.

Meningeal-racemose cysticercosis takes the form of thin-walled, large, cystic structures in the basal or Sylvian cisterns. When these begin to degenerate, they initiate an inflammatory reaction leading to occlusion of blood vessels located therein. Thus, not infrequently, imaging presentations on meningeal-racemose cysticercosis includes cerebral infarction.

Serological Diagnosis

Detection of specific antibodies to *T. solium* confirms the diagnosis. The enzyme-linked immunoelectrotransfer blot assay (EITB, Western Blot) provides specific confirmation of the diagnosis and complements neuroimaging.[14] Specificity of this assay is 100%, and its sensitivity in cases with viable parasites is estimated to be over 95%,[14] although it may be significantly lower in patients with a single cyst, a single degenerating parasite, or in the calcified stage.[15] Commercial antibody-detection enzyme-linked immunosorbent assays (ELISAs) using crude or semipurified antigens are much less sensitive and specific. Parasitic antigen assays are available using monoclonal antibody-based ELISA that are more specific but less sensitive than antibody detection. Detection in the CSF is highly sensitive and specific.

TREATMENT

Whereas, it is widely assumed that cysticercosis outside the nervous system is a benign condition that does not merit specific treatment, NCC presents a very different scenario, with significant morbidity and occasional mortality. Until 1978, the only available therapeutic approaches were restricted to surgery for cyst excision, ventricular shunts, or corticosteroids to mitigate inflammation. The discovery in Mexico that praziquantel (PZQ) was effective for porcine cysticercosis and its subsequent use in human NCC provided for the first time an effective specific drug against this parasitic disease.[16,17] Later, albendazole (ABZ) provided a cheaper and more effective drug to kill the parasites.[18-20] Despite a long-standing controversy, the current consensus is that the resolution of parenchymal

NCC cysts using antiparasitic agents leads to faster and improved chances of resolution and reduces the likelihood of seizure relapses.

Albendazole is a benzimidazole with primary action through selective degeneration of parasite cytoplasmic microtubules, leading to decreased adenosine triphosphate (ATP) formation and energy depletion. It has antimitotic activity (binds to tubulin), disrupting cell division. It also causes loss of transport of secretory vesicles alter glucose intake, leading to parasite starvation. Peak plasma concentrations of its metabolite, ABZ sulfoxide occur 2–3 hours after administration. It has very good penetration in CSF (43% of plasma levels).[21,22]

Praziquantel is a pyrazino-isoquinoline derivative with primary effects leading to muscle contraction, paralysis, and tegumentary damage to the parasite. Other effects include changes in carbohydrate metabolism, decrease in enzymatic activities, and alterations in surface membranes. Peak plasma concentrations occur 1½–2 hours after administration. PZQ penetrates well into CSF, although less than ABZ (24% of plasma concentration at steady state).[23,24]

The combination of ALB and PZQ is much more efficacious in resolving multiple-cyst NCC, although in one large study no difference was found compared to ABZ alone for patients with only one or two lesions.[25,26] Concomitant use of PZQ significantly increases plasma levels of ABZ sulfoxide, without increased side effects, although the increased efficacy seems to involve additional synergistic effects, not only due to increased plasma ABZ sulfoxide levels.

Besides antihelminthic treatment, two groups of therapeutic agents are useful in the management of parenchymal NCC: (i) Corticosteroids and (ii) antiseizure medications. Corticosteroids reduce inflammation and hence are useful in the transitional stages of NCC. When there are multiple parenchymal cysts with cerebral edema, the administration of corticosteroids is imperative as this reduces the intracranial tension. In addition, the administration of corticosteroids reduces the chances of inflammatory exacerbation associated with degenerating cysts in consequence of administration of antihelminthic agents. Hence, it is standard practice to coadminister corticosteroids along with antihelminthic treatment for NCC. All patients with parenchymal cysticercosis with seizures should receive antiseizure medications. The choice of antiseizure medications is somewhat unclear. Both carbamazepine and phenytoin are known to induce the metabolism of PZQ and ABZ. This may reduce the effectiveness of their antihelminthic action. An antiseizure medication, which does not induce the hepatic microsomal enzyme system, e.g., levetiracetam may be preferred under such circumstances.

Apart from medical management, resort to surgery is required in some cases. The indications for and modalities of surgical intervention are rapidly changing. Shunt surgery was commonly required in cases of hydrocephalus. Nowadays, resort to endoscopic third ventriculostomy may obviate this requirement. Endoscopic surgery has also come to play a major role in the treatment of intraventricular cysticercosis, especially with free-floating cysts. When, however, the cysts are stuck with considerable ependymitis, resort to ventricular drainage might be best.

CONCLUSION

Neurocysticercosis, which is the infestation of the human brain by the larval stage of the pork tapeworm, *Taenia solium* is a testimony to poverty, lack of sanitation and poor hygiene. Efforts are on to improve diagnosis and treatments this might reduce the disease burden. Eventually, however, eradication of the tapeworm through preventative approaches, including improved sanitation, pork production and meat hygiene as well as personal hygiene will be the key to reducing the global burden of neurocysticercosis.

REFERENCES

1. Commission on Tropical Diseases of the International League Against Epilepsy. Relationship between epilepsy and tropical diseases. Commission on Tropical Diseases of the International League Against Epilepsy. Epilepsia. 1994;35:89-93.
2. Garcia HH, Gilman RH, Martinez M, Tsang VC, Pilcher JB, Herrera G, et al. Cysticercosis as a major cause of epilepsy in Peru. The Cysticercosis Working Group in Peru (CWG). Lancet. 1993;341 (8839):197-200.
3. Medina MT, Rosas E, Rubio-Donnadieu F, Sotelo J. Neurocysticercosis as the main cause of late-onset epilepsy in Mexico. Arch Intern Med. 1990;150(2):325-7.
4. Dixon HB, Lipscomb FM. Cysticercosis: An Analysis and Follow-up of 450 Cases. London: Medical Research Council; 1961.
5. Schenone H, Villarroel F, Rojas A, Ramirez R. Epidemiology of human cysticercosis in Latin America. In: Flisser A, Willms K, Laclette JP, Larralde C, Ridaura C, Beltran F (Eds). Cysticercosis: Present State of Knowledge and Perspectives. New York: Academic Press; 1982.
6. White AC Jr. Neurocysticercosis: a major cause of neurological disease worldwide. Clin Infect Dis. 1997;24:101-13.
7. Tsang VCW, Wilson M. *Taenia solium* cysticercosis: An underrecognized but serious publica health problem. Parasitol Today. 1995;11(3):124-6.
8. Nash TE, Neva FA. Recent advances in the diagnosis and treatment of cerebral cysticercosis. N Engl J Med. 1984;311(23):1492-6.
9. Garcia HH, Del Brutto OH; Cysticercosis Working Group in Peru. Neurocysticercosis: updated concepts about an old disease. Lancet Neurol. 2005;4(10):653-61.
10. Escobar A. The pathology of neurocysticercosis. In: Palacios E, Rodriguez-Carbajal J, Taveras JM, (Eds). Cysticercosis of the Central Nervous System. Springfield: Charles C. Thomas; 1983. pp. 27-54.

11. Rabiela MT, Rivas A, Flisser A. Morphological types of *Taenia solium* cysticerci. Parasitol Today. 1989;5(11):357-9.
12. White AC Jr, Coyle CM, Rajshekhar V, Singh G, Hauser WA, Mohanty A, et al. Diagnosis and Treatment of Neurocysticercosis: 2017 clinical practice guidelines by the Infectious Diseases Society of America (IDSA) and the American Society of Tropical Medicine and Hygiene (ASTMH). Clin Infect Dis. 2018;66(8):1159-63.
13. Del Brutto OH, Nash TE, White AC Jr, Rajshekhar V, Wilkins PP, Singh G, et al. Revised diagnostic criteria for neurocysticercosis. J Neurol Sci. 2017;372:202-10.
14. Tsang VC, Brand JA, Boyer AE. An enzyme-linked immunoelectrotransfer blot assay and glycoprotein antigens for diagnosing human cysticercosis *(Taenia solium)*. J Infect Dis. 1989;159(1):50-9.
15. Robles C, Chavarría M. [A case of successfully treated cerebral cysticercosis]. Gac Med Mex. 1980;116(2):65-71.
16. Botero D, Castaño S. Treatment of cysticercosis with praziquantel in Colombia. Am J Trop Med Hyg. 1982;31(4):811-21.
17. Sotelo J, Escobedo F, Rodriguez-Carbajal J, Torres B, Rubio-Donnadieu F. Therapy of parenchymal brain cysticercosis with praziquantel. N Engl J Med. 1984;310:1001-7.
18. Escobedo F, Penagos P, Rodriguez J, Sotelo J. Albendazole therapy for neurocysticercosis. Arch Intern Med. 1987;147(4):738-41.
19. Sotelo J, Escobedo F, Penagos P. Albendazole vs praziquantel for therapy for neurocysticercosis. A controlled trial. Arch Neurol. 1988;45(5):532-4.
20. Garcia HH, Pretell EJ, Gilman RH, Martinez SM, Moulton LH, Del Brutto OH, et al; Cysticercosis Working Group in Peru. A trial of antiparasitic treatment to reduce the rate of seizures due to cerebral cysticercosis. N Engl J Med. 2004;350(3):249-58.
21. Jung H, Hurtado M, Sanchez M, Medina MT, Sotelo J. Plasma and CSF levels of albendazole and praziquantel in patients with neurocysticercosis. Clin Neuropharmacol. 1990;13(6):559-64.
22. Dayan AD. Albendazole, mebendazole and praziquantel. Review of non-clinical toxicity and pharmacokinetics. Acta Trop. 2003;86 (2-3):141-59.
23. Mohamed AE, Yasawy MI, Al Karawi MA. Combined albendazole and praziquantel versus albendazole alone in the treatment of hydatid disease. Hepatogastroenterology. 1998;45(23):1690-4.
24. Guo DM, Xie SP, Jia JP. [Therapeutic efficacy of praziquantel, albendazole and a combination of the two drugs in cysticercosis]. Zhongguo Ji Sheng Chong Xue Yu Ji Sheng Chong Bing Za Zhi. 2003;21:187-8.
25. Garcia HH, Gonzales I, Lescano AG, Bustos JA, Zimic M, Escalante D, et al; Cysticercosis Working Group in Peru. Efficacy of combined antiparasitic therapy with praziquantel and albendazole for neurocysticercosis: a double-blind, randomised controlled trial. Lancet Infect Dis. 2014;14:687-95.
26. Garcia HH, Lescano AG, Lanchote VL, Pretell EJ, Gonzales I, Bustos JA, et al; Cysticercosis Working Group in Peru. Pharmacokinetics of combined treatment with praziquantel and albendazole in neurocysticercosis. Br J Clin Pharmacol. 2011;72:77-84.

59 CHAPTER

Acute Viral Encephalitis

UK Misra, Jayantee Kalita

INTRODUCTION

Viral encephalitis refers to inflammation of the brain parenchyma by a viral infection and is a serious global public health problem. There are over 100 neurotropic viruses that may have neuroinvasion. Herpes simplex virus (HSV) is the most common sporadic focal encephalitis and arbovirus encephalitis is the leading cause of endemic encephalitis. HSV encephalitis is especially important because it is treatable by specific antiviral therapy. Japanese encephalitis (JE) is the most common endemic encephalitis globally, especially in South East Asia. West Nile virus (WNV) is the most widespread virus. In many regions, several viral encephalitis cocirculate such as JE, dengue, Zika, and chikungunya (CHIK).

EPIDEMIOLOGY

Globally, 1,444,720 incident cases, 89,900 deaths, and 4.80 million disability-associated life in years (DALYs) were related to encephalitis in 2019. The age-standardized incidence rate and age-standardized mortality rate (ASMR) decreased from 23.17 and 2.18 to 19.33 and 1.19 per 100,000 person-years respectively over the past 30 years. Although the global burden of encephalitis has decreased in the past 30 years, a further decline stopped from 2011 to 2013.[1] There is marked variation in the incidence of encephalitis in different regions which ranked fifth in south Asia and 14th in Australasia, Western Europe, and high-income North America.[2] JE is the single largest cause of viral encephalitis at the global level, while HSV is the most common cause of infective encephalitis in western countries. The incidence of viral encephalitis is much lower than that in developing countries where rabies, JE, dengue, and CHIK virus account for many-fold larger annual occurrence. The incidence of encephalitis was 5.23 cases/100,000/year in England, but it was as high as 185 cases/100,000 in a rural population of Nepal during an outbreak of JE.[3] It is sometimes difficult to diagnose and a specific etiology could be established in <50% of cases. Although several studies have assessed the frequency of various pathogens in encephalitis in western countries but such studies have been lacking in Asian populations. A large number of viruses can produce encephalitis which belongs to DNA or RNA viruses and the common viruses are mentioned in **Box 1**.

BOX 1 Causes of acute viral encephalitis.

- *Arbovirus*: Japanese encephalitis, West Nile encephalitis, dengue, eastern and western equine encephalitis, Venezuelan equine encephalitis, St Louis encephalitis, and Murray valley encephalitis
- *Reovirus*: Colorado tick fever encephalitis
- *Bunyavirus*: Californian encephalitis
- *Herpes virus*: Herpes simplex virus I and herpes simplex virus II, varicella zoster, human herpes virus 6, B-virus, Epstein–Barr, and cytomegalo
- *Myxo and paramyxo*: Measles, mumps, influenza, parainfluenza, and Nipah virus
- Adeno, parvo, and rhabdovirus

CLINICAL FEATURES

The diagnosis of viral encephalitis is suspected in the context of fever, headache, and altered level of sensorium. The other symptoms and signs of cerebral dysfunction include four groups of abnormalities: (1) Cognitive dysfunction (acute memory disturbances), (2) Behavioral changes (disorientation, hallucinations, psychosis, personality changes, and agitation), (3) Focal neurological abnormalities (anomia, dysphasia, hemiparesis, hemianopia, etc.), and (4) Seizures. Once the diagnosis of encephalitis is suspected, history and careful general and neurological examinations are required.

HISTORY

Medical history can be obtained from the caregiver because the patient may be confused, or comatose. The geographical location and the recent travel history may provide cues about the causative pathogens, which may be prevalent in certain geographical regions. JE is prevalent in South East Asia, West Nile in the Middle East or Europe and America, and *Nipah virus* in Malaysia, Singapore, and India. The seasonal occurrence can give clues—mumps in spring, and dengue and JE in postmonsoon period in India. Patient's occupations, e.g., forestry workers are prone to Lyme disease. Contact with animals, such as farm animals may be reservoirs for certain viruses, e.g., West Nile. History of insect or animal bites can be relevant for arbovirus infection as well as rabies, respectively. Past contact with an individual afflicted by an infective condition is important, certain viral and nonviral pathogens cause encephalitis only or much more frequently in immunosuppressed individuals such as acquired immunodeficiency syndrome (AIDS) or those who are on immunosuppressive medications. The mode of disease course may provide clues to the etiology, e.g., enterovirus infection has a typical biphasic course. An associated abnormality outside the nervous system (bleeding tendency in hemorrhagic fever, the hydrophobia in rabies patients) may also point to a specific pathogen.

GENERAL EXAMINATION

Viral infection of the nervous system may be a part of a generalized systemic disease. The other organs therefore may be involved prior to or in association with the central nervous system (CNS) manifestations. Evidence for such involvement should be obtained by history or examination. Skin rashes are sometimes seen in encephalitis, e.g., dengue, West Nile, and herpes zoster encephalitis. Parotitis may be associated with mumps, gastrointestinal signs with enteroviral disease and upper respiratory findings may accompany influenza virus infection and HSV-1 encephalitis.

Neurological Examination

The neurological findings relate to those of disruption of brain function and associated meningitis. The signs of brain dysfunction are altered sensorium, focal neurological signs, and seizures. Additional signs may include autonomic and hypothalamic disturbances, diabetes insipidus, and hyponatremia due to inappropriate antidiuretic hormone secretion and cerebral salt wasting. The symptoms and signs are nonspecific and do not help in differentiating the causative virus. Similarly, the evolution of the clinical signs and their severity depend on host immunity and age (very young and the very old have the most extensive and serious signs of encephalitis).

DIFFERENTIAL DIAGNOSIS

Viral encephalitis can be confused with a number of nonviral infections (bacterial, fungal, parasitic, and spirochaetal), vasculitis, pseudomigraine with sterile cerebrospinal fluid (CSF) pleocytosis, and a number of metabolic encephalopathies including mitochondrial disease. The difference between encephalitis and encephalopathy is resented in the **Table 1**.

INVESTIGATIONS

Peripheral blood counts and cellular morphology may help in differentiating viral from nonviral infections. Normal or low leukocyte counts with predominant lymphocytes in the peripheral blood are common in viral encephalitis. Thrombocytopenia, coagulopathy, and liver and kidney function abnormality may be associated with dengue, Zika, and CHIK. Erythrocyte sedimentation rate is a nonspecific test that is usually normal. Electroencephalography (EEG) and neuroimaging are supportive, and microbiological tests and histopathology are diagnostic.

Electroencephalography

The EEG is an early, sensitive but nonspecific indicator of cerebral function. EEG shows background slowing prior to the parenchymal involvement on neuroimaging. Focal abnormalities in the form of slowing or epileptiform activities may be seen in EEG. During the acute phase, the severity of EEG abnormalities does not usually correlate with the extent of the disease. However, a rapidly improving EEG indicates a good prognosis, while lack of improvement of the EEG suggests an unfavorable prognosis. There may be seizures in the acute phase; interictal epileptiform EEG activity is rarely seen except in HSV encephalitis. The EEG abnormalities usually subside more slowly than the clinical symptoms. In

TABLE 1: Differentiating features between encephalitis and encephalopathy.

Parameters	Encephalopathy	Encephalitis
Fever	Uncommon	Common
Headache	Uncommon	Common
Focal sign	Absent	May present
Seizure	Generalized	Focal/generalized
CSF pleocytosis	Uncommon	Common
EEG	Diffuse slowing	Diffuse/focal
Cranial MRI/CT	Normal	Abnormal

(CSF: cerebrospinal fluid; CT: computed tomography; EEG: electroencephalography; MRI: magnetic resonance imaging)

Source: Adapted from Misra UK, et al (2022).[15]

herpes simplex encephalitis (HSE), EEG abnormalities are seen in 80% of the patients. In addition to the background slowing there is temporal showing, and periodic lateralized epileptiform discharges during 2–14 days of encephalitis **(Figs. 1A and B)**. In JE and dengue, the changes are nonspecific and reveal generalized slowing of background activity and sometimes epileptiform discharges. The background slowing is more marked in JE than other viral encephalitides **(Fig. 2)**.

Computed Tomography and Magnetic Resonance Imaging

These investigations help in demonstrating brain involvement in encephalitis. Brain magnetic resonance imaging (MRI) is more sensitive than computed tomography (CT) scan. A typical MRI protocol includes T1 and T2 spin-echo sequences, a fluid-attenuation inversion recovery (FLAIR) sequence, and latter is considered more sensitive in

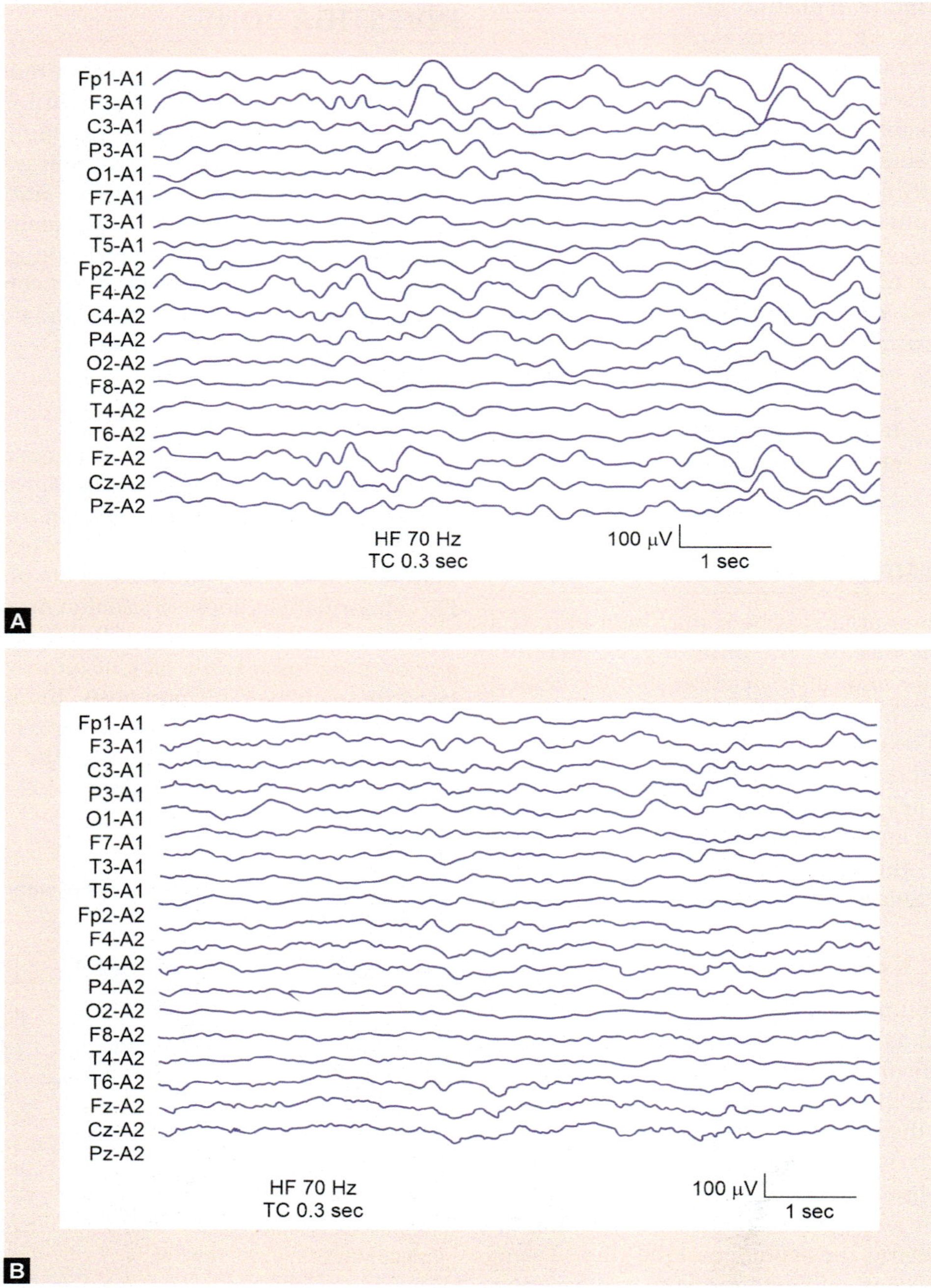

FIGS. 1A AND B: Electroencephalography findings in two patients with herpes simplex encephalitis. (A) Periodic lateralized epileptiform discharges over frontotemporal areas with background slowing. (B) There is background slowing which is more prominent in frontotemporal areas.

Image courtesy: With permission EEG Book.

detecting subtle changes in the early stage of encephalitis. Gradient echo imaging is also useful in detecting small areas of hemorrhages. In HSE, CT scan may be normal in the early stage, and may reveal low density lesion involving the temporal lobe and insula with occasional hemorrhagic changes. Contrast enhancement is a late feature. Cranial CT scans 1–2 weeks after onset of HSE reveal progressively increasing abnormalities with the involvement of contra lateral temporal lobe, insula, and cingulate gyri. The early MRI findings in HSE include gyral edema on T1-weighted imaging (T1WI) and high signal intensity in the temporal lobe and cingulate gyrus on T2WI and FLAIR **(Figs. 3A and B)**. Diffusion-weighted imaging (DWI) may show restricted diffusion in the early stage. There may be evidence of hemorrhage. Neonatal HSV-2 infection often causes more widespread signal abnormalities than HSV-1 encephalitis, with periventricular white matter involvement and sparing of the medial temporal and inferior frontal lobes. Varicella zoster infection may reveal MRI evidence of myelitis, encephalitis, large- and small-vessel stroke, and ventriculitis depending on the clinical presentation. Large vessel arteritis presents with ischemic/hemorrhagic infarctions.

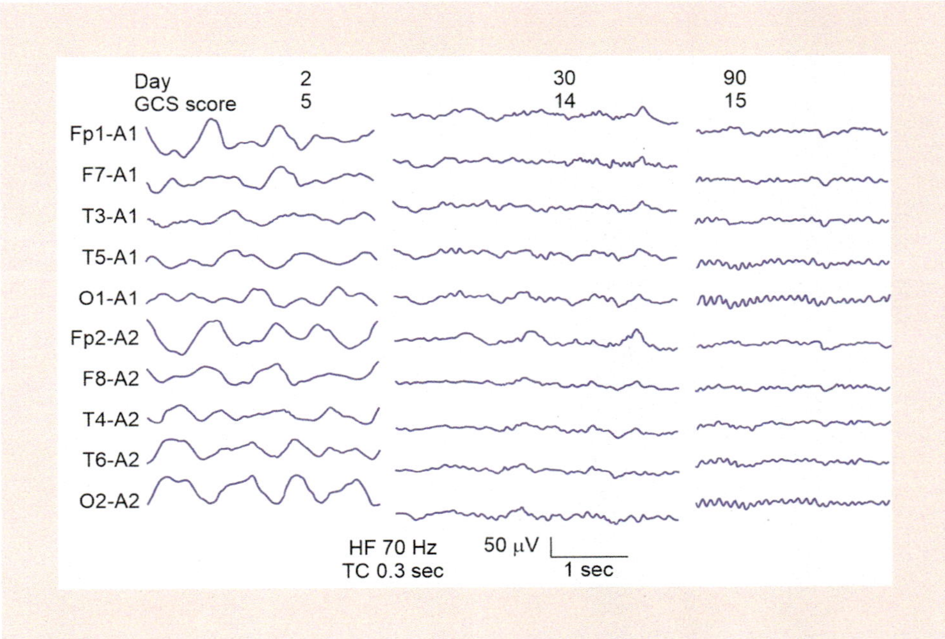

FIG. 2. Electroencephalography findings of a patient with Japanese encephalitis on day 2, 30, and 90. There is delta slowing which has improved to theta slowing at 1 month and normal alpha at 3 months.

Image courtesy: With permission from Misra UK, Kalita J. Clinical Electroencephalography, 2nd Edition. India: Elsevier; 2018.

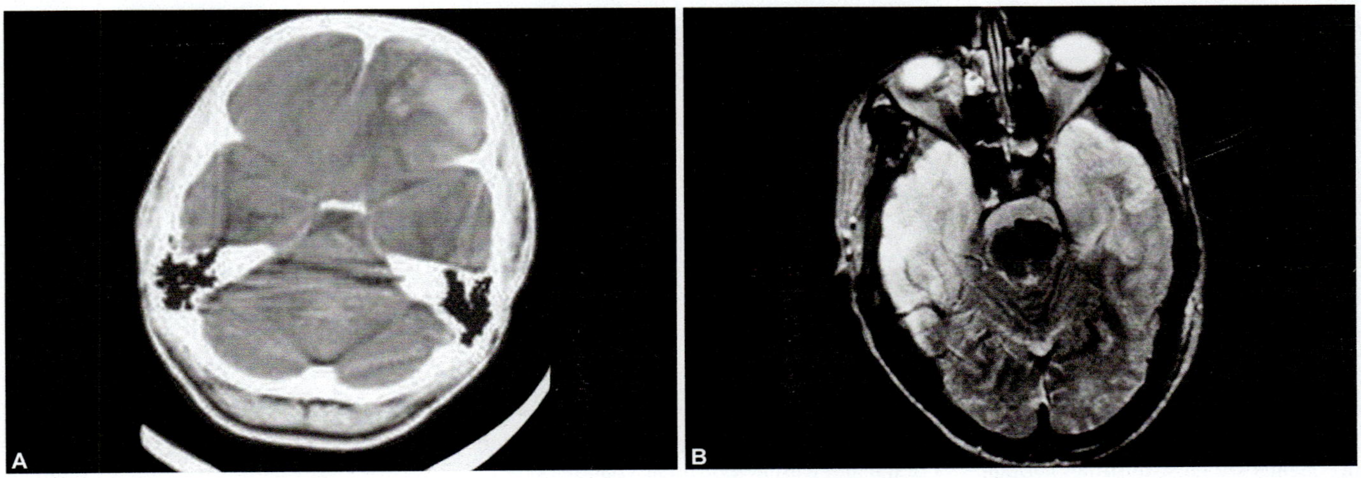

FIGS. 3A AND B: Computed tomography (CT) and magnetic resonance imaging (MRI) findings of a patient with herpes simplex encephalitis. (A) The temporal hypodensity on CT scan (B) more marked revealing hyperintensity of temporal lobes bilaterally on T2 MRI.

MRI of arbovirus encephalitis such as Japanese and Equine encephalitis reveals involvement of thalamus, basal ganglia, and midbrain which are hyperintense on T2 and FLAIR, and hypointense on T1. Occasionally, there lesions may be hemorrhagic **(Figs. 4A to F)**. West Nile encephalitis shows more frequent substantia nigra involvement than thalamus and basal ganglia involvement. Spinal cord involvement is more prominent in JE than West Nile encephalitis **(Figs. 5A to E)**. Dengue and CHIK show nonspecific changes. In polio and Coxsackievirus (CV) encephalitis, T2-weighted MRI may show hyperintensities in the midbrain and anterior horn of the spinal cord

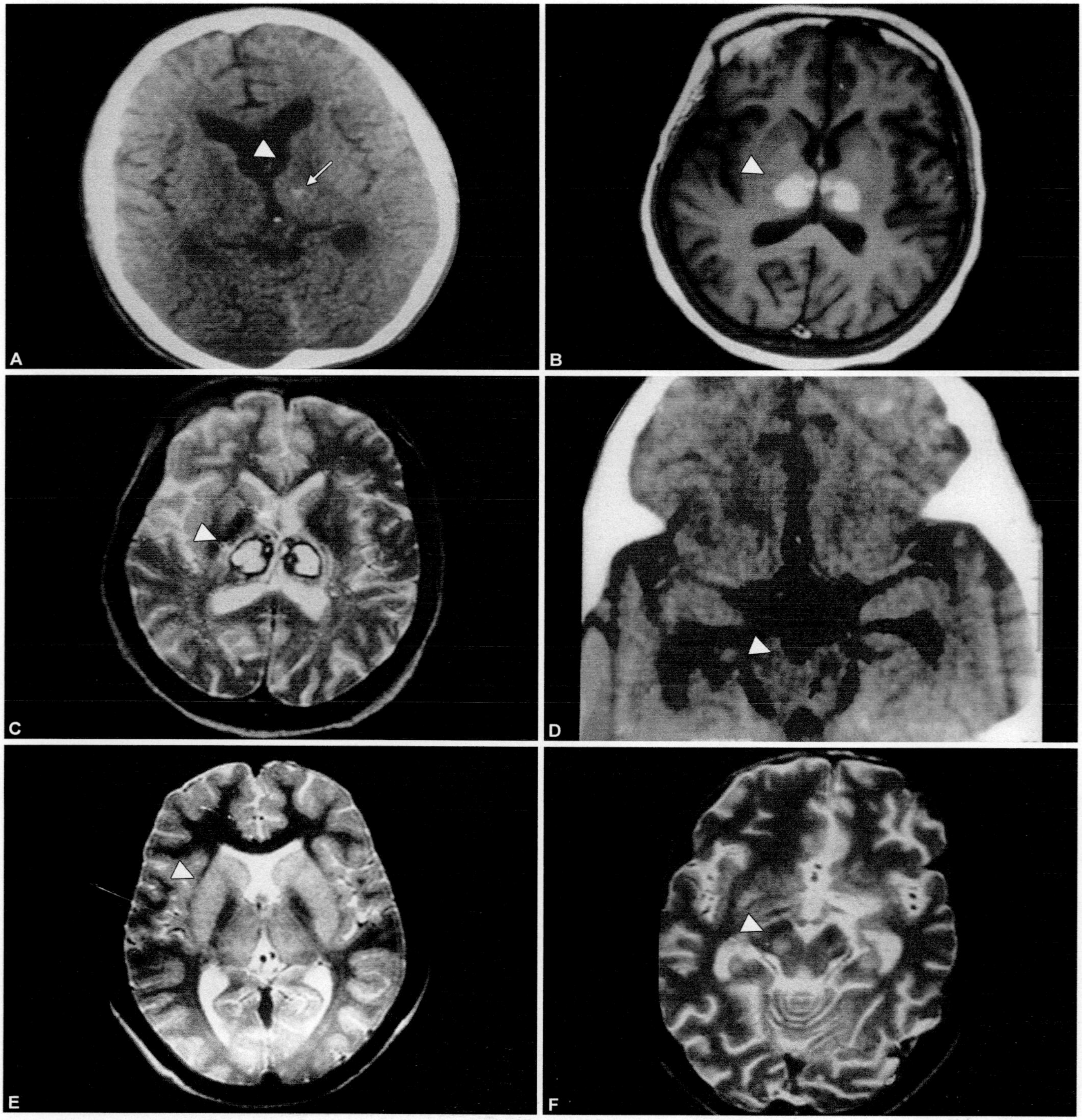

FIGS. 4A TO F: Cranial computed tomography (CT) and magnetic resonance imaging (MRI) findings of two patients with Japanese encephalitis. (A) CT scan shows hypodensity of thalami with hemorrhagic change on left. (B) T1 MRI shows hyperintense and (C) T2 image shows mixed intense thalamic lesions suggestive of hemorrhagic changes. (D) CT scan of another patient shows hypodensity in mid brain. (E) MRI of same patient on T2 sequence shows bilateral thalamic, and basal ganglia involvement, and (F) mid brain involvement.

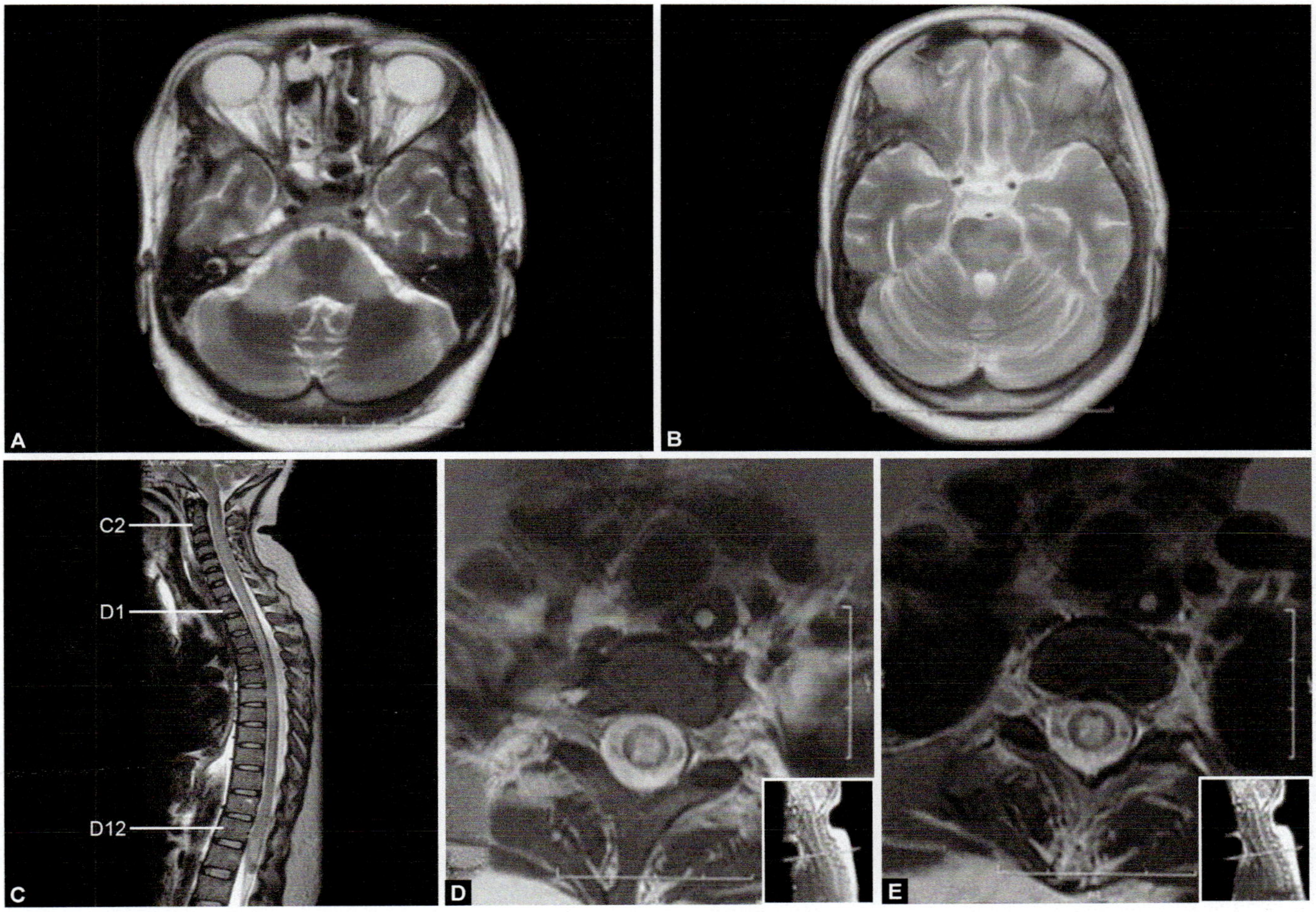

FIGS. 5A TO E: Craniospinal MRI in T2 sequence shows hyperintense signal changes in (A) middle cerebellar peduncle bilaterally, (B) central pons, (C) whole of spinal cord. (D and E) Axial sections of spinal cord show hyperintense signal changes in the central part.

Source: With permission from Kalita J, Vibhute A, Kumar M, Misra UK. Myelopathy in West Nile virus encephalitis: Report of a case and review of literature. J Spinal Cord Med. 2020;43(4):444-8.

VIROLOGICAL TESTS

The gold standard of diagnosis in encephalitis is virus isolation in cell culture, which is now replaced by the detection of specific nucleic acid sequence from CSF or brain using polymerase chain reaction (PCR). Intrathecal antibody production to a specific virus is also strong evidence for etiological diagnosis. Virus detection from throat, stool, urine, or blood as well as systemic serological responses like seroconversion or a specific immunoglobulin M (IgM) provides less strong evidence. CSF is the convenient specimen and is recommended for the diagnosis of viral encephalitis. Routine analysis of CSF reveals lymphocytic pleocytosis (10–500/mm^3) with mild to moderate rise in protein and normal glucose except in HSE there may be low glucose and red blood cell (RBC). The choice of the test is determined by types of infection [plasma or serum in dengue, CHIK, and CSF PCR or IgM enzyme-linked immunosorbent assay (ELISA) in HSE or JE] and time of specimen collection (serum antigen in dengue within 1–4 days, PCR in HSE, and JE first week and IgM both in serum and CSF, respectively after first week of illness). Brain biopsy is invasive and is not used in routine clinical practice. At autopsy, brain specimens may be obtained for virus isolation, nucleic acid and antigen detection as well as for immunohistochemistry and in situ hybridization.

Viral Culture

Viral culture from CSF and brain tissue as well as from throat and stool specimens are performed in four different cell lines: The cells are evaluated for cytopathic effect and the findings are confirmed by a neutralizing or an immunofluorescence antibody test. Viral cultures from CSF are positive in young children with enteroviral infection but only rarely by probes or by gel electrophoresis. Respiratory viruses could be detected by PCR of throat samples, although these do not confirm the etiology of encephalitis. CSF PCR is highly sensitive and specific in HSE, the sensitivity is 96% and the specificity 99% when CSF is studied between 2 and 10 days from the onset of symptoms. Instead of single PCR tests, multiplex PCR is being used in diagnostics. The sensitivity has been improved and it approaches that of the single PCR and the specificities are equal. Real-time PCR makes it possible to get the result in a short time while observing the yield cycle by cycle. The usage of microarrays for the detection of viral nucleic acid is expensive and not widely available, but has the possibility to become a regular diagnostic technique. This technique, however, has high false positivity and detection of the clinically irrelevant infective agent. Several microbes can be studied at the same time and identification of the genotype will be easier than using the current conventional tests for measles, mumps, and rubella are only occasionally needed in countries with effective vaccination programs.

Histopathology

The histopathological changes in encephalitis include the triad of (1) damage to the parenchyma (usually neuronal damage or loss, and demyelination), (2) reactive gliosis, and (3) inflammatory cellular infiltration by hematogenous elements in the immunocompetent host. These changes are associated with (multi) nodular encephalitis, as in the majority of viral encephalitides consisting of cell death, neuronophagia, focal or nodular proliferation of astroglia and microglia, and focal/nodular infiltration by lymphocytes and eventually macrophages. Thus, the classical encephalitic nodules are composed of a mixture of microglia, astrocytes, and lymphocytes usually around affected neuron(s).

Immunohistochemistry and In Situ Hybridization

The techniques of immunohistochemistry (IHC), in situ hybridization (ISH), and PCR have significantly impacted the neuropathological diagnosis of viral encephalitis with high sensitivity and specificity,[4] but a detailed discussion is beyond the scope of this chapter. Nevertheless, there are situations in which these investigations may not be diagnostic, e.g., the virus may have burnt out, faulty tissue preservation, and contamination or latent infection.

TREATMENT

Antiviral Therapy

Specific antiviral therapy has a role in HSE, HZV, and cytomegalovirus encephalitis. In two randomized controlled trials, acyclovir (10 mg/kg every 8 hours given intravenously for 10 days) was more effective than vidarabine (15 mg/kg/day) in improving the survival of adult biopsy-proven HSE patients. In view of good tolerability, acyclovir is recommended treatment for viral encephalitis even before confirmation of the diagnosis of HSE.[5] Acyclovir if given early before coma sets in, it can reduce mortality and morbidity. Acyclovir is also the treatment of choice for neonatal HSE; the daily dose of acyclovir for neonatal HSE is 60 mg/kg because of high excretion in urine (80% of circulating acyclovir). Renal impairment can precipitate acyclovir toxicity; therefore, its doses should be adjusted according to the creatinine clearance. Short duration of treatment (below 10 days) may result in relapse of HSE, in weeks to months; therefore treatment for 14 days in immunocompetent adults and 21 days in immune-suppressed patients and neonates has been recommended. The use of vidarabine for HSE is limited to the rare patients who cannot be given acyclovir.

Besides HSV, acyclovir is also effective against VZV. In CMV encephalitis, combination therapy with ganciclovir (5 mg/kg IV twice daily) with foscarnet (60 mg/kg IV every 8 hours or 90 mg/kg every 12 hours) is recommended. Antiretroviral therapy must be added or continued in human immunodeficiency virus (HIV)-infected patients. Valacyclovir seems to be promising in HSV and VZV encephalitis but remains to be evaluated in formal trials. Pleconaril is a broad-spectrum antiviral with the potential for use in enteroviral encephalitis.

Corticosteroids

The role of dexamethasone as an adjunct treatment in viral encephalitis is controversial. Occasionally, HSE is associated with severe, vasogenic edema with evidence of midline shift on CT or MRI, in them a high-dose corticosteroids may have a role. Steroid pulse therapy with methylprednisolone has been observed to be beneficial in a small number of patients with acute viral encephalitis who had progressive disturbances of consciousness.[6] The best evidence for steroid therapy is in VZV encephalitis. Primary VZV infection may cause severe encephalitis in immunocompetent children due to cerebral vasculitis. Based on available data, combined acyclovir/steroid treatment may be advised in immunocompetent individuals with severe VZV encephalitis and probably in other cases of acute viral encephalitis where progressive cerebral edema is documented on CT/MRI. The duration of dexamethasone or methyl prednisone treatment should be 3–5 days in order to minimize adverse effects. Present authors, however, generally avoid corticosteroids in viral encephalitis because of side effects and lack of evidence.

Cerebral slat wasting is more common than syndrome of inappropriate secretion of antidiuretic hormone (SIADH) and hyponatremia requires salt supplementation—hypertonic saline for serve hyponatremia (<126 mEq/L) and normal saline and oral salt 8–11 g daily through nasogastric tube for mild hyponatremia. Attention should be paid not to do rapid correction. Fluid restriction is generally not recommended unless there is definite evidence of SIADH.

GENERAL MEASURES

All cases of acute encephalitis ideally should be managed in neurointensive care unit (NICU) with access to mechanical ventilation (MV). Irrespective of the etiology, care of comatose patients includes care of airway, cardiovascular support, and maintenance of nutrition, fluid, and electrolyte balance. Care should be taken to prevent aspiration, infection, deep venous thrombosis, and pressure sore. Status epilepticus can be controlled with intravenous lorazepam/midazolam/diazepam, sodium valproate, levetiracetam, or lacosamide. Discrete seizure may be treated with oral or nasogastric antiepileptic drugs. Raised intracranial pressure may be treated with carbonic acid anhydrase inhibitor, mannitol, or corticosteroid. Secondary bacterial infections may require appropriate antibiotics. The patients with encephalitis do not require isolation except for severely immunosuppressed patients, rabies encephalitis, patients with exanthematous encephalitis, and those with a contagious viral hemorrhagic pathology.

In the following section, a few encephalitides will be discussed briefly.

Herpes Simplex Encephalitis

Herpes simplex encephalitis occurs due to two closely related human viruses HSV-1 an HSV-2, which produce infection only in humans. HSV-2 virus generally causes aseptic meningitis and rarely encephalitis. HSV-1 is widely prevalent and nearly half the people have antibodies against HSV-1 by the age of 15 years and 90% by adulthood. HSE is a rare complication of HSV-1 infection, and is the most common sporadic focal encephalitis in the world. During primary infection, HSV-1 is transported by retrograde transport through trigeminal sensory nerves and lies dormant in the sensory ganglia. HSE has a typical clinical picture because of specific localization in orbitofrontal and medial temporal cortex. The localization of HSV-1 to limbic cortex is attributed to the cytochemical characteristics of the brain and the spread of the virus from cell to the cell from the base of the brain to the anterior and middle cranial fossa.[7] The pathological changes in HSE are inflammation, necrosis, and inclusion bodies. HSE in adults may as well be due to the reactivation of HSV in the trigeminal ganglia. The meninges of the anterior and middle cranial fossa are innervated by the trigeminal nerve and the mechanism of spread of HSV has been confirmed in experimental studies in which selective retrograde spread of HSV occurs along the V3 division of trigeminal nerve following inoculation of the tooth by HSV resulting in ipsilateral temporal lobe infection.

Herpes simplex encephalitis has no seasonal variation or gender preference. It is primarily a disease of adults but has a bimodal distribution, about one-third patients are below 20 years of age and 50% are older than 50 years. The age preference in HSE may be due to primary infection in the young age and reactivation in the elderly. Clinical features of HSE have an insidious to fulminant course. About 30–60% of patients have an upper respiratory or gastrointestinal disturbance prior to encephalitis. Fever (40–41°C) and headache are the common and early symptoms. The clinical picture is determined by frontotemporal involvement leading to personality change and behavioral alterations. The typical clinical findings include fear, hallucination, and anosmia. Seizures occur in 70% of patients, which are often focal. Early seizures occur in 40% of patients. Focal seizures and focal neurological symptoms occur in 75% of patients, hemiparesis in one-third, and aphasia, and superior quadrantanopia may also occur. Status epilepticus is more common in HSE compared to JE (75% vs. 54%).[8] An opercular syndrome characterized by weakness in pharyngeal, laryngeal, tongue, and masticatory muscles may also occur. Rapidly developing coma may occur in some patients with few or no focal neurological signs. Some patients may have atypical clinical picture, which can be diagnosed by PCR only.[5,9] The MRI, EEG, and treatment are described earlier.

In modern era, about 15% patients with HSE die, 20% have a severe deficit, and 65% have a favorable outcome.[10]

Varicella Zoster

Varicella zoster virus (VZV) is a double-stranded DNA virus from the *Herpesviridae* family. After primary infection, the virus establishes latency principally in dorsal root ganglia and cranial sensory ganglia which are the sources of reactivation when cellular immunity declines. VZV reactivation may be complicated by local, neurological, or disseminated involvement. The most important triggers for the reactivation of VZV are age and immune depression. Amongst the neurological complications, VZV can cause peripheral (5th, 7th, and 9th cranial nerves, radiculopathy) and CNS involvement (meningitis, meningoencephalitis, myelitis, stroke, VZV vasculopathy, and necrotizing retinitis). Varicella vasculopathy presents as an ophthalmic zoster followed by acute contralateral hemiplegia or headache, mental status changes, or focal deficit, and these deficit may appear up to 1 year after herpes zoster.[11] Several studies have reported a potential role of VZV in neurocognitive impairment in giant cell arteritis. Neurological manifestations can precede or even occur without skin lesions of HZ "zoster sine herpete". Involvement of the CNS, and especially myelitis or cerebral vasculitis, was described in association with immunosuppression, but data are controversial as it has not been shown by more recent studies.[12]

JAPANESE ENCEPHALITIS

Japanese encephalitis was first reported from Japan, in 1933, and since then there has been an increase in number and area of distribution of JE. JE primarily reported from the Asian countries including Japan, China, Taiwan, Korea, Burma, Bangladesh, Sri Lanka, Nepal, Thailand, Vietnam, and India. In many parts of India, low-level transmission occurs round the year, but epidemics occur during postmonsoon period. In the 1970s, patients with JE were reported from south India, and from 1973 onward outbreaks were reported from West Bengal, Bihar, Uttar Pradesh, Assam, Andhra Pradesh, and Karnataka. JE is usually a disease of rural areas affecting people of lower socioeconomic status. For every one patient with JE, there may be about 1,000 subclinical infections. JE epidemics are related to rainfall, flood, paddy cultivation, pig farming, and mosquito breeding. JE is a zoonotic disease that is transmitted by JE virus-infected female *Culex* mosquito bite. The humans are the dead-end host. Pigs are amplifying host and JE virus life cycle is maintained by pig-mosquito-pig cycle. *Culex tritaeniorhynchus* is the most important and efficient vector for JE virus transmission. The incubation period of JE virus in humans is 6–16 days, following which either viremia subsides or there may be clinical symptoms. In the endemic region, children are commonly affected because adults escape because of herd immunity.

Clinical Features

The clinical course of JE includes three stages—(1) prodromal, (2) encephalitis, and (3) convalescent phases. The prodromal stage includes fever, headache, nausea, vomiting, and anorexia, which last for 3-4 days in 75%, and many patients may recover without progressing to the encephalitic stage. The encephalitic stage includes headache, altered sensorium, behavioral abnormality, seizures, and focal signs. The severely affected patients may lapse into deep coma with extensor posturing. Seizures occur in <10% of adults and in 60–80% of children, which may be focal or secondary generalized. The focal signs in JE include hemiplegia, quadriplegia, lower motor neuron signs (focal reflex loss and muscle wasting), and rarely cerebellar signs. Cranial nerve palsy in JE is rare. Tremulous eye movements have been described in JE. JE is an encephalomyelitis and anterior horn cell involvement simulates polio myelitis-like illness. In the acute stage, there may be focal reflex loss and focal wasting with neurogenic changes on electromyography due to anterior horn cell involvement.[13] As the patients recover from coma, and present with a wide variety of movement disorders such as parkinsonian features, choreoathetosis, tremor, and dystonia **(Fig. 6)**. In children, dystonia is more common than in adults.[8] The movement disorders in JE have a regressive course and subside over months to years. Cognitive and focal weaknesses are sequelae in some patients.[14]

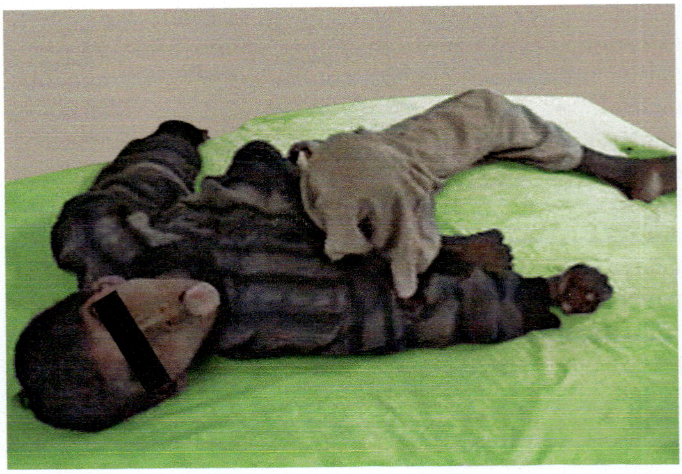

FIG. 6: Generalized dystonia with oromandibular dystonia in a patient with Japanese encephalitis at 3 months follow-up.

Dengue

Dengue is an important member of Flaviviridae family which spreads following the bite of infected *Aedes aegypti* mosquito. Dengue infection presents as dengue fever (DF), dengue hemorrhagic fever (DHF), and dengue shock syndrome (DSS). In 2009, WHO has classified dengue infection as:

- Dengue without warning signs
- Dengue with warning signs
- Severe dengue

Dengue fever is a self-limiting disease of 2–7 days manifesting with fever, headache, myalgia, arthralgia, conjunctivitis, retro-orbital pain, nausea, and vomiting. There may be skin rash on the 3rd or 4th day. DHF manifests with additional hemorrhagic complication such as mucosal bleeding, epistaxis, and gastric hemorrhage; in dengue, virus infection, thrombocytopenia, and evidence of plasma leakage (edema, interstitial edema, pulmonary edema, ascites, pleural effusion, and pericardial effusion) may also occur. DSS is similar to DHF with additional features of circulatory failure and shock. In DSS, hypotension and plasma leakage lead to multiorgan dysfunction. The patients with DSS need close monitoring because of short interval of few hours between warning signs and development of shock and a few minutes between cardiac failure and cardiac arrest. Secondary dengue infection may be associated with DSS due to antibody-dependent immune enhancement.

Pathophysiology

Thrombocytopenia, coagulopathy, and increased vascular permeability are responsible for the complications of dengue. Vascular leak in DHF/DSS, which occurs following secondary heterotypic dengue virus (DENV) infection is attributed to antibody-dependent enhancement, complement activation product, and is present during acute phase of DENV infection. DENV NS1 antigen adheres to endothelial cells making these vulnerable to complement-mediated injury or as a result of direct attack by anti-NS1. In secondary heterotypic DENV infection, T cells, monocytes, and macrophages result in the release of cytokines and chemokines, which may lead to cytokine storm. DENV may also lead to viral protein toxicities (direct endothelial damage).[15]

Neurological Complications

Initially, dengue was considered as non-neurotropic virus, however, increasing number of neurological manifestations have been reported. Direct CNS invasions of dengue virus have been demonstration by demonstrating viral proteins, ribonucleic acid (RNA), and immunoglobulins. The main neurological manifestations of dengue are dengue encephalopathy, encephalitis, and immune mediate neurological syndrome and muscle involvement.

Dengue Encephalopathy

Dengue encephalopathy is the most common neurological manifestation of DENV infection. It may present with altered sensorium, behavioral abnormality, and seizures. Dengue encephalopathy may occur in DF, DHF, and DSS. Dengue encephalopathy is attributed to hypoxia, shock, cerebral edema, electrolyte imbalance, renal or hepatic failure, and systemic or intracerebral hemorrhage. The patients with dengue encephalopathy have normal CSF.

Dengue encephalitis: The clinical picture of dengue encephalitis is similar to dengue encephalopathy. Seizures may occur in up to half of these patients. Dengue is the cause of acute encephalitis syndrome (AES) in South East Asia in 5–20% patients. Autopsy studies on dengue patients have revealed positive PCR or dengue antigen on immunostaining; however, there is a paucity of histopathological evidence of encephalitis raising doubts about direct viral CNS injury. In a recent autopsy study of three patients, a microscopic examination of the brain revealed cerebral edema, inflammation, and hemorrhage.[16]

Cranial MRI or CT scan in dengue is usually normal but may reveal nonspecific abnormality especially in the patients with hypotension, shock, or bleeding diathesis. Coinfection with JE also may result in MRI abnormality. In a study on MRI changes in 21 dengue patients, thalamic or basal ganglia lesion was seen in three, focal cerebral lesion in three, white matter abnormality in two, and meningeal enhancement in three patients. Seven of these patients had CSF pleocytosis.[17] Dengue encephalitis patients also have systemic features making it difficult to differentiate from encephalopathy, especially when CSF is not possible because of coagulopathy or thrombocytopenia. However, the differentiation between encephalopathy and encephalitis is not clinically important as the management of the two conditions is similar.

Dengue immune-mediated neurological syndromes: The immune-mediated syndromes manifest after 1–2 weeks of infection and include Guillain–Barré syndrome, acute disseminated encephalomyelitis, transverse myelitis, neuromyelitis optica, peripheral mononeuropathy, plexopathy, and cranial nerve palsy. The treatment of postinfectious dengue immune-mediated syndrome is similar to that of any immune-mediated syndrome. Ischemic and hemorrhagic strokes are rarely reported in dengue.

Dengue-associated transient muscle dysfunction (DATMD): Myalgia is common in dengue infection. Muscle weakness in dengue although was earlier reported as myositis, but it is more appropriate to call it as DATMD because of transient muscle weakness and lack of inflammatory changes in muscle biopsy. DATMD is associated with raised serum creatinine kinase (CK), myalgia, and/or muscle weakness. In a study on 31 patients from India, 16 patients had varying degrees of muscle weakness with high serum CK and 15 had only raised CK. The majority patients have mild-to-moderate proximal weakness but rarely weakness may be severe leading to respiratory failure. In the majority of patients, serum CK is moderately elevated but may rarely go up to 100,000 IU/L in the patients who have rhabdomyolysis. Dengue may also be associated with myocarditis. The EMG findings in dengue are subtle and nonspecific.[18] There is no spontaneous activity and the motor unit potentials are normal to small size. These findings are in contrast to inflammatory myopathy. Muscle biopsy in three patients with the DATMD revealed interstitial edema and hemorrhage, and there was a paucity of inflammatory infiltrates **(Figs. 7A to C)**. In

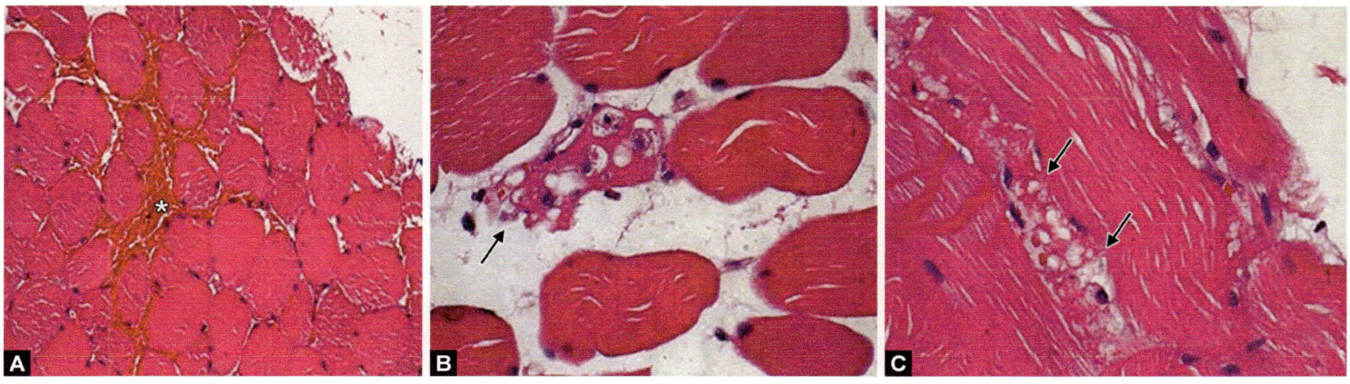

FIGS. 7A TO C: Muscle biopsy of a patient with dengue-associated transient muscle dysfunction. His platelet count was 68,000/mm^3 and creatine kinase (CK) was 1,562 IU/L. Vastus lateralis muscle biopsy on the 12th day of illness revealed mild endoneurial edema, (A, asterisk) a small focus of interstitial hemorrhages (B and C, arrows) with evidence of scattered necrotic fibers with myophagocytosis. There was no inflammatory infiltrates. Hematoxylin and Eosin (H&E) staining, magnification 9120; B H&E staining, × 200; C × 320.

Source: With permission from Misra UK, et al (2012).[19]

patients with DSS, there were occasional myonecrosis, myophagocytosis, and inflammatory cells around necrotic fibers. The patients with DATMD improve completely by 2 weeks.[19] Patients with DATMD may have associated encephalopathy and/or encephalitis. These patients have a more severe illness. Muscle weakness in DENV infection may also be due to hypokalemia which responds to potassium supplementation. The hypokalemic paralysis in dengue is attributed to shift of potassium and renal tubular dysfunction leading to high urinary potassium excretion.

The treatment of dengue is volume management. Hypotension in dengue is treated with fluid and not with inotropes. For details of management, readers may refer to a book by Misra UK and Kalita J—Diagnosis and Management of Neurological Disorders, Wolters Kluwer.[20]

Chikungunya

Chikungunya is a single-stranded RNA virus which spreads by *Aedes* mosquitoes. The first outbreak of CHIK in India was reported in Calcutta in 1960, and the virus was isolated in 2005. CHIK outbreaks have been reported throughout India. The majority of patients infected with CHIK show clinical illness and only 3% patients are asymptomatic. The symptoms develop after 2–4 days of mosquito bite and include fever and ocular pain similar to dengue infection. The clinical differentiating features between CHIK, dengue, and scrub typhus are summarized in **Table 2**. Polyarthralgia including axial pain is typical of CHIK infection. There may be mild mucosal bleeding. In the chronic stage, the patients may have polyarthralgia which persists for weeks to years. The neurological manifestations of CHIK are rare but encephalitis with pupillary abnormality has been reported. Following CHIK infection, various immune-mediated syndromes including Guillain–Barré syndrome, transverse myelitis, and stimulus sensitive myoclonus have been reported. In a study on 30 CHIK patients with neurological manifestations, 12 had encephalitis, and 12 encephalomyelitis.[21] The CSF in CHIK infection is usually normal and MRI is either normal or reveals nonspecific changes. Autopsy studies have shown radiculopathy, brain swelling, and subarachnoid hemorrhage. On microscopy, there were inflammatory infiltrations in periventricular and basal ganglia region, and small foci of demyelination.[22] Treatment is symptomatic. Aspirin and nonsteroid anti-inflammatory drugs should be avoided in dengue, CHIK, and those with coagulopathy and thrombocytopenia.

TABLE 2: Differentiating points between dengue, Chikungunya, and scrub typhus.

Parameters	Dengue	Chikungunya	Scrub typhus
Fever	+	+	+
Rash	3–7 days	1–4 days	Eschar from beginning
Retro-orbital pain	+	–	–
Myalgia	+++	+	++
Polyarthritis	–	+++	–
Tenosynovitis	–	+	–
Hypotension	+	+	–
Thrombocytopenia	+++	+	++
Bleeding	+	–	+

(+: present; –: absent)

Source: With permission from Misra UK, et al (2022).[15]

West Nile Virus Encephalitis

West Nile virus is an arthropod-born single-stranded RNA virus belonging to family Flaviviridae. The name of WNV is derived from West Nile district of Uganda where this virus was first isolated in 1937. WNV is prevalent in Africa, America, Middle East, and Asia. WNV spreads by the bite of *Culex* mosquitoes and is maintained by bird-mosquito-bird cycle. In India WNV was first reported in 1952 and subsequently has been reported from nearly all the parts of India. After an incubation period of 2–15 days, WNV infection results in mild self-limiting illness in >80% subjects. The remaining 20% patients have fever, headache, fatigue, meningitis, myalgia, weakness, gastrointestinal symptoms, and morbilliform and rash. The rash in WNE is nonitching, presents on trunk and extremities sparing palms and soles. The neurological illness occurs in <1% patients and manifests with meningitis, encephalitis, and acute flaccid paralysis simulating poliomyelitis. The patients with WNV may have neck stiffness, altered sensorium, fever, myoclonus, and parkinsonian features. There may be cranial nerve palsy, myelitis, polyradiculopathy, optic neuritis, or seizures. WNV infection may be more severe in elderly (>55 years) and immune-compromised patients. Rarely it may lead to pancreatitis, myocarditis, or hepatic dysfunction. There are reports of Guillain–Barré syndrome, axonal type of neuropathy, polyradiculopathy, and plexopathy in WNV infection. MRI findings have been described in previous section. CSF findings are similar to JE, but may have systemic manifestations such as derangement of liver function. Myelitis in WNE may be associated with pyramidal, spinothalamic, and posterior column involvement with or without anterior horn cell involvement. There is no specific treatment, and the majority of the patients improve. The sequelae may of WNE be due to myelitis.

Enterovirus

Enteroviruses (EV) are RNA viruses of the family *Picornaviridae*, and include >100 serotypes, which have a single positive-strand genomic RNA. *Enterovirus* infection occurs in summer and autumn in temperate region and round the year in tropical and subtropical countries. Neonates and infants infected with Coxsackie virus develop myocarditis, meningitis, and encephalitis with mortality of 10%. In south India, 4.7% patients with a clinical signs of AES were positive for EV 75, and in northern Indian children with AES ECV 21 were identified as a causative agent in 51.8% isolates, followed by ECV 1, CV B1, EV 75, CV B5, and ECV 19. Echoviruses (ECHO-Vs) causing aseptic meningitis in young children. *Enterovirus* can invade the CNS during viremic phase affecting the anterior horn cells of the spinal cord, motor cortex, cerebellum, thalamus, hypothalamus, midbrain, and medulla causing neuronal death and paralysis. Antibodies are produced within the first 7–10 days in the lymphatic system of the gastrointestinal tract before the invasion of the CNS tissue.

Clinical Features

Most EV infections are asymptomatic or result in non-specific fever or mild upper respiratory symptoms. However, EVs can also cause a wide variety of clinical illnesses, which are mild to potentially life threatening. CV infection during pregnancy is associated with spontaneous abortions, fetal myocarditis, and neurodevelopmental delay in the new born. Enterovirus can cause various diseases in the nervous system, including aseptic meningitis, encephalitis, meningoencephalomyelitis, poliomyelitis like illness, opsoclonus-myoclonus syndrome, benign intracranial hypertension, and brainstem (rhombencephalitis). Some cases are mild and reversible but severe cases present with myoclonus followed by rapid onset of respiratory distress due to neurogenic, pulmonary hemorrhage, cyanosis, shock, coma, and apnea and if appropriate interventions are delayed, there may be sudden death. Other systemic complications of enteroviral encephalitis include neonatal sepsis like illness, viral myocarditis, and dilated cardio-myopathy. Destruction of beta cells in CV B infections leads to juvenile onset diabetes mellitus.

For the diagnosis of enteroviral encephalitis, rectal swab, throat swab, serum, and CSF samples are required. For enteroviral neurologic disease other than EV71-associated disease, the sensitivity of EV-PCR of CSF is 76–100%.[23] In EV71, CSF viral culture is positive in 0–3% cases only because of low concentration of virus in the CSF. CV and Echovirus are readily isolated from CSF.

Diagnosis of enteroviral encephalitis is said to be:

- Definitive if either (1) virus is detected by PCR or culture in CSF or (2) by viral detection in both rectal and throat swabs as well as in blood by PCR and absence of other viruses in CSF.
- *Probable encephalitis*: If virus is detected in both rectal and throat swabs by PCR and absence of other viruses in CSF.
- Possible enteroviral infection is diagnosed when virus is detected in either rectal or throat swab by PCR and absence of other in CSF.

Neuroimaging of enterovirus encephalitis reveals the involvement of posterior portion of the medulla oblongata, posterior portion of the pons, midbrain, bilateral dentate nuclei of the cerebellum, and spinal cord. Rhombencephalitis is caused by EV71 shows characteristic lesions in the posterior portions of the medulla oblongata and pons in MRI.

There is no specific antiviral drug but ribavirin, pleconaril, and intravenous immunoglobulin (IVIg) have been used with possible improvement.[23]

Nipah Virus

The name "Nipah" comes from a Malaysian village, where the first outbreak was reported in 1998–1999. Nipah is a RNA virus, which has been a major cause of encephalitis outbreaks with high mortality in Malaysia–Singapore and Indo-Bangladesh regions. The Malaysia–Singapore outbreak was attributed to contact with pigs. Whereas, the Philippines outbreak was associated with horse slaughter. The Indo-Bangladesh outbreaks were associated with consumption of raw date palm sap contaminated by fruit bats. In 2018, Nipah outbreak was reported form Kerala. The patients usually manifest with fever, encephalitis with or without respiratory involvement, and acute respiratory distress syndrome (ARDS). About 50% patients may have thrombocytopenia, leukopenia, and elevated transaminases. Nipah encephalitis may present with relapse or residual deficits in survivors. Relapse of encephalitis occurs after months to years after recovery from acute infection. Psychiatric and neurological complications may occur as sequelae. The MRI in acute Nipah encephalitis shows multifocal discrete T2 high-signal-intensity is disseminated throughout the brain. In relapse or late-onset Nipah encephalitis, MRI characteristically shows multiple areas of patchy and confluent cortical involvement. The diagnosis can be confirmed by isolation and nucleic acid amplification in the acute phase or antibody detection during the convalescent phase. There is no specific treatment and is limited to supportive care. Ribavirin, monoclonal antibody, and favipiravir are the only antiviral with some activity against *Nipah virus*. Standard precautions, hand hygiene, and personal protective equipment are needed for prevention.[24]

Changing Spectrum of AES and Diagnostic Challenge in India

The AES in 1990 was dominated by malaria and JE, which were especially noted in the postmonsoon period. In 1990s and early 2000s, the encephalitis patients were associated with systemic manifestations such as thrombocytopenia, liver, and kidney dysfunction, and these patients turned out to be due to dengue. In the subsequent years, lack of improvement in some of these patients resulted in further investigation and scrub typhus was found to be responsible. Scrub typhus although simulated dengue infection by systemic manifestations such as thrombocytopenia, liver and kidney dysfunction, elevated serum CK, encephalitis, and encephalopathy, but leukocytosis and the muscle involvement in scrub typhus are due to vasculitis as opposed to DATMD. However, a group of investigators considered *Enterovirus* infection being another etiological agent. Coinfection of *Flavivirus* infection, malaria, and scrub typhus is possible and has been reported. In the initial stage, the laboratory confirmatory tests are not easily available or may take a long time to be of clinical significance.

The AES patients may be categorized into pure neurological AES (JE, HSE, and WN), in which cranial CT/MRI revealing frontotemporal lesion is consistent with HSE, or thalamic, and basal ganglia lesions which are consistent with JE. CSF PCR or IgM antibody for JE and HSE is confirmatory. Presence of frontotemporal involvement on MRI indicates acyclovir treatment pending virological confirmation. In systemic AES (dengue, malaria, scrub typhus, and *Leptospira*), CT/MRI, PCR for HSE and JE, and acyclovir therapy may not be useful, rather treatable etiologies such as malaria, scrub typhus, and leptospirosis should be investigated and treated. If smear or antigen for malaria is positive, should receive antimalarial; if negative doxycycline and ceftriaxone should be started pending serological confirmation of scrub typhus, *Leptospira*, or dengue. A syndromic approach of AES based on the prevalent infection in a geographical region may be developed, which may be cost-effective **(Flowchart 1)**.

CONCLUSION

There are numerous viruses producing encephalitis with a geographical and climatic predilection. Arthropod borne viruses are the most frequent cause in the tropical regions. HSE is the most important cause of focal encephalitis without any regional or climatic variation. The diagnosis of encephalitis is based on differentiating infectious form noninfectious causes and then categorizing the treatable etiologist which should be differentiated from those for which only supportive treatment is needed. One should be careful about variation in the clinical picture and emerging virus as a cause of encephalitis.

ACKNOWLEDGMENT

We thank to Mr Shakti Kumar for secretarial help.

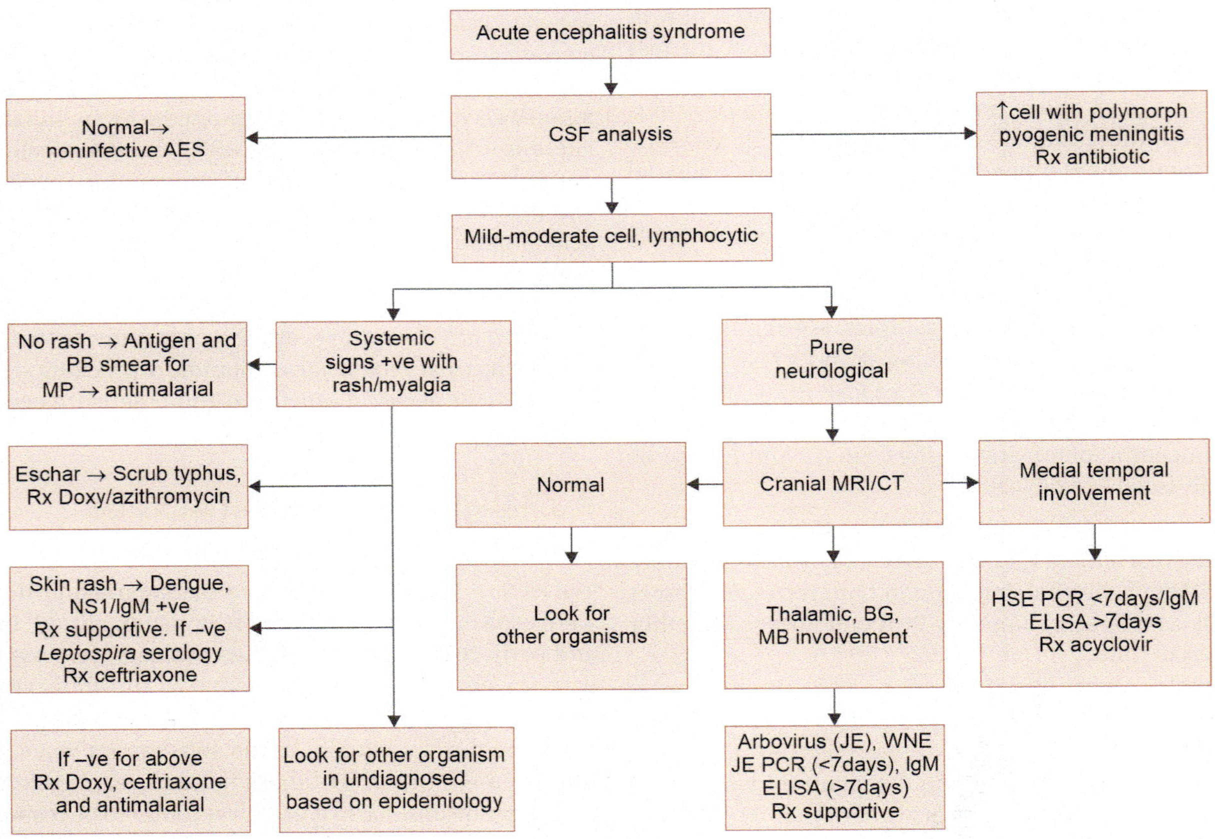

FLOWCHART 1: Showing approach to a patient with acute encephalitis syndrome.

(AES: acute encephalitis syndrome; BG: basal ganglia; CT: computed tomography; CSF: cerebrospinal fluid; ELISA: enzyme-linked immunosorbent assay; HSE: herpes simplex encephalitis; JE: Japanese encephalitis; MP: malarial parasite; MRI: magnetic resonance imaging; PB: peripheral blood; PCR: polymerase chain reaction)

Source: With permission from Misra UK, et al (2022).[15]

REFERENCES

1. Wang H, Zhao S, Wang S, Zheng Y, Wang S, Chen H, et al. Global magnitude of encephalitis burden and its evolving pattern over the past 30 years. J Infect. 2022;84(6):777-87.
2. GBD 2016 Neurology Collaborators. Global, regional, and national burden of neurological disorders, 1990-2016: a systematic analysis for the Global Burden of Disease Study 2016. Lancet Neurol. 2019;18(5):459-80.
3. Jmor F, Emsley HC, Fischer M, Solomon T, Lewthwaite P. The incidence of acute encephalitis syndrome in Western industrialised and tropical countries. Virol J. 2008;5:134.
4. Budka H. Viral infections. In: Garcia JH, Budka H, McKeever PE, Sarnat HB, Sima AAF (eds). Neuropathology—The Diagnostic Approach. St Louis: Mosby; 1997; pp. 353-91.
5. Chaudhuri A, Kennedy PG. Diagnosis and treatment of viral encephalitis. Postgrad Med J. 2002;78(924):575-83.
6. Nakano A, Yamasaki R, Miyazaki S, Horiuchi N, Kunishige M, Mitsui T. Beneficial effect of steroid pulse therapy on acute viral encephalitis. Eur Neurol. 2003;50(4):225-9.
7. Damasio AR, Van Hoesen GW. The limbic system and the localisation of herpes simplex encephalitis. J Neurol Neurosurg Psychiatry. 1985;48:297-301.
8. Kalita J, Misra UK, Pandey S, Dhole TN. A comparison of clinical and radiological findings in adults and children with Japanese encephalitis. Arch Neurol. 2003;60:1760-4.
9. Fodor PA, Levin MJ, Weinberg A, Sandberg E, Sylman J, Tyler KL. Atypical herpes simplex virus encephalitis diagnosed by PCR amplification of viral DNA from CSF. Neurology. 1998;51:554-9.
10. Raschilas F, Wolff M, Delatour F, Chaffaut C, De Broucker T, Chevret S, et al. Outcome of and prognostic factors for herpes simplex encephalitis in adult patients: results of a multicenter study. Clin Infect Dis. 2002;35(3):254-60.
11. Sreenivasan N, Basit S, Wohlfahrt J, Pasternak B, Munch TN, Nielsen LP, et al. The short- and long-term risk of stroke after herpes zoster - a nationwide population-based cohort study. PLoS One. 2013;8(7):e69156.
12. Corral C, Quereda C, Muriel A, Martínez-Ulloa PL, González-Gómez FJ, Corral Í. Clinical spectrum and prognosis of neurological complications of reactivated varicella-zoster infection: the role of immunosuppression. J Neurovirol. 2020;26(5):696-703.
13. Misra UK, Kalita J. Anterior horn cells are also involved in Japanese encephalitis. Acta Neurol Scand. 1997;96:111-7.
14. Misra UK, Kalita J. Overview: Japanese encephalitis. Prog Neurobiol. 2010;91:108-20.
15. Misra UK, Kalita J. Changing Spectrum of Acute Encephalitis Syndrome in India and a Syndromic Approach. Ann Indian Acad Neurol. 2022;25(3):354-66.
16. Rathi KR, Arora MM, Sahai K, Tripathi S, Singh SP, Raman DK, et al. Autopsy findings in fatal dengue hemorrhagic fever—06 cases. Med J Armed Forces India. 2013;69(3):254-9.
17. Bhoi SK, Naik S, Kumar S, Phadke RV, Kalita J, Misra UK. Cranial imaging findings in dengue virus infection. J Neurol Sci. 2014;342:36-41.
18. Kalita J, Misra UK, Maurya PK, Shankar SK, Mahadevan A. Quantitative electromyography in dengue-associated muscle dysfunction. J Clin Neurophysiol. 2012;29:468-71.
19. Misra UK, Kalita J, Maurya PK, Kumar P, Shankar SK, Mahadevan A. Dengue-associated transient muscle dysfunction: Clinical, electromyography and histopathological changes. Infection. 2012;40:125-3.
20. Misra UK. Kalita J. Diagnosis and Management of Neurological Disorders. India: Wolters Kluwer Health; 2011; pp. 429.
21. Robin S, Ramful D, Le Seach' F, Jaffar-Bandjee MC, Rigou G, Alessandri JL. Neurologic manifestations of pediatric chikungunya infection. J Child Neurol. 2008;23:1028-35.
22. Ganesan K, Diwan A, Shankar SK, Desai SB, Sainani GS, Katrak SM. Chikungunya encephalomyeloradiculitis: Report of 2 cases with neuroimaging and 1 case with autopsy findings. AJNR Am J Neuroradiol. 2008;29:1636-7.
23. Jain S, Patel B, Bhatt GC. Enteroviral encephalitis in children: clinical features, pathophysiology, and treatment advances. Pathog Glob Health. 2014;108(5):216-22.
24. Banerjee S, Gupta N, Kodan P, Mittal A, Ray Y, Nischal N, et al. Nipah virus disease: A rare and intractable disease. Intractable Rare Dis Res. 2019;8(1):1-8.

60 CHAPTER

Pyogenic Meningitis

SP Gorthi, Dulari Gupta, Mahadevan Kumar

INTRODUCTION

Meningitis and encephalitis are inflammatory conditions of the central nervous system (CNS) that can lead to high rates of mortality and disability. Meningitis, defined as inflammation of the meninges surrounding the brain and spinal cord, is typically characterized by headache, neck stiffness, and cerebrospinal fluid (CSF) pleocytosis.

ETIOLOGY

The causative organism of acute pyogenic meningitis is age-determined. Pneumococcal meningitis is caused by the lancet-shaped facultative anaerobic gram-positive coccus. *Streptococcus pneumoniae* is the most common cause of bacterial meningitis in adults. Predisposing factors include pneumonia, otitis media, sinusitis, head trauma, CSF leaks, sickle cell disease, splenectomy, diabetes mellitus, alcoholism, and hypogammaglobulinemia. The second most common cause of meningitis is gram-negative diplococcus, *Neisseria meningitidis*. It is a part of normal nonpathogenic flora in the nasopharynx of up to 8–25% of adults. It colonizes and infects only humans. Congenital terminal complement deficiency (C5–C8) predisposes to meningococcemia and is commonly encountered in military recruits' barracks and in other community dwellings which promote overcrowding. The gram-negative encapsulated *Haemophilus influenzae* is commonly isolated in older adults with pyogenic meningitis and spreads via respiratory droplets predisposed by immunocompromised status, chronic lung disease, splenectomy, leukemia, and sickle cell disease. The gram-positive bacillus *Listeria monocytogenes* causes meningitis in immunocompromised individuals and listeria outbreaks are associated with the consumption of unpasteurized dairy, soft cheeses, meat, and sea foods. Other predisposing factors are impaired cell-mediated immunity in old age, organ transplantation, malignancy, immunosuppressant therapies, and pregnancy. The same factors may predispose to *Brucella melitensis*. The gram-positive coccus, *Staphylococcus aureus* is responsible for acute pyogenic meningitis following neurosurgical procedures like ventriculoperitoneal shunts and head trauma. It can also spread from various infectious foci such as pneumonia, endocarditis, urinary tract infection, or skin infections. Other risk factors are intravenous drug abuse, cirrhosis, and immunosuppressed states.

Recurrent community-acquired meningitis is caused by *S. pneumoniae*. Causative organisms are different for community-acquired as compared to nosocomial meningitis. Gram-negative bacilli are the most frequent causes of nosocomial infections. Enterobacteriaceae, *Proteus*, *Escherichia coli*, *Klebsiella*, *Serratia*, and *Enterobacter* cause meningitis in adults with alcoholism, malignancy, diabetes, congestive heart failure, and hepatic or renal insufficiency.

PATHOGENESIS

The intact blood–brain barrier protects the CNS from bacterial invasion. But due to the special surface properties of bacteria and host immune deficiencies, at times bacterial invasion occurs and any of the nervous system compartments such as epidural space, dura, subdural space, leptomeninges, subarachnoid space, and brain parenchyma can get infected. After the bacterial invasion the following may result-epidural abscess, pachymeningitis, subdural empyema, leptomeningitis, and brain abscess. The invasion also triggers an intense inflammatory response that engulfs the entire cerebrospinal axis. The source of pathogens could be a direct invasion from the spine, skull, or hematogenous from the heart, lung, ear, or oral cavity. Predisposing factors for nosocomial infections are primarily caused by openings into the CNS. Predisposing factors in 404 single episodes of bacterial meningitis are listed in **Table 1**.[1]

TABLE 1: Predisposing factors in 404 single episodes of bacterial meningitis.

Factor	Community acquired % ($n = 253$)	Nosocomial % ($n = 151$)
Acute otitis media	19	01
Chronic otitis media	07	00
Sinusitis	12	04
Pneumonia	15	08
Endocarditis	07	01
Head Injury	09	13
Recent Neurosurgery	00	68
Neurosurgical devices	01	32
Altered immune Status	19	31
Diabetes mellitus	10	06
Alcoholism	18	05
Cerebrospinal fluid leak	08	13

Source: With permission from Durand ML, et al (1991).[1]

PATHOPHYSIOLOGY

The pathophysiology and clinical features are similar in all patients with acute pyogenic meningitis, regardless of the causative organisms. The first step in meningitis is nasopharyngeal colonization by a new organism. Subsequently, local invasion and bacterial replication follow. Inflammation starts in the subarachnoid space. Increased blood flow across the blood–brain barrier results in vasogenic edema. Inflammation in subarachnoid space leads to cerebral vasculitis and/or infarction. Increased CSF outflow resistance leads to hydrocephalus and interstitial edema. Increased intracranial pressure is secondary to vasogenic edema, cytotoxic edema, and interstitial edema. Cranial nerve palsies can occur due to the accumulation of purulent exudates at the base of the brain. The same pathology can also block the CSF pathways causing obstructive hydrocephalus. The exudate of leptomeningeal inflammation spreads over the convexities of the cerebral cortex causing arterial or venous thrombosis with infarction and hemorrhage resulting in focal neurological deficits. The meninges and blood vessels are thickened by inflammatory cells. This leads to rheological disturbances and thrombosis which results in cerebral infarction and focal neurological deficits. Virchow-Robin spaces are an extension of the subarachnoid spaces and often inflammation extends into these perivascular parenchymal spaces.[2]

CLINICAL FEATURES[3]

A diffuse erythematous maculopapular rash is present in over 50% of patients with meningococcemia. The rash in the form of petechiae and purpura appears on the trunk and lower extremities. The petechiae may appear on mucous membranes and conjunctiva but never in the nail beds. The rash of staphylococcal endocarditis involves nail beds in addition to the mucus membranes and the extremities.

The classical triad of meningitis includes fever, neck stiffness, and altered mental status. But meningitis can occur even in the absence of these findings. The main predisposing factors are diabetes mellitus, otitis media, pneumonia, sinusitis, and chronic alcoholism. Symptoms due to systemic infection are fever, chills, myalgias, and rash. Symptoms due to CNS involvement are photophobia, headache, nausea, vomiting, focal neurological deficits, and altered sensorium. Findings of meningeal inflammation include neck stiffness, Kernig sign, Brudzinski sign, jolt accentuation, and cranial nerve palsies. Focal neurological findings and seizures are due to secondary cerebral vasculitis resulting from meningeal inflammation. Elevated intracranial pressure (ICP) is secondary to meningeal inflammation and cytotoxic edema. Raised ICP causes altered sensorium, headache, seizures, and cranial nerve palsies. *Neck stiffness* is tested by gentle forward flexion of the neck with the patient in the supine position. *Kernig's sign* is elicited by flexing the knee 90° in the supine position and the sign is considered positive when extension of the knee elicits resistance or pain in low back or thigh. *Brudzinski sign* is positive when in supine position passive neck flexion results in voluntary flexion of knees and hips. *Jolt accentuation test* consists of having the patient turn his head horizontally at a frequency of 2–3 rotations per second and this sign is considered positive if the headache worsens. Severe meningeal irritation leads to a *tripod position* in which knees and hips are flexed, back arched lordotically, neck extended, and arms support back **(Figs. 1A to E)**.

The various clinical features were studied in 14 retrospective and 2 prospective studies; the results of which are summarized in **Table 2**. There was significant heterogeneity in studies in respect of patient population and definitions. A highly sensitive test rules out the disease if it is negative and a highly specific test rules in the disease if it is positive. The likelihood ratio (LR) suggests how much more (LR > 1) or less (LR < 1) likely the disease is (LR = 1 no effect; LR = 3–10 disease is more likely LR: 0.3–0.1 disease less likely). Data from the pooled retrospective studies suggest that the absence of fever, neck stiffness, and altered mental status cannot rule out meningitis. Jolt accentuation headache may be helpful (LR+ 2.4 LR– 0.5). So, the bottom line from retrospective studies is the absence of the classic triad of fever, neck stiffness, and altered mental status does not rule out meningitis (sensitivity = 0.46).[4,5]

Seizures are seen in 40% of cases. Generalized seizures occur due to fever, metabolic derangements, or toxic factors (example alcohol withdrawal). Focal seizures are more likely to occur after 4–10 days and are caused by arterial thrombosis, cortical vein thrombosis, or abscess formation. Cranial nerve palsies (CN III, IV, VII, and VIII) are due to purulent exudates in the arachnoid sheaths of specific cranial nerves. Cerebral edema and increased intracranial pressure may be due to noncommunicating hydrocephalus

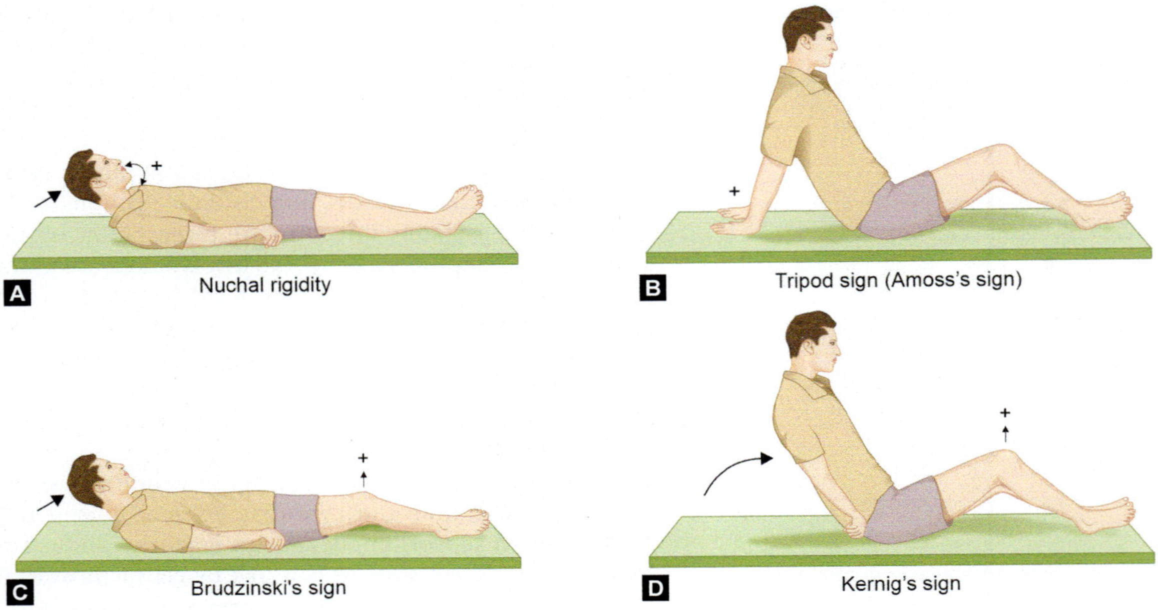

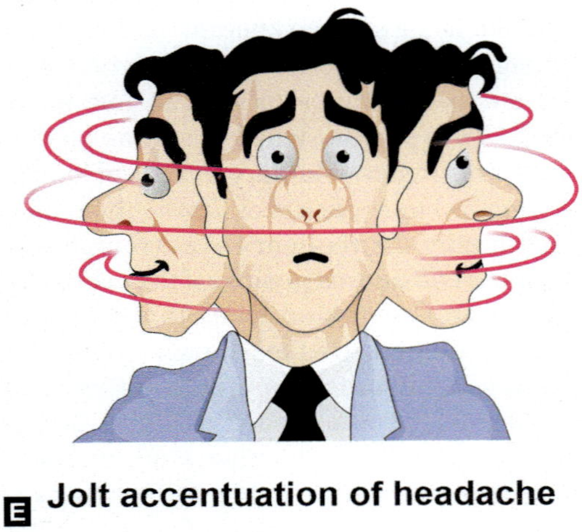

FIGS. 1A TO E: (A) Nuchal rigidity, (B) Kernig's sign, (C) Brudzinski's sign, (D) Tripod sign (Amoss's sign), and (E) Head jolt test.

TABLE 2: Classical signs of meningitis. Likelihood ratios in prospective studies.

Finding	LR+ (95% CI)	LR– (95% CI)
Nausea/vomiting	1.3 (1.1–1.6)	0.64 (0.44–0.92)
Headache	1.1 (1.0–1.3)	0.43 (0.19–0.96)
Neck Stiffness	1.1 (0.82 = 1.4)	0.95 (0.74–1.2)
Fever	0.82 (0.62–1.1)	1.2 (0.94–1.5)
Kerning sign	4.2 (0.23–77)	0.92 (0.81–1.0)
Brudzinski sign	0.97 (0.26–3.5)	1.0 (0.94–1.1)
Jolt accentuation	2.4 (1.4–4.2)	0.05 (0.01 = 0.38)

caused by basilar exudates and exudates in the Virchow-Robin space.

Certain clinical features point toward particular etiologies. Meningococcal meningitis heralds itself with meningococcemia and a macular erythematous rash which rapidly evolves into petechiae and purpuric form. The similar rash may be encountered in echovirus type 9, *Acinetobacter*, Rocky Mountain spotted fever and other rickettsia fevers, *S. aureus* endocarditis, sepsis, thrombotic thrombocytic purpura, and vasculitis. A suppurative focus like pneumonia, otitis media, or sinusitis is seen in about 30% of patients with pneumococcal or *H. influenzae* meningitis. Staphylococcal pneumoniae is seen in meningitis secondary to CSF rhinorrhea or otorrhea.

DIAGNOSIS

Apart from routine investigations, blood culture and CSF examination are the most important investigations. Approximately, 6 mL of CSF is required for analysis including measurement of CSF opening pressure, and gross assessment for turbidity and color. The characteristic CSF picture in pyogenic meningitis includes an elevated CSF pressure >20 cmH_2O, neutrophilic leukocytosis, hypoglycorrhachia (blood sugar <40 mg/dL) and an increased CSF protein >45 mg/dL. In patients suspected of having immunosuppression, history of CNS disease, mass lesion, stroke, focal infection, patients presenting with new onset seizures, papilledema, and abnormal levels of consciousness or focal neurological deficits, CSF examination is differed till neuroimaging rules out any abnormality. The CSF should be collected in numbered bottles and the fourth bottle should be taken to the laboratory immediately for cell count. In cases of human immunodeficiency virus (HIV)-positive individuals CSF should be tested with Gram stain, acid-fast bacillus (AFB) stain, India ink stain, and cryptococcal antigen as polymicrobial and mixed infections are commonly encountered. CSF Gram stain has sensitivity up to 90% but decreases drastically after oral antibiotics. The presence of $<10^3$ colony forming units per mL (CFU/mL) concentration of bacteria is associated with a positive Gram stain in 25%; 10^3–10^5 CFU/mL has a positive Gram stain in 60% and if CFU/mL is $>10^5$ then Gram stain is positive in 97%. Latex agglutination test with a sensitivity ranging from 50 to 100% is useful in suspected cases of meningitis who received antibiotic therapy when Gram stain and culture are negative. Limulus lysate assay detects 10^3-gram-negative bacteria/mL of CSF and as little as 0.1 ng/mL of endotoxin. Polymerase chain reaction has almost 100% sensitivity and specificity. CSF lactate concentration of >4.2 mmol/L has a sensitivity of 98% and specificity of 100%. Serum C reactive protein (CRP) has a sensitivity of 96% and specificity of 96% and a negative predictive value of 99%. That means normal CRP rules out bacterial meningitis. A bacterial meningitis score has been conceived with important parameters and is shown in **Table 3**. Similarly, Thwaites criteria are used to differentiate bacterial meningitis from tubercular meningitis. Thwaites' index is obtained by adding up the weighted diagnostic index scores for dichotomized clinical variables including age, blood white cell count, duration of illness, CSF total white cell count, and neutrophil percentage. A score of 4 or more is suggestive of pyogenic meningitis **(Table 4)**.[6-9]

Neuroimaging before CSF is advocated if the cerebral herniation is threatened and is recommended. Diffuse meningeal enhancement especially in cerebral convexity, subdural empyema, brain abscess, and infarcts is common findings. The pyogenic source may also be detected such as sinusitis, otorrhea, CSF rhinorrhea, and basal skull fracture.

TABLE 3: Bacterial meningitis index.

Parameter	Score
Positive Gram stain	1
CSF WBC >10,000 cells/mm^3	1
CSF protein >80 mg	1
Peripheral WBC count >10,000/mm^3	1
History of seizure	1
A score of 1 or >1 is associated with pyogenic meningitis	

(CSF: cerebrospinal fluid; WBC: white blood cell)

TABLE 4: Thwaites diagnostic criteria for differentiating tubercular meningitis from bacterial meningitis.

Variable	Cut off for each variable	Score
Age (years)	≥36 years, <36 years	2, 0
Blood WBC (mL)	≥15,000, <15,000	4, 0
History of illness	≥6, <6	–5, 0
CSF total WBC (mL)	≥900, <900	3, 0
CSF% neutrophils	≥75, <75	4, 0
If score is < 4 it suggests tubercular meningitis > bacterial meningitis		

(CSF: cerebrospinal fluid; WBC: white blood cell)

DIFFERENTIAL DIAGNOSIS

Febrile encephalopathy syndrome in the tropics is commonly due to cerebral malaria, pyogenic meningitis, and viral encephalitis. Important noninfectious causes include heat stroke, neuroleptic malignant syndrome, and serotonin syndrome. Patients with subarachnoid hemorrhage seeking medical attention after 48 hours may mimic pyogenic meningitis as they develop fever due to the presence of blood products in CSF.

COMPLICATIONS

The profound inflammation involving the meninges and blood vessels results in convulsions, cranial nerve palsies, focal cerebral abscess, damage to the spinal cord or nerve roots, and hydrocephalus. Patients may suffer from deafness, ocular palsies, blindness, changes in sensorium, seizures, subdural empyema, and brain abscess. Sudden deterioration may be due to brain herniation secondary to raised intracranial pressure. The other complications encountered during the course of illness include intravascular coagulation, meningococcemia, panophthalmitis, arthritis, purpura, pericarditis, epididymitis, albuminuria, herniation, and Waterhouse–Fredrickson syndrome due to adrenal hemorrhage.

TREATMENT[10]

Empirical antibiotic therapy must be given before the organism is isolated. The choice of antibiotic depends on patients' age and associated comorbidities like post-neurosurgery status, immunodeficiency, etc. Gram staining of the organism if available will guide the choice of antibiotic. To achieve optimal levels of CSF, all antibiotics are to be administered intravenously. The guidelines for empirical antibiotics are given in **Table 5**. Suggested specific antibiotic therapy is given in **Table 6**.

TABLE 5: Empirical antibiotic therapy for pyogenic meningitis depending on age and comorbidities.

Age group/comorbidities	Antimicrobial agent
Neonates	Ampicillin plus cefotaxime
Infants and Children and Adults	Third generation cephalosporins (cefotaxime or ceftriaxone plus vancomycin)
Older adults	As in 2 above plus ampicillin
Neurosurgical procedures	Ceftazidime plus vancomycin
Immunocompromised state	Ampicillin plus third-generation cephalosporins plus vancomycin
Neutropenic state	Cefepime

TABLE 6: Specific antibiotic therapy depending on microorganisms responsible for pyogenic meningitis.

Organism	Antimicrobial agent	Duration
Streptococcus pneumoniae • Sensitive to penicillin • Resistant to penicillin	• Penicillin G, ampicillin • Vancomycin plus third-generation cephalosporins	10–14 days
Neisseria meningitidis	Penicillin G, Ampicillin	7 days
H. influenzae • β-lactamase negative • β-lactamase positive	• Ampicillin • Third-generation cephalosporins	7–10 days
Enterobacteriaceae	Third-generation cephalosporins	21 days
Pseudomonas aeruginosa	Cefepime/ meropenem	21 days
Listeria monocytogenes	Ampicillin or Penicillin G	21 days
Staphylococcal aureus • Methicillin sensitive • Methicillin resistant	• Nafcillin or oxacillin • Vancomycin	7–10 days
Staphylococcus epidermidis	Vancomycin	

Adjunctive Therapy and Supportive Care

- Dexamethasone 0.15 mg/kg every 6 hours for 4 days for children, 12 mg every 12 hours for adults. Dexamethasone decreases sensory neuronal hearing loss and improves neurological outcomes. It should be started shortly before giving the first dose of intravenous antibiotics, so that it can inhibit the production of inflammatory cytokines. It has been found to be most useful in pneumococcal and meningococcal infections.
- *Supportive care*:
  - Fluid and electrolyte imbalance [monitor for syndrome of inappropriate antidiuretic hormone secretion (SIADH)]
  - Loss of autoregulation, so maintain normal SBP
  - Treatment for ICP—elevate head to 30°, hyperventilation till $PaCO_2$ drops to 27–30 mm Hg, hyperosmolar agents (mannitol and glycerol)

PROGNOSIS

The mortality rate for treated cases of acute bacterial meningitis remains significant because of the numerous potential complications (increase ICP, hydrocephalus, focal neurological deficits, seizures, brain abscess, subdural empyema, and sepsis). Factors associated with significantly higher overall mortality rates are age >60, obtundation on admission and seizures occurring within 24 hours of admission.

PREVENTION

Vaccination for Acute Bacterial Meningitis[11]

Vaccines are now available for *H. influenzae* type b (Hib), *N. meningitidis*, and *S. pneumoniae*.

- *Recommendation for Hib vaccine in children >5 years*: Vaccinate if risk factors like asplenia, sickle cell disease, immune deficiency, or immunosuppression
- Recommendation for meningococcal and pneumococcal vaccine.
  - During epidemic outbreaks
  - Travel to hyperendemic areas
  - High-risk immunodeficiency groups (terminal coagulant deficiency and properdin deficiency)
- Recommendation for pneumococcal vaccine—(1) all adults >65 years old, (2) individuals with chronic cardiorespiratory conditions, Chronic alcoholics, asplenia, multiple myeloma, HIV infection, Wiskott-Aldrich syndrome, diabetes mellitus, and hepatic and renal dysfunction
- The close household, and medical personnel contacts for meningococcal and *H. influenzae* meningitis be treated with rifampicin prophylactically.
- In April 2008, the National Technical Advisory Group on Immunization (NTAGI) in India had advised *H. influenzae* and pneumococcal vaccination to be rolled out in India in a phased manner.[12] Currently, *H. influenzae* vaccination (since 2013) and pneumococcal vaccination (since 2017) are both available under the National Immunization Program of the Government of India.[13]

Case Vignette of *Brucella* Meningitis (Figs. 2 and 3)

A 45-year-old male, a farmer by profession presented to the hospital with complaints of altered sensorium, fever, and headache for 1 day. He had a history of arthralgia for the past 4 months. On CSF examination, protein was raised (346 mg/dL) and sugar was reduced (15 mg/dL) with total nucleated cells 120 and 65% polymorphs suggestive of pyogenic meningitis. Magnetic resonance imaging (MRI) brain showed leptomeningeal enhancement suggestive of meningitis. CSF smear showed a few pus cells with a few gram-negative coccobacilli. The culture grew gram-negative coccobacilli which were nonmotile, catalase, and oxidase positive, identified as *B. melitensis* by automated identification system Vitek 2 compact, (Biomerieux). The patient was treated with doxycycline and ceftriaxone for 6 weeks. His sensorium improved and he was discharged against medical advice after 5 days of admission. Blood culture remained negative even after 14 days of incubation. On follow-up, he was advised to take rifampicin and doxycycline for 12 weeks.

[*Case courtesy*: Dr (Col) Mahadevan Kumar Professor Microbiology and Head AMSP Dr Aishwarya Babu Krishna Kumar Assistant Professor, Dr Sunita Bhatawadekar Associate Professor Bharati Vidyapeeth (DTU) Medical College.]

Case Vignette of Enterococcal Meningitis (Figs. 4 to 6)

A 37-year-old male sustained a depressed frontal bone fracture in a road traffic accident. He underwent surgery for repair of the CSF leak with ventriculoperitoneal shunting. Postoperatively, he developed meningitis due to

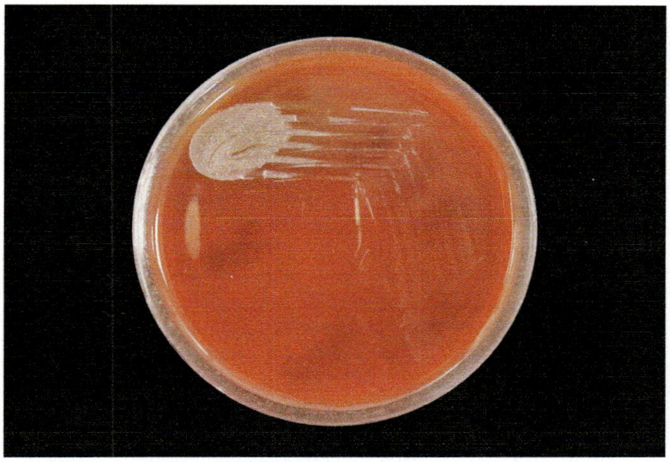

FIG. 2: Colonies of *Brucella melitensis* on blood agar.

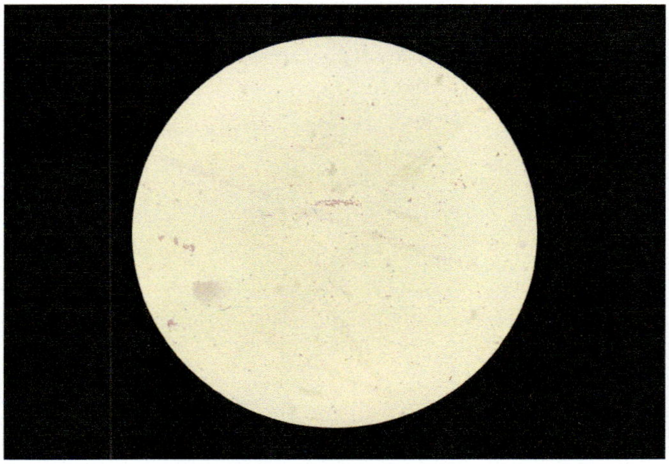

FIG. 3: Gram-negative bacilli on direct smear from cerebrospinal fluid.

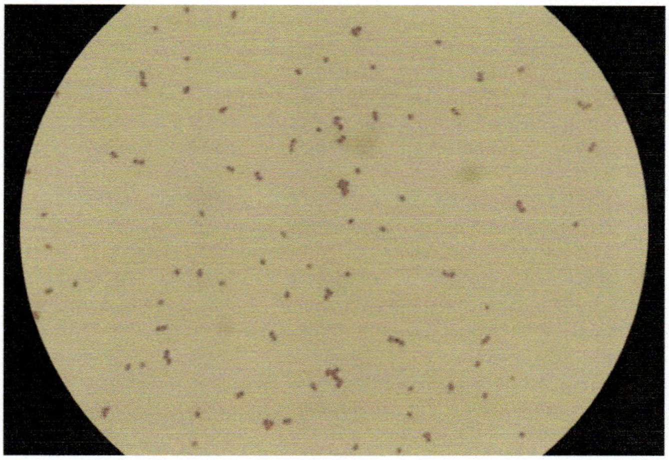

FIG. 4: *Enterococcus faecium* on Gram-stain.

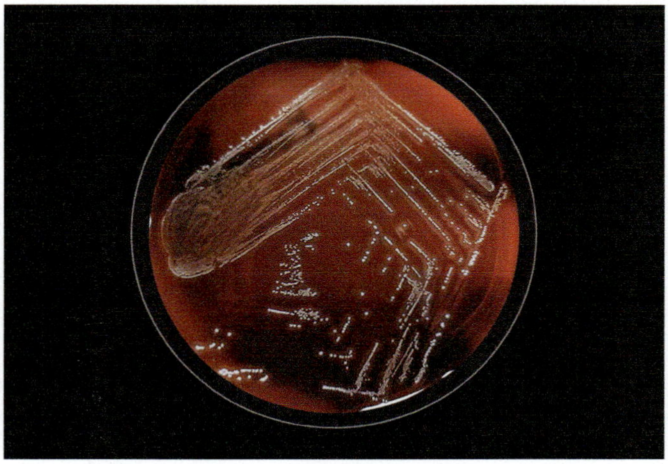

FIG. 5: *Enterococcus faecium* isolated on blood agar.

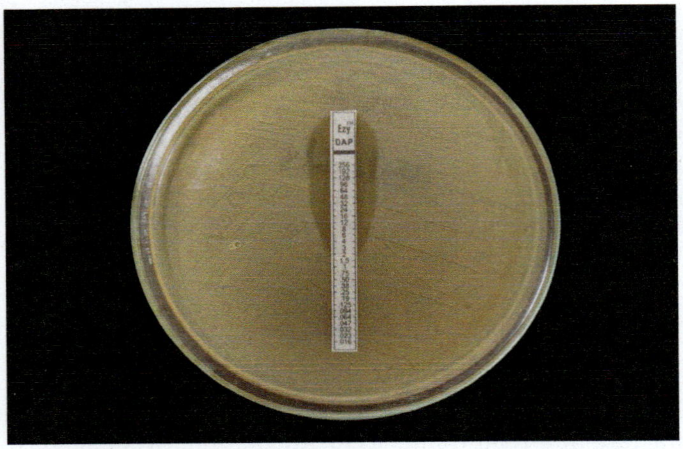

FIG. 6: Susceptibility of daptomycin (MIC 2 mg/L) for *Enterococcus faecium* on Mueller Hinton Agar.

Enterococcus faecium [vancomycin-resistant *Enterococcus* (VRE). He was treated with linezolid and discharged. He reported back with the persistence of VRE in CSF resistant to linezolid. He was then treated successfully with daptomycin and tigecycline.

[*Images courtesy*: Dr Aishwarya Babu Krishna Kumar Assistant Professor Dr Sunita Bhatawadekar Associate Professor Bharati Vidyapeeth (DTU) Medical College.]

CONCLUSION

Pyogenic meningitis requires instant and astute care to achieve good outcomes. Modern microbiological support is necessary for the decision-making process. Time is of the essence and timely appropriate therapy is often rewarded with the reversal of the condition.

REFERENCES

1. Durand ML, Calderwood SB, Weber DJ, Miller SI, Southwick FS, Caviness VS Jr, et al. Acute bacterial meningitis in adults. A review of 493 episodes. N Eng J Med. 1993;328:21-8.
2. Scheldt VM, Whitney RJ, Marra CM. Infection of the central nervous system, 3rd edition. Philadelphia: Lippincott Williams & Williams; 2004.
3. Van de Beek D, de Gan's J, Spaniard L, Weisfelt M, Reitsma JB, Vermeulen M. Clinical features and prognostic factors in adults with bacterial meningitis. N Engl J Med. 2004;351:1849-59.
4. Thomas KE, Hasbun R, Jekel J, Quagliarello VJ. The diagnostic accuracy of Kernigs sign, Brudzinski sign and Nuchal rigidity in adults with suspected meningitis. Clinical Infect Dis. 2002;35(1): 46-51.
5. Atta J, Attala R, Cook DJ, Wing JG. Does this patient have acute meningitis? The Rational Clinical Examination. JAMA. 1999;282 (2):175-81.
6. Costerm JM, Brower MC, Sprengen MES, Roosendaal SD, van der Ende A, van de Beek D. Cranial CT, lumbar puncture and clinical determinants in bacterial meningitis: A nationwide cohort study. Clini Infect Dis. 2018;67(6):920-6.
7. Garden LV, Jorgensen PE, Nexø E, Wang P. C-Reactive protein and Bacterial meningitis. A Meta-analysis. Scand J Clin Lab Invest. 1998;58:383-93.
8. Nigranc LE, Kupperman N, Maccas CG, Cannavino CR, Moro-Sutherland DM, Schremmer RD, et al. Clinical prediction rule for identifying children with CSF pleocytosis at very low risk of bacterial meningitis. JAMA. 2007:297:32-60.
9. Suleman T, Sai Medi, H. Erdem, Senbayrak S, Ozturk-Engin D, Inan A, et al. The Diagnostic utility of the Thwaites system and the lancet consensus scoring system in tuberculous vs. non-tuberculous subacute and chronic meningitis. Multicenter analysis of 395 patients. BMJ Infect Dis. 2020;20:788.
10. Turkel AR, Hartman BJ, Kaplan SL, Kaufman BA, Roos KL, Scheld WM, et al. Practice guidelines for the management of Bacterial meningitis. Clinical Infect Dis. 2004;39:1267-84.
11. Gorthi SP, Nagpal AK. Meningococcal vaccine: Which, when and for whom? MJAFI 2010;66(1):2-3.
12. Advisory Committee on Vaccines and Immunization Practices, Indian Academy of Pediatrics. (2019). IAP Guidebook on Immunization 2018–2019. [online] Available fromhttps://iapindia.org/pdf/124587-IAP-GUIDE-BOOK-ON-IMMUNIZATION-18-19.pdf [Last accessed December, 2022].
13. NHM. (2018). National Immunization Schedule. [online] Available from http://www.nhm.gov.in/New_Updates_2018/NHM_Components/Immunization/report/National_%20Immunization_Schedule.pdf [Last accessed December, 2022].

61
CHAPTER

Fungal Meningitis

Chandrashekhar Meshram, Prafulla Shembalkar, Nitin Chandak

INTRODUCTION

Fungi are eukaryotic organisms and generally develop from spores. There at least one and a half million fungal species. But 70,000 of them had been formally described and only 300 of those cause virulence in humans. About 10–15% cause central nervous system (CNS) infections.[1] Most pathological fungi are dimorphic, that is, they are capable of existing in yeast and a filamentous or mold state. In the yeast state, they are unicellular, round to elongated, and reproduce by budding. In the filamentous or mold state, they grow by extension of their tips to form tubular filamentous structures called hypha. Parts of the hypha can form reproductive elements called spores, conidia, or arthroconidia that are capable of becoming air-borne. Humans acquire infection by inhalation of the fungal spores[2] **(Box 1)**.

Fungi can reach the CNS with different modalities—(1) hematogenous spread; (2) direct focal extension from anatomical regions such as paranasal sinuses, ear, or orbits; and (3) traumatic introduction. Fungal meningitis is a serious syndrome with a high burden of morbidity and mortality, generally presenting as subacute or chronic meningitis.

BOX 1 Fungal species responsible for meningitis.

- *True yeast:*
    - *Cryptococcus*
    - Histoplasmosis
    - Blastomycosis
    - Coccidiosis
- *Pseudohyphae:*
    - *Candida*
- *True hyphae:*
    - Septate—*Aspergillus* and *Fusarium*
    - Nonseptate—*Rhizopus, Rhizomucor*, and *Mucor*

EPIDEMIOLOGY

Fungal meningitis is an uncommon cause of meningitis, often not suspected and difficult to diagnose. The symptoms are nonspecific, the course is prolonged and confused with other causes of chronic meningitis like tuberculous meningitis.[3]

In 2006, there were >72,000 meningitis-related hospitalizations in the United States; more than half (54.6%) of all meningitis-related hospitalizations were attributed to a virus, while bacterial meningitis accounted for 21.8% of all meningitis-related hospital stays. Funguses and other microorganisms were noted in only 7.3% of all hospitalizations related to meningitis. All remaining meningitis-related hospitalizations did not specify a causative microorganism (17.2%).[4] This pattern would not have changed much since then.

In another study conducted in the United States between 2000 and 2012 among fungal meningitis, the most common causative organism was *Cryptococcus* species (70.1% of cases), followed by *Coccidioides* species (16.4%), *Histoplasma capsulatum* (6.0%), and *Candida* species (7.6%).[5] When considering the incidence estimates it should be considered that fungal meningitis is often underdiagnosed due to nonspecific symptoms and a low index of suspicion.

The incidence of fungal infections is increasing with greater numbers of infections noted among immunosuppressed patients. However, some fungi, such as *Cryptococcus, Coccidioides*, and *Histoplasma*, can also cause infection in immunocompetent patients.

In the USA, it was estimated that invasive mycoses caused by *Candida* species are responsible for 72–228 infections per million population annually, while *Cryptococcus neoformans* is responsible for 30–66 infections and *Aspergillus* species, 12–34 infections per million population.[6]

The most common CNS fungal infection worldwide is cryptococcal meningoencephalitis **(Table 1)**[7,8].

TABLE 1: Central nervous system involvement with invasive fungal infection.[7,8]

Fungus	%
Cryptococcosis	67–84
Invasive *Candida*	3–64
Disseminated blastomycosis	40
Disseminated coccidioidomycosis	25
Disseminated histoplasmosis	5–20
Invasive aspergillosis	4–6
Zygomycosis	12
Dematiaceous	100

BOX 2 Predisposing factors.

- HIV/AIDS
- Solid organ transplantation
- Leukemia and lymphoma
- Systemic lupus erythematosus
- Chronic granulomatous disease
- Corticosteroid therapy
- Cytotoxic agents
- Inherited immunodeficiency
- IV drug abuse
- Trauma, surgery
- Alcoholism
- Diabetes mellitus
- Idiopathic CD4 lymphopenia
- Autosomal dominant hyper-IgE syndrome
- Coronavirus disease 2019 (COVID-19) infection

(AIDS: acquired immunodeficiency syndrome; HIV: human immunodeficiency virus; IgE: immunoglobulin E)

The data on the burden of opportunistic mycoses in India is not clear though the climate is well suited for a wide variety of fungal infections. An increased incidence of invasive candidiasis, aspergillosis, and zygomycosis is reported in India.[8] Invasive candidiasis is the most common opportunistic mycosis followed by invasive aspergillosis. Though the exact prevalence of aspergillosis is not known, high prevalence is expected in Indian hospitals where often construction activities continue in the hospital vicinity without a proper impervious barrier.[9]

India has the highest burden of mucormycosis with 140 cases per million. In the coronavirus disease 2019 (COVID-19) pandemic, there has been an increased incidence of this fungal infection with more than fivefold rise in hospital admissions due to *Mucor*[10] **(Box 2)**.

CLINICAL FEATURES

Because of the low specificity of symptoms in most patients, any CNS-related symptoms should prompt a diagnostic work-up in patients at risk, particularly in those with clinical signs of a primary infection outside the CNS (e.g., fungal pneumonia or sinusitis).

Cryptococcus

Central nervous system infections with *Cryptococcus* usually present with meningoencephalitis, and are mostly caused by *C. neoformans* and, less frequently, by *C. gattii*. These infections commonly arise from a primary lung infection, either as primary dissemination or reactivation of a latent infection. Patients infected with *C. gattii* and immunocompetent individuals more frequently develop space-occupying CNS cryptococcomas than immunocompromised individuals or patients infected with other *Cryptococcus* species.[11]

By far the most common presentation, representing up to 90% of HIV-related cryptococcal disease, is cryptococcal meningitis (CM), which caused an estimated 223,100 cases and 181,100 deaths among people living with HIV in 2014 and accounted for 15% of all the people dying from HIV-related deaths globally.[12] Mortality from CM remains highest in low-income countries. The estimated 1-year mortality of people living with HIV who receive care for CM is 70% in low-income countries versus 20–30% for high-income countries. A major reason for this high mortality is a delay in diagnosis, largely as a result of limited access to lumbar puncture (LP) and rapid diagnostic assays. Further contributing factors are the limited availability and high cost of currently recommended antifungal drugs and intensive care.[13]

Cryptococcal meningitis has been reported as the most common opportunistic infection of the CNS in patients with HIV/AIDS in India accounting for 2–7% of all opportunistic infections.[14,15]

Risk Factors and Clinical Manifestations

About 50% of infections are HIV related, up to one-third are solid organ transplant patients and the remaining one-third have other risk factors such as steroid use, sarcoid, and hepatorenal failures **(Box 2)**. Some patients have no known underlying immunocompromising conditions (13–18%). In such patients, fever and meningeal signs may be absent resulting in delayed diagnosis and high mortality (up to 35–50%).[16] *C. gattii* has been associated with antigranulocyte-monocyte colony-stimulating factor (GM-CSF) autoantibodies. This autoimmune reaction has a key role in promoting infections with *Cryptococcus* species in otherwise healthy individuals through a reduction of the endogenous activity of GM-CSF.

The fungus inhabits the soil and uses the virulence factor laccase to protect itself from phytotoxins in its role as a plant pathogen of seedlings. In humans, it uses this laccase as a neurotropic virulence factor, oxidizing neurocatecholamines within dopaminergic tracts, particularly the basal ganglia, to produce immunosuppressive compounds such as melanin.[16]

Cryptococcus has a tropism for dopaminergic tracts. This may explain a propensity toward subcortical pathologies, including gait disturbances and dementias during chronic infections. Presentations with mental status changes, seizures, or meningeal signs may occur. In the absence of fever, these presentations make the diagnosis of the cryptococcal disease difficult. Cranial neuropathies affecting cranial nerves II through VIII may occur. These are secondary to raised intracranial pressure (ICP), inflammation, or direct fungal invasion. Hydrocephalus may lead to visual and hearing loss, cognitive impairment, and gait ataxia with or without urinary incontinence. These may persist if the diagnosis is delayed.

Headache, altered mental status, nausea, vomiting, deterioration of vision, and sixth nerve palsy (often from increased CSF opening pressure) are common signs and symptoms in patients with CNS cryptococcosis.

Clinical symptoms in patients with uncontrolled HIV infections might be absent or subtle before initiation of antiretroviral therapy (ART); however, these symptoms can precipitate or worsen after a response to antifungal therapy due to immune reconstitution inflammatory syndrome (IRIS) following ART.[11] Similarly, a rapid reduction of immunosuppressive pharmacotherapy (cessation of calcineurin inhibitors) to restore an adequate immune response in patients with solid organ transplantation and cryptococcosis can also result in IRIS.[17]

Spinal arachnoiditis can occur following antifungal therapy and mycological response in patients with cryptococcal meningoencephalitis who are HIV-negative. This complication has been found to be associated with increased inflammatory biomarkers in the CSF (soluble CD 27 and soluble CD21) and responds to corticosteroids.[18]

DIAGNOSIS

In CNS cryptococcosis, magnetic resonance imaging (MRI) may show meningeal enhancement, hydrocephalus, dilated Virchow–Robin spaces or intracerebral lesions, or nodules (cryptococcomas) and pseudocysts.

Cerebrospinal Fluid Study

The ICP should be measured at the time of the initial LP. Patients suspected of having increased ICP and/or CNS mass lesions should first have neuroimaging to rule out the presence of a space-occupying lesion.

Cerebrospinal fluid (CSF) opening pressure is often elevated. Characteristic CSF parameters showed elevated white cell count, with lymphocyte predominance, elevated CSF protein, and low CSF glucose. In HIV-associated CM, the CSF white cell count is lower and can often be normal (Williamson et al.). Diagnosis is established by India ink staining **(Figs. 1 and 2)**, cryptococcal antigen (CrAg) testing and CSF fungal culture. India ink examination of the CSF has a variable sensitivity of 30–90%. Fungal culture has high sensitivity and specificity though growth often takes several days.[11] CrAg test has high sensitivity and specificity in CSF as well as blood. The diagnosis of CM can be established

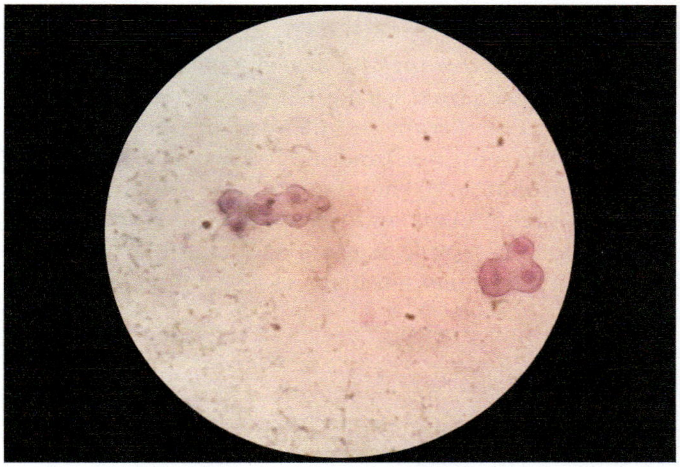

FIG. 1: *Cryptococcus* cerebrospinal fluid (CSF) cytospin preparation-Giemsa stain.

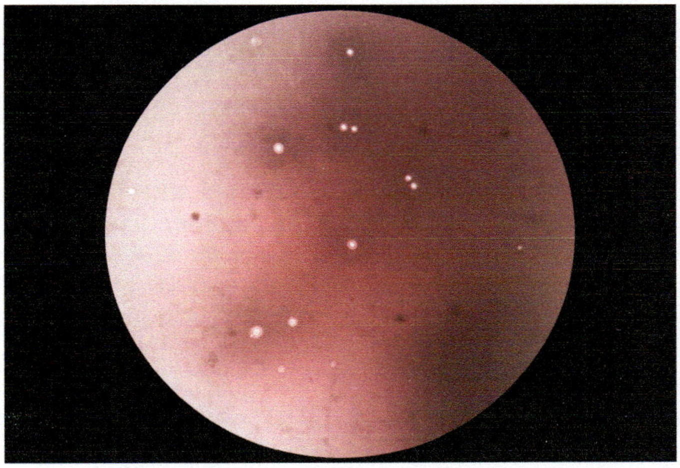

FIG. 2: *Cryptococcus* cerebrospinal fluid (CSF) India ink preparation.

rapidly by CrAg test. Rapid CrAg assay in CSF, serum, plasma, or whole blood (depending on access to LP) is preferred based on the much higher diagnostic accuracy of these rapid CrAg assays versus the India ink test and the fact that these rapid assays depend less on the healthcare provider's skills. Advantages of the lateral-flow assay over the latex agglutination assay include its rapid (<10 minutes) turnaround time, cost-effectiveness, minimal training requirements, and laboratory infrastructure, no need for refrigerated storage and higher clinical and analytical sensitivity.[13]

TREATMENT

Therapy of CM is divided into primary therapy (induction and consolidation) and maintenance (suppressive) therapy. Treatment strategies are based on whether the patient is HIV infected, an organ transplant recipient or a non-HIV-infected, nontransplant patient.[19]

HIV Infected Patients (Table 2)[20,21]

- *Consolidation therapy*—for 8 weeks following induction therapy, fluconazole 800 mg/day
- *Maintenance therapy*—until immune reconstitution (CD4 > 200 cells/mm^3) and suppression of viral loads on ART, fluconazole 200 mg/day

In resource-limited settings, routine LP after 2 weeks of induction therapy to confirm CSF sterilization is not indicated if the patient has had a clear clinical response to treatment.

Non-HIV Patients

Non-HIV-infected patients are treated with amphotericin B (0.7–1 mg/kg/day), plus flucytosine (100 mg/kg/day in four divided doses) for at least 4 weeks for patients with meningitis without neurological complications and with negative CSF yeast culture results after 2 weeks of therapy. Induction therapy can be extended for a total of 6 weeks in patients with neurological complications. Induction therapy is followed by consolidation therapy with fluconazole 400 mg/day for 8 weeks.

Organ Transplant Patients

Organ transplant recipients are treated with liposomal amphotericin B (3–4 mg/day) or amphotericin B lipid complex (5 mg/kg/day), plus flucytosine for at least 2 weeks followed by fluconazole (400–800 mg) (6–12 mg/kg/day) for 8 weeks, then fluconazole (200–400 mg/day) for 6–12 months.

Complications of Cryptococcal Meningitis

Over half of patients will develop intracranial hypertension and hydrocephalus, which is treated by repeated therapeutic LPs. Patients with rapid deterioration in mental status signaling high ICP are at a very high risk of death within days of presentation. Patients with elevated ICP should undergo daily large-volume LPs to reduce the opening pressure to normal.[22]

Surgical shunting may be needed if the pressure continues to be high. Cryptococcal infection is not a contraindication for surgery as this fungus does not form biofilms on CNS catheters. However, there is a risk of recurrent obstruction from infected debris and may require shunt revision.[18]

When to initiate ART—for patients with cryptococcal meningoencephalitis, it is suggested that ART may be started between 2 and 10 weeks after antifungal therapy has been initiated. The potential advantage of early immune recovery against the risk of developing IRIS must be considered. There is improved survival with delayed than early initiation of ART in patients undergoing treatment for cryptococcal meningoencephalitis.[23]

PROGNOSIS

The prognosis depends on nature of the underlying immunosuppression and/or the concurrent disease. For example, relapse rates among solid organ transplant recipients are very low.[24]

The mortality is high in HIV-associated CM—17% at 2 weeks and 34% at 10 weeks. In one series, overall mortality was 41% in those followed for 1 year.[25]

Positive India ink examination of the CSF; initial CSF or serum CrAg titer >1:32; CSF white blood cell count <20/μL and/or high opening pressure on LP, altered mental status, and rate of clearance of infection predict acute mortality in HIV-associated CM.[23]

Other factors conferring poor prognosis include positive India ink examination of the CSF; CSF white blood cell count <20/μL; initial CSF or serum CrAg titer >1:32; and/or high opening pressure on LP.

PREVENTING SYMPTOMATIC DISEASE

The best way to prevent cryptococcal disease in individuals with HIV is through early initiation of ART even at high CD4 counts.

TABLE 2: Induction phase (WHO recommendation 2022).[13,20,21]

Option	Drug	Week 1	Week 2
1	LAmB available	Single dose of 10 mg/kg LAmB + flucytosine 100 mg/kg/day in four divided daily doses + fluconazole 1,200 mg/day	Flucytosine 100 mg/kg/day + fluconazole 1,200 mg/day
2	LAmB not available	DAmB (1 mg/kg/day + flucytosine 100 mg/kg/day in four divided daily doses	Fluconazole 1,200 mg/day
3	AmB not available	Flucytosine 100 mg/kg/day + fluconazole 1,200 mg/day	Flucytosine 100 mg/kg/day + fluconazole 1,200 mg/day
4	Flucytosine not available	LAmB 3–4/mg/kg/day + fluconazole 1,200/day	LAmB 3–4/mg/kg/day + fluconazole 1,200/day
5	LAmB and flucytosine not available	DAmB 1 mg/kg/day + fluconazole 1,200 mg/day	DAmB 1 mg/kg/day + fluconazole 1,200 mg/day

(DAmB: amphotericin deoxycholate; LAmB: liposomal amphotericin B)

However, in patients with a low CD4 count, a strategy involving serum or plasma CrAg screening and antifungal therapy in addition to ART may further reduce the risk of developing CM. CrAg is detectable in serum at least 3 weeks prior to the onset of neurologic symptoms.

Screening with serum CrAg and treatment with antifungal therapy may reduce the risk of developing CM in patients who are at high risk for developing the disease. A recent World Health Organization (WHO) international guideline recommends screening for serum CrAg, and giving preemptive antifungal therapy among CrAg-positive individuals for prevention of invasive cryptococcal disease before ART initiation for those living with HIV who have a CD4 cell count <100 cells/mm.[20]

Future Needs

Although there is a reduction in the estimated absolute global burden of HIV-associated CM compared with 2014, likely to be due to ART expansion, the cryptococcal disease still accounts for 19% of AIDS-related deaths, similar to 2014 estimates.[26]

This suggests that earlier diagnosis, more rapidly fungicidal amphotericin-based regimens, and prompt immune reconstitution with ART are priorities for improving outcomes.

To end CM deaths by 2030, cryptococcal diagnostics, meningitis treatments, and implementation of preventive screening are urgently needed.[26]

Candidiasis

Although *Candida* species are responsible for the majority of hospital-acquired fungal infections *Candida* CNS infection is uncommon.

There is a relative increase in the proportion of non-albicans *Candida* (NAC) isolates such as *Candida glabrata, Candida parapsilosis, Candida tropicalis,* and *Candida krusei.* They are virulent and often associated with treatment failures.[27] In a study of candidemia among ICU patients from India, *C. tropicalis* (72%) was more common as compared to *Candida albicans* (28%). *C. parapsilosis* which has the tendency to cause device-related infections were isolated in nearly 10%.[27] Most cases of CNS *Candida* infection occur with *C. albicans*, though uncommon other *Candida* species causing CNS disease is known.[22] India, being a tropical country, experiences a high prevalence of invasive candidiasis. Contributory factors include—favorable climatic conditions (warm and humid), a large population of immunocompromised hosts (high prevalence of diabetes, autoimmune disease, poor nutrition, and retroviral infection) and over-the-counter access to antibiotics and steroids.[9]

Diagnosing invasive candidiasis in the early stages entails a high index of suspicion. A primary risk factor for disseminated candidiasis is neutropenia. Clinical presentation is often nonspecific and overlaps with those of bacterial infections.

Central nervous system infections caused by *Candida* species usually arise from hematogenous spread. Acute meningitis is the most common presentation, but infection can be more indolent and associated with chronic meningitis, brain abscess formation, ventriculitis, mycotic aneurysms, vasculitis with cerebral infarctions, and spinal infections. Thus, the presence of CNS symptoms should raise the suspicion of a *Candida* infection of the CNS in patients with specific risk factors especially in premature infants and postneurosurgical patients. Clinical signs of disseminated *Candida* infection (e.g., septic skin lesions) should prompt appropriate diagnostic interventions, including the ophthalmological examination.[28] CNS involvement should be considered in particular in premature infants and postneurosurgical patients. MRI may show meningeal enhancement and small cerebral microabscesses (<3 mm) with reduced diffusion.

The CSF may only show elevated CSF protein. CSF cultures are more likely to be positive in patients with acute meningitis and often are negative in those with the slower course of meningitis. At present there are no rapid diagnostic assays specific for *Candida* species in the CSF. CSF 1,3-β-D-glucan (BDG), (not specific for *Candida*, can be positive with other fungal infections) is a useful adjunct diagnostic test for *Candida* meningitis.[22]

Treatment is with liposomal amphotericin B at 5 mg/kg daily, with or without oral flucytosine.[29] Fluconazole 400–800 mg (6–12 mg/kg) daily is recommended after response to the initial treatment as step-down therapy after the patient has responded to initial treatment and should be continued until symptoms have been resolved such as the radiological abnormalities and CSF pleocytosis. Infected devices, including ventriculostomy drains and shunts, should be removed.[29] The preferred regimen for neonates is amphotericin B deoxycholate (DAmB), 1 mg/kg intravenous daily with liposomal amphotericin B (LAmB), 5 mg/kg daily, as an alternative. The step-down treatment is recommended with fluconazole, 12 mg/kg daily, if the clinical isolate is susceptible. Although echinocandins (such as caspofungin, micafungin, and anidulafungin) are the standard initial therapy in disseminated *Candida* infections, their levels are undetectable in the CSF and only 10–20% in the brain parenchyma, and are not effective in CNS candidiasis. Therefore it is important to diagnose CNS involvement during fungemia.

Mortality in patients with CNS involvement is high even after antifungal treatment, with some studies showing a 30–50% mortality rate.[22]

Aspergillus Meningitis

Central nervous system infections are well recognized manifestations of disseminated aspergillosis observed in about 10% of immunocompromised patients and with mortality rates > 90%. Intracranial spread may occur in 10–20% of cases, with focal masses being more common than meningoencephalitis. By contrast, *Aspergillus* meningitis is rare and is found more frequently in immunocompetent rather than in immunocompromised hosts with a case fatality rate up to 72%.[30] The most frequent causative agent is *Aspergillus fumigatus* **(Figs. 3 and 4)** followed by *Aspergillus flavus* and *Aspergillus terreus*. The respiratory tract is usually the portal of entry, with subsequent hematogenous dissemination to the CNS. However, direct inoculation of CNS or paraspinal tissue as a result of surgery, trauma, intravenous drug use, or contaminated medical supplies may also occur in immunocompetent persons.[31]

An outbreak of *A. fumigatus* meningitis occurred in five healthy women following spinal anesthesia for cesarean section in Colombo, Sri Lanka.[32] The source of infection was syringes contaminated with *A. fumigatus*. There is also a case report from India of a 28-year-old immunocompetent lady with *A. fumigatus* meningitis possibly following spinal anesthesia for cesarean section.[33]

The diagnosis of *Aspergillus* meningitis is very difficult and challenging. In fact, a diagnosis during life was obtained only in 55.9% of patients although with a much higher frequency among immunocompetent patients (69.2%).[30] The most common clinical presentation is acute meningitis, followed by meningoencephalitis. It is characterized by CSF neutrophil pleocytosis in 68% of cases and hypoglycorrhachia in 62% of cases. Cultures of CSF are positive only in one-third of cases, but the GM antigen test (*Aspergillus* galactomannan antigen-GM) can be useful, with a sensitivity reaching 87%.[30]

The PCR performed on CSF in subjects with hematologic disorders showed good sensitivity (100%) and specificity (93%) but it is not widely implemented.

Voriconazole has good CNS penetration and is the first-line treatment in the majority of cases that are due to *A. fumigatus*, with 35–47% response and 31–43% overall 1-year survival.[16]

Higher-dose liposomal amphotericin B is an alternative option. The treatment duration should be tailored according to treatment response and clinical improvement. In case of focal lesions or signs of intracranial hypertension, a neurosurgical intervention is needed.

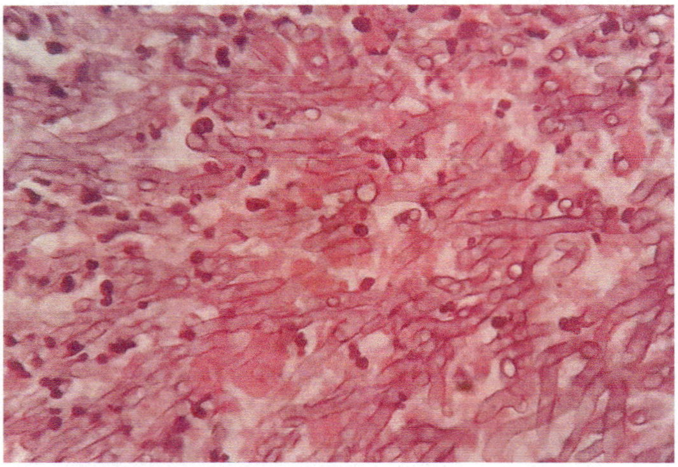

FIG. 3: *Aspergillus* histopathological examination (HPE).

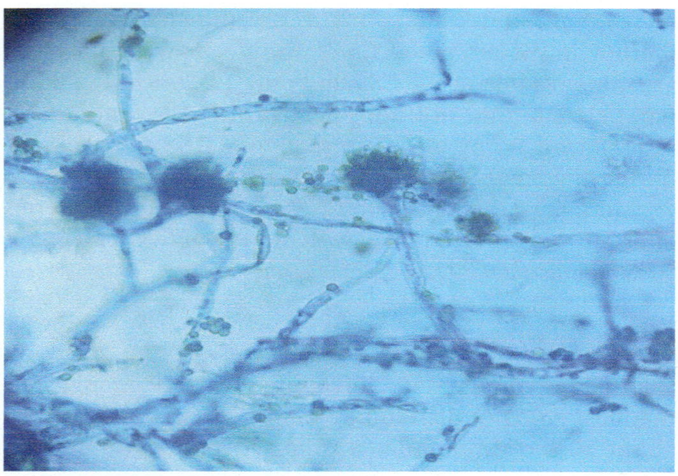

FIG. 4: *Aspergillus* wet preparation.

Coccidioidomycosis

Coccidioidomycosis is caused by the aerosolization and inhalation of two species of fungi which are soil dwellers, *Coccidioides immitis* and *Coccidioides posadasii*. Following spore exposure, 60% of individuals remain asymptomatic, while the rest develop mild to severe pneumonia. Only 1% of exposed individuals develop the disseminated disease, which can involve the skin, bones, visceral organs, and the CNS in up to 30% of cases.[22] Coccidioidomycosis is rare in India, there are case reports from India in patients who have traveled/worked in endemic areas in USA.[34]

Disseminated coccidioidomycosis occurs amongst high-risk groups like those in late pregnancy, and those who are immunocompromised because of AIDS or transplant recipients. CNS coccidioidomycosis manifests as meningitis, intraparenchymal abscesses, strokes, or spinal cord lesions. Meningitis is the most common presentation.

Central nervous system involvement presents as chronic basal meningitis with headache, low-grade fever, weight loss, and mental status changes. A granulomatous and suppurative meningitis occurs around the basilar cisterns, and appears as leptomeningeal enhancement of the basilar cisterns and middle cerebral artery cisterns on MRI.[35] This may mimic the radiographic appearance of other etiologies of basilar meningitis, including tuberculous meningitis. Hydrocephalus and ischemic vasculitis may complicate cases. Leptomeningeal enhancement of the basilar cistern is observed in 91% of cases and hydrocephalus in 78%.[35] Up to 26% of patients will have evidence of cerebral infarction due to vasculitis of small and medium vessels. The spinal imaging shows high frequency of intraspinal disease that may be asymptomatic—37% nerve root clumping, 16% intramedullary and spinal cord hyperintensity on T2 signal, and 16% with intradural masses.[35] This suggests the need to make both intracranial and spinal imaging for patients with coccidioidal meningitis even in the absence of back pain or radiculopathy.

Diagnosis

A CSF lymphocytic pleocytosis is most common, though a neutrophilic predominant profile may also be seen. 15% of patients exhibit CSF eosinophilia.[36] CSF eosinophilia is a unique feature of coccidioidomycosis infection and if present differentiates it from tuberculous meningitis. CSF glucose is low in approximately 70% of patients, and protein is elevated in 89%.

The definite diagnosis requires culture and isolation of *Coccidioides* species from CSF but it is positive in less than one-third of cases.

Several nonculture techniques like complement fixation coccidioidal antibody tests based on a complement-fixing methods or immunodiffusion can be employed to diagnose coccidioidal meningitis. The positivity rates of CSF antibody vary from 41 to 91%. The high false negative rate of CSF antibodies and culture emphasizes the importance of tests for serum antibodies. Systemic evaluation for disseminated coccidioidomycosis disease through serum anti-*Coccidioides* antibodies and urine *Coccidioides* antigen assay can aid in diagnosis and management decisions.[36]

Treatment

Aggressive management is required and includes antifungal medication, therapeutic LPs, and consideration of shunt placement if the ICP is refractory to multiple therapeutic LPs. Hydrocephalus with transependymal flow may require shunting.

The updated Infectious Diseases Society of America (IDSA) guidelines recommend oral fluconazole 400 mg daily or itraconazole 200 mg twice or three times per day as initial therapy when fluconazole is not tolerated.[37]

Intrathecal amphotericin B deoxycholate is recommended for patients in the first trimester of pregnancy to avoid the teratogenic effects of azoles. Relapse is nearly universal if treatment is discontinued, sometimes occurring years after discontinuation of treatment.[36] Hence, following clinical improvement, lifelong suppressive therapy with fluconazole (400 mg) should be continued to prevent relapse.

In those whose disease is identified early and who remain on a lifelong treatment with azoles, the prognosis is typically good.[36]

Histoplasmosis

Histoplasmosis is a disease caused by inhalation of spores of the fungus *H. capsulatum* that thrives in nitrogen-rich soil replete with bat or bird droppings.

The disease is highly endemic in some regions of North America, Central America, and South America but it is also reported in certain countries of Asia such as China, India, and Thailand.[30]

Histoplasmosis often involves subjects with underlying medical conditions and in particular people living with HIV, however, one-third of subjects affected by CNS histoplasmosis have no underlying medical conditions leading to immunosuppression.[38] The majority of *Histoplasma* infections are asymptomatic. Among symptomatic patients, 80% present with self-limiting pulmonary histoplasmosis.[39] However, in immunocompromised patients, extrapulmonary dissemination of histoplasmosis occurs. Risk factors for CNS histoplasmosis are exposure to chicken coops, CD4 count <150/μL, transplant recipients, those receiving immunosuppressive medications, and patients with hematological malignancies.[38,39]

Central nervous system involvement occurs in 5–10% of disseminated histoplasmosis cases.[38] The most frequent clinical features are brain abscesses, chronic meningitis, relapsing meningitis, and isolated spinal cord lesions.[40] Unlike other dimorphic fungal CNS infections, up to 98% of CNS histoplasmosis patients exhibit fevers over 38°C.[40] Additional symptoms of CNS histoplasmosis include headache (17–56%), decreased level of consciousness (26–44%), confusion (17–44%), and focal cranial nerve deficits (17–28%), followed by seizures, personality changes, ataxia, and clonus.[40]

Magnetic resonance imaging may show solitary or multifocal small (<2 cm), round, ring-enhancing mass lesions located most commonly subcortically, at the gray-white junction, posterior fossa structures, or the brainstem.

CSF shows a lymphocytic pleocytosis in 50% of cases, a neutrophilic preponderance in 11% of cases and low glucose level (<40 mg/dL) in 53% of patients.[40]

Histoplasma can be isolated from fungal culture of CSF in approximately 25% of cases and often multiple high volume sampling is needed to increase yield. Moreover, the slow growing nature of this fungus often causes a treatment delay.[38] The most sensitive test for diagnosis is based on the detection of antibody and antigen in the CSF. According to a recent study the sensitivity of *Histoplasma* antigen detection in CSF was 78% with a specificity of 93%,[41] whereas sensitivity for anti-*Histoplasma* immunoglobulin G (IgG) or immunoglobulin M (IgM) antibody was 82% of cases and the specificity was 93%. The combination of both the assays leads to an accuracy of 98% in detecting CNS histoplasmosis' cases.[41] The sensitivity of antigen detection was better among immunocompromised patients (81%) than those not immunocompromised (31%) and in patients with more severe disease (93% vs. 55%).[38] Serum tests for *Histoplasma* antigen and antibody, as well as urine antigen testing, are useful in establishing diagnoses of disseminated histoplasmosis.

The IDSA 2007 guidelines suggest initial antifungal management with liposomal amphotericin B at 3–5 mg/kg daily for 4–6 weeks followed by itraconazole for 12 months or until normalization of CSF and *Histoplasma* antigen levels; surgical excision of contrast enhancing lesions is often not necessary.[42]

Blastomycosis

Of extrapulmonary blastomycosis cases, 5–10% involve the CNS. CNS blastomycosis occurs in both immunocompetent and immunocompromised patients with similar frequencies but blastomycosis infections in immunocompromised hosts are more aggressive. CNS blastomycosis manifests as meningitis, intracranial, and epidural abscesses. However, dissemination to the CNS from the lung is accompanied by spread to more common sites, such as the skin, bone, and genitourinary tract. There may be concomitant purulent vertebral osteomyelitis.

Central nervous system involvement presents with headache (63–86%) and focal neurologic deficits (56%), followed by altered mental status, seizures, and vision changes with variable duration of symptom onset to diagnosis (median of 90 days).[43] MRI may show diffuse meningeal enhancement or mass lesions in the basal ganglia or cerebellum.

Brain abscesses are seen in about 56% of CNS blastomycosis and may be solitary or multiple commonly involving the cerebellum, midbrain, and the pituitary stalk.[5,43] Diagnosis through CSF analysis is difficult. CSF shows pleocytosis with either lymphocytic or neutrophilic predominance and elevated CSF protein.

The definite diagnosis is obtained by the isolation of the fungus from a sterile site such as blood or CSF. But CSF fungal cultures in CNS blastomycosis patients are often negative. Culture of serial high-volume CSF sampling may be needed and ventricular fluid sampling may be more sensitive than lumbar fluid sampling.[16] A presumptive diagnosis could be inferred by the positivity of *Blastomyces dermatitidis* antigen in serum and urine. These have a sensitivity of 81% (serum) and 82% (urine) but their specificity is impeded by cross-reactivity with other fungal infections including histoplasmosis (21).

Diagnosis is often definitively made by the histological examination of tissues in disseminated diseases with the help of silver or periodic acid–Schiff (PAS).[43]

Treatment is with Liposomal amphotericin B for the initial phase of 4–6 weeks followed by prolonged treatment with azoles for at least 12 months. In those subjects with underlying immune systems disorders a life-long antifungal treatment should be considered.[43,44]

FUTURE DIRECTIONS

There are practical difficulties in establishing diagnosis of CNS fungal infections. Diagnosis depends on positive fungal culture and if negative then on examination of tissue. But fungal culture is not sensitive and the turnaround time is long. Repeated high volume CSF samples increases yields but are not always feasible. Samples for histopathology are difficult to obtain because of anatomical location of the lesion and overall risk of procedure. Therefore, there is a need for better diagnostic tests. Nucleic acid-based diagnostic techniques are the fastest growing and most promising segment of fungal diagnostics. The polymerase chain reaction (PCR) can be species or genus specific or can target multiple species. Species or genus-specific PCR assays only target a narrow spectrum of pathogens, and therefore can only be used if there is strong suspicion for the infection with a certain pathogen. Panfungal real-time PCR on the other hand enables the unspecific detection and quantification of all fungal DNA present in a sample through the use of universal fungal primers. Panfungal PCR is a promising and highly sensitive diagnostic test for screening of patients suspected to have fungal infections. A recent study from India evaluated utility of panfungal PCR in patients of febrile neutropenia with suspected invasive fungal infections and found it highly sensitive (82.76%) and specific (90.48%).[45] The use of panfungal PCR assay in combination with other diagnostic modalities can be helpful, especially in a country like India where the resources are limited and can direct the appropriate use of antifungal therapy.

Metagenomic next-generation sequencing (mNGS) is a hypothesis-free approach which evaluates all the nucleic acid present in a sample. mNGS of CSF or brain tissue screens for nearly all potential CNS infections and can identify novel or unexpected pathogens. mNGS may be particularly well suited for fungal CNS infections. A case series of patients with diagnostically challenging subacute or chronic meningitis using mNGS of CSF identified four fungi (*C. neoformans, Aspergillus oryzae, H. capsulatum,* and *Candida dubliniensis*) among the seven patients.[46] This included the first reported case of CNS vasculitis caused by *A. oryzae*, and the fourth reported case of *C. dubliniensis* meningitis. The mNGS may be helpful in supporting the presence or exclusion of CNS infection when a coinfection is suspected in an immunosuppressed patient.

CONCLUSION

Fungal meningitis though uncommon is important as its morbidity and mortality is high. Collective efforts are needed to generate the database about clinical presentation, diagnosis, treatment, complications, and outcome. A public health approach leading to the prevention, earlier diagnosis, and improved treatment of fungal meningitis and its complications is critical to reducing the incidence and associated high mortality of fungal meningitis in low- and middle-income countries.

REFERENCES

1. Góralska K, Blaszkowska J, Dzikowiec M. Neuroinfection caused by fungi: Infection. 2018;46:443-59. https://doi.org/10.1007/s15010-018-1152-2
2. Roos KL. Meningitis fungal. In: Encyclopedia of the Neurological Sciences, Volume 2. Philadelphia: Elsevier; 2014.
3. Hesarur N, Seshagiri DV, Nagappa M, Rao S, Santosh V, Chandrashekar N, et al. Case report: Chronic fungal meningitis masquerading as tubercular meningitis. Am J Trop Med Hyg. 2020;103(4):1473-9.
4. Holmquist LC. Allison Russo CA, Elixhauser A. (2006). Meningitis-related hospitalizations in the United States. [online] Available from https://pubmed.ncbi.nlm.nih.gov/21735578/ [Last accessed December, 2022].
5. Charalambous LT, Premji A, Tybout C, Hunt A, Cutshaw D, Elsamadicy AA, et al. Prevalence, healthcare resource utilization and overall burden of fungal meningitis in the United States. J Med Microbiol. 2014;67(2):215-27.
6. Pfaller MA, Pappas PG, Wingard JR. Invasive fungal pathogens: current epidemiological trends. Clin Infect Dis. 2006;43(Suppl): S3-S14.
7. Kethireddy S, Andes D. CNS pahrmacokinetics of anti-fungal agents. Expert Opin Drug Metab Toxicol. 2007;3:573-81.
8. Murthy JMK, Sundaram C. Fungal infections of the central nervous system. In. Biller J, Ferro JM (eds). Handbook of clinical neurology. New York: Elsevier; 2014. pp. 1383-401.
9. Chakrabarti A, Chatterjee SS, Shivaprakash MR. Overview of opportunistic fungal infections in India. Nihon Ishinkin Gakkai Zasshi. 2008;49(3):165-72.
10. Kulkarni R, Pujari SS, Gupta D, Ojha P, Dhamne M, Bolegave V, et al. Cerebrovascular involvement in mucormycosis in COVID-19 pandemic. J Stroke Cerebrovasc Dis. 2022;31(2):106231.
11. Williamson PR, Jarvis JN, Panackal AA, Fisher MC, Molloy SF, Loyse A, et al. Cryptococcal meningitis: Epidemiology, immunology, diagnosis and therapy. Nat Rev Neurol. 2017;13:13-24.
12. Rajasingham R, Smith RM, Park BJ, Jarvis JN, Govender NP, Chiller TM, et al. Global burden of disease of HIV-associated cryptococcal meningitis: an updated analysis. Lancet Infect Dis. 2017;17(8): 873-81.
13. World Health Organization. (2022). Guidelines for diagnosing, preventing and managing cryptococcal disease among adults, adolescents and children living with HIV. [online] Available from https://www.who.int/publications/i/item/9789240052178 [Last accessed January, 2023].
14. Shankar SK, Mahadevan A, Sundaram C, Sarkar C, Chacko G, Lanjewar DN, et al. Pathobiology of fungal infections of the central nervous system with special reference to the Indian scenario. Neurol India. 2007;55(3):198-215.
15. Satishchandra P, Mathew T, Gadre G, Chandramukhi A, Mahadevan A, Shankar SK. Cryptococcal meningitis: clinical, diagnostic and therapeutic overviews. Neurol India. 2007;55: 226-32.
16. Panackal AA, Williamson PR. Fungal infections of the central nervous system. Continuum (Minneap Minn). 2015;21(6 Neuroinfectious Disease):1662-78.
17. Sun HY, Alexander BD, Huprikar S, Forrest GN, Bruno D, Lyon GM, et al. Predictors of immune reconstitution syndrome in organ transplant recipients with cryptococcosis: implications for the management of immunosuppression. Clin Infect Dis. 2015;60:36-44.
18. Panackal AA, Komori M, Kosa P, Khan O, Hammoud DA, Rosen LB, et al. Spinal arachnoiditis as a complication of cryptococcal meningoencephalitis in non-HIV previously healthy adults. Clin Infect Dis. 2017;64:275-83.
19. Perfect JR, Dismukes WE, Dromer F, Goldman DL, Graybill JR, Hamill RJ, et al. Clinical practice guidelines for the management of cryptococcal disease: 2010 update by the infectious diseases society of America. Clin Infect Dis. 2010;50(3):291-322.
20. World Health Organization. (2018). Guidelines for the diagnosis, prevention and management of cryptococcal disease in HIV-infected adults, adolescents, and children. [online] Available from http://apps.who.int/iris/bitstream/handle/10665/260399/9789241550277-eng.pdf [Last accessed January, 2023].
21. Jarvis JN, Lawrence DS, Meya DB, Kagimu E, Kasibante J, Mpoza E, et al; Ambition Study Group. Single-dose liposomal amphotericin B treatment for Cryptococcal meningitis. N Engl J Med. 2022;386(12):1109-20.
22. Jia DT, Thakur K. Fungal infections of the central nervous system. Semin Neurol. 2019;39(3):343-57.
23. Cox GM, Perfect JR. (2022). *Cryptococcus neoformans* meningoencephalitis in patients with HIV: Treatment and prevention. [online] Available from https://www.uptodate.com/contents/cryptococcus-neoformans-meningoencephalitis-in-persons-with-hiv-treatment-and-prevention [Last accessed January, 2023].
24. Singh N, Lortholary O, Alexander BD, Gupta KL, John GT, Pursell KJ, et al. Antifungal management practices and evolution of infection in organ transplant recipients with *Cryptococcus neoformans* infection. Transplantation. 2005;80(8):1033-9.
25. Jarvis JN, Bicanic T, Loyse A, Namarika D, Jackson A, Nussbaum JC, et al. Determinants of mortality in a combined cohort of 501 patients with HIV-associated Cryptococcal meningitis: implications for improving outcomes. Clin Infect Dis. 2014;58(5): 736-45.
26. Rajasingham R, Govender NP, Jordan A, Loyse A, Shroufi A, Denning DW, et al. The global burden of HIV-associated cryptococcal infection in adults in 2020: a modelling analysis. Lancet Infect Dis. 2022:S1473-3099(22)00499-6.
27. Ahmad S, Kumar S, Rajpal K, Sinha R, Kumar R, Muni S, et al. Candidemia among ICU patients: Species characterization, resistance pattern and association with *Candida* score: A prospective study. Cureus. 2022;14(4):e24612.
28. Schwartz S, Kontoyiannis DP, Harrison T, Ruhnke M. Advances in the diagnosis and treatment of fungal infections of the CNS. Lancet Neurol. 2018;17(4):362-72.
29. Pappas PG, Kauffman CA, Andes DR, Clancy CJ, Marr KA, Ostrosky-Zeichner L, et al . Clinical practice guideline for the management of candidiasis: 2016 update by the Infectious Diseases Society of America. Clin Infect Dis. 2016;62(4):e1-50.
30. Antinori S, Corbellino M, Meroni L, Resta F, Sollima S, Tonolini M, et al. *Aspergillus* meningitis: a rare clinical manifestation of central nervous system aspergillosis. Case report and review of 92 cases. J Infect. 2013;66(3):218-38.
31. McCarthy M, Rosengart A, Schuetz AN, Kontoyiannis DP, Walsh TJ. Mold infections of the central nervous system. N Engl J Med. 2014;371(2):150-60.
32. Gunaratne P, Wijeyaratne C, Seneviratne H. *Aspergillus* meningitis in Sri Lanka—A post-Tsunami effect? N Engl J Med. 2007;356: 754-6.
33. Rathish B, Wilson A, Warrier A, Pillay R, Thomas J. *Aspergillus fumigatus* meningitis in an immunocompetent young woman. Indian J Pathol Microbiol. 2020;63(3):488-90.
34. Verghese S, Arjundas D, Krishnakumar KC, Padmaja P, Elizabeth D, Padhye AA, et al. Coccidioidomycosis in India: Report of a second imported case. Med Mycol. 2002;40(3):307-9.
35. Lammering JC, Iv M, Gupta N, Pandit R, Patel MR. Imaging spectrum of CNS coccidioidomycosis: Prevalence and significance of concurrent brain and spinal disease. AJR Am J Roentgenol. 2013;200(6):1334-46.

36. Drake KW, Adam RD. Coccidioidal meningitis and brain abscesses: analysis of 71 cases at a referral center. Neurology. 2009;73(21): 1780-6.
37. Galgiani JN, Ampel NM, Blair JE, Catanzaro A, Geertsma F, Hooveret SE, et al. Infectious Diseases Society of America (IDSA) clinical practice guideline for the treatment of coccidioidomycosis. Clin Infect Dis. 2016;63(6):e112-46.
38. Wheat J, Myint T, Guo Y, Kemmer P, Hage C, Terry C, et al. Central nervous system histoplasmosis: Multicenter retrospective study on clinical features, diagnostic approach and outcome of treatment. Medicine (Baltimore). 2018;97(13):e0245.
39. Assi MA, Sandid MS, Baddour LM, Roberts GD, Walker RC. Systemic histoplasmosis: a 15-year retrospective institutional review of 111 patients. Medicine (Baltimore). 2007;86(3):162-9.
40. Wheat LJ, Batteiger BE, Sathapatayavongs B. *Histoplasma capsulatum* infections of the central nervous system. A clinical review. Medicine (Baltimore). 1990;69(04):244-60.
41. Bloch KC, Myint T, Raymond-Guillen L, Hage CA, Davis TE, Wright PW, et al. Improvement in diagnosis of *Histoplasma* meningitis by Combined testing for histoplasma antigen and immunoglobulin G and immunoglobulin M Anti-*Histoplasma* antibody in cerebrospinal fluid. Clin Infect Dis. 2018;66(1):89-94.
42. Wheat LJ, Freifeld AG, Kleiman MB, Baddley JW, McKinsey DS, Loyd JE, et al; Infectious Diseases Society of America. Clinical practice guidelines for the management of patients with histoplasmosis: 2007 update by the Infectious Diseases Society of America. Clin Infect Dis. 2007;45(7):807-25.
43. Bariola JR, Perry P, Pappas PG, Proia L, Shealey W, Wright PW, et al. Blastomycosis of the central nervous system: a multicenter review of diagnosis and treatment in the modern era. Clin Infect Dis. 2010;50(6):797-804.
44. Chapman SW, Dismukes WE, Proia LA, Bradsher RW, Pappas PG, Threlkeld MG, et al; Infectious Diseases Society of America. Clinical practice guidelines for the management of blastomycosis: 2008 update by the Infectious Diseases Society of America. Clin Infect Dis. 2008;46(12):1801-12.
45. Srinivas S, Kumari P, Gupta DK. Utility of Panfungal PCR in the diagnosis of invasive fungal infections in febrile neutropenia. J Family Med Prim Care. 2021;10:2533-40.
46. Wilson MR, O'Donovan BD, Gelfand JM, Sample HA, Chow FC, Betjemann JP, et al. Chronic meningitis investigated via metagenomic next-generation sequencing. JAMA Neurol. 2018;75(8):947-55.

62 CHAPTER

Leprosy

Kiran Katoch

INTRODUCTION

Leprosy continues to affect the population in a few countries of the world, namely India, some countries in Southeast Asia, and Brazil. The disease is characterized by the appearance of raised/flat, erythematous/hypopigmented lesions with a variable loss of sensation, and is usually associated with thickened peripheral or local cutaneous nerves. Leprosy is primarily considered a skin and nerve disease, although the nasal mucosa, eyes, and reticuloendothelial system are the other common sites of clinical manifestation. However, *Mycobacterium leprae* affects nearly all body organs though they are not primarily manifested clinically. The clinical and pathological manifestations are determined by the natural resistance of the host to *M. leprae* and the immunological response of the host.

EPIDEMIOLOGY

The epidemiology of any disease is dependent on the factors pertaining to the infective organism, host factors, and also to some extent on the environmental factors and genetic factors of the host population. The same is true for leprosy as well. India attained the global elimination target of the prevalence of the disease of less than 1 per 10,000 population in December 2005. Presently, its diagnosis and control have been merged with other diseases under the National Health Mission. Although both the prevalence [prevalence ratio (PR): Total leprosy cases/10,000 population] and the annual new case detection rate (ANCDR: New leprosy case/100,000 population per year) have shown a gradual declining trend; nevertheless, this is more or less stationary for the past 10–15 years, as seen in **Figure 1**. Other factors and transmission

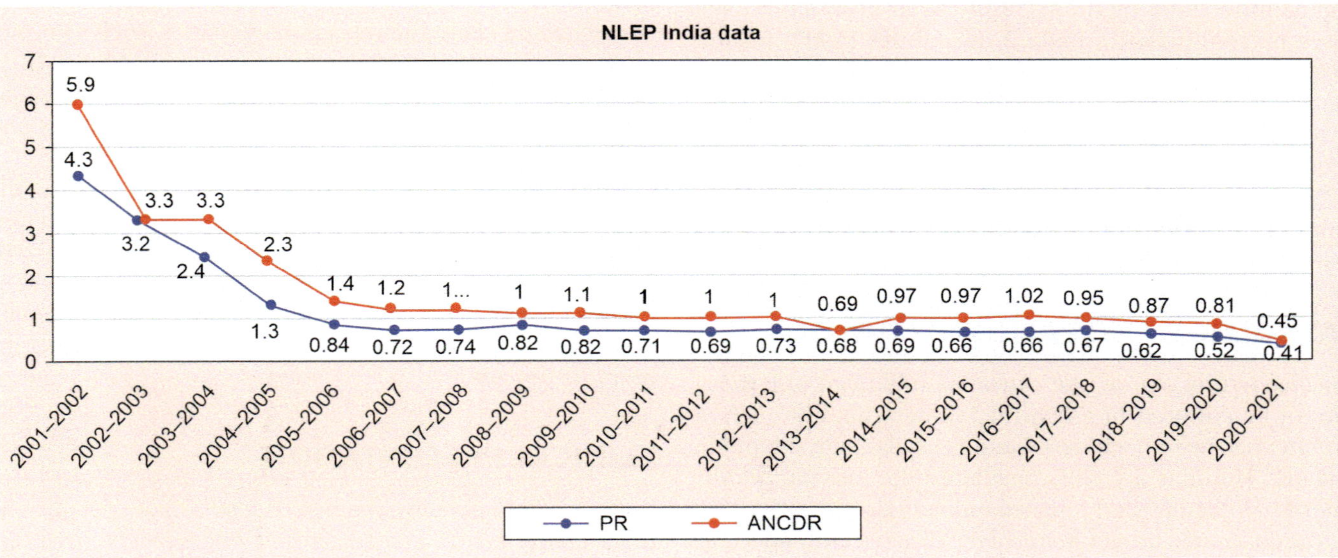

FIG. 1: Trends of leprosy reporting in the NLEP, India.

(ANCDR: annual new case detection rate; NLEP: National Leprosy Eradication Program; PR: prevalence ratio)

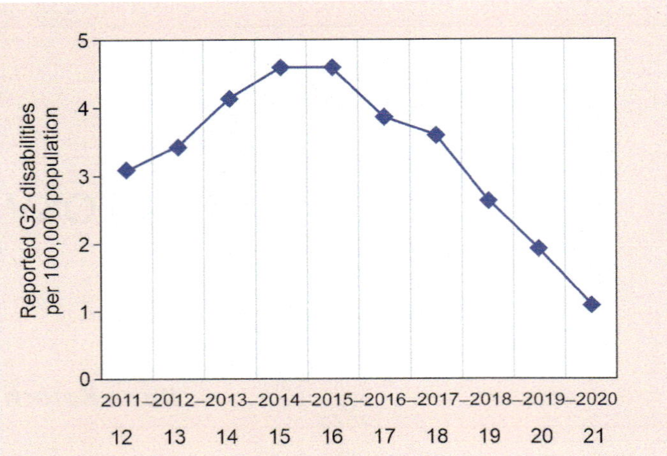

FIG. 2: G2 disability rates in new leprosy cases in the NLEP, India. (G2: grade 2; NLEP: National Leprosy Eradication Program)

dynamics of the disease need to be studied and tackled to control the occurrence and spread of the disease. The fall in the number of reported cases during the COVID-19 pandemic (2019–2021) could be due to the engagement of health staff in the more serious health-related issues of the pandemic.

Epidemiologically, a shift is seen in the type of leprosy cases that are being reported, and more multibacillary (MB) cases are being reported as compared to the paucibacillary (PB) cases. The neural involvement remains more or less the same, although patients presenting with only neural leprosy are missed many a time, both in the health systems and at the tertiary care centers.

Leprosy is one of the infectious diseases which involve the nervous system. If left untreated or inadequately treated it leads to sensory as well as motor damage to the tissue/organs innervated by them, resulting in disabilities. New cases presenting with grade 2 disabilities (G2D) (visible disabilities) are reported in the program, and **Figure 2** shows the reported G2D over the years in the National Leprosy Eradication Program (NLEP), India. The more recent decline, from 2019 onward, could be partially due to the COVID-19 pandemic and subsequent lesser reporting in the program. Moreover, most tertiary care institutions have not seen a decline in the G2D rate.

PATHOLOGY AND PATHOPHYSIOLOGY

Mycobacterium leprae, the causative organism of leprosy, cannot be cultured in any artificial medium, although its genome has been deciphered and is available in the public domain. Humans are still considered the most important source of infection, and infected individuals are responsible for the continued transmission of the disease. Only about 1% of the population who are exposed to the organism manifest the disease[1] in their lifetime. The manifestations as well as the pathology of the disease are influenced by the host immune response, and several genes and genomic regions have been implicated in the complex genetic mechanism controlling host susceptibility to the disease.

Mycobacterium leprae enters the body through the skin and naso-oral routes and establishes infection in the dendritic cells (DCs), monocytes, and macrophages of the skin as well as the Schwann cell of the nerve. The uptake of *M. leprae* by the DCs and subsequent local production of cytokines and chemokines regulate inflammation and influence the course of the adaptive cell-mediated immunity into a Th1 or Th2 response.

The Schwann cell, which is primarily a nonimmune target, actually protects the *M. leprae* and helps it to evade the immune response of the host.[2] The bacillary load in the Schwann cell is an important determinant of subsequent immune pathology as well as dissemination to other tissues.[3] This affects the myelinated and unmyelinated fibers as well as the autonomic fibers. It is believed that *M. leprae* triggers the reprogramming of the adult Schwann cells, which it has invaded, to progenitor/stem-like cells (pSLCs), which induce migratory and immunostimulatory properties which promote bacterial dissemination.[2] It has also been observed that unmyelinated Schwann cells at nerve terminals and neurosynaptic junction can modulate the synapse formation, its repair, and also a response to neurotransmitter signaling and nerve conduction.[4]

The Schwann cell infection, growth of *M. leprae* in it, and dissemination to other tissues as well as the host response result in demyelination and axonal atrophy, accompanied with edema and characteristic inflammation. This usually heals with the replacement of functional tissue by connective tissue and resulting fibrosis.[5]

Another factor that may be playing a role in nerve damage is the nerve growth factor (NGF), which is endogenously produced as proNGF by the peripheral effector cells, such as keratinocytes, melanocytes, smooth muscle cells, fibroblasts, and Schwann cells. The release of cytokines, such as tumor necrosis factor alpha (TNF-α), interleukin 6 (IL-6), and IL-17 as a result of NGF (also produced by Schwann cells) may also be contributing to the evolution of neural lesions and disabilities associated with leprosy.[6]

Besides the direct involvement of nerves by the organism, damage to the nerve is also seen during both type 1 and 2 reactions by the release of cytokines in response by the host, to the invading organism. This can be induced by the organism itself or even by some antigens which remain after the death of *M. leprae* in the body, which can trigger the immune process.

CLINICAL PRESENTATION

Like the skin, nerve involvement is also usually patchy, and the sensory, motor, and autonomic fibers can be involved. Clinical presentations involving the sensory nerves are the most common symptoms seen and are one of the cardinal signs of diagnosis of the disease.

Dermal Nerve

Dermal nerve involvement leads to impaired/altered and/or loss of sensation in the lesion and areas innervated by it. The involvement of intracutaneous dermal nerves results in loss of thermal sensation as the initial deficit and then involves other modalities such as pain and touch.[7] The autonomic fibers are usually involved simultaneously, while the motor fibers may be involved simultaneously or later on as the disease progresses. Importantly, more than 50% of the fibers are involved before this can be discerned by clinical examination. The disease damages both the myelinated and the unmyelinated nerve fibers, as a result of both direct invasion of the Schwann cell and by the involvement of the vascular endoneurium. These nerves can be palpated as they are thickened around the skin lesion, close to the margin of the lesion.

Peripheral Nerves

The most commonly involved peripheral nerves are shown in **Figure 3** and are namely the ulnar, median, greater auricular, superficial radial, common fibular, superficial fibular, common peroneal, and posterior tibial nerves. These can be palpated in the locations shown in **Figure 3**. Besides these, other peripheral nerve trunks, like supraorbital, and radial nerves may also be involved. They are palpable, thickened, and more rigid and cord-like at the tubercular spectrum of the disease, while softer at the lepromatous end of the disease. These nerve enlargements are usually adjacent to the skin lesions in the tuberculoid spectrum and more widespread with several nerve trunk involvement toward the lepromatous spectrum of the disease. Peripheral nerve involvement is assessed by the palpation of the nerve trunks in the places as marked in **Figure 3**. These may be tender and/or also may present as acute neuritis with pain and inflammation locally as well as in the nerve trunk. One or more nerve trunks can be involved, are painful, and are usually seen in both type 1 and erythema nodosum leprosum (ENL) reactions in which both the sensory and the motor fibers are involved. It requires immediate treatment to prevent irreversible nerve damage to the fibers. Sometimes due to repeated involvement and neurological injury, hyperactive host response, nerve abscess may be formed along the nerve trunks. This may be acute and painful or may remain as cystic lesions in more chronic cases. It is due to caseation necrosis as a result of unregulated immune activation by the host.

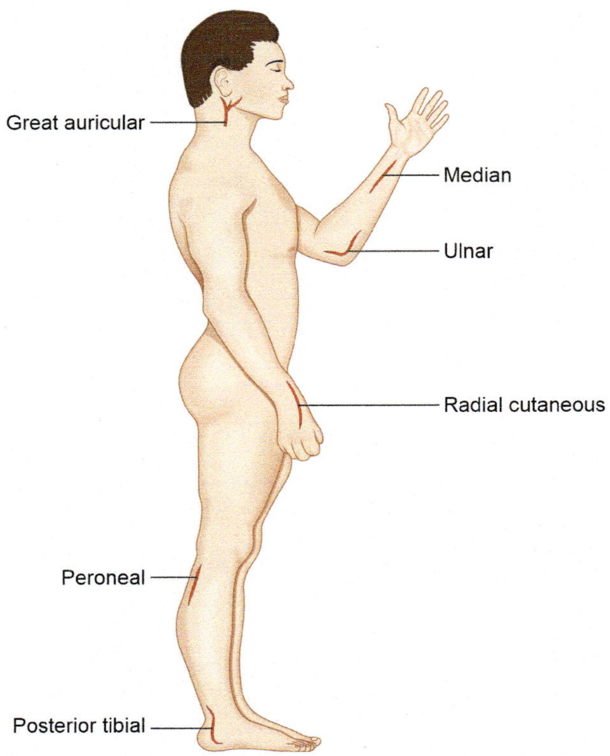

FIG. 3: Anatomical position of involvement of the peripheral nerves in leprosy.

After leprosy treatment, the nerve may gradually shrink, but they remain abnormally firm/soft respectively in PB and MB diseases, and are thick and palpable. Their consistency varies according to the type of leprosy, i.e., firm and hard at the tuberculoid pole and enlarged and soft at the lepromatous pole of the disease **(Figs. 4A and B)**.

Motor nerve involvement leads to neural impairment, paresis, and later paralysis of the innervated part and disabilities, if not adequately treated. The most common motor nerve involvement is of the ulnar nerve, leading to ulnar claw, median nerve loss of opposition of the thumb, wrist drop due to involvement of radial nerve, foot drop due to involvement of lateral popliteal nerve, clawing of toes due to involvement of the posterior tibial nerve, lagophthalmos, and deviation of the jaw due to facial nerve involvement. All these are the known complications of leprous neuropathy.

Usually, the skin and the nerves are involved simultaneously. However, in 4–7% of cases (as observed in India), a pure *neuritic* form of leprosy is also seen, wherein only nerves are involved without any involvement/symptomatology of the skin. This is known as the pure neuritic leprosy (PNL) and can present as single nerve involvement (mononeuritic) and two or more than two peripheral nerve involvement (polyneuritic). When skin lesions are never observed during the course of the disease it is also known as primary neuritic leprosy, and in patients whose skin lesions have subsided and regressed, while only nerve trunk thickening is observed, it is known as secondary neuritic leprosy.[8]

In about 40% of patients with acute neuritis, neuropathic pain may persist for a longer time in the nerve trunks and is referred to as *chronic neuritis*. This is more often seen in patients with repeated reactions and long-standing disease. This may continue even after successful completion of the course of multidrug therapy (MDT) and is believed to be due to small fiber involvement of the nerve **(Figs. 5 and 6)**.

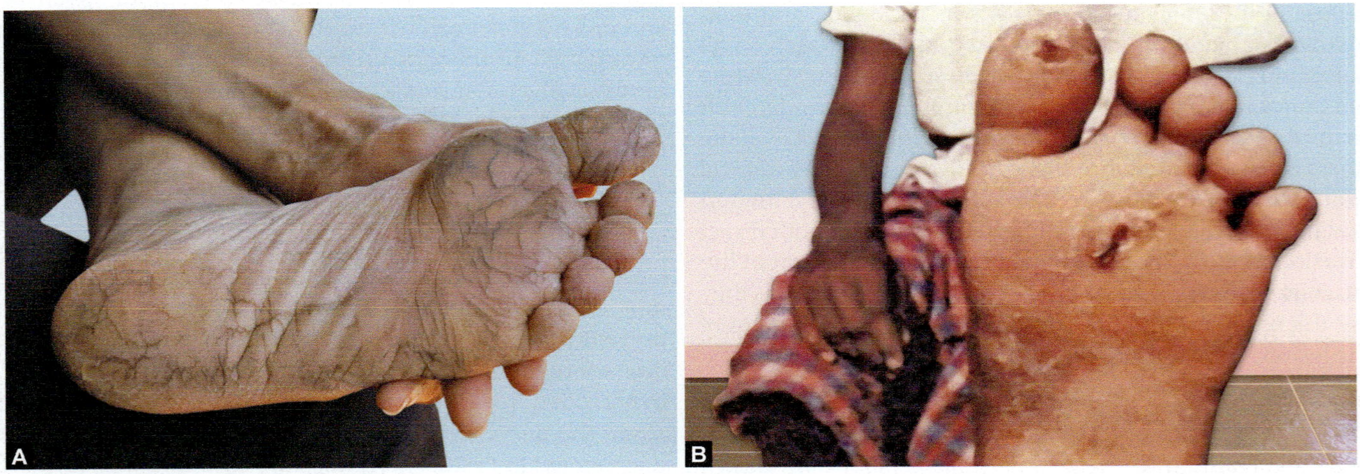

FIGS. 4A AND B: Involvement of (A) autonomic and (B) sensory nerves, respectively.

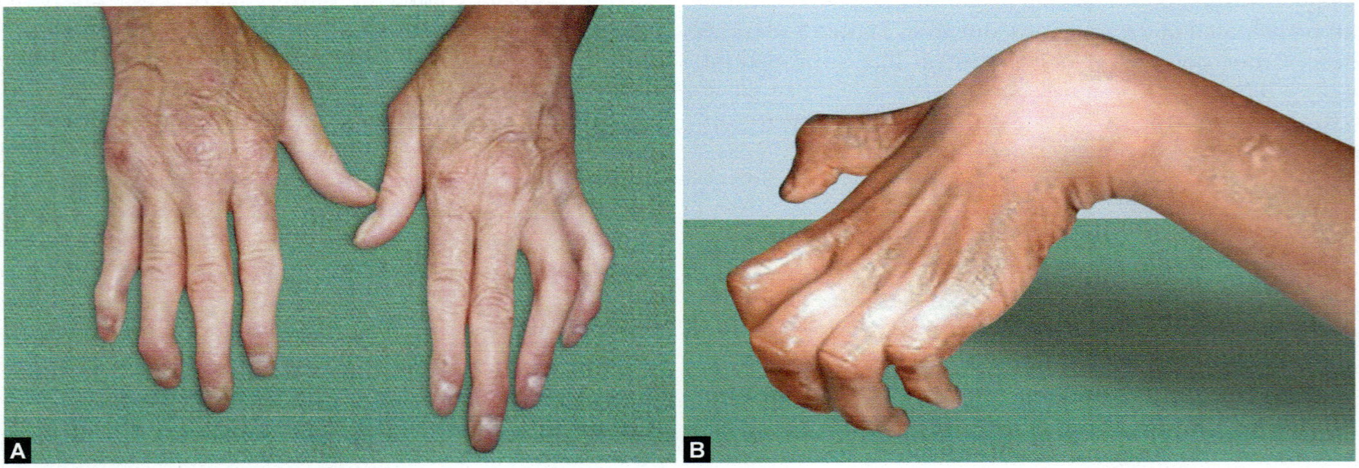

FIGS. 5A AND B: Involvement of the nerves of the hand and resulting disabilities due to motor involvement.

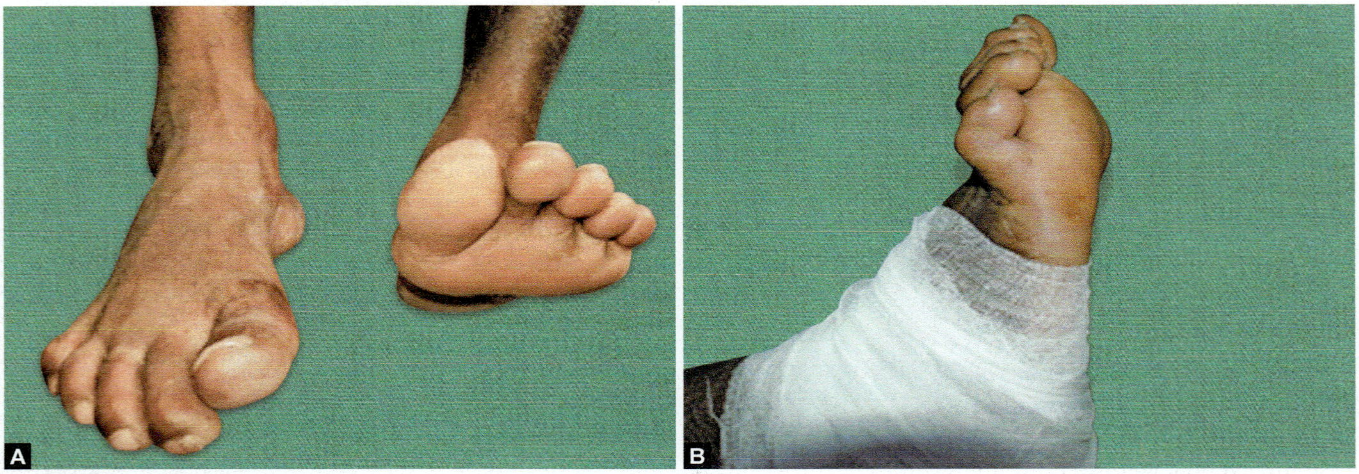

FIGS. 6A AND B: Disabilities resulting after involvement of the motor nerve fibers of the nerves innervating the foot.

Silent Neuritis or Quiet Nerve Paralysis

Silent neuritis is another term, frequently used, observed, and reported now. Here, the patient develops nerve damage and disabilities without any pain and overt inflammation. It is usually seen in patients after completion of MDT, or those who have taken MDT irregularly.[9] It is characterized by the occurrence of disabilities/loss of motor function suddenly without any pain and signs of inflammation. Its frequency varies according to the cohort observed and investigated. This condition is also called leprosy late-onset neuropathy (LLON)[5] and is probably related to the immune process of the host in response to the persisting *M. leprae* antigens.

Autonomic Nerves

Loss of sweating or profuse patchy/generalized sweating, ichthyosis, and dryness of the skin are due to involvement of the autonomic fibers,[10] which is usually due to the damage to small unmyelinated fibers.[11] This also tends to be regional with involvement of the peripheral nerves and results in loss of vasomotor and sudomotor functions, confined to the innervating territory. Later, with the spread of the disease, it leads to widespread involvement, which may affect the eyes, cardiovascular system, central nervous system (CNS), adrenal glands, etc., leading to dysautonomia.[10] Some studies have reported autonomic nerve lesions about as frequent as somatic lesions and are believed to be related to the immune-inflammatory reaction against *M. leprae*. The parasympathetic system is believed to be involved first, followed by the sympathetic system. In a series of 25 leprosy patients, the RR interval (in the electrocardiogram) variations were found to be reduced during both resting and deep forced hyperventilation.[12] The authors concluded that sensory nerve damage is accompanied by autonomic involvement. The autonomic functions are significantly more altered in MB patients than the PB patients.

Complex regional pain syndrome [(CRPS)/Sudeck's dystrophy] is a painful and disabling condition seen in some patients in which a triad of autonomic, sensory, and motor symptoms is seen, which is usually disproportionate to what is commonly observed.[5]

Cranial Nerves

Cranial nerve involvement in leprosy is observed in a substantial number of cases.[13] Among the cranial nerves, the involvement of the facial nerve is most commonly reported and observed followed by olfactory, trigeminal, auditory, and VI cranial nerves. Besides, sometimes presenting as the first presenting symptom, these nerves are also involved in type 1 reactions. Rarely, more than one cranial nerve may also be involved. Trigeminal neuralgia leads to impaired/loss of tear formation, leading to dryness of the cornea and resulting injuries. Involvement of the facial nerve leads to lagophthalmos and the inability to close the eyelids, leading to frequent injuries and variable loss of vision. The involvement of the other cranial nerves as mentioned above is seen in a variable number of patients by different investigators.

Central Nervous System

Leprosy is considered a disease of the peripheral nervous system, but CNS involvement has also been reported. Earlier studies, as well as autopsies conducted in the pre-MDT era, do show involvement of the medulla oblongata and spinal cord. This was documented,[14] and it was believed that this was because of long-standing untreated disease. Hyperreflexia and spastic paralysis have also been noted by few workers due to leprosy[15,16] due to CNS involvement. Recently too, *M. leprae* has been documented in the neurons of medulla oblongata and spinal cord using molecular methods.[17] Brain and spinal cord lesions have also been demonstrated using magnetic resonance imaging.[18] Studies using molecular methods, i.e., gene sequencing and polymerase chain reaction (PCR) amplification, have demonstrated the involvement of the frontal cortex of the brain in a leprosy patient.[19] These observations do point toward the CNS involvement in leprosy, but this is much less than the involvement of the skin and peripheral nervous system.

INVESTIGATIONS AND DIAGNOSIS

The diagnosis of leprosy is essentially by clinical examination. The presence of any two of the signs/symptoms is required for the diagnosis of the disease. These are namely the presence of flat hypopigmented/raised erythematous lesion with impaired sensations, the presence of a thickened dermal nerve near the lesion or thickened peripheral nerve, and the demonstration of acid-fast bacilli (AFB) on slit skin smear (SSS) examination after Ziehl–Neelsen (ZN) staining. Thickened and palpable dermal nerves with varied degree of impaired sensation are the hallmark for clinical diagnosis of the disease. However, the patient may also present with reactions (both type 1 and 2), which may camouflage the salient features listed above, although AFB may be seen in the lesions and other prominent sites. Therein too, besides the signs of inflammation, thickened peripheral nerves are present.

Palpation, feeling of the nerve, testing of sensations, locating and delineating the area with impaired/altered sensation, history of symptoms, assessing the pain threshold, etc., are important signs to be elicited and recorded. Overt inflammation and tenderness, if any, are the key indicators to test for leprosy neuropathy and monitor the disease progression as well as reactions due to the disease.

Laboratory Tests and Other Investigations

The presence of AFB in SSS and/or in biopsy and fine needle aspiration cytology (FNAC) specimens and/or its specific antigens/products, by immunohistochemistry in the biopsied skin or nerve specimen, is the definitive diagnostic tool. However, a biopsy is not always possible, and at times the results may be misleading/inconclusive if the biopsy is not taken properly and not from an appropriate active disease site. Diagnosis of pure neural leprosy can be aided by FNAC from the cutaneous nerve/abscess and demonstration of AFB or specific *M. leprae* antigen from the tissue for definitive diagnosis.

Monofilament Testing

The use of graded Semmes-Weinstein monofilaments (MFs) for semiquantitative testing of sensory sensations is a useful tool[20] for diagnosis as well as monitoring disease activity. For sensory evaluation, MFs ranging from 2 to 399 g are used at points supplied by major nerve trunks in the upper and lower extremities. Details of the sites where one is to be tested for diagnosis and monitoring of the disease are detailed in the IAL Textbook of Leprosy.[20] Touch sensibility is tested by using a standard test of Semmes-Weinstein MF with sufficient force to bend the filament and recorded. The application scores range from scores 1 to 5 (5 mg—score 5, 200 mg—score 4, 2 g—score 3, 4 g—score 4, 300 g—score 1). These have been shown to correlate with the neurophysiological abnormalities. These can be periodically tested to monitor the disease and the response to treatment.

Voluntary Muscle Testing

Assessment is done using the modified Medical Research Council (MRC) 6-point scale ranging from 0 to 5, wherein 5 represents normal strength and 0 complete paralysis. The muscles tested include eyelid closure, little finger abduction, palmer abduction of the thumb, wrist extension, foot dorsiflexion, etc., and are graded on the MRC scale.[20] Muscle strength testing is also done by some researchers using dynamometry.[21]

Besides the assessment for warm and cold sensations, vibration perception thresholds are also measured for the proprioceptive sensation assessment using a standard tuning fork.

Earlier autonomic nervous system affection was also studied using intradermal injection of 0.1 mL of carbachol and measuring the sweating response in the area.[22]

Nerve Conduction Studies

Nerve conduction studies are done on the nerve trunks and help to establish the functional assessment of the tested peripheral nerve.[20] In the upper extremities, the ulnar, median, and radial nerves are tested, while in the lower limb the common peroneal and sural nerves are tested. Parameters usually assessed in these nerves are the distal motor latency, sensory peak latency, compound muscle action potential amplitude, sensory nerve action potential amplitude, and motor and sensory conduction velocities. These can be periodically repeated to assess the progress of the disease. The abnormalities noted in these, if any, can be due to both axonal and demyelination of the nerve fibers.

Quantitative Sensory Testing

Quantitative sensory testing (QST) involves evaluation of C fibers and A-delta fibers that are involved early in leprosy.[21] The stimuli are delivered through a test electrode, which is in contact with the examinee's skin. The subject is asked to report the change in thermal temperature and/or pain, which is recorded and analyzed.

Peripheral Nerve High-resolution Sonography

Peripheral nerve high-resolution sonography is an important tool. The nerve ultrasound (12–18 MHz) is used for the assessment of long segments of major peripheral nerves. It has been found to correlate with the clinical parameters and grade of thickening, sensory loss, and motor weakness. The abnormalities of nerve echo structure, fascicular architecture, endoneural flow, nerve edema, nerve abscesses, and cross-sectional area of nerve[23] are measured and correlated with the clinical findings. It is currently extensively used for diagnosis as well as monitoring of the disease and can be undertaken at district and subdistrict levels. The ulnar, median, and radial nerves as well as the superficial radial cutaneous nerve and ulnar cutaneous nerves can be visualized and assessed in the upper extremities. In the lower extremities the distal sciatic nerve, bifurcation of the common peroneal nerve, posterior tibial nerve, and sural nerve are usually assessed and examined.

Doppler Imaging

Doppler imaging is used to assess the increase in endoneural vascularity, especially during reactions. *Doppler flow velocimetry* is used to evaluate small unmyelinated fibers as well as vasomotor reflexes. These are accomplished using magnetic resonance and computerized tomography (CT) imaging.

Infrared Thermography

Infrared thermography is used to evaluate peripheral autonomic function. It maps the skin temperature in areas in both upper and lower limbs and assesses the microcirculation flow changes in the limbs.[24]

Molecular Methods

With the deciphering of the *M. leprae* genome molecular methods using *M. leprae*-specific PCR are available for confirmation of the diagnosis in skin smears,[25] biopsies, and FNAC aspirates including those from nerves.

Differential Diagnosis

Leprosy is one of the infectious neuropathies and important leading causes of neuropathy in India. Clinical diagnosis is usually made after history taking, a careful clinical examination of the skin and nerves. In a few cases, only the nerve is involved and therefore the consideration and exclusion of other causes are necessary. Other causes of neuropathies must be considered in the differential diagnosis, which include other infectious diseases such as diphtheria and human immunodeficiency virus (HIV); metabolic diseases such as diabetes mellitus (DM); toxic neuropathies due to arsenic, mercury, lead, organophosphorus poisoning; nutritional deficiencies alone or in combination with other diseases and chronic alcoholism and/or tobacco intake; autoimmune diseases such as rheumatoid arthritis, systemic lupus erythematosus (SLE); hereditary diseases, etc.[26,27]

Metabolic Diseases

It is important to look for DM, impaired glucose tolerance test, dyslipidemia, glycated hemoglobin (HbA1c), and microvascular and macrovascular complications of DM. These usually clinch the diagnosis of polyneuropathies due to DM. DM neuropathies are often associated with low nerve conduction velocities. The other risk factors associated with DM are long-standing disease, high consumption of alcohol and chronic alcoholism, and tobacco smoking and chewing.

Uremic polyneuropathy, especially associated with chronic kidney disease (CKD), affects all levels of the nervous system as well as the peripheral nerves. The elevated blood urea and creatinine with a history of renal disease clinch the diagnosis in favor of CKD.

Neurosarcoidosis is a chronic inflammatory granulomatous disease, which may present as a small fiber neuropathy. It usually presents with multifocal peripheral hyperalgesia and allodynia (extreme sensitivity to pain) and also the involvement of the facial nerve. It can be differentiated by its substantial systemic involvement, as well as observation of noncaseating granulomas in the lymph nodes and various other organs in biopsy specimens.

Immunoglobulin amyloidosis (AL) occurs as either a primary disorder or associated with multiple myeloma, macroglobulinemia, and non-Hodgkin's lymphoma. The polyneuropathy in these disorders is due to small fiber disease with peripheral loss of pain and temperature sensations. It is also associated with peripheral nerve thickening and dysfunction. The presence of amyloid material in biopsies on histopathological examination clinches the diagnosis.

Infectious Diseases

Guillain-Barré syndrome may be associated with peripheral as well as cranial nerve involvement. However, a history of fever, diarrhea, and symptoms of upper respiratory tract infection usually precede the neuropathic systems. Patients usually start developing ascending paralysis involving the feet and hand and move toward the trunk. The autonomic nervous system is also involved.

Human immunodeficiency virus associated polyneuropathy is one of the many neurological complications of HIV. Distal sensory polyneuropathy is the most common presentation, associated with HIV neuropathies. HIV enzyme-linked immunosorbent assay (ELISA) and other tests clinch the diagnosis.

Diphtheritic neuropathy: One of the severe complications of diphtheria is diphtheritic polyneuropathy (DP). It can be easily recognized by the salient clinical and laboratory features of diphtheria.

Autoimmune-related Neuropathies

Chronic dysimmune neuropathies are a clinically heterogeneous group of polyneuropathies due to immunemediated etiology. The demyelinating polyneuropathy is recognized by a combination of clinical, electrophysiological, pathological, and immunological features beyond 8 weeks of the onset of the clinical syndrome. In rheumatoid arthritis and SLE, vasculitis and neuropathy usually present with painful mononeuropathies or asymmetric polyneuropathy of acute or subacute onset. The clinical features of these respective autoimmune diseases help to distinguish them from neuropathies of leprosy.

Paraneoplastic neuropathy is usually observed in a few patients with carcinoma. This neuropathy may be due to treatment toxicity, tumorous infiltration, metabolic disturbances, or terminal cachexia and can be easily distinguished due to the underlying disease.

Toxin-induced Neuropathy

Chronic *arsenic* exposure and *lead* exposure may be responsible for the chronic nerve-related pain in areas and occupations prone to these metal exposures. Chronic symptoms are also seen due to environmental pollution. Nerve conduction velocity studies usually reveal subclinical motor neuropathy in a few patients. Estimation of blood levels of these metals is raised, with changes/reduced compound motor action potential (CMAP) on nerve conduction studies.

In acute exposure to high-level mercury vapors, besides clinical signs and symptoms of bronchitis, interstitial pneumonitis, pulmonary edema, and renal insufficiency, signs of chronic intoxication include behavioral changes; postural tremor, insidious onset of stocking distribution of sensory loss, presence of Romberg sign, absent ankle reflexes, postural tremors with mild motor involvement are also seen. Specific signs and symptoms of mercury inhalation differentiate it from leprosy neuritis.

Organophosphorus poisoning: The clinical manifestations include miosis, impaired consciousness, muscular fasciculations, convulsions, delirium, and paralysis. Late symptoms of neurotoxicity include severe distal weakness due to axonal neuropathy. History of poisoning clinches the diagnosis.

Alcoholic neuropathy: Polyneuropathy has been reported to be present in 13–66% of chronic alcoholics. The pathophysiology of alcoholic polyneuropathy is usually a combination of the toxic effect of alcohol with deficiency of thiamine. This neuropathy is mainly of axonal type and is characterized by painful sensory symptoms and weakness in the distal lower extremities. Autonomic dysfunction is often associated with the above symptoms. Detailed history taking and examination for other signs of alcoholism are usually seen.

Nutrition Deficiency Neuropathy

Nutrition deficiency neuropathy is usually seen with severe malnutrition and thiamine deficiency and is associated with other signs of deficiencies. This is also seen in patients who are on long-term isoniazid therapy.

Hereditary Neuropathies

Charcot–Marie–Tooth (CMT) disease is a degenerative neuropathy involving both the sensory and the motor systems. It manifests in early adulthood, as a part of multisystem disorder characterized by muscle weakness and atrophy, decreased sensation, and hammer toes with high foot arches. Involvement of multiple organs distinguishes it from leprous neuropathy.

Porphyria is an inherited metabolic syndrome caused by specific enzyme deficiencies in the heme biosynthesis pathway, affecting its metabolism. Porphyric neuropathy is a motor-predominant axonal neuropathy involving the upper limbs and then the lower limbs, which may lead to quadriparesis. The affection of the respiratory system can be fatal. Occasionally, and less commonly, it may present with wrist and/or foot drop. Sensory symptoms are usually absent. Patients of this disorder can have proximal motor neuropathy in combination with psychiatric symptoms and abdominal pain, which may be associated with orthostatic hypotension, paroxysmal hypertension, and tachycardia.

MANAGEMENT

Despite several advances made in deciphering the genome of *M. leprae,* and also understanding its entry into the peripheral nerves, challenges remain in the treatment of neuropathy due to leprosy. The main pillars still remain prompt diagnosis and complete treatment of the disease.[28] *Complete and prompt MDT* is the mainstay of treatment of all types of leprosy including the neuropathies. According to the latest guidelines for treatment of leprosy a three-drug regimen consisting of daily dapsone and clofazimine combined with monthly rifampicin is given for 6 months and 12 months for PB and MB leprosy patients, respectively.[29] Prompt treatment of both type 1 and 2 reactions, judicious use of anti-inflammatory agents, reconstructive surgery, physiotherapy, and rest to the affected part are the main pillars of management of neuritis and neuropathies of leprosy.

Although MDT is effective as it kills *M. leprae,* neuritis and neuropathies of leprosy are also associated and triggered by some antigens of the organism, which take a longer time to clear from the tissues and may provoke and precipitate reactions and nerve damage. Live bacilli lodged in the nerves, smooth muscles, Schwan cells, and macrophages can also precipitate reactions as well as nerve damage and require measures to control it.

Anti-inflammatory Agents

Corticosteroids are used for the treatment of acute neuritis in varying doses and duration for the treatment for both type 1 and 2 reactions as well as acute neuritis. Corticosteroids have both anti-inflammatory action and antisuppressant effects. There is increased expression of anti-inflammatory proteins and decreased production of proinflammatory proteins with their use.[28]

In the ALERT MDT Field Evaluation Study, 300 MB and 294 PB cases were followed over a period of 10 years in which steroids were used for both MB and PB patients. In patients with no impairment at the start of the study, treatment with steroids resulted in full recovery in 88% with acute neuropathy and in about 51% of those with chronic or recurrent neuropathy.[30] The median time required for full recovery from acute neuropathy was approximately 6 months. However, in patients with acute neuropathy that were not treated with steroids, 42% were found to have fully recovered.

The NLEP recommends its usage (corticosteroids) in adequate dosages and for varying durations (20–32 weeks) for the treatment of acute neuritis, and prevention of nerve function impairment (NFI). This is combined with rest to the part as well as active exercises after the subsidence of the acute episode. Its role in chronic neuritis is however not clear and is also overshadowed by the side effects of steroids when given for longer duration. It is recommended that steroids should be used with MDT even after completion of the MDT schedule. MDT will take care of any active and live bacilli, which remain after treatment and may be responsible for triggering the chronic reaction and neuritis.

Studies have also shown that when prophylactic low-dose steroids are given with MDT, the incidence of new reactions and NFI were reduced in the short-term, but the effect was not sustainable in the long term.[31]

Other anti-inflammatory agents such as thalidomide, cyclosporine, methotrexate, azathioprine, and others have been used in the control of reactions (mainly ENL and type 2 reactions) and have been shown to control the reaction and neuritis associated with it. This is so especially in patients who suffer from long-term side effects of the intake of long duration of corticosteroids. These agents can also be used to taper off corticosteroids, and the low maintenance dose relieves the symptoms of chronic neuritis.

Clofazimine directly acts on *M. leprae* but also acts as an anti-inflammatory agent and has shown its anti-inflammatory effect by reducing the incidence of reactions as well as the neuropathy associated with the disease.[32,33] There was a significant decrease in reactions, NFI, and also silent neuritis in patients who received an initial dose of clofazimine (for 12 weeks) before starting the standard

MDT, as compared to the control group that did not receive clofazimine.[34] In the study on PB patients,[35] it was observed that there was no change in NFI in these patients, although only a small sample size was included, and furthermore, there was no follow-up of the patients. As nerve damage is reported and does occur during as well as after stoppage of treatment, a longer follow-up is required to assess the results. However, it may be noted that the World Health Organization (WHO) in its guidelines for diagnosis treatment and prophylaxis of leprosy 2018[29] has recommended the use of clofazimine in PB patients as well. They contemplate that as this dose of clofazimine is well accepted and tolerated; it will decrease the morbidity of the disease.

Immunomodulators such as *Mycobacterium indicus pranii (MIP)*, previously also known as Mw, have been tried with MDT to reduce the incidence and severity of reactions and neuritis and pain associated with it. This immunomodulator is a rapidly growing nonpathogenic mycobacterium, is used as dead bacilli, and shares several antigens with *M. leprae*.[36] It is available in the market; the Drugs Controller General of India (DCGI) has approved it as an immunomodulator. It is safe, well accepted, cost-effective, and used by several workers in India, and is effective in reducing the incidence of reactions and NFI in all types of leprosy patients when combined with MDT.[37-40] Other immunomodulators such as levamisole and zinc have also been used with dapsone therapy for control of reactions and neuritis, with benefit. However, their effect on MDT has not been reported.

For *chronic pain* simple nonsteroidal anti-inflammatory drugs (NSAIDs) have been used, although usually not very effective. Several studies were conducted using opioids, tricyclic antidepressants (TCAs) such as nortriptyline, amitriptyline; anticonvulsants such as carbamazepine (400–600 mg daily), gabapentin, and pregabalin have sometimes proven effective in relieving the chronic pain of neuropathies.

In late-onset neuritis without pain (silent neuritis/quiet nerve paralysis) a fresh course of MDT along with steroids is usually recommended to take care of the dormant bacilli to reverse the condition. This needs to be supported with active exercises and physiotherapy.

Surgery: Drainage of nerve abscess and release of entrapment of the nerve are recommended to relieve the pain in acute and subacute neuritis. Reconstructive surgery is usually done to improve the function as well as correct the disability caused by neuritis and arrests the damage caused by it. This needs to be followed with care of the part as well as appropriate active physiotherapy to maintain the functionality.[41]

CONCLUSION

In leprosy too, prevention is better than cure and therefore proper emphasis needs to be given to prompt an adequate treatment to prevent neuritis caused by the disease.

Neuritis in leprosy increases the morbidity of the disease and is due to a multitude of factors, some understood and others still not known. It causes disability and is the main cause of stigma associated with the disease. Tools for its early detection are now more widely available, and it needs to be tackled promptly both at the health systems level and in tertiary care centers. Some treatment modalities are available, and combined immunotherapy (with MIP) with MDT is quite promising and also cost-effective.[40]

REFERENCES

1. Gulia A, Fried I, Massone C. New insights in the pathogenesis and genetics of leprosy. F1000 Med Rep. 2010;2:30.
2. Masaki T, Qu J, Chole-Waclaw J, Burr K, Raaum R, Rambukkhara A. Reprogramming adult Schwann cells to stem-like cells by leprosy bacilli promotes dissemination of infection. Cell. 2013;1562:31-67.
3. Miko TL, Le Maitre C, Kinfu Y. Damage and regeneration of peripheral nerves in advanced treated leprosy. Lancet. 1993;342:521-5.
4. Armati PJ, Mathey EK. An update on Schwann cell biology—immunomodulation, neural regulation, and other surprises. J Neurol Sci. 2013;33:68-72.
5. Nascimento OJM. Leprosy neuropathy: clinical presentations. Arq Neuropsiquiatr. 2013;71:661-6.
6. Aarao TLS, DeSousa JR, Falcao ASC, Falcao LFM, Quaresma JAS. Nerve growth factor and pathogenesis of leprosy: review and update. Front Immunol. 2018;9:939-45.
7. Dastur DK. Cutaneous nerves in leprosy: the relationship between histopathology and cutaneous sensibility. Brain. 1995;78:615-33.
8. Wilder-Smith EP. Diagnosis of pure neuritic leprosy. Neurol J Southeast Asia. 2002;7:61-3
9. Jena S, Mishra S, Mohanty G. Silent neuropathy in leprosy. Indian J Dermatol Veenereol Leprol. 2002;68:84-5.
10. Katoch K. Autonomic nerve affection in leprosy. Indian J Lepr. 1996;68:49-54.
11. Caryon A. Investigation into the physiopathology of the nerve in leprosy. Int J Lepr. 1971;39:238-94.
12. Soysal A, Atay T, Ozu T, Arpaci B. Lectrophysiological evaluation of peripheral and autonomic involvement in leprosy. Can J Neurol Sci. 2004;31:357-61.
13. Gourie-Devi M. Cranial neuropathy in patients with leprosy. Neurol India. 2006;54:248-9.
14. Mistuda K. Atlas of Leprosy. Okayama, Japan: Chotokai Foundation; 1952.
15. Brody JA, Yase Y, Chennier G, Philippe Y. Hyperreflexia and spastic paralysis among New Caledonian leprosy patients. American J Trop Med. 1969;18:132-7.
16. Katoch K. Central nervous system involvement in leprosy. Indian J Lepr. 1984;56:813-8.
17. Aung T, Kitajima S, Nomoto M, En J, Yonezawa S, Arikawa I, et al. *Mycobacterium leprae* in neurons of the medulla oblongata and spinal cord in leprosy. Exp Neurol. 2007;66:284-94.

18. Polvarapu K, Prateesh-Kumar V, Vengalil S, Nashi S, Lavania M, Bhattacharya K, et al. Brain and spinal cord lesions in leprosy: a magnetic resonance imaging-based study. Amer J Trop Med Hyg. 2019;100:92-9.
19. Lee KR, Moon KS, Yun SJ, Won YH, Lee HK, Lee MC, et al. Brain involvement by leprosy presenting as a frontal cystic lesion. J Neurosurg. 2014;121:184-8.
20. Narsimha Rao P, Sunetha SK, Ebenzer GJ. Neuritis: definition, clinio-pathological manifestations, and proforma to record nerve impairment in leprosy. In: Kumar B, Kar HK (Eds). IAL Textbook of Leprosy, 2nd edition. New Delhi: Jaypee Brothers Medical Publishers; 2016. pp. 397-415.
21. Vijayan J, Wilder-Smith EP. Neurological manifestations of leprosy. In: Scollard DM, Gillis TP (Eds). The International Textbook of Leprosy. Greenville: American Leprosy Missions; 2016.
22. Mathur NK, Pasricha JS, Pal D, Singh N. Comparison of the cutaneous, autonomic, and somatic nervous functions in the lesions of leprosy. Int J Lepr. 1971;39:146-50.
23. Jain S, Visser LH, Praveen LN, Narsimha Rao P, Surekha T, Ellati R, et al. High-resolution sonography, a new technique to detect nerve damage in leprosy. PLOS Negl Trop Dis. 2009;3(8)e498.
24. Tiago LMP, Santos DF, Antuines DE, Tiago LMP, Goaulart IMB. Assessment of neuropathic pain in leprosy patients with relapse or treatment failure by infrared thermography: a cross-sectional study. PLoS Negl Trop Dis. 2021;15(9)e0009794.
25. Naaz F, Katoch K, Mohanty PS, Chauhan DS, Yadav VS , Kumar A, et al. Use of RLEP-PCR as a molecular tool and definitive laboratory test from skin smear scrapings for early diagnosis of leprosy in field situations. Indian J Lepr. 2016;88:199-207.
26. Shah B. Differential diagnosis of neurological disorders in relation to leprosy. In: Kumar B, Kar HK (Eds). IAL Textbook of Leprosy, 2nd edition. New Delhi: Jaypee Brothers Medical Publishers; 2016. pp. 316-27.
27. Trivedi S, Pandit A, Ganguly G, Das SK. Epidemiology of peripheral neuropathy: an Indian perspective. Ann Indian Acad Neurol. 2017;20:173-84.
28. Ebenzer GJ, Scollard DM. Treatment and evaluation of advances in leprosy neuropathies. Neurotherapeutics. 2021;18(4):2337-50.
29. World Health Organization. (2018). Guidelines for the diagnosis, treatment and prevention of leprosy. [online] Available from https://apps.who.int/iris/bitstream/handle/10665/274127/9789290226383-eng.pdf. [Last accessed January, 2023].
30. Saunderson P, Gebre K, Desta P, Byass P, Lockwood DN. The pattern of leprosy-related neuropathy in the AMFES patients in Ethiopia: definitions, incidence, risk factors, and outcome. Lepr Rev. 2020;71:(3):285-308.
31. Smith WC, Anderson AM, Withington SG, van Brakel WH, Croft RP, Nicholls PG, et al. Steroid prophylaxis for prevention of nerve function impairment in leprosy: randomized placebo-controlled trial (TRIPOD 1). BMJ. 2004;328:(7454):1459.
32. Pfaltzgraff RE. The control of neuritis in leprosy with clofazimine. Int J Lepr. 1978;40:392-8.
33. Venkatesan K. Clinical pharmacokinetic considerations in the treatment of patients with leprosy. Clin Pharmacokinet. 1989;16: 365-86.
34. Arunthathi S, Kumar SK. Does clofazimine have a prophylactic role against neuritis. Lepr Rev. 1997;68:233-41.
35. Poulidar CB, Chaudhari ND, Khatu SS. Effect of clofazimine on nerve function impairment in pauci-bacillary leprosy patients. Int J Res Dermatol. 2019;5:110-5.
36. Mustafa AS, Talwar GP. Early and late reactions in tuberculoid and lepromatous leprosy patients with lepromins from *Mycobacterium leprae* and five selected cultivable mycobacteria. Lepr India. 1978;50:566-71.
37. Sharma P, Mishra RS, Kar HK, Mukherjee A, Poricha D, Kaur H, et al. *Mycobacterium w.* vaccine, a useful adjuvant to multidrug therapy in multibacillary leprosy: a report on hospital-based immunotherapeutic clinical trials with a follow-up of 1–7 years after treatment. Lepr Rev. 2000;71:179-92.
38. Kaur I, Dogra S, Kumar B, Radotra BD. Combined 12-month WHO/MDT MB regimen and *Mycobacterium w.* vaccine in multibacillary leprosy: a follow-up of 136 patients. Int J Lepr Other Mycobact Dis. 2002;70:174-81.
39. Kamal R, Natrajan M, Katoch K, Arora M. Clinical and histopathological evaluation of the effect of addition of immunotherapy with Mw vaccine to standard chemotherapy in borderline leprosy. Indian J Lepr. 2017;84:287-306.
40. Muniyandi M , Singh M , Singh M, Rajshekhar K, Katoch K. Cost-effectiveness of incorporating *Mycobacterium indicus pranii* vaccine to multidrug therapy in newly diagnosed leprosy cases for better treatment outcomes and immunoprophylaxis in contacts, as leprosy control measures for National Leprosy Eradication Program in India. Indian J Med Res. 2021;154:121-31.
41. Srinivasan H, Palande D, World Health Organization. (1996). Action program for elimination of leprosy. Essential surgery in leprosy: techniques for district hospitals. [online] Available from http://apps.who.int/iris/handle/10665/63357. [Last accessed January, 2023].

Part 4C: Epilepsies

63

CHAPTER

Epileptogenesis: Pathophysiology, Diagnosis, and Therapeutic Approaches

Sudhir Chandra Sarangi, Soumya Sucharita Pattnaik, Ratnav Singh

INTRODUCTION

Epileptogenesis refers to the process involving the complex artificial changes in the brain after a brain insult which converts the normal brain into an epileptic brain, i.e., brain incapacitated by spontaneous recurrent seizures (SRSs). The recent evidence depicts that epileptogenesis is stretched beyond the period of latency, i.e., from the occurrence of precipitating insult to the onset of the first unprovoked seizure episode.[1] The current hypothesis suggests that the pathogenesis of epilepsy involves three stages such as (1) the initial precipitating event, (2) the latent period where no seizure occurs, and (3) the chronic period with SRSs **(Fig. 1)**.[2] The initial insult can be due to exogenous stimuli or endogenous homeostasis alteration. It can be but is not limited to perturbation in ion channels, blood–brain barrier (BBB), excitotoxic neurodegeneration, neuroapoptosis, altered proteins, epigenetic or genetic dysregulation, inflammation, and gliosis. In the latent period, there may be aggravation of the insult-related pathology or resultant changes such as neurodegeneration, neurogenesis, neuroinflammation, neural reorganization, hyperexcitability, and altered structural/functional/plasticity of neurons. All these changes can lead to SRSs with features like hyperexcitable neuronal system, reactive gliosis, hippocampal sclerosis, mossy fiber sprouting, altered cognition and behaviors, and spontaneous electroencephalogram (EEG) changes.[3]

Epileptogenesis often accompanies the alterations and comorbid conditions of overlapping neural networks[4] and/or resulted in SRSs. Thus, epilepsy treatment should focus on both antiepileptogenesis and comorbidity modification. Antiepileptogenesis is thus a process to counteract the pathways of epileptogenesis which aim for prevention, modification, and ultimately cure of seizures. Prevention can be complete in terms of end to the development of epilepsy or partial which can delay the development of epilepsy or reduce its severity, duration, and frequency (seizure modification). Antiepileptogenesis, to some extent, could also modulate the progression of epilepsy even after its occurrence. Cure of epilepsy represents an absolute and enduring reversal of epilepsy pathology which will not need any future antiepileptic treatment. Thus, antiepileptogenic treatment may be administered irrespective of seizure

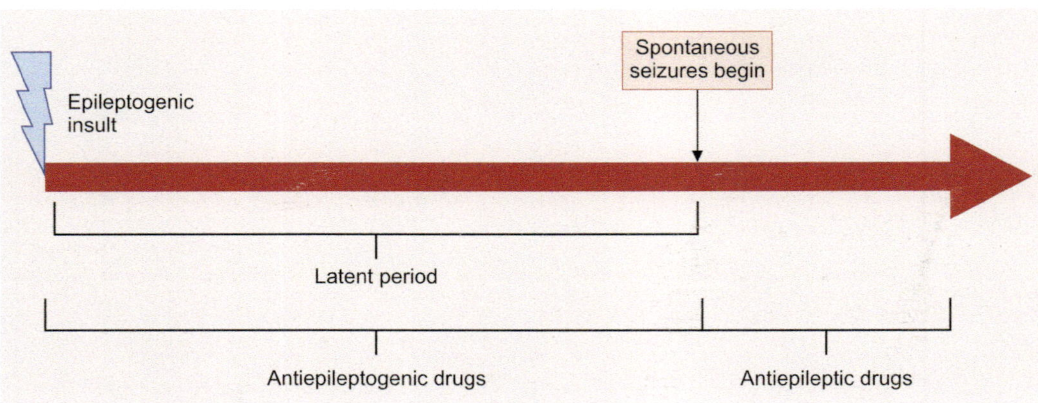

FIG. 1: Epileptogenesis process: Latent period and spontaneous recurrent seizures.

onset time, i.e., both pre- and postseizure onset. However, the insult modification approach directly modifies the insult itself along with the potential to alter epileptogenesis by modifying the insult itself. In either case, progression may be reduced along with SRSs occurrence. Treatment provided postseizure onset may assuage the seizures' properties, but lacks insult modification capacity. The agents targeting epilepsy comorbidity modify symptoms and progression of related comorbidities, such as cognitive decline, neuropsychiatric disorders, and somatomotor impairment.[5,6] Thus the combination of treatments targeting antiepileptogenesis and comorbidity-modification can also alleviate the symptoms and reverse epilepsy-associated pathology.

PATHOPHYSIOLOGICAL CHANGES IN EPILEPTOGENESIS

Structural and Morphological Changes

Neurogenesis and Altered Quality of Neurons

Adult *neurogenesis* is normally confined to two brain regions, i.e., subgranular zone (SGZ) of the hippocampal dentate gyrus (DG) and the subventricular zone (SVZ) of the forebrain lateral ventricles. This is essential for learning and memory and is also implicated in neuropsychiatric diseases including epilepsy. This has been observed in the brains of various epilepsy models and hippocampal tissue from temporal lobe epilepsy (TLE) subjects

The severity of status epilepticus (SE) influences long-term outcomes, i.e., survival of dentate granule cells (DGCs) rather than short-term neurogenesis. Adult neurogenesis is correlated with the severity of initial epileptogenic insult, epileptogenesis stage, and the aging status of the brain. Neurogenesis is exaggerated in the early part of epilepsy and the recent onset of seizures, which comes down may be below the baseline value even after one month of seizure onset. This may be explained due to the rapid turnover and use of the neural stem cell (NSC) pool or the changed availability of special support for NSCs.[7]

In addition to quantitative change, there is a change in the quality of the DGCs as well. Normally, the neuronal cells appear with one dendrite; however, the DGCs affected by seizures are with sprouting and present with additional hilar basal dendrites (HBDs). EEG findings have shown that these HBDs receive additional recurrent inputs from neighboring granule cells **(Fig. 2)**.

Ectopic neurogenesis such as increased neuroblast migration to the olfactory bulb and nonolfactory forebrain regions is also observed during prolonged seizures and epileptogenesis in the adult rat. The human epileptic brain also shows ectopic DGCs with CA3 pyramidal cells, and this is proepileptogenic.

Interventions like antimitotic agent Ara-C, cyclooxygenase (COX)-2 inhibitors, levetiracetam, genetic ablation of Nestin-TK, and ephrin-B3 have reduced the frequency and severity of seizures.[7]

Low-dose radiation suppressed hippocampal adult neurogenesis in the TLE kindling model. However, radiation and antimitotic drugs have nonspecific effects. A transgenic cell ablation strategy was used to ablate adult neurogenesis and has shown a reduction of SRSs. These data suggest that neurogenesis is an inherent part of epileptogenesis, though its role in later phases (chronic) epilepsy remains to be studied.

Focal Cortical Dysplasia

Complicated neuronal interactions and imbalances in neurotransmitters are the base of epileptogenesis in *focal cortical dysplasia (FCD)*, which is identified with the presence of dysregulated neuronal structure in white matter, laminar degeneration, and abnormal balloon cells in the brain. Alpha-amino-3-hydroxy-5-methyl-4-isoxazolepropionic acid (AMPA) and N-methyl-D-aspartate (NMDA) receptor overexpression, abnormal gamma-aminobutyric acid (GABA) receptor subunits, neurodevelopmental migratory defects leading to perturbed pyramidal neurons synaptic inhibition, and misplaced interneurons cause decreased inhibitory activity in the brain. FCD type II and tuberous sclerosis share some common features due to mammalian target of rapamycin (mTOR) pathway overactivity leading to irregular cell growth with cytomegalic neurons, unusual synaptogenesis, and connections between neurons. All these features in FCD lead to epileptogenesis.[8]

Altered plasticity of neurons occurs in TLE with hippocampal *sclerosis* where excitatory loops are created between normal and ectopic DGC due to granule cell axon *(mossy fiber) sprouting* **(Fig. 1)**. The hippocampal DG contains three layers—(1) molecular layer (cell-free), (2) granule cell layer (dense granule cells), and (3) polymorphic layer (hilus). The mossy fibers project to the hilar mossy cells and also synapse onto CA3 region pyramidal neurons. The hilar region mossy cell axons also raise projections to the dendrites of contralateral granule cells present in the molecular layer and also to the inhibitory basket cells of the granule cell layer. These neuronal circuits act to reduce neuronal excitability, i.e., excitatory input generated in the entorhinal cortex reaches the DGC and extends to mossy cells, which in turn inhibit the DGC. In epilepsy, with the loss of mossy cells in hilus, the mossy fibers sprout and innervate the molecular layer. Mossy fiber sprouting is initiated as a result of excitatory mossy cells degeneration, loss of reelin expression, loss of GABA-ergic and neuropeptidergic hilar interneurons, and increased expression of several factors [neuromodulin, brain-derived neurotrophic factor (BDNF), extracellular matrix proteins] by granule cells, and mTOR activation. The role of mossy fiber sprouting in epileptogenesis is supported by evidence from experimental and human TLE. Development of epilepsy and cognitive

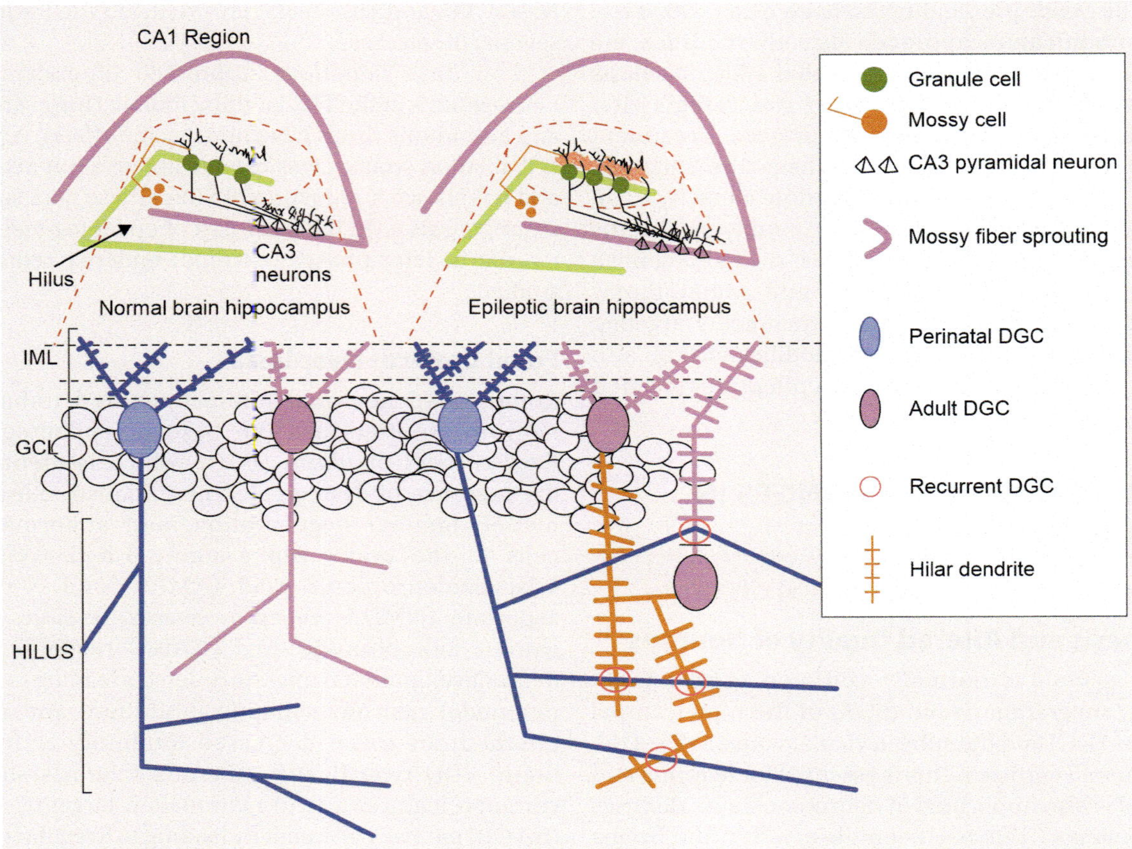

FIG. 2: Altered quality (maturation and integration) of adult—dentate granule cells.
(CA1, and CA3 region: CA1 and CA3 regions of the hippocampus, DGC: dentate granule cell; GCL: granule cell layer; IML: inner molecular layer)

deficits is found to be abridged after a reduction in abnormal neurogenesis in rodents. Rapamycin (an mTOR inhibitor) suppressed mossy fiber sprouting in the kainic acid or pilocarpine-induced epilepsy model, though spontaneous seizure frequency is reduced only in the kainic acid model. Currently, there is a lack of any specific drugs targeting mossy fiber sprouting, which limits the exact data interpretation of this pathway.[9]

Reactive gliosis has been found in the epileptogenic area of brain tissue obtained from subjects having surgery for epilepsy and from genetic and injury-induced epilepsy in experimental animal models. Morphological changes in the glial cell (mainly comprising microglia, astrocytes, and oligodendrocytes) are causally correlated to epileptogenesis. *Microglia activation* occurs as an initiating cellular event within minutes of SE onset. This activation is precipitated by adenosine triphosphate (ATP), high mobility group box 1 (HMGB1), blood-circulating molecules, and the neurotransmitters released from functionally triggered viable or damaged cells. Microglia have a role in seizure-induced neurodegeneration, as evidenced through nonlesional seizures in animals like Unverricht-Lundborg's progressive myoclonus epilepsy (induced by cystatin B gene mutations). Microglial activation paves the way for astrocyte activation and myoclonus, which follows neuronal activity modulation in epilepsy. Neuronal release of chemokine CX3CL1 (fractalkine) stimulates microglial CXC-chemokine receptor 1 (CXCR1), which promotes neurogenesis, neuronal survival, and synaptic plasticity. Activated microglia and astrocytes liberate cytokines [interleukin (IL)-1β and tumor necrosis factor (TNF)-α], chemokines, and danger signals (like HMGB1 and ATP), which direct neuronal hyperexcitability, aberrant neurogenesis, and tissue remodeling contributing to epileptogenesis. However, in one study minocycline (a potent microglia inhibitor) dosing in a pilocarpine-induced SE model in rats had no antiepileptogenic effects, but attenuated learning impairment, spontaneous seizures, and neuronal loss. Microglia have both physiological and pathological functions; so selective blockade of unfavorable microglia functions is needed for antiepileptogenic response.[10]

Blood-brain barrier dysfunction common finding in epilepsy (both patients and experimental epilepsy models) and results from reactive gliosis or endothelial cells dysfunction/activation by adenosine kinase (AK), released adhesion molecules from circulating leukocytes. Altered BBB permeability is commonly found in drug-resistant epilepsy (DRE), SE, or neurotrauma. Neuroinflammatory mediators disturb the paracellular tight junctional pathway and endothelial cells mediated pinocytosis and phagocytosis. Consequently, serum protein (specifically albumin) exposure to brain tissue led to inflammation in perivascular astrocytes. Several pathophysiological changes are shared between the process of BBB dysfunction and epileptogenesis such as endothelial cell dysfunction, neuronal damage through inflammatory cytokines, aberrant tight junctions, edema, oxidative stress, increased matrix metalloproteinases, altered pericytes, micropinocytosis, and maladaptive angiogenesis.[11]

Neurodegeneration

Neurodegeneration is the progressive transformation of neuronal activity that may include neuronal loss. Though the causal association of neurodegeneration and epilepsy has not been established, the neurodegeneration observed in the epileptic brain of patients and experimental models with acquired/secondary epilepsy may be the product of neurotrauma or a consequence of frequent epileptic seizures. The development of acquired epilepsy may be due to neurodegenerative changes in the limbic structures. Mesial TLE has morphological changes including hippocampal loss of neurons, sclerosis, synaptic rearrangement, and reactive gliosis, which produces altered neuroplasticity in the DG and ultimately neuronal hyperexcitability. A flow of changes occurs including increased intracellular Ca^{2+}, oxidative stress, and apoptotic signals including activated Bcl, P53, and caspase. These factors lead to reactive gliosis. In contrast to these, there is evidence that even adequate neuroprotection failed to attenuate SRSs in SE or neurotrauma models. Also febrile seizures animal models are devoid of neurodegeneration. These facts point out that neuronal loss/neurodegeneration is not a prerequisite or preceding factor of epileptogenesis.[12]

Functional

Neurotransmitter Changes

Gamma-aminobutyric Acid

The role of GABA in epileptogenesis and other neurological disorders is because of its presynaptic inhibitory action primarily through GABA A ($GABA_A$) receptor. Bicuculline ($GABA_A$ antagonist) increased the neuronal firing of the hippocampus and thereby enhanced seizure activity in conscious animals, whereas pretreatment with a $GABA_A$ agonist muscimol before bicuculline administration prevented seizures development.

There is increased epileptic activity of limbic seizures or generalized seizures from the thalamic nucleus Glutamate and the $GABA_A$ antagonist. GABA receptor trafficking from synaptic to extrasynaptic sites and overexpression of drug efflux protein (glycoprotein P) are associated with benzodiazepine resistance in SE. GABA neurotransmission is regulated by several candidate genes (21 no.s). The role of $GABA_B$ receptors in epileptogenesis is not clear; in the hippocampus, its antagonist causes an increase in seizure susceptibility. Moreover, its agonists induce anticonvulsant or proconvulsant effects in rats, which is dependent upon the age of the animals **(Fig. 3)**.[13]

Glutamate

It is the principal excitatory neurotransmitter. NMDA antagonists act on the synaptic membrane to antagonize the action of NMDA and AMPA receptors; these receptors have relocated to the synaptic membrane from subsynaptic sites. Vesicular glutamate transporters are identified to be expressed in the thalamus and cortex brain regions of both convulsive and nonconvulsive rodents. Glutamate uptake is significantly reduced and vesicular glutamate transporters

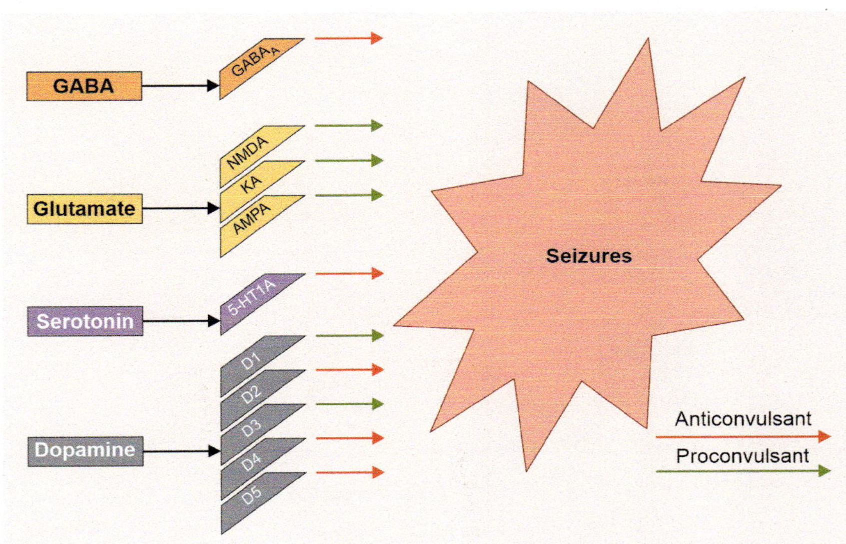

FIG. 3: Neurotransmitters involved in epileptogenesis.
(AMPA: alpha-amino-3-hydroxy-5-methyl-4-isoxazole propionic acid; GABA: gamma-aminobutyric acid; NMDA: N-methyl-D-aspartate)

are more expressed in the cortical regions of rats with induced epilepsy, suggesting an imbalance in the glutamate-mediated pathway.

Hippocampal neuronal death has been correlated with the influx of Ca^{2+} through the NMDA glutamate receptor. In the other key areas of the brain, i.e., amygdala and hippocampal tissue, there is also impairment of balance between the excitatory glutamatergic and inhibitory GABAergic systems which are the result of brain insults like trauma or SRSs or SE.

In autosomal dominant temporal epilepsy, the glutamate and AMPA-mediated neurotransmission are controlled by LGI1-associated proteins. *LGI1* gene polymorphisms are also a known fact, which can have an association with the progression of epileptogenesis **(Fig. 3)**.[13]

Serotonin

Selective serotonin reuptake inhibitors (SSRIs) activating 5-HT1A receptors reduce the occurrence of seizures. Mice with multiple-PDZ domain protein, which blocks $5\text{-}HT_{2C}$ receptor and $GABA_B$ receptors, show less severe convulsions. Agonists of 5-HT7 increase seizure threshold and need an increased dose of proconvulsant picrotoxin **(Fig. 3)**.[13]

Dopamine

Studies have demonstrated increased seizure severity and decreased seizure threshold with stimulation of D1-like receptors (D1 and D3). In contrast, there are reduced seizures with stimulation of D2-like receptors (D2, D3, and D4). The proconvulsive effect was noted through genetic inhibition of these receptors. The distribution of D2-like receptors has quite a variation in the epileptic brain, as evidenced by genetic epilepsy in rats with frontal and parietal cortices having a higher concentration of receptors and less abundance in the hippocampal CA3 region. Alteration in dopamine turnover in the frontal cortex and hippocampus of rats has been observed following pilocarpine-induced SE. GBR-12,909, a selective dopamine reuptake inhibitor, has shown antiseizure potential at a higher dose in limbic seizures **(Fig. 3)**.[13,14]

Neuropeptides

Neuropeptides play a major role in the pathogenesis of various neurological disorders including epilepsy and act as either excitatory or inhibitory agents in SE and generalized onset epilepsy. Inhibitory neuropeptides having anticonvulsant action such as somatostatin, dynorphin, neuropeptide Y, and galanin were reduced and proconvulsant neuropeptides such as neurokinin B and substance P were elevated during epilepsy. The level of adrenocorticotropic hormone (ACTH) increased during seizures and remains elevated after the seizure terminates. It is an approved therapy for generalized childhood epilepsy, i.e., atypical absence seizures. The renin–angiotensin system markers such as hyperactivation of angiotensin II and lower levels of Ang-(1-7), Ang IV, almandine, and MAS receptors were correlated in epilepsy pathology. Corticotropin-releasing hormone (CRH) administration has shown a proconvulsive effect in the kainic-acid model of seizures. In generalized epilepsy, elevated CRH levels have been observed in the case of generalized seizures. Prodynorphin knockout animals have shown structural and functional changes in the hippocampus with neuronal loss following kainic-acid injection which opines that Kappa receptor agonist may have antiepileptic potential. Substance P accumulation and its receptor-expressing cell activation in the hippocampus of epileptic patients led to increased dendritic branching and synapse formation. This substantiates the potential role of substance P antagonists in the treatment of epilepsy by reduction of susceptibility to seizures and self-recurring SE **(Fig. 4)**.[13,15]

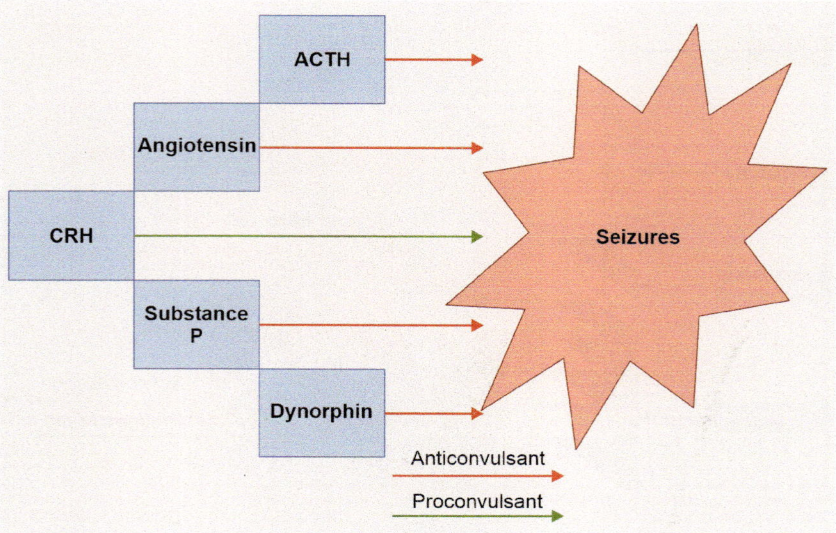

FIG. 4: Neuropeptides involved in epileptogenesis.
(ACTH: adrenocorticotropic hormone; CRH: corticotropin-releasing hormone)

Neuropsychiatric Association

Acquired epilepsy, especially TLE, has more association with neuropsychiatric disorders such as depression, anxiety, and neurocognition abnormalities that gradually worsened over time. The underlying pathogenesis may be related to the progression of epilepsy and its influence on the functionality of the different regions of the brain that are involved in cognition. The epilepsy duration correlates with the amount of cortical atrophy, hippocampal sclerosis, and decreased psychometric activities in some studies.[12]

Channelopathies and Electrolyte Imbalance

Several mutations and BBB dysfunction lead to alter electrolytes level inside the brain, which is a precipitating factor for a lower seizure threshold **(Table 1)**.[16]

Blood–brain Barrier and Astrocytes

Blood–brain barrier dysfunction causes serum albumin extravasation in perivascular brain tissue, which activates transforming growth factor (TGF) receptor 2 and related SMAD2 signaling, altering astrocyte function. It leads to hyperexcitability of neuronal network accompanied by downregulated gap junction connexins, potassium channels, aquaporin 4 channels, glutamate transporters, and altered cation-chloride cotransporters expression. Also, there is disruption of the balance between glutamate and GABA due to decreased production of glutamine synthetase (that converts glutamate into glutamine) in the brain and there is increased activity of AK in astrocytes that regulates the adenosine levels. All these mechanisms can lead to the generation of seizures and epileptogenesis. TGF signaling

TABLE 1: Channelopathies involved in various types of epilepsy.

Gating category	Function	Gene mutated	Phenotype
Na^+ channel	Generation and propagation of action potential	*SCN1A*	• SME • PE and/or FS+ • GE and/or FS+
		SCN1B	• EFS+ • IE • PS • SME
		SCN2A	• BFNS • FS and GEFS+ • EE
		SCN3A	CPS
		SCN8A	EE
		SCN9A	• SME • FS and FS+
K^+ channel	Regulation of outward K^+ current and action potentials, modulation of neurotransmitter release	*KCNA2*	EEE
		KCNB1	EE
		KCNC1	PME
		KCND2	• EE and autism • TLE
		KCND3	GE
		KCNH2	Epilepsy with LQT2
		KCNH5	EE
		KCNQ2	BFNS
		KCNQ3	• BFNS • BECTS • IE • EE
		KCNV2	• PS • EE

Continued

Continued

Gating category	Function	Gene mutated	Phenotype
Ca^{2+} channel	React to membrane potential depolarization by opening and provide an elevation of Ca^{2+} ions to drive many processes	*CACNA1A*	• EE • IGE
		CACNA1H	• CAE • MAE • IGE
		CACNA2D2	EE
		CACNB4	• JME • IGE
Cl^- channel	Maintenance of resting membrane potential and regulation of cell volume	*CLCN2*	• JME • GTCS • IGE • IE
		CLCN4	EE

(BECTS: benign epilepsy of childhood with centrotemporal spikes; BFNS: benign familial neonatal seizures; CAE: childhood absence epilepsy; CPS: complex partial seizure; EE: epileptic encephalopathy; FS: febrile seizure; GE: generalized epilepsy; GEFS: generalized epilepsy with febrile seizures plus; IE: idiopathic epilepsy; IGE: idiopathic generalized epilepsy; JME: juvenile myoclonic epilepsy; LQT2: long QT syndrome type 2; MAE: myoclonic-astatic epilepsy; PE: partial epilepsy; PEFS: partial epilepsy with febrile seizures plus; PS: partial seizure; SME: severe myoclonic epilepsy; TLE: temporal lobe epilepsy)

inhibitors, such as losartan (the angiotensin receptor 2 antagonists) have shown the potential to prevent these dysfunctions and epilepsy and the occurrence and frequency of spontaneous seizures in animal models.[11]

Molecular

Neuroinflammation in Epilepsy

Neuroinflammation plays a critical role in the epileptogenesis process. Aberrant inflammatory responses affect the function of normal cells and lead to BBB dysfunctions, which may induce the seizures' progression and lead to refractory epilepsy. These changes are mediated by a multitude of factors such as interrupted ion channel function, inflammatory agents (such as IL-1B and IL-10) release, and abnormal uptake and release of excitatory neurotransmitters such as glutamate.

Activation of inflammatory markers such as HMGB1, S100 calcium-binding protein B (S100B), TGF-β, IL-1β, COX-1, and COX-2, and prostaglandins lead to a significant alteration in the functions of the neuronal and glial cell, and BBB in brain cells that leads to the development of epileptogenesis.

Increased cytokine expression, abnormal leukocyte infiltration, and reactive gliosis which are manifestations of chronic inflammation have been observed in brain tissue from human subjects with DRE. There are extensive applications for the inflammation pathway in epileptogenesis as the pathways are broad and have multiple targets, so can be used for therapeutic, preventive, and disease-modifying indications. Several anti-inflammatory agents have been studied and some like corticosteroids and ACTH have been used in epilepsy treatment including infantile spasms.[17,18]

Alpha-amino-3-hydroxy-5-methyl-4-isoxazolepropionic Acid

Alpha-amino-3-hydroxy-5-methyl-4-isoxazolepropionic acid receptor is a subunit of glutamate receptor and has a role in the major and swift excitatory synaptic transmission in the brain. It leads to an abnormal hyperexcitable circuit which develops seizures and is also associated with neurodegeneration and apoptosis by more calcium uptake.

Perampanel reduces intracellular Ca^{2+} level which is raised due to AMPA receptor stimulation and thereby decreases excitability. In the SE model, this drug treatment led to attenuation of neuronal cell damage in the hippocampus and the piriform cortex, but it did not have antiepileptogenic effects as there was no significant reduction in SRSs. Other AMPA antagonists have also shown similar kinds of neuroprotective effects **(Figs. 5A to C)**.[12]

Adenosine Pathway

Adenosine exerts anticonvulsant potential by acting through A1 receptors. Depletion of A1 receptors in seizure-generating areas in the brain of animals contributed to epileptogenesis. Moreover, astrogliosis is related to persistent AK (that degrades adenosine) hyperactivity reducing adenosine levels. Studies showed that delivery of adenosine or AK inhibitors reduced seizures in an animal model of epilepsy. However, there is limited clinical therapeutic usefulness due to the adverse effects of adenosine on peripheral systems **(Figs. 5A to C)**.[19]

Amyloid-β Protein

Deposition of amyloid-β enhances neuronal excitability and hyperactivation which leads to epileptogenesis. Amyloid-β deposits lead to excess release of dopamine that results in

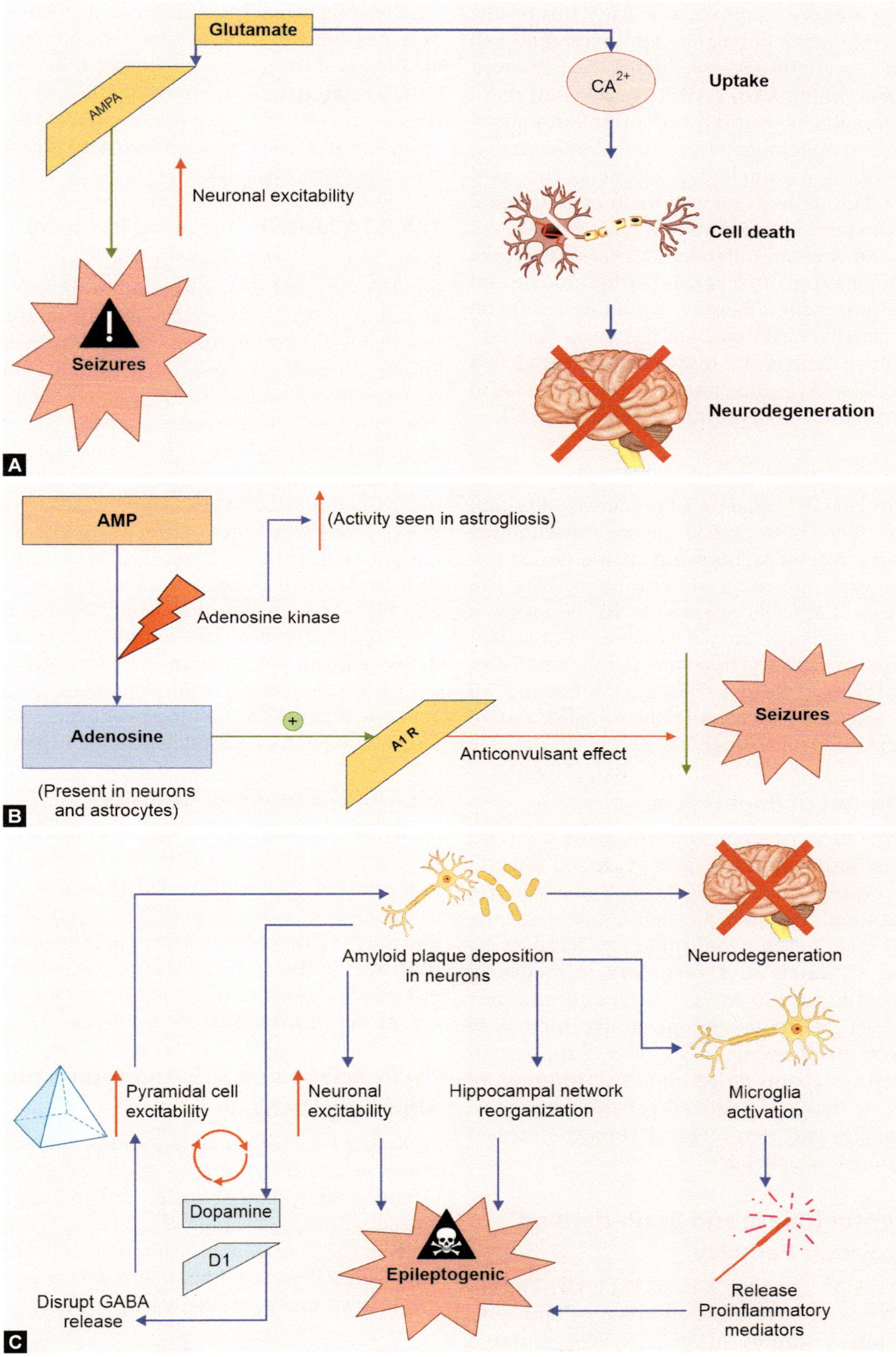

FIGS. 5A TO C: Role of molecular markers [(A) Alpha-amino-3-hydroxy-5-methyl-4-isoxazolepropionic acid (AMPA), (B) adenosine, and (C) amyloid-β] in epileptogenesis.
(AMP: adenosine monophosphate; GABA: gamma-aminobutyric acid)

disruption of the GABAergic inhibitory activity. This results in an excitatory/inhibitory imbalance and pyramidal cell hyperexcitability. As a consequence, there are increased amyloid-β deposits which form a vicious cycle and there is enhanced microglia activation and proinflammatory markers that lead to epileptogenesis. Studies have shown increased expression of amyloid-β in the cortex and hippocampus of TLE patients as well as in experimental epilepsy models. In mice epilepsy models having the excess presence of amyloid-ß, some antiepileptic drugs (AEDs) like valproate, lamotrigine, and other agents like bexarotene had reduced amyloid production thereby temporary reduction in epileptiform activity. Levetiracetam has been shown to reverse the cognitive deficits and hippocampal remodeling in an animal model and in some animal models it has also reduced the overproduction of amyloid-ß **(Figs. 5A to C)**.[12]

Tau Protein

Tau protein is involved in axonal transport and stabilization of microtubules. There is enhanced neuronal excitability due to unstable microtubules following altered tau pathology. Tau phosphorylation reduced neuronal activity and decreased seizures. Surgically resected brain tissues from drug-resistant TLE patients and FCD have pathological evidence of hyperphosphorylated tau. It has been also found in cerebrospinal fluid in patients following SE and convulsive seizures which indicates a higher risk of developing epilepsy and poor prognosis.[12]

Mammalian Target of Rapamycin

Mammalian target of rapamycin signaling plays a crucial role in epileptogenesis pathways such as axonal regeneration and sprouting, neurogenesis, cellular proliferation and migration, synaptic plasticity, and dendritic morphology. It also affects neuronal excitability by modulating ion channels and receptors in neurons. Hyperactivation of this pathway is observed in tuberous sclerosis complex (TSC) patients and animal models of acquired epilepsy and genetic TSC model. Suppression of mTOR activity by rapamycin resulted in disruption of epileptogenesis in terms of reduced seizure frequency, neuronal pathology, and neurological comorbidities in several animal models of epilepsy.[12]

Tyrosine Receptor Kinase and Brain-derived Neurotrophic Factor Pathway

Activation of tyrosine receptor kinase B (TrkB) and an increase in BDNF level have been observed in both preclinical and clinical studies of TLE. BDNF-mediated activation of TrkB induces phosphorylation of certain intracellular signaling pathways which modulate neuronal activity. Activation of TrkB induces two major signaling pathways—(1) phosphorylation of Y515 leading to binding of the adaptor protein, SHC, and (2) phosphorylation of Y816 leading to binding and activation of the enzyme PLCγ1. This has been shown to meditate epileptogenesis. This further produces structural changes in the hippocampal DGC similar to those identified in the epileptic brain. It also regulates GABA-mediated inhibition. BDNF promotes long-term potentiation in terms of increased efficacy of excitatory synapses **(Figs. 6A to D)**.[14]

JAK/STAT-BDNF Signaling Pathway

Janus kinase (JAK)–signal transducers and activators of transcription (STAT) expression are involved in the proliferation of NSCs, synaptic plasticity, neuron survival and death, glial differentiation, and neurogenesis in adults. Studies showed that there is an activation of the JAK2/STAT3 pathway after 1 hour of SE induction in the hippocampus of experimental animals; subsequently, activation of STAT3 regulated genes that are involved in modulation of type A GABA receptor subunit, cell proliferation, and survival. JAK2/STAT3 pathway activation after SE also leads to elevated BDNF levels which act on the TrkB receptor and activate certain pathways such as IP3/DAG, mitogen-activated protein (MAP)/extracellular signal-regulated kinase (ERK), and PI3/Akt leading to enhanced NF-κB transcription, the release of cytokines, and neuroinflammation. Moreover, BDNF leads to neuronal firing by increased calcium influx which further leads to epileptogenesis. Administration of WP1066, a JAK/STAT inhibitor reduced SRSs following the latent phase in the SE model induced by pilocarpine.[14]

MEK/ERK Signaling Pathway

MEK/ERK signaling pathway regulates the function of neurons by phosphorylation of transcription factors, following the influence of certain stimuli and conditions such as an influx of calcium, epilepsy, and brain ischemia. This pathway regulates synaptic excitability and neurogenesis that are induced by seizures by phosphorylation of eukaryotic translation initiation factor 4E and NMDA receptors **(Figs. 6A to D)**.[14]

Cyclic Adenosine 3′,5′-monophosphate Signaling Pathway

Following the binding of neurotransmitters or neuromodulators to the G-protein coupled receptors, there is the elevation of cyclic adenosine 3′,5′-monophosphate level and subsequent activation of protein kinase A and ERK. This leads to CREB protein phosphorylation which activates the c-fos gene. During seizures, this serves as a transcription factor for various genes in the hippocampus **(Figs. 6A to D)**.[14]

JNK Signaling Pathway

The MAP kinases include p38, c-Jun NH2-terminal kinase (JNK), and ERK lead to the activation of activator protein 1 (AP-1). JNK is a protein having pleiotropic effects such as cell differentiation and survival, cell death and apoptosis, inflammation, gene expression, and DNA repair. Transcription factor AP-1 consisted of c-Jun and c-Fos which are having DNA binding action and role in oxidative stress. JNK signaling pathway triggered phosphorylation of c-Jun leads to neuronal apoptosis and plasticity. In the kainic acid seizures model, there is an alteration of the AP-1 activity by JNK phosphorylation. AP-1 influences apoptosis, whereas kainic acid (which causes epilepsy) influences AP-1 activity via JNK phosphorylation. In this model, valproate has shown seizure protection potential through inhibition of AP-1 activity and the JNK signaling pathway **(Figs. 6A to D)**.[14,20]

Wnt Signaling Pathway

The Wnt/β-catenin signaling pathway may have a crucial role in neural plasticity, cell polarity, neuronal homeostasis, and apoptosis (through regulation of genes such as c-Myc and cyclin D1), and its alteration has been observed in several neurological disorders including epilepsy. Following seizures, there is increased expression of Wnt signaling components, as well as increased neurogenesis and neuronal death. There is increased expression of β-catenin and *Wnt2* gene in new neurons of rat hippocampus following electroconvulsive seizures.

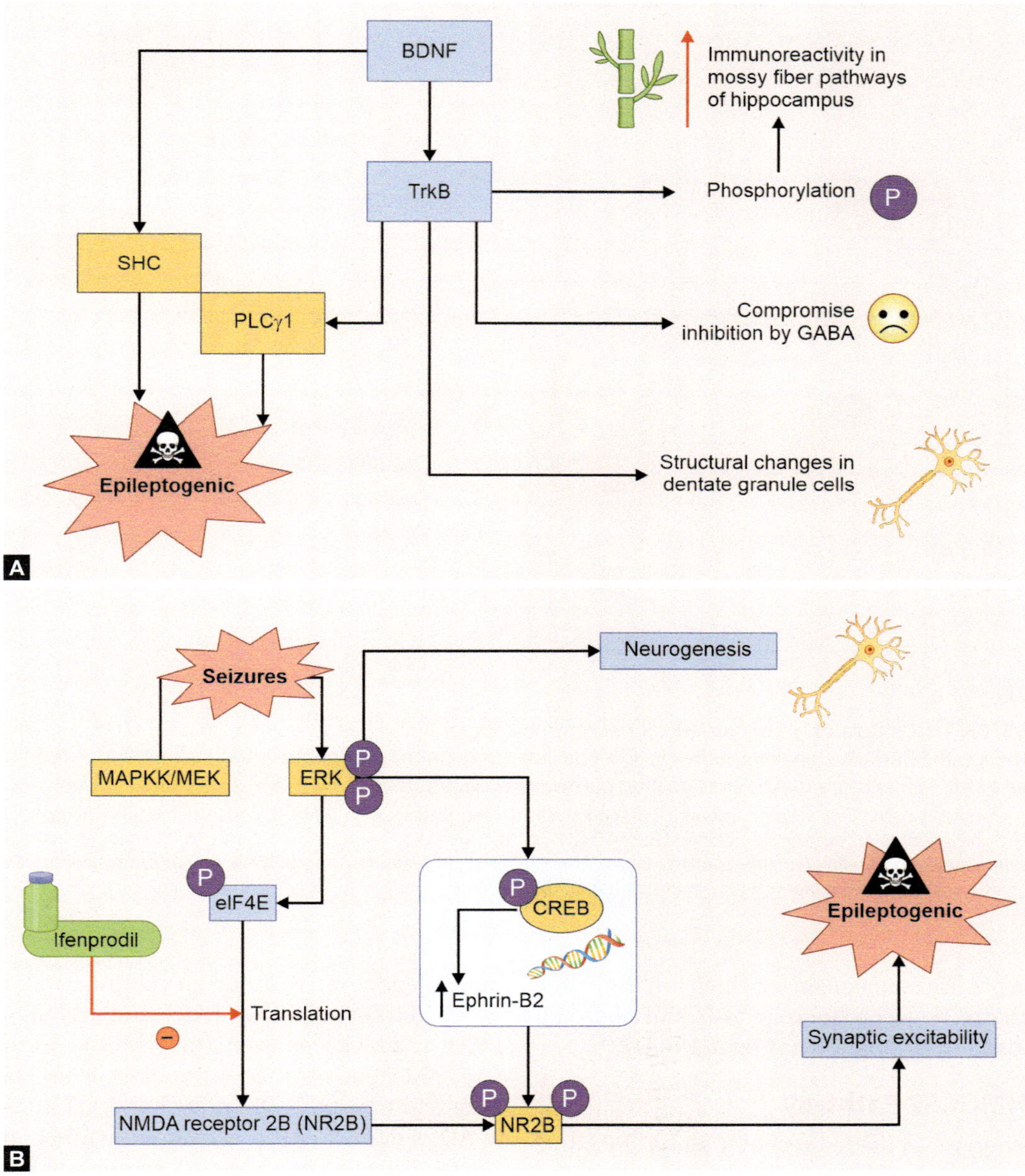

FIGS. 6A TO D: *Continued*

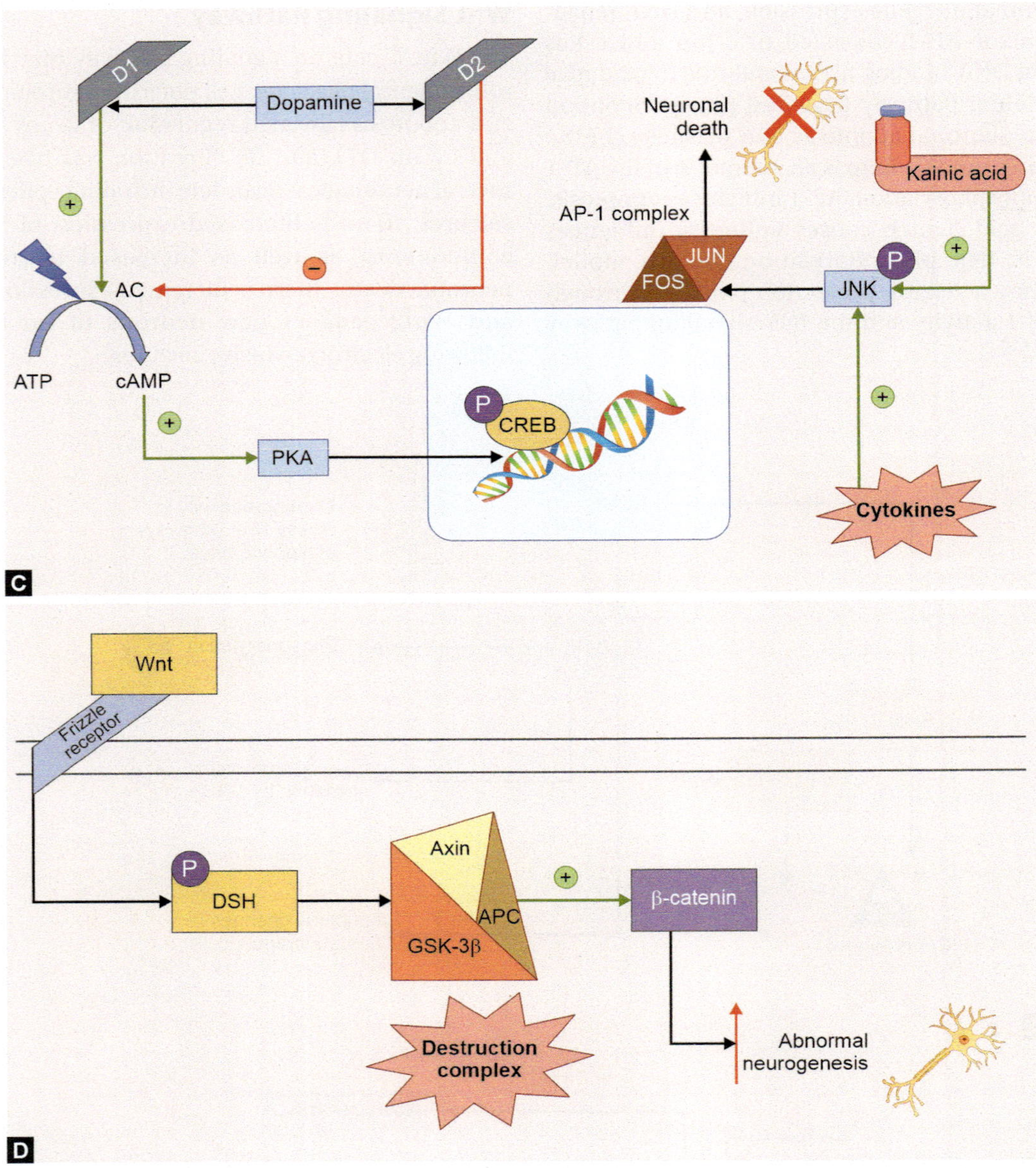

FIGS. 6A TO D: Role of (A) brain-derived neurotrophic factor (BDNF) and tyrosine kinase B (TrkB) signaling pathway, (B) ERK/MEK signaling pathway, (C) Cyclic adenosine monophosphate (cAMP), and c-Jun N-terminal kinase (JNK) signaling, and (D) Wnt signaling pathway in epileptogenesis.

(AC: adenylyl cyclase; AP-1: activator protein 1; ATP: adenosine triphosphate; CREB: cAMP-response element binding protein; DSH: dishevelled; eIF4E: eukaryotic initiation factor 4E; GSK-3β: glycogen synthase kinase 3 beta; MEK/ERK: mitogen-activated protein kinases/extracellular signal-regulated kinase; NR2B: N-methyl-D-aspartate receptor 2B; PLCγ1: phospholipase Cγ1; SHC: Src homology and collagen; Wnt: wingless/integrated)

However, the precise mechanism by which Wnt signaling causes an imbalance between neurogenesis and neuronal death in epileptogenesis is unknown **(Figs. 6A to D)**.[14]

PPAR-α and HMGCS2 Pathway

Peroxisome proliferator-activated receptor alpha (PPAR-α) modulates the expression of genes coding proteins involved in cholinergic/dopaminergic signaling and glutamate homeostasis in the brain. PPARs are altered in several neurodegenerative/neurodevelopmental diseases such as Alzheimer's disease (AD) and psychiatric disorders. PPAR-α downregulation may hinder anti-inflammatory and antioxidative processes and may alter lipid metabolism, fatty acid transport, and mitochondria function in the brain of AD patients PPAR-α activates the mitochondrial enzyme hydroxyl methyl glutaryl-CoA synthase 2 (HMGCS2), a key enzyme required for the generation of ketone bodies. The ketone bodies such as acetoacetate and β-hydroxybutyrate produced by astrocytes in the brain protect the neurons from damage by inducing the fundamental changes in glutamate metabolism by a process called "neuron-glia metabolic coupling". A recent study reported that alteration in the PPAR-α/HMGCS2 signaling pathway may result in hindering the process of ketogenesis, thereby, damaging the neuronal cells. This leads to the development of epileptogenesis and predisposes the risk of seizures. Some preclinical studies and one pilot clinical study reported that fenofibrate, a PPAR-α agonist, has shown neuroprotective effects such as anticonvulsant, anti-inflammatory, and antioxidant action **(Fig. 7)**.[21,22]

Ketone Bodies

The ketogenic diet has shown potential benefits in controlling seizures in epilepsy, especially in DRE. A recent study found reduced seizure frequency in 60% of patients whereas 38% of patients reported >50% seizure reduction, and a seizure-free period was achieved in 13%. Ketone bodies and polyunsaturated fatty acids may exert anticonvulsant action through modulation of ion channels, neurotransmitters, oxidative stress, and brain energy metabolism **(Fig. 7)**.[23,24]

Neurosteroids

Studies showed that neurosteroids may have a role in chronic epilepsy. There were reduced synaptic currents and a reduction in $GABA_A$ receptors in the DG. A marked reduction in δ subunit-containing $GABA_A$ receptors was noticed in the SE model in the DG, which suggests the effect of neurosteroids on nonsynaptic $GABA_A$ receptors may be reduced. Neurosteroids are being used for the prevention of seizures caused by pilocarpine, pentylenetetrazole (PTZ), and bicuculline. Treatment with finasteride increased epileptogenesis in the hippocampus-kindling model, which may be due to a decrease in allopregnanolone and other neurosteroids.[18]

Progesterone

Progesterone has shown potential anticonvulsant activity in experimental and clinical studies. In the kindling model of epilepsy, progesterone inhibited evoked seizures and hindered the progression of epileptogenesis.[18]

Oxidative Stress

Oxidative stress plays a crucial role in the epileptogenesis process. Activation of TLRs leads to oxidative stress by the formation of reactive nitrogen species (RNS) and reactive oxygen species (ROS) thereby generating spontaneous seizures in chronic epilepsy. Oxidative stress activates thioredoxin, an antioxidant protein that further activates the NLRP3 inflammasome. Animal studies have shown that less oxidative stress resulted in improved cognitive functions and less neuronal damage following SE. Administration of N-acetyl-cysteine, an antioxidant resulted in hindered seizure progression by blocking ROS generation, activating transcription factor NRF2. Similarly, inhibition of NOS during the initial stage of epileptogenesis in the SE model effectively reduced spontaneous seizures, neuro-

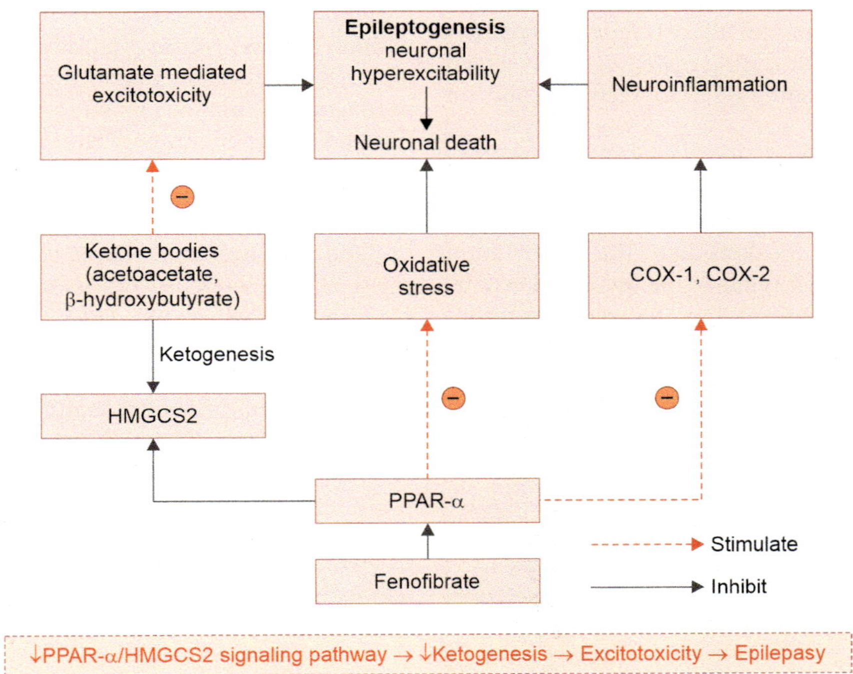

FIG. 7: Role of PPAR-α/HMGCS2 pathway and ketone bodies in epileptogenesis.
(HMGCS2: mitochondrial enzyme hydroxyl methyl glutaryl-CoA synthase 2; PPAR-α: peroxisome proliferator-activated receptor alpha)

degeneration, and neuroinflammation. The functions of glutathione peroxidase and superoxide dismutase are altered in myoclonic epilepsy in humans.[17]

Genetics

Neuroinflammation and Genetic Epilepsy

There is scarce evidence regarding the study of neuroinflammation and oxidative stress in the experimental model of genetic epilepsies as most of the studies are conducted in an animal model of epilepsy with acquired brain injuries (e.g., central nervous system infection, SE, or neurotrauma). However, some studies were conducted in a genetic model of epilepsy such as "Genetic Absence Epilepsy Rats from Strasbourg (GAERS)" and inbred "Wistar Albino Glaxo Rats from Rijswijk (WAG/Rij)" rat models and cystatin B knocked out mice. These showed that neuroinflammation and oxidative stress have been observed before the development of seizures. In WAG/Rij and GAERS model, spike-and-wave discharges (SWDs) were enhanced by inflammation and reduced following administration of the anti-inflammatory drug VX-765. In another study conducted in a genetic model of absence seizures, IL-1β levels were elevated before the development of SWD suggesting the possible role of IL-1β in the development of absence seizures.[17]

Transcriptomic and Epigenetic Modifications

Transcriptomic modification such as upregulation of T-type calcium channels promotes seizures during epileptogenesis whereas deletion of CACNA1H which encodes for the channel resulted in reducing spontaneous seizures and neuronal damage in the SE model. There is induction of RE1-silencing transcription factor during epileptogenesis which alters the expression of encoding genes for receptors and ion channels.

Epigenetic mechanisms such as microRNA (miRNA) expression, DNA methylation, and histone modification also regulate gene expression during epileptogenesis as evident from experimental and clinical studies. The methylation hypothesis of epileptogenesis refers to the increased activity of DNMT enzymes and subsequent hypermethylation. Hence, novel therapeutics targeting these pathways may also hinder the epileptogenesis progression.

Inhibitors of histone deacetylase, e.g., valproate reduced neurogenesis and neuronal damage in the SE model but did not control the seizures whereas there was increased histone acetylation in the cerebral cortex and hippocampus of mice by inhibitor sodium butyrate.

Based on some literature, miRNAs may serve as a biomarker for epileptogenesis before the onset of seizures and hence have the potential therapeutic target for antiepileptogenic therapies. Targeting-specific miRNA resulted in the regulation of neuroinflammatory mediators and thereby inhibited epileptogenesis in the experimental model of seizures. However, further studies are needed to establish any definitive conclusion.[25]

RELEVANCE OF EPILEPTOGENESIS IN THE DIAGNOSIS OF EPILEPSY

Biomarkers

A biomarker is a characteristic that can be measured to determine normal biologic processes, pathogenic processes, or responses to an exposure or intervention, including therapeutic interventions.

The sensitive and specific marker for epilepsy can be designated based on the goal being fulfilled by it, i.e., risk assessment markers identifying a given epilepsy syndrome, prognosis anticipating markers, e.g., timeline after secondary insult developing epilepsy, and diagnostic markers which can accurately identify the ongoing epileptogenesis process with or without background data of the previous insult.

Evidence suggests that HMGB1, changes in blood cytokine levels and T2 MRI may be biomarkers for predicting the risk of developing epilepsy in patients. An increased blood level of HMGB1 was observed during epileptogenesis following SE in an animal model of epilepsy. Similarly, a clinical study reported a higher level of HMGB1 level in patients following neurotrauma, and this predicted the mortality and adverse neurological outcomes assessed after 1 year of follow-up. In another study, the ratio of CSF IL-1β levels to blood levels the following neurotrauma in the 1st week of injury served as a predictive biomarker of posttraumatic epilepsy after 3 years. Another study reported a significantly elevated level of IL-6, IL-1 RA, IL-1, and IL-8 within 72 hours of onset of febrile SE in children compared to children with fever but not having seizures. T2 hyperintensity in magnetic resonance imaging (MRI) is also a predictor of mesial TLE in patients with febrile SE.[26]

Electroencephalography

Epileptic seizures themselves can be served as a specific biomarker of epileptogenesis and epileptogenicity. Ictal electroencephalography (EEG) is not considered to be ideal due to its cost issues, time consumption, and risk of evaluation. Interictal EEG is gaining more relevance because it contains certain transient features like interictal EEG spikes and sharp waves (IIS), high-frequency oscillations (HFOs) (80–600 Hz), and advanced features like "microseizures" and "microperiodic epileptiform discharges" which are EEG seizure-like events and focal periodic epileptiform discharges (on submillimeter spatial scales). Interictal EEG within 24 hours of seizure has 51% importance compared to later EEG (34%). The presence of HFOs and microseizures as recorded through the placement of microelectrodes in cerebral tissue has enhanced the diagnostic approaches before surgery (presurgical evaluation). These also increased the understanding of spatial and temporal scales for identifying abnormal brain electrical signals. In MTLE patients, atrophy of the hippocampus region and reduced neuron densities has been correlated with HFOs and fast ripple frequency.[27]

ROLE OF THERAPEUTICS ON EPILEPTOGENESIS

Although a wide range of AEDs is available for the management of epilepsy, nearly 30% of people with epilepsy (PWE) remain pharmacoresistant. None of the currently available AEDs has the disease-modifying/antiepileptogenic potential; rather they provide only symptomatic relief. Moreover, treatment with them exerts several adverse effects such as depression, anxiety, and cognitive decline which further deteriorate the quality of life in PWE. AEDs exert their therapeutic benefits in seizures by several mechanisms such as the inhibition of voltage-gated calcium or sodium channels, blocking excitatory events associated with glutamate, enrichment of GABA-mediated inhibition, and being ligands for synaptic vesicle proteins (SVA2). Apart from the effect on seizure control, evidence also suggests the neuroprotective potential of some AEDs (e.g., valproate, phenobarbitone, levetiracetam, topiramate, lamotrigine, benzodiazepines, and vigabatrin). Hence, the question arises whether these AEDs have the potential in modifying neurodegeneration which plays a crucial role in the pathway of epileptogenesis. The effect of currently available AEDs repurposed drugs, and other potential therapeutic candidates on neurodegeneration, seizure control status and cognitive deficits in the experimental model of epilepsy are summarized in **Tables 2, 3, and 4**, respectively.[28]

TABLE 2: Therapeutic potential of approved and commonly used antiepileptic drugs (AEDs) for modification of epileptogenesis.

Name of AED	Model	Treatment duration	Effect on spontaneous recurrent seizures (SRS)	Effect on neurodegeneration	Effect on neurobehavioral abnormalities	References
Valproate	Electrically status epilepticus (SE)	28 days	Not reduced	Neuroprotective effect	No effect	29
	Kainic acid-induced SE	40 days	Reduced	Neuroprotective effect	No effect	30
	Pilocarpine-induced SE	21 days	No reduction	No neuroprotective effect	Not studied	31
Carbamazepine	Electrically-induced SE	14 days	No effect	No neuroprotective effect	No effect	32
	Pilocarpine-induced SE	56 days	25% reduction in SRS	Moderate neuroprotective effect	Not studied	33
	Methylazoxymethanol (MAM) and pilocarpine-induced SE	60 days	No effect	No neuroprotective effect	Not studied	34
Phenobarbitone	Kainic acid-induced SE	117 days	No reduction in SRS	No neuroprotective effect	Aggravation of behavioral abnormalities	35
	Kainic acid-induced SE	40 days	No reduction in SRS	No neuroprotective effect	No effect	30
	Pilocarpine-induced SE	14 days	Reduction in frequency, but no reduction in duration and severity	No neuroprotective effect	No effect	36
	PTZ-induced seizure	16 days	Reduced the severity	• Prevented glutamate • Mediated neurotoxicity	Not studied	37
Phenytoin	Flurothyl-induced seizures	28 days	No effect	Not studied	Not studied	38
Diazepam	Electrically-induced SE	Single-dose	Reduction in development and severity of seizures	Less hippocampal damage and mossy fiber sprouting	Not studied	39
	Pilocarpine-induced SE	Single-dose	No effect	Significant neuronal loss in the hippocampus	Not studied	40

Continued

Continued

Name of AED	Model	Treatment duration	Effect on spontaneous recurrent seizures (SRS)	Effect on neurodegeneration	Effect on neurobehavioral abnormalities	References
Levetiracetam	Pilocarpine-induced SE	5 days	No effect	Significant neuroprotection in dentate gyrus, hilus, CA1 and CA3 areas	Not studied	41
	Electrically-induced SE	35 or 56 days	No effect	No neuroprotection	No effect	42
	Kainte-induced SE		Reduced	Neuroprotective effect: suppression of seizure-induced neurogenesis.	Not studied	43
	Pilocarpine-induced SE	Single-dose	No change in ictal discharge in EEG	Less neuronal damage	Transient attenuation of ictal behavior in epileptic rats,	44
Topiramate	Pilocarpine-induced SE	6 days	No effect	Moderate neuroprotection	Not studied	40
	Pilocarpine-induced SE	7 days	No effect	Neuroprotection in the CA1 and CA3 region	Not studied	45
	Pilocarpine-induced SE	3 doses	Reduced	Not studied	Not studied	46
Lacosamide	Pilocarpine-induced SE	3 doses	Reduced	Not studied	Not studied	46
	Electrically-induced SE	23 days	No effect	Dose-dependent neuroprotection	Not studied	47
	Electrically-induced SE	23 days	• Early treatment: Reduced no of SRS • Late treatment: No effect	Not studied	Not studied	48
Lamotrigine	Pentylenetetrazole (PTZ) kindling model	For 15 days (alternate day)	Reduced	No effect	Not studied	49
	Electrically-induced SE	44 days	No effect	No effect	Not studied	50
Perampanel	Pilocarpine-induced SE	Single-dose	Reduced	Neuroprotective effect	Attenuation of behavioral abnormalities	51
	Genetic (WAG/Rij rat model of epileptogenesis: a model of absence seizures)	68 days	Reduced	Not studied	Partially reduced	52
	Kindling model	Single-dose	Reduced in a dose-dependent manner	Not studied	Not studied	53
Brivaracetam	Controlled cortical impact (CCI) injury model	Single-dose	Reduced	Not studied	Not studied	54

TABLE 3: Repurposed drugs for epileptogenesis.

Drug	MOA	Type of study	Finding	Reference
Anakinra	IL-1 receptor antagonist	Preclinical	• ↓ duration and frequency of SRS • Prevent behavioral impairment and neuronal loss.	55
		Clinical (case report)	↓ seizure frequency	56
Anakinra + canakinumab	Anti-IL-1+ monoclonal antibody	Clinical (case report)	↓ seizure, improved quality of life	57

Continued

Continued

Drug	MOA	Type of study	Finding	Reference
N-acetyl-cysteine	Antioxidant	Clinical	↓ seizure frequency	58
Ibuprofen	COX inhibitor	Clinical (RCT)	No effect	59
Aspirin	COX inhibitor	Clinical	↓ seizure frequency	60, 61
Adalimumab	Anti-TNF monoclonal antibody	Clinical pilot study	• ↓ seizure frequency in 5/11 patients • 3 patients had no further neurocognitive deterioration in 3 patients	62
Tocilizumab	IL-6 receptor inhibitor	Clinical	Termination of status epilepticus in 6/7 patients	63
Minocycline	Tetracycline antibiotics	Clinical (Case report)	↓ seizure frequency	64
Natalizumab	Anti-alpha 4 integrin antibody	Clinical (Case report)	↓ seizure frequency	65
Fingolimod	Sphingosine-phosphate receptors (S1PRs) analog	Preclinical	• ↓ chronic seizure activity, neuroprotective and antibiotic effects, and reduced cytotoxic T cell infiltrate • Temporary reduction in seizures; positive effects on cognitive decline • ↓ SRS • ↓ neuronal loss and decreased microglial activation	66-68
Losartan	Antihypertensive		• ↓ severity, frequency, and duration of seizures • ↑ threshold and delayed the onset of seizures • delayed the onset of seizures, ↓frequency, and duration of epilepsy • Neuroprotection in CA1 of the hippocampus, attenuated seizures induced behavioral deficits • ↓ reduction in the incidence of delayed seizures from 59.1 to 5.56% • ↓ BBB breakdown	69-71 72
Isoflurane	Anesthetic	Preclinical	• ↓ SRS; did not affect duration and severity • No effect on SRS; significant neuroprotection	73, 74
Statins (lovastatin, atorvastatin, rosuvastatin, simvastatin)	Hypolipidemic drug (HMG CoA reductase inhibitors)	Preclinical	• No effect • Significant ↓ pro-inflammatory cytokines (IL-1β, TNF-α, IL-6) and ↑ anti-inflammatory cytokines IL-10	75-80
		Clinical	• ↓ in development of epilepsy • No effect	
Rapamycin and other mTOR inhibitors		Preclinical	• ↓ SRS, mossy fiber sprouting, cell death, BBB leakage, and gliosis • No effect on SRS	81-84
		• Clinical (Pilot study) • Case report • Clinical trial	• ↓seizure frequency and duration • Discontinuation of everolimus resulted in a relapse of seizures	85-87
Saroglitazar	Dual PPARα/γ Agonist	Preclinical	↓ seizures and oxidative stress	88
Fenofibrate	peroxisome proliferator-activated receptor alpha (PPARα)	Clinical	↓ seizure frequency; control of motor–behavioral seizures.	89
		Preclinical	↓ frequency of large inhibitory postsynaptic currents (IPSCs)	

(COX: cyclooxygenase; BBB: blood–brain barrier; HMG: high mobility group; IL: interleukin; MOA: Mechanism of action; RCT: randomized controlled trial; SRS: spontaneous recurrent seizure; TNF: tumor necrosis factor)

TABLE 4: Potential therapeutic candidate for modification of epileptogenesis.

Molecules	MOA	Model	Finding	Reference
PQR620	mTOR inhibitor	Kainate-induced SE	No effect on seizures, effect on reduction in anxiety	90
PQR530	A phosphoinositide-3 kinase (PI3K)-Akt/mTOR pathway inhibitor	Kainate-induced SE	No effect on seizures	
Z-944	T-type calcium channel antagonist	Kainate-induced SE	Decreased no. of convulsion and positive effect on behavioral abnormalities	91
Adenosine	inhibition of hippocampal DNA methylation	Kainate-induced SE	Decreased seizures and mossy fiber sprouting	92
Antagomir	Antisense Oligonucleotide (targets microRNA-134)	Kainate-induced SE	Cessation of SRS and reduction in hippocampal astrogliosis	93
1NMPP1	TrkB inhibitor	Kainate-induced SE	Reduction of SRS and anxiety-like behaviors	94

(MOA: mechanism of action; mTOR: mammalian target of rapamycin; SRS: spontaneous recurrent seizure; SE: status epilepticus)

REFERENCES

1. Pitkänen A, Lukasiuk K, Dudek FE, Staley KJ. Epileptogenesis. Cold Spring Harb Perspect Med. 2015;5(10):a022822.
2. Reddy DS, Kuruba R. Experimental models of status epilepticus and neuronal injury for evaluation of therapeutic interventions. Int J Mol Sci. 2013;14(9):18284-318.
3. Pitkänen A, Ndode-Ekane XE, Lapinlampi N, Puhakka N. Epilepsy biomarkers—toward etiology and pathology specificity. Neurobiol Dis. 2019;123:42-58.
4. Kanner AM, Mazarati A, Koepp M. Biomarkers of epileptogenesis: Psychiatric comorbidities (?). Neurotherapeutics. 2014;11(2): 358-72.
5. Pitkänen A, Nehlig A, Brooks-Kayal AR, Dudek FE, Friedman D, Galanopoulou AS, et al. Issues related to development of antiepileptogenic therapies. Epilepsia. 2013;54 Suppl 4(0 4):35-43.
6. Pitkänen A, Engel J Jr. Past and present definitions of epileptogenesis and its biomarkers. Neurotherapeutics. 2014;11(2):231-41.
7. Chen L, Wang Y, Chen Z. Adult neurogenesis in epileptogenesis: An update for preclinical finding and potential clinical translation. Curr Neuropharmacol. 2020;18(6):464-84.
8. Tahta A, Turgut M. Focal cortical dysplasia: etiology, epileptogenesis, classification, clinical presentation, imaging, and management. Childs Nerv Syst. 2020;36(12):2939-47.
9. Hendricks WD, Westbrook GL, Schnell E. Early detonation by sprouted mossy fibers enables aberrant dentate network activity. Proc Natl Acad Sci U S A. 2019;116(22):10994-9.
10. Lee JW, Chun W, Lee HJ, Kim SM, Min JH, Kim DY, et al. The Role of Microglia in the Development of Neurodegenerative Diseases. Biomedicines. 2021;9(10):1449.
11. Löscher W, Friedman A. Structural, molecular, and functional alterations of the blood-brain barrier during epileptogenesis and epilepsy: A cause, consequence, or both? Int J Mol Sci. 2020;21(2): 591.
12. Casillas-Espinosa PM, Ali I, O'Brien TJ. Neurodegenerative pathways as targets for acquired epilepsy therapy development. Epilepsia Open. 2020;5(2):138-54.
13. Werner FM, Coveñas R. Classical neurotransmitters and neuropeptides involved in generalized epilepsy: a focus on antiepileptic drugs. Curr Med Chem. 2011;18(32):4933-48.
14. Gautam V, Rawat K, Sandhu A, Kumari P, Singh N, Saha L. An insight into crosstalk among multiple signaling pathways contributing to epileptogenesis. Eur J Pharmacol. 2021;910:174469.
15. Krasniqi S, Daci A. Role of the angiotensin pathway and its target therapy in epilepsy management. Int J Mol Sci. 2019;20(3):726.
16. Bartolini E, Campostrini R, Kiferle L, Pradella S, Rosati E, Chinthapalli K, et al. Epilepsy and brain channelopathies from infancy to adulthood. Neurol Sci. 2020;41(4):749-61.
17. Vezzani A, Balosso S, Ravizza T. Neuroinflammatory pathways as treatment targets and biomarkers in epilepsy. Nat Rev Neurol. 2019;15(8):459-72.
18. Clossen BL, Reddy DS. Novel therapeutic approaches for disease-modification of epileptogenesis for curing epilepsy. Biochim Biophys Acta Mol Basis Dis. 2017;1863(6):1519-38.
19. Masino SA, Kawamura M Jr, Ruskin DN. Adenosine receptors and epilepsy: current evidence and future potential. Int Rev Neurobiol. 2014;119:233-55.
20. Hsieh CL, Lin JJ, Chiang SY, Su SY, Tang NY, Lin GG, et al. Gastrodia elatamodulated activator protein 1 via c-Jun N-terminal kinase signaling pathway in kainic acid-induced epilepsy in rats. J Ethnopharmacol. 2007;109(2):241-7.
21. Wójtowicz S, Strosznajder AK, Jeżyna M, Strosznajder JB. The novel role of PPAR alpha in the brain: promising target in therapy of Alzheimer's disease and other neurodegenerative disorders. Neurochem Res. 2020;45(5):972-88.
22. Bayoumy NMK, El-Shabrawi MM, Younes S, Omar HH. PPARα receptor expression in patients with metabolic syndrome. Diabetes Metab Syndr. 2018;12(5):711-4.
23. Jagadish S, Payne ET, Wong-Kisiel L, Nickels KC, Eckert S, Wirrell EC. The ketogenic and modified atkins diet therapy for children with refractory epilepsy of genetic etiology. Pediatr Neurol. 2019;94: 32-7.
24. Green SF, Nguyen P, Kaalund-Hansen K, Rajakulendran S, Murphy E. Effectiveness, retention, and safety of modified ketogenic diet in adults with epilepsy at a tertiary-care centre in the UK. J Neurol. 2020;267(4):1171-8.
25. Conboy K, Henshall DC, Brennan GP. Epigenetic principles underlying epileptogenesis and epilepsy syndromes. Neurobiol Dis. 2021;148:105179.
26. Engel J Jr, Pitkänen A. Biomarkers for epileptogenesis and its treatment. Neuropharmacology. 2020;167:107735.
27. Gotman J. Can EEG abnormalities be a biomarker of epileptogenesis? Epilepsy Curr. 2021;21(3):157-8.

28. Trojnar MK, Małek R, Chrościńska M, Nowak S, Błaszczyk B, Czuczwar SJ. Neuroprotective effects of antiepileptic drugs. Pol J Pharmacol. 2002;54(6):557-66.
29. Brandt C, Gastens AM, Sun Mz, Hausknecht M, Löscher W. Treatment with valproate after status epilepticus: effect on neuronal damage, epileptogenesis, and behavioral alterations in rats. Neuropharmacology. 2006;51(4):789-804.
30. Bolanos AR, Sarkisian M, Yang Y, Hori A, Helmers SL, Mikati M, et al. Comparison of valproate and phenobarbital treatment after status epilepticus in rats. Neurology. 1998;51(1):41-8.
31. Klitgaard H, Matagne A, Vanneste-Goemaere J, Margineanu DG. Pilocarpine-induced epileptogenesis in the rat: impact of initial duration of status epilepticus on electrophysiological and neuropathological alterations. Epilepsy Res. 2002;51(1-2):93-107.
32. Halonen T, Nissinen J, Pitkänen A. Effect of lamotrigine treatment on status epilepticus-induced neuronal damage and memory impairment in rat. Epilepsy Res. 2001;46(3):205-23.
33. Capella HM, Lemos T. Effect on epileptogenesis of carbamazepine treatment during the silent period of the pilocarpine model of epilepsy. Epilepsia. 2002;43 Suppl 5:110-1.
34. Nobili P, Cattalini A, de Grazia U, Cagnoli C, de Curtis M, Battaglia GS, et al. Early chronic carbamazepine-in-food administration to MAM/pilocarpine rats does not affect convulsive motor seizures. Front Pharmacol. 2020;11:181.
35. Mikati MA, Holmes GL, Chronopoulos A, Hyde P, Thurber S, Gatt A, et al. Phenobarbital modifies seizure-related brain injury in the developing brain. Ann Neurol. 1994;36(3):425-33.
36. Brandt C, Nozadze M, Heuchert N, Rattka M, Löscher W. Disease-modifying effects of phenobarbital and the NKCC1 inhibitor bumetanide in the pilocarpine model of temporal lobe epilepsy. J Neurosci. 2010;30(25):8602-12.
37. Silva Brum LF, Elisabetsky E. Antiepileptogenic properties of phenobarbital: behavior and neurochemical analysis. Pharmacol Biochem Behav. 2000;67(3):411-6.
38. Applegate CD, Samoriski GM, Ozduman K. Effects of valproate, phenytoin, and MK-801 in a novel model of epileptogenesis. Epilepsia. 1997;38(6):631-6.
39. Pitkänen A, Kharatishvili I, Narkilahti S, Lukasiuk K, Nissinen J. Administration of diazepam during status epilepticus reduces development and severity of epilepsy in rat. Epilepsy Res. 2005;63(1):27-42.
40. Rigoulot MA, Koning E, Ferrandon A, Nehlig A. Neuroprotective properties of topiramate in the lithium-pilocarpine model of epilepsy. J Pharmacol Exp Ther. 2004;308(2):787-95.
41. Santana-Gómez CE, Valle-Dorado MG, Domínguez-Valentín AE, Hernández-Moreno A, Orozco-Suárez S, Rocha L. Neuroprotective effects of levetiracetam, both alone and combined with propylparaben, in the long-term consequences induced by lithium-pilocarpine status epilepticus. Neurochem Int. 2018;120:224-32.
42. Brandt C, Glien M, Gastens AM, Fedrowitz M, Bethmann K, Volk HA, et al. Prophylactic treatment with levetiracetam after status epilepticus: lack of effect on epileptogenesis, neuronal damage, and behavioral alterations in rats. Neuropharmacology. 2007;53(2):207-21.
43. Sugaya Y, Maru E, Kudo K, Shibasaki T, Kato N. Levetiracetam suppresses development of spontaneous EEG seizures and aberrant neurogenesis following kainate-induced status epilepticus. Brain Res. 2010;1352:187-99.
44. Zheng Y, Moussally J, Cash SS, Karnam HB, Cole AJ. Intravenous levetiracetam in the rat pilocarpine-induced status epilepticus model: Behavioral, physiological and histological studies. Neuropharmacology. 2010;58(4-5):793-8.
45. André V, Dubé C, François J, Leroy C, Rigoulot MA, Roch C, et al. Pathogenesis and pharmacology of epilepsy in the lithium-pilocarpine model. Epilepsia. 2007;48(Suppl 5):41-7.
46. Shishmanova-Doseva M, Peychev L, Yoanidu L, Uzunova Y, Atanasova M, Georgieva K, et al. Anticonvulsant effects of topiramate and lacosamide on pilocarpine-induced status epilepticus in rats: A role of reactive oxygen species and inflammation. Int JMolSci. 2021;22(5):2264.
47. Licko T, Seeger N, Zellinger C, Russmann V, Matagne A, Potschka H. Lacosamidetreatment following status epilepticus attenuates neuronal cell loss and alterations in hippocampal neurogenesis in a rat electrical status epilepticus model. Epilepsia. 2013;54(7): 1176-85.
48. Wasterlain CG, Stöhr T, Matagne A. The acute and chronic effects of the novel anticonvulsant lacosamide in an experimental model of status epilepticus. Epilepsy Res. 2011;94(1-2):10-7.
49. Chen Y, He X, Sun Q, Fang Z, Zhou L. Effect of lamotrigine on seizure development in a rat pentylenetetrazole kindling model. Brain Behav. 2017;7(7):e00727.
50. Nissinen J, Large CH, Stratton SC, Pitkänen A. Effect of lamotrigine treatment on epileptogenesis: an experimental study in rat. Epilepsy Res. 2004;58(2-3):119-32.
51. Mohammad H, Sekar S, Wei Z, Moien-Afshari F, Taghibiglou C. Perampanel but not amantadine prevents behavioral alterations and epileptogenesis in pilocarpine rat model of status epilepticus. Mol Neurobiol. 2019;56(4):2508-23.
52. Citraro R, Leo A, Franco V, Marchiselli R, Perucca E, De Sarro G, et al. Perampanel effects in the WAG/Rij rat model of epileptogenesis, absence epilepsy, and comorbid depressive-like behavior. Epilepsia. 2017;58(2):231-8.
53. Dupuis N, Enderlin J, Thomas J, Desnous B, Dournaud P, Allorge D, et al. Anti-ictogenic and antiepileptogenic properties of perampanel in mature and immature rats. Epilepsia. 2017;58(11):1985-92.
54. Ling DSF, Yang L, Goodman JH. Brivaracetam prevents the development of epileptiform activity when administered early after cortical neurotrauma in rats. Epilepsia. 2022;63(4):992-1002.
55. Dyomina AV, Zubareva OE, Smolensky IV, Vasilev DS, Zakharova MV, Kovalenko AA, et al. Anakinra Reduces Epileptogenesis, Provides Neuroprotection, and Attenuates Behavioral Impairments in Rats in the Lithium-Pilocarpine Model of Epilepsy. Pharmaceuticals (Basel). 2020;13(11):340.
56. Mochol M, Tauбøll E, Sveberg L, Tennøe B, Berg Olsen K, Heuser K, et al. Seizure control after late introduction of anakinra in a patient with adult onset Rasmussen's encephalitis. Epilepsy Behav Rep. 2021;16:100462.
57. DeSena AD, Do T, Schulert GS. Systemic autoinflammation with intractable epilepsy managed with interleukin-1 blockade. J Neuroinflammation. 2018;15(1):38.
58. Ben-Menachem E, Kyllerman M, Marklund S. Superoxide dismutase and glutathione peroxidase function in progressive myoclonus epilepsies. Epilepsy Res. 2000;40(1):33-9.
59. van Stuijvenberg M, Derksen-Lubsen G, Steyerberg EW, Habbema JD, Moll HA. Randomized, controlled trial of ibuprofen syrup administered during febrile illnesses to prevent febrile seizure recurrences. Pediatrics. 1998;102(5):E51.
60. Lance EI, Sreenivasan AK, Zabel TA, Kossoff EH, Comi AM. Aspirin use in Sturge-Weber syndrome: side effects and clinical outcomes. J Child Neurol. 2013;28(2):213-8.
61. Godfred RM, Parikh MS, Haltiner AM, Caylor LM, Sepkuty JP, Doherty MJ. Does aspirin use make it harder to collect seizures during elective video-EEG telemetry? Epilepsy Behav. 2013;27(1):115-7.
62. Lagarde S, Villeneuve N, Trébuchon A, Kaphan E, Lepine A, McGonigal A, Roubertie A, et al. Anti-tumor necrosis factor alpha therapy (adalimumab) in Rasmussen's encephalitis: An open pilot study. Epilepsia. 2016;57(6):956-66.
63. Jun JS, Lee ST, Kim R, Chu K, Lee SK. Tocilizumab treatment for new onset refractory status epilepticus. Annf Neurol. 2018;84(6): 940-5.
64. Nowak M, Strzelczyk A, Reif PS, Schorlemmer K, Bauer S, Norwood BA, et al. Minocycline as potent anticonvulsant in a patient with astrocytoma and drug resistant epilepsy. Seizure. 2012;21(3):227-8.

65. Sotgiu S, Murrighile MR, Constantin G. Treatment of refractory epilepsy with natalizumab in a patient with multiple sclerosis. Case report. BMC neurology. 2010;10(1):10:84.
66. Pitsch J, Kuehn JC, Gnatkovsky V, Müller JA, van Loo KMJ, de Curtis M, et al. Anti-epileptogenic and anti-convulsive effects of fingolimod in experimental temporal lobe epilepsy. Mol Neurobiol. 2019;56(3):1825-40.
67. Leo A, Citraro R, Amodio N, De Sarro C, Gallo Cantafio ME, Constanti A, et al. Fingolimod exerts only temporary antiepileptogenic effects but longer-lasting positive effects on behavior in the WAG/Rij rat absence epilepsy model. Neurotherapeutics. 2017;14(4):1134-47.
68. Gao F, Liu Y, Li X, Wang Y, Wei D, Jiang W. Fingolimod (FTY720) inhibits neuroinflammation and attenuates spontaneous convulsions in lithium-pilocarpine induced status epilepticus in rat model. Pharmacol Biochem Behav. 2012;103(2):187-96.
69. Bar-Klein G, Cacheaux LP, Kamintsky L, Prager O, Weissberg I, Schoknecht K, et al. Losartan prevents acquired epilepsy via TGF-β signaling suppression. Ann Neurol. 2014;75(6):864-75.
70. Nozaki T, Ura H, Takumi I, Kobayashi S, Maru E, Morita A. The angiotensin II type I receptor antagonist losartan retards amygdala kindling-induced epileptogenesis. Brain Res. 2018;1694:121-8.
71. Tchekalarova JD, Ivanova NM, Pechlivanova DM, Atanasova D, Lazarov N, KortenskaL, et al. Antiepileptogenic and neuroprotective effects of losartan in kainate model of temporal lobe epilepsy. Pharmacol Biochem Behav. 2014;127:27-36.
72. Bar-Klein G, Lublinsky S, Kamintsky L, Noyman I, Veksler R, Dalipaj H, et al. Imaging blood-brain barrier dysfunction as a biomarker for epileptogenesis. Brain. 2017;140(6):1692-705.
73. Bar-Klein G, Klee R, Brandt C, Bankstahl M, Bascuñana P, Töllner K, et al. Isoflurane prevents acquired epilepsy in rat models of temporal lobe epilepsy. Ann Neurol. 2016;80(6):896-908.
74. Swissa E, Bar-Klein G, Serlin Y, Weissberg I, Kamintsky L, Eisenkraft A, et al. Midazolam and isoflurane combination reduces late brain damage in the paraoxon-induced status epilepticus rat model. Neurotoxicology. 2020;78:99-105.
75. Funck VR, de Oliveira CV, Pereira LM, Rambo LM, Ribeiro LR, Royes LF, et al. Differential effects of atorvastatin treatment and withdrawal on pentylenetetrazol-induced seizures. Epilepsia. 2011;52(11):2094-104.
76. Gouveia TL, Scorza FA, Iha HA, Frangiotti MI, Perosa SR, Cavalheiro EA, et al. Lovastatin decreases the synthesis of inflammatory mediators during epileptogenesis in the hippocampus of rats submitted to pilocarpine-induced epilepsy. Epilepsy Behav. 2014;36:68-73.
77. Oliveira CV, Grigoletto J, Canzian JM, Duarte MMMF, Duarte T, Furian AF, et al. Effect of atorvastatin on behavioral alterations and neuroinflammation during epileptogenesis. Epilepsy Behav. 2018;78:109-17.
78. Vitturi BK, Gagliardi RJ. The influence of statins on the risk of post-stroke epilepsy. Neurol Sci. 2020;41(7):1851-7.
79. Guo J, Guo J, Li J, Zhou M, Qin F, Zhang S, et al. Statin treatment reduces the risk of poststroke seizures. Neurology. 2015;85(8):701-7.
80. Hsieh PF, Tung H, Lin CH. Statin effects on post-stroke epilepsy and mortality - Taiwan population-based study. Neurol Res. 2020;42(5):422-9.
81. Zeng LH, Rensing NR, Wong M. The mammalian target of rapamycin signaling pathway mediates epileptogenesis in a model of temporal lobe epilepsy. J Neurosci. 2009;29(21):6964-72.
82. Huang X, McMahon J, Yang J, Shin D, Huang Y. Rapamycin down-regulates KCC2 expression and increases seizure susceptibility to convulsants in immature rats. Neuroscience. 2012;219:33-47.
83. Buckmaster PS, Lew FH. Rapamycin suppresses mossy fiber sprouting but not seizure frequency in a mouse model of temporal lobe epilepsy. J Neurosci. 2011;31(6):2337-47.
84. Barker-Haliski M, Knox K, Zierath D, Koneval Z, Metcalf C, Wilcox KS, et al. Development of an antiepileptogenesis drug screening platform: Effects of everolimusand phenobarbital. Epilepsia. 2021;62(7):1677-88.
85. Samueli S, Abraham K, Dressler A, Gröppel G, Mühlebner-Fahrngruber A, Scholl T, et al. Efficacy and safety of Everolimus in children with TSC - associated epilepsy - Pilot data from an open single-center prospective study. Orphanet J Rare Dis. 2016;11(1):145.
86. Krueger DA, Wilfong AA, Holland-Bouley K, Anderson AE, Agricola K, Tudor C, et al. Everolimus treatment of refractory epilepsy in tuberous sclerosis complex. Ann Neurol. 2013;74(5):679-87.
87. Mingarelli A, Vignoli A, La Briola F, Peron A, Giordano L, Banderali G, et al. Dramatic relapse of seizures after everolimus withdrawal. Eur J Paediatr Neurol. 2018;22(1):203-6.
88. Panigrahy SR, Pradhan S, Maharana CS. Amelioration of oxidative stress and neuroinflammation by Saroglitazar, a dual PPARα/γ agonist in MES induced epileptic rats. Biomed Pharmacol J. 2019;12(04):1985-91.
89. Puligheddu M, Melis M, Pillolla G, Milioli G, Parrino L, Terzano GM, et al. Rationale for an adjunctive therapy with fenofibrate in pharmacoresistant nocturnal frontal lobe epilepsy. Epilepsia. 2017;58(10):1762-70.
90. Gericke B, Brandt C, Theilmann W, Welzel L, Schidlitzki A, Twele F, et al. Selective inhibition of mTORC1/2 or PI3K/mTORC1/2 signaling does not prevent or modify epilepsy in the intrahippocampal kainate mouse model. Neuropharmacology. 2020;162:107817.
91. Casillas-Espinosa PM, Shultz SR, Braine EL, Jones NC, Snutch TP, Powell KL, et al. Disease-modifying effects of a novel T-type calcium channel antagonist, Z944, in a model of temporal lobe epilepsy. Prog Neurobiol. 2019;182:101677.
92. Williams-Karnesky RL, Sandau US, Lusardi TA, Lytle NK, Farrell JM, Pritchard EM, et al. Epigenetic changes induced by adenosine augmentation therapy prevent epileptogenesis. J Clin Invest. 2013;123(8):3552-63.
93. Reschke CR, Silva LFA, Vangoor VR, Rosso M, David B, Cavanagh BL, et al. Systemic delivery of antagomirs during blood-brain barrier disruption is disease-modifying in experimental epilepsy. Mol Ther. 2021;29(6):2041-52.
94. Liu G, Gu B, He XP, Joshi RB, Wackerle HD, Rodriguiz RM, et al. Transient inhibition of TrkB kinase after status epilepticus prevents development of temporal lobe epilepsy. Neuron. 2013;79(1):31-8.

64

CHAPTER

New-onset Epilepsy: A Diagnostic Approach and Special Epilepsies in India

Jasmine Parihar, Sanjeev V Thomas, Manjari Tripathi

INTRODUCTION

Epilepsy is one of the most common diseases that neurologists and physicians come across. Seizures account for 1–2% of patients presenting to the emergency department.[1] The challenges lie in diagnosing and managing patients with new-onset seizures and deciding whether they fulfill the diagnosis of epilepsy. Over the past decade, there have been advances in the diagnosis of epilepsy with the new definition of epilepsy being one important development.[2] A comprehensive evaluation will determine the likelihood of recurrence of seizures in a patient presenting with new-onset seizures. This will further guide the decision on initiation and choice of antiseizure medications (ASMs).

This chapter reviews the diagnostic approach to a patient who has new-onset seizures by establishing the diagnosis of epilepsy, ruling out seizure mimics, discussing initial workup, and selecting appropriate ASMs for the management of such patients.

DEFINITIONS

Epilepsy

The International League Against Epilepsy (ILAE) revised the definition of epilepsy in 2014 for early identification and timely management of patients with epilepsy.[2]

Epilepsy is defined as when any of the following exists:

- At least two unprovoked seizures occurring >24 hours apart
- One unprovoked seizure and a probability of further seizures similar to the general recurrence risk after two unprovoked seizures (e.g., ≥60%) occurring over the next 10 years
- Diagnosis of an epilepsy syndrome

The second criterion was added by the ILAE working group in 2014 and emphasizes the importance of neuroimaging and electroencephalography (EEG) in the evaluation of patients with a first-time seizure, as some of these patients will meet the criteria for epilepsy at the time of a first seizure.

Unprovoked Seizure

Unprovoked seizure refers to a seizure of unknown etiology as well as one that occurs about a preexisting brain lesion or progressive nervous system disorder. Unprovoked seizures that are determined to be due to an underlying brain lesion or disorder are also referred to as remote symptomatic seizures. They carry a higher risk of future epilepsy compared with acute symptomatic seizures.

Acute Symptomatic Seizure

Acute symptomatic seizure refers to a seizure that occurs at the time of a systemic insult or in close temporal association with a documented brain insult.[3] Such insults include metabolic derangements, drug or alcohol withdrawal, and acute neurologic disorders such as stroke, encephalitis, or acute head injury.

The time window within which a seizure may be considered acute symptomatic has not been clearly defined and may vary based on the type of insult.

EPIDEMIOLOGY

With an increasing approach to health care the number of patients who are diagnosed with new-onset epilepsy is increasing. However, due to the lack of proper registries, the data on the epidemiology of epilepsy in India is scarce.

The rate of hospitalization, mortality, and expenditure is higher in patients who have new-onset epilepsy than those with chronic epilepsy, making it a significant public health issue.

There are more than 10 million persons with epilepsy (PWE) in India with a prevalence of 1%.[4] Various studies report overall prevalence between 5.6 and 10 per 1,000 populations.[4-7] The incidence of epilepsy is less studied with a very few studies available from India. An Indian study from Kolkata, India has reported an incidence of 27.3 per 100,000 per year.[8] Other studies have reported an incidence of 0.2–0.6 per 1,000 per year.[9-11]

RISK FACTORS

Risk factors for the development of new-onset epilepsy vary with the age of onset. **Box 1** mentions risk factors according to the age of presentation.

CLINICAL PRESENTATIONS

The initial presentation of epilepsy may occur at any age and with any seizure semiology. Usually, generalized epilepsies, epilepsies due to congenital structural deformity of the brain, and metabolic syndromes have an earlier age of onset whereas acquired diseases such as trauma, vascular causes, and neoplastic etiologies have onset in adulthood. Epilepsies of unknown etiology can present at any age. The clinical presentation and semiology of seizures are essential to establish the diagnosis of epilepsy and characterizing the epilepsy type.

Establishing the Diagnosis of Epilepsy

Patients who present with new-onset seizures should be evaluated for the possibility of epilepsy. According to the ILAE, patients should have two unprovoked seizures to fulfil the diagnosis of epilepsy. We know that not all patients with a single unprovoked seizure are equally likely to have a second seizure. Under the new ILAE definition, a patient who has a single unprovoked seizure and a likelihood of seizure recurrence of >60% can also be diagnosed as having epilepsy. This probability of another seizure can be established by abnormal brain imaging, abnormal EEG findings, and the presence of focal neurological deficits. In a systematic review assessing the risk of seizure recurrence following a single unprovoked seizure, between 21% and 45% of patients had another unprovoked seizure within the first 2 years.[12] From a practical standpoint, four risk factors have been identified that approximately double a patient's risk of seizure recurrence: prior brain injury, abnormal neuroimage findings that correspond to the suspected seizure focus, focal or generalized epileptiform discharges on EEG, or a nocturnal seizure.[13-16]

Acute symptomatic seizures and seizure mimics should be ruled out before establishing the diagnosis of epilepsy. An acute symptomatic seizure is defined as a clinical seizure occurring at the time of a systemic insult or in close temporal association with a documented brain insult.[3] These seizures are a result of acute insults and may not recur if the primary abnormality is corrected. These patients do not fulfil the criteria of epilepsy. **Table 1** lists the causes of acute symptomatic seizure.[17]

Seizure mimics are clinical conditions that may be erroneously diagnosed as epilepsy. These should be identified to provide the right treatment and prognosis and

BOX 1 **Risk factors for development of new-onset epilepsy.**

- *Neonatal*: Perinatal hypoxia, CNS infections, inborn errors of metabolism, congenital anomalies, genetic disorder
- *Infants and children*: Genetic disorder, CNS infections, trauma, developmental disorder
- *Adolescent*: Head injury, CNS infections, epilepsy syndrome, brain tumors, illicit drug use
- *Adults*: Head injury, CNS infections, brain tumors
- *Elderly*: Stroke, tumors, dementias, trauma (SDH)

(CNS: central nervous system; SDH: subdural hematoma)

TABLE 1: Possible causes of acute symptomatic seizures.[3,17]

Insult	Clinical features
Illicit drugs	Amphetamine-like drugs, cocaine, crack, angel dust (phencyclidine); less likely for heroin or cannabis
Infections	• Within • Viral encephalitis • Bacterial meningitis • Degenerative phase of neurocysticercosis
Medication	Chlorpromazine, clozapine, maprotiline, clomipramine, bupropion, meperidine, flumazenil, cyclic antidepressants, theophylline, isoniazid, alkylating antineoplastic agents, ciclosporin, overdose of medication
Metabolic	• Renal or hepatic dysfunction, especially rapid changes • Hyperammonemia (35 mM) • Na <115 mg/dL (<5 mM) • Mg <0.8 mg/dL (<0.3 mM) • Ca <5 mg/dL (<1.2 mM) • Creatinine >10 mg/dL • Glucose <36 mg/dL (2.0 mM) or 450 mg/dL (25 mM) • Associated with ketoacidosis
Traumatic	• Within • Associated with hemorrhage
Vascular	• Subarachnoid bleeding • Ischemic stroke (<7 days) • Intracerebral hemorrhage • Cerebral vein thrombosis
Withdrawal, deficiency	• Alcohol • Benzodiazepine • Barbiturate • Rarely vitamin B12 • Vitamin B6 (young children)
Other	• Posterior reversible encephalopathy syndrome • Cerebral anoxia • Eclampsia • Multiple sclerosis within 7 days of relapse

prevent unnecessary ASM-related side effects. Syncope and psychogenic attacks are the most common seizure mimics that are managed as epilepsy. Various mimics and chameleons of epilepsy are listed in **Table 2**.

Characterizing the Epilepsy Type

Prognosis and the choice of ASM depends on the type of epilepsy a patient has. The type of epilepsy can be established based on clinical semiology, brain imaging findings, and EEG findings.

The ILAE in 2017 revised the classification of epilepsy design to work with the classification of seizure types. It has three levels of diagnosis: seizure type, epilepsy type, and epilepsy syndrome. Based on the seizure type,[18] epilepsy may be classified as focal, generalized, combined focal, and unknown onset[19] **(Fig. 1 and Flowchart 1)**. Other than this, the patient may fit into epilepsy syndrome. The

TABLE 2: Differential diagnosis of seizures.

Diagnosis	Symptoms
Cardiac events with falls and loss of consciousness	Not necessarily with prodromes, due to cardiac arrhythmia, or carotid sinus hypersensitivity (see also below under syncope)
Migraine	• Progression of neurologic symptoms > 5–15 minutes followed by headaches (but not always) • Personal and/or family history of migraine • *Basilar migraine*: Confusion, bilateral blindness; headache may be minimal or absent
Movement disorders	Rare, specific syndrome, like paroxysmal dyskinesia
Psychogenic	• Is not equal to absence of "organic" findings → positive psychiatric history or findings mandatory • *Semiology suggestive of psychogenic onset*: Eyes closed, resistant to forceful opening, eye fluttering, rhythmic horizontal head movement, pelvic thrusting • Paradoxical response to antiepileptic drug introduction ("even worse") or no change at all
Syncope	• Brief loss of consciousness, with rapid recovery • *Typical prodromes*: Nausea, "spots before the eyes," sweating, light-headedness, cardiac palpitations • Muscle jerks at the end of event, usually less rhythmic, only few ("convulsive syncope") • Precipitating circumstances often identifiable • *Cave in the elderly*: Recovery may take 10–60 minutes in the elderly, mimicking postictal state • Loss of consciousness left often; syncope may present as transient ischemic attack (e.g., speech difficulties)
Transient global amnesia	More often in patients >50 years; prolonged duration (several hours) without alteration of consciousness, isolated memory deficit excluding long-term memory before onset of the symptoms
Transient ischemic attack	• More often in patients >50 years • Rather negative symptoms (e.g., weakness and aphasia), but usually no loss of consciousness

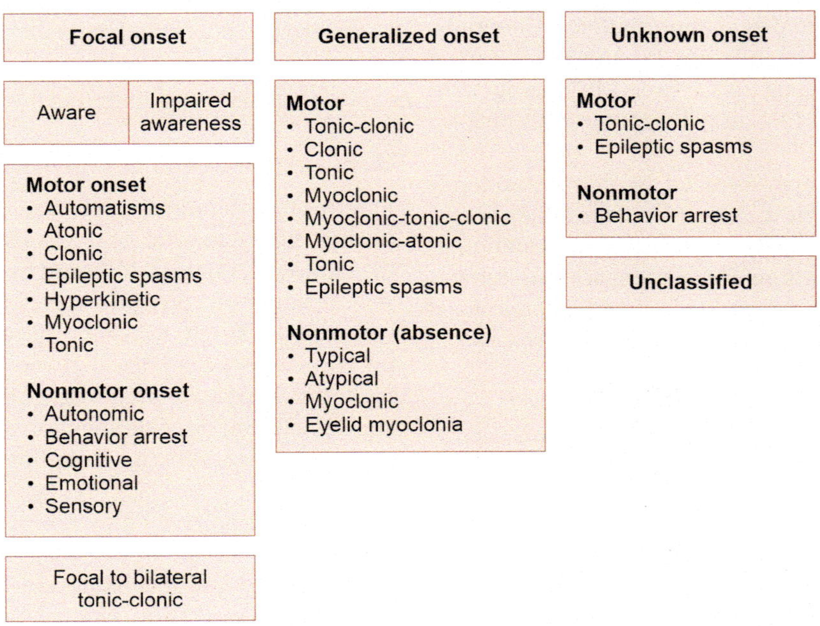

FIG. 1: Classification of seizure types expanded version[17] [International League Against Epilepsy (ILAE) 2017] (ILAE 2017).

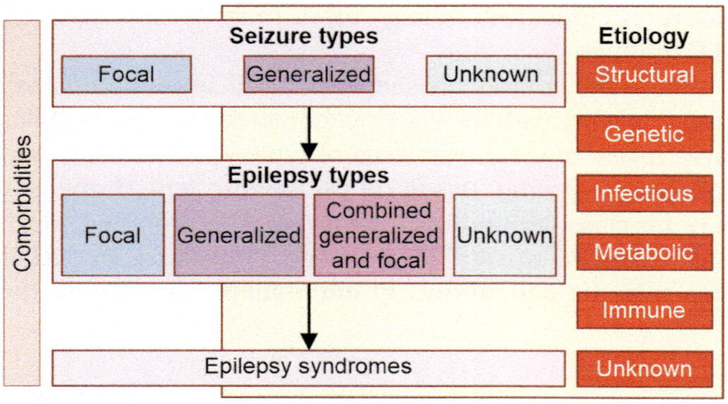

FLOWCHART 1: Framework of classification of the epilepsies [International League Against Epilepsy (ILAE) 2017].[18]

new classification also incorporates etiology at each stage, emphasizing the treatment implications.

A patient with generalized seizure may present with myoclonic, atonic, or initial bilateral tonic/tonic-clonic activity, etc. A patient can be said to have a focal seizure if there are the following clinical symptoms and signs:

- Lateralized motor or sensory symptoms
- Forced head or eye deviation to one side
- Automatisms
- Aura
- Language disturbances
- Postseizure Todd's palsy

However, in new-onset seizures the focality cannot be easily established, and patients may present with bilateral tonic-clonic movements that may or may not have a focal onset. The presence of a focal lesion in brain imaging can suggest focal onset. EEG is another modality that can be used to establish focal or generalized onset depending on the type of discharges. It should be carried out as early as possible after the seizure to detect abnormalities. Generally, a single routine EEG is insufficient for the detection of epileptiform discharges, and up to three EEGs, long-term EEG, and sleep-deprived EEG may be required to pick up abnormal discharge.[20-22]

Unknown-onset epilepsy is used to denote epilepsy where the clinician is unable to determine if the epilepsy type is focal or generalized because of insufficient information or noncontributory investigations.[19] A patient with unknown-onset epilepsy may later be categorized as focal or generalized if seizure semiology is clearer in subsequent seizures.

DIAGNOSIS

Clinical Diagnosis

The diagnosis of epilepsy is primarily based on history and examination. All efforts should be made to find out the description of events from the patient as well as the witness of seizures. Leading questions should be asked regarding the preictal status (the circumstances in which the seizure happened, any aura), the ictal phase (type of activity, eye deviation, head turning, frothing from the mouth, tongue bite, consciousness level), and postictal phase (incontinence, level of consciousness, confusion, amnesia, drowsiness, postictal paralysis). The duration of the event should be inquired about. If available, a video recording of the event should be seen. Substance abuse, treatment history, past medical history, and family history should be inquired for. The examination is generally normal unless carried out during a seizure or immediately in the postictal period. The clinician should look for any focal deficit, pupillary dilatation, and positive Babinski sign during the episode. Tongue bite, fractures, and trauma-related injuries should be looked for.

Brain Imaging

Neuroimaging is recommended in all patients who present with new-onset epilepsy. Although a magnetic resonance imaging (MRI) brain is the investigation of choice in epilepsy, it is not readily available and may not be affordable to all. In all circumstances MRI brain should be preferred over a computed tomography (CT) brain. However, CT may be done in an emergency setting to rule out acute brain hemorrhage and in the setting of acute brain trauma. MRI should be carried out with epilepsy protocol that includes the following:

- Standard T1-weighted images
- Three-dimensional (3D) volumetric T1-weighted images
- Axial and coronal T2-weighted [T2/short tau inversion recovery (STIR)] imaging
- Axial and coronal fluid-attenuated inversion recovery (FLAIR) sequences
- Axial T2 gradient echo or susceptibility-weighted sequences
- Various etiologies that can be clearly identified on MRI brain epilepsy protocol include mesial temporal sclerosis, cortical dysplasia, brain tumors, vascular malformations, stroke, and central nervous system (CNS) infections [including neurocysticercosis (NCC)].

Electroencephalography

Electroencephalography is an important investigation during the evaluation of new-onset epilepsy, especially if the etiology is unclear. It should be carried out as near to the seizure activity as possible to pick up maximum discharges. Generally, a single EEG recording is not sufficient to pick up the discharges. Up to three EEG recordings have a higher pickup rate than a single EEG record. EEG should be conducted with sleep deprivation and provocative measures such as hyperventilation and photic stimulation to increase the yield.

An abnormal EEG may not only aid in confirming the diagnosis of epilepsy but also help in categorizing the epilepsy type and localizing the epileptic focus. It is also essential investigation when considering nonconvulsive status epilepticus and in cases of evaluation of drug refractory epilepsies. A negative EEG recording however does not rule out epilepsy.

Other Investigations

Depending on the scenario, a patient may require laboratory investigations including electrolyte levels, renal and hepatic function tests, and toxicology screen. In patients with suspected syncope/arrhythmias, an electrocardiogram should be performed. The elevated serum prolactin level in the immediate postictal period may help to differentiate seizures from psychogenic nonepileptic seizures (PNES). However, it is not recommended routinely.

Advanced Investigations

- *Lumbar puncture*: It should be carried out in patients in whom CNS infections are suspected. In other circumstances, cerebrospinal fluid analysis is not very useful.
- *Long-term video EEG recording*: This is useful in cases of evaluation of drug-refractory epilepsy and where the diagnosis of epilepsy is in doubt.
- Diffusion tensor imaging MRI improves the detection of hippocampal sclerosis and cortical dysplasia.
- Susceptibility-weighted MRI is an advanced MRI sequence that is very sensitive in detecting blood products, iron, and calcium contents in the brain and can help in detecting calcified lesions, hemorrhages, and cavernous malformations.
- Functional MRI (fMRI) maps brain activity depending on the blood flow and oxygenation levels in different areas of the brain. It is a noninvasive investigation to map the eloquent motor sensory and language cortex. It is routinely used as part of surgical planning in epilepsy surgeries.
- *18F-fluorodeoxyglucose positron emission tomography (FDG-PET) brain*: This is an imaging modality that demonstrates the glucose uptake in the brain depending on cerebral metabolism. It is generally performed as a part of the presurgical evaluation. Interictal FDG-PET can localize the epileptogenic focus in the form of reduced metabolism.
- *Single-photon emission CT (SPECT)*: In SPECT, the regional cerebral blood flow can be imaged using radiotracers 99mTc-hexamethyl propylene amine oxime or 99mTc ethyl cysteinate dimer (ECD). Both ictal and interictal SPECTs are required during the workup of drug-refractory epilepsy to identify an epileptogenic focus.
- *Magnetoencephalography (MEG)*: It records the magnetic fields generated by neuronal electric currents in the brain. It is similar to EEG, but the brain activity is not significantly affected by the intervening tissue layer and has a more clinically reliable localization of the epileptic activities. It also finds its utility in cases of drug refractory requiring epilepsy surgery.

MANAGEMENT

In a patient who presents with new-onset seizures the decision to start ASM should be individualized based on the likelihood of subsequent seizures. Since ASM comes with side effects, these should not be started in all patients who present with new-onset seizures. In other words, establishing the diagnosis of epilepsy decides the need for ASM. The risk of subsequent seizures should be explained to the patient and the family members, and the decision to start ASM should take into account the patient's preferences after knowing the risk and benefits, job profile, and risk-taking ability. Not all patients may agree to wait for another seizure before starting ASM. Though the decision to start ASM can be debated after the first unprovoked seizure, in a patient presenting with a second unprovoked seizure ASM should be started without hesitation.

In patients with acute symptomatic seizure the decision to start ASM depends on the severity and expected duration of the underlying illness. ASM may be started if there is a risk of recurrence of acute symptomatic seizure.

The factors that increased the risk of seizure recurrence include abnormal neuroimaging, abnormal EEG, abnormal neurological examination, and nocturnal seizure. In patients presenting with their first unprovoked seizure immediate ASM treatment reduces the risk of seizure recurrence by 35% over the next 1–2 years.[23-25] However, the long-term risk of seizures is not affected by early initiated or delayed treatment start.[23,24,26,27]

The goal of epilepsy treatment in patients with new-onset epilepsy is to control seizures with a minimal number of ASMs (preferably monotherapy) and minimize the adverse defects. More than half of the patients may become seizure-free with monotherapy.[28,29]

Although there are many ASMs available, the choice depends on epilepsy type, medication availability, and cost as well as comorbidities. Here, we briefly discuss the literature regarding the choice of ASMs in various epilepsy types. The SANAD (Standard and New Antiepileptic Drugs) trials are the largest individual randomized trials examining the different ASMs as monotherapy in epilepsy. The first SANAD trial was conducted in 2007 including 1,721 patients with focal epilepsy and 716 patients with generalized epilepsy. The SANAD II trial included 990 patients with focal epilepsy and 520 patients with generalized epilepsy.[30,31]

Selecting the Antiseizure Medication in Focal Epilepsy

The SANAD trial, published in 2007, was a seminal study of 1,721 patients with focal epilepsy randomized to treatment with carbamazepine, gabapentin, lamotrigine, oxcarbazepine, or topiramate. The primary outcome was time to treatment failure, defined as discontinuation of the drug due to uncontrolled seizures or adverse effects.

Lamotrigine was significantly better than carbamazepine, gabapentin, and topiramate, and nonsignificantly better than oxcarbazepine. For time to 12-month remission, however, carbamazepine was significantly better than gabapentin and nonsignificantly better than lamotrigine, topiramate, and oxcarbazepine. The results of the SANAD trial suggest that lamotrigine is the best first-line treatment for focal epilepsy due to its combination of efficacy and tolerability, with carbamazepine as a reasonable alternative in patients who can tolerate it. Multiple new ASMs have been launched after the SANAD trial, including levetiracetam, zonisamide, lacosamide, and eslicarbazepine. Levetiracetam is the most studied and widely prescribed ASM in patients with focal epilepsy owing to its favorable side effect profile, wide spectrum of epilepsy management, ease of titration, and wide availability. However, it should be used with caution in patients who have a history of psychiatric illness. In patients with psychiatric illness lamotrigine and carbamazepine are better options as the first line.

Selecting the Antiseizure Medication in Generalized Epilepsy

The 2007 SANAD trial included 716 patients with generalized epilepsy or epilepsy that could not be definitively classified at the time of treatment initiation. This trial found that valproate was significantly better than topiramate in terms of time to treatment failure in the overall analysis, and significantly better than both topiramate and lamotrigine in patients with a confirmed diagnosis of generalized epilepsy. For time to 12-month remission, valproate was significantly better than lamotrigine in both groups, but not significantly different from topiramate in either group. Thus, valproate appeared to have the best combination of efficacy and tolerability of the three drugs studied. Similar results in favor of valproate were published in the SANAD II trial, suggesting valproate as the most effective ASM for generalized or unclassified epilepsy. However, the side-effect profile of valproate does not practically make it a drug of choice in generalized epilepsy. Valproate is contraindicated in women of childbearing age due to teratogenicity and long-term neurocognitive deficits in children. Weight gain, hair loss, polycystic ovarian syndrome, hyperammonemia, and hepatic encephalopathy are additional side effects of valproate.

Levetiracetam has emerged as the most extensively studied new antiepileptic drug (AED) for generalized epilepsy as well. In the KOMET (Keppra vs. Older Monotherapy in Epilepsy Trial) study, levetiracetam was found to be equivalent to valproate for both treatment withdrawal rate and time to the first seizure.[32] None of the new AEDs have been studied as monotherapy in patients with generalized epilepsy.

The choice of ASM depends on the seizure type, syndrome, age, gender, comorbidities, and comedications. The general recommendations according to expert opinion are as follows:[33]

- *Initial treatment of focal epilepsy*: Levetiracetam, carbamazepine, oxcarbazepine, lamotrigine, lacosamide
- *Generalized tonic-clonic seizure*: Levetiracetam, lamotrigine, topiramate, valproate, zonisamide
- *Absence seizure*: Ethosuximide, valproate, lamotrigine
- *Myoclonic seizure*: Valproate; avoid carbamazepine.
- *Comorbid psychiatric illness*: Lamotrigine, oxcarbazepine, valproate, or lacosamide; avoid levetiracetam and perampanel.
- *Women of childbearing age/pregnancy*: Levetiracetam and lamotrigine; avoid valproate.

Counseling the Patient with New-onset Epilepsy

In addition to seizure control, the quality of life of PWE is determined by factors such as disability, mental status, ASM side effects, injuries, social stigma, and access to education, employment, and travelling/driving. This section briefly describes the comorbidities for which PWE should be evaluated and the various aspects of counseling that the treating physician should be aware of when dealing with patients with new-onset epilepsy.

The most common comorbidity is psychiatric illness. Depression, anxiety, and suicidal tendencies are seen more commonly in PWE compared to the general population. These may be directly related to epilepsy in terms of being labelled "epileptic," degree of seizure control, fear of having a seizure, loss of independence, number of ASM burden or their side-effects, or due to stigmatization. The stigma associated with epilepsy is deep-rooted. A child may be bullied at school, may not be included in sports or other events at school, and may be left out of parties or trips. Adults may face difficulty in getting married, maintaining relations, bearing children, finding jobs, etc. The PWE may also suffer from learning disabilities that may be due to uncontrolled seizures or as a part of disorders like cerebral palsy. The other comorbidities in PWE include migraine, obesity, and poor bone health due to ASM like phenytoin. Identifying the comorbidities and encouraging the patients to talk about these can help in timely management. Prophylactic replacement of calcium and vitamin D is mostly sufficient to prevent fractures.

It is obvious that a seizure while driving could have catastrophic consequences. The inability to drive can affect a patient's independence, job, and personal responsibilities and increase the financial burden for the patient and family. PWE should be informed that Indian laws do not allow driving in any PWE irrespective of seizure control. Seizures may cause injuries due to falls, fractures, shoulder dislocation, dental injuries, vertebral compression fractures, and tongue lacerations. They can also lead to burns, drowning, and concussions. Hence, unsafe activities such as driving, cooking without supervision, and swimming should be strictly avoided. Electricians, construction workers, drivers, pilots, and heavy machinery workers should be advised to seek alternate jobs.

Excessive emphasis on safety precautions may also discourage people with epilepsy from participating in activities that are part of a healthy lifestyle, such as physical exercise and easy sports. Children should not be barred from education in context of epilepsy. The teachers and schoolmates should be informed about the disease and ideally be trained on the emergency seizure management protocols. Most PWE do not transmit the disease to their children. However, some very rare forms may have genetic risks, and counseling for such individuals should ideally be taken up by a geneticist or epileptologist.

SPECIAL FEATURES OF EPILEPSY IN THE INDIAN CONTEXT

The prevalence of epilepsy in India is 1%[4] As there is a high treatment gap and scarcity of neurologists in India, it is highly likely that the reported prevalence is much less than the actual prevalence. The prevalence in males has been reported to be double than that in females. Cultural and social factors may play a role in male predominance reported in epilepsy in India.

Neurocysticercosis

Neurocysticercosis is commonly found to be the cause of chronic epilepsy in India. NCC is also commonly present with new-onset epilepsy. In a study from rural north India, of 79 patients with first-onset seizure, 43 (54.4%) were diagnosed with NCC based on MRI findings.[34] The radiological findings generally lead to the diagnosis where NCC may be found in different stages. Other than initial steroids and anthelmintic treatment, the management of NCC is not different from other types of epilepsies.

Central Nervous System Tuberculosis

Epilepsy is common in patients with CNS tuberculosis, especially brain tuberculomas. Since the prevalence of tuberculosis in India is high,[35] physicians and neurologists see a large number of patients with new-onset epilepsy attributable to brain tuberculomas. In these patients antitubercular treatment along with ASMs is needed to control the disease. Generally, after the resolution of CNS tuberculosis ASMs can be withdrawn.

Eating Epilepsy

Eating epilepsy is a distinct type of reflex focal epilepsy where seizure is trigged by the act of eating either during or immediately after meals. The focus is likely related to the involvement of perisylvian neuronal circuits.[36] It has been widely reported from the Indian subcontinent.[37-39] The maximum prevalence had been reported in Sri Lanka (5.6% of all epilepsy cases) with prevalence in India <1%.[37,38] It has the usual age of onset in the second decade with male predominance.[40] Giving clobazam half prior to meals in addition to other ongoing ASMs has been reported to be beneficial in controlling epilepsy.[40]

Hot Water Epilepsy

Hot water epilepsy (HWE) is a unique kind of reflex epilepsy, which has been reported from south India where pouring hot water rapidly over the head may induce seizure. Its prevalence has been reported to be 1.14–2.99/1,000 population.[41-44] The exact mechanism of HWE is not known but is likely related to increased sympathetic activity.[45]

CONCLUSION

To conclude, for a patient with new-onset seizures it is essential to rule out acute symptomatic causes. Extensive workup may be needed, and each case of new-onset epilepsy must be visualized. In addition to proper history examination and initial investigations such as EEG and brain imaging, the advanced investigation may be reserved for specific/drug-resistant cases. The choice of ASMs depends on the prominent seizure type in epilepsy and hence should be carefully chosen. Thorough evaluation and management of comorbidities and detailed counseling should also be an integral part of epilepsy management.

REFERENCES

1. Huff JS, Morris DL, Kothari RU, Gibbs MA. Emergency department management of patients with seizures: a multicenter study. Acad Emerg Med. 2001;8(6):622-8.
2. Fisher RS, Acevedo C, Arzimanoglou A, Bogacz A, Cross JH, Elger CE, et al. ILAE official report: a practical clinical definition of epilepsy. Epilepsia. 2014;55(4):475-82.
3. Beghi E, Carpio A, Forsgren L, Hesdorffer DC, Malmgren K, Sander JW, et al. Recommendation for a definition of acute symptomatic seizure. Epilepsia. 2010;51(4):671-5.
4. Sridharan R, Murthy BN. Prevalence and pattern of epilepsy in India. Epilepsia. 1999;40(5):631-6.
5. Gourie-Devi M, Gururaj G, Satishchandra P, Subbakrishna DK. Prevalence of neurological disorders in Bangalore, India: a community-based study with a comparison between urban and rural areas. Neuroepidemiology. 2004;23(6):261-8.
6. Sridharan R. (2002). Epidemiology of epilepsy. [online] Available from http://www.jstor.org/stable/24106692. [Last accessed January, 2023].

7. Goel D, Agarwal A, Dhanai J, Semval VD, Mehrotra V, Saxena V, et al. Comprehensive rural epilepsy surveillance program in Uttarakhand state of India. Neurol India. 2009;57(3):355.
8. Banerjee TK, Ray BK, Das SK, Hazra A, Ghosal MK, Chaudhuri A, et al. A longitudinal study of epilepsy in Kolkata, India. Epilepsia. 2010;51(12):2384-91.
9. Saha SP, Bhattachrya S, Roy BK, Basu A, Roy T, Das SK, et al. A prospective incidence study of epilepsy in a rural community of West Bengal, India. Neurol Asia. 2008;13:41-8.
10. Sawhney IMS, Singh A, Kaur P, Suri G, Chopra JS. A case control study and one year follow-up of registered epilepsy cases in a resettlement colony of North India, a developing tropical country. J Neurol Sci. 1999;165(1):31-5.
11. Mani KS, Rangan G, Srinivas HV, Kalyanasundaram S, Narendran S, Reddy AK. The Yelandur study: a community-based approach to epilepsy in rural South India—epidemiological aspects. Seizure. 1998;7(4):281-8.
12. Krumholz A, Wiebe S, Gronseth GS, Gloss DS, Sanchez AM, Kabir AA, et al. Evidence-based guideline: management of an unprovoked first seizure in adults: report of the guideline development subcommittee of the American Academy of Neurology and the American Epilepsy Society. Neurology. 2015;84(16):1705-13.
13. Hauser WA, Rich SS, Annegers JF, Anderson VE. Seizure recurrence after a 1st unprovoked seizure: an extended follow-up. Neurology. 1990;40(8):1163-70.
14. Chen T, Si Y, Chen D, Zhu L, Xu D, Chen S, et al. The value of 24-hour video-EEG in evaluating recurrence risk following a first unprovoked seizure: a prospective study. Seizure. 2016;40:46-51.
15. Kho LK, Lawn ND, Dunne JW, Linto J. First seizure presentation: do multiple seizures within 24 hours predict recurrence? Neurology. 2006;67(6):1047-9.
16. Bora I, Seçkin B, Zarifoglu M, Turan F, Sadikoglu S, Ogul E. Risk of recurrence after first unprovoked tonic-clonic seizure in adults. J Neurol. 1995;242(3):157-63.
17. Delanty N, Vaughan CJ, French JA. Medical causes of seizures. Lancet (London, England). 1998;352(9125):383-90.
18. Fisher RS, Helen Cross J, French JA, Higurashi N, Hirsch E, Jansen FE, et al. Operational classification of seizure types by the International League Against Epilepsy: position paper of the ILAE commission for classification and terminology. Epilepsia. 2017;58(4):522-30.
19. Scheffer IE, Berkovic S, Capovilla G, Connolly MB, French J, Guilhoto L, et al. ILAE classification of the epilepsies: position paper of the ILAE commission for classification and terminology. Epilepsia. 2017;58(4):512-21.
20. Burkholder DB, Britton JW, Rajasekaran V, Fabris RR, Cherian PJ, Kelly-Williams KM, et al. Routine vs. extended outpatient EEG for the detection of interictal epileptiform discharges. Neurology. 2016;86(16):1524-30.
21. Geut I, Weenink S, Knottnerus ILH, van Putten MJAM. Detecting interictal discharges in first seizure patients: ambulatory EEG or EEG after sleep deprivation? Seizure. 2017;51:52-4.
22. Baldin E, Hauser WA, Buchhalter JR, Hesdorffer DC, Ottman R. Yield of epileptiform electroencephalogram abnormalities in incident unprovoked seizures: a population-based study. Epilepsia. 2014;55(9):1389-98.
23. Leone MA, Giussani G, Nolan SJ, Marson AG, Beghi E. Immediate antiepileptic drug treatment, versus placebo, deferred, or no treatment for first unprovoked seizure. Cochrane database Syst Rev. 2016;2016(5):CD007144.
24. Marson A, Jacoby A, Johnson A, Kim L, Gamble C, Chadwick D. Immediate versus deferred antiepileptic drug treatment for early epilepsy and single seizures: a randomized controlled trial. Lancet (London, England). 2005;365(9476):2007-13.
25. Musicco M, Beghi E, Bordo B, Viani F. Randomized clinical trial on the efficacy of antiepileptic drugs in reducing the risk of relapse after a first unprovoked tonic-clonic seizure. First Seizure Trial Group (FIRST Group). Neurology. 1993;43(3 Pt 1):478-83.
26. Musicco M, Beghi E, Solari A, Viani F. Treatment of first tonic-clonic seizure does not improve the prognosis of epilepsy. First Seizure Trial Group (FIRST Group). Neurology. 1997;49(4):991-8.
27. Leone MA, Solari A, Beghi E. Treatment of the first tonic-clonic seizure does not affect long-term remission of epilepsy. Neurology. 2006;67(12):2227-9.
28. Brodie MJ, Kwan P. Staged approach to epilepsy management. Neurology. 2002;58(8 Suppl 5):S2-8.
29. Kwan P, Brodie MJ. Early identification of refractory epilepsy. N Engl J Med. 2000;342(5):314-9.
30. Marson A, Burnside G, Appleton R, Smith D, Leach JP, Sills G, et al. The SANAD II study of the effectiveness and cost-effectiveness of valproate versus levetiracetam for newly diagnosed generalized and unclassifiable epilepsy: an open-label, noninferiority, multicenter, phase 4, randomized controlled trial. Lancet (London, England). 2021;397(10282):1375-86.
31. Marson A, Burnside G, Appleton R, Smith D, Leach JP, Sills G, et al. The SANAD II study of the effectiveness and cost-effectiveness of levetiracetam, zonisamide, or lamotrigine for newly diagnosed focal epilepsy: an open-label, noninferiority, multicenter, phase 4, randomized controlled trial. Lancet (London, England). 2021;397(10282):1363-74.
32. Trinka E, Marson AG, Van Paesschen W, Kälviäinen R, Marovac J, Duncan B, et al. KOMET: an unblinded, randomized, two parallel-group, stratified trial comparing the effectiveness of levetiracetam with controlled-release carbamazepine and extended-release sodium valproate as monotherapy in patients with newly diagnosed epilepsy. J Neurol Neurosurg Psychiatry. 2013;84(10):1138-47.
33. Shih JJ, Whitlock JB, Chimato N, Vargas E, Karceski SC, Frank RD. Epilepsy treatment in adults and adolescents: expert opinion, 2016. Epilepsy Behav. 2017;69:186-222.
34. Mital AK, Choudhary P, Jain RB. Prevalence and risk factors for neurocysticercosis in children with a first-onset seizure in rural North India. Paediatr Int Child Health. 2020;40(3):158-65.
35. Muralidharan V, Nair BR, Rajshekhar V. Changing trends of presentation of central nervous system tuberculosis: relative prevalence of cranial and spinal tuberculosis and drug resistance patterns. Neurol India. 2019;67(3):792.
36. Patel M, Satishchandra P, Saini J, Bharath RD, Sinha S. Eating epilepsy: phenotype, MRI, SPECT, and video-EEG observations. Epilepsy Res. 2013;107(1-2):115-20.
37. Seneviratne U, Seetha T, Pathirana R, Rajapakse P. High prevalence of eating epilepsy in Sri Lanka. Seizure. 2003;12(8):604-5.
38. Singh P, Bansal AR, More A, Bhuyan S, Garg A. Eating epilepsy in north India: case series and its management. J Epilepsy Res. 2019;9(2):152.
39. Mandal DK, Bandyopadhyay S, Tarafdar J, Mukherjee A, Chaudhury S, Deb A, et al. Eating epilepsy: a study of twenty cases. J Indian Med Assoc. 1992;90(1):9-11.
40. Senanayake N. Eating epilepsy—a reappraisal. Epilepsy Res. 1990;5(1):74-9.
41. Satishchandra P, Sinha S. Hot-water epilepsy: from bench to bedside. Ann Indian Acad Neurol. 2013;16(2):137-43.
42. Mani KS, Mani AJ, Ramesh CK. Hot-water epilepsy—a peculiar type of reflex epilepsy: clinical and EEG features in 108 cases. Trans Am Neurol Assoc. 1974;99:224-6.
43. Mani KS, Gopalakrishnan PN, Vyas JN, Pillai MS. "Hot-water epilepsy"—a peculiar type of reflex epilepsy. A preliminary report. Neurol India. 1968;16(3):107-10.
44. Gururaj G, Satishchandra P. Correlates of hot water epilepsy in rural south India: a descriptive study. Neuroepidemiology. 1992;11(4-6):173-9.
45. Satishchandra P, Ullal GR, Shankar SK. Hot water epilepsy. Adv Neurol. 1998;75:283-93.

65 CHAPTER

Drug-resistant Epilepsy

Chaturbhuj Rathore, Kurupath Radhakrishnan

INTRODUCTION

Treatment with antiseizure medicines (ASMs) remains the cornerstone of epilepsy management. However, approximately one-third of the patients with newly diagnosed epilepsy continue to have seizures despite adequate ASM therapy. These patients with drug-resistant epilepsy (DRE) face multiple medical, social, and economical problems which adversely affect their quality of life. Management of these patients, either medically or surgically, is very challenging. It also requires a multidisciplinary approach with the involvement of several specialties. Despite many diagnostic and therapeutic advances in recent years, the outcome of the patients with DRE has not greatly changed. Nonetheless, many upcoming developments have the potential to change the current situation. In this chapter, we discuss the current concepts in the diagnosis and management of patients with DRE and highlight the potential future therapeutic opportunities.

DEFINING DRUG-RESISTANT EPILEPSY

A universally agreed definition of DRE is essential for establishing an early diagnosis, guiding treatment decisions, and for comparing patient outcomes from different centers. Early diagnosis of drug resistance is important to plan intervention at an early stage so as to avoid long-term psychosocial consequences of uncontrolled seizures. However, due to the diverse underlying etiologies of epilepsy, variable seizure manifestations, and varied outlooks of the patients and their caregivers, it is difficult to develop and apply a uniform definition of DRE in clinical practice.

Practically, one can define drug resistance as the failure of optimal medical therapy to produce long-term seizure freedom. However, the concepts of optimal medical treatment and duration of seizure freedom are subjective which have resulted in various definitions of DRE in the literature. Nonetheless, some evidence-based information is available to guide the clinicians. Many long-term longitudinal studies have reported that approximately one-third of patients with new-onset epilepsy do not respond to optimal medical therapy.[1-3] At the same time, these studies have also shown that the chances of sustained seizure freedom with medical therapy after the failure of two appropriate ASM trials are <5%.[1,3] The International League Against Epilepsy (ILAE) has given a consensus definition of DRE based on this data.[4] The broad framework of this definition consists of two hierarchical levels. Level I is basically focused on categorizing the outcome of each therapeutic intervention (ASM trial) as seizure freedom or treatment failure on the basis of certain standard criteria. If the patient has failed to respond to an adequate trial of an ASM given for a sufficient period, then the outcome is classified as treatment failure. However, if the information is insufficient for determining the efficacy of an intervention, then the outcome is categorized as undermined. Based on Level I assessment, DRE is defined as "failure of adequate trials of two tolerated and appropriately chosen and used antiepileptic drug (AED) schedules (whether as monotherapy or in combination) to achieve sustained seizure freedom." Sustained seizure freedom is defined as seizure freedom for a minimum of 12 months or for a period three times the previous longest seizure-free period, whichever is longer. It is important to realize that drug resistance cannot be defined in the presence of inadequate and suboptimal AED trials, use of inappropriate drugs, and drug failure due to idiosyncratic reactions. The definition places a great emphasis on seizure freedom as it is the only outcome that can lead to sustained improvement in quality of life.

Although the ILAE definition serves as a useful guide, one should have a pragmatic approach while defining drug resistance. Many patients with uncontrolled seizures might not meet the ILAE criteria for drug resistance.[5] The

ILAE definition also does not consider seizure severity and other epilepsy-related complications while defining drug resistance. Apart from the frequency of seizures, their severity and impact on patient's social and occupational life should also be considered. A patient with very infrequent but life-threatening seizures may still be classified as having drug resistance although seizure frequency may be low. Another important consideration is the adverse effects of the ASMs while achieving seizure freedom. If a patient is seizure-free only with doses causing intolerable side effects, then it may also be considered a treatment failure.

EPIDEMIOLOGY

The various studies evaluating the incidence and prevalence of DRE have been heterogeneous with regard to the definition of drug resistance, study settings (whether population-based or hospital-based), and populations studied (adults *vs.* children). This is further complicated by the inclusion of many patients with pseudoresistance. Henceforth, it is difficult to ascertain the accurate epidemiology of DRE. Many long-term hospital-based longitudinal studies have suggested that approximately one-third of the patients with newly diagnosed epilepsy do not respond to ASM therapy.[1-3] In the Glasgow cohort of 1,036 patients, 36% were not seizure-free during the last year of follow-up.[3] This obviously is an overestimate as many patients with mild epilepsy may not come to the hospital, more so in developing countries.

A population-based study of 360 prevalent cases from France identified DRE in 56 (15.5%) cases which corresponded to a prevalence of 0.94 per 1,000 [95% confidence interval (CI) 0.69–1.19].[6] In this study, DRE was defined as the failure of two first-line ASM to produce seizure control with a seizure frequency of one per month or more. By using the ILAE definition of one seizure per year, DRE was identified in 22.2% of cases. The point prevalence of DRE in other population-based studies has varied from 0.08 to 0.1 per 100.[7] In a meta-analysis of 35 observational studies which included 13,080 patients with epilepsy and 3,941 patients with DRE, the pooled prevalence proportion of patients with DRE was 0.30 (95% CI 0.19–0.42).[7] Among the 19 studies which evaluated the incidence proportion of DRE, the pooled incidence proportion was 0.20 (95% CI 0.14–0.27).[7] However, in this analysis, studies were quite heterogeneous and only 12% of the studies met the ILAE criteria of DRE. In a recent meta-analysis involving 103 studies, the cumulative incidence of DRE was 25.0% (95% CI 6.8–34.3) in studies in children, while it was 14.6% in adults. Among people with epilepsy, the prevalence of DRE was 13.7% (95% CI 9.2–19.0) in population-based studies while it was 36.3% (95% CI 30.4–42.4) in clinic-based studies.[8]

RISK FACTORS FOR DRUG-RESISTANT EPILEPSY

Early identification of patients with DRE may help in planning timely intervention without waiting for the trial of unnecessary medicines with resultant side effects. In their widely cited study, Kwan and Brodie showed that response to the first ASM is the major factor that predicts seizure freedom.[1,3] If the patient does not respond to the first ASM, then the chances of subsequent seizure freedom are <25%.[1,3] Other factors consistently associated with DRE in different studies are symptomatic etiology, focal epilepsy, presence of neurological deficit, and an abnormal electroencephalogram (EEG).[8,9] In a large study involving 2,200 patients, Semah and colleagues reported that the clinical course is largely determined by the underlying epilepsy syndrome.[10] In focal epilepsies, etiology is the most important factor in determining the prognosis with mesial temporal sclerosis and focal cortical dysplasia being associated with the highest risk of (80–90%) of developing DRE. Various other factors found to be associated with DRE are early onset of epilepsy, longer disease duration, female sex, presence of status epilepticus, presence of polymorphic seizures, large numbers of seizures before treatment, complex febrile seizures or febrile status epilepticus, developmental delay, and generalized epileptiform discharges on scalp EEG[8,9] **(Box 1)**.

Idiopathic generalized epilepsies are usually considered to be drug-responsive syndromes. However, about one-third of the patients with juvenile myoclonic epilepsy do not adequately respond to ASMs.[11] Presence of psychiatric comorbidity, a combination of all three seizure types (myoclonic jerks, absence seizures, and generalized tonic-clonic seizures), and presence of focal features and generalized paroxysmal fast activity (GPFA) on EEG are the factors associated with drug resistance in juvenile myoclonic epilepsy.[11]

BOX 1 Risk factors for drug-resistant epilepsy.

- Symptomatic epilepsy
- Neurological deficit
- Intellectual disability
- Structural lesion on MRI
- High initial seizure frequency
- Poor response to first antiseizure medicine
- Abnormal EEG
- Polymorphic seizures
- Neonatal seizures
- Status epilepticus
- Febrile seizures
- Psychiatric comorbidity

(EEG: electroencephalogram; MRI: magnetic resonance imaging)

CELLULAR MECHANISMS OF DRUG RESISTANCE

Despite the ongoing research for the last five decades, the underlying cellular mechanisms of drug resistance in epilepsy remain poorly understood. This indicates that drug resistance is likely to be multifactorial in origin and mechanisms may vary depending upon the epilepsy syndrome, genetic profile, epilepsy site, and the type of ASMs used. The cellular mechanisms of drug resistance have been studied mainly in animal models and also in the resected brain tissue in patients with DRE undergoing surgery. In humans, it is very difficult to obtain brain tissue from nonresistant epilepsy cases for comparison. Hence, although many hypotheses regarding putative mechanisms of drug resistance have been proposed, the preclinical and clinical evidence is mostly lacking.[12] It should be noted that these hypotheses are not mutually exclusive but multiple mechanisms may be operational in a given patient. Genetic variations with respect to absorption, metabolism, transfer across blood–brain barrier, target of action in the brain, and elimination of ASMs are being increasingly incriminated in the etiopathogenesis of drug resistance. The proposed mechanisms for drug resistance in epilepsy are illustrated in **Figure 1** and are discussed here.

Alteration of Drug Targets in the Brain (Target Hypothesis)

This hypothesis proposes that the brain targets of ASMs become less sensitive to medicines as a result of structural and functional alterations. The ASMs exert their antiseizure effect by acting on various targets in the brain, which include voltage-gated ion channels, neurotransmitter receptors, and enzymes or transporters involved in the metabolism of neurotransmitters. The strongest evidence for the target hypothesis has come from human studies showing that carbamazepine-induced blockade of voltage-gated sodium channels in hippocampal dentate granule cells is completely absent in patients with DRE.[13] In addition, carbamazepine-induced blockade of fast recovery from depolarization is also significantly reduced in these patients. This effect has also been shown with phenytoin and in hippocampal CA1 neurons in animal models.[14] However, such loss of sodium channel blockade by lamotrigine was not observed in the same studies. These changes have been shown to result from the alteration of various subunits of sodium channels. In addition to voltage-gated sodium channels, experimental evidence has shown that other targets of ASMs are also affected in patients with DRE. Animal studies have demonstrated alteration in various subunits of γ-aminobutyric acid type A ($GABA_A$) receptors, internalization of $GABA_A$ receptors, and change in functions from adult type hyperpolarizing $GABA_A$ receptors to neonatal depolarizing receptors during the process of epileptogenesis.[12,15] All these mechanisms reduce the sensitivity of $GABA_A$ receptors to benzodiazepines and phenobarbitone. However, a major limitation of the target hypothesis is that majority of the patients with DRE are resistant to all the drugs acting through various targets, thereby indicating that mechanisms of drug resistance are not specific for individual ASM. Although plausible, the evidence for the target hypothesis is imperfect, especially for ASMs other than carbamazepine and phenobarbitone.

Alteration of Drug Uptake in the Brain (Transporter Hypothesis)

This hypothesis proposes that the transport of ASMs across the blood–brain barrier and toward their targets is reduced due to increased expression of the multidrug efflux transporters in patients with DRE. Multidrug transporters such as P-glycoprotein (Pgp), multidrug resistance protein (MRP), and breast cancer-related protein (BCRP) are located in the capillary endothelial cells which form the blood–brain barrier and reduce the penetration of multiple drugs.[16] These ATP-binding cassette (ABC) transmembrane proteins remove various substrates from the cell back into the capillary lumen against the concentration gradient and thus maintain the integrity of the blood–brain barrier. It has been shown in human tissues as well as in animal models that Pgp is overexpressed in

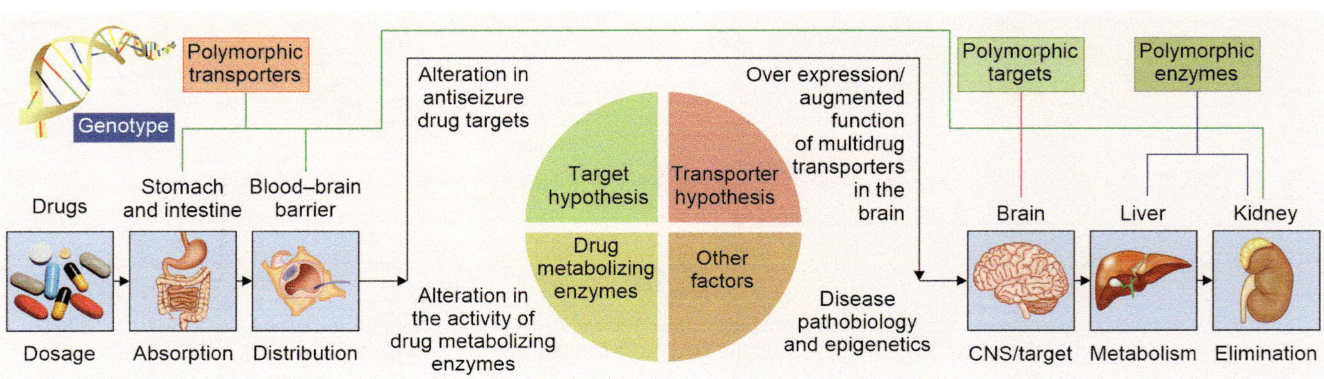

FIG. 1: Genetic influences on the absorption, distribution, metabolism, and targets of action of antiseizure medicines and their implications on drug-resistance.

epileptic tissue.[17,18] Additionally, recent studies have shown overexpression of an intracellular transporter protein, major vault protein (MVP), in the brain tissues of patients with focal DRE, which can be another substrate for drug resistance.[19,20] It has also been shown that at least some ASMs are transported by these membrane transporters and their overexpression is associated with lower brain levels of ASMs **(Figs. 2A and B)**.[17,21] In addition, inhibition of Pgp by tariquidar is associated with increased brain levels of ASMs and can counter the ASM resistance.[22] Positron emission tomography (PET) studies in humans using verapamil, which is a substrate of Pgp, have shown increased expression of Pgp in patients with DRE as compared to normal controls and patients with drug-responsive epilepsy.[23] Pgp is encoded in the *ABCB1* gene, and polymorphism of *ABCB1* gene has been associated with DRE in humans.[24,25] All these facts indicate a substantial role of Pgp and other transporters in causing drug resistance in epilepsy.

However, the direct evidence for the transporter hypothesis in humans is lacking. The most important limitation is that many drugs may not be the substrates for Pgp.[26] Additionally, whether Pgp overexpression is a cause of DRE or effect of repeated seizures is unclear. There is overexpression of Pgp in animal models immediately after a seizure.[12,21] Despite these limitations, Pgp overexpression is a plausible hypothesis and many new drugs targeting Pgp or strategies to bypass Pgp are being explored as potential therapeutic options in patients with DRE.

Neuronal Network Hypothesis

This hypothesis proposes that structural and functional alterations in the form of neurogenesis and astrogliosis during the process of epileptogenesis lead to the development of abnormal neuronal networks with reduced intrinsic inhibitory mechanisms and overexpression of excitatory mechanisms.[27] The most important evidence for this has come from patients with hippocampal sclerosis who demonstrate mossy fiber sprouting and axonal loss in CA1 and CA4 regions. This is further corroborated by the fact that many patients become either seizure-free or pharmacoresponsive after the surgical resection of the sclerosed hippocampus. However, not all the patients with abnormal neural networks develop DRE, and hence the direct validity of this hypothesis in causing drug resistance is rather limited.

Pharmacokinetic Hypothesis

This hypothesis is based on the assumption that there is increased expression of multidrug transporters within peripheral tissues including the gastrointestinal system, liver, and kidneys which prevent the entry or enhanced elimination of ASMs in the blood resulting in low-serum levels of ASMs.[12,21] There are few reports in patients with epilepsy showing low levels of phenytoin in spite of high doses which was associated with increased expression of peripheral drug transporters.[28] However, the majority of the patients with DRE do achieve therapeutic plasma levels of ASMs, and hence this hypothesis is not considered as a major contributor to drug resistance.

Intrinsic Severity Hypothesis

This hypothesis states that people with DRE have intrinsically severe disease and common neurobiological factors contribute to disease severity and drug resistance.[12,21] The hypothesis is based on the observation that a higher number of seizures at the disease onset are associated with

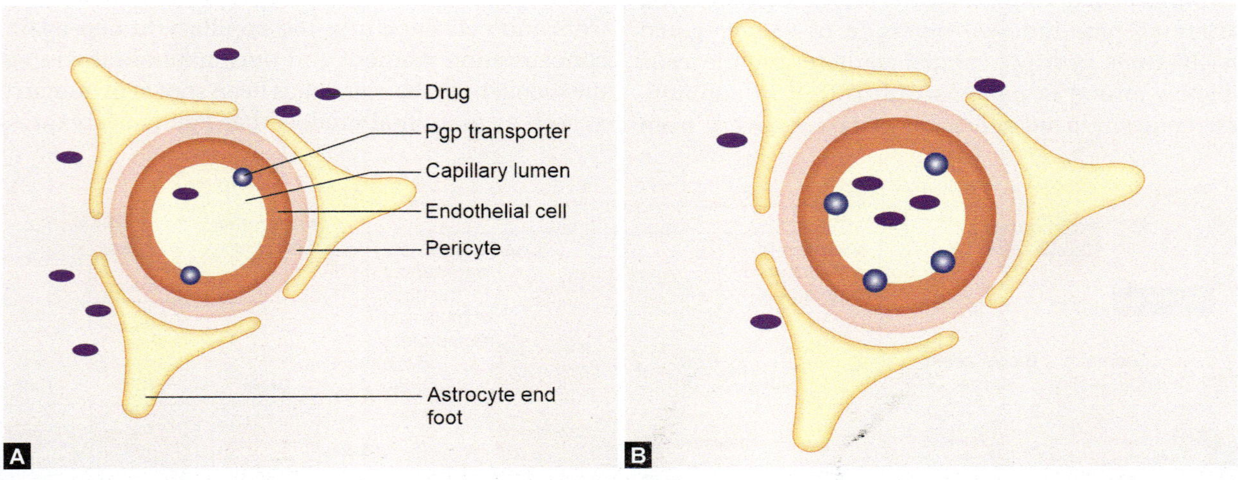

FIGS. 2A AND B: Schematic representation of transporter hypothesis: (A) Normal expression of Pgp transporter at capillary endothelial cells is associated with normal levels of the drug in extravascular space and within target cells; (B) Increased expression of Pgp transporter at capillary endothelial cells transports the drug back into capillary lumen and is associated with lower levels of the drug in the extravascular space.

(Pgp: P-glycoprotein)

the development of DRE.[1] However, many patients with epilepsy have a fluctuating and evolving course and are not resistant from the beginning.[3]

Gene Variant Hypothesis

This hypothesis states that variation in the genes associated with ASM pharmacokinetics and pharmacodynamics can cause drug resistance. This includes genes encoding for enzymes that metabolize ASMs and those encoding channels and receptor targets of ASMs. The evidence for this has come from the studies showing that polymorphisms in genes encoding CYP2C9 (an enzyme that metabolizes phenytoin) are associated with reduced serum levels of phenytoin.[29] Additionally, polymorphism in *SCN1A*, *SCN2A*, and *SCN8A* genes is associated with decreased response to carbamazepine and phenytoin.[12,21] There have been many studies suggesting that *ABCB1* gene polymorphism is associated with increased expression of Pgp in epileptic tissue and drug resistance.[25] However, results from these all studies are inconsistent and the evidence at present is rather feeble. Improvement in genomic technology and its widespread availability at an affordable cost may result in the application of pharmacogenomics in the personalized selection of ASMs, as currently happening in cancer chemotherapy.

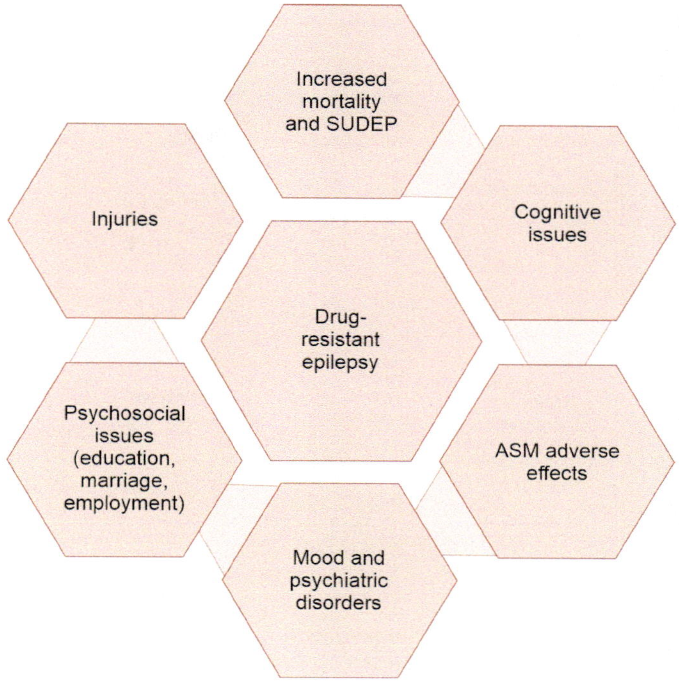

FIG. 3: The comorbidities confronted by patients with drug-resistant epilepsy.
(ASM: antiseizure medicine; SUDEP: sudden unexplained death in epilepsy)

Epigenetic Hypothesis

This hypothesis states that apart from the genome, variations in other "omes" such as epigenome, transcriptome, proteome, and microbiome can be associated with drug resistance.[12,21] Several micro-RNAs have been found to be associated with the development of temporal lobe epilepsy (TLE), but the cause-effect relationship has not been very clear. Similarly, there is emerging evidence linking gut microbiota, response to the ketogenic diet, and development of DRE.[30]

Other Hypotheses

Other putative mechanisms of drug resistance in patients with epilepsy include neuroinflammation, mitochondrial oxidative stress dysfunction, autoantibodies, and electrical coupling through gap junctions in neurons.[12,21] These mechanisms represent the potential areas of future research that may open new avenues for specific therapies.

COMPLICATIONS AND COMORBIDITIES OF DRUG-RESISTANT EPILEPSY

Continuing seizures and medication side effects can cause considerable impairment in daily activities, education, employment, and social interaction in patients with DRE[31,32] **(Fig. 3)**. Repeated or prolonged seizures can cause adverse psychological and behavioral effects. Depression, anxiety, and psychosis are more common in patients with DRE and in those with a longer duration of epilepsy.[31,33] Additional morbidity of uncontrolled seizures includes accidental injury, cognitive decline, and sudden unexplained death in epilepsy (SUDEP).[34] Multiple studies have suggested a progressive decline in memory and cognitive functions in patients with drug-resistant TLE.[35] Quality of life is significantly impaired in these patients with restrictions on driving and socializing. Rates for employment, marriage, and fertility are considerably lower in patients with poorly controlled seizures.[36,37] A long period of inadequate seizure control can produce profound psychosocial problems, including poor academic achievement, diminished self-esteem, dependent behavior, and a restricted lifestyle, all of which lead to impaired quality of life.[36,37] Patients whose seizures are inadequately controlled by AEDs account for 80% of the annual cost attributable to epilepsy.[38]

MANAGEMENT OF DRUG-RESISTANT EPILEPSY

Management of DRE is quite challenging and requires considerable expertise and experience. A multidisciplinary and holistic approach is required while managing patients with DRE because of disease heterogeneity and multiple associated comorbidities and psychosocial issues **(Fig. 4)**. Ideally, all the patients with apparent DRE should be referred to and managed at a compressive epilepsy care center by a multidisciplinary team. As an initial step, a diagnosis of true drug resistance should be established.

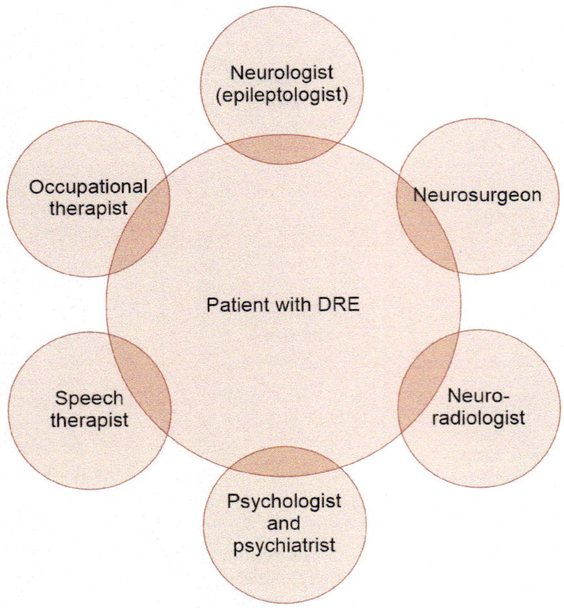

FIG. 4: Multidisciplinary organization in the management of patients with drug-resistant epilepsy (DRE).

All the patients with true DRE should undergo a basic presurgical evaluation as resective surgery, if feasible, offers the best chance of sustained seizure freedom in this group of patients. Continued medical therapy has limitations in these patients but becomes necessary when surgical treatment is not possible. Although seizure freedom is the ultimate treatment goal in all epilepsy patients, it may not be possible in many patients with DRE where the goal should be "minimal seizures with minimal ASM side effects and improved quality of life." It should be noted that the quality of life in these patients who cannot achieve seizure freedom is largely determined by the adverse effects of the ASMs and hence drug overload should be avoided at all costs. Palliative therapies can be offered in selected patients to reduce seizure burden and to improve the quality of life. These basic principles of management are discussed in more detail in the following sections and represented in **Flowchart 1**.

Ruling Out Pseudoresistance

Approximately 20–30% of the patients evaluated at comprehensive epilepsy care centers do not have true DRE due to

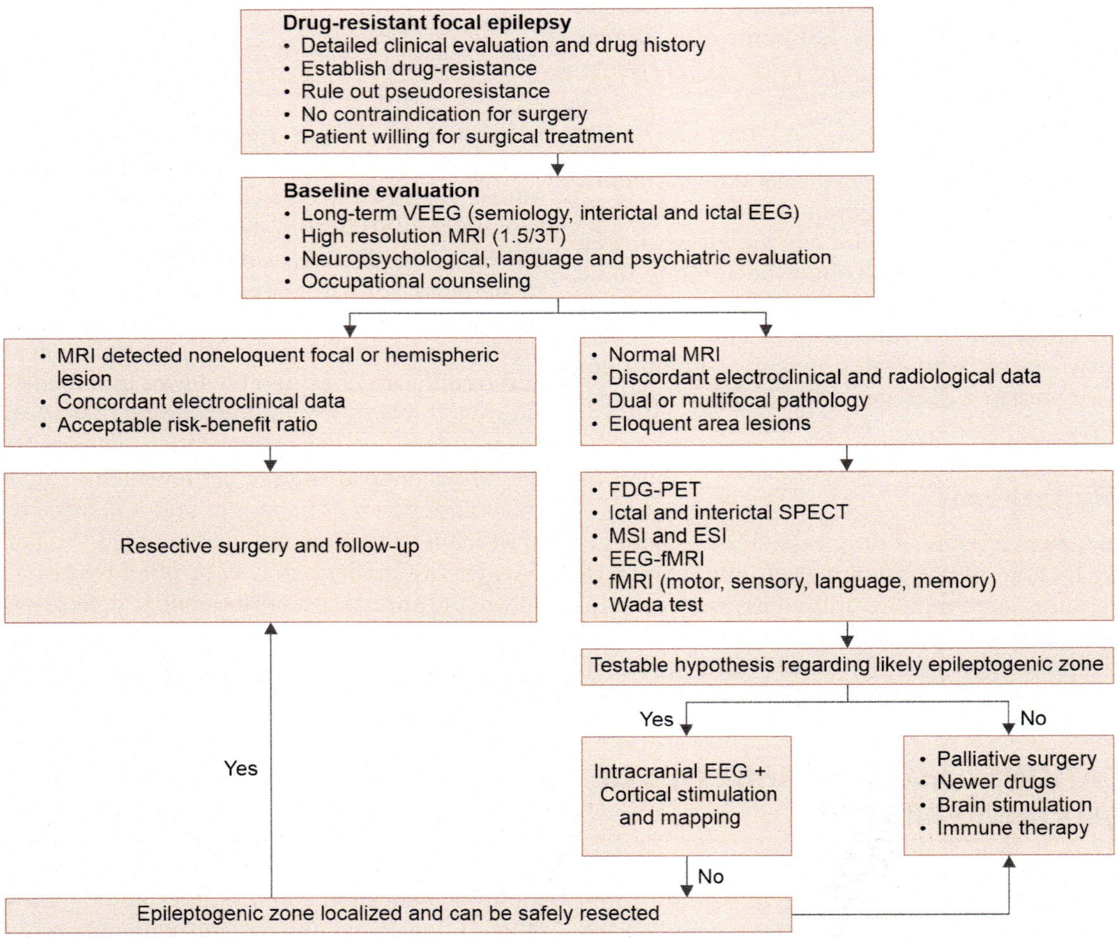

FLOWCHART 1: Step-wise approach to the evaluation and management of patients with drug-resistant epilepsy.

(EEG-fMRI: electroencephalogram–functional MRI; ESI: electrical source imaging; MSI: magnetic source imaging; SPECT: single-photon emission computed tomography; VEEG: video-electroencephalogram)

Source: Adapted from Rathore C, et al (2015).[48]

TABLE 1: Causes of pseudo-drug resistance in epilepsy.

Wrong diagnosis	Other conditions misdiagnosed as epilepsy especially psychogenic nonepileptic events, syncope, parasomnia, etc.
Wrong drug(s)	Inappropriate drug for the epilepsy syndrome, e.g., carbamazepine in patients with juvenile myoclonic epilepsy; pharmacokinetic or pharmacodynamic interactions
Wrong dose	Inadequate dose; frequent changes; dose-limiting side effects
Wrong lifestyle	Poor compliance, sleep disturbances, drug or alcohol abuse

a variety of reasons[39] **(Table 1)**. The most important reason for the pseudoresistance is the wrong diagnosis of epilepsy. Approximately 10–20% of patients admitted for presurgical evaluation have psychogenic nonepileptic events, either in isolation or in combination with true seizures.[39] The other condition commonly misdiagnosed as seizures in adults is syncope, either vasovagal or cardiogenic. A careful analysis of history and video-EEG monitoring will help in establishing the diagnosis of nonepileptic events. Video-EEG monitoring is an essential part of the evaluation of patients with DRE. This may also be helpful in confirming the syndromic diagnosis of epilepsy in difficult cases that can help in choosing the appropriate ASM. A careful evaluation of history and all the past medical records should be undertaken to confirm that the patient has received appropriate medical therapy, at adequate doses, and for the proper duration. Finally, an inquiry should be made about lifestyle issues such as noncompliance, and alcohol and drug abuse which can precipitate seizures in a patient with otherwise well-controlled epilepsy.

Surgical Treatment of Drug-resistant Epilepsy

Resective surgery offers the best chance of sustained seizure freedom in patients with true DRE and hence all the patients with DRE should undergo presurgical evaluation. The process of selecting patients for surgery is quite complex and should be undertaken at a well-equipped comprehensive epilepsy care center under the guidance of an experienced multidisciplinary team.

Surgery for epilepsy is one of the most underutilized therapeutic interventions in spite of its proven efficacy. Three randomized controlled trials and numerous long-term cohort studies have conclusively proven the safety and efficacy of surgery over the continued medical treatment in the selected patients with DRE.[40-44] Surgical therapy with subsequent seizure freedom has been shown to improve the employment rates and lessen the adverse psychosocial consequences leading to an overall improvement in quality of life.[40,45] The above factors clearly suggest that continued medical therapy is not an optimal treatment for certain forms of DRE.

Surgically Remediable Epilepsy Syndromes

With the recognition that certain forms of epilepsy with well-defined pathophysiologic substrates have a poor prognosis after the failure of a few ASMs and an excellent surgical prognosis, the concept of surgically remediable epileptic syndromes was introduced to promote early surgical intervention for these groups of epilepsies[46] **(Box 2; Figs. 5A to F)**. Mesial temporal lobe epilepsy associated with hippocampal sclerosis (MTLE-HS) is the prototype of surgically remediable epileptic syndromes. It is the most common type of focal epilepsy in adults and one that is most resistant to medical treatment and easiest to tackle surgically. Anterior temporal lobectomy (ATL) with amygdalohippocampectomy is the most commonly performed epilepsy surgery, constituting about 60–70% of surgeries in any epilepsy surgery series. Epilepsies associated with cortical dysplasias, benign tumors like ganglioglioma, those with vascular malformations, and certain pediatric epilepsies associated with hemimegalencephaly and Rasmussen's encephalitis also fall in this category. In endemic areas, calcified cysticercus granuloma can be a cause for DRE amenable to surgical treatment.

Early Epilepsy Surgery

With epilepsy surgery becoming safer and less invasive, more emphasis is being placed on the early identification of DRE. Surgical treatment of epilepsy should not be considered as the last resort after all combinations of ASMs have been tried. Preoperative duration of epilepsy ranges from 12 to 20 years in both developed and developing countries.[43,47] Continuing frequent seizures during childhood, adolescence, and early adult life can produce

BOX 2 Surgically remediable epilepsy syndromes.*

- Mesial temporal lobe epilepsy associated with hippocampal sclerosis
- *Circumscribed epileptogenic lesions (not near eloquent areas):*
  - *Benign neoplasms:*
    - Ganglioglioma
    - Dysembryoplastic neuroepithelial tumor
    - Low-grade astrocytoma
    - Oligodendroglioma
  - Vascular malformations
  - Atrophic scars (gliosis)
- *Large unihemispheric epileptogenic lesions (for hemispherotomy):*
  - Hemiconvulsion–hemiplegia–epilepsy syndrome
  - Sturge–Weber syndrome
  - Rasmussen's encephalitis
  - Hemimegalencephaly
- *Epileptic encephalopathies and multifocal disease (for corpus callosotomy):*
  - Lennox–Gastaut syndrome

*Adapted from Rathore C, et al (2015).[48]

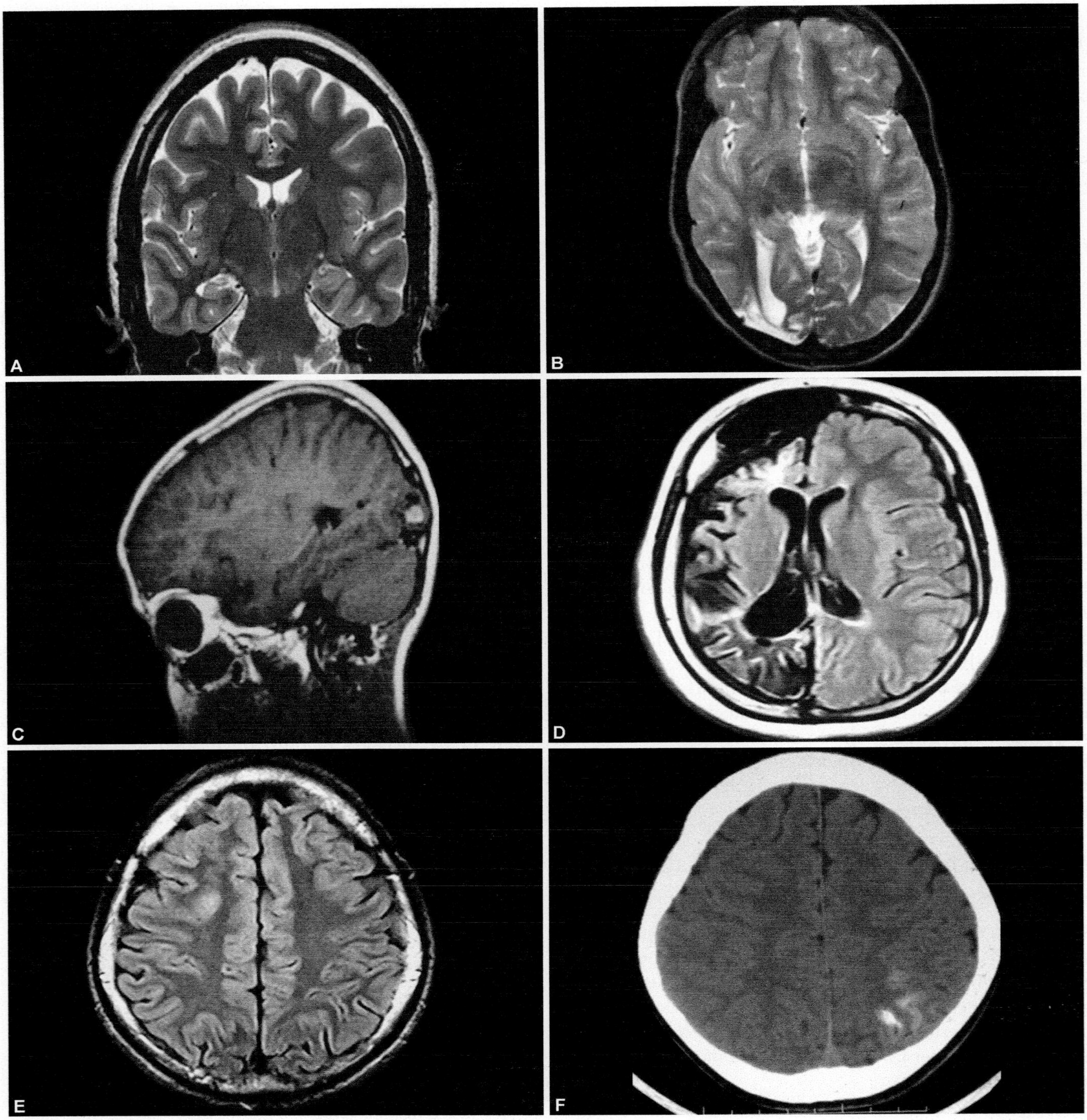

FIGS. 5A TO F: Common surgically remediable syndromes; (A) Right mesial temporal sclerosis; (B) Right occipital gliosis; (C) Left occipital ganglioglioma; (D) Right hemispheric gliosis; (E) Right frontal focal cortical dysplasia; (F) Sturge–Weber syndrome involving left parieto-occipital region.

devastating psychosocial, familial, educational, and occupational sequelae. Once the lifestyle gets fixed, surgical treatment undertaken to successfully terminate seizures may have very little influence on the quality of life of the individual. Referral to a comprehensive epilepsy program should be considered as soon as a trial of two ASM regimens fails to control seizures. One randomized controlled trial has shown the efficacy of early epilepsy surgery over continued medical treatment. However, the trial was prematurely terminated due to difficulty in recruiting patients suggesting a reluctance among the patients and physicians to consider early epilepsy surgery.[41]

Concept and Process of Presurgical Evaluation

The main objective of the presurgical evaluation is to identify an abnormal area of cortex from which the seizures originate and to determine whether it can be removed without producing any significant functional impairment.[48] The final success of epilepsy surgery depends upon the accurate localization and complete removal of the "*epileptogenic zone*," which is defined as the area necessary and sufficient for initiating seizures, and whose removal or disconnection is necessary for the abolition of seizures. The various modalities used for the localization of presumed epileptogenic zone are high-resolution MRI, video-EEG monitoring, neuropsychological testing, interictal PET, single-photon emission computed tomography (SPECT), magnetoencephalography (MEG), and electrical source imaging (ESI) **(Box 3)**. These can be further supplemented by identifying the important functional areas using functional MRI, cortical stimulation and mapping (functional deficit zone), and Wada testing. Few selected patients will require intracranial monitoring for final localization. As all the different modalities provide different information and the information provided by none of the modalities is absolute, chances of surgical success increase with increasing concordance between different modalities.[48] Presurgical evaluation is usually performed in a step-wise manner, with more difficult cases requiring more invasive and complex investigations to define the epileptogenic zone.

BOX 3 **Different modalities used during presurgical evaluation.**

Basic evaluation:
- Detailed clinical evaluation
- Long-term scalp video-EEG monitoring (semiology, interictal, and ictal EEG)
- 1.5T/3T MRI
- Neuropsychological evaluation
- Psychosocial and psychiatric evaluation
- Language evaluation
- Occupational evaluation and counseling

Additional evaluation (in selected cases):

For source localization:
- Novel MRI contrasts and postprocessing
- Interictal and ictal SPECT coregistered to MRI
- FDG–PET
- EEG–fMRI
- Magnetic source imaging
- Electrical source imaging
- Electrocorticography
- Intracranial EEG

For predicting and minimizing postoperative deficits:
- Functional MRI (motor, sensory, language, and memory)
- Wada test
- Diffusion tensor imaging (DTI) and tractography
- Cortical stimulation and mapping

(SPECT: single photon emission computed tomography; FDG–PET: 18-flourodeoxyglucose–positron emission tomography; fMRI: functional MRI)

Source: Adapted from Rathore C, et al (2015).[48]

Outcomes of Epilepsy Surgery

Seizure freedom is the most important outcome following epilepsy surgery. The proportion of patients becoming seizure-free varies depending upon the type and site of surgery **(Table 2)**. Overall, 70–80% of the patients become seizure-free after temporal resections and hemispheric surgeries while 50–60% become seizure-free following extratemporal resections.[40,43,44,49,50] ASMs can be stopped in 40–50% of patients following temporal resections and in 25–30% of patients following extratemporal resections.[43,51] Quality of life and chances of meaningful employment improve following successful epilepsy surgery.[45,52] Epilepsy surgery is very safe and the chances of major complications after resective epilepsy surgery are <1%.[53] There is 10–15% risk of minor decline in verbal memory following dominant temporal lobe resections which can be minimized by proper selection of the patients.[54] Limited data suggest that mortality risk is also reduced after successful epilepsy surgery.[55]

Palliative Surgery and Other Palliative Procedures

Palliative surgery is an option in those patients with DRE where resective and curative epilepsy surgery is not possible due to various reasons. The aim of palliative surgery is to reduce the burden of disabling seizures and thus improve the quality of life of the patients. Corpus callosotomy is reserved for patients with refractory severe epilepsy resulting in frequent generalized seizures and injurious drop attacks with no focal substrate for epilepsy. Lennox–Gastaut syndrome with drop attacks remains the best indication with approximately 80% of patients becoming free of drop attacks.[56] Neurostimulation procedures including vagal nerve stimulation, deep brain stimulation of the subthalamic nucleus, and responsive

TABLE 2: Seizure and antiseizure medicine-related outcomes following different types of epilepsy surgeries.

Type of surgery	Seizure-free outcome	Antiseizure medicine-free outcome
Temporal resections	66–80%	30–50%
Extratemporal resections	50–60%	25–30%
Hemispherotomy	70–80%	50–70%
Corpus callosotomy*	80%	Nil
VNS, DBS, and RNS#	50%	Nil

* Patients free of drop attacks.

50% responder rate.

(DBS: deep brain stimulation; RNS: responsive neurostimulation; VNS: vagus nerve stimulation) neurostimulation have been shown to reduce seizures frequency in 50% of the patients.[57]

The ketogenic diet has proven efficacy in reducing seizure burden in children and adolescents with DRE. Randomized controlled trials have shown that it reduces seizure frequency by 50% in half of the patients after 1 year of diet.[58] However, its efficacy in adult patients needs further evidence. The major problem is the tolerability of high-fat unpleasant dietary regimens and the need for close supervision. The Modified Atkins diet is a potential alternative in less supervised settings. In a pilot study, probiotic therapy was shown to reduce seizure frequency in 30% of the patients but it needs further proof.[59]

Optimizing Antiseizure Medicine Therapy

Many long-term follow-up studies of patients with new-onset epilepsy have shown that the chances of seizure freedom with further ASM trials after the failure of two AED regimens are very low.[1-3] The situation has not changed much after the introduction of newer ASMs in recent years. The long-term follow-up of Glasgow cohort has shown that the proportion of patients becoming seizure-free with ASM therapy has remained the same over the last 20 years.[1,3] However, many recent studies have shown that approximately 20% of the patients with DRE patients with DRE can become seizure-free with further ASM trials, though a majority (70%) of them relapse on long-term follow-up.[60,61] The studies have also shown that seizure frequency can be reduced by 50% in 20–70% of these patients. These data provide hope for these patients with DRE who otherwise are destined to live with continued seizures and call for continued ASM trials in patients with disabling seizures.

There is no definite evidence or guidelines to help in the choice of ASMs after the failure of two ASM regimens and treatment needs to be individualized. There are no studies that have compared the different drugs or drug combinations in patients with DRE mainly due to logistic reasons. Efficacy data for the majority of the ASMs come from the phase III efficacy trials where one ASM is compared against a placebo in patients with DRE. This data does not provide information regarding the comparative efficacy of different ASMs. Extrapolating this data with an aim of indirect comparison between different drugs or through network meta-analysis has its limitations as placebo response varies between different studies. Secondly, these studies typically do not use seizure freedom as the primary outcome. The primary outcome of these trials is either decrease in the median monthly seizure frequency or a 50% responder rate (proportion of patients with >50% reduction in seizure frequency). Finally, these trials include only one seizure type in the outcome analysis and not all the seizures a patient is having. All these limitations preclude any meaningful analysis of the comparative efficacy of various ASMs.

In the absence of vigorous data, the clinicians usually follow the principle of rationale polytherapy or the pharmacomechanistic approach, although direct evidence for such an approach is not robust. This is based on the principle that combining ASMs with different mechanisms of action may produce a better or synergistic effect as compared to combining drugs with the same mechanism of action. The evidence for this approach has come from a few observational controlled studies in adults. Cereghino and colleagues in 1975 first reported that combining two drugs with the same mechanism of action may not be useful. They reported that combining phenobarbitone with phenytoin was more effective than combining phenytoin and carbamazepine in 47 cognitively impaired patients.[62] A comprehensive review of all the animal and human studies showed that combining sodium channel blockers with drugs having GABAergic action is particularly useful.[63] In clinical studies, the combination of valproate and lamotrigine has been consistently shown to have a probable synergistic effect in both focal and generalized epilepsies.[64,65] Other combinations, believed to be synergistic, are ethosuximide and valproate for the absence seizures, carbamazepine and clobazam for focal seizures, and lamotrigine with topiramate for the broad range of seizures.[66-68] The combinations of stiripentol with clobazam and cannabidiol with clobazam are also thought to be particularly useful in patients with Dravet syndrome.[68,69] Combining the drugs with the different mechanisms of action also decreases the risk of adverse effects. In the pooled analysis of lacosamide data, the rate of adverse events doubled when it was combined with another sodium channel-blocking agent as compared to its combination with drugs with a different mechanism of action.[70]

Recent results from SANAD (Standard vs. newer antiepileptic drugs) trials have shown that certain ASMs are more effective than others. Valproate remains the most effective drug in patients with generalized epilepsies.[71] Recent data in patients with drug-resistant juvenile myoclonic epilepsy have shown that valproate and lamotrigine combination is the most effective duo therapy in these patients and it should be tried in all the patients with drug-resistant genetic generalized epilepsies.[11] The chances of seizure freedom after the failure of the valproate and lamotrigine combination are remote. Still, these patients can be tried on topiramate, zonisamide, and perampanel if seizures are disabling. In patients with focal epilepsy, carbamazepine remains the most effective drug, although it may be associated with more adverse reactions.[72] We usually combine carbamazepine with clobazam as initial duo therapy in patients with drug-resistant focal epilepsy. In nonresponders, we try to switch over to a combination of valproate and lamotrigine due to its proven efficacy. In cases resistant to valproate and lamotrigine, all the other possible combinations can be tried, though the chances of seizure freedom are remote.

Certain side effects and side benefits of various ASMs should be kept in mind while selecting a drug for a patient with DRE. In patients with associated mood disorders and psychiatric problems, drugs such as levetiracetam and perampanel can be avoided while other mood-stabilizing drugs such as carbamazepine and valproate can be preferred. Similarly, valproate and topiramate may be preferred in patients with associated migraine. Topiramate and zonisamide may be preferred in patients with obesity. Such an approach of individuating the treatment approach offers the best chance of improving the quality of life of these patients.

Seizure freedom is an elusive goal in these patients. One should avoid too frequent changes in ASM therapy before trying one medicine in sufficient doses and for a sufficient duration. The quality of life in these patients is also determined by the adverse reaction to drugs especially those affecting cognition, coordination, and mood.[73] Rationalizing the therapy and reducing the drug load are likely to improve the quality of life in patients with DRE. One should not keep on adding drugs in the hope that more drugs will produce better seizure control. Ineffective drugs should be removed at each step while adding a new drug. The goal of therapy should be clearly explained to the patients and sometimes continuing the same therapy for minor nondisabling seizures may be the best option. The principles of drug therapy in DRE are summarized in **Box 4 and Flowchart 2**.

Autoimmune Epilepsy and Immune Therapy

Autoimmune epilepsies can present with purely drug-resistant seizures without other manifestations. It has been shown that many patients with DRE have underlying immune mechanisms and benefit from immune therapy.[74] While the role of immune therapy in certain childhood epileptic encephalopathies and autoimmune encephalitis is well established, it should also be considered in patients

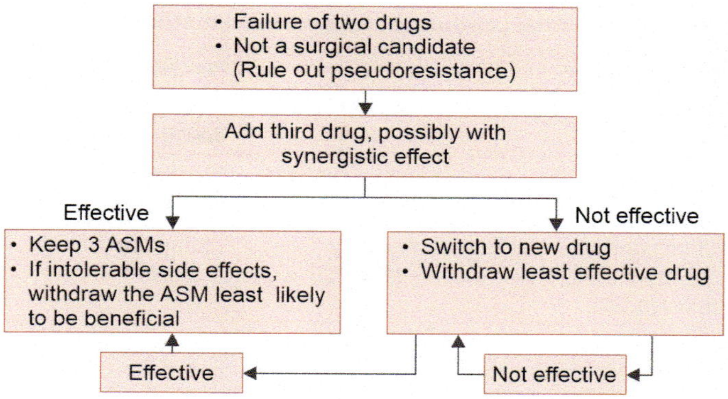

FLOWCHART 2: Step-wise approach to the medical management of the patients with drug-resistant epilepsy.

with medically and surgically refractory epilepsy especially if the patient has an explosive onset, multifocal seizures, and associated mild cognitive changes.

Novel Antiseizure Medicines

Although the currently available ASMs have not been able to change the outcome of DRE to a great extent, there is a hope that this scenario might change with the availability of a few newer drugs in near future. Cenobamate has been recently approved by the Food and Drug Administration (FDA) for the treatment of partial seizures in adults. Clinical trials of this drug have shown that it produced seizure freedom in 20% of the patients with DRE which is highly impressive.[75] Cenobamate acts through a dual mechanism of sodium channel blockade and enhancement of GABA transmission. Similar impressive results have been obtained with fenfluramine, a serotonin agonist which acts on 5HT2B/C receptors, in patients with Dravet syndrome where it produced long-term seizure freedom in 25% of the patients.[76] Padsevonil is a new molecule that is undergoing phase III trials to test its efficacy in patients with DRE.[77] It also has dual mechanism as it acts on the presynaptic SV2 proteins as well as on postsynaptic $GABA_A$ receptors. The preclinical results with this drug have shown a good effect on seizure control. With the availability of these new drugs, the chances of seizure freedom in patients with DRE are likely to improve.

Precision Medicine

It is a treatment approach in which disease treatment is tailored according to the individual's unique genetic structure, lifestyle, and environment. Although clinicians have been individualizing the treatment according to a patient's unique characteristics, the scenario has changed with the recent advances in genomic techniques. With the identification of many causative genes and underlying mechanisms and biology for various epilepsies, rationale

BOX 4 **Principles of medical management in drug-resistant epilepsy.**

- Make sure each drug regimen is given a fair chance to work:
  - Try each drug in optimal doses before discarding
  - Give sufficient time for the efficacy to be known
- Avoid overdosing, toxicity, and inadequate polypharmacy:
  - Remove unnecessary drugs at each step
- Choose add-on drugs by virtue of their efficacy, tolerability, and possible side benefits
- CBZ + CLB and VPA + LTG are probable synergistic combinations
- Keep trying and do not loose heart in patients with disabling seizures
- Know and accept when progress is unlikely

(CBZ: carbamazepine; CLB: clobazam; LTG: lamotrigine; VPA: valproic acid)

TABLE 3: Potential candidates for precision medicine therapy in epilepsy.

Mutated gene	Protein function	Epilepsy syndrome	Potentially useful treatment
Aldehyde dehydrogenase 7 family member A1 (ALDH7A1)	Aldehyde dehydrogenase	Pyridoxin-dependent epilepsy	Pyridoxine (B6 vitamin)
Cholinergic receptor nicotinic alpha 4 subunit (CHRNA4)	Nicotinergic acetylcholine receptor	Nocturnal frontal lobe epilepsy	Acetazolamide, zonisamide, and nicotine patches
Glutamate ionotropic receptor N-methyl-D-aspartate (NMDA) type subunit 2A and 2B (GRIN2A, 2B)	Glutamate (NMDA) receptor	Focal epilepsy and speech disorder ± mental retardation	Memantine, dextromethorphan
Potassium voltage-gated channel subfamily A member 2 (KCNA2)	Voltage-gated potassium channel	EIEE	4-aminopyridine
Potassium voltage-gated channel subfamily Q member 2 (KCNQ2)	Potassium channel	Benign familial neonatal convulsions; EIEE	Retigabine/ezogabine
Potassium sodium-activated channel subfamily T member 1 (KCNT1)	Potassium channel	EIEE	Quinidine
Protocadherin 19 (PCDH19)	Cell adhesion molecule	EIEE	Potassium bromide, clobazam
Phospholipase C beta 1 (PLCB1)	Unclassified enzyme	EIEE	Inositol
Pyridoxamine 5'-phosphate oxidase (PNPO)	PNP oxidase	PNP oxidase deficiency	Pyridoxal-5-phosphate
Proline-rich transmembrane protein 2 (PRRT2)	Unclassified enzyme	Benign familial infantile seizures with paroxysmal choreoathetosis	Carbamazepine, oxcarbazepine
Sodium voltage-gated channel alpha subunit 1 (SCN1A)	Voltage-gated sodium channel	Dravet syndrome	GABAergic drugs, fenfluramine, cannabidiol
Sodium voltage-gated channel alpha subunit 2 (SCN2A)	Voltage-gated sodium channel	Benign familial infantile seizures; EIEE	High-dose phenytoin, levetiracetam
Sodium voltage-gated channel alpha subunit 2 (SCN2A)	Voltage-gated sodium channel	EIEE	Lidocaine, acetazolamide
Sodium voltage-gated channel alpha subunit 8 (SCN8A)	Voltage-gated sodium channel	Benign familial infantile seizures; EIEE	Phenytoin, carbamazepine, amitriptyline, nilvadipine, carvedilol
Solute carrier family 2 member 1 (SLC2A1)	Transporter	GLUT-1 deficiency	Ketogenic diet
Syntaxin-binding protein 1 (STXBP1)	Membrane trafficking	EIEE	Levetiracetam, folinic acid, vigabatrin
TSC (tuberous sclerosis complex) subunits 1 and 2 (TSC1 and 2)	Unclassified; mutations cause increased mTOR activity	Tuberous sclerosis	Everolimus

(EIEE: early infantile epileptic encephalopathy)

treatment strategies have been devised, sometimes with dramatic results. The best example is Dravet syndrome which results from the mutations in *SCN1A* gene and where drugs acting through sodium channel blockers are either ineffective or counterproductive. Many new pathogenic variations in different genes have been identified, especially in early onset epileptic encephalopathies that can be targeted with a specific therapy[12] **(Table 3)**. However, many of such case reports are anecdotal and precision therapy with a theoretically ideal molecule has not been effective. Still, it represents an exciting area in epilepsy therapy and has the potential to change the outcome of many patients with DRE.

IMPROVING OUTCOMES AND FUTURE PERSPECTIVES

Although the outcomes in DRE epilepsy have not changed over the last three decades, the recent and upcoming developments do offer some hope. Improving the outcomes in DRE is an ongoing process and research is being done at multiple levels. Consistent with multifactorial mechanisms of DRE, it is prudent to conclude that no single approach is likely to be useful in greatly changing the outcomes. It is the combination of medical, surgical, immune, and genetic therapies that can improve outcomes in these patients. On the medical front, the development of newer ASM with multiple mechanisms of action has the potential to improve seizures control in patients with DRE. Similarly, drugs targeting the potential mechanisms of drug resistance are being explored as new therapies in patients with DRE. Verapamil, a competitive inhibitor of Pgp, has been shown to be of benefit in animal studies and an open-label pilot study.[78] During the process of epileptogenesis, there is a reversal of inhibitory GABAergic transmission to an excitatory GABAergic transmission probably due to the intracellular accumulation of chlorine by the overexpression of sodium/potassium/chlorine exchanger NKCC1. Bumetanide, an inhibitor of NKCC1, has shown promising results in animal studies and, along with other NKCC1 inhibitors, is a promising future treatment.[79] Considering the role of inflammation in drug resistance, cyclooxygenase-2 inhibitors and interleukin-1 inhibitors are being explored as potential therapeutic options.[80] However, all these are only a few of the approaches being explored for improving the management of DRE.

On the surgical front, acceptance of stereo-EEG world over has helped in improving outcomes of epilepsy surgery and has resulted in the surgical treatment of more difficult cases with resultant improvement in seizure control.[81] This along with further advances in structural and functional imaging techniques including 7T MRI is likely to improve the selection of many patients for epilepsy surgery.[82] Better delineation of EEG signals using quantitative EEG techniques, delineation of epilepsy networks using functional MRI techniques, and exploration of high-frequency oscillation as surrogate markers of epileptogenicity have the potential to refine the outcomes following epilepsy surgery.[83] There have been further developments in palliative treatment options with pilot studies showing benefits with transcranial magnetic stimulation and trigeminal nerve stimulation.[57] As discussed above, with advances in genetic technologies and the identification of many causative genes in DREs, precision medicine and gene therapy are potential future options.

INDIAN SCENARIO

With an epilepsy prevalence of 0.5%, there are more than one million people with DRE in India, and half of them are potential surgical candidates. However, only <2% of these patients undergo a comprehensive evaluation and presurgical assessment.[84] There are only 53 centers in India that offer comprehensive epilepsy care, video-EEG monitoring, and epilepsy surgery.[85] Annually, <1,000 epilepsy surgeries are performed in India.[84,85] These data indicate a large gap in the evaluation and management of patients with DRE in India and call for comprehensive action at multiple levels for increasing the awareness regarding proper assessment and epilepsy surgery for DRE in India. There are large waiting lists for video-EEG monitoring and epilepsy surgery in major government centers in India while the evaluation at private hospitals is expensive.[84] There is a need for the development of innovative and cost-effective models for the assessment and management of patients with DRE in India.

CONCLUSION

Approximately one-third of patients with epilepsy do not respond to adequate trials of ASMs and the management of these patients with DRE poses inimitable challenges. Due to the multiple comorbidities, management of these patients requires a multidisciplinary and holistic approach. Once the pseudoresistance is ruled out, all the patients with DRE should be evaluated for epilepsy surgery as resective surgery in carefully selected patients offers the best chance of long-term seizure freedom in these patients. Few patients with disabling seizures can benefit from palliative surgery. Although chances of seizure freedom with further ASMs trials are low, adequate trials of ASMs should be given to all the patients with disabling seizures while avoiding drug overload. Newer developments in the medical, surgical, and genetic fields offer new hopes for many patients with DRE.

REFERENCES

1. Kwan P, Brodie MJ. Early identification of refractory epilepsy. N Engl J Med. 2000;342:314-9.
2. Sillanpaa M, Schmidt D. Natural history of treated childhood-onset epilepsy: prospective, long-term population-based study. Brain. 2006;129:617-24.
3. Chen Z, Brodie MJ, Liew D, Kwan P. Treatment outcomes in patients with newly diagnosed epilepsy treated with established and new antiepileptic drugs: A 30-year longitudinal cohort study. JAMA Neurol. 2018;75:279-86.
4. Kwan P, Arzimanoglou A, Berg AT, Brodie MJ, Allen Hauser W, Mathern G, et al. Definition of drug resistant epilepsy: consensus proposal by the ad hoc Task Force of the ILAE Commission on Therapeutic Strategies. Epilepsia. 2010;51:1069-77.
5. Zaccara G, Mula M, Ferrò B, Consoli D, Elia M, Giallonardo AT, et al. Do neurologists agree in diagnosing drug resistance in adults with focal epilepsy? Epilepsia. 2019;60:175-83.
6. Picot MC, Baldy-Moulinier M, Daurès JP, Dujols P, Crespel A. The prevalence of epilepsy and pharmacoresistant epilepsy in adults: a population-based study in a Western European country. Epilepsia. 2008;49:1230-8.
7. Kalilani L, Sun X, Pelgrims B, Noack-Rink M, Villanueva V. The epidemiology of drug-resistant epilepsy: A systematic review and meta-analysis. Epilepsia. 2018;59:2179-93.
8. Sultana B, Panzini MA, Veilleux Carpentier A, Comtois J, Rioux B, Gore G, et al. Incidence and prevalence of drug-resistant epilepsy: A systematic review and meta-analysis. Neurology. 2021;96:805-17.
9. Xue-Ping W, Hai-Jiao W, Li-Na Z, Xu D, Ling L. Risk factors for drug-resistant epilepsy: A systematic review and meta-analysis. Medicine (Baltimore). 2019;98:e16402.
10. Semah F, Picot MC, Adam C, Broglin D, Arzimanoglou A, Bazin B, et al. Is the underlying cause of epilepsy a major prognostic factor for recurrence? Neurology. 1998;51:1256-62.

11. Baheti N, Rathore C, Bansal AR, Shah S, Veedu HK, Prakash S, et al. Treatment outcomes in drug resistant juvenile myoclonic epilepsy: Valproate resistance may not be the end of the road. Seizure. 2021;92:112-7.
12. Löscher W, Potschka H, Sisodiya SM, Vezzani A. Drug resistance in epilepsy: Clinical impact, potential mechanisms, and new innovative treatment options. Pharmacol Rev. 2020;72:606-38.
13. Remy S, Gabriel S, Urban BW, Dietrich D, Lehmann TN, Elger CE, et al. A novel mechanism underlying drug resistance in chronic epilepsy. Ann Neurol. 2003;53:469-79.
14. Remy S, Urban BW, Elger CE, Beck H. Anticonvulsant pharmacology of voltage-gated Na^+ channels in hippocampal neurons of control and chronically epileptic rats. Eur J Neurosci. 2003;17:2648-58.
15. Coulter DA. Mossy fiber zinc and temporal lobe epilepsy: pathological association with altered "epileptic" gamma-aminobutyric acid A receptors in dentate granule cells. Epilepsia. 2000;41 (Suppl 6):S96-9.
16. König J, Müller F, Fromm MF. Transporters and drug-drug interactions: important determinants of drug disposition and effects. Pharmacol Rev. 2013;65:944-66.
17. Tishler DM, Weinberg KI, Hinton DR, Barbaro N, Annett GM, Raffel C. MDR1 gene expression in brain of patients with medically intractable epilepsy. Epilepsia. 1995;36:1-6.
18. Liu JY, Thom M, Catarino CB, Martinian L, Figarella-Branger D, Bartolomei F, et al. Neuropathology of the blood-brain barrier and pharmaco-resistance in human epilepsy. Brain. 2012;135:3115-33.
19. Balan S, Lekshmi S, Radha K, Vijai J, Banerjee M, Radhakrishnan K. Major vault protein (MVP) gene polymorphisms and drug resistance in mesial temporal lobe epilepsy with hippocampal sclerosis. Gene. 2013;526:449-53.
20. Liu B, Wang T, Wang L, Wang C, Zhang H, Gao GD. Up-regulation of major vault protein in the frontal cortex of patients with intractable frontal lobe epilepsy. J Neurol Sci. 2011;308:88-93.
21. Tang F, Hartz AMS, Bauer B. Drug-resistant epilepsy: multiple hypotheses, few answers. Front Neurol. 2017;8:301.
22. Brandt C, Bethmann K, Gastens AM, Löscher W. The multidrug transporter hypothesis of drug resistance in epilepsy: proof-of-principle in a rat model of temporal lobe epilepsy. Neurobiol Dis. 2006;24:202-11.
23. Feldmann M, Asselin MC, Liu J, Wang S, McMahon A, Anton-Rodriguez J, et al. P-glycoprotein expression and function in patients with temporal lobe epilepsy: a case-control study. Lancet Neurol. 2013;12:777-85.
24. Siddiqui A, Kerb R, Weale ME, Brinkmann U, Smith A, Goldstein DB, et al. Association of multidrug resistance in epilepsy with a polymorphism in the drug-transporter gene ABCB1. N Engl J Med. 2003;348:1442-8.
25. Bournissen FG, Moretti ME, Juurlink DN, Koren G, Walker M, Finkelstein Y. Polymorphism of the MDR1/ABCB1 C3435T drug-transporter and resistance to anti-convulsant drugs: a meta-analysis. Epilepsia. 2009;50:898-903.
26. Baltes S, Gastens AM, Fedrowitz M, Potschka H, Kaever V, Löscher W. Differences in the transport of the antiepileptic drugs phenytoin, levetiracetam and carbamazepine by human and mouse P-glycoprotein. Neuropharmacology. 2007;52:333-46.
27. Fang M, Xi ZQ, Wu Y, Wang XF. A new hypothesis of drug refractory epilepsy: neural network hypothesis. Med Hypotheses. 2011;76:871-6.
28. Lazarowski A, Czornyj L, Lubienieki F, Girardi E, Vazquez S, D'Giano C. ABC transporters during epilepsy and mechanisms underlying multidrug resistance in refractory epilepsy. Epilepsia. 2007;48 (Suppl 5):140-9.
29. van der Weide J, Steijns LS, van Weelden MJ, de Haan K. The effect of genetic polymorphism of cytochrome P450 CYP2C9 on phenytoin dose requirement. Pharmacogenetics. 2001;11:287-91.
30. Olson CA, Vuong HE, Yano JM, Liang QY, Nusbaum DJ, Hsiao EY. The gut microbiota mediates the anti-seizure effects of the ketogenic diet. Cell. 2018;173:1728-41.
31. Hauser WA, Hesdorffer DC. Epilepsy: Frequency, Causes and Consequences. New York City: Demos Press; 1990.
32. Quintas R, Raggi A, Giovannetti AM, Pagani M, Sabariego C, Cieza A, et al. Psychosocial difficulties in people with epilepsy: a systematic review of literature from 2005 until 2010. Epilepsy Behav 2012;25:60-7.
33. Torta R, Keller R. Behavioral, psychotic, and anxiety disorders in epilepsy: etiology, clinical features, and therapeutic implications. Epilepsia. 1999;40 (Suppl 10):S2-20.
34. Sperling MR, Feldman H, Kinman J, Liporace JD, O'Connor MJ. Seizure control and mortality in epilepsy. Ann Neurol. 1999;46:45-50.
35. Hwang G, Hermann B, Nair VA, Conant LL, Dabbs K, Mathis J, et al. Brain aging in temporal lobe epilepsy: Chronological, structural, and functional. Neuroimage Clin. 2020;25:102183.
36. Varma NP, Sylaja PN, George L, Sarma PS, Radhakrishnan K. Employment concerns of people with epilepsy in Kerala, South India. Epilepsy Behav. 2007;10:250-4.
37. Santosh D, Kumar TS, Sarma PS, Radhakrishnan K. Women with onset of epilepsy prior to marriage: disclose or conceal? Epilepsia. 2007;48:1007-10.
38. Begley CE, Famulari M, Annegers JF, Lairson DR, Reynolds TF, Coan S, et al. The cost of epilepsy in the United States: an estimate from population-based clinical and survey data. Epilepsia. 2000;41:342-51.
39. Benbadis SR, Agrawal V, Tatum WO. How many patients with psychogenic nonepileptic seizures also have epilepsy? Neurology. 2001;57:915-7.
40. Wiebe S, Blume WT, Girvin JP, Eliasziw M; Effectiveness and Efficiency of Surgery for Temporal Lobe Epilepsy Study Group. A randomized, controlled trial of surgery for temporal lobe epilepsy. N Engl J Med. 2001;345:311-8.
41. Engel J Jr, McDermott MP, Wiebe S, Langfitt JT, Stern JM, Dewar S, et al.; Early Randomized Surgical Epilepsy Trial (ERSET) Study Group. Early surgical therapy for drug-resistant temporal lobe epilepsy: a randomized trial. JAMA. 2012;307:922-30.
42. Dwivedi R, Ramanujam B, Chandra PS, Sapra S, Gulati S, Kalaivani M, et al. Surgery for drug-resistant epilepsy in children. N Engl J Med. 2017;377:1639-47.
43. Rathore C, Panda S, Sarma PS, Sapra S, Gulati S, Kalaivani M, et al. How safe is it to withdraw antiepileptic drugs following successful surgery for mesial temporal lobe epilepsy? Epilepsia. 2011;52:627-35.
44. Jain P, Tomlinson G, Snead C, Sander B, Widjaja E. Systematic review and network meta-analysis of resective surgery for mesial temporal lobe epilepsy. JNNP. 2018;89:1138-44.
45. Siriratnam P, Foster E, Shakhatreh L, Neal A, Carney PW, Jackson GD, et al. The effect of epilepsy surgery on productivity: A systematic review and meta-analysis. Epilepsia. 2022;63(4):789-811.
46. Engel J Jr. Surgery for seizures. N Engl J Med. 1996;334:647-52.
47. Haneef Z, Stern J, Dewar S, Engel Jr J. Referral pattern for epilepsy surgery after evidence-based recommendations: a retrospective study. Neurology. 2010;75:699-704.
48. Rathore C, Radhakrishnan K. Concept of epilepsy surgery and presurgical evaluation. Epileptic Disord. 2015;17:19-31.
49. Téllez-Zenteno JF, Dhar R, Wiebe S. Long-term seizure outcomes following epilepsy surgery: a systematic review and meta-analysis. Brain. 2005;128:1188-98.
50. Hu WH, Zhang C, Zhang K, Shao XQ, Zhang JG. Hemispheric surgery for refractory epilepsy: a systematic review and meta-analysis with emphasis on seizure predictors and outcomes. J Neurosurg. 2016;124:952-61.
51. Menon R, Rathore C, Sarma SP, Radhakrishnan K. Feasibility of antiepileptic drug withdrawal following extratemporal resective epilepsy surgery. Neurology. 2012;79:770-6.

52. Hamiwka L, Macrodimitris S, Tellez-Zenteno JF, Metcalfe A, Wiebe S, Kwon CS, et al.; CASES Investigators. Social outcomes after temporal or extratemporal epilepsy surgery: a systematic review. Epilepsia. 2011;52:870-9.
53. Brotis AG, Giannis T, Kapsalaki E, Dardiotis E, Fountas KN. Complications after anterior temporal lobectomy for medically intractable epilepsy: A systematic review and meta-analysis. Stereotact Funct Neurosurg. 2019;97:69-82.
54. Sherman EM, Wiebe S, Fay-McClymont TB, Tellez-Zenteno J, Metcalfe A, Hernandez-Ronquillo L, et al. Neuropsychological outcomes after epilepsy surgery: systematic review and pooled estimates. Epilepsia. 2011;52:857-69.
55. Téllez-Zenteno JF, Dhar R, Hernandez-Ronquillo L, Wiebe S. Long-term outcomes in epilepsy surgery: antiepileptic drugs, mortality, cognitive and psychosocial aspects. Brain. 2007;130:334-45.
56. Chan AY, Rolston JD, Lee B, Vadera S, Englot DJ. Rates and predictors of seizure outcome after corpus callosotomy for drug-resistant epilepsy: a meta-analysis. J Neurosurg. 2018;1:1-10.
57. Starnes K, Miller K, Wong-Kisiel L, Lundstrom BN. A review of neurostimulation for epilepsy in pediatrics. Brain Sci. 2019;9: 283.
58. Sourbron J, Klinkenberg S, van Kuijk SMJ, Lagae L, Lambrechts D, Braakman HMH, et al. Ketogenic diet for the treatment of pediatric epilepsy: review and meta-analysis. Childs Nerv Syst. 2020;36: 1099-109.
59. Gómez-Eguílaz M, Ramón-Trapero JL, Pérez-Martínez L, Blanco JR. The beneficial effect of probiotics as a supplementary treatment in drug-resistant epilepsy: a pilot study. Benef Microbes. 2018;9: 875-81.
60. Luciano AL, Shorvon SD. Results of treatment changes in patients with apparently drug-resistant chronic epilepsy. Ann Neurol. 2007;62:375-81.
61. Callaghan B, Schlesinger M, Rodemer W, Pollard J, Hesdorffer D, Allen Hauser W, et al. Remission and relapse in a drug-resistant epilepsy population followed prospectively. Epilepsia. 2011;52: 619-26.
62. Cereghino JJ, Brock JT, Van Meter JC, Penry JK, Smith LD, White BG. The efficacy of carbamazepine combinations in epilepsy. Clin Pharmacol Ther. 1975;18:733-41.
63. Deckers CL, Czuczwar SJ, Hekster YA, Keyser A, Kubova H, Meinardi H, et al. Selection of antiepileptic drug polytherapy based on mechanisms of action: the evidence reviewed. Epilepsia. 2000;41:1364-74.
64. Brodie MJ, Yuen AW. Lamotrigine substitution study: evidence for synergism with sodium valproate? 105 Study Group. Epilepsy Res. 1997;26:423-32.
65. Poolos NP, Warner LN, Humphreys SZ, Williams S. Comparative efficacy of combination drug therapy in refractory epilepsy. Neurology. 2012;78:62-8.
66. Rowan AJ, Meijer JW, de Beer-Pawlikowski N, van der Geest P, Meinardi H. Valproate-ethosuximide combination therapy for refractory absence seizures. Arch Neurol. 1983;40:797-802.
67. Stephen LJ, Sills GJ, Brodie MJ. Lamotrigine and topiramate may be a useful combination. Lancet. 1998;351:958-9.
68. Chen Z, Brodie MJ, Kwan P. What has been the impact of new drug treatments on epilepsy? Curr Opin Neurol. 2020;33:185-90.
69. Lattanzi S, Trinka E, Striano P, Zaccara G, Del Giovane C, Nardone R, et al. Cannabidiol efficacy and clobazam status: A systematic review and meta-analysis. Epilepsia. 2020;61:1090-8.
70. Sake JK, Hebert D, Isojärvi J, Doty P, De Backer M, Davies K, et al. A pooled analysis of lacosamide clinical trial data grouped by mechanism of action of concomitant antiepileptic drugs. CNS Drugs. 2010;24:1055-68.
71. Marson A, Burnside G, Appleton R, Smith D, Leach JP, Sills G, et al.; SANAD II Collaborators. The SANAD II study of the effectiveness and cost-effectiveness of valproate versus levetiracetam for newly diagnosed generalised and unclassifiable epilepsy: an open-label, non-inferiority, multicentre, phase 4, randomised controlled trial. Lancet. 2021;397:1375-86.
72. Marson AG, Al-Kharusi AM, Alwaidh M, Appleton R, Baker GA, Chadwick DW, et al.; SANAD Study group. The SANAD study of effectiveness of carbamazepine, gabapentin, lamotrigine, oxcarbazepine, or topiramate for treatment of partial epilepsy: an unblinded randomised controlled trial. Lancet. 2007;369: 1000-15.
73. Perucca P, Carter J, Vahle V, Gilliam FG. Adverse antiepileptic drug effects: toward a clinically and neurobiologically relevant taxonomy. Neurology. 2009;72:1223-9.
74. Husari KS, Dubey D. Autoimmune epilepsy. Neurotherapeutics. 2019;16:685-702.
75. Krauss GL, Klein P, Brandt C, Lee SK, Milanov I, Milovanovic M, et al. Safety and efficacy of adjunctive cenobamate (YKP3089) in patients with uncontrolled focal seizures: a multicentre, double-blind, randomised, placebo-controlled, dose-response trial. Lancet Neurol. 2020;19:38-48.
76. Lagae L, Sullivan J, Knupp K, Laux L, Polster T, Nikanorova M, et al. Fenfluramine hydrochloride for the treatment of seizures in Dravet syndrome: a randomised, double-blind, placebo-controlled trial. Lancet. 2019;394:2243-54.
77. Bialer M, Johannessen S, Koepp M, Levy RH, Perucca E, Tomson T, et al. Progress report on new antiepileptic drugs: A summary of the Fourteenth Eilat Conference on New Antiepileptic Drugs and Devices (EILAT XIV). I. Drugs in preclinical and early clinical development. Epilepsia. 2018;59:1811-41.
78. Borlot F, Wither RG, Ali A, Wu N, Verocai F, Andrade DM. A pilot double-blind trial using verapamil as adjuvant therapy for refractory seizures. Epilepsy Res. 2014;108:1642-51.
79. Pressler RM, Boylan GB, Marlow N, Blennow M, Chiron C, Cross JH, et al.; NEonatal seizure treatment with Medication Off-patent (NEMO) consortium. Bumetanide for the treatment of seizures in newborn babies with hypoxic ischaemic encephalopathy (NEMO): an open-label, dose finding, and feasibility phase 1/2 trial. Lancet Neurol. 2015;14:469-77.
80. Schlichtiger J, Pekcec A, Bartmann H, Winter P, Fuest C, Soerensen J, et al. Celecoxib treatment restores pharmacosensitivity in a rat model of pharmacoresistant epilepsy. Br J Pharmacol. 2010;160: 1062-71.
81. Steriade C, Martins W, Bulacio J, Morita-Sherman ME, Nair D, Gupta A, et al. Localization yield and seizure outcome in patients undergoing bilateral SEEG exploration. Epilepsia. 2019;60:107-20.
82. Park JE, Cheong EN, Jung DE, Shim WH, Lee JS. Utility of 7 Tesla Magnetic Resonance Imaging in Patients with Epilepsy: A Systematic Review and Meta-analysis. Front Neurol. 2021;12: 621936.
83. Park CJ, Hong SB. High frequency oscillations in epilepsy: detection methods and considerations in clinical application. J Epilepsy Res. 2019;9:1-13.
84. Rathore C, Radhakrishnan K. Epidemiology of epilepsy surgery in India. Neurol India. 2017;65(Supplement):S52-9.
85. Baheti N, Rathore C, Bansal AR, Kannan L, Gopinath S, Pillai A, et al. Current practices in epilepsy monitoring units (EMU) in India. Seizure. 2021;93:13-9.

66 CHAPTER

Psychogenic Nonepileptic Seizures

Parthvi Ravat, Karan Desai, Sangeeta H Ravat

INTRODUCTION

Psychogenic nonepileptic seizures (PNES) are episodes of altered subjective experience, involuntary movements, and lack of self-control that can resemble epilepsy, syncope, or other paroxysmal disorders. However, rather than being caused by neuronal hypersynchronization (as in epilepsy), or cerebral hypoperfusion (as in convulsive syncope), PNES are the result of a complex neuropsychiatric dysfunction.[1]

This entity is known by multiple names: Dissociative seizures, nonepileptic attack disorder (NEAD), PNES, psychogenic epilepsy, psychogenic nonepileptic episodes (PNEEs), nonepileptic seizures, functional seizures, and "pseudoseizures." The International League Against Epilepsy (ILAE) has identified PNES as one of the 10 key neuropsychiatric issues associated with epilepsy. In the Diagnostic and Statistical Manual of Mental Disorders (DSM)-V, PNES is listed in the section of somatic symptom disorder as "conversion disorder" or "functional neurological symptom disorder with attacks."[2] The vast amount of literature on this subject uses varying terminology. For example, the International Classification of Diseases (ICD)-10 is in favor of dissociative convulsions; some authors suggest PNES as the standard usage.[3] Usage of the term "seizure" does confuse the patient's and relative's understanding of the diagnosis. At the same time, the prefix psycho in a person's diagnosis might be misinterpreted or stigmatized by society. We suggest the use of the term NEAD since it is nonjudgmental.

The approach to this disorder requires a multidisciplinary approach, starting with the neurologist's keen analysis of the history, an exhaustive review of investigations such as magnetic resonance imaging (MRI) and video electroencephalogram (VEEG) for confirmation of diagnosis followed by appropriate psychopharmacology, and psychological support.

EPIDEMIOLOGY

Psychogenic nonepileptic seizure has an annual incidence of at least 1.5–6.17/100,000.[1] The prevalence of PNES in the general population has been estimated at 2–50/100,000.[1,4,5] Generally, PNES makes up for 10% of all seizure emergencies and around 30% of cases in epilepsy monitoring units (EMUs). In neurology outpatient departments (OPDs), they make up 2% of new references, and in seizure clinics, they comprise approximately 15% of the diagnoses. Women make up 60–80% of all PNES patients, although the gender disparity decreases with increasing age.[1,6] Second- and third-decade onsets are common in females whereas the age of onset in males with PNES is higher.[6] It can be seen in children of 8–10 years of age, and amongst the geriatric population (age 70–80 years). Like epilepsy, PNES is also diagnosed more frequently in the lower socioeconomic class and those with intellectual disabilities.[6]

PATHOLOGY AND PATHOPHYSIOLOGY

Amongst the many hypotheses proposed as a pathophysiological model for PNES, a comprehensive thinking model is proposed known as the integrative cognitive model (ICM).[7] This model proposes that a range of internal and external events can trigger an affective–cognitive–behavioral cascade that leads to the manifestation of a seizure-like episode. An awareness of the pathophysiological pathways in this model allows us to understand how the relevant risk factors and comorbidities of an individual eventually lead to the manifestation of PNES.

Triggers **(Fig. 1)** in the above model include a "perceived threat" and/or "conditioned cues," which are facilitated by the failure of the inhibitory systems. This model proposes a hypothetical entity which is called a "seizure scaffold,"

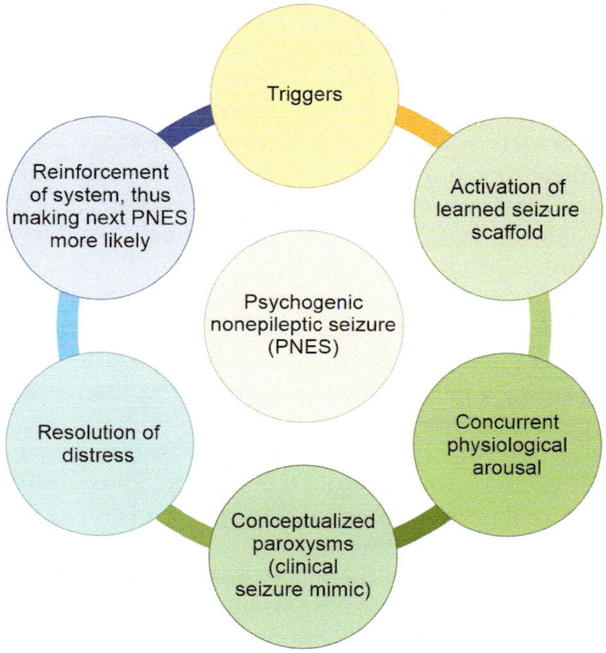

FIG. 1: Integrative cognitive model—self-fulfilling prophecy.

which is the psychological representation of PNES. It is a learned mental model combining various aspects such as:

- Instinctive automatisms (freezing, thrashing of limbs, pelvic thrusting, etc.)
- Personal experiences, either of the illness itself (epilepsy, syncope), childhood traumatic experiences (sexual, physical, or psychological abuse or neglect), or stressful life events (death of a parent, kidnapping, etc.)[8,9]
- In certain cases, the personal experience of an epileptic seizure (ES)

The suppression of intolerable memories has long been presumed to be a primary function of such dissociative attacks according to Pierre Janet, or in Freudian terms, the "primary gain" of "conversion." PNES can serve as an allostatic mechanism that relieves distress, especially when other coping mechanisms are unavailable or have been overwhelmed.[9] This reinforces the entire cycle of finding solace in the seizure-like behavior by way of "detachment from reality," and the secondary gains of public attention. The vicious cycle thus continues.

Neurobiologically, PNES could be the culmination of dysfunction in specific brain networks and their connectivity. Although imaging studies in patients with PNES have so far failed to converge on any concrete pathognomonic structural abnormalities, altered fronto-limbic connectivity and reduced gray matter in limbic and prefrontal areas (areas responsible for abnormal stress and emotion regulation) have been demonstrated in some cases.[10]

COMORBIDITIES

In an individual PNES patient, it is difficult to establish whether a co-occurring condition is a true comorbidity, a predisposition, or the underlying cause. Some of the common comorbidities include the following:

- *Epilepsy*: Comorbid epilepsy occurs in roughly 10% of adults and up to 30% of children with PNES.[11] There may be predisposing conditioning that occurs with every true seizure in epilepsy patients, or patients with a family history of epilepsy leading to PNES. One of the common causes of pseudo-refractory epilepsy is a "mixed seizure disorder," i.e., the co-occurrence of PNES and ES. When there is a change in the seizure semiology or a sudden increase of seizures on the same dosage of antiseizure medication (ASM), one must keep in mind the possibility of PNES. Keeping a high level of vigilance for the same is crucial to avoid overmedication, potential delay in diagnosis, and eventually avoiding poor outcomes. One hypothesis that can explain the co-occurrence of ES and PNES is the role of experience-dependent neuroplasticity of the brain, or the ability of the brain to change in response to the environment.[11] This theory is better encapsulated in children, with studies unraveling a higher volume of the supplementary motor areas in children with a faster emotion-identification reaction time.[12] In contrast to that, no significant differences were noted in the basal ganglia, thalamus, or cerebellum of subjects with a functional neurological disorder, suggesting that a decrease in gray matter in these areas may be related to the duration of symptoms.[13] Thus, more longitudinal neuroimaging would be needed to validate the role of experience-dependent neuroplasticity response to adverse life events and to subsequently find any genetic predisposition to develop functional neurological symptoms.
- *Psychiatric disorders*: Psychiatric comorbidities are common, particularly dissociative disorders, mood disorders (depression, anxiety, and posttraumatic stress disorder), and personality disorders (especially borderline personalities). In congruence with the ICM, as described above, a history of trauma and stressful life events is frequently but not invariably reported. Interpersonal relationships are often characterized by insecure attachment. Indian studies have shown comorbid depressive disorders in almost 90% of patients.[14]
- *Migraine*: A study conducted on almost 1,000 Indian migraineurs reported a very high rate of PNES (especially swoon-type reactions) accompanying severe migraine attacks in women (13% of girls and 23% of women), but almost no PNES events in men (0% of boys, 1% of men).[15] PNES patients report more frequent and longer-lasting migraine attacks than those with epilepsy.[16] The pathophysiology for this can be explained by the triggers. Severe pain along with the uncertainty and associated worry about the attack duration and intensity can serve as a potent trigger while sensorimotor and cognitive aura symptoms can be a part of the learned.

- Various other comorbidities such as chronic pain, sleep problems, asthma, and history of head injury are found at higher rates in patients with PNES than in the general population.[7]

DIAGNOSTIC CRITERIA FOR PSYCHOGENIC NONEPILEPTIC SEIZURES

A sound clinical assessment with the use of appropriate investigations is usually adequate in formulating a diagnosis of PNES. However, the DSM-V diagnostic criteria **(Box 1)** and "ILAE levels of diagnosis" **(Table 1)**[17] are useful in varying clinical scenarios.

CLINICAL FEATURES

Seizure symptoms and history in patients with ES are usually produced by the witness, and the patient volunteers the information about the aura (if any). However, the PNES patient would talk more about the preceding circumstances and the consequences of the event, rather than the event itself.[18] During interviewing a PNES suspect, one must remember to tolerate the silences and use continuers (mmm, right, etc.), gaze, and head nodding to form a conclusive impression.[19]

BOX 1 **Diagnostic and Statistical Manual of Mental Disorders (DSM)-V diagnostic criteria for conversion disorder.**

- One or more symptoms of altered voluntary motor or sensory function
- Clinical findings can provide evidence of incompatibility between the symptom and recognized neurological or medical conditions
- Another medical or mental disorder does not better explain the symptom or deficit
- Symptom or deficit results in clinically significant distress or impairment in social, occupational, or other vital areas of functioning or warrants medical evaluation

In the clinic, some salient clinical features on history and examination help in clinching an early diagnosis of PNES. Due to the abovementioned unreliability of the patient's account of his/her symptoms, history taken directly from the eyewitness is crucial. Requesting the eyewitness to mimic the semiology, or to furnish a home video (details in subsequent sections) of the events, helps hasten the process.

Some motor features that may strongly support the suspicion of PNES include the following:

- *Swoons*: A relaxed fall to the ground without injury, followed by lying still without convulsion, with eyes closed for various periods, feigning unconsciousness, but usually followed by rapid recovery without postictal confusion **(Video 1)**
- *Tantrums*: The patient emits a cry, falls, thrashes about with a convulsive struggle if restrained, kicks, and may bite (either himself or spectators), and is often noisy, shouting, roaring, or crying.
- *Abreactive attacks*: There may be initial overbreathing, which may pass unrecognized, followed by sudden movement and stiffening of the body, which is followed by breath-holding, gasping, uncoordinated jerking of the body with pelvic thrusting, and back arching.
- Motor features may also include phasic clonic activity, asynchronous limb movements, side-to-side head movements, intermittent shaking movements with episodes of inactivity, restless body turning (jactitation), forward pelvic thrusting, and opisthotonos posturing (arc de cercle) **(Video 2)**. Vocalization and verbalization at the onset, violent behavior, biting **(Video 3)**, slapping, and very rarely whole-body rigidity may be seen.

Other nonmotor accompaniments of PNES include hyperventilation (HV), dizziness, paresthesias, emotional outbursts, weeping at the end, avoiding eye contact, directed violence, preictal pseudosleep [confirmed by electroencephalogram (EEG)], ictal stuttering, and a postictal whispering tone. *Tongue bite* in PNES is rare, and if present, is found at the tip or on the lips as opposed to that on the lateral border in ES. Some ocular features suggestive of PNES include rapid eye flutter, erratic blinking,

TABLE 1: ILAE levels of diagnosis.[17]

Diagnostic level	History	Witnessed event	EEG
Possible	+	By witness or self-report/description	No epileptiform activity in routine or sleep-deprived interictal EEG
Probable	+	By clinician who reviewed video recording or in person, showing semiology typical of PNES	No epileptiform activity in routine or sleep-deprived interictal EEG
Clinically established	+	By clinician experienced in diagnosis of seizure disorders (on video or in person), showing semiology typical of PNES, while not on EEG	No epileptiform activity in routine EEG or ambulatory ictal EEG, capturing a typical ictus
Documented	+	By clinician experienced in diagnosis of seizure disorders, showing semiology typical of PNES, while on video EEG	No epileptiform activity immediately before, during, or after ictus captured on ictal video EEG with typical PNES semiology

(EEG: electroencephalogram; ILAE: International League Against Epilepsy; PNES: psychogenic nonepileptic seizures)

TABLE 2: Semiologic features differentiating PNES from ES.

Signs favoring PNES	Signs favoring ES	Indeterminate signs
Usually in an awake state, crowded places	Onset during physiologic sleep/ nocturnal seizures	Gradual onset
Long duration, fluctuating course	Postictal confusion	Nonstereotyped events
Asynchronous movements, side-to-side head/body movements	Stertorous breathing	Flailing or thrashing movements
Pelvic thrusting	Self-injury	Opisthotonos
Forced eye closure	Cyanosis	Tongue biting
Ictal crying		Urinary incontinence
Memory recall		Fecal incontinence
Directed violence		

(ES: epileptic seizures; PNES: psychogenic nonepileptic seizures)

TABLE 3: Clinical differentiators.

	Frontal lobe seizures	PNES
Occurrence	Sleep	Wakefulness
Duration	<1 minute	Several minutes
Semiology	Stereotypic	Variable and bizarre
Posturing	Arms in abduction, turning to prone position	Opisthotonus (video reference at the end of the chapter)
Thrashing	Leg movements are more common, bipedaling, cycling movements	Side-to-side movements of the head, trunk
Vocalization	Monotonous, with/ without emotional content	Frequently with emotional content
Awareness	Minimal loss	Variable
Scalp EEG	Usually no change, or movement artifact. Intracortical electrodes are required	Movement artifact

(ES: epileptic seizures; PNES: psychogenic nonepileptic seizures)

and geotropic (downward) eye deviation (as opposed to the usual uprolling of eyeballs) **(Table 2)**. Adolescents and adults who bring stuffed toys to the EMU were more likely to be diagnosed with PNES and this has been referred to as the "teddy bear sign."[20] The reliability of this sign is not established.

The abovementioned signs can be called highly suggestive, but not pathognomonic to PNES without clinical, and in many cases EEG/radiological, correlation (details in later sections). A prolonged duration of events, lasting for 45–60 minutes or more, often rules in the favor of PNES. It may not be possible to separate ES from PNES purely based on the stereotype of events.[21]

The closest epileptic differential to PNES in clinical practice is the hypermotor seizure originating in the frontal lobes. Some of the key differentiators between the two are mentioned in **Table 3**.

When the patient is being assessed during the attack, either in the hospital or in the VEEG room, the following points **(Table 4)** are useful to differentiate between true seizure and PNES.

TABLE 4: Examination clinchers.

Examination procedure (during the attack)	Findings in psychogenic nonepileptic seizures (PNES)
Drop the patient's hand over their face	Hand falls to the side
If eyes are closed, attempt to open them	Resistance to eye-opening
If eyes are open, place a mirror in front of the patient	*Evidence of visual fixation*: Look for evidence of convergent gaze and fixation on the reflection. This method is also useful for stopping the seizure
If eyes are open, roll the patient from one side to the other	At the start, eyes will often deviate to the ground. The patient should then be rolled onto the other side and a note taken if the eyes are still directed toward the ground (Henry and Woodruff sign)
Corneal reflex	Intact
Plantar reflex	Flexor

The findings in the first three tests suggest some preservation of intact awareness and volition. As a cautionary note, some patients may learn to produce the "correct" neurological response with any of these examinations.

APPROACH TO DIAGNOSIS IN THE EMERGENCY ROOM

Making a clinical diagnosis in the emergency room (ER) is more nuanced as the risk of missing an organic pathology is higher. This point holds true especially in cases without any known psychiatric comorbidities and in de novo presentations. The first presentation of PNES directly to the ER is a disturbing event for the family. In such cases, when a patient appears to feign unconsciousness or PNES is suspected, the use of noxious agents like spirit, or ammonia smells near the nose of the patient, is strongly discouraged due to it being insensitive and lacking in empathy. Admission to the ER and a swift workup to rule out organicity are needed in such cases. In cases that already have an established diagnosis of PNES or mixed epilepsy, the approach is reversed as repeated admissions and investigations in the ER can accentuate the "neurocognitive PNES scaffold" or attention-seeking tendency. Such patients should be quickly sent back home after giving reassurance to the caregivers and the patient, and if needed, a reinforcement of psychopharmacology and psychological support services is ensured.

DIFFERENTIAL DIAGNOSIS OF PSYCHOGENIC NONEPILEPTIC SEIZURES

Any paroxysmal event, either physiological or pathological, may mimic PNES. Differentiating between most of them is usually possible on clinical grounds; however, investigations may be necessary for some. The below-mentioned conditions are not an exhaustive list, but both neurological and non-neurological conditions should be considered when evaluating a patient with suspected PNES.

Syncope and Nonneurological Conditions

- *Syncope and other cardiac conditions*: It remains the closest nonneurological mimic of PNES. It often has a nonspecific aura (e.g., visual blurring, nausea, and light-headedness), and is seldom associated with convulsive movements as well.[22] Other symptoms depend on the mechanism of syncope, either vasovagal, arrhythmogenic (prolonged QT syndrome), or structural causes (valvular disease or congenital anomalies).[22] The age of the patient and the confounding circumstances usually aid in clinching the diagnosis. For events preceded by diaphoresis or that occur shortly after standing up, a cardiac etiology or vasovagal syncope is likely.[23]
- *Metabolic conditions*: Hypoglycemia, hyponatremia, or hypocalcemia can cause episodic weakness, tingling, focal spasms, cramps, and dizziness that may be misinterpreted as PNES.[24,25] The frequency of this medical misdiagnosis is not widely published.

Neurological Disorders

- *True epilepsy*: Many focal epilepsies such as frontal lobe epilepsies arising from the cingulate cortex and mesial temporal lobe epilepsies may have semiological traits (e.g., kissing, spitting, crying, laughing, and irrelevant talks) that may raise suspicion of PNES. A detailed consideration of the clinical differences, as mentioned in the earlier sections of this review, needs consideration.
- *Sleep disorders*: Conditions such as night terrors and sleep talking can appear like PNES. Nonrapid eye movement (NREM) parasomnias are usually associated with confusional arousal, which may be a clue. But sleep talking, or somnambulism, may often be confusing. Rapid eye movement (REM) sleep behavioral disorder (RBD) is classically associated with dream-enactment-like behavior and also thrashing movements. Certain periodic limb movements during sleep can also be very stereotypical and jerky in nature. The timing of occurrence of these events and postictal awareness may be a clue. In rare cases, there may be a need for EEG correlation.
- Neurological disorders such as limb-shaking transient ischemic attacks (TIAs), benign positional vertigo, paroxysmal movement disorders, cataplexy, and episodic ataxias with intermittent, fleeting neurological symptoms need careful consideration before labeling someone with the diagnosis of PNES.[26]

Nonpsychogenic Nonepileptic Seizure Psychiatric Disorders

Altered states of behavior, under the influence of drug abuse and some axis-1 psychiatric illnesses (e.g., schizophrenia or psychotic depression), should be considered when patients present with intermittent positive sensory phenomena or bizarre, repetitive movements. These events are frequently complex in nature, nonstereotypical, and often more prolonged (>5 minutes in duration).[27]

INVESTIGATIONS

Home Videos

With the recent advent of smartphones with image resolutions at par with the best EMUs and far superior portability, home videos have become a boon for the early diagnosis of PNES. Since the assessment of ictal semiology is a key part of diagnosing epilepsy/PNES, a good quality video is worth a thousand descriptions of the event by even the most reliable witnesses. One retrospective study reviewing the events captured in the EMU revealed that video data alone (without EEG), reviewed by an experienced epileptologist, provided excellent sensitivity (93%) and specificity (94%) in distinguishing ES from PNES.[28] A similar "out of EMU" retrospective study was done in North India that also showed a similar range of accuracy for diagnosing PNES.[29,30] A key to validation depends on the epileptologist rating the videos, as nonexperienced neurologists may not deliver such high accuracy. Another limiting factor is the quality of home videos in terms of adequate coverage of the semiology, as outpatient video recordings may miss the exact moment of onset, also missing the phenomenology that truly represents the essence of the PNES. Nevertheless, in a low-resource setting like ours, the demonstration of ictal semiology on home videos can enhance the diagnostic level of certainty as per the ILAE's staged approach to the diagnosis of PNES.[31]

Video Electroencephalogram

Video electroencephalogram is the gold standard investigation for confirmation of the clinical suspicion of PNES. 20–50% of individuals admitted to an EMU as a part of drug-refractory epilepsy evaluation have PNES.[32] Up to 40% of patients with clinical suspicion of seizures, who are seen in general neurology clinics, have PNES.[33] Capturing the "habitual" event confirmed by the relative is crucial. VEEG recordings that capture the habitual PNES features, with a normal corresponding background EEG, during and after an event, strongly support the diagnosis of PNES. The presence of superimposed movement artifacts during the events is expected. Any ictal slowing and amplitude dampening on EEG may be indicative of another differential such as a syncope, TIA, and rarely even migraine. To ensure that cardiac differentials are captured, the electrocardiogram tracing recorded during standard VEEG monitoring should be reviewed. In the case of multiple semiologies, one must ensure that a potentially true epileptogenic semiology is not missed. In patients on long-term ASM treatment who have been diagnosed with PNES, a longer VEEG may be needed with the latter part of the record taken after tapering off the ASM.

Caveats and Pearls in Video Electroencephalogram Interpretation

Nearly 30% of patients with epilepsy may have normal routine interictal EEGs at presentation, and over 10% of healthy individuals may have nonspecific abnormalities or benign variants (waveforms that are subtly different from the more common, normal waveforms, but are not pathological in nature).[34] Rhythmic shaking movements associated with PNES can cause artifacts in the delta, theta, and alpha ranges that may mimic epileptiform discharges, but unlike true seizures, these discharges do not display any spatiotemporal evolution.[35] PNES often has a "stuttering" pattern of rhythmic motor activity, where "rest periods" between the periods of motor activity correspond to normal background electrical activity on EEG.[35] This "on-off-on" pattern of motor activity (alternating periods of rest and rhythmic motor movement) during a seizure is common in patients with PNES, but it is incompatible with ES. The absence of ictal or interictal correlates on EEG does not rule out a true ES with certainty in all cases. The knowledge that an ES can arise from a very small pool of neuronal tissue, events that may clinically resemble an epilepsia partialis continua (EPC), may not demonstrate ictal epileptiform correlate on scalp EEG.[36] Similarly, in clinical scenarios where the seizure originates from deep orbitofrontal/interhemispheric cortices and hypothalamic hamartomas, the ictal EEG epileptiform correlate can frequently be subtle, falsely lateralizing, or undiscernible due to contaminating artifacts. Seizures coming from these areas may clinically also be very brief, with minimal postictal confusion. These above-nuanced concepts underscore the importance of a careful history-taking and bedside ictal/peri-ictal physical examination of patients undergoing evaluation for drug-refractory epilepsy in the EMU.

Role of Induction Protocols

The majority of the patients with PNES in the EMU will spontaneously experience a habitual event within 2 days after admission.[37] But in a resource-limited setting like ours, a 2–3-day recording may not be feasible, so the use of a provocative technique during short-term outpatient VEEG studies can be very effective.[38] There is currently no standardized provocative technique, with each EMU having their protocols. The patients and/or their relatives are explained about the induction tests and explained that they may experience their habitual events. Explaining that at most, these procedures may produce some discomfort without any harm or lasting effect is vital. If patients or relatives do not give consent, they should not be performed. Some commonly used induction tests include compression of the temple region, verbal suggestion, tuning fork application, moist swab application at the temple, torch light stimulation, and saline injection. Due to ethical concerns, saline injection is generally the least preferred one although it has been proven to be quite effective. Often after precipitating the event with a suggestion, it is further suggested that the VEEG machine will stop the event and prevent its recurrence in the future, which works as therapy in some patients. The success rate of induction tests is higher in village dwellers, homemakers, and less-educated patients. Interpretation and explanation of the outcomes of a successful induction in cases with mixed epilepsy are as crucial as the continuation of ASM for epilepsy. The use of induction tests has raised ethical concerns as it may be associated with deception, violation of patient autonomy, and undermining of the doctor–patient relationship.[39] The intention to do good by the patient (beneficence) and do no harm to the patient (malfeasance) usually supersedes these concerns, particularly if proper consent is taken. It may be more harmful and financially burdensome to miss the diagnosis of PNES. In a study of patients with PNES, there was an average delay of 7.2 years in reaching the diagnosis.[40] A delay in the diagnosis may lead to potential exposure to ASM toxicity, and rare intubations for psychogenic status epilepticus. Yet provocative studies are not uniformly used across all centers. Some of these ethical concerns can be circumvented by incorporating only routine EEG activation procedures such as HV and photic stimulation (PS) as provocative measures along with some verbal suggestions, thereby avoiding the use of a placebo.

Noninvasive Imaging

Magnetic resonance imaging studies with a ≥1.5 Tesla scanner and epilepsy-specific sequences usually confirm any major focal lesions responsible for ES.[41] Patients with PNES can also have MRI abnormalities; in one study, up to 30% of patients with PNES were identified as having MRI abnormalities (nonspecific gliosis and postoperative changes were most common.)[42] Patients with PNES and patients with ES can both have normal brain MRI findings, suggesting that MRI may not differentiate between these two types of seizures. Single-photon emission computed tomography (SPECT) is commonly employed during presurgical evaluation of patients with epilepsy, as it can help identify the ictal focus through imaging cerebral blood flow. Nevertheless, the capability of SPECT to differentiate between PNES and ES remains unknown.

Psychiatric and Neuropsychological Evaluation

A psychiatric comorbidity is common in patients with PNES.[40] The types of comorbid psychiatric disorders most often present in patients with PNES are depression, anxiety, posttraumatic stress disorder (PTSD), and personality disorders.[43] A psychiatric evaluation can identify conflicts or traumatic experiences that might aid the diagnosis of PNES that would not be routinely addressed in a neurological evaluation. Appropriate neuropsychological batteries based on DSM-V criteria are performed when deemed appropriate.

Blood Tests

There is an increase in serum protein levels in some ES. Serum prolactin levels can rise to >500 IU/mL in ≥90% of patients following a generalized convulsion, and in ≥60% of patients following a focal seizure.[44] The involvement of the limbic regions is responsible for the elevation in prolactin levels during the ES.[45] Serum prolactin levels that are measured 10–20 minutes postictally may help to differentiate between convulsive/complex partial ES and PNES. They cannot distinguish between ES and syncope.[45] Other serum proteins such as neuron-specific enolase and creatine kinase are not sensitive markers of ES and do not help to reliably discriminate between these seizures and PNES.[46]

MANAGEMENT OF PSYCHOGENIC NONEPILEPTIC SEIZURES

Management involves a multidisciplinary approach where the neurologist, mental health professionals (psychiatrist and psychologists), social worker, and occupational therapists should work in collaboration in planning treatment. Treatment of PNES involves effective communication of the diagnosis, assessment for other psychiatric and psychiatric comorbidities, supervised tapering of ASMs, psychotropic medications, and cognitive behavioral therapy (CBT). There are no universally accepted guidelines about the type or duration of treatment of PNES. These patients are a heterogeneous population, so treatment protocols may vary on a case-to-case basis. The concept of these four phases of treatment may apply to each case.[47]

First Phase: Diagnosis Delivery

It is usually the neurologist who communicates the diagnosis of PNES. There is mounting evidence that the process of communicating the diagnosis is a crucial therapeutic step in the management of patients with PNES. Having family members present during the conversation augments a better understanding of the condition, as often the patient's underlying psychological condition may lead to misunderstandings and delays in effective intervention.[48] Terms such as "pseudoseizures," "hysteria," and "conversion" are avoided, and sticking to a uniform term "PNES" or "NEAD" is important. Explaining that although the events are not originating because of epileptic discharges from the brain, they still arise from the cognitive and emotional networks of the brain helps in reassuring the patients and family. The possibility of there being an underlying psychological or psychiatric issue underneath the surface needs to be delicately handled. Provision of letters to referring clinicians or supplementary written/multimedia information on PNES for the patient and family consolidates the process of effective communication.

Second Phase: Engagement of Psychiatry and Psychology Services

For many patients and families with a prolonged label of drug refractory epilepsy, abrupt removal of the "seizure" label may be difficult to accept. In our country, due to the stigma involved with mental illness, patients rarely volunteer activities to participate in mental health treatment immediately after they receive the diagnosis. Ideally, immediately after delivering the diagnosis, but latest at the first follow-up after communicating the diagnosis, patients must understand their diagnosis. A second opinion may be offered if there is still a lack of clarity at the patient's end. Contact with a mental health provider is initiated.[49]

Third Phase: Acute Intervention

After formal psychiatric and psychological assessment is performed, the predisposing, precipitating, and perpetuating factors should be unraveled. Individualized psychotherapeutic and psychopharmacological treatment plans should be formulated. This phase has a primary goal of reduction of the ictal frequency. The secondary goals are improvement in the psychiatric comorbidities and quality of life. It usually involves a combination of CBT and psychopharmacology. Other potential psychotherapeutic interventions include psychodynamic therapy and group therapies (e.g., family therapy in the case of dysfunctional families).[48] During this transition to mental healthcare follow-up, the roles of the neurologists include: (1) limiting invasive investigations of other symptoms for which a medical cause has been ruled out, (2) supervising the taper of ASMs, and (3) being available for evaluation and management of newly arisen symptoms that are suspicious of epilepsy.

Psychologic Treatment of Psychogenic Nonepileptic Seizures

In cases where a major psychiatric illness is not at the root cause of the PNES, CBT may be the first-line psychological treatment. Two CBT-based approaches have undergone pilot randomized controlled trials, with significant seizure reductions. One is a conventional CBT approach, while the other is a multimodality CBT-informed psychotherapy based on a workbook used by therapists and patients to treat either ES or PNES.[7,50,51] There is no robust evidence of the efficacy of other psychological interventions. Some of the different psychotherapy methods that may help in the management of PNES include:

- *Psychodynamic therapy*: It aims at enabling patients with PNES who are aware of maladaptive behavioral patterns.
- *Mindfulness-based therapy (MBT)*: MBT is efficacious in the management of various neuropsychiatric conditions. Mindfulness can be defined as "paying attention in a particular way: on purpose, in the present moment, and nonjudgmentally."
- *Acceptance commitment therapy (ACT)*: ACT is a hybrid therapy that derives its components from both CBT and MBT.
- *Psychoeducation-based therapeutic approach*: It is a treatment modality comprising a flexible model based on the confluence of therapeutic and educational interventions. This approach focuses on imparting illness-related information along with managing the surrounding circumstances.
- *Prolonged exposure therapy*: A diagnosis of PNES is often accompanied by a comorbid diagnosis of PTSD. It is an empirically validated treatment modality to treat patients with a dual diagnosis of PNES and PTSD. This therapy targets avoidance strategies adopted by patients to curb anxiety triggered by cues related to trauma or by flashbacks of the experience itself.
- *Eye movement desensitization and reprocessing (EMDR)*: EMDR is an empirically validated treatment for PTSD. The core principle involved in EMDR is an emphasis on the information processing system. Thus, this eight-phase model focuses on reprocessing memories of events related to underlying current symptoms to bring the patient back to a psychologically healthy state.
- *Hypnotherapy*: Hypnosis is one of the oldest therapeutic approaches for conversion disorders since the time of seminal practitioners such as Jean Charcot and Sigmund Freud. The latest neuroimaging findings reveal that the neural processes involved in conversion symptoms and hypnotic mechanisms are the same.
- *Paradoxical intention therapy (PIT)*: PIT builds upon a deliberate undertaking of the targeted activity or behavior to identify, and eventually remove it. It is indicated specifically for psychiatric cases with low patient opposition and a lack of control of symptoms. Hence, PIT is well suited for PNES.
- *Novel integrative psychotherapy*: Up to 93% of PNES diagnosis is often accompanied by another comorbid psychiatric diagnosis.[52] Every patient has exclusive semiology, triggering or maintaining factors. Hence, a uniform therapeutic approach might not be efficacious for all patients. Novel integrative psychotherapy is based on a biopsychosocial approach to treatment, aimed at providing individualized case-specific treatment to each patient.

TABLE 5: Pharmacotherapy.

Molecule	Usual starting dose (mg)	Low starting dose (mg)	Therapeutic dose (daily) (mg)
Paroxetine	20	5–10	20–60
Sertraline	50	12.5–25	50–250
Fluvoxamine	50	25	100–300
Fluoxetine	20	5–10	20–60
Citalopram	20	10	20–40
Escitalopram	10	10	20–40
Venlafaxine	37.5	37.5	37.5–300

Pharmacological Treatment of Psychogenic Nonepileptic Seizures[48]

Despite the lack of more robust clinical data, there is enough evidence in the form of smaller studies and anecdotal reports that appropriate psychopharmacology may help in cases of PNES based on their underlying psychiatric comorbidities. Antidepressants may be useful in adults and the elderly with PNES and concomitant anxiety, depression, or adjustment disorders **(Table 5)**. Additional management of substance abuse, insomnia, and further augmentation strategies for more severe psychiatric comorbidities are beyond the scope of this discussion. A list of some commonly used molecules in the management of comorbid mood disorders is mentioned in **Table 5**.

Final Phase: Long-term Interventions

For patients who remain symptomatic after the acute intervention phase, ongoing care is pertinent to ensure adequate functional recovery. Individualized interventions include long-term psychotherapy, ongoing psychotropic management of psychiatric comorbidities, and the involvement of social workers and occupational therapists. The neurologist may follow them for 6 months after discontinuing the ASMs. This recommendation is for a very small subset of patients with mixed epilepsy that may be missed during the initial evaluations. Usually, by this time, the patient is out of follow-up with the neurologist, except in cases with additional neurological comorbidities. Patients with mixed epilepsy should be treated with the lowest effective ASM dose for ES.

PROGNOSIS

The overall prognosis of PNES is poor. Complete remission of the PNES events is reported to occur in about 40% of patients over time. Nearly a third of patients experience a modest reduction in event frequency, while the remaining third of patients continue to have a chronically intractable course.[53] The assessment of PNES outcomes should also encompass psychosocial comorbidities, functionality, and overall quality of life.[54] One study tried to consider all these factors and revealed that 44% of patients were not seizure-free and remained dependent (poor outcome), 40% of patients were either seizure-free but dependent or not seizure-free but independent (intermediate outcome), and only 16% of patients were seizure-free and independent (good outcome).[54] An important prognostic factor highlighted consistently is the duration of illness, thus highlighting the importance of an early diagnosis.[28] The abovementioned figures suggest that despite an early diagnosis, the outcome of PNES is not as robust as that of newly diagnosed epilepsy. Factors associated with better overall outcomes among adults include higher educational status, younger age at both time of seizure onset and time of diagnosis, seizures with a less dramatic semiology, and milder psychological comorbidities.[52,55] The lack of robust Indian data on PNES outcomes needs consideration before generalizing the abovementioned data as the psychosocial factors in our population are very heterogenous and diverse from some of the western literature.

INDIAN PERSPECTIVES

In India, there is a recent increase in the number of publications on PNES. In terms of social and cultural beliefs and stressors, there remain unique challenges due to the diverse groups of patients. Delays in diagnosis are also higher due to a lack of timely access to a tertiary care level EMU. The advent of smartphone videos may be useful in circumventing this gap to some extent. Similar challenges also occur on the treatment front as the stigma of acceptance of psychiatric/psychological comorbidity is high. Additionally, in many cases, the social structures at the root of the PNES may be difficult to modify. The lack of trained healthcare professionals to cater to the large population, and cope with the urban and rural populations of the country, is of concern.

CONCLUSION

Psychogenic nonepileptic seizures are characterized by paroxysmal changes in responsiveness, movements, or behaviors that may mimic ES but lack the neurobiological and electrophysiological origins of ES. They remain a considerable chunk of referrals to EMUs across the country and are often missed even by referring clinicians. A high index of suspicion in all cases of drug-refractory epilepsy with atypical features must be maintained. Diagnosis of PNES depends on an astute clinical sense and is supported by a multidisciplinary evaluation. The neurobiology of PNES is still poorly understood despite recent work based on functional MRI (fMRI) and other functional neuroimaging models. Despite access to the best EMUs, fewer than 40% of cases with PNES remain event-free at 5 years after the diagnosis.[53] An errant diagnosis of epilepsy in cases of PNES subjects the patient to unnecessary ASMs, delays the address to the underlying psychopathology, and timely delivery of appropriate treatment. The financial burden on the healthcare system and the individual is significant. On the opposite end of this spectrum, timely diagnosis is extremely rewarding to both the patient/caregivers and treating physicians.

VIDEO LEGENDS

Video 1: Swoon. This nonepileptic attack disorder (NEAD) video shows the neurologist giving a "suggestion" to the patient using the tuning fork as an induction protocol. This is a swoon as described in our text. This patient had no postictal confusion and a very rapid recovery.

Video 2: This nonepileptic attack disorder (NEAD) video shows the posturing of opisthotonus, also called "arc de cercle" as seen in NEAD. This nonepileptic spell also stopped when suggested to the patient.

Video 3: This nonepileptic attack disorder (NEAD) episode shows ictal biting, bipedaling movements, side-to-side head movements. His electroencephalogram (EEG) during this record was also without any epileptiform discharges. The patient's ictus stopped on giving suggestion.

REFERENCES

1. Duncan R, Oto M. Psychogenic nonepileptic seizures in patients with learning disability: comparison with patients with no learning disability. Epilepsy Behav. 2008;12:183-6.
2. Peeling JL, Muzio MR. Conversion Disorder. In: StatPearls [Internet]. Treasure Island (FL): StatPearls Publishing; 2022.
3. Benbadis SR. Psychogenic nonepileptic "seizures" or "attacks"? It's not just semantics: attacks. Neurology. 2010;75:84-6.
4. Benbadis SR, Allen Hauser W. An estimate of the prevalence of psychogenic nonepileptic seizures. Seizure. 2000;9:280-1.
5. Kanemoto K, LaFrance WC, Duncan R, Gigineishvili D, Park SP, Tadokoro Y, et al. PNES around the world: where we are now and how we can close the diagnosis and treatment gaps—an ILAE PNES task force report. Epilepsia Open. 2017;2:307-16.
6. Goldstein LH, Robinson EJ, Reuber M, Chalder T, Callaghan H, Eastwood C, et al. Characteristics of 698 patients with dissociative seizures: a UK multicenter study. Epilepsia. 2019;60(11):2182-93.
7. Popkirov S, Asadi-Pooya AA, Duncan R, Gigineishvili D, Hingray C, Miguel Kanner A, et al. The etiology of psychogenic nonepileptic seizures: risk factors and comorbidities. Epileptic Disord. 2019;21:529-47.
8. Brown RJ, Syed TU, Benbadis S, LaFrance WC, Reuber M. Psychogenic nonepileptic seizures. Epilepsy Behav. 2011;22:85-93.
9. Michaelis R, Tang V, Wagner JL, Modi AC, Lafrance WC, Goldstein LH, et al. Psychological treatments for people with epilepsy. Cochrane Database Syst Rev. 2017;10(10):CD012081.
10. Mcsweeney M, Reuber M, Levita L. Neuroimaging studies in patients with psychogenic nonepileptic seizures: a systematic meta-review. Neuroimage Clin. 2017;16:210-21.
11. Fobian AD, Elliott L. A review of functional neurological symptom disorder etiology and the integrated etiological summary model. J Psychiatry Neurosci. 2019;44(1):8-18.

12. Kozlowska K, Griffiths KR, Foster SL, Linton J, Williams LM, Korgaonkar MS. Gray matter abnormalities in children and adolescents with functional neurological symptom disorder. Neuroimage Clin. 2017;15:306-14.
13. Langer N, Hänggi J, Müller NA, Simmen HP, Jäncke L. Effects of limb immobilization on brain plasticity. Neurology. 2012;78:182-8.
14. Patidar Y, Gupta M, Khwaja G, Chowdhury D, Batra A, Dasgupta A. Clinical profile of psychogenic nonepileptic seizures in adults: a study of 63 cases. Ann Indian Acad Neurol. 2013;16:157.
15. Chakravarty A, Mukherjee A, Roy D. Migraine, epileptic seizures, and psychogenic nonepileptic seizures: observations in Indian patients in a clinic-based study. Neurol India. 2010;58:631.
16. Shepard MA, Silva A, Starling AJ, Hoerth MT, Locke DEC, Ziemba K, et al. Patients with psychogenic nonepileptic seizures report more severe migraine than patients with epilepsy. Seizure. 2016;34:78-82.
17. Lafrance WC, Baker GA, Duncan R, Goldstein LH, Reuber M. Minimum requirements for the diagnosis of psychogenic nonepileptic seizures: a staged approach. Epilepsia. 2013;54:2005-18.
18. Wolf P, Benbadis S, Dimova PS, Vinayan KP, Michaelis R, Reuber M, et al. The importance of semiological information based on epileptic seizure history. Epileptic Disord. 2020;22:15-31.
19. Plug L, Sharrack B, Reuber M. Conversation analysis can help to distinguish between epilepsy and nonepileptic seizure disorders: a case comparison. Seizure. 2009;18:43-50.
20. Kim SH, Kim H, Lim BC, Chae JH, Kim KJ, Hwang YS, et al. Paroxysmal nonepileptic events in pediatric patients confirmed by long-term video-EEG monitoring—single tertiary center review of 143 patients. Epilepsy Behav. 2012;24:336-40.
21. Hubsch C, Baumann C, Hingray C, Gospodaru N, Vignal JP, Vespignani H, et al. Clinical classification of psychogenic nonepileptic seizures based on video-EEG analysis and automatic clustering. J Neurol Neurosurg Psychiatry. 2011;82:955-60.
22. Aydin MA, Salukhe TV, Wilke I, Willems S. Management and therapy of vasovagal syncope: a review. World J Cardiol. 2010;2:308.
23. McKeon A, Vaughan C, Delanty N. Seizure versus syncope. Lancet Neurol. 2006;5:171-80.
24. Zenenberg RD, Carluccio AL, Merlin MA. Hyponatremia: evaluation and management. Hosp Pract (1995). 2010;38:89-96.
25. Rozance PJ, Hay WW. Describing hypoglycemia—definition or operational threshold? Early Hum Dev. 2010;86:275.
26. Walters AS. Clinical identification of the simple sleep-related movement disorders. Chest. 2007;131:1260-6.
27. Elliott B, Joyce E, Shorvon S. Delusions, illusions, and hallucinations in epilepsy: 1. elementary phenomena. Epilepsy Res. 2009;85:162-71.
28. Chen DK, LaFrance WC. Diagnosis and treatment of nonepileptic seizures. Continuum (Minneap Minn). 2016;22:116-31.
29. Ramanujam B, Dash D, Tripathi M. Can home videos made on smartphones complement video-EEG in diagnosing psychogenic nonepileptic seizures? Seizure. 2018;62:95-8.
30. Dash D, Sharma A, Yuvraj K, Renjith A, Mehta S, Vasantha PM, et al. Can home video facilitate diagnosis of epilepsy type in a developing country? Epilepsy Res. 2016;125:19-23.
31. Scheffer IE, Berkovic S, Capovilla G, Connolly MB, French J, Guilhoto L, et al. ILAE classification of the epilepsies: position paper of the ILAE commission for classification and terminology. Epilepsia. 2017;58:512-21.
32. King DW, Gallagher BB, Murvin AJ, Smith DB, Marcus DJ, Hartlage LC, et al. Pseudoseizures: diagnostic evaluation. Neurology. 1982;32:18-23.
33. Bazil CW, Kothari M, Luciano D, Moroney J, Song S, Vasquez B, et al. Provocation of nonepileptic seizures by suggestion in a general seizure population. Epilepsia. 1994;35:768-70.
34. Gregory RP, Oates T, Merry RTG. Electroencephalogram epileptiform abnormalities in candidates for aircrew training. Electroencephalogr Clin Neurophysiol. 1993;86:75-7.
35. Cragar DE, Berry DTR, Fakhoury TA, Cibula JE, Schmitt FA. A review of diagnostic techniques in the differential diagnosis of epileptic and nonepileptic seizures. Neuropsychol Rev. 2002;12:31-64.
36. Alsaadi TM, Thieman C, Shatzel A, Farias S. Video-EEG telemetry can be a crucial tool for neurologists experienced in epilepsy when diagnosing seizure disorders. Seizure. 2004;13:32-4.
37. Gogia B, Rai PK, Matthys SA, Mong ER, Rodriguez R, Yassin A, et al. Use of noninvasive induction techniques in the diagnosis of PNES. Epilepsy Behav. 2019;99:106491.
38. Zanzmera P, Sharma A, Bhatt K, Patel T, Luhar M, Modi A, et al. Can short-term video-EEG substitute long-term video-EEG monitoring in psychogenic nonepileptic seizures? A prospective observational study. Epilepsy Behav. 2019;94:258-63.
39. Leeman BA. Provocative techniques should not be used for the diagnosis of psychogenic nonepileptic seizures. Epilepsy Behav. 2009;15:110-4.
40. Brown RJ, Reuber M. Psychological and psychiatric aspects of psychogenic nonepileptic seizures (PNES): a systematic review. Clin Psychol Rev. 2016;45:157-82.
41. Devinsky O, Gazzola D, Lafrance WC. Differentiating between nonepileptic and epileptic seizures. Nat Rev Neurol. 2011;7:210-20.
42. Craven I, Kotsarini C, Hoggard N. Recent advances in imaging epilepsy. Postgrad Med J. 2010;86:552-9.
43. Martino I, Bruni A, Labate A, Vasta R, Cerasa A, Borzì G, et al. Psychopathological constellation in patients with PNES: a new hypothesis. Epilepsy Behav. 2018;78:297-301.
44. Sperling MR, Pritchard PB, Engel J, Daniel C, Sagel J. Prolactin in partial epilepsy: an indicator of limbic seizures. Ann Neurol. 1986;20:716-22.
45. Chen DK, So YT, Fisher RS. Use of serum prolactin in diagnosing epileptic seizures: report of the therapeutics and technology assessment subcommittee of the American Academy of Neurology. Neurology. 2005;65:668-75.
46. Willert C, Spitzer C, Kusserow S, Runge U. Serum neuron-specific enolase, prolactin, and creatine kinase after epileptic and psychogenic nonepileptic seizures. Acta Neurol Scand. 2004;109:318-23.
47. Asadi-Pooya AA. Psychogenic nonepileptic seizures: a concise review. Neurol Sci. 2017;38:935-40.
48. Lafrance WC, Reuber M, Goldstein LH. Management of psychogenic nonepileptic seizures. Epilepsia. 2013;54:53-67.
49. Baslet G, Dworetzky B, Perez DL, Oser M. Treatment of psychogenic nonepileptic seizures: updated review and findings from a mindfulness-based intervention case series. Clin EEG Neurosci. 2015;46:54-64.
50. Kamil SH, Qureshi M, Patel RS. Cognitive behavioral therapy (CBT) in psychogenic nonepileptic seizures (PNES): a case report and literature review. Behav Sci (Basel). 2019;9(2):15.
51. Phakey N, Godara K, Garg D, Sharma S. Psychogenic nonepileptic seizures and psychosocial management: a narrative review. Ann Indian Acad Neurol. 2021;24:146-54.
52. Durrant J, Rickards H, Cavanna AE. Prognosis and outcome predictors in psychogenic nonepileptic seizures. Epilepsy Res Treat. 2011;2011:1-7.
53. Bowman ES. Nonepileptic seizures: psychiatric framework, treatment, and outcome. Neurology. 1999;53:S84-8.
54. Reuber M, Pukrop R, Bauer J, Helmstaedter C, Tessendorf N, Erich Elger C. Outcome in psychogenic nonepileptic seizures: 1 to 10-year follow-up in 164 patients. Ann Neurol. 2003;53:305-11.
55. Walther K, Volbers B, Erdmann L, Dogan Onugoren M, Gollwitzer S, Kasper BS, et al. Psychological long-term outcome in patients with psychogenic nonepileptic seizures. Epilepsia. 2019;60:669-78.

Part 4D: Demyelinating and Immunological Diseases

67 CHAPTER

Multiple Sclerosis

Tapas Kumar Banerjee, Joydeep Biswas

INTRODUCTION

Multiple sclerosis (MS) is a chronic autoimmune disease of the central nervous system (CNS). The core pathology is inflammatory demyelination coupled with axonal degeneration, the later perhaps often not being emphasized. The disease is more prevalent in females than males and the onset usually is in the 20–40 years age group. MS generally takes a relapsing-remitting course with remissions following acute attacks of neurological dysfunction; relapse occurs after a varying periods of remission. A proportion of individuals has progressive course of illness right from the beginning. Incidentally, cases have been reported with the disease remaining clinically silent in life and only identified at autopsy. More often, however, MS is a disabling neurological illness and affects people in their most productive years of life.

EPIDEMIOLOGY

The most up-to-date epidemiological data is derived from the Atlas of MS 2020.[1] It has been estimated that 2.8 million people worldwide suffer from MS, meaning thereby that the prevalence worldwide is 1 in 3,000 people. MS is mostly seen in Europe and North America. San Marino and Germany have the highest prevalence with 337 per 100,000 and 303 per 100,000, respectively. In contrast, the prevalence is low in Africa and Western Pacific countries, where it is estimated to be around 5 per 100,000. In South and Southeast Asian countries, including India, the prevalence is about 9 (range, 0–25) per 100,000.[1] A study from South India found the crude prevalence rate of MS to be 8.3 per 100,000.[2]

The global annual incidence rate is 2.1 per 100,000 persons. Eighty-five percent of people initially present with relapsing-remitting course of the disease, whereas in 12% it is primary progressive. In 3%, the disease type is unknown. Globally, the average age of onset of MS is 32 years. About 1.5% of all MS occur in individuals under the age of 18 years.[1]

Data indicate that people living in countries closer to the equator have a lower risk of MS, whilst those living in countries closer to the poles are at greater risk.[3] It has been postulated that there is less sunlight with consequent low vitamin D levels in higher geographical latitudes and vitamin D deficiency increases the propensity for MS. In general, the female/male ratio of MS is 2:1. But in Western Pacific and South-East Asia, females are affected three to four times more than males.

Comprehensive and accurate global epidemiological data on MS is yet not available, because of paucity of information from Africa and other resource-limited countries. The Atlas of MS 2020[1] collected data from 115 countries covering 87% of the world's population. But a more comprehensive information that included incidence rate, pediatric MS, types of MS, etc., could be collected from only 75 countries, i.e., 65% of 115 responding countries.

ETIOPATHOGENESIS

Multiple sclerosis is an autoimmune disease of the CNS where genetic and environmental factors both contribute. Monozygotic twins have 25% chance of developing MS; first degree relatives have a slightly higher risk of 2–5%.[4] The HLA-DRB1*15:01, DQA1*0102, and DQB1*0602 alleles in the class II major histocompatibility complex (MHC-II) are the important MS risk factors.[5,6] Putative environmental agents include viral infection, vitamin D deficiency, obesity, smoking, etc. There is a likely connection between Epstein–Barr virus and MS. Vitamin D and ultraviolet rays are protective whereas smoking increases the susceptibility. Gut microbiome may have influence in the development of autoimmunity. Epidemiologically, it has been observed that those who migrate from low-risk to high-risk countries before adolescence have higher propensity for MS and *vice versa*.

In MS, the peripherally circulating autoreactive T and B lymphocytes cross the blood-brain barrier and accumulate in the CNS. The CD4+ T helper cell subtypes (Th1 and Th17) liberate damaging cytokines. CD8+ T cells initiate destruction of oligodendrocytes, myelin, and axons.[4] B lymphocytes lead to antibody production via plasma cells. Besides, the MHC-II on B cells present the appropriate antigens to T cells to activate the latter. The autoreactive T and B cells work in tandem and also function independently in the pathogenesis of MS. In addition to this, the regulatory lymphocytes that in healthy subjects keep the immune reactions under control become attenuated in this illness. Subsequently, macrophages and microglial cells in the CNS also get activated under the influence of autoreactive T and B cells. The net result is CNS inflammation and consequent demyelination. In the early stages, the nerve fibers after demyelination get repaired through the process of remyelination and the patient recovers clinically. Subsequently, the CNS resident immune cells, i.e., microglia and astrocytes, as well as B lymphocytes form ectopic germinal centers in brain parenchyma and meninges; these contribute to neurodegeneration and progressive and enduring disability.[7] Both immune-dependent and immune-independent (mitochondrial injury, oxidative stress, and glutamate excitotoxicity) mechanisms interplay in progressive CNS degeneration. *In summary, the T lymphocytes are the key drivers in relapsing MS whereas B lymphocytes are one of the principal movers in progressive disease.*

CLINICAL PRESENTATIONS

Demyelinating lesions are widely distributed in the CNS. The clinical presentation of an acute attack depends upon the site of the active lesion/s. The wide range of presenting clinical manifestations in MS include:

- *Optic neuritis*: Typically, unilateral optic neuritis is observed with acute blurring of vision and pain during eye movement. The visual blurring is partial; optic disk is mostly appeared normal (retro-bulbar neuritis) or may be swollen (papillitis) on fundoscopic examination. Bilateral simultaneous optic neuritis is less common. Visual impairment reaches its peak in 1–2 weeks. In very mild cases, color vision alone is impaired but visual acuity remains intact. Severe form of disease with complete blindness and loss of light perception is rare. Presentation with severe continuous orbital pain with blindness or progressive visual loss is a "red flag" for a diagnosis of MS.
- *Brain stem/cerebellar dysfunction*: Cerebellar ataxia, unilateral or bilateral internuclear ophthalmoplegia (INO), horizontal or vertical multidirectional nystagmus, and 5th, 6th, or 7th cranial neuropathies may be frequently encountered.
- *Spinal cord dysfunction*: Myelopathy leading to sensory or motor long tract signs can occur. Partial myelopathy is more common than complete transverse myelitis. Sphincter and erectile dysfunctions may be observed. Paresthesia or pain (deafferentation pain) in limbs or trunk may occur due to posterior column demyelination. Occasionally, there may be segmental sensory loss of pain and temperature sensation. But a sharp sensory level with deficit of all modalities of sensation is uncommon in MS. Some patients experience a girdle-like sensation around chest or abdomen with intensities varying from tightening feeling to actual pain; this is termed as "MS hug".
- *Cerebral hemispheric dysfunction*: There may occur hemiparesis or homonymous hemianopia in MS. The prevalence of seizures in MS is around 3%, as against 0.27–1.7% in general population.[8] Seizure semiology is focal in over 85%.[9] Acute encephalopathy (drowsiness, headache, and vomiting) in children or adolescent is an extremely rare feature of MS and rather, points toward "acute disseminated encephalomyelitis (ADEM)".[10,11]
- A *true "relapse" of MS* is defined as an acute exacerbation of symptoms and signs that last at least for 24 hours; the underlying pathology being appearance of new inflammatory demyelinating lesion in CNS. On the other hand, increase in core body temperature secondary to fever, exposure to hot weather, or exercise may temporarily lead to exacerbation of symptoms. This is *"pseudo-relapse"* (Uhthoff's phenomenon) and the underlying mechanism is not new demyelination but transient worsening conduction abnormality in an already demyelinated fiber.
- *Fatigue:* This is fairly common in MS with lifetime prevalence of 80%.[12] Fatigue has two components—(1) peripheral and (2) central. The peripheral fatigue is the consequence of motor weakness. Central fatigue, presumed to be an outcome of CNS dysfunction, is manifested by reduced motivation and vitality, typically worsening in the evening time.[13] Fatiguability impairs performance of cognitive tasks. Fatigue is aggravated during sleep disturbances, emotional stress, depression, or along with presence of cognitive impairment.[14,15]
- *Cognitive decline:* Slowing of cognitive processing and decline in episodic memory are the two principal cognitive issues in MS.[16] Attention span, verbal fluency, conceptual reasoning, and visuo-spatial perceptions may also be affected.[17]
- *Psychiatric manifestations:* Depression is common. 10% of MS suffer from manic-depressive bipolar disorder and paranoia. A rare condition "laughing-weeping syndrome" may occur in severe cases, characterized by inappropriate euphoria or despair that is contrary to the individuals actual emotional state and is often associated with brain-stem demyelination.
- *Paroxysmal attacks:* These are recurrent, very short-lasting (seconds to minutes duration) nonepileptic events. Good response to anticonvulsants (e.g.,

carbamazepine) is a feature of these paroxysmal events. These include:
- Lhermitte's phenomenon, where neck flexion induces an electric shock-like sensation radiating down the spine and often spreading to arms and legs.
- Painful tonic spasm or paroxysmal dystonia may occur, characterized by brief stereotyped, at times, short-lasting, painful unilateral dystonic spells.[18]
- Trigeminal neuralgia is observed at times. MS comprises 18% of those rare cases, which manifest with bilateral trigeminal neuralgia.[19]
- Paroxysmal dysarthria or ataxia.

DIAGNOSTIC CRITERIA OF MS AND MS SUBTYPES

Classification of MS

In 1996, the International Advisory Committee on Clinical Trials in MS described four subtypes based on the course of illness **(Figs. 1A to D)**. These four MS subtypes are:[20]
1. Relapsing-remitting MS (RRMS)
2. Secondary progressive MS (SPMS)
3. Primary progressive MS (PPMS)
4. Progressive relapsing MS (PRMS)

Relapsing-remitting Multiple Sclerosis

This is the most common type of MS, accounting for 70–80%. This is characterized by well-defined recurrent attacks of neurological deficits with full or partial recovery and without any disease progression between the relapses. Incidentally, clinically isolated syndrome (CIS) is a single clinical episode of inflammatory demyelination of CNS, lasting beyond 24 hours. Some individuals with CIS cases do not go on to develop MS with recurrent clinical events; hence CIS was not considered MS in the 1996 classification.

Secondary Progressive Multiple Sclerosis

Prior to the advent of disease-modifying therapies (DMTs), it was estimated that after 10 years, 50% of RRMS and after 25 years 90% of RRMS would convert to SPMS.[21] In SPMS, the disease becomes progressive with or without intermittent relapses.

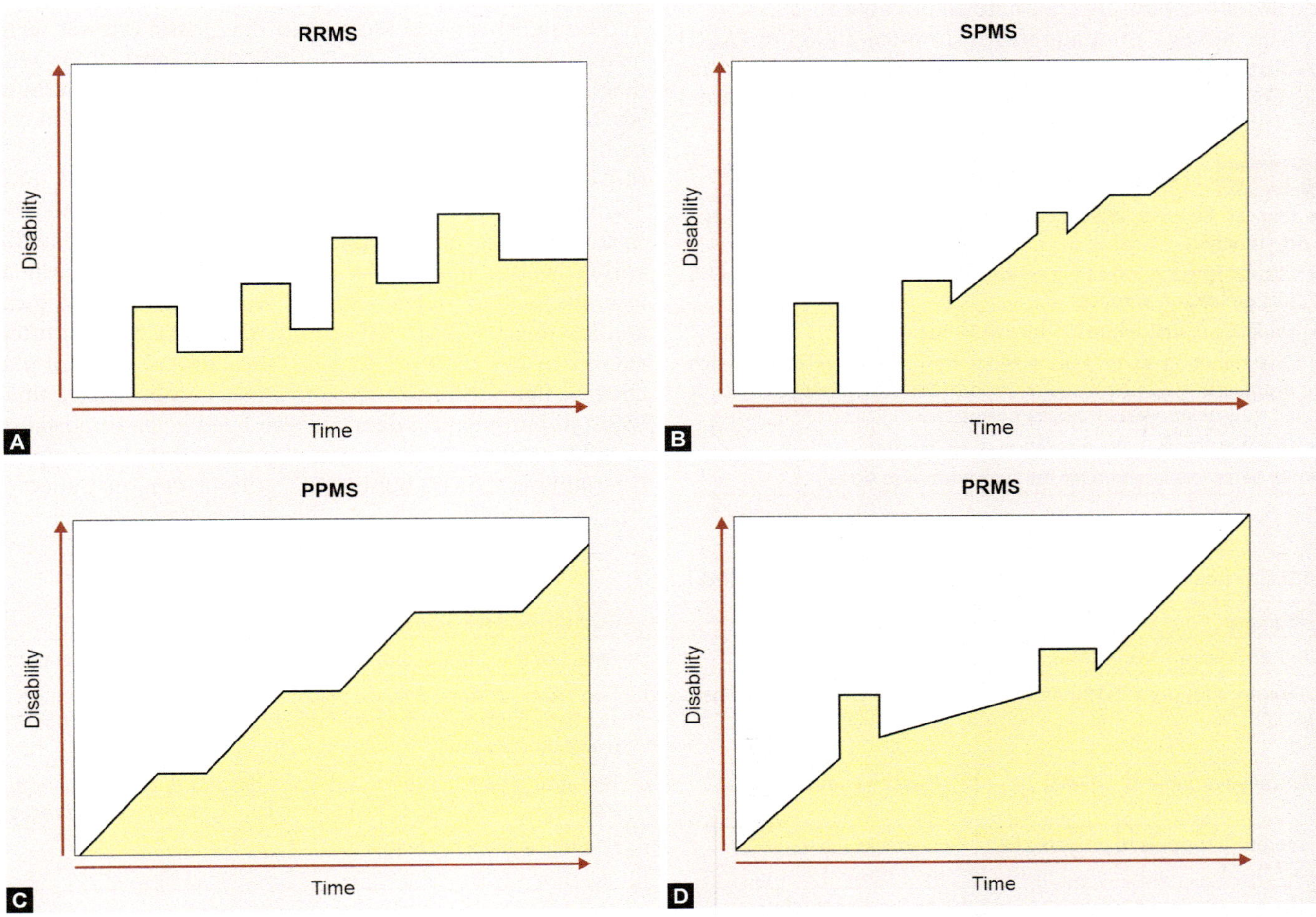

FIGS. 1A TO D: Clinical courses of MS subtypes— (A) Relapsing remitting MS; (B) Secondary progressive MS; (C) Primary progressive MS; and (D) Progressive relapsing MS.

Primary Progressive Multiple Sclerosis

Approximately, 15–20% of MS are of this type. Here, the disease is progressive right from onset with short periods of nonprogression and occasionally even having transient minor improvement.

Progressive Relapsing Multiple Sclerosis

A special category of PPMS, in which, there are clear-cut relapses on the background of a progressive illness. Nearly 5% of MS belong to this group.

Diagnostic Criteria of MS

Diagnosis of MS requires white matter symptoms and signs fulfilling both "dissemination in space (DIS)" and "dissemination in time (DIT)" criteria. DIS indicates occurrence of lesions at two or more distinct anatomical sites in the CNS. On the other hand, DIT means new lesions appearing in CNS at different time points. On the basis of mainly clinical parameters, Schumacher's criteria[22] (summarized in **Box 1**) were introduced in 1965 for MS. Subsequently, Poser's criteria came into existence in 1983, in which, evoked potential studies and cerebrospinal oligoclonal band (OCB) were added to the clinical criteria.[23] The Poser's criteria are summarized in **Table 1**.

The advent of magnetic resonance imaging (MRI) revolutionized the diagnostic work-up of MS and has become an indispensable tool.[24,25] Currently, the McDonald criteria are widely followed for the diagnosis of MS, in which a combination of clinical and cerebrospinal MRI findings are utilized. The aim is, through the aforementioned data, to establish DIS and DIT.

As per the McDonald criteria, two clear attacks typical of MS, documented by objective evidence of two lesions separated in time and separated in space may be sufficient to make an MS diagnosis solely on clinical grounds. No additional tests may be needed. However, even in the absence of a second clinical attack, serial MRI scans may be sufficient to diagnose MS in many CIS cases by applying the MRI diagnostic criteria. The MRI diagnostic criteria have undergone several modifications since the first version[26] in 2001 as in 2005,[27] 2010,[28] and 2017.[29] The McDonald MRI diagnostic criteria 2001 and 2005 for RRMS are summarized in **Table 2**. The DIS criteria of McDonald in 2001 and 2005 were derived from the earlier observations of Berkhof[30] and Tintore.[31] The subsequent revision in McDonald criteria in 2010 simplified the process of DIS and DIT on MRI scans and made it even possible to establish DIS/DIT from a single imaging study, thus obviating the need for multiple or serial imaging studies. The criteria improved diagnostic sensitivity of MS significantly without reducing specificity. The McDonald 2010 criteria drew inspiration from the published works of MAGNIMS research group.[32,33]

The latest revised McDonald diagnostic criteria were introduced in 2017.[29] McDonald 2010 and 2017 MRI diagnostic criteria for RRMS are summarized in **Table 3**, where the subtle differences between the two criteria are highlighted. Based upon MAGNIMS 2016 observations,[34,35] McDonald 2017 included both symptomatic and asymptomatic MRI lesions for determination of DIS and DIT. In addition, instead of juxta-cortical lesion mentioned in the earlier McDonald criteria, the term cortical-juxtacortical lesion is used in McDonald 2017. In fact, histopathological studies reveal that in MS, the juxtacortical lesions often extend to the cortex.[36] In fact, intracortical and subpial cortical demyelination also do exist. cerebrospinal fluid (CSF) immunological data has also been given importance in the McDonald 2017; the panel proposed that in a typical CIS fulfilling the DIS but not DIT criteria, demonstration of

BOX 1 Schumacher criteria of multiple sclerosis.

- Clinical features indicative of central nervous system (CNS) dysfunction
- Clinical features indicative of affection in ≥2 distinct areas of CNS (dissemination in space)
- Evidence of CNS white matter involvement
- Dissemination in time as evident from (1) ≥2 relapses—each event lasting ≥24 hour and ≥1 month interval between attacks, or (2) slow or stepwise disability progression
- Onset of illness in the age range of 10–50 years
- No better explanation for the symptoms and signs

TABLE 1: Poser diagnostic criteria for multiple sclerosis (MS).

Diagnosis	Clinical presentation	Additional data required
Clinically definite MS (CDMS)	≥ Two attacks*	Two clinical evidence; one clinical and one paraclinical evidence**
Laboratory supported definite MS (LSDMS)	≥ One attack and oligoclonal band	Two attacks and one evidence (clinical or paraclinical); one attack and two clinical evidences; one attack, and one clinical and one paraclinical evidence
Clinically probable MS (CPMS)	At least one attack	Two attacks and one clinical evidence; one attack and two clinical evidences; one attack, one clinical, and one paraclinical evidences
Laboratory supported probable MS (LSPMS)	Two attacks	No more evidence is required

*Each attack lasting ≥24 hours with ≥1 month interval between attacks.
**Paraclinical evidence is that derived from evoked potential studies.

TABLE 2: McDonald MRI diagnostic criteria (2001) and revised McDonald criteria (2005) for RRMS.

McDonald 2001	McDonald 2005
DIS criteria: Any three of below: 1. ≥ One gadolinium enhancing (Gd+) lesion or 9 T2 hyperintense lesion if no Gd+ lesion 2. ≥ One infratentorial lesion 3. ≥ One juxtacortical lesion 4. ≥ One periventricular lesion *Note*: One spinal may replace one cerebral lesion.	*DIS criteria:* Any three of below: 1. ≥ One gadolinium enhancing (Gd+) lesion or 9 T2 hyperintense lesion if no Gd+ lesion 2. ≥ One infratentorial lesion 3. ≥ One juxtacortical lesion 4. ≥ One periventricular lesion *Note*: One spinal may replace one infratentorial lesion; one Gd+ spinal equivalent to one Gd+ cerebral lesion; individual spinal lesion may be added to individual cerebral lesion to fulfil the total of nine lesions.
DIT criteria: • If the first scan done ≥3 months after clinical onset, the presence of ≥1 Gd+ lesion at a site separate from that in original clinical event. If no Gd+ lesion at this time, a follow-up scan after at least 3 months needed. If new T2 lesion or Gd+ lesion in second scan, this indicates DIT • If first scan done <3 months of clinical onset, a second scan done ≥3 months after clinical event showing new Gd+ lesion confirms DIT. If no Gd+ lesion in second scan, a further scan ≥3 months after the first scan showing a new T2 lesion or Gd+ lesion will fulfill the criteria of DIT	*DIT criteria*: • Gd+ lesion ≥3 months after the onset of clinical attack, if at a site different from that corresponding to initial event • New T2 lesion if it appears at any time compared to a reference scan done at least 30 days after the onset of clinical attack

(DIT: dissemination in time; RRMS: relapsing-remitting multiple sclerosis)

TABLE 3: McDonald MRI diagnostic criteria of 2010 and of 2017 for RRMS *(differences between the 2 criteria)*.

McDonald 2010	McDonald 2017
DIS criteria: ≥ One T2 lesion in at least two of four MS—typical areas of the CNS (periventricular, *juxtacortical*, infratentorial, or spinal cord)	*DIS criteria:* ≥ One T2 lesion in at least two of the four MS—typical areas of the CNS (periventricular, cortical-juxtacortical, infratentorial, or spinal cord)
DIT criteria: Simultaneous existence of *asymptomatic* Gd+ lesion and T2 lesion in the scan, or a new T2 or Gd+ lesion in follow-up MRI irrespective of timing of baseline scan	*DIT criteria:* Simultaneous existence of Gd+ lesion and T2 lesion *(either symptomatic or asymptomatic)* in the scan, or a new T2 or Gd+ lesion in follow-up MRI irrespective of timing of baseline scan

(CNS: central nervous system; DIS: dissemination in space; MRI: magnetic resonance imaging; RRMS: relapsing-remitting multiple sclerosis)

BOX 2 McDonald 2017 diagnostic criteria of PPMS.

Retrospectively or prospectively determined progressive disability over 1 year, plus any two of the followings:

1. ≥ *One T2-hyperintense lesions in ≥1 of following cerebral lesion*: Periventricular, cortical/juxtacortical, or infratentorial
2. ≥ Two T2-hyperintense lesions in the spinal cord
3. Presence of CSF-specific oligoclonal bands

(CSF: cerebrospinal fluid; PPMS: progressive relapsing multiple sclerosis)

CSF OCB (in the absence of atypical CSF findings) allows a diagnosis of MS to be made. McDonald 2001, 2005, and 2010 diagnostic criteria of PPMS also exist. The McDonald 2017 diagnostic criteria of PPMS are summarized in **Box 2.**[29]

Revised Classification of MS

In 2013, the new classification of MS[37] has been introduced and takes into account the MRI and laboratory findings in addition to clinical features. In this current classification, the term *"active"* indicates (1) clinical relapse followed by full or partial recovery and/or (2) MRI evidence of contrast-enhancing T1 lesion or new/unequivocally enlarging T2 hyperintense lesion. The term *"progressive"* indicates steadily increasing clinical deterioration without unequivocal recovery. When there are periods where the neurological dysfunction remains static the condition is termed *"non-progressive"*. According to the 2013 classification, the new subtypes of MS are:

- Clinically isolated syndrome
- Relapsing-remitting MS
- Secondary progressive MS
- Primary progressive MS

Clinically Isolated Syndrome

This condition is now included in the ambit of MS and categorized into "active" and "not active". MRI evidence of DIS/DIT identifies cases of MS among those who have single clinical event, fulfilling the McDonald criteria. These latter cases are termed "active CIS", and warrants treatment with disease-modifying treatment.

Relapsing-remitting Multiple Sclerosis

This is divided into "active" and "not active". Those who have new gadolinium-enhanced lesion on MRI are "active". Conversely, those RRMS are "inactive" who within the assessment period did not show clinical relapse or new/enlarged T2 lesion/s or contrast enhanced lesion/s.

Secondary Progressive Multiple Sclerosis

This has been categorized into four groups—(1) active, progressive; (2) active, not progressive; (3) not active, progressive; and (4) not active, not progressive. The progression of the disease is determined by history or objective measure of progression in disability over a span of one year.

Primary Progressive Multiple Sclerosis

This can also be categorized, using the above-mentioned criteria, into four groups—(1) active, progressive; (2) active, not progressive; (3) not active, progressive; (4) not active, not progressive. Of note, the term PRMS is no more used.

DIFFERENTIAL DIAGNOSIS

A wide range of disorders are to be considered in the differential diagnosis of MS. These may be categorized as follows:

- *Idiopathic inflammatory demyelinating disorders*:
  - Acute disseminated encephalomyelitis
  - Neuromyelitis optica spectrum disorders (NMOSD)
  - Myelin oligodendrocyte glycoprotein (MOG)-associated disorders (MOGAD)
- Cerebral neoplasm, particularly cerebral lymphoma
- *Idiopathic inflammatory nondemyelinating disorders*:
  - Neuro-Behçet's disease
  - Systemic lupus erythematosus
  - Sjögren syndrome
  - Wegener granulomatosis
  - Isolated CNS vasculitis
  - Antiphospholipid syndrome
  - Susac's syndrome
  - Clipper syndrome
  - Sarcoidosis

In CIS manifesting with acute optic neuritis, the differential diagnoses include (1) ischemic optic neuropathy, (2) infections-tuberculosis, neurosyphilis, postviral neuritis, and Lymes disease, (3) infiltrative (e.g., sarcoid and lupus), (4) toxic/nutritional, and (5) chronic recurrent inflammatory optic neuropathy (CRION).

In the differential diagnoses of CIS manifesting as acute myelitis, there are (1) compressive myelopathies, (2) ischemic, (3) infective [e.g., tuberculosis, neurosyphilis, human immunodeficiency virus (HIV), and human T-cell lymphotropic virus type 1 (HTLV-1)], and (4) toxic/nutritional/metabolic (e.g., vitamin B12 deficiency and copper deficiency).

INVESTIGATIONS

There is no single, specific confirmatory test for MS. The diagnosis is essentially based upon clinical findings, cerebrospinal MRI, and CSF.

Magnetic Resonance Imaging

With advancement in imaging techniques over the last four decades, MRI has become the single most important diagnostic tool for MS. This investigation has played a crucial role in establishing the McDonald diagnostic criteria for this disorder (see above). The standard protocol warrants MRI (at magnetic field strength of 1.5T or 3T) of both brain and spinal cord using several sequences—T1-weighted pre- and postgadolinium, T2-weighted and fluid-attenuated inversion recovery (FLAIR) or short-tau inversion recovery (STIR). T2 hyperintense lesions, radially-oriented and adjacent to the lateral ventricles are classical imaging features in MS, often called the "Dawson's fingers" **(Fig 2)**. Presence of a central vein within a T2 hyperintense white matter lesion ("central vein sign") is highly specific for MS.[38] Chronic small hypointense lesion/s, or the "black holes" **(Fig. 3)**, are occasionally visible in supratentorial region indicative of severe irreversible axonal loss in addition to demyelination. The demyelinating plaques are generally oval/ovoid shaped, >5 mm in diameter; but at times the lesion may be tumefactive **(Figs. 4A and B)**, which implies that the shape and size mimics a tumor.[39] Rarely, the lesion/s take the shape of concentric multilayered rings of varying intensities, representing bands of demyelination alternating with bands of relative myelin preservation, termed as, Balo's concentric sclerosis.[40] Gadolinium enhancement may be homogenous but is typically of the "open-ring pattern".[41] In untreated MS, brain atrophy occurs at a rate of 0.5–1.0% per year. Atrophy of brain is more strongly related to physical and cognitive impairment in MS, compared to the standard metrics

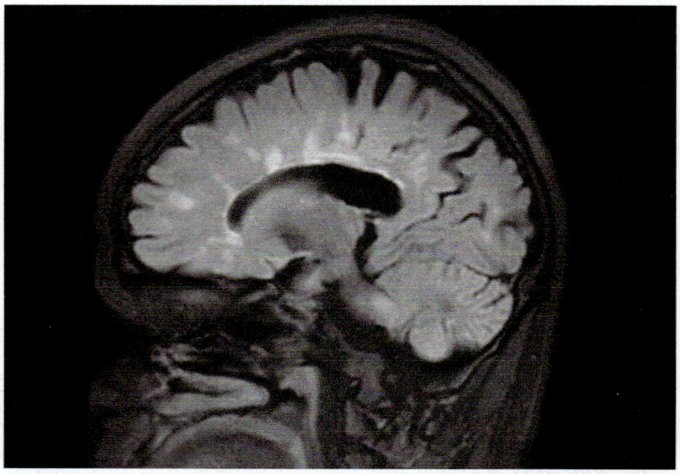

FIG. 2: Sagittal fluid-attenuated inversion recovery (FLAIR) sequence of brain showing the "Dawson's fingers".

(T1 hypointense, T2 hyperintense, and gadolinium-enhancing plaques) and is an important prognostic indicator.[42] Fully automated computer segmentation techniques relying on high-resolution T1-weighted images are reliable tools to measure cerebral atrophy. Advanced techniques, i.e., magnetic resonance spectroscopy (MRS), magnetization transfer ratio (MTR), and diffusion tensor imaging (DTI) offer the potential to improve pathological imaging in MS.

In MS manifesting as optic neuritis, thin, fat-suppressed STIR sequences reveal characteristic short hyperintense lesion/s; the lesion may enhance on contrast. Demyelinating lesions in the spinal cord are of short segment (limited to two vertebrae or less), peripherally located in the white matter and occupy < half the cross-sectional area of cord.

Cerebrospinal Fluid

The routine analysis is normal with cell counts typically ≤50 cells/μL; only 1–2% of MS have cell counts >50. On differential cell count, lymphocytes account for >90%. The diagnostic biomarkers of MS are (1) quantitatively elevated IgG, or the IgG index, and (2) detection of OCB by isoelectric focusing technique. The sensitivity of OCB positivity (95%) is far superior to immunoglobulin G (IgG) index (60%). The diagnostic specificity is between 60 and 90%. In order to establish that IgG is synthesized intrathecally, OCB tests from both serum and CSF should be simultaneously performed. Positive OCB means either selective occurrence in CSF or more bands in CSF than in serum.[43]

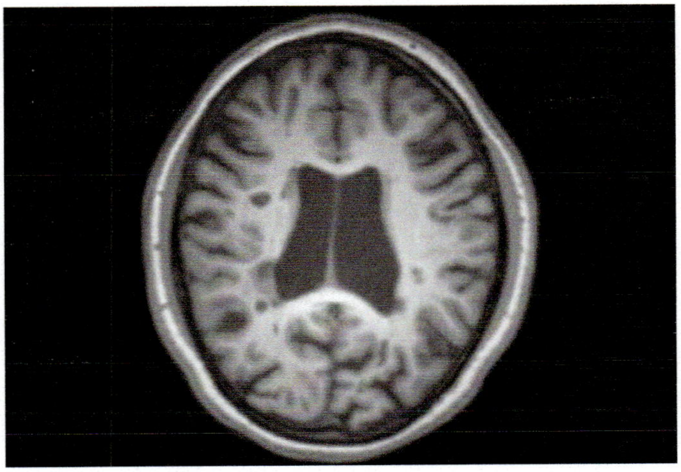

FIG. 3: T1 sequence showing "black holes" in brain.

Serum Neurofilament Light Chain

This is indicative of inflammation-driven axonal damage. This is not a specific biomarker of MS, since elevated level may occur in other postinflammatory neuroaxonal degenerative disorders. However, high serum neuro-filament light chain (sNfL) level is strongly predictive of progression or future relapses in MS.[44] Serum NfL is an important predictor for conversion of CIS to MS.[45]

Optical Coherence Tomography

This is a noninvasive tool to obtain cross-sectional image/s of retina. Spectral-domain optical coherence tomography (SDOCT) measures thickness of individual retinal layers. This test indicates axonal and ganglion cell loss. Atrophy of retinal nerve fiber layer (RNFL), particularly of inner and outer layers as determined by SDOCT are more severe in progressive MS than RRMS.[46]

TREATMENT

The pharmacotherapy of MS can be classified into (1) treatment of acute attack, (2) symptomatic therapy, and (3) DMT to arrest disease progression.

- *Treatment of acute attack:* Pulse methylprednisolone (MP) shortens the attack duration and accelerates the process of remission in RRMS. The dose is 500–1,000 mg intravenous infusion daily for 3–5 days.

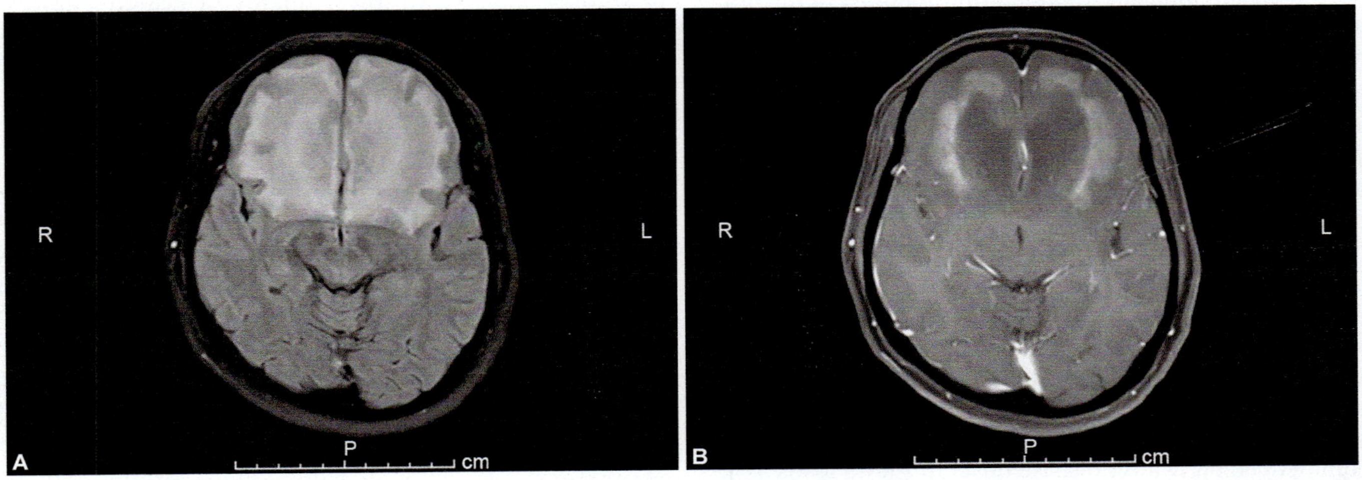

FIGS. 4A AND B: "Tumefactive" cerebral lesion in MS—(A) Fluid-attenuated inversion recovery (FLAIR) sequence; (B) T1-weighted image revealing peripheral contrast enhancement.

- *Symptomatic therapies:* These are required for the alleviation of various symptoms in MS. For spasticity—baclofen and tizanidine; for overactive bladder syndrome—oxybutynin and mirabegron; and for pain and paresthesia—pregabalin, duloxetine, gabapentin, and venlafaxine are required. Botulinum toxin (BoNT) injection can be useful for spasticity. Intravesicular BoNT injection in urinary bladder wall and in the external urinary sphincter is required in severe overactive bladder syndrome and detrusor-sphincter dyssynergia, respectively. Amantadine or modafinil is beneficial to overcome the symptom of fatigue in MS. For oscillopsia, gabapentin, memantine, or levetiracetam may be tried. Dalfampridine (4-aminopyridine) blocks the voltage-dependent potassium channels in demyelinated axons and restores nerve conduction. This property of dalfampridine is utilized to improve walking ability in MS.
- *DMTs to arrest disease progression:* In 1993, a new era of DMT for RRMS began with the Food and Drug Administration (FDA) approval of interferon β-1b.[47] In the subsequent 5 years, interferon β-1a and glatiramer came into use. The DMT landscape has greatly widened over the previous 10 years and includes a large number of drugs both as platform therapy and as high-efficacy therapy (HET). The aim of DMT in RRMS is to achieve "no evidence of disease activity" (NEDA)[48] Early institution of DMT is strongly advocated to significantly alter the natural history of the illness.[49] Data has revealed that the risk of increasing "expanded disability status scale"(EDSS) score escalates by *7.4% for every year of delay* in DMT initiation after MS onset.[50]

The platform drugs (so-called first-line drugs) have moderate efficacy with annualized relapse rate (ARR) reductions in the range of 30–50%. The adverse effects of these drugs are usually mild. These platform DMTs include interferon-beta 1b (IFNβ-1b 250 μg/500 μg subcutaneously daily), IFNβ-1a (22 μg/44 μg subcutaneously thrice a week), IFNβ-1a (30 μg intramuscular, weekly), pegylated IFNβ-1a (125 μg subcutaneously, every 2 weeks), glatiramer (20 mg subcutaneously, daily), teriflunomide (14 mg orally daily), dimethyl fumarate (240 mg orally twice daily), and fingolimod (0.5 mg orally daily). On the other hand, HET has the potential to reduce ARRs far >50%,[51] but the adverse effects are also more and often severe. HETs for MS include alemtuzumab, natalizumab, rituximab, ocrelizumab, ofatumumab, ponesimod, ozanimod, and cladribine.

In the conventional "escalation approach" to RRMS, treatment typically commences with platform DMTs. In those cases where the drugs show "suboptimal" efficacy, HET may be introduced. On the contrary, "induction" approach implies treatment initiation with HET to achieve maximum benefit; therapy may subsequently be maintained with platform drugs to mitigate risk of major side-effects. Studies have now shown that HET, when commenced early after disease onset in RRMS leads to less disability after 6–10 years compared to when used late in the course of illness.[52] A paradigm shift in DMT is now being considered since the long-term outcome of RRMS has been demonstrated to be better with the "induction approach" than with the "escalation approach".[53] This advantage, however, needs to be balanced with the propensity of HETs to cause serious adverse effects.

Highly active MS, i.e., rapidly evolving severe RRMS or aggressive MS is characterized by frequent relapses with several gadolinium enhanced T1 lesions on MRI scans.[54] If at onset, the disease appears to be highly active, induction approach with HET is advocated to prevent substantial physical and cognitive deficits.[55] In this situation, autologous hematopoietic stem cell transplantation (AHSCT) may be considered as a therapeutic option. AHSCT has the potential to suppress MS in 70–80% of patients for 4–5 years, and in this regard is superior to many HETs. Since 2005, the mortality associated with procedure has dropped from 4 to 0.3%.[56]

The general perception thus far has been that beyond a certain degree of disability (EDSS > 4), the benefit from DMT is unsatisfactory.[57] Recent data have, however, challenged this perception. It is now being observed that even at a more advanced stage of MS, DMTs might be beneficial. In fact, ocrelizumab has shown to slow deterioration of PPMS with 25% reduction in disability progression at 12 and 24 weeks compared to controls.[58] Siponimod is likely to be useful in the treatment of SPMS.[59]

It is incorrect to consider progressive MS as only neuro-degeneration; there are, in addition, significant inflammatory processes involved.[60] So the message should be that while ideally DMT should be started soon after the onset of MS to obtain the best outcome, it should not necessarily be abandoned in patients at the progressive stage.[61]

Incidentally, the above mentioned DMTs are "on-label" or in other words, approved for use in the western nations. Affected individuals from about 70% of low- and low-middle income countries have no access to the on-label DMTs.[62] Several other drugs, e.g., azathioprine, rituximab, mitoxantrone methotrexate, cyclophosphamide, and mycophenolate mofetil have also shown efficacy in RRMS in studies, albeit with lower quality of evidence. These represent "off-label" DMTs for treatment of MS. Because of low cost, easy availability, and good efficacy, off-label DMTs, e.g., azathioprine[63] and rituximab[64,65] are widely used in low- and low-middle income countries.[62]

SPECIAL FEATURES IN THE INDIAN CONTEXT

Multiple sclerosis was once considered to be extremely rare in the Indian subcontinent except among the Parsi community. In the small Parsi community of 70,000, the estimated prevalence was about 25 per 100,000.[66,67] In contrast, in the 1970s, among the non-Parsi Indians, hospital-based registry derived prevalence rates ranged from 0.17 to 1.33 per 100,000.[68] The current prevalence of MS in India is at least eightfold higher.[2] Better awareness of the disease with improved investigational facilities rather than a true increase in prevalence rates has contributed significantly to this change. Previous literature from Asia noted that the vast majority of the Asian MS presented with bilateral optic nerve affection, myelopathy, and painful tonic spasms and that cerebral or cerebellar involvements were rare. So, it was considered that opticospinal form of MS (labelled as OS-MS) predominated in Asia, as phenotypically distinct from the western hemisphere.[69] However, most of these are now recognized to be neuromyelitis optica-spectrum disorder with the introduction of serum aquaporin-4 IgG (AQP4-IgG) test/s and based upon the current definition.[70] But still the nomenclature OSMS is retained since a few could be MS with the characteristic MS type lesions on the brain MRI.[71]

The current data indicates that the age of onset and clinical presentations of MS in India are similar to that observed in the Western countries.[72] Pediatric MS has also been reported from India.[73] Vitamin D levels are substantially lower among MS cases than among the matched controls.[74] Khadilkar et al. has demonstrated through case-control study that childhood mumps, autoimmune disease, and smoking have strong association with MS in India.[75]

The genetic susceptibility factors for MS in India is similar to that in the western nations. HLA-DRB1*15:01/02 and HLA-DQB1*06:02 are significantly associated with Indian MS cohorts also.[76] However, a study from Mumbai demonstrated two novel alleles DRB1*1506 and DRB1*1508 in association with MS.[77]

Banerjee et al. conducted a prospective study over a 7-year period on a CIS cohort. Out of 82 individuals, 36 (44%) converted to MS. In 24 months, the conversion rate was 38%. The predictors for conversion to MS were earlier age of onset of CIS and demonstration of CSF-OCB, load of total T2 lesions cerebral lesions, and the presence of periventricular and juxta-cortical locations of lesions on baseline studies.[78] Our conversion rate is lower than that from the European countries (55–85%)[79] but higher than that from China.[80] The predictors for conversion to MS in India are similar to that observed in the western literature.[81,82]

CONCLUSION

There have been enormous diagnostic and therapeutic advances MS over the past decade. These have fueled deeper insights into the disease process. Three decades ago, one used to approach this disease with certain amount of pessimism. A paradigm shift has now occurred in the treatment of MS and perhaps we are looking forward to a curative therapy by the next decade. Awareness of MS has grown in India and a substantial number of cases now seem to exist. Several original research papers pertaining to MS have come from India. It is now high time that we have a nationwide epidemiologic data on MS that also covers the disease profile, risk factors, and response to therapy.

REFERENCES

1. MS International Federation. (2020). Atlas of MS 3rd edition. [online] Available from https://www.msif.org/wp-content/uploads/2020/10/Atlas-3rd-Edition-Epidemiology-report-EN-updated-30-9-20.pdf [Last accessed April, 2023].
2. Pandit L, Kundapur R. Prevalence and patterns of demyelinating central nervous system disorders in urban Mangalore, South India. Mult Scler. 2014;20(12):1651-3.
3. Simpson S Jr, Wang W, Otahal P, Blizzard L, van der Mei IAF, Taylor BV. Latitude continues to be significantly associated with the prevalence of multiple sclerosis: an updated meta-analysis. J Neurol Neurosurg Psychiatry. 2019;90(11):1193-200.
4. Baecher-Allan C, Kaslow BJ, Weiner HL. Multiple sclerosis: Mechanisms and immunotherapy. Neuron. 2018;97(4):742-68.
5. Mosca L, Mantero V, Penco S, Mantia LL, Benedetti SD, Marazzi MR, et al. HLA-DRB1*15 association with multiple sclerosis is confirmed in a multigenerational Italian family. Funct Neurol. 2017;32(2):83-8.
6. Hillert J. Human leukocyte antigen studies in multiple sclerosis. Ann Neurol. 1994;36:S15-17.
7. Lehmann-Horn K, Kronsbein HC, Weber MS. Targeting B cells in the treatment of multiple sclerosis: recent advances and remaining challenges. Ther Adv Neurol Disord. 2013;6(3):161-73.
8. Uribe-San-Martin R, Ciampi-Diaz E, Suarez-Hernández F, Vásquez-Torres M, Godoy-Fernández J, Cárcamo-Rodriguez C. Prevalence of epilepsy in a cohort of patients with multiple sclerosis. Seizure. 2014;23(1):81-3.
9. Benjaminsen E, Myhr KM, Alstadhaug KB. The prevalence and characteristics of epilepsy in patients with multiple sclerosis in Nordland county, Norway. Seizure. 2017;52:131-5.
10. Tenembaum SN. Acute disseminated encephalomyelitis. Hanb Clin Neurol. 2013;112:1253-62.
11. Brass SD, Caramanos Z, Santos C, Dilenge ME, Lapierre Y, Rosenblatt B. Multiple sclerosis vs acute disseminated encephalomyelitis in childhood. Pediatr Neurol. 2003;29(3):227-31.
12. Krupp LB, Serafin DJ, Christodoulou C. Multiple sclerosis-associated fatigue. Expert Rev Neurother. 2010;10(9):1437-47.
13. Tedeschi G, Dinacci D, Lavorgna L, Prinster A, Savettieri G, Quattrone A, et al. Correlation between fatigue and brain atrophy and lesion load in multiple sclerosis patient independent of disability. J Neurol Sci. 2007;263(1-2);15-9.
14. Heesen C, Nawrath L, Reich C, Bauer N, Schulz KH, Gold SM. Fatigue in multiple sclerosis: an example of cytokine mediated sickness behaviour? J Neurol Neurosurg Psychiatry. 2006;77(1):34-9.
15. Schneider S, Stone AA, Schwartz JE, Broderick JE. Peak and end effects in patients' daily recall of pain and fatigue: a within-subjects analysis. J Pain. 2011;12(1):228-35.
16. Sumowski JF, Benedict R, Enzinger C, Filippi M, Geurts JJ, Hamalainen P, et al. Cognition in multiple sclerosis: State of the field and priorities for the future. Neurology. 2018;90:278-88.
17. Rao SM, Leo GJ, Bernardin L, Unverzagt F. Cognitive dysfunction in multiple sclerosis: I: frequency, patterns, and prediction. Neurology. 1991;41:685-91.
18. El Otmani H, Benmansour Y, Araqi-Houssaini A, Benkirane N, Dany F, Rafai MA, et al. Paroxysmal dystonia and multiple sclerosis. Rev Neurol (Paris). 2014;170(2):119-23.
19. Brisman R. Bilateral trigeminal neuralgia. J Neurosurg. 1987;67(1):44-8.

20. Lublin FD, Reingold SC. Defining the clinical course of multiple sclerosis: results of an international survey. National multiple sclerosis society (USA) advisory committee on clinical trials of new agents in multiple sclerosis. Neurology. 1996;46:907-11.
21. Trojano M, Paolicelli D, Bellacosa A, Cataldo S. The transition from relapsing-remitting MS to irreversible disability: clinical evaluation. Neurol Sci. 2003;24(suppl 5):S268-70.
22. Schumacher GA, Beebe G, Kibler RF, Kurland LT, Kurtzke JF, Mcdowell F, et al. Problems of experimental trials of therapy in multiple sclerosis. Report by the panel on the evaluation of experimental trials of therapy in multiple sclerosis. Ann NY Acad Sci. 1965;122:522-68.
23. Poser CM, Paty DW, Scheinberg L, McDonald WI, Davis FA, Ebers GC, et al. New diagnostic criteria for multiple sclerosis: guidelines for research protocols. Ann Neurol. 1983;13(3):227-31.
24. Young IR, Hall AS, Pallis CA, Legg NJ, Bydder GM, Steiner RE. Nuclear magnetic resonance imaging of the brain in multiple sclerosis. Lancet. 1981;2(8255):1063-6.
25. Cohen JA, Rae-Grant A. Diagnosing multiple sclerosis. In: Handbook of Multiple Sclerosis. 2nd edition. London, England: Springer Healthcare; 2012:15-27.
26. McDonald WI, Compston A, Edan G, Goodkin D, Hartung HP, Lublin FD, et al. Recommended diagnostic criteria for multiple sclerosis: guidelines from the International Panel on the diagnosis of multiple sclerosis. Ann Neurol. 2001;50(1):121-7.
27. Polman CH, Reingold SC, Edan G, Filippi M, Hartung HP, Kappos L, et al. Diagnostic criteria for multiple sclerosis: 2005 revisions to the "McDonald Criteria". Ann Neurol. 2005;58(6):840-6.
28. Polman CH, Reingold SC, Banwell B, Clanet M, Cohen JA, Filippi M, et al. Diagnostic criteria for multiple sclerosis: 2010 revisions to the McDonald criteria. Ann Neurol. 2011;69(2):292-302.
29. Thompson AJ, Banwell BL, Barkhof F, Carroll WM, Coetzee T, Comi G, et al. Diagnosis of multiple sclerosis: 2017 revisions of the McDonald criteria. Lancet Neurol. 2018;17(2):162-73.
30. Barkhof F, Filippi M, Miller DH, Scheltens P, Campi A, Polman CH, et al. Comparison of MR imaging criteria at first presentation to predict conversion to clinically definite multiple sclerosis. Brain. 1997;120:2059-69.
31. Tintorè M, Rovira A, Martinez M, Rio J, Díaz-Villoslada P, Brieva L, et al. Isolated demyelinating syndromes: comparison of different MR imaging criteria to predict conversion to clinically definite multiple sclerosis. Am J Neuroradiol. 2000;21:702-6.
32. Swanton JK, Rovira A, Tintorè M, Altmann DR, Barkhof F, Filippi M, et al. MRI criteria for multiple sclerosis in patients presenting with clinically isolated syndromes: a multicenter retrospective study. Lancet Neurol. 2007;6(8):677-86.
33. Montalban X, Tintorè M, Swanton J, Barkhof F, Fazekas F, Filippi M, et al. MRI criteria for MS in patients with clinically isolated syndromes. Neurology. 2010;74(5):427-34.
34. Filippi M, Rocca MA, Ciccarelli O, Stefano ND, Evangelou N, Kappos L, et al. MRI criteria for the diagnosis of multiple sclerosis: MAGNIMS consensus guidelines. Lancet Neurol. 2016;15:292-303.
35. Filippi M, Preziosa P, Meani A, Ciccarelli O, Mesaros S, Rovira A, et al. Prediction of a multiple sclerosis diagnosis in patients with clinically isolated syndrome using the 2016 MAGNIMS and 2010 McDonald criteria: a retrospective study. Lancet Neurol. 2018;17(2):133-42.
36. Geurts JJG, Barkhof F. Gray matter pathology in multiple sclerosis. Lancet Neurol. 2008;7:841-51.
37. Lublin FD, Reingold SC, Cohen JA, Cutter GR, Sørensen PS, Thompson AJ, et al. Defining the clinical course of multiple sclerosis: the 2013 revisions. Neurology. 2014;83:278-86.
38. Hemond CC, Bakshi R. Magnetic Resonance imaging in Multiple Sclerosis. Cold Spring Harb Perspect Med. 2018;8(50):a028969.
39. Sanchez P, Chan F, Hardy TA. Tumefactive demyelination: updated perspectives on diagnosis and management. Expert Rev Neurother. 2021;21(9):1005-17.
40. Harandi AA, Esfandani A, Pakdaman H, Abbasi M, Sahraian MA. Balo's concentric sclerosis: an update and comprehensive literature review. Rev Neurosci. 2018;29(8):873-82.
41. Minneboo A, Uitdehaag BMJ, Ader HJ, Barkhof F, Polman CH, Castelijns JA. Patterns of enhancing lesion evolution in multiple sclerosis are uniform within patients. Neurology. 2005;65(1):56-61.
42. Radue EW, Barkhof F, Kappos L, Sprenger T, Häring DA, de Vera A, et al. Correlation between brain volume loss and clinical and MRI outcomes in multiple sclerosis. Neurology. 2015;84(8):784-93.
43. Deisenhammer F, Zetterberg H, Fitzner B, Zetti UK. The cerebrospinal fluid in multiple sclerosis. Front Immunol. 2019;10:726.
44. Bittner S, Oh J, Havrdova EK, Tintorè M, Zipp F. The potential of serum neurofilament as biomarker for multiple sclerosis. Brain. 2021;144(10):2954-63.
45. Costa GD, Martinelli V, Sangalli F, Moiola L, Colombo B, Radaelli M, et al. Prognostic value of serum neurofilaments in patients with clinically isolated syndromes. Neurology. 2019;92(7):e733-41.
46. Behbehani R, Al-Hassan AA, Al-Salahat A, Sriraman D, Oakley JD, Alroughani R. Optical coherence tomography segmentation analysis in relapsing remitting versus progressive multiple sclerosis. PLoS One. 2017;12(2):e0172120.
47. Interferon β-1b is effective in relapsing-remitting multiple sclerosis. I: Clinical results of a multicenter, randomized, double-blind, placebo-controlled trial. The IFNB Multiple Sclerosis Study Group. Neurology. 1993;43:655-61.
48. Ziemssen T, Derfuss T, de Stafano N, Giovannoni G, Palavra F, Tomic D, et al. Optimizing treatment success in multiple sclerosis. J Neurol. 2016;263(6):1053-65.
49. Jeffery DR. Early intervention with immunomodulatory agents in the treatment of multiple sclerosis. J Neurol Sci. 2002;197(1-2):1-8.
50. Kavaliunas A, Manouchehrinia A, Stawiarz L, Ramanujam R, Agholme J, Hedström AK, et al. Importance of early treatment initiation in the clinical course of multiple sclerosis. Mult Scler. 2017;23:1233-40.
51. Samjoo IA, Worthington E, Drudge C, Zhao M, Cameron C, Häring DA, et al. Efficacy classification of modern therapies in multiple sclerosis. J Comp Eff Res. 2021;10(6):495-507.
52. He A, Merkel B, Brown JWL, Ryerson LZ, Kister I, Malpas CB, et al. Timing of high-efficacy therapy for multiple sclerosis: a retrospective observational cohort study. Lancet Neurol. 2020;19(4):307-16.
53. Spelman T, Magyari M, Piehl F, Svenningsson A, Rasmussen PV, Kant M, et al. Treatment escalation vs immediate initiation of highly effective treatment for patients with relapsing-remitting multiple sclerosis: Data from 2 different national strategies. JAMA Neurol. 2021;78(10):1197-204.
54. Diaz C, Zarco LA, Rivera DM. Highly active multiple sclerosis: An update. Mult Scler Relat Disord. 2019;30:215-24.
55. FernándezÓ. Is there a change of paradigm towards more effective treatment early in the course of apparent high-risk MS? Mult Scler Relat Disord. 2017;17:75-83.
56. Muraro PA, Martin R, Mancardi GL, Nicholas R, Sormani MP, Saccardi R. Autologous haematopoietic stem cell transplantation for treatment of multiple sclerosis. Nat Rev Neurol. 2017;13(7):309-405.
57. Coles AJ, Cox A, Le Page E, Jones J, Trip SA, Deans J, et al. The window of therapeutic opportunity in multiple sclerosis: evidence from monoclonal antibody therapy. J Neurol. 2006;253:98-108.
58. Montalban X, Hauser SL, Kappos L, Arnold DL, Bar-Or A, Comi G, et al. Ocrelizumab versus placebo in secondary progressive multiple sclerosis. N Engl J Med. 2017;376:209-20.
59. Kappos L, Bar-Or A, Cree BAC, Fox RJ, Giovannoni G, Gold R, et al. Siponimod versus placebo in secondary progressive multiple sclerosis (EXPAND): a double-blind, randomised phase 3 study. Lancet. 2018;391(10127):1263-73.
60. Steinman L, Zamvil SS. Beginning of the end of two-stage theory purporting that inflammation then degeneration explains

pathogenesis of progressive multiple sclerosis. Current Opin Neurol. 2016;29:340-4.

61. Cerqueira JJ, Compston DAS, Geraldes R, Rosa MM, Schmierer K, Thompson A, et al. Time matters in multiple sclerosis: can early treatment and long-term follow-up ensure everyone benefits from the latest advances in multiple sclerosis? J Neurol Neurosurg Psychiatry. 2018;89(8):844-50.
62. Laurson-Doube J, Rijke N, Helme A, Baneke P, Banwell B, Viswanathan S, et al. Ethical use of off-label disease-modifying therapies for multiple sclerosis. Mult Scler. 2021;27(9):1403-10.
63. Massacesi L, Tramacere I, Amoroso S, Battaglia MA, Benedetti MD, Filippini G, et al. Azathioprine versus beta interferons for relapsing-remitting multiple sclerosis: a multicentre randomized non-inferiority trial. PLoS One. 2014;9(11):e113371.
64. Chisari CG, Sgarlata E, Arena S, Toscano S, Luca M, Patti F. Rituximab for the treatment of multiple sclerosis: a review. J Neurol. 2022;269(1):159-83.
65. Mathew T, John SK, Kamath V, Murgod U, Thomas K, Baptist AA, et al. Efficacy and safety of rituximab in multiple sclerosis: Experience from a developing country. Scler Relat Disord. 2020;43:102210.
66. Bharucha NE, Bharucha EP, Wadia NH, Singhal BS, Bharucha AE, Bhise AV, et al. Prevalence of multiple sclerosis in the Parsis of Bombay. Neurology. 1988;38:727-9.
67. Wadia NH, Bhatia K. Multiple sclerosis is prevalent in the Zoroastrians (Parsis) of India. Ann Neurol. 1990;28:177-9.
68. Singhal BS. Multiple Sclerosis—Indian experience. Ann Acad Med Singapore. 1985;14:32-6.
69. Kuroiwa Y, Hung TP, Landsborough D, Park CS, Singhal BS. Multiple Sclerosis in Asia. Neurology. 1977;27(2):188-92.
70. Wingerchuk DM, Banwell B, Bennett JL, Cabre P, Carroll W, Chitnis T, et al. International consensus diagnostic criteria for neuromyelitis optica spectrum disorders. Neurology. 2015;85(2):177-89.
71. Singhal BS, Advani H. Multiple sclerosis in India: An overview. Ann Indian Acad Neurol. 2015;18(Suppl 1):S2-5.
72. Singhal A, Bhatia R, Srivastava MV, Prasad K, Singh MB. Multiple sclerosis in India: An institutional study. Mult Scler Relat Disord. 2015;4:250-7.
73. Banerjee TK, Mukherjee A, Bhargava A. Childhood multiple sclerosis – report of two Indian cases. J Assoc Physicians India. 2002;50:1091-2.
74. Pandit L, Ramagopalan SV, Malli C, D'Cunha A, Kunder R, Shetty R. Association of vitamin D and multiple sclerosis in India. Mult Scler. 2013;19:1592-6.
75. Khadilkar S, Sahni AO, Agarwal SA. A case control study of environmental risk factors in Indians with multiple sclerosis. Neurophasia. 2005;10:47-52.
76. Vinoy N, Sheeja N, Kumar S, Biswas L. Class II HLA (DRB1, & DQB1) alleles and IL7R (rs6897932) variants and the risk for Multiple Sclerosis in Kerala, India. Mult Scler Relat Disord. 2021;50:102848.
77. Kankonkar S, Jeyanthi G, Singhal BS, Shankarkumar U. Evidence for novel DRB1*15 allele association among clinically definite multiple sclerosis patients from Mumbai, India. Hum Immunol. 2003;64:478-82.
78. Banerjee TK. Conversion of clinically isolated syndrome to multiple sclerosis: a prospective multi-center study in Eastern India. Mult Scler J Exp Transl Clin. 2019;5(2):2055217319849721.
79. D'Alessandro R, Vignatelli L, Lugaresi A, Baldin E, Granella F, Tola MR, et al. Risk of multiple sclerosis following clinically isolated syndrome: a 4-year prospective study. J Neurol. 2013;260:1583-93.
80. Liu Y, Duan Y, Yu C, Qin W, Chen H, Dong H, et al. Clinical isolated syndrome: a 3-year follow-up study in China. Clin Neurol Neurosurg. 2011;113:658-60.
81. Tintorè M, Rovira A, Rio J, Otero-Romero S, Arrambide G, Tur C, et al. Defining high, medium and low impact prognostic factors for developing multiple sclerosis. Brain. 2015;138:1863-74.
82. Morrissey SP, Miller DH, Kendall BE, Kingsley DP, Kelly MA, Francis DA, et al. The significance of brain magnetic resonance imaging abnormalities at presentation with clinically isolated syndromes suggestive of multiple sclerosis: a 5-year follow-up study. Brain. 1993;116:135-46.

68

CHAPTER

Neuromyelitis Optica and Myelin Oligodendrocyte Glycoprotein Antibody-associated Disorder

Lekha Pandit

INTRODUCTION

Inflammatory diseases of the central nervous system (CNS) are a heterogeneous group of disorders manifesting in monophasic or recurrent attacks, characterized by mono- or polysymptomatic neurologic dysfunction, of varying severity and affecting all age groups. Broadly they include antibody-mediated CNS disorders with identifiable biomarkers, CNS inflammatory diseases without known biomarkers, and systemic inflammatory diseases with secondary CNS involvement. Antibody-mediated demyelinating disorders may constitute 10–15% of all demyelinating disorders and particularly in the pediatric population.[1] They respond well to immunotherapy making it important for early diagnosis and intervention.[2,3] This chapter will focus on neuromyelitis optica spectrum disorders (NMOSDs) and myelin oligodendrocyte glycoprotein antibody-associated disorders (MOGADs), which are typical examples of antibody-mediated demyelinating CNS disorders with identifiable biomarkers. A review of epidemiology, clinical presentations, diagnostic evaluation, treatment, and outcome of these two disorders will be presented.

NEUROMYELITIS OPTICA SPECTRUM DISORDERS

Neuromyelitis optica spectrum disorders are a group of autoimmune diseases affecting the CNS, predominantly targeting the optic nerve and spinal cord. Our understanding of the etiology, the clinical spectrum of the disease, and treatment has evolved over time and particularly so in the last decade. Most of the descriptions of NMOSD in recent times have revolved around the discovery of aquaporin-4 immunoglobulin G (AQP4-IgG), a pathogenic autoantibody targeting the AQP4 water channel.

The earliest reports of neuromyelitis optica (NMO) came from the clinicopathological case series of Antoine Portal (1804), Giovanni Pescetto (1844), and Jacob Clarke (1856) who described cases with simultaneous visual loss and myelitis.[4] Sir Clifford Albutt[5] has often been credited for the first clinical case report that he published in 1870 under the title "On the Ophthalmoscopic Signs of Spinal Disease". In 1894, Eugene Devic and Fernand Gault[6,7] coined the term "neuromyélite optique aiguë" when they presented a case which had concurrent optic neuritis (ON) and myelitis and also reviewed other 16 cases from existing literature. More than a century later, the first modern classification of NMO was proposed in 1999 by Wingerchuk et al.[8] and included ON, longitudinally extensive transverse myelitis (LETM) defined as spinal cord magnetic resonance imaging (MRI) showing signal abnormality extending three or more vertebral segments, among the major diagnostic criteria. A subsequent revision in 2005[9] incorporated the newly discovered AQP4-IgG, a serum antibody targeting AQP4 water channel.[10] Soon, it became apparent that patients could have limited forms of AQP4-IgG positive (AQP4-IgG+) NMOSD such as monophasic/recurrent LETM or recurrent ON which were associated at times with systemic autoimmune disorders. The term "neuromyelitis optica spectrum disorders" was coined for these conditions.[11] As the clinical spectrum expanded, a variety of presentations unfolded and included protracted vomiting, narcolepsy, brainstem syndromes, and symptomatic brain lesions. Approximately 25% of patients meeting the criteria for NMOSD are not AQP4-IgG+. In 2015, another revision of the diagnostic criteria was made to accommodate patients with atypical presentations as well as those who were seronegative for AQP4-IgG. It was named as the international consensus diagnostic criteria for NMOSDs[12] **(Box 1)**, otherwise known as an International Panel for NMO Diagnosis (IPND) criteria.

BOX 1 International consensus diagnostic criteria for NMOSD.

NMOSD diagnostic criteria for adult patients

Diagnostic criteria for NMOSD with AQP4-IgG:
1. At least 1 core clinical characteristic
2. Positive test for AQP4-IgG using best available detection method (cell-based assay strongly recommended)
3. Exclusion of alternative diagnosis

Diagnostic criteria for NMOSD without AQP4-IgG or NMOSD with unknown AQP4-IgG status:
1. At least 2 core clinical characteristics occurring as a result of one or more clinical attacks and meeting all of the following requirements:
   a. At least 1 core clinical characteristic must be optic neuritis, acute myelitis with LETM, or area postrema syndrome
   b. Dissemination in space (2 or more different core clinical characteristics)
   c. Fulfillment of additional MRI requirements, as applicable
2. Negative tests for AQP4-IgG using best available detection method, or testing unavailable
3. Exclusion of alternative diagnoses

Core clinical characteristics:
1. Optic neuritis
2. Acute myelitis
3. Area postrema syndrome: Episode of otherwise unexplained hiccups or nausea and vomiting
4. Acute brainstem syndrome
5. Symptomatic narcolepsy or acute diencephalic clinical syndrome with NMOSD-typical diencephalic MRI lesions
6. Symptomatic cerebral syndrome with NMOSD-typical brain lesions

Additional MRI requirements for NMOSD without AQP4-IgG and NMOSD with unknown AQP4-IgG status:
1. *Acute optic neuritis*—requires brain MRI showing (A) normal findings or only nonspecific white matter lesions, *or* (B) optic nerve MRI with T2-hyperintense lesion or T1-weighted gadolinium-enhancing lesion extending over >1/2 optic nerve length or involving optic chiasm **(Fig. 1)**
2. *Acute myelitis*—requires associated intramedullary MRI lesion extending over ≥3 contiguous segments (LETM) *or* ≥3 contiguous segments of focal spinal cord atrophy in patients with history compatible with acute myelitis **(Fig. 1)**
3. *Area postrema syndrome*—requires associated dorsal medulla/area postrema lesions
4. *Acute brainstem syndrome*—requires associated periependymal brainstem lesions

(AQP4: aquaporin-4; IgG: immunoglobulin G; LETM: longitudinally extensive transverse myelitis; MRI: magnetic resonance imaging; NMOSD: neuromyelitis optica spectrum disorder)

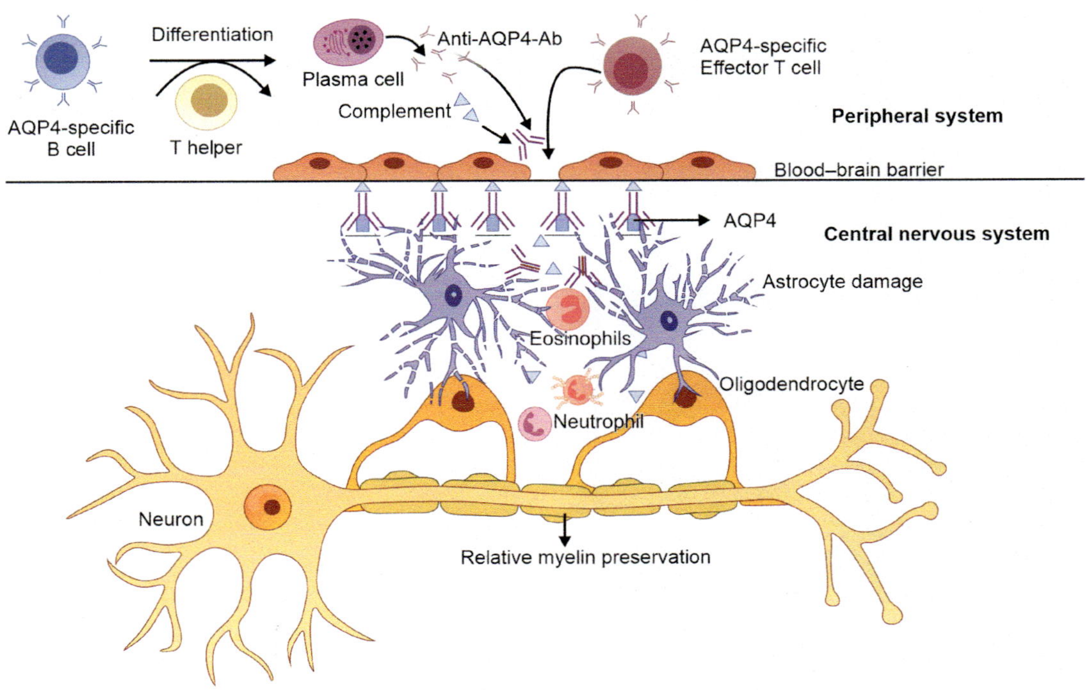

FIG. 1: Immunopathogenesis of AQP4-IgG-associated NMOSD. AQP4-specific B cells transform in the periphery into plasmablasts-secreting anti-AQP4 Ab, enter the CNS, and target AQP4 protein located densely on astrocyte foot processes, compliment activation results in profound astrocytic damage and axonal loss with relative myelin preservation. Inflammatory infiltrates are composed of CD4+ > CD8+ T cells, eosinophils, and neutrophils with compliment and immunoglobulin deposition.

(Ab: antibody; AQP4: aquaporin-4; CNS: central nervous system; NMOSD: neuromyelitis optica spectrum disorder)

Pathogenesis and Immunopathology

About 3% of NMOSD patients have a familial clustering.[13] Human leukocyte antigen (HLA) association studies from India have shown an association with HLA DRB1*03.[14] This has been noted in some western studies too.[15-17] Very little is understood about the environmental factors related to this disease. The intestinal microbiota has recently emerged as a significant environmental factor for NMOSD.[18,19] In a study from southern India,[18] gut microbiome sequencing showed an abundance of *Clostridium bolteae,* a gram-negative pathogen that shared sequence similarity with a highly immunogenic AQP4 peptide (p92-p104).

The concentration of serum AQP4-IgG is nearly 500 times that in cerebrospinal fluid (CSF) suggesting that the antibody production takes place peripherally and then enters the CSF through the breached blood–brain barrier (BBB) **(Fig. 1)**. Evidence indicates that AQP4-IgG enters the CNS at areas of increased BBB permeability by endothelial transcytosis and binds selectively to AQP4 (the main water channel protein in the CNS) and results in impairment of water homeostasis.[20] There is the activation of complement present in astrocytes, which leads to a further increase in BBB permeability and infiltration of peripheral leukocytes, mainly eosinophils and neutrophils. The combined effect of complement-mediated injury and cellular infiltration causes the death of astrocytes, oligodendrocytes, and neurons. NMOSD lesions **(Figs. 2A to D)** are characterized by demyelination of both gray and white matter and occasionally necrosis and cavitations of the optic nerve and spinal cord. The inflammatory infiltrate is typically composed of neutrophils and eosinophils and blood vessels are thickened and hyalinized. Immunopathological

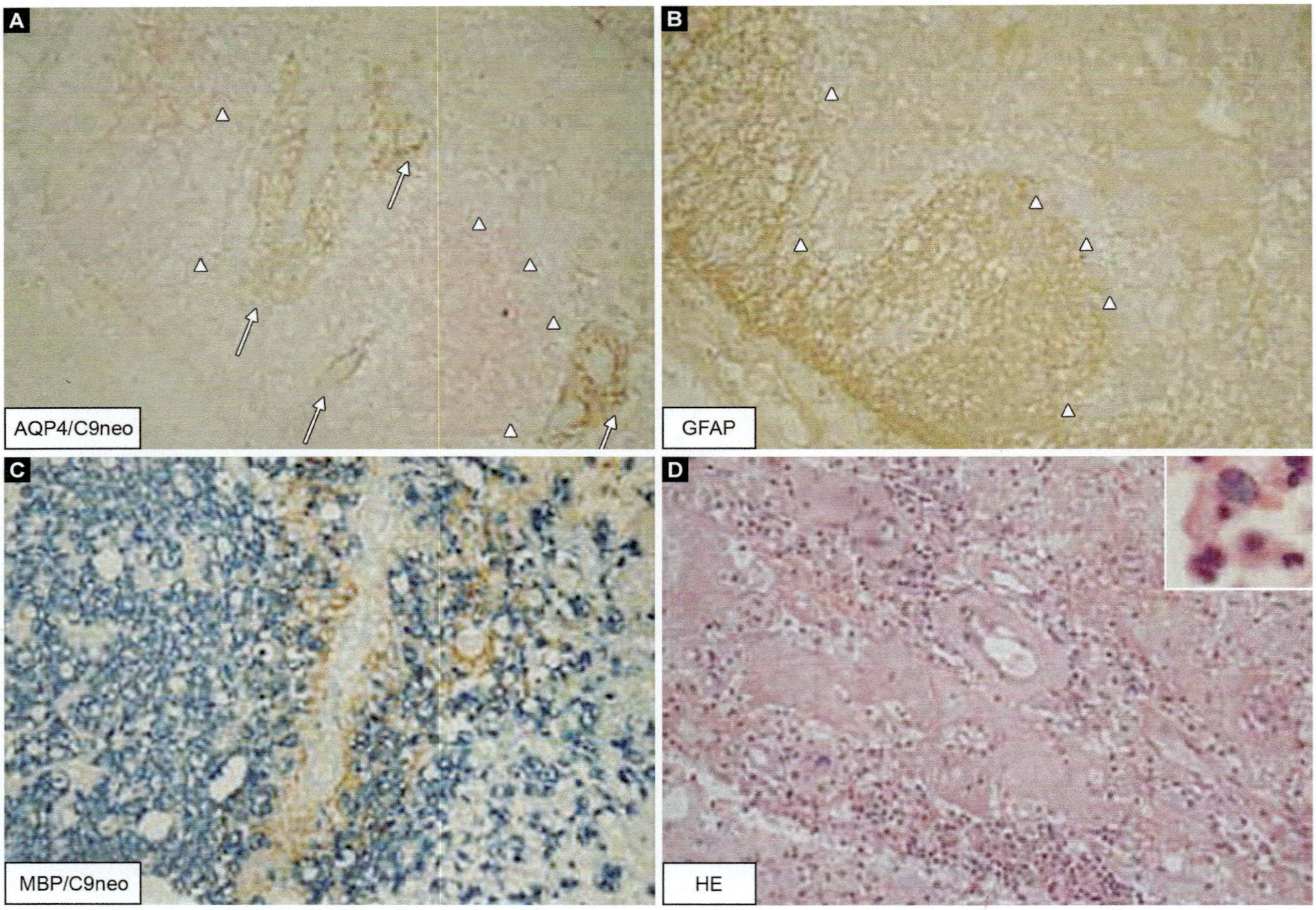

FIGS. 2A TO D: Neuropathology of aquaporin-4 immunoglobulin G (AQP4-IgG) positive NMOSD. (A) Double staining of aquaporin-4 (AQP4—pink) and active complement (C9neo—brown). This is the vasculocentric pattern deposition of C9neo (arrows) surrounded by loss of AQP4 (arrow heads located at the border). (B) Section stained with glial fibrillary acidic protein (GFAP is an astrocytic protein). GFAP staining is diminished in the areas lacking AQP4. (C) Double staining of myelin basic protein (MBP) and C9neo. In contrast to pattern of AQP4, MBP immunostaining is relatively preserved indicating preservation of myelin. (D) In hematoxylin and eosin staining, there are lot of dilated vessels at the necrotic NMOSD lesion, infiltrated by massive number of neutrophils (upper right corner) and macrophages.

(NMOSD: neuromyelitis optica spectrum disorder)

Image courtesy: Tatsuro Misu, MD, PhD, Department of Multiple Sclerosis Therapeutics and Neurology, Tohoku University Graduate School of Medicine.

examination reveals a vasculocentric rim and rosette pattern composed of immunoglobulins and complement components in active lesions, which are seen in the end feet of astrocytes where AQP4 is maximally expressed. NMOSD lesions typically show decreased AQP4 expression and selective loss of astrocyte markers such as glial fibrillary acidic protein (GFAP).[20]

Epidemiology

Epidemiological studies in the past have been confounded by differences in methodology, diagnostic criteria for NMOSD, different assays for AQP4-IgG assays, and composition of populations studied. European countries have shown a prevalence of 0.7–4/100,000, while studies from Asia have reported 2.6 and 3.65/100,000 from India and Japan,[21] respectively. The only exception was a population-based study that compared the incidence and prevalence of NMO/NMOSD among Afro-Caribbeans in Martinique and a well-defined population in Olmsted County, Minnesota in the USA. The incidence of NMO/NMOSD in Martinique versus Olmsted county (7.3 *vs.* 0.7/10000) and prevalence (10 *vs.* 3.9/100,000) were strikingly different.[22] Ethnicity-specific prevalence was similar in Martinique and Olmsted County: 11.5 and 13/100,000 in blacks, and 6.1 and 4.0/100,000 in whites respectively, suggesting that the disease is likely to be more common among people of nonwhite ancestry. A more recent systematic review of epidemiological studies that selected patients fulfilling 2015 IPND criteria and AQP4-IgG testing showed that the global prevalence was <5/100,000.[23] A discernible bias was seen in favor of nonwhite and indigenous populations.[24]

Clinical Features

The disease is more common in women among AQP4-IgG+ patients, the female-to-male ratio ranging from 2:1 to 10:1 and median age from 32 to 41 years. More than 90% of patients have a relapsing course. A set of six core clinical characteristics involving optic nerve, spinal cord, area postrema (dorsal medulla), diencephalon, brainstem, and cerebrum has been identified for the diagnosis of NMOSD.[12]

Optic Neuritis

Optic nerve involvement in AQP4-IgG+ NMOSD may be unilateral or bilateral and is typically characterized by severe visual loss and/or poor recovery after steroid therapy. The involvement of the optic nerve is often lengthy (involves >50% of length), affecting the chiasm and prechiasmatic regions. While ON is often unilateral, sequential and bilateral simultaneous ON can occur and is suggestive of NMOSD.

Transverse Myelitis

Transverse myelitis (TM) in AQP4-IgG+ NMOSD typically manifests as LETM and commonly affects the cervical cord with the occasional confluence with caudal brainstem lesions **(Fig. 3)**. The onset may be acute or subacute and may be heralded or accompanied by vomiting[25] (due to accompanying caudal brainstem lesions), Lhermitte's sign, and/or tonic spasms.[26] At times, the clinical manifestations of spinal cord dysfunction may be subtle and in contrast with the extensive spinal cord involvement seen on imaging. Occasionally, AQP4-IgG+ myelitis may show short-segment[27] involvement and may even be asymptomatically detected[28] during the course of the evaluation.

Brain and Brainstem Syndromes

- *Area postrema syndrome*: Patients may present with intractable hiccups or nausea/vomiting.[25] If accompanied by MRI lesions in the dorsal medulla, these symptoms qualify for the diagnosis of area postrema syndrome within 2 days of onset and after 7 days if MRI is normal.
- *Acute brainstem symptoms*: These include motor, sensory, or cerebellar dysfunction associated with parenchymal or ependymal lesions. Brainstem involvement may lead to acute neurogenic respiratory failure and death.
- *Hypothalamic lesions*: Narcolepsy, hypersomnolence, and autonomic dysfunction including hypotension, bradycardia, and hypothermia are some of the manifestations of diencephalic syndrome and are associated with MRI lesions in the thalamus, hypothalamus, or third ventricular region.
- *Hyponatremia*: Hyponatremia secondary to syndrome of inappropriate antidiuretic hormone secretion (SIADH) or due to cerebral salt wasting syndrome.

Symptomatic cerebral lesions may cause hemiparesis, hemisensory loss, encephalopathy, or cortical visual loss. Pain is a common feature of NMOSD[29] and impacts the quality of life. Neuropathic pruritis has been described.[30] Cognitive impairment has been detected on formal testing in >50% of NMOSD patients with brain lesions. Memory, attention, verbal fluency, processing speed, and executive functions are particularly affected.[31,32] The last trimester of pregnancy and the postpartum period are particularly vulnerable to relapses.[33]

Seronegative NMOSD

After extracting patients who are seropositive for either AQP4-IgG or MOG-IgG, there still remain patients who are without a known biomarker. It ranges from 27 to 36%.[34,35] Whether the seronegativity of this group is due to a lack of sensitivity of current antibody assays or the presence of uncharacterized immune responses needs to be ascertained. They show no gender preponderance, commonly present as isolated LETM or relapsing disease with LETM as the first manifestation. Most importantly, the Expanded Disability Status Scale (EDSS) is comparable with that of AQP4-IgG+ NMOSD.

Pediatric NMOSD

Studies in the pediatric population are few and have shown a low prevalence of NMOSD. NMOSD appears to increase with age and increasing sex ratio after the age of 11 years (females > males), suggesting that hormonal changes at puberty may influence disease frequency at a later age.[36] The female-to-male ratio is 3:1 as compared to 9:1 in adults.[37] It is worth noting that pediatric LETM may not have a close association with NMOSD. In the pediatric age group, LETM may be seen in a variety of other conditions including acute disseminated encephalomyelitis (ADEM) and in 15% of multiple sclerosis (MS) patients during a relapse.

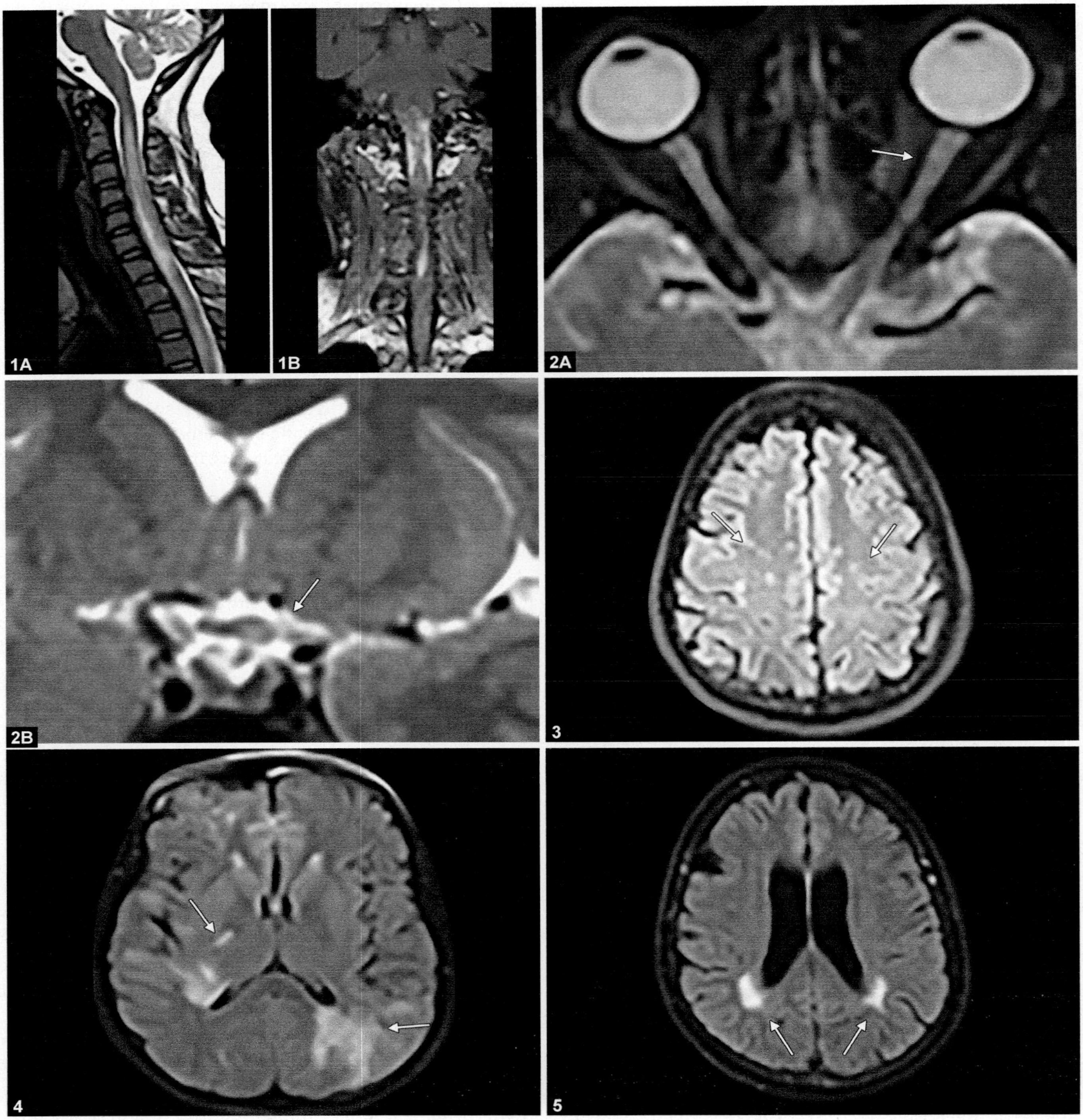

FIG. 3: *Continued*

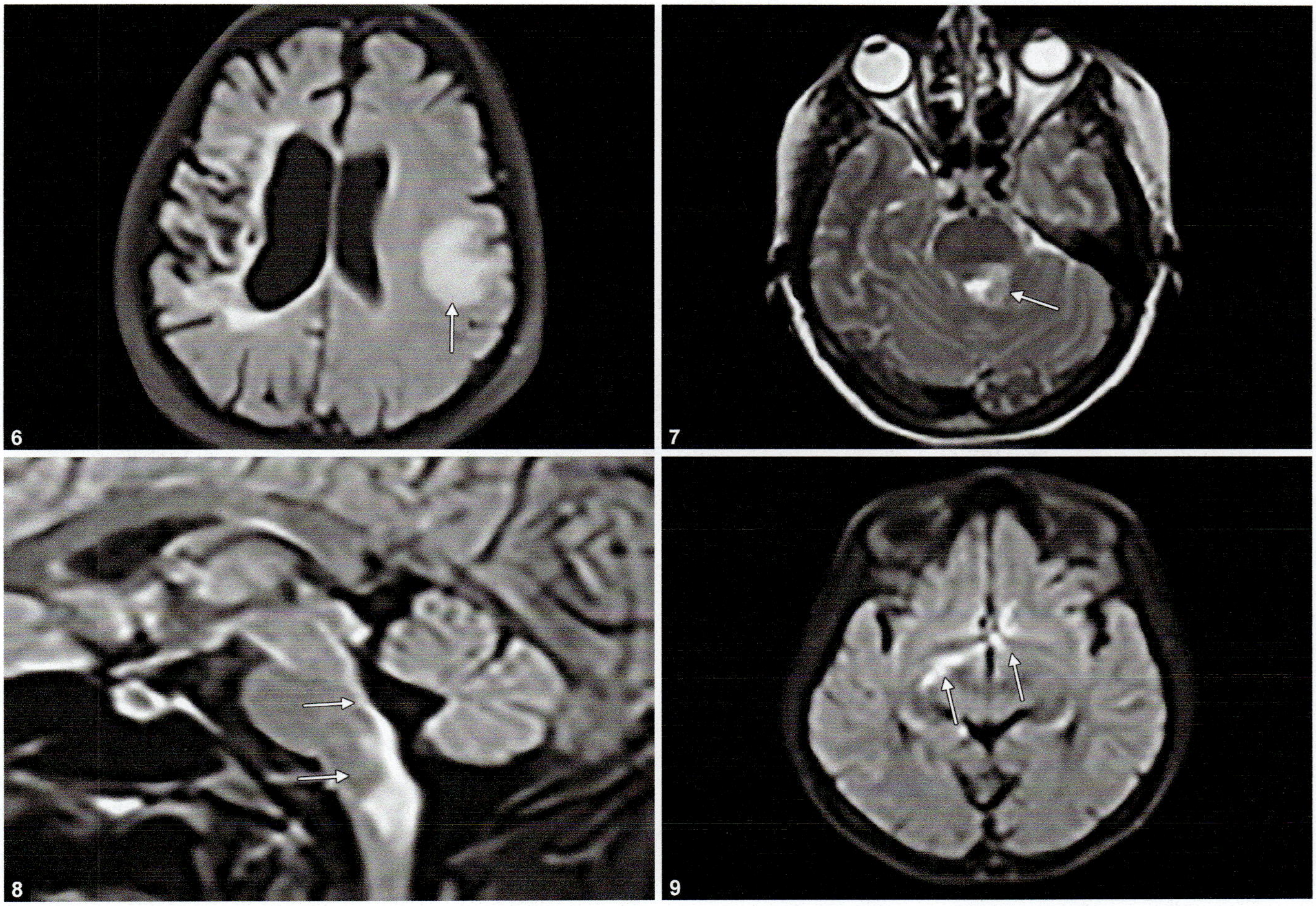

FIG. 3: Radiology of AQP4-IgG positive NMOSD. (1A) Sagittal T2W image of cervical spine showing LETM extending >3 vertebral segments; (1B) coronal FLAIR showing cervical LETM extending into medulla; (2A) FAT-SAT image of orbit revealing long-segment optic nerve atrophy (arrow); (2B) optic neuritis involving chiasm; axial FLAIR images showing (3) punctuate/dot like lesions in the brain; (4) "cloud like" subcortical brain lesion and pyramidal tract (arrow) involvement; (5) periependymal lesions; (6) tumefactive lesion (arrow) and gliosis on opposite side; (7) brainstem lesion involving dorsal medulla extending into cerebellum; (8) dorsal brainstem lesion extending into floor of 4th ventricle in area postrema syndrome; (9) hypothalamic involvement (arrow)

(FAT-SAT: fat-saturation; FLAIR: fluid-attenuated inversion recovery; LETM: longitudinally extensive transverse myelitis; NMOSD: neuromyelitis optica spectrum disorder)

NMOSD in the Context of Other Autoimmune Disorders

Concomitant autoimmune disorders and nonorgan-specific autoantibodies are seen in a third of NMOSD patients particularly those associated with AQP4-IgG.[33,38] Thyroid disease (the most common coexisting autoimmune disorder), myasthenia gravis, and celiac disease are known to occur. NMOSD patients frequently have a family history of autoimmune disease.[38]

Diagnosis

The diagnostic criteria published in 2015[12] titled "International Consensus Diagnostic Criteria for Neuromyelitis Spectrum Disorders" (IPND criteria) divided NMOSD with and without AQP4-IgG based on serologic testing. NMOSD with AQP4-IgG can be diagnosed when one of the six typical core syndromes is recognized—ON, acute myelitis, area postrema syndrome, acute brainstem syndrome, symptomatic narcolepsy or acute diencephalic clinical syndrome with NMOSD-typical diencephalic MRI lesions, and symptomatic cerebral syndrome with NMOSD-typical brain lesions **(Box 1)**. They must be associated with seropositivity for AQP4-IgG detected by the best available method when alternative diagnoses are excluded. Two core clinical features are required if the patient is seronegative and all of the following conditions are met: (1) at least one core clinical feature must be NMO-typical (ON, acute myelitis with LETM, or area postrema syndrome); (2) there must be clinically proven dissemination in space (two or more different core clinical syndromes) with additional MRI requirements specific for each clinical syndrome. The IPND criteria have been validated by different groups,[39,40] which confirms that the new criteria have increased the diagnostic rates. Additionally, they confirm that all AQP4-IgG+ NMOSDs have the same prognosis irrespective of the clinical presentation.[35]

Magnetic Resonance Imaging

The new diagnostic criteria have opened up the clinical phenotypes of NMOSD that go beyond ON and LETM allowing particularly AQP4-IgG+ patients with limited disorders (and often accompanying radiological features) to be diagnosed.

MRI brain: About 60% of patients with NMOSD accumulate asymptomatic white matter lesions on a longitudinal study. As many as 16% may fulfill Barkhof criteria for MS.[41] Detection of brain MRI white matter lesions compatible with MS does not exclude the diagnosis of NMOSD but is considered a red flag, indicating that additional evidence may be required to confidently distinguish NMOSD from MS in individual cases. The distribution of lesions is common in areas that have high AQP4 concentration[42,43] but can be seen elsewhere too **(Fig. 3)**. Nonspecific findings are most common and include punctate/dot lesions and small patchy subcortical lesions on T2-weighted (T2W) and fluid-attenuated inversion recovery (FLAIR) sequences. The so-called "NMOSD typical lesions" are located in the dorsal medulla, periependymal surfaces of the third and fourth ventricle, hypothalamus, thalamus, and corticospinal tracts. Large tumefactive subcortical lesions are occasionally seen.

Optic nerve: In AQP4-IgG+ NMOSD, optic nerve involvement may be unilateral or bilateral, lengthy lesions, commonly involving posterior portions and optic chiasm. They may show increased T2W signals or gadolinium enhancement. Similar findings have been described in MOG-IgG+ NMOSD except that long-segment involvement is in the anterior portions of the optic nerve and predominantly in the retro-orbital and prechiasmatic regions.[44]

Spinal cord: In the acute phase, LETM associated with NMOSD shows hyperintense signals on sagittal T2W, proton density, or short tau inversion recovery (STIR) sequences extending over three or more vertebral segments and hypointense signals on T1W images in the corresponding regions. Lesions are typically in the central cord with >70% of the lesion residing within the gray matter of the cord. Lesions may show variable patterns of enhancement in about 70% of patients. In the chronic phase, long-segment atrophy of the cord extending >3 vertebral segments with or without T2W signal changes may be seen.

Optical Coherence Tomography

An optical coherence tomography (OCT) is a noninvasive tool for evaluating afferent visual pathways in NMOSD and helps to quantify damage to the retina, including the ganglion cells and their axons. Numerous studies have shown peripapillary retinal nerve fiber layer (pRNFL) thinning and decreased total macular volume (TMV) in NMOSD, not just in the clinically affected eye but also in the unaffected eye.[45] Till recently, subclinical optic nerve involvement was described only in MS. In NMOSD, it is suggested that subclinical disease may be consequent to damage to Müller cells that are richly present in the retina and contain an abundance of AQP4 channels.[46] Though OCT is not used routinely for diagnosis, its high sensitivity suggests a role for longitudinal evaluation of visual functions after ON, as a predictor for visual recovery, and as a marker for evaluating therapeutic interventions. Other visual evaluation tools such as visual evoked potential (VEP) studies are supportive of the diagnosis of ON.

Cerebrospinal fluid: CSF pleocytosis with cell counts >50 cells/mm^3 (high proportion of neutrophils) and raised protein (100–500 mg/dL) may be common. Oligoclonal IgG bands are present in <15–30% of AQP4-IgG+ NMOSD.

Biomarkers (Autoantibodies) Associated with NMOSD

Autoantibodies Against Aquaporin-4

Early detection of AQP4-IgG is important for the diagnosis of seropositive NMOSD, predicting future relapses and influence attack-related disability and treatment choices.[40] Comparative studies[47,48] have shown that assays with the highest sensitivity involve detection of AQP4-IgG binding to cells expressing recombinant AQP4 either quantitatively with flow cytometry or visual observation using cell-based assay (CBA) with a mean sensitivity of 76.7% (range 55.6–96.7%). A CBA developed and standardized in southern India,[49] in Mangalore, **(Fig. 4)** had a sensitivity of 81.6% in patients fulfilling IPND criteria for NMOSD. In high-risk syndromes suggestive of NMOSD (such as isolated or recurrent LETM and long-segment ON), sensitivity varied from 0 to 70%. The Mangalore assay showed a sensitivity of 29.4% underscoring the fact that the latter may have a heterogeneous etiology. Testing for AQP4-IgG should be done during an attack and before treatment. It is noteworthy that the commercial assay (EUROIMMUN, Germany) while showing high specificity lags in sensitivity compared to live CBA. A small number of patients may test positive for MOG-IgG (detailed later in this chapter). Double positive samples are unusual and should be retested with live CBA and preferably in a different laboratory.

Treatment

It is worth remembering that NMOSD has a relapsing course if left untreated. Relapse is defined similarly to MS—new or worsening neurological symptoms lasting >24 hours without fever or infection and occurring 30 days after the previous attack. Unlike MS, NMOSD relapses are often severe and

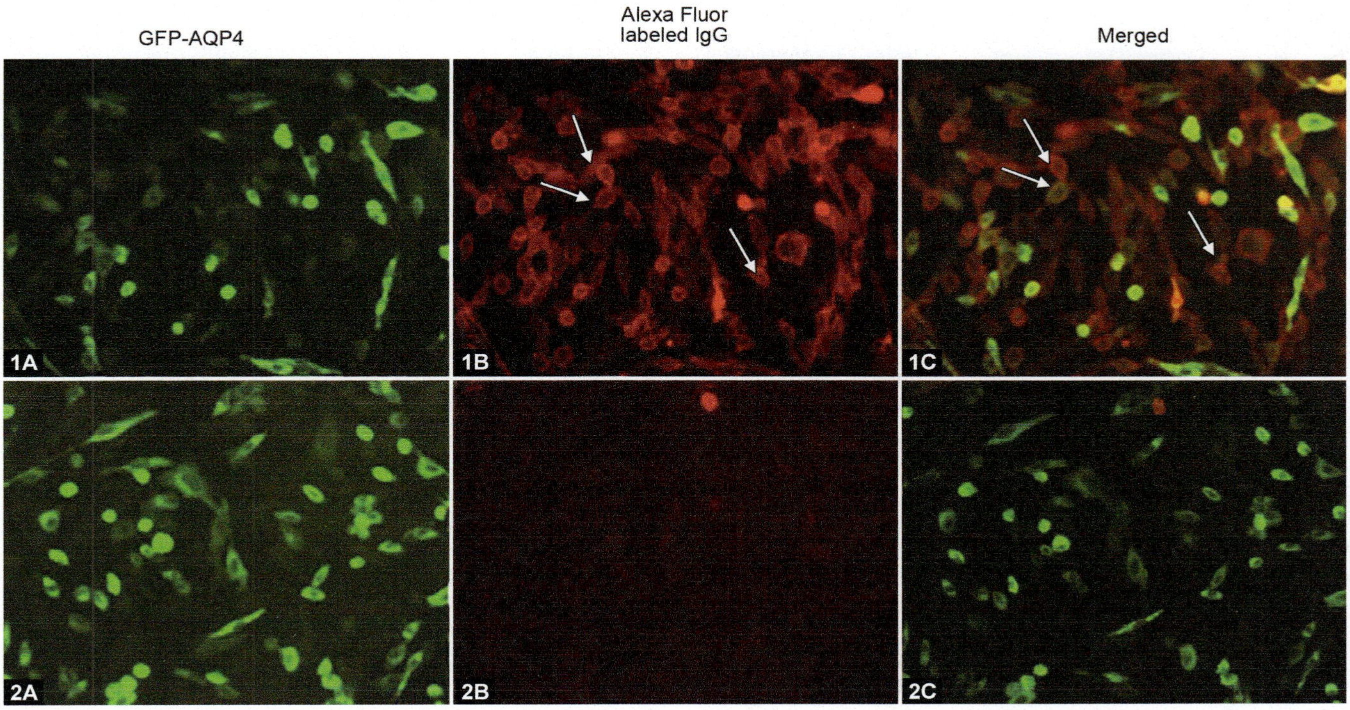

FIG. 4: Cell-based assay for AQP4-IgG (Mangalore assay). Serum from patient when incubated with Chinese hamster ovary (CHO) cells transfected with AQP4 expressing plasmids (1A), a positive reaction was seen (1B) as red fluorescence of Alexa Fluor tagged secondary antibody (anti-human IgG) marked with arrows, better appreciated after merging of a and b images (1C) marked with arrows. Healthy control when similarly tested showed (2A to C) an absence of the same.

(AQP4-IgG: aquaporin-4 immunoglobulins G)

only partially reversible. This may result in severe visual loss, paralysis, neuropathic pain, bladder dysfunction, and sometimes even altered sensorium or respiratory failure. MS disease-modifying should be avoided.

Acute Therapy

Steroids: Intravenous corticosteroids in the form of methylprednisolone (IVMP) (1 g daily for 5 days) are the standard first-line treatment.[50] Early administration of steroids has been shown to protect retinal nerve fiber layers in NMOSD.[51] However, parenteral steroids may be more effective in MS than NMOSD and may be more beneficial during the first attack.[52]

Plasma exchange (PLEX): Escalating therapy to PLEX improves chances of remission[53] and must be offered particularly for severe TM and ON unresponsive to steroids. Time from onset of relapse to starting of PLEX is a strong predictor of complete remission. Nearly 40% of patients will respond if PLEX is initiated within 2 days after relapse, in contrast to <5% responding after 6 days of relapse.[54] Patients who show no response within 3–5 days after initiating parenteral steroids should be offered PLEX or immunoadsorption. In severe TM, PLEX may be administered as first-line therapy. Usually, a course of seven exchanges on alternate days is given. PLEX is not only useful in AQP4-IgG+ patients where it is shown to reduce antibody titers, but it is also beneficial for seronegative patients. Factors favoring good response after PLEX include shorter disease duration with fewer past attacks and lower pre-existing disability.[55] If the patient cannot be initiated on PLEX, the second course of IVMP at a higher dose of up to 2 g for 5 days may be given.[56] There is insufficient data on the efficacy of intravenous immunoglobulin in the treatment of relapse in NMOSD and the only randomized trial planned was abandoned due to recruitment problems.[57]

Maintenance Therapy

In the last 3 years, several phase 111 clinical trials of NMOSD-specific drugs showed a significant reduction in relapse rates in AQP4-IgG+ NMOSD when compared to placebo and have been approved by food and drug administration (FDA). These include satralizumab[58,59] (SAkuraSKy and SAkuraStar studies), an interleukin-6 receptor (IL-6) inhibitor, inebilizumab[60] (N-MOmentum study), an antibody against CD19+ B cells, and eculizumab[61] (PREVENT study), an antibody-blocking C5 component of complement.

All three drugs are relatively safe **(Table 1)**. The risk of meningococcal infection is associated with eculizumab and meningococcal vaccination is advised before starting therapy. Patients in the trial had higher rates of upper

TABLE 1: Maintenance therapy for NMOSD.

Therapy	Dosing/Day	Optimizing therapy	Side effects	Monitoring requirement
AZA PO	2–3 mg/kg/day	• Measure TPMT activity • Target dose adjusted by—Absolute lymphocyte count 600–1,000/μL, total count ≥3,000, mean corpuscular volume increase >5% of baseline • Add oral steroids (0.5 mg/kg) × 6 months	Hepatotoxicity, GI side effects, fatigue, leuko- and lymphopenia, infections, bone marrow suppression, and malignancies with long term	Hemoglobin, total count, differential count, absolute lymphocyte count, and liver functions
MMF PO	1,500–3,000 mg	• Absolute lymphocyte count 1,000–1,500/μL • MMF plasma levels: 1–2 μg/mL • Add oral steroids (0.5 mg/kg) × 4–6 months	GI side effects, hypercholesterolemia, elevation of transaminases, bone marrow suppression and infections, including progressive multifocal leukoencephalopathy (PML) rarely	Differential count, liver functions
RTX IV	1 g at 2 weekly intervals every 6 months or after B-cell monitoring	• B-cell monitoring—CD19+ or CD20+ B cells >0.1% of total lymphocytes, CD27+ memory • B cells >0.05% of peripheral blood mononuclear cells	Allergic reactions (preventive premedication is obligatory), infections, low IgG/IgM levels, and late-onset neutropenia, PML	• CD19+/20+ cells and CD27+ cells • Allergic reactions during infusion • Monitoring serum immunoglobulins
Satralizumab SC	120 mg on day 1, 14th, 28th, then every 4 weeks	Neutrophil counts	Hepatotoxicity, upper respiratory infection, headache	• Blood counts • LFT every 4 weeks for 3 months and every 3 months then on
Eculizumab IV	900 mg/week for 4 weeks, then 1,200 mg every 2 weeks	Meningococcal vaccination prior to therapy (at least 2 weeks before)	Headache, nasopharyngitis, backache, cough, fatigue	RFT, blood counts, LFT, haptoglobin levels, compliment activity assays
Inebilizumab IV	300 mg at day 1 and 15, then 300 mg every 6 months	Monitoring of immunoglobulins	Urinary tract infection, arthralgia, backache	Quantitative estimation of serum immunoglobulins

(AZA: azathioprine; GI: gastrointestinal; IV: intravenous; LFT: liver function test; MMF: mycophenolate mofetil; NMOSD: neuromyelitis optica spectrum disorder; PO: per oral; RFT: renal function test; RTX: rituximab; SC: subcutaneous; TPMT: thiopurine methyltransferase)

respiratory tract infection and headache when compared to the placebo arm. In the N-MOmentum study, patients receiving inebilizumab had a higher frequency of urinary tract infection, arthralgia, and back pain compared to those on placebo. Apart from injection site skin irritation, no significant side effects were observed with satralizumab. While no concerns were found during and after pregnancy, more data is required to establish safety during pregnancy. Currently, these drugs are recommended for AQP4-IgG+ NMOSD but not for seronegative NMOSD and in adult patients only. Prohibitive costs and lack of availability in developing countries make it less likely that these drugs will be frequently prescribed outside of high-income countries.

"Off-label" treatments are still the mainstay of therapy available for NMOSD. These therapies include azathioprine (AZA), mycophenolate mofetil (MMF), and rituximab (RTX). International guidelines[62,63] for the use of these drugs are based on expert opinions and small retrospective studies.

Patients need careful counseling about potential risks including infections, cytotoxicity, and malignancy. They should be willing for frequent monitoring over time and women of childbearing age should have effective contraception. Pregnancy and chronic infections, particularly HIV, hepatitis B and C, and tuberculosis, should be excluded before the start of therapy. The dosing, optimization of therapy, precautions, and specific remarks about individual drugs are mentioned in **Table 1**.

Azathioprine: It is a purine inhibitor and inhibits both T- and B-cell proliferation. It is the cheapest of all and the first drug tried in NMOSD. Combination of AZA (2.5–3 mg/kg/day) with oral prednisolone[64] (0.5–1 mg/kg/day) followed by a gradual taper of steroids by the 6 month will reduce the risk of relapse. Prior testing for thiopurine methyltransferase enzyme activity may be useful as patients with low activity are at higher risk for severe side effects.[65] Retrospective studies have shown that AZA may be the least effective in relapse prevention and that breakthrough relapses were more severe when compared to RTX.[66] Kleiter et al.[67] have suggested hematological parameters which are indicative of optimal AZA therapy and these include a reduction in total lymphocyte count to 600–1,000/μL, a leukocyte count, which should remain at >3,000/μL, and the mean corpuscular volume, which should increase by about 5% from baseline.

Mycophenolate mofetil: MMF through its active metabolite mycophenolic acid inhibits lymphocyte proliferation by suppression of guanosine nucleotide biosynthesis. Several retrospective studies have evaluated the beneficial effects of MMF therapy in mostly AQP4$^+$ NMOSD, in the reduction of relapse rates by 80–93% and improvement in EDSS over a follow-up of 20–27 months.[65,66,68,69] These studies also showed that in comparison with RTX, there was no difference in risk of relapse, though breakthrough relapses were more severe. MMF is titrated to a dose of 1,500–3,000 mg/day. The effect of treatment usually starts within 2–3 months and, hence, it is advisable to add oral steroids for the initial few months.

Rituximab: RTX is a chimeric anti-CD20 monoclonal antibody that depletes both naïve and memory B cells. Cree et al.,[70] in an open-labeled study, confirmed the utility of RTX in NMOSD. These preliminary results were confirmed in several case series that reported a reduction of the annualized relapse rate of 87–96%, relapse-free state of 44–72%, and improvement in disability in 80–100% of patients.[71-73] The high efficacy of RTX suggests that in severe NMOSD, it could be used as a first line rather than as an escalating therapy. There is no standard dosing regimen recommended for RTX. Infusions may be given as two doses of 1 g each at 2-week intervals or follow practices for oncology indications wherein weekly dosing at 375 mg/m^2 body surface area is preferred. More than 80% of patients remain B-cell depleted for 6 months and this is the basis for 6 monthly redosing with the drug. However, this runs the risk of relapse in the minority in whom repopulation of B cells may occur earlier. Re-infusion with RTX based on periodic B-cell counts[73] (CD19+ or CD20+ B cells >0.1% of total lymphocytes, CD27+ memory B cells >0.05% of peripheral blood mononuclear cells) may be more accurate, in determining dosing intervals. Another reason for repopulation is a genetic polymorphism in the fragment c gamma receptor 3A (FcgR3A) allele which is associated with insufficient memory B-cell depletion and an elevated risk of attacks during RTX treatment.[74] Relapses may also occur in the immediate period after an infusion probably due to elevated proinflammatory cytokines in the background of a relapse. It is preferable to vaccinate patients before initiating therapy or at the tail end of an infusion cycle with the resumption of medication after 4–6 weeks following vaccinations. Live vaccines are contraindicated.

Other Therapies

Combination therapies may be attempted when breakthrough relapses occur despite adequate immunosuppression. Combining RTX with MMF is one such example. Cyclophosphamide (intravenous infusion) has been associated with breakthrough relapses in several studies[75] and, hence, may not be an initial consideration for the treatment of NMOSD. Mitoxantrone, methotrexate, cyclosporin, and tacrolimus have been used with limited success in a small number of patients. Monthly intravenous immunoglobulin G (IVIg) and periodic PLEX have been used as adjuvant therapy, in a few patients with modest benefit. New and promising therapies under development include aquaporumab, which is a nonpathogenic recombinant monoclonal antibody that blocks the binding of AQP4-IgG, bortezomib, a protease inhibitor, ravulizumab, a new-generation C5 antibody, and sivelestat, a neutrophil elastase inhibitor. There is limited data on the use of hematopoietic stem cell transplantation (HSCT) in patients with NMOSD.

MYELIN OLIGODENDROCYTE GLYCOPROTEIN ANTIBODY-ASSOCIATED DISORDER

Introduction

Myelin oligodendrocyte glycoprotein (MOG) is present on the surface of oligodendrocytes and may act as a cell adhesion molecule, regulate microtubule stability, and modulate immune interactions. It is a member of the immunoglobulin superfamily and, hence, highly immunogenic, its location on the outermost part of the myelin sheath in the CNS making it a potential target for MOG antibodies.[76] In 2017, a study using MOG self-antigen tetramers detected by radioimmunoassay technique detected MOG-IgG in a subset of patients with ADEM.[77] Serum antibody against MOG was later reported in patients with atypical MS, seronegative NMOSD, and isolated ON. There is a growing need for distinguishing MOGAD from AQP4-IgG+ NMOSD. The IPND diagnostic criteria for NMOSD recognize approximately 30% of patients with MOGAD alone. The new international proposed criteria for MOGAD have been published recently.[78]

Pathology and Pathophysiology

In animal models, MOG antibody induces demyelination in experimental autoimmune encephalomyelitis (EAE) models immunized with MOG.[79] When human MOG antibodies were injected intrathecally in rodents with myelin reactive T cells, MOG-IgG was found to be directly pathogenic causing demyelination and complement deposition. Tissue injury is likely to be triggered by MOG-IgG and/or augmentation of inflammation is likely mediated by MOG-reactive T cells **(Fig. 5)**. Human autopsy studies[80] show perivenous and confluent demyelination **(Figs. 6A to O)**. Cortical lesions are frequent and subcortical demyelinating lesions are prominent. A predominantly CD4-positive inflammatory response and complement deposition are noted, with some

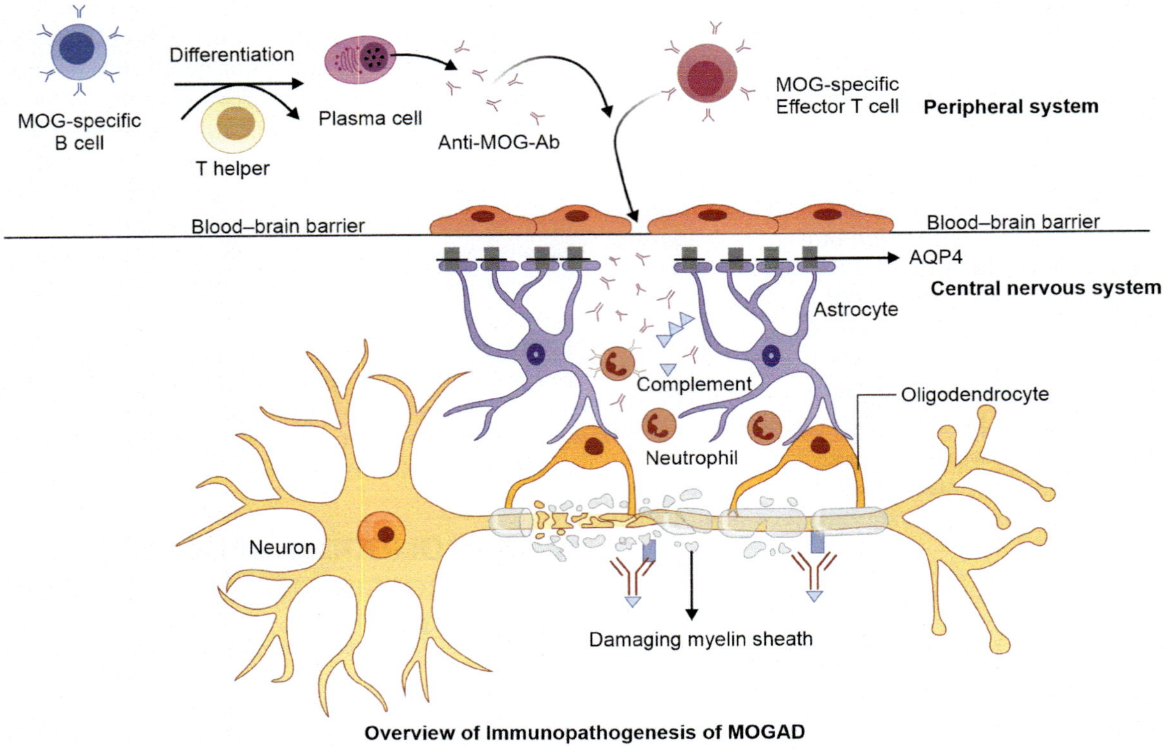

FIG. 5: Immunopathogenesis of MOGAD. MOG-specific B-cells transform into anti-MOG Ab producing cells in the periphery, enter the CNS through a breached blood–brain barrier (BBB), target MOG and induce complement mediated damage to oligodendrocytes with resultant myelin sheath damage, relative preservation of astrocytes and axons. Immune cell infiltrate is composed of CD4+ T cells, granulocytes with complement and immunoglobulin deposition.

(Ab: antibody; CNS: central nervous system; MOG: myelin oligodendrocyte glycoprotein; MOGAD: myelin oligodendrocyte antibody-associated disorder)

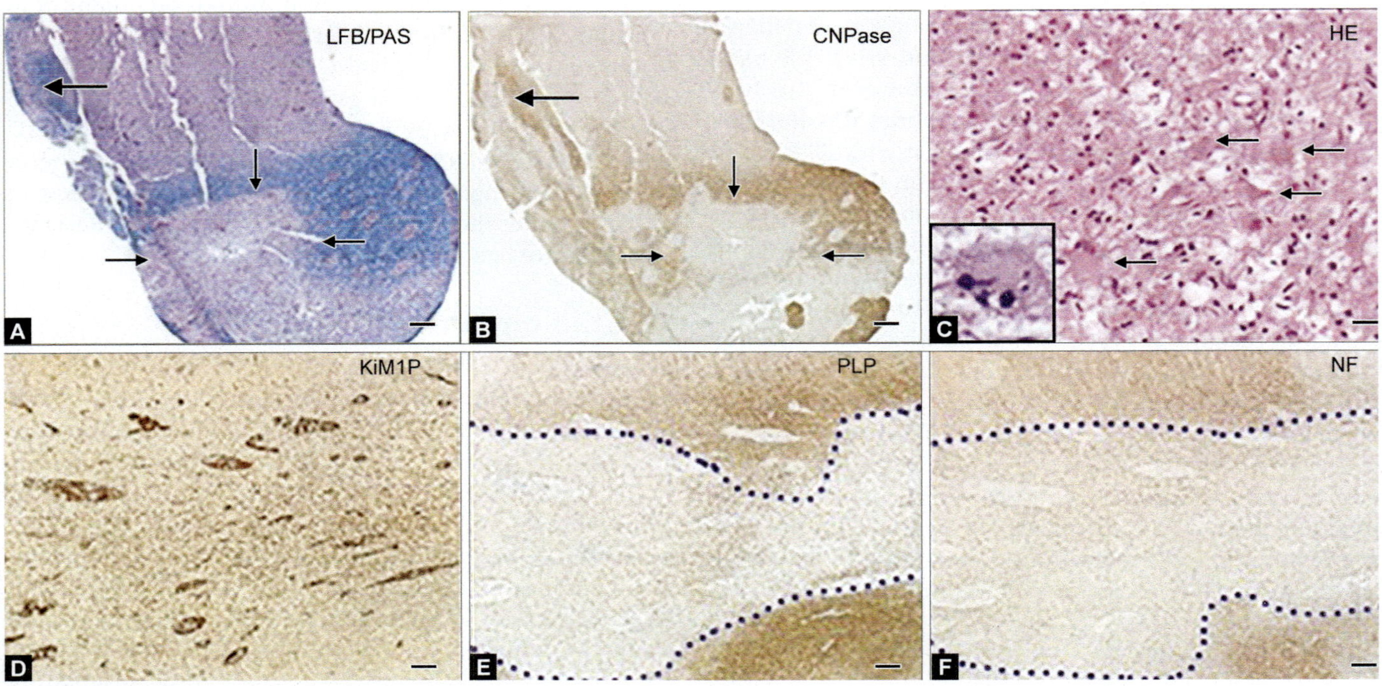

FIGS. 6A TO O: *Continued*

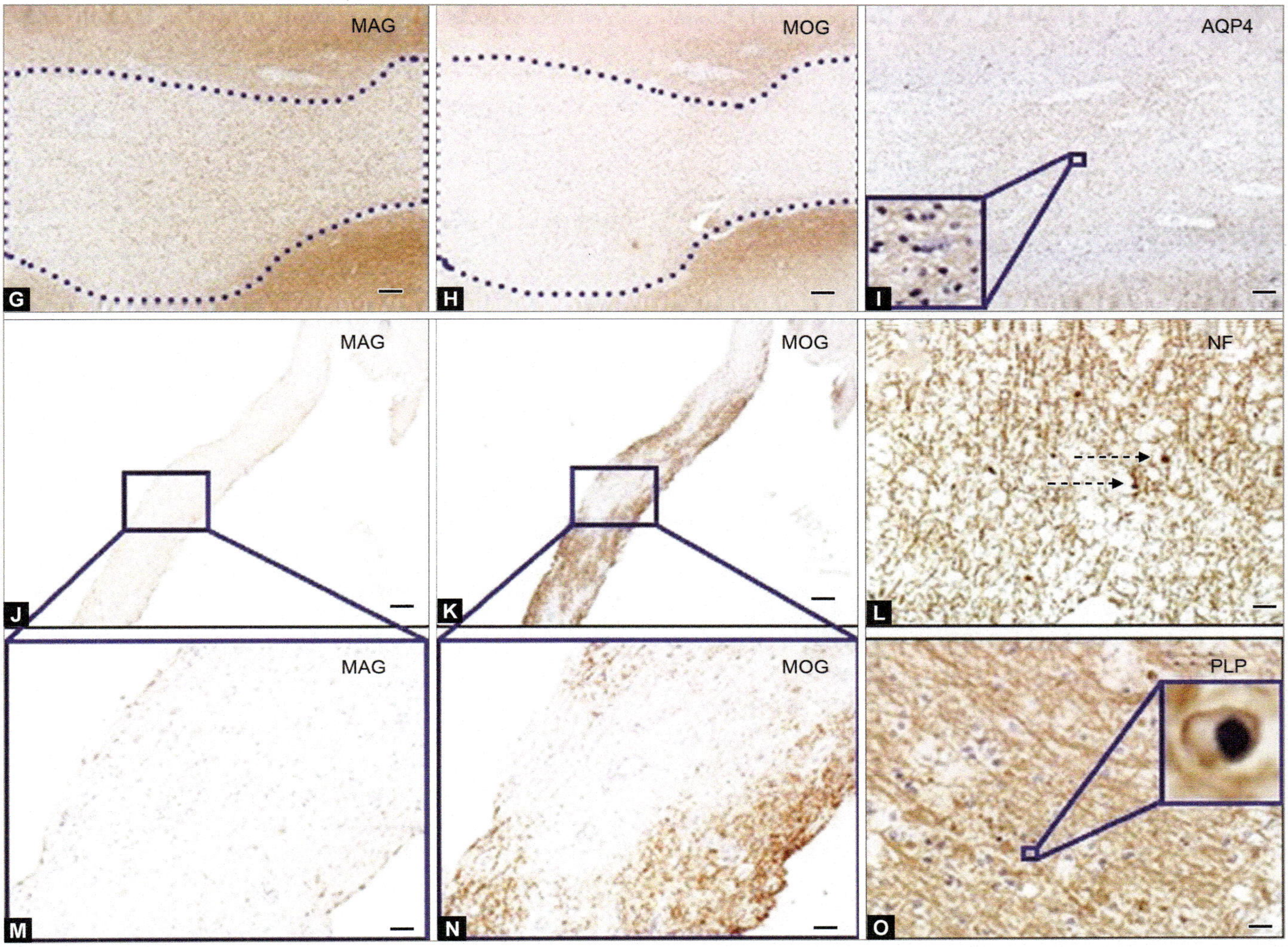

FIGS. 6A TO O: Neuropathology of MOGAD. Brain biopsy: White matter pathology of MOGAD. (A) LFB/PAS stain and myelin protein CNPase immunohistochemistry (B) on consecutive sections show perivenous (thick arrows) and confluent (arrows) demyelination that coexists in the subcortical white matter, (C) H&E stain shows marked hypertrophic reactive astrocytes in the white matter lesion and Creutzfeldt-Peters cells are occasionally noted (box). (D) KiM1P immunohistochemistry shows extensive microglia/macrophage infiltration in the white matter. The blue dotted lines contour the demyelinating lesion (E) with relative preserved axons (F). The loss of minor myelin protein MAG (G) and MOG (H) are equal. AQP4 is preserved in the lesion (I) Preferential MAG loss (J and M) with relative MOG preservation (K and N) is seen (L) Mild axonal damage characterized by axonal spheroid (indicated with dashed arrows) is present in the demyelinating lesions. (O) Apoptotic oligodendrocytes with condensed nucleus (highlighted in the box) are seen in the lesions.

(AQP4: aquaporin-4; CNPase: cyclic-nucleotide phosphodiesterase; H&E: hematoxylin and eosin stain; LFB: Luxel fast blue; MAG: myelin-associated glycoprotein; MOGAD: myelin oligodendrocyte glycoprotein antibody-associated disease; NF:neurofilament; PAS: periodic acid-Schiff; PLP: proteolipid protein)

Source: With permission form Höftberger R, et al (2020).[80]

studies reporting overlap with pattern II MS pathology. Expression of AQP4 is preserved and astrocyte damage is not prominent.

Epidemiology

There are limited epidemiological studies from Europe which show a disease incidence ranging from 1.6 to 3.4 per million per year and a prevalence of 20 per million [95% confidence interval (CI) 11–34].[81,82] MOGADs have been reported globally including from India,[83,84] and more than half of these are among children. Some geographic differences have been highlighted in some publications from Sri Lanka[85] and the United Kingdom,[86] in that, MOGAD was more frequently reported than NMOSD in these regions.

Clinical Features

Most common presentations include ON—unilateral or bilateral,[87] ADEM,[88] and TM.[89] Other less common manifestations include NMOSD phenotype that fulfills IPND criteria[12] for seronegative NMOSD, cortical encephalitis,[90] and brainstem involvement.[91] Attacks may develop over several days and may plateau with variable recovery if untreated. Unlike other acquired demyelinating disorders, >50% of MOGAD has a monophasic course. There are no real indicators for a potentially relapsing course, but most relapsing cases do so within a median follow-up of 3 years.[91] Typically, they may be preceded by an infection or vaccination.

Optic Neuritis

Optic neuritis may present as the initial presentation or often during relapses. Clinically symptoms are similar to that of AQP4-IgG-associated ON. Visual loss is typically central and severe. One feature that distinguishes MOGAD-ON is disk edema that may be seen in up to 85% of patients and is occasionally associated with peripapillary hemorrhage, unlike with NMOSD and MS **(Fig. 5)**. Recovery of visual loss is good in the majority with <15% suffering severe visual loss (≤20/200). Nearly half of these patients develop relapse and some have glucocorticoid dependence.

Acute Disseminated Encephalomyelitis

This is the most common presentation in >65% children and is characterized by altered sensorium accompanied by seizures and/or polysymptomatic presentation and supported by MRI features. Occasionally, there may be "ADEM-like" presentations wherein clinical and MRI features are typical but without encephalopathy. Recurrence of ADEM known as multiphasic ADEM may be seen in 30–50% of MOGAD-ADEM.

Transverse Myelitis

Transverse myelitis may be an isolated event during the patient's lifetime or occur with ADEM or ON. It presents as a subacute quadriparesis/paraparesis and with a severity similar to AQP4-IgG-associated NMOSD. Significant bladder and erectile dysfunction may remain as sequelae, more oftener than motor deficits.[89] Lhermittes or Uthoff phenomenon may occur.

Other less common presentations: NMOSD (AQP4-IgG negative)–MOGAD accounts for a third of all seronegative NMOSD. Cortical encephalitis[90] is a newly characterized syndrome described with MOGAD and may be unilateral in the majority of cases. Clinical manifestations include seizures, aphasia, stroke-like presentations, and headache. Unilateral encephalitis is otherwise known by the acronym FLAMES (FLAIR-hyperintense lesions in anti-MOG antibody associated encephalitis with seizures). Isolated brainstem and cerebellar features are less common than in MS. Ataxia and diplopia are the most common presentations. Area postrema syndrome is less frequently seen.[91] Cranial neuropathy (3rd, 5th, and 8th) has been reported alongside CNS disease and may be due to the involvement of myelin surrounding the intra-axial portion of these cranial nerves.[92] Myelitis may extend into proximal parts of the cauda equina nerve roots and produce a myeloradiculitis presentation. Isolated peripheral nervous system involvement is unlikely and MOG-IgG testing should be repeated with live CBA and in higher dilutions (detailed below in section on testing for MOG-IgG) in such situations.

Pediatric MOGAD

Children account for approximately 50% of MOGAD and MOG-IgG is positive in nearly a third of all acquired demyelinating disorders.[1] The most common phenotype is ADEM particularly in the very young followed by ON and myelitis or a combination of both as children get older. A leukodystrophy-like MRI pattern has been described following ADEM in some instances.[88]

Coexisting Autoantibodies and Autoimmune Disease

In contrast to AQP4-IgG-associated NMOSD, coexisting autoimmunity either in the form of serological or clinical evidence of disease is not common.[38,93] Patients may develop N-methyl-D-aspartate receptor (NMDAR) encephalitis before or after having MOGAD.[94] These patients may develop clinical and prominent MRI features of demyelination preceded by anti-NMDAR encephalitis simultaneously or have an initial demyelinating illness with brainstem or demyelinating syndromes suggestive of MOGAD followed by encephalitis. A similar relationship has been seen with AQP4-IgG-associated NMOSD and anti-NMDAR encephalitis too.

Diagnosis

Recommendations for the diagnosis of MOGAD were made initially in 2018.[95] Currently, an international panel of experts has formulated inclusive criteria based on the recent understanding of MOGAD.[78] At the very core of the diagnosis is detection of MOG-IgG by a sensitive CBA, supported by typical clinical presentations as outlined above and MRI supportive of the diagnosis **(Table 2)**.

Testing for MOG-IgG

The biological specimen that is currently recommended for testing is serum. Cell-based assays are highly recommended for optimal detection of MOG-IgG.[96,97] Live CBA using MOG in its full-length conformational form is specific and superior to fixed CBA available from commercial sources.[98] In addition to greater specificity of live CBA, false positive results could be eliminated by testing serial dilutions of patient samples (low titers disappear with higher dilutions of samples). In one such study,[98] 50% of patients with low titers (1:20 to 1:40) were false positive, 18% with moderate titers (1:100) were false positive, while titers of ≥1,000 were associated with zero false positive results. In the commercial (EUROIMMUN) assay, dilution is set at 1 in 10 and serial

TABLE 2: International MOGAD panel classification.

<table>
<tr><th colspan="4">Diagnosis of MOGAD (requires fulfillment of A, B, and C)</th></tr>
<tr><td>(A) Core clinical demyelinating event*</td><td colspan="3">• Optic neuritis*
• Myelitis
• ADEM
• Cerebral monofocal or polyfocal deficits
• Brainstem or cerebellar deficits
• Cerebral cortical encephalitis often with seizures</td></tr>
<tr><td rowspan="4">(B) Positive MOG-IgG test</td><td rowspan="4">Cell-based assay: serum</td><td>Clear positive**</td><td>No additional supporting features required</td></tr>
<tr><td>Low positive</td><td rowspan="3">• AQP4-IgG seronegative
• ≥1 supporting clinical or MRI feature</td></tr>
<tr><td>Positive without reported titer</td></tr>
<tr><td>Negative but CSF positive</td></tr>
<tr><td>Supporting clinical or MRI features</td><td>Optic neuritis</td><td colspan="2">• Bilateral simultaneous clinical involvement
• Longitudinal optic nerve involvement (>50% length of the optic nerve)
• Perineural optic sheath enhancement
• Optic disk edema</td></tr>
<tr><td></td><td>Myelitis</td><td colspan="2">• Longitudinally extensive myelitis
• Central cord lesion or H-sign
• Conus lesion</td></tr>
<tr><td></td><td>Brain, brainstem, or cerebral syndrome</td><td colspan="2">• Multiple ill-defined T2 hyperintense lesions in supratentorial and often infratentorial white matter
• Deep gray matter involvement
• Ill-defined T2-hyperintensity involving pons, middle cerebellar peduncle, or medulla
• Cortical lesion with or without lesional and overlying meningeal enhancement</td></tr>
<tr><td colspan="4">(C) Exclusion of better diagnoses including multiple sclerosis</td></tr>
</table>

*Clinical features should match typical presentations as described in text.

**MOG-IgG titers required for diagnosis are outlined in text.

(ADEM: acute disseminated encephalomyelitis; AQP4-IgG: aquaporin-4 immunoglobulins G; MOGAD: myelin oligodendrocyte glycoprotein-associated disorders; MRI: magnetic resonance imaging)

dilutions are not performed routinely. The international MOGAD panel classification has categorized MOG-IgG titer as follows—clear positive/low positive when tested by live CBA depending on individual laboratory cut off values [e.g., Mangalore MOGAD assay (*under submission*) recognizes a clear positive result if MOG-IgG is detected at dilutions >1:320, low titer if >1:160–320 dilutions, and negative if titer <1:160]. When tested by fixed CBA (EUROIMMUN) method, a titer >1:100 is considered as clear positive, while a titer >1:10 but <1:100 is deemed to be low positive. When MOG-IgG test titers are low or MOG-IgG is positive only in CSF but not serum or when test reports do not mention assay titers, additional criteria are required.[78]

The highest likelihood for MOG-IgG seropositivity is when testing is done at the time of the attack and before treatment with steroids or PLEX. If serum was obtained after treatment interventions, it is ideal to test samples 3 months later. In other circumstances, seroconversion of an initially negative result to a positive is extremely uncommon. MOG-IgG titers may wane over time, but may also persist for several years in some. Onset serum MOG-IgG titers do not have a prognostic value for recovery or subsequent relapse. Currently, there are no guidelines about serial MOG-IgG titer screening outside of a research setting.

Magnetic Resonance Imaging

Brain MRI: Brain MRI may be normal (particularly with isolated ON or TM), show clinically silent lesions, or manifest with clinical signs **(Fig. 7)**. Supratentorial lesions are ill-defined, often bilateral and large, involving deep gray matter seen with ADEM and ADEM-like presentations. Cerebral cortical encephalitis is accompanied by unilateral or bilateral FLAIR-hyperintense lesions. A leukodystrophy-like MRI pattern may occur in a small number of patients.[88] Leptomeningeal enhancement may be seen in <10% of adults and ~33% of children.[92] In the brainstem, pontine lesions are common and large middle cerebellar peduncle lesions with ill-defined margins are very characteristic. Diffuse brainstem lesions involving medulla, pons, or midbrain account for 20% of infratentorial lesions. Peri 4th ventricular lesions may be seen. Area postrema and midbrain lesions can occasionally be associated with persistent nausea and vomiting, reported in a small number.

MRI spinal cord: Most TM attacks have corresponding T2W hyperintense lesions on spinal MRI, though 10% may be normal.[99] Patients may have asymptomatic spinal cord lesions during nonspinal cord attacks and silent brain lesions with clinical myelitis. Myelitis may be typically LETM, short segment, or a combination of both. Conus myelitis is more common in MOGAD (30–40%) as compared to AQP4-IgG+ NMOSD (12–15%). Thickening and enhancement of dorsal roots have been described.[100] On axial scans, lesions are usually central and confined to the gray matter and a third of these may show an axial H pattern (H sign) or a sagittal line **(Fig. 7)**. Over time, there may be significant spinal cord atrophy.

MRI optic nerve: MRI of the orbit including fat suppression and postcontrast images are useful. Optic nerve hyperintensity and contrast enhancement typically involve >50% of the optic nerve which is often prechiasmatic. Bilateral optic nerve enhancement is seen in 50% of cases of MOGAD-ON and occasionally the nerve sheath alone shows enhancement (optic perineuritis) that extends into the orbital fatty tissue **(Fig. 7)**.

Cerebrospinal Fluid Evaluation

Routine testing may reveal mild pleocytosis in 50% of patients while a small number may have counts >100 white blood cells/high-power field. The latter is more common during an attack and more frequently with ADEM and TM. Elevated proteins may occur in nearly a third of patients and oligoclonal bands are present in <20%. Oligoclonal bands may be transiently present. Isolated detection of MOG-IgG in CSF has been reported,[95] but the diagnostic significance is uncertain.

Optical Coherence Tomography

During an acute attack of ON, OCT shows pRNFL thickening **(Fig. 8)** consistent with optic disk edema that is commonly associated with MOGAD. In the next 3–6 months after ON, thinning of pRNFL **(Fig. 8B)** and macular ganglionic cell and

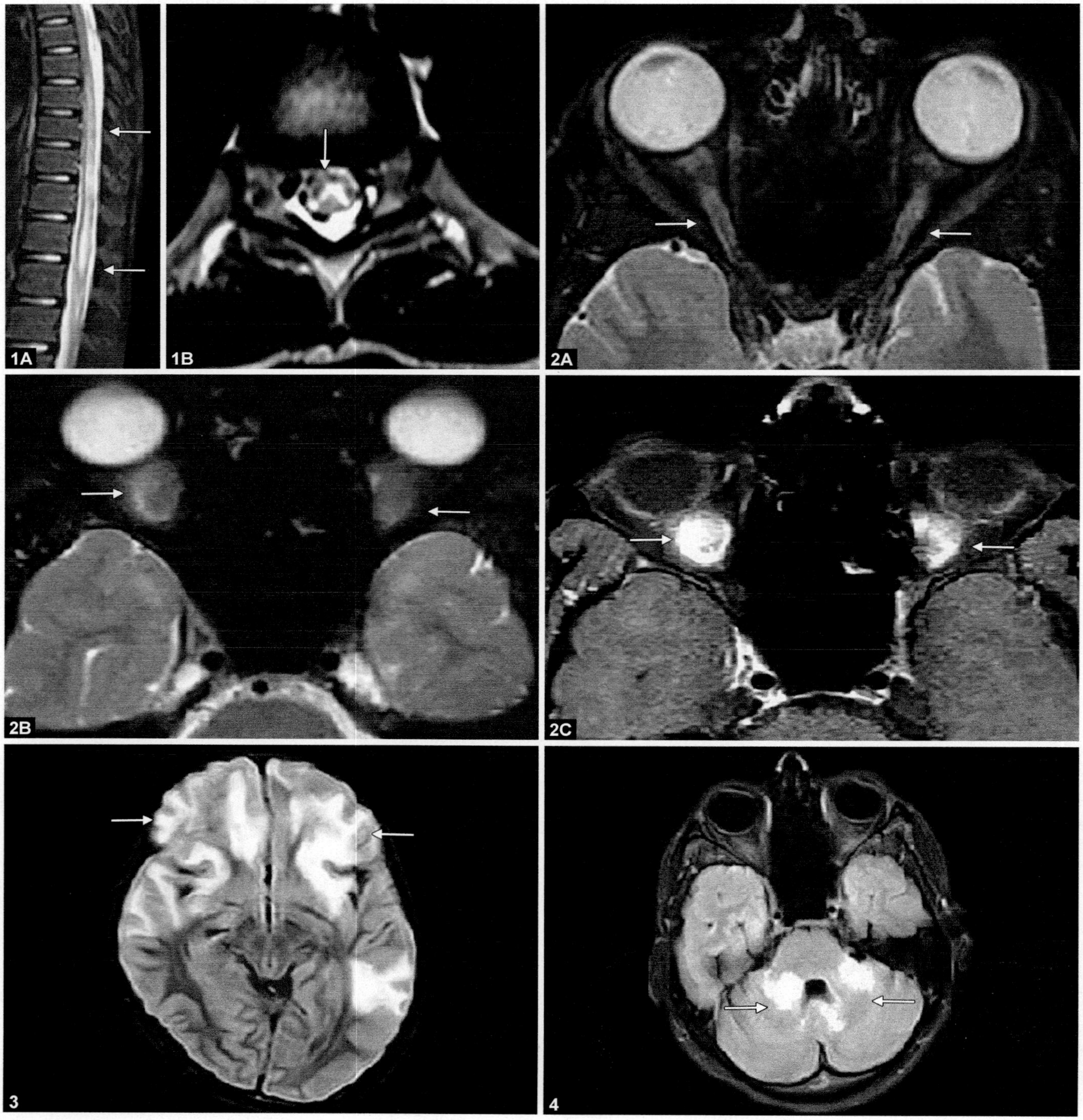

FIG. 7: *Continued*

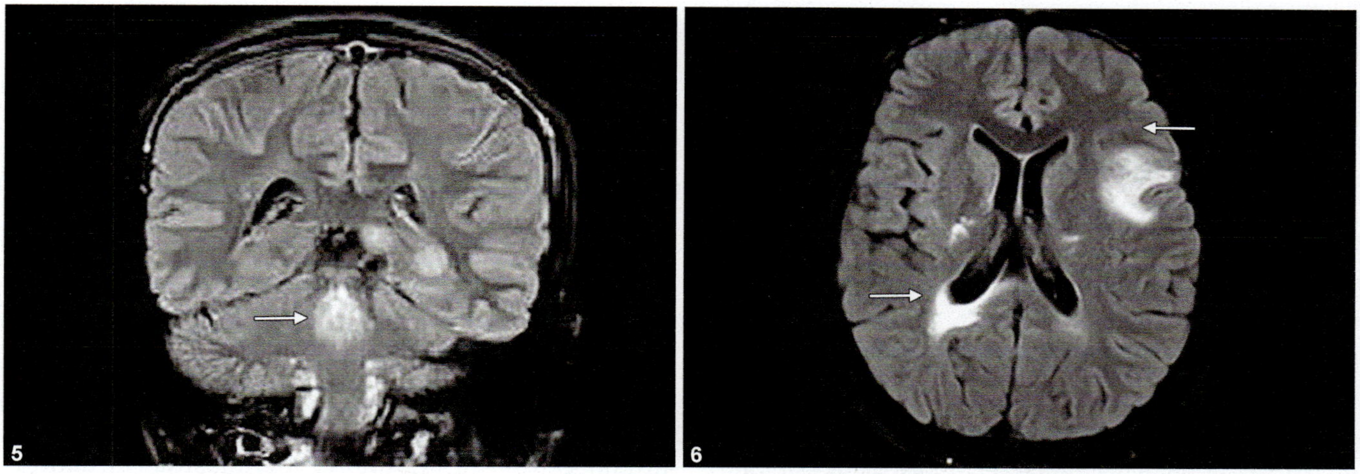

FIG. 7: Radiology of MOGAD. (1A) showing T2 FLAIR MRI sagittal images of dorsal cord showing LETM extending to include the conus (arrows), axial image showing "H sign" (1B). (2A) MRI of orbit axial fat suppressed image showing hyperintensity of both optic nerves sparing the chiasm, axial images showing bilateral optic nerve sheath and periorbital fat hyperintense signals (2B), with enhancement in postgadolinium scans (2C). Axial FLAIR brain images in a patient presenting with cortical encephalitis showing dramatic cortical swelling bilaterally (3), large T2 FLAIR images with ill-defined margins in bilateral middle cerebellar peduncles and adjoining cerebellum (4), diffuse lesion with ill-defined margins in the brainstem (arrow) and diencephalon (5), axial FLAIR brain imaging showing asymptomatic lesions in a patient presenting with MOGAD myelitis (6).

(FLAIR: fluid-attenuated inversion recovery; LETM: longitudinally extensive transverse myelitis; MOGAD: myelin oligodendrocyte glycoprotein antibody-associated disorder; MS: multiple sclerosis)

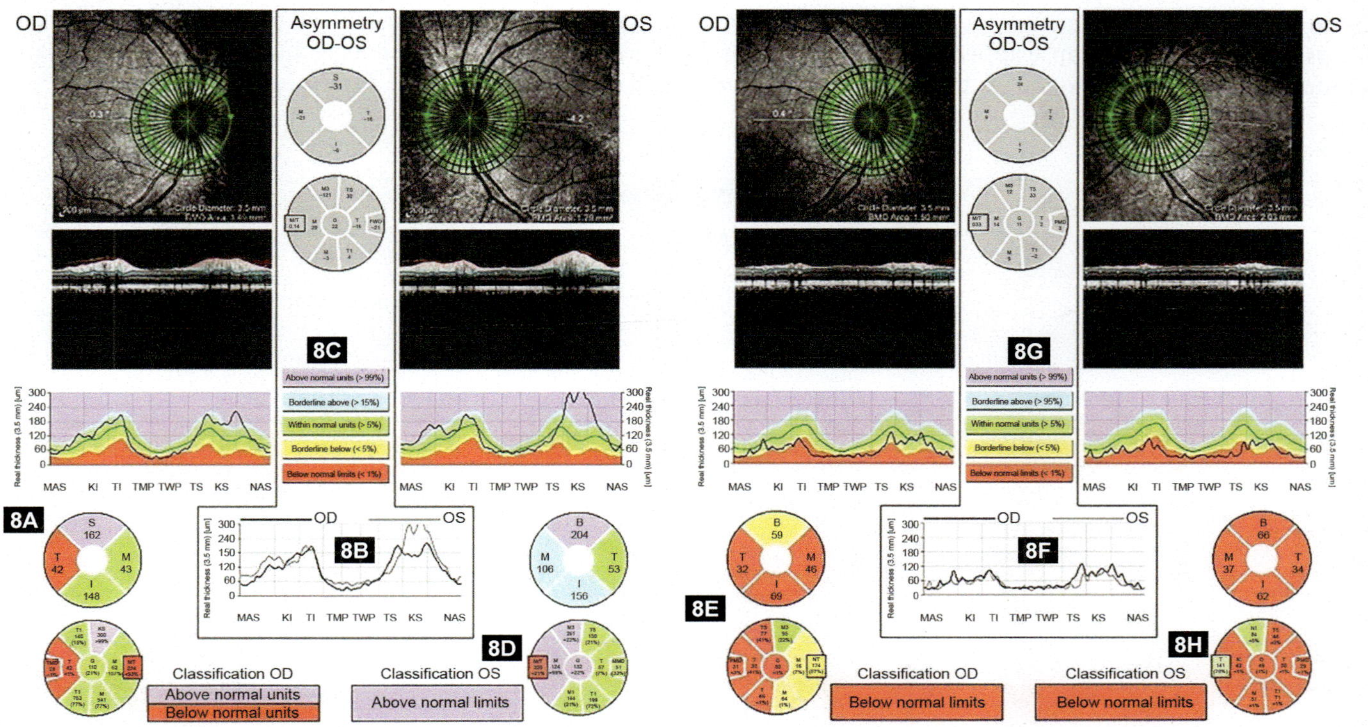

FIG. 8: Optical coherence tomography in MOGAD associated optic neuritis. During an attack of bilateral optic neuritis (8A–D), OCT images show RNFL thickening (color coded in mauve) of right (OS) > left (OD) eye. After 6 months, RNFL thinning (8E–H) is seen (color coded in red).

(MOGAD: myelin oligodendrocyte glycoprotein antibody-associated disorder; OCT: optical coherence tomography; RNFL: retinal nerve fiber layer) inner plexiform layer (mGCIPL) is most often seen and may be accompanied by optic atrophy clinically **(Fig. 8)**. In the non-ON eye, subclinical thinning of pRNFL and mGCIPL may be seen.[83] While the severity of optic nerve thinning is similar in both AQP4-IgG and MOG-IgG disorders, visual loss is more severe in the former.

Treatment

Treatment of MOGAD is highly variable **(Fig. 9)** and there are no standard recommendations.[101] More than 50% of patients have a monophasic course and there are no reliable predictors of clinical course. After the first attack, low-dose steroids alone for 3–6 months may be sufficient and is often recommended.[102] Intravenous immunoglobulins and PLEX have been used.[103] Most often disability is attack related. Therefore, acute treatment at the very onset, without delay is important. In patients with relapsing MOGAD, a decision to give long-term treatment has to be taken after weighing risk versus benefit in individual patients **(Fig. 9)**. The severity and degree of recovery after relapses and persistence of MOG-IgG positivity may influence decisions on maintenance treatment.[103] Long-term therapies are based on observational studies.[86,101,102] It is important to differentiate relapses in relation to steroid tapering or cessation, most often seen in doses <20 mg/day in adults and <0.5 mg/kg per day in children.[104] Duration of treatment before tapering steroids impacts relapse risk. The risk of relapse appeared higher for therapy <3 months as compared to longer therapy.[102] While there are no comparative studies on the efficacy of different immunosuppressants, MMF, AZA, and RTX may be considered for long-term immunosuppression.

DIFFERENTIAL DIAGNOSIS OF MOGAD AND AQP4-IgG-POSITIVE NMOSD

The most important differentiation is between the two disorders and MS **(Table 3)**. Low-titer/false positive MOG-IgG may occur and derail the diagnostic process in a variety of settings including MS, brain injury, and encephalitis. In broader terms, disorders that present with optic nerve and spinal cord diseases should be considered in the differential diagnosis and include a variety of genetic, inflammatory/autoimmune, neoplastic, structural, and metabolic disorders.[105] A progressive course, an acute onset with maximum deficits within hours, lack of improvement with steroids/PLEX, persistent enhancement of lesions >3 months, and silent accrual of lesions on MRI should raise red flags against the diagnosis of NMOSD and MOGAD.

CONCLUSION

The definitions, clinical spectrum of disease, investigative profile, and therapeutic paradigms of these group of disorders are continuously evolving. Early diagnosis and therapy have helped in reducing the impact of these diseases and associated disability.

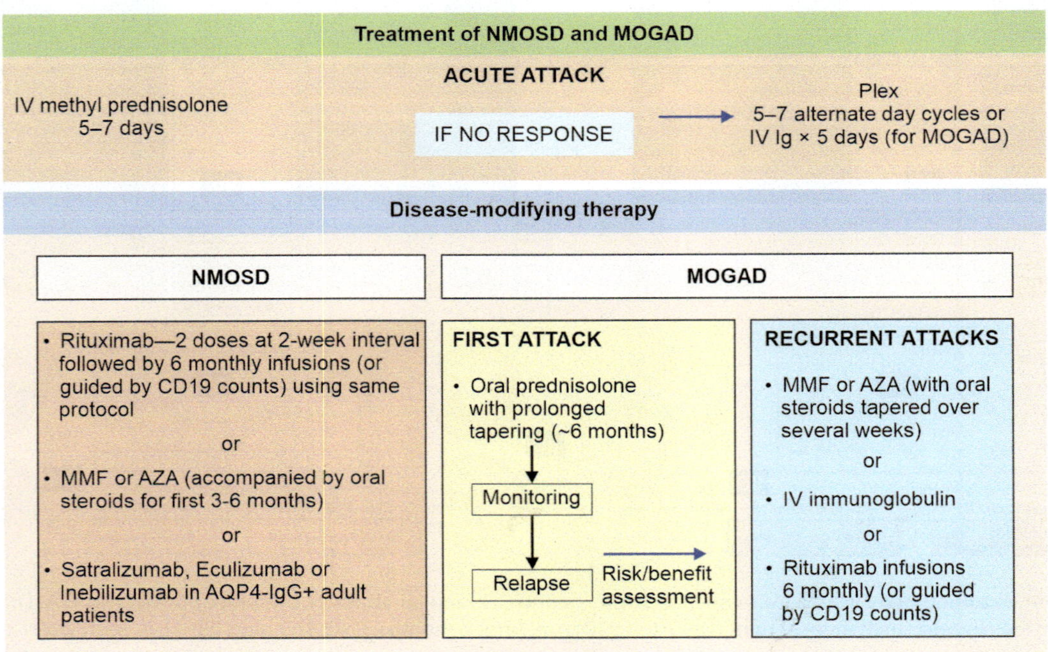

FIG. 9: Treatment algorithm for NMOSD and MOGAD.
(NMOSD: neuromyelitis optica spectrum disorder; MOGAD: myelin oligodendrocyte glycoprotein antibody-associated disorder)

TABLE 3: Differences between MS, MOGAD, and NMOSD.

	MS	NMOSD	MOGAD
Antecedent infection/ vaccination	Rare	Rare	Common
Common age at onset	20–30 years	>40 years	More often in children
Gender F:M	3:1	8–9:1	1–2:1
Clinical manifestations	ON, TM (partial cord), BS attacks	ON, TM (complete spinal cord dysfunction), BS attacks	ADEM, ON, TM, autoimmune encephalitis
Course	Mostly relapsing remitting from onset with later secondary progression	Relapsing, but no secondary progression	Monophasic or relapsing, no secondary progression
MRI brain	Multiple well-defined focal lesions adjoining lateral ventricles, Dawson's finger, U-fiber involvement, T1W-hypointense lesions	• Atypical for MS/brainstem lesions • No brain lesions	Atypical for MS, ill-defined fluffy lesions, "ADEM like", brainstem or no brain lesions
MRI spinal cord	Short-segment eccentric lesions predominantly in cervical cord. Contrast enhancement frequent	Long-segment lesions in cervical and dorsal cord (central). Contrast enhancement frequent	Long- and/or short-segment lesions (central), conus involvement seen. H-sign present. Contrast enhancement infrequent
MRI optic nerve	Short-segment, most often unilateral, intra-orbital lesions. Contrast enhancement frequent	Long-segment lesions, bilateral more often, posterior optic pathway involving optic chiasm	Long-segment lesions predominantly prechiasmatic, most often bilateral
CSF oligoclonal bands	80–90%	<10%	<10%
Prognosis	Majority ambulatory if treated with optimal DMD from onset. Progressive phase associated with disability	Attack-related accumulation of disability	Disability mostly with onset attack. Persistent MOG-IgG titer may suggest further relapse

(ADEM: acute disseminated encephalomyelitis; BS: brainstem; CSF: cerebrospinal fluid; DMD: Duchenne muscular dystrophy; MS: multiple sclerosis; MOGAD: myelin oligodendrocyte antibody-associated disorder; NMOSD: neuromyelitis optica spectrum disorder; ON: optic neuritis; TM: transverse myelitis)

REFERENCES

1. Longoni G, Levy DM, Yeh EA. The changing landscape of childhood inflammatory central nervous system disorders. J Pediatr. 2016;179:24-32.e2.
2. Varley J, Taylor J, Irani SR. Autoantibody-mediated diseases of the CNS: structure, dysfunction and therapy. Neuropharmacol. 2018;132:71-82.
3. Ranshoff RM, Scafer D, Vincent A, Blachère NE, Bar-Or A. Neuroinflammation: ways in which the immune system affects the brain. Neurotherapeutic. 2015;12:896-909.
4. Jarius S, Wildeman B. The history of neuromyelitis optica. J Neuroinflammation. 2013;10:797.
5. Jarius S, Wildemann B. The case of the Marquis de Causan (1804): an early account of visual loss associated with spinal cord inflammation. J Neurol. 2012;259:1354-7.
6. Allbutt T. On the ophthalmoscopic signs of spinal disease. Lancet. 1870;95:76-8.
7. Devic E. Myelite Aigue compliquee de nevrite optique. Bull Med (Paris). 1894;8:1033-4.
8. Wingerchuk DM, Hogancamp WF, O'Brien PC, Weinshenker BG. The clinical course of neuromyelitis optica (Devic's Syndrome). Neurology. 1999;53:1107-14.
9. Wingerchuk D, Lennon V, Pittock S, Lucchinetti CF, Weinshenker BG. Revised diagnostic criteria for neuromyelitis optica. Neurology. 2006;66:1485-9.
10. Lennon V, Wingerchuk D, Kryzer T, Pittock SJ, Lucchinetti CF, Fujihara K, et al. A serum autoantibody marker of neuromyelitis optica: distinction from multiple sclerosis. Lancet. 2004;364: 2106-12.
11. Wingerchuk DM, Lennon VA, Lucchinetti CF, Pittock SJ, Weinshenker BG. The spectrum of neuromyelitis optica. Lancet Neurol. 2007;6:805-15.
12. Wingerchuk DM, Banwell B, Bennett JL, Cabre P, Carroll W, Chitnis T, et al. International consensus diagnostic criteria for neuromyelitis optica spectrum disorders. Neurology. 2015;85:177-89.
13. Matiello M, Kim HJ, Kim W, Brum DG, Barreira AA, Kingsbury DJ, et al. Familial neuromyelitis optica. Neurology. 2010;75:310-5.
14. Pandit L, Malli C, D'Cunha A, Mustafa S. Human leukocyte antigen association in Neuromyelitis Optica in Indian population. Mult Scler. 2015;21:1217-8.
15. Brum DG, Barreira AA, Dos Santos AC, Kaimen-Maciel DR, Matiello M, Costa RM, et al. HLADRB association in neuromyelitis optica is different from that observed in multiple sclerosis. Mult Scler J. 2010;16:21-9.
16. Deschamps R, Paturel L, Jeannin S, Chausson N, Olindo S, Béra O, et al. Different HLA class II (DRB1 and DQB1) alleles determine either susceptibility or resistance to NMO and multiple sclerosis among the French Afro-Caribbean population. Mult Scler. 2011;17:24-31.
17. Zéphir H, Fajardy I, Outteryck O, Blanc F, Roger N, Fleury M, et al. Is neuromyelitis optica associated with human leukocyte antigen? Mult Scler. 2009;15:571-9.
18. Pandit L, Cox LM, Malli C, D'Cunha A, Rooney T, Lokhande H, Willocq V, et al. Clostridium bolteae is elevated in neuromyelitis optica spectrum disorder in India and shares sequence similarity with AQP4. Neurol Neuroimmunol Neuroinflamm. 2020;8(1):e907.
19. Cree BA, Spencer CM, Varrin-Doyer M, Baranzini SE, Zamvil SS. Gut microbiome analysis in neuromyelitis optica reveals

overabundance of Clostridium perfringens. Ann Neurol. 2016;80:443-7.
20. Papadopoulos MC, Verkman AS. Aquaporin 4 and neuromyelitis optica. Lancet Neurol. 2012;11:535-44.
21. Papp V, Magyari M, Aktas O, Berger T, Broadley SA, Cabre P, et al. Worldwide Incidence and Prevalence of Neuromyelitis Optica: A Systematic Review. Neurology. 2021;96:59-77.
22. Flanagan EP, Cabre P, Weinshenker BG, Sauver JS, Jacobson DJ, Majed M, et al. Epidemiology of aquaporin-4 autoimmunity and neuromyelitis optica spectrum. Ann Neurol. 2016;79:775-83.
23. Pandit L, D'Cunha A, Mallapur PU. Incidence and prevalence of neuromyelitis optica spectrum disorders in the background of international consensus diagnostic criteria – A Systematic Review. Neurol India. 2022;70(5):1771-9.
24. Bukhari W, Clarke L, O'Gorman C, Khalilidehkordi E, Arnett S, Prain KM, et al. The clinical profile of NMOSD in Australia and New Zealand. J Neurol. 2020;267:1431-43.
25. Apiwattanakul M, Popescu BF, Matiello M, Weinshenker BG, Lucchinetti CF, Lennon VA, et al. Intractable vomiting as the initial presentation of neuromyelitis optica. Ann Neurol. 2010;68:757-61.
26. Kim SM, Go MJ, Sung JJ, Park KS, Lee KW. Painful tonic spasm in neuromyelitis optica: incidence, diagnostic utility, and clinical characteristics. Arch Neurol. 2012;69:1026-31.
27. Flanagan EP, Weinshenker BG, Krecke KN, Lennon VA, Lucchinetti CF, McKeon A, et al. Short myelitis lesions in aquaporin-4-IgG-positive neuromyelitis optica spectrum disorders. JAMA Neurol. 2015;72:81-7.
28. Flanagan EP, Weinshenker BG, Krecke KN, Pittock SJ. Asymptomatic myelitis in neuromyelitis optica and autoimmune aquaporin-4 channelopathy. Neurol Clin Pract. 2015;5:175-7.
29. Zhao S, Mutch K, Elsone L, Nurmikko T, Jacob A. Neuropathic pain in neuromyelitis optica affects activities of daily living and quality of life. Mult Scler. 2014;20:1658-61.
30. Nethravathi M, Saini J, Mahadevan A, Hari-Krishna B, Yadav R, Pal PK, et al. Is pruritus an indicator of aquaporin-positive neuromyelitis optica? Mult Scler. 2017;6:810-7.
31. Blanc F, Noblet V, Jung B, Rousseau F, Renard F, Bourre B, et al. White matter atrophy and cognitive dysfunctions in neuromyelitis optica. PLoS One. 2012;7:e33878.
32. Meng H, Xu J, Pan C, Cheng J, Hu Y, Hong Y, et al. Cognitive dysfunction in neuromyelitis optica: a systematic review and meta-analysis. J Neurol. 2017;264(8):1549-58.
33. Wingerchuk DM. Neuromyelitis optica spectrum disorders. Continuum (Minneap Minn). 2010;16(5 Multiple Sclerosis):105-21.
34. Pandit L, Sato DK, Mustafa S, Takahashi T, D'Cunha A, Malli C, et al. Serological markers associated with neuromyelitis optica spectrum disorders in South India. Ann Indian Acad Neurol. 2016;19:505-9.
35. Sepúlveda M, Armangué T, Sola-Valls N, Arrambide G, Meca-Lallana JE, Oreja-Guevara C, et al. Neuromyelitis optica spectrum disorders: Comparison according to the phenotype and serostatus. Neurol Neuroimmunol Neuroinflamm. 2016;3:e225.
36. Chitnis T, Ness J, Krupp L, Waubant E, Hunt T, Olsen CS, et al. Clinical features of neuromyelitis optica in children: US Network of Pediatric MS Centers report. Neurology. 2016;86:245-52.
37. Collongues N, Marignier R, Zephir H, Papeix C, Fontaine B, Blanc F, et al. Long-term follow-up of neuromyelitis optica with a pediatric onset. Neurology. 2010;75:1084-8.
38. Malli C, Pandit L, D'Cunha A, Sudhir A. Coexistence of autoantibodies and other autoimmune diseases with Multiple Sclerosis and related disorders – Experience from the Mangalore Demyelinating Disease Registry (MANDDIR). Ann Indian Acad Neurol. 2021;24:740-4.
39. Hamid SH, Elsone L, Mutch K, Solomon T, Jacob A. The impact of 2015 neuromyelitis optica spectrum disorders criteria on diagnostic rates. Mult Scler. 2017;23:228-33.
40. Hyun JW, Jeong IH, Joung A, Kim SH, Kim HJ. Evaluation of the 2015 diagnostic criteria for neuromyelitis optica spectrum disorder. Neurology. 2016;86:1772-9.
41. Matthews L, Marasco R, Jenkinson M, Küker W, Luppe S, Leite MI, et al. Distinction of seropositive NMO spectrum disorder and MS brain lesion distribution. Neurology. 2013;80:1330-7.
42. Pittock SJ, Weinshenker BG, Lucchinetti CF, Wingerchuk DM, Corboy JR, Lennon VA. Neuromyelitis optica brain lesions localized at sites of high aquaporin 4 expression. Arch Neurol. 2006;63:964-8.
43. Kim W, Park MS, Lee SH, Kim SH, Jung IJ, Takahashi T, et al. Characteristic brain magnetic resonance imaging abnormalities in central nervous system aquaporin-4 autoimmunity. Mult Scler. 2010;16:1229-36.
44. Sato DK, Callegaro D, Lana-Peixoto MA, Waters PJ, de Haidar Jorge FM, Takahashi T, et al. Distinction between MOG antibody-positive and AQP4 antibody-positive NMO spectrum disorders. Neurology. 2014;82:474-81.
45. Ratchford J, Quigg M, Conger A, Frohman T, Frohman E, Balcer LJ, et al. Optical coherence tomography helps differentiate neuromyelitis optica and MS optic neuropathies. Neurology. 2009;73:302-8.
46. Syc SB, Saidha S, Newsome SD, Ratchford JN, Levy M, Ford E, et al. Optical coherence tomography segmentation reveals ganglion cell layer pathology after optic neuritis. Brain. 2012;135:521-33.
47. Prain K, Woodhall M, Vincent A, Ramanathan S, Barnett MH, Bundell CS, et al. Australian and New Zealand NMO Collaboration. AQP4 antibody assay sensitivity comparison in the era of the 2015 diagnostic criteria for NMOSD. Front Neurol. 2019;10:1028.
48. Waters PJ, McKeon A, Leite MI, Rajasekharan S, Lennon VA, Villalobos A, et al. Serologic diagnosis of NMO: a multicenter comparison of aquaporin-4-IgG assays. Neurology. 2012;78:665-71.
49. Pandit L, Malli C, D'Cunha A, Sudhir A. Overcoming the challenges in diagnosis of AQP4-IgG positive neuromyelitis optica spectrum disorders in resource poor settings using an indigenized and cost effective cell based assay. J Neuroimmunol. 2021;360:577706.
50. Kira J-i, Yamasaki R, Yoshimura S, Fukazawa T, Yokoyama K, Fujihara K, et al. Efficacy of methylprednisolone pulse therapy for acute relapse in Japanese patients with multiple sclerosis and neuromyelitis optica: A multicenter retrospective analysis – 1. Whole group analysis. Clin Exp Neuroimmunol. 2013;4:305-17.
51. Nakamura M, Nakazawa T, Doi H, Hariya T, Omodaka K, Misu T, et al. Early high-dose intravenous methylprednisolone is effective in preserving retinal nerve fiber layer thickness in patients with neuromyelitis optica. Graefe's Arch Clin Exp Ophthalmol. 2010;248:1777-85.
52. Yamasaki R, Matsushita T, Fukazawa T, Yokoyama K, Fujihara K, Ogino M, et al. Efficacy of intravenous methylprednisolone pulse therapy in patients with multiple sclerosis and neuromyelitis optica. Mult Scler. 2016;22:1337-48.
53. Kleiter I, Gahlen A, Borisow N, Fischer K, Wernecke KD, Wegner B, et al. Neuromyelitis optica: evaluation of 871 attacks and 1153 treatment courses. Ann Neurol. 2016;79:206-16.
54. Stiebel-Kalish H, Hellmann MA, Mimouni M, Paul F, Bialer O, Bach M, et al. Does time equal vision in the acute treatment of a cohort of AQP4 and MOG optic neuritis? Neurol Neuroimmunol Neuroinflamm. 2019;6:e572.
55. Lim YM, Pyun SY, Kang BH, Kim J, Kim KK. Factors associated with the effectiveness of plasma exchange for the treatment of NMO-IgG-positive neuromyelitis optica spectrum disorders. Mult Scler. 2013;19:1216-8.
56. Trebst C, Jarius S, Berthele A, Paul F, Schippling S, Wildemann B, et al. Update on the diagnosis and treatment of neuromyelitis optica: recommendations of the Neuromyelitis Optica Study Group (NEMOS). J Neurol. 2014;261:1-16.

57. Absoud M, Gadian J, Hellier J, Brex PA, Ciccarelli O, Giovannoni G, et al. Protocol for a multicentre randomiSed controlled TRial of IntraVEnous immunoglobulin versus standard therapy for the treatment of transverse myelitis in adults and children (STRIVE). BMJ Open. 2015;5:e008312.
58. Yamamura T, Kleiter I, Fujihara K, Palace J, Greenberg B, Zakrzewska-Pniewska B, et al. Trial of satralizumab in neuromyelitis optica spectrum disorder. N Engl J Med. 2019;381:2114-24.
59. Traboulsee A, Greenberg BM, Bennett JL, Szczechowski L, Fox E, Shkrobot S, et al. Safety and efficacy of satralizumab monotherapy in neuromyelitis optica spectrum disorder: a randomised, double-blind, multicentre, placebo-controlled phase 3 trial. Lancet Neurol. 2020;19:402-12.
60. Cree BAC, Bennett JL, Kim HJ, Weinshenker BG, Pittock SJ, Wingerchuk DM, et al. N-MOmentum study investigators. Inebilizumab for the treatment of neuromyelitis optica spectrum disorder (N-MOmentum): a double-blind, randomised placebo-controlled phase 2/3 trial. Lancet. 2019;394:1352-63.
61. Pittock SJ, Berthele A, Fujihara K, Kim HJ, Levy M, Palace J, et al. Eculizumab in Aquaporin-4-positive neuromyelitis optica spectrum disorder. N Engl J Med. 2019;381:614-25.
62. Sellner J, Boggild M, Clanet M, Hintzen RQ, Illes Z, Montalban X, et al. EFNS guidelines on diagnosis and management of neuromyelitis optica. Eur J Neurol. 2010;17:1019-32.
63. Pandit L, Mustafa S. Optimizing the management of Neuromyelitis Optica and Spectrum disorders in resource poor settings: Experience from the Mangalore demyelinating disease registry. Ann Ind Academy Neurol. 2013;16:572-6.
64. Costanzi C, Matiello M, Lucchinetti CF, Weinshenker BG, Pittock SJ, Mandrekar J, et al. Azathioprine: Tolerability, efficacy, and predictors of benefit in neuromyelitis optica. Neurology. 2011;77:659-66.
65. Mealy MA, Wingerchuk DM, Palace J, Greenberg BM, Levy M. Comparison of relapse and treatment failure rates among patients with neuromyelitis optica: Multicenter study of treatment efficacy. JAMA Neurol. 2014;71:324-30.
66. Jeong IH, Park B, Kim SH, Hyun JW, Joo J, Kim HJ. Comparative analysis of treatment outcomes in patients with neuromyelitis optica spectrum disorder using multifaceted endpoints. Mult Scler. 2016;22:329-39.
67. Kleiter I, Gold R. Present and future therapies in neuromyelitis optica spectrum disorders. Neurotherapeutics. 2016;13:70-83.
68. Jacob A, Matiello M, Weinshenker BG, Wingerchuk DM, Lucchinetti C, Shuster E, et al. Treatment of neuromyelitis optica with mycophenolate mofetil: retrospective analysis of 24 patients. Arch Neurol. 2009;66:1128-33.
69. Mealy Huh SY, Kim SH, Hyun JW, Joung AR, Park MS, Kim BJ, et al. Mycophenolate mofetil in the treatment of neuromyelitis optica spectrum disorder. JAMA Neurol. 2014;71:1372-8.
70. Cree BA, Lamb S, Morgan K, Chen A, Waubant E, Genain C. An open label study of the effects of rituximab in neuromyelitis optica. Neurology. 2005;64:1270-2.
71. Kim SH, Huh SY, Lee SJ, Joung A, Kim HJ. A 5-year follow-up of rituximab treatment in patients with neuromyelitis optica spectrum disorder. JAMA Neurol. 2013;70:1110-7.
72. Bedi GS, Brown AD, Delgado SR, Usmani N, Lam BL, Sheremata WA. Impact of rituximab on relapse rate and disability in neuromyelitis optica. Mult Scler. 2011;17:1225-30.
73. Kim SH, KimW, Li XF, Jung IJ, Kim HJ. Repeated treatment with rituximab based on the assessment of peripheral circulating memory B cells in patients with relapsing neuromyelitis optica over 2 years. Arch Neurol. 2011;68:1412-20.
74. Kim SH, Jeong IH, Hyun JW, Joung A, Jo HJ, Hwang SH, et al. Treatment outcomes with rituximab in 100 patients with neuromyelitis optica: Influence of FCGR3A polymorphisms on the therapeutic response to rituximab. JAMA Neurol. 2015;72:989-95.
75. Kim Bichuetti DB, Oliveira EM, Boulos Fde C, Gabbai AA. Lack of response to pulse cyclophosphamide in neuromyelitis optica: evaluation of 7 patients. Arch Neurol. 2012;69:938-9.
76. John TG, Bernard CC. The structure and function of myelin oligodendrocyte glycoprotein. J Neurochem. 1999;72:1.
77. O'Connor KC, McLaughlin KA, De Jager PL, Chitnis T, Bettelli E, Xu C, et al. Self-antigen tetramers discriminate between myelin autoantibodies to native or denatured protein. Nat Med. 2007;13:211.
78. Banwell B, Bennett JL, Marignier R, Kim HJ, Brilot F, Flanagan EP, et al. Diagnosis of myelin oligodendrocyte glycoprotein antibody-associated disease: International MOGAD Panel proposed criteria. Lancet Neurol. 2023;22(3):268-82.
79. Spadaro M, Winklmeier S, Beltrán E, Macrini C, Höftberger R, Schuh E, et al. Pathogenicity of human antibodies against myelin oligodendrocyte glycoprotein. Ann Neurol. 2018;84:315.
80. Höftberger R, Guo Y, Flanagan EP, Lopez-Chiriboga AS, Endmayr V, Hochmeister S, et al. The pathology of central nervous system inflammatory demyelinating disease accompanying myelin oligodendrocyte glycoprotein autoantibody. Acta Neuropathol. 2020;139:875.
81. O'Connell K, Hamilton-Shield A, Woodhall M, Messina S, Mariano R, Waters P, et al. Prevalence and incidence of neuromyelitis optica spectrum disorder, aquaporin-4 antibody-positive NMOSD and MOG antibody-positive disease in Oxfordshire, UK. J Neurol Neurosurg Psychiatry. 2020;91:1126-8.
82. De Mol CL, Wong Y, van Pelt ED, Wokke B, Siepman T, Neuteboom RF, et al. The clinical spectrum and incidence of anti MOG associated acquired demyelinating syndromes in children and adults. Mult Scler. 2020;26:806-14.
83. Pandit L, Mustafa S, Nakashima I, Takahashi T, Kaneko K. MOG-IgG-associated disease has a stereotypical clinical course, asymptomatic visual impairment and good treatment response. Mult Scler J Exp Transl Clin. 2018;4:1-9.
84. Netravathi M, Bollampalli HK, Bhat MD, Ganaraja VH, Prasad S, Mahadevan A, et al. Clinical, neuroimaging and therapeutic response in AQP4-positive NMO patients from India. Mult Scler Relat Disord. 2019;30:85-93.
85. Senanayake B, Jitprapaikulsan J, Aravinthan M, Wijesekera JC, Ranawaka UK, Riffsy MT, et al. Seroprevalence and clinical phenotype of MOG-IgG-associated disorders in Sri Lanka. J Neurol Neurosurg Psychiatry. 2019;90:1381-3.
86. Jurynczyk M, Messina S, Woodhall MR, Raza N, Everett R, Roca-Fernandez A, et al. Clinical presentation and prognosis in MOG-antibody disease: a UK study. Brain. 2017;140:3128-38.
87. Mader S, Gredler V, Schanda K, Rostasy K, Dujmovic I, Pfaller K, et al. Complement activating antibodies to myelin oligodendrocyte glycoprotein in neuromyelitis optica and related disorders. J Neuroinflamm. 2011;8:184.
88. Armangue T, Olivé-Cirera G, Martínez-Hernandez E, Sepulveda M, Ruiz-Garcia R, Muñoz-Batista M, et al. Associations of paediatric demyelinating and encephalitic syndromes with myelin oligodendrocyte glycoprotein antibodies: a multicentre observational study. Lancet Neurol. 2020;19:234-46.
89. Marriano R, Messina S, Kumar K, Kuker W, Leite MI, Palace J. Comparison of clinical outcomes of transverse myelitis among adults with myelin oligodendrocyte glycoprotein antibody vs aquaporin-4 antibody disease. JAMA Netw Open. 2019:2:e1912732.
90. Ogawa R, Nakashima I, Takahashi T, Kaneko K, Akaishi T, Takai Y, et al. MOG antibody-positive, benign, unilateral, cerebral cortical encephalitis with epilepsy. Neurol Neuroimmunol Neuroinflamm. 2017;4:e322.
91. Kunchok A, Krecke KN, Flanagan EP, Jitprapaikulsan J, Lopez-Chiriboga AS, Chen JJ, et al. Does area postrema syndrome occur in myelin oligodendrocyte glycoprotein-IgG-associated disorders (MOGAD)? Neurology. 2020;94:85-8.

92. Cobo-Calvo A, Ayrignac X, Kerschen P, Horellou P, Cotton F, Labauge P, et al. Cranial nerve involvement in patients with MOG antibody-associated disease. Neurol Neuroimmunol Neuroinflamm. 2021;8:1.
93. Kunchok A, Flanagan EP, Snyder M, Saadeh R, Chen JJ, Weinshenker BG, et al. Coexisting systemic and organ specific autoimmunity in MOG-IgG1 associated disorders versus AQP4-IgG+ NMOSD. Mult Scler. 2021;27:630-5.
94. Titulaer MJ, Höftberger R, Iizuka T, Leypoldt F, McCracken L, Cellucci T, et al. Overlapping demyelinating syndromes and anti–N-methyl-D-aspartate receptor encephalitis. Ann Neurol. 2014;75:411-28.
95. Jarius S, Paul F, Aktas O, Asgari N, Dale RC, de Seze J, et al. MOG encephalomyelitis: international recommendations on diagnosis and antibody testing. J Neuroinflammation. 2018;15:134.
96. Reindl M, Schanda K, Woodhall M, Tea F, Ramanathan S, Sagen J, et al. International multicenter examination of MOG antibody assays. Neurol Neuroimmunol Neuroinflamm. 2020;7(2):e674.
97. Waters PJ, Komorowski L, Woodhall M, Lederer S, Majed M, Fryer J, et al. A multicenter comparison of MOG-IgG cell-based assays. Neurology. 2019;92:e1250-5.
98. Sechi E, Buciuc M, Pittock SJ, Chen JJ, Fryer JP, Jenkins SM, et al. Positive predictive value of myelin oligodendrocyte glycoprotein autoantibody testing. JAMA Neurol. 2021;78:741-6.
99. Sechi E, Krecke KN, Pittock SJ, Dubey D, Lopez-Chiriboga AS, Kunchok A, et al. Frequency and characteristics of MRI-negative myelitis associated with MOG autoantibodies. Mult Scler. 2021;27:303-8.
100. Dubey D, Pittock SJ, Krecke KN, Morris PP, Sechi E, Zalewski NL, et al. Clinical, radiologic and prognostic features of myelitis associated with myelin oligodendrocyte glycoprotein autoantibody. JAMA Neurol. 2019;76:301-9.
101. Jurynezyk M, Jacob A, Fujihara K, Palace J. Myelin oligodendrocyte glycoprotein (MOG) antibody associated disease: practical considerations. Pract Neurol. 2019;19:187-95.
102. Juryezyk, Hegen H, Rendl M. Recent developments in MOG-igG associated neurological disorders. Ther Adv Neurol Disord. 2020;13:1-20.
103. Cobo-Calvo A, Ruiz A, Maillart E, Audoin B, Zephir H, Bourre B, et al. Clinical spectrum and prognostic value of CNS MOG autoimmunity in adults: the MOGADOR study. Neurology. 2018;90:e1858-69.
104. Hacohen Y, Mankad K, Chong WK, Barkhof F, Vincent A, Lim M, et al. Diagnostic algorithm for relapsing acquired demyelinating syndromes in children. Neurology. 2017;89:269-78.
105. Ramanathan S, Mohammed S, Tantsis E, Nguyen TK, Merheb V, Fung VSC, et al. Clinical course, therapeutic responses and outcomes in relapsing MOG antibody associated demyelination. J Neurol Neurosurg Psychiatry. 2018;89:127-37.

69

CHAPTER

Uncommon Demyelination Syndromes

Kamakshi Dhamija, Maya Bhat, Netravathi M

INTRODUCTION

The diagnosis of multiple sclerosis (MS), the most commonly acquired demyelination syndrome, is relatively straightforward if the clinical and radiological findings unequivocally suggest the etiology. However, clinical uncertainties exist when the presentations are atypical, and the patient does not fit into either MS or one of the allied demyelinating disorders such as acute disseminated encephalomyelitis (ADEM), neuromyelitis optica spectrum disorder (NMOSD), or myelin oligodendrocyte glycoprotein antibody disease (MOGAD). Given the rarity of such demyelination, the knowledge about the clinical approach and therapeutics of these disorders remains limited. The discovery of anti-myelin oligodendrocyte glycoprotein (MOG) immunoglobulin has helped in the characterization of a few of these atypical demyelination syndromes under its rubric; nevertheless a major chunk remains unclassified. This chapter aims to review the spectrum of these uncommon syndromes with emphasis on their clinical and radiological features as well as the therapeutic aspects.

SPECTRUM OF ATYPICAL DEMYELINATION SYNDROMES

The atypical demyelination syndromes have been included lately under the category of atypical idiopathic inflammatory demyelinating lesions (AIIDLs).[1] The common pathology among these disorders is demyelination; however, atypicality with respect to MS exists both clinic-radiologically and histopathologically. The atypicality may be in the form of a larger size, unusual morphology, atypical contrast enhancement, or other unusual characteristics that do not fit into the clinical or radiological description of MS and NMOSD.

We propose the classification of these AIIDLs based on their historical analogy to MS, although there is significant overlap between the two categories:

1. Atypical MS phenotypes
2. Non-MS phenotypes

1. *Atypical MS phenotypes*:
   - Balo's concentric sclerosis (BCS)
   - Marburg's variant
   - Schilder's diffuse myelinoclastic sclerosis
2. *Non-MS phenotypes:*
   - Tumefactive demyelination (TD)
   - Acute hemorrhagic leukoencephalitis (AHL) (Hurst's disease)

ATYPICAL MULTIPLE SCLEROSIS PHENOTYPES

Balo's Concentric Sclerosis

As illustrated in the name itself, the disease is characterized pathologically by alternating areas of damaged and preserved myelin, which gives a typical "onion-bulb"-like appearance to the lesion. The initial description of BCS comes from the clinicopathological description of an index case described by Hungarian neuropathologist Josef Balo in 1928 who called this entity as "leukoencephalitis periaxialis concentrica."[2] In this seminal report, the disease was described pathologically to cause white matter destruction in concentric layers in a manner that leaves the axon cylinder intact. The condition was postulated to resemble acute MS or Schilder's disease; however, features differing from the two entities were also simultaneously highlighted.

Given the rarity of the condition, our major understanding of the disease process comes from either single case reports or case series.

Balo's concentric sclerosis occurs most commonly at an average age of 34 years, with an age range of 3–62 years.[3] Pediatric cases, both with monophasic and relapsing-remitting character, have been described in the literature.[4] BCS is seen to be slightly more common in males than females, and younger males may be more predisposed to the condition.[5] A predilection for the South-East Asian population has been reported previously.[3]

Clinically, the symptoms are referable to the location of the lesion in the supratentorium, and patients present with a combination of symptoms such as headache, seizures, and cognitive or behavioral changes. Focal disturbances are attributable to the area of involvement and can present with aphasia or motor weakness, among others.[6] The onset is relatively acute, and rapid progression over days to weeks is seen.[7] Although the most common site of involvement is the white matter of cerebral hemispheres, atypical locations such as basal ganglia, brainstem, cerebellum, spinal cord, optic chiasm, and spinal cord have been reported in the literature.[3]

The histopathological characteristics of BCS have generated much curiosity and speculation among researchers. Akin to MS, the primary demyelination is believed to begin around a central venule. Centrifugally the disease process spreads peripherally in a radial manner, the inflammatory activity being periodically interrupted and leaving areas of intact or even remyelinated fibers in between, to be subsequently followed by the next wave of susceptible oligodendrocytes, hence the typical concentric ring appearance of the lesion.[8] Another theory proposed is hypoxia theory, which suggests that the active zones of demyelination have histopathological features of hypoxia-induced tissue injury, which is subsequently shielded by a zone of neuroprotective factors as heat shock protein-70 and hypoxia inducible factor 1 alpha which may lead to this zone of preserved myelin, only to be followed by next layer of susceptible oligodendroglial tissue.[9] **Figure 1** gives a pictorial representation of the presumed pathogenesis of BCS. A stronger link to ischemic theory also comes given its association with cerebral autosomal dominant arteriopathy with subcortical infarcts and leukoencephalopathy (CADASIL),[10] which further strengthens the notion that vascular factors can modulate the process of demyelination process involved in BCS. However, pathogenetically its correlation with MS remains unclear and is still a matter of debate. Whether it represents an "acute" form of MS was a long-perceived thought since the previously published case reports witnessed a relatively acute and fulminant course of the disease. However, with the advent of magnetic resonance imaging (MRI), patients are identified in their "earlier" stages. Hence, BCS does not carry a uniformly fulminant and poor prognosis as initially thought. To complicate the understanding, nevertheless, cases evolving finally into MS,[11] as well as patients having the concurrent presence of MS, have been well described in the literature.[3] A case of a patient with BCS and aquaporin-4 positivity has also been reported.[12]

Radiology of Balo's Concentric Sclerosis

Computed tomography (CT) brain in BCS can be normal or reveal areas of hypoattenuation. However, with the advent of MRI, clinicians can diagnose the condition earlier. On MRI, the concentric pattern which gives the appearance of "onion rings or whorled pattern" constitutes the hallmark feature of BCS. Acute BCS, on T2 sequences, appears as alternate rings of hyper- and hypointensity, which corresponds to

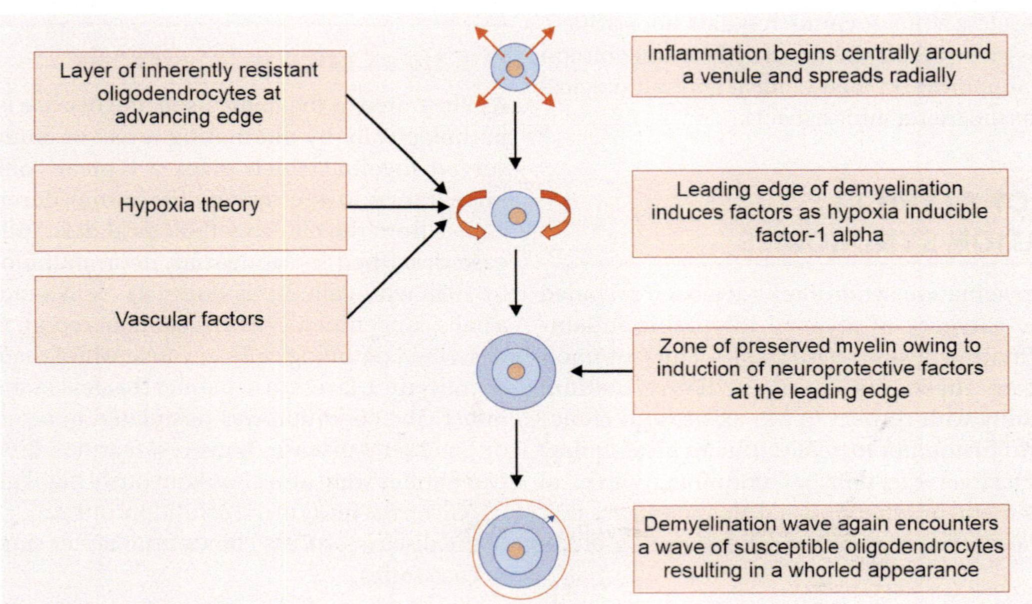

FIG. 1: Diagrammatic representation of presumed pathogenesis behind concentric ring formation of Balo's concentric sclerosis.

areas of inflammatory demyelination and areas of preserved myelin, respectively. On T1 sequences, these corresponding areas appear hypo- and isointense.[6] Sequential diffusion-weighted imaging (DWI) has helped to identify the natural course of the disease. Initially, on DWI, the area of restricted diffusion is seen to begin centrally, which later on follows a centrifugal pattern and progresses to take a concentric ring appearance. This evolves into a concentric appearance of restricted diffusion along T2 hyperintense areas alternating with rings of facilitated diffusion.[13] However, as compared to T2 images, DWI may show lesser rings because of the inherent lower spatial resolution of diffusion images.[6] Over time, these areas of restricted diffusion tend to facilitate. The sequential patterns on DWI provide insight into an ischemic theory behind Balo's pathogenesis.[14] On contrast T1 scan, the concentric ring enhancement may be seen. MR spectroscopy (MRS) in acute BCS shows decreased N-acetylaspartate (NAA) peak (which signifies neuronal loss), increased lactate (signifying impaired aerobic metabolism), and elevated choline and lipid peaks (suggestive of increased lipid membrane turnover).[6]

There exists evidence of the coexistence of MS-typical lesions along with Balo's lesions,[6,15] and also that BCS lesions may either regress on follow-up or transform into lesions typical of MS over time.[16] **Figures 2A and B** illustrate the regression of BCS lesions in one of our patients observed on two sequential MRIs.

Cerebrospinal Fluid Findings in Balo's Concentric Sclerosis

Cerebrospinal fluid (CSF) usually reveals a mononuclear lymphocytosis and only occasional oligoclonal bands.[6] Whether the presence of oligoclonal bands (OCBs) in CSF favors the evolution of BCS into MS subsequently is one school of thought. However, even with reports of the coexistence of MS-like lesions in patients with BCS, OCBs have been observed in two-thirds of patients only.[17] The role of OCBs in BCS and its relationship to MS is an intriguing area of research.

Treatment of Balo's Concentric Sclerosis

Given the rarity of the disease, the treatment of BCS is largely case- and experience-based. Corticosteroids remain the mainstay of therapy; however, in the event of failure of steroids, plasma exchange and intravenous immunoglobulin (IVIG)[18] have been tried with variable success. Since there is some pathological evidence that BCS may have a predominance of type III MS pattern of immunopathology,[19] it may not be robustly responsive to plasmapheresis.[20]

There has been a suggestion that even in the BCS group, there may be the heterogeneity of presentation which may help guide the clinical decisions.[21] Tzanetakos D et al. proposed a classification of BCS in three groups, which tend

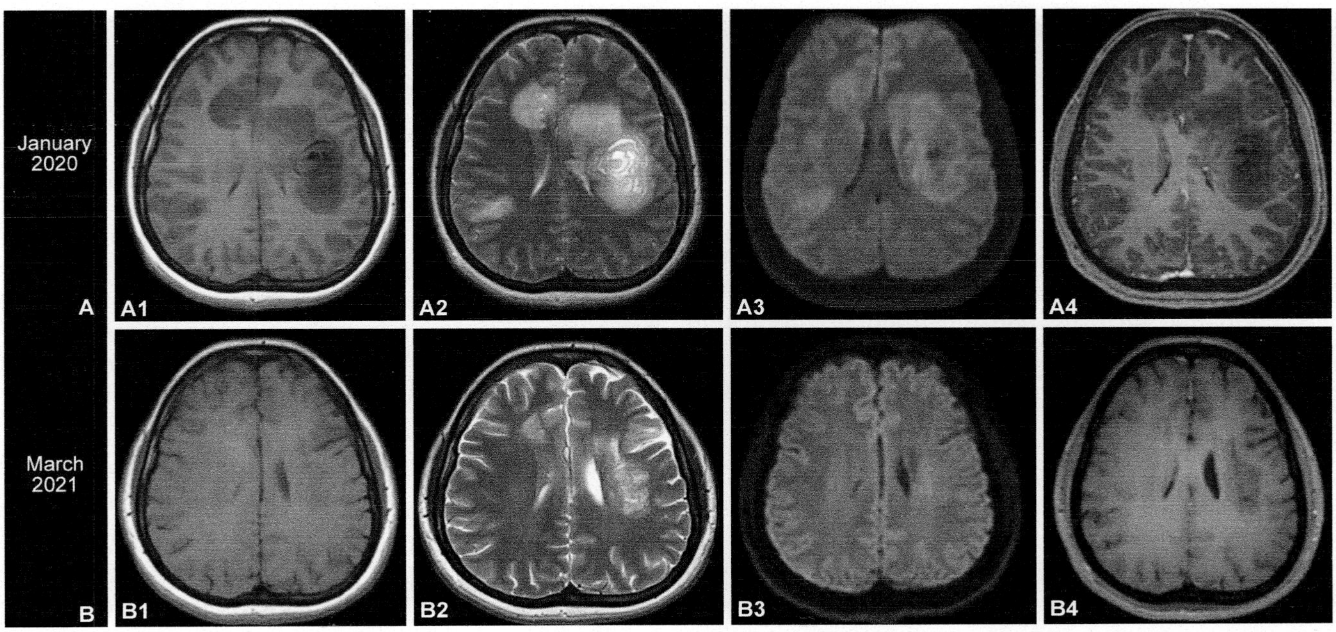

FIGS. 2A AND B: A case of (BCS). (A) MRI brain images of the patient as of January 2020: (A1) Axial T1 image reveals alternate zones of hypo- and isointense rings in a typical BCS lesion; (A2) Axial T2 image reveals alternate zones of hyper- and hypointense rings in the lesion; (A3) Axial diffusion images have some evidence of ring formation, not as pronounced as in T2 images; (A4) Axial T1 contrast images do not show contrast enhancement. (B) MRI brain images of the patient as of March 2021: (B1) Axial T1 image reveals marked resolution of the previous abnormality; (B2) Axial T2 image reveals improved but persistent ring pattern of BCS lesion; (B3) Axial diffusion images depict near complete resolution of diffusion abnormality; (B4) Axial T1 contrast images do not show any abnormality.

(BCS: Balo's concentric sclerosis; MRI: magnetic resonance imaging)

to have a significant clinical, pathologic, and therapeutic correlate.

Group 1: The first group constitutes patients of BCS with or without coexisting nonspecific white matter changes, which do not amount to a diagnosis of MS, respond poorly to steroids, and require aggressive immunomodulation as cyclophosphamide and mitoxantrone at the onset. Plasmapheresis also seems not to help the acute disease course, and may even exacerbate the disability given the lack of autoantibody-dependent responses in this pattern.

Group 2: The second group constitutes patients with coexisting MS typical lesions. They are usually well responsive to steroids, and conventional disease-modifying therapies (DMTs) for MS are effective in subsequent control of the disease as well. Many authors have reported successful use of interferons,[18] dimethyl fumarate,[19] natalizumab,[21] glatiramer,[22] and fingolimod in such patients.

Group 3: The third group although has typical MS-like lesions concurrently, it however constitutes patients who are poor responders to steroids and behave more closely to tumefactive MS. Such patients usually respond to B-cell depletion therapies such as rituximab.

Thus, the therapeutic options for BCS may be guided by the clinical and radiological phenotypes and given the lack of sufficient treatment evidence, the management remains an individual case to the case-based decision.

Marburg's Variant of Multiple Sclerosis

This presumably fulminant form of demyelination was first described in a postmortem study by Marburg in 1906.[23] The presentation is usually fulminant with a relentless monophasic course or a stepwise deterioration that reflects the involvement of cerebral white matter, infratentorium, and spinal cord. Since the lesions are typically large and tumefactive in nature, patients can have a polysymptomatic nature of the presentation, including but not limited to encephalopathy, seizures, and focal deficits. Brainstem involvement often leads to herniation and mortality. The usual natural history of the disease is death within a year of onset; however, stabilization and clinical remission have been reported rarely.[24-27] The readily available neuroimaging as well as advances in neurocritical care might potentially be responsible for the increasing number of cases being reported with a good outcome.

Pathologically, the disease is characterized by a destructive and fulminant form of MS with areas of profound macrophage activation resulting in inflammatory demyelination, necrosis, and axonal damage. Cases with perivascular infiltration and fibrinoid necrosis may suggest some overlap with central nervous system (CNS) vasculitis as well.[25,28,29] The lesions tend to be widely spread across the neuroparenchyma, and the degree of inflammatory demyelination is severe. Rare cases of meningeal and gray matter involvement have been reported.[30] It is postulated that some patients are inherently susceptible to the occurrence of widespread demyelination by the presence of a less cationic and more vulnerable isoform of myelin basic protein (MBP).[23]

Radiology of Marburg's Variant of Multiple Sclerosis

The lesions in Marburg's variant are multifocal, often tumefactive, and widely spread across, hence "multifocal tumefactive demyelination" is an appropriate acronym. Involvement of cerebral white matter across periventricular and juxtacortical areas, with frequent involvement of the brainstem and spinal cord, is seen. Patients with acute, nontumefactive, widespread diffusion-restricting lesions with a typical topography of MS have been reported.[27] Close differential happens to be ADEM; however, unlike in ADEM, here the lesions tend to be of different ages. There is the presence of outer ring enhancement[30] with corresponding areas of peripherally restricted diffusion signifying advancing edges of demyelination with broken blood–brain barrier and zones of cytotoxic edema. A case report of more than 100 contrast-enhancing lesions has been reported.[26]

Cerebrospinal Fluid Findings in Marburg's Variant of Multiple Sclerosis

Cerebrospinal fluid in Marburg's MS variant often reveals a normal or slightly raised cell count and increased protein. The presence of OCBs is less common as compared to MS.[31]

Treatment of Marburg's Variant of Multiple Sclerosis

The treatment of this entity can be quite challenging and tasking for clinicians. Intravenous (IV) steroids and plasmapheresis are the cornerstones of management, but usually the response to them is suboptimal and poor, requiring quick escalation to higher immunosuppression. Most of the case reports favor the use of cyclophosphamide[32] and mitoxantrone;[24,25,27,29,33] however, successful treatment with ocrelizumab[34] and alemtuzumab[26] has been reported.

Schilder's Diffuse Myelinoclastic Sclerosis

This entity, also known as myelinoclastic diffuse sclerosis or encephalitis periaxialis diffusa, was first described in 1912 by Austrian psychiatrist Paul Ferdinand Schilder, hence the acronym. In the initial histopathological description by Schilder, he observed two well-demarcated areas of demyelination with complete sparing of axons and subcortical U fibers in a 14-year-old girl with signs of raised intracranial pressure. When further cases were described, it was realized that many of the previous cases described as Schilder's disease were actually adrenoleukodystrophy or subacute sclerosing panencephalitis. However, in the current era of aquaporin-4 and MOG antibody-mediated disorders, the previously described cases might well have been a manifestation of these entities as well. We will limit our discussion to the historical descriptions of the disease.

The description of this entity is majorly limited to the pediatric population, most commonly between 5 and 14 years of age,[35] with an equal gender predilection. Thought to be a relatively acute form of MS, it usually presents with alteration of sensorium, seizures, and focal deficits owing to a larger size as compared to typical MS lesions. Poser's criteria for the disease emphasized the importance of ruling out adrenoleukodystrophy and ADEM.[36] Hence, strict clinical criteria included: "(1) clinical symptoms and signs atypical for an early course of multiple sclerosis (MS)-like bilateral optic nerve involvement, signs of intracranial hypertension, aphasia, psychiatric manifestation, (2) a normal cerebrospinal fluid (CSF) or atypical for MS, (3) one or two symmetrical bilateral plaques measuring at least 3 × 2 cm and involving the centrum semiovale of the cerebral hemispheres on brain scans, (4) no fever, viral or mycoplasma infection, or vaccination preceding the symptomatology, and (5) a normal serum concentration of very-long-chain fatty acids."[37]

Radiology of Schilder's Diffuse Myelinoclastic Sclerosis

As defined by Poser et al.,[36] this entity is defined radiologically by the presence of one or two roughly symmetrical plaques larger than 2 cm in size. Since the pathology is demyelination, the lesion characteristics favor the appearance of TD involving the white matter of frontoparietal lobes, often with corpus callosum. The lesions minimally enhance, are usually cystic, do not cause mass effect, and the brainstem is usually spared.[38] Chronic plaques may cause considerable difficulty in distinguishing from leukodystrophies. Especially the involvement of bilateral parieto-occipital lobes (butterfly pattern) may resemble Loes pattern-1 of adrenoleukodystrophy.[39] Since such lesions have common differentials as abscess, ischemia, or mass lesions, few radiological pointers may help in differentiating these lesions from demyelination (described ahead under TD).

Bacigaluppi et al.[37] have proposed noninvasive diagnostic criteria supplementing the historical Poser's criteria in the diagnosis of Schilder's disease. The criteria include:

- No signs of intracranial hypertension
- Presence of one or two subcortical cyst-like lesions with eventually open ring sign at CT/MR
- Exclusion of ischemia, abscess, and metastasis by classical neuroradiological means and further of primary neoplasm using perfusion MR and consideration of abnormal glutamate/glutamine elevation on short-echo time MRS

Given the rarity of the condition and the lack of a uniform consensus on the existence, and evaluation of this entity, we do not have definite treatment options. Corticosteroids have been the cornerstone of therapy with good improvement.[40] A case report mentions the positive role of IVIGs as well.[41]

NON-MULTIPLE SCLEROSIS PHENOTYPES

Tumefactive Demyelination

Often there occurs a situation when a patient presents with signs and symptoms referable to cortical dysfunction, and a solitary large lesion resembling a neoplastic process is seen on an MRI scan. TD remains a broader class, which can be seen in patients with MS, as a part of ADEM, NMOSD, or MOGAD, or as a standalone lesion when it poses the most difficult diagnostic and therapeutic challenges, often necessitating biopsy to effectively rule out neoplastic process. Notably, TD is not synonymous with tumefactive MS. In the coronavirus disease-19 (COVID-19) era, there have been reports of its association with COVID-19[42] and post-COVID-19 vaccinal association as well.[43,44]

The clinical features are guided by the size and location of the lesion. The lesions can be solitary or multiple. Since TD is characterized by its large size, usually the symptoms include impaired consciousness, seizures, cognitive deficits, and focal deficits. Cases of isolated relapsing-remitting TD have been reported.[45]

Pathology has evidence of demyelination with relative axonal sparing, although areas of widespread axonal damage can occur. There is reactive astrocytosis and the presence of foamy macrophages.[23] An acute demyelinating lesion may mimic a glioma with the presence of reactive astrocytes (like Creutzfeldt–Peters cells). Immunohistochemical stains for macrophages and myelin may help in differentiation from a neoplastic process.[46]

Radiology of Tumefactive Demyelination

Computed tomography head usually reveals the presence of a hypodense rim around the lesion, which can serve as a useful diagnostic tool in differentiation from mass lesions.[46] On MRI, a tumefactive lesion has a size defined by more than 2 cm in size. Clues in favor of demyelinating lesions on MRI are a rim of surrounding hypointensity on T2 sequences, open or closed ring enhancement, minimal surrounding edema, and peripheral diffusion restriction, especially at the contrast-enhancing rim zone. A typical acute demyelinating lesion restricts in the periphery as compared to the core of the lesion in abscess and ischemia. Utilization of MR perfusion scan can help in its differentiation from mass lesion. On the perfusion scan, demyelination shows decreased perfusion by intact vasculature, in contrast to increased perfusion in primary brain tumors. Conventional MRS reveals show decreased NAA peak, increased lactate, and elevated choline and lipid peaks,[6] as illustrated previously. This MRS finding is also found in mass lesions. However, once chronicity sets in for demyelination, decreased NAA persists, but other peaks tend to normalize. This is contrary to mass lesions, which will continue to show raised lactate, choline, and lipid peaks at follow-up. Some authors have advocated a follow-up MRS after the initiation of anti-inflammatory treatment to show improvement in MRS parameters.[46] Another interesting observation in MRS of demyelination is the presence of elevated glutamate/glutamine peak using short-echo time proton MRS.[47] On positron emission tomography (PET)-CT, neoplasms have greater metabolic uptake than TD, and the combined use of MRS and PET-CT may have a greater role in differentiating the two entities.[48] **Figure 3** highlights characteristic MRI features of a TD lesion.

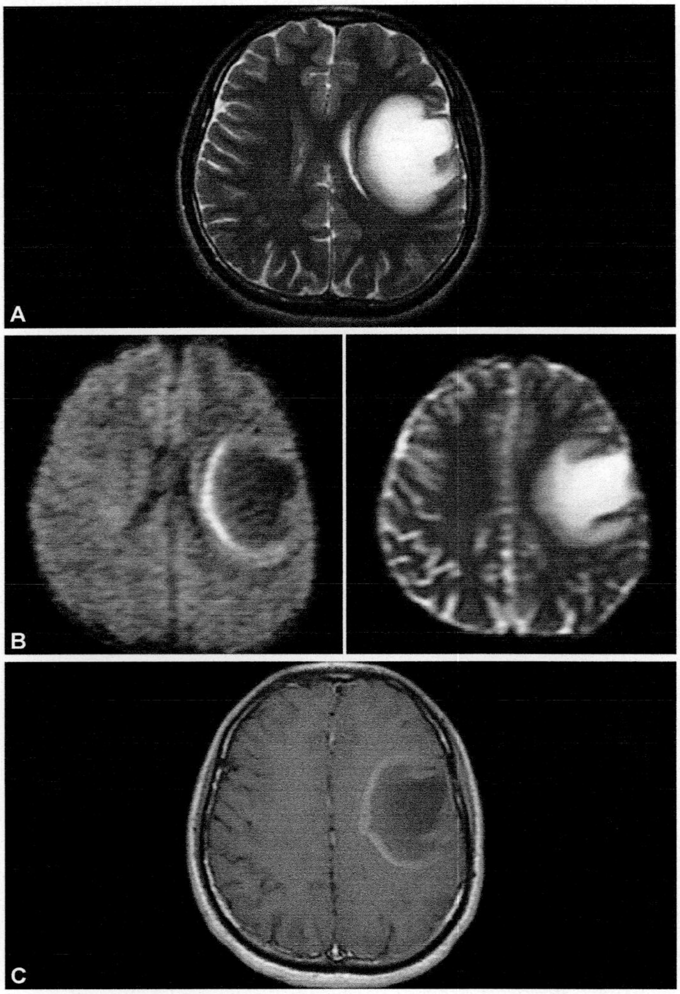

FIGS. 3A TO C: MRI characteristics of a typical tumefactive demyelinating lesion. (A) Axial T2 image showing a tumefactive lesion in left frontal region with surrounding hypointense rim; (B) Axial DWI and ADC images showing rim of diffusion restriction at the periphery of lesion; (C) Axial T1 contrast images depicting peripheral contrast enhancement corresponding to edges with diffusion restriction.

(ADC: apparent diffusion coefficient; DWI: diffusion-weighted imaging; MRI: magnetic resonance imaging)

Based on the radiological features, the MAGNIMS (magnetic resonance imaging in MS) group[49] has proposed that AIIDLs can be classified into either of the four types **(Figs. 4A to D)**:

1. *Infiltrative*: The demyelination zone has large ill-defined areas of T2 hyperintensity with contrast uptake being absent or inhomogeneous.
2. *Megacystic*: The lesions in this form are large, with tumefactive quality, being ≥3 cm in diameter and are cystic, with expansion often seen along the cortical ribbon with an incomplete ring of enhancement.
3. *Balo's like*: The typical appearance of concentric rings of alternating T2 hypo- and hyper-intensities within the lesion
4. *Ring-like*: Rounded lesions (≥2 cm) having a ring-like contrast enhancement with perilesional edema

Cerebrospinal Fluid Findings in Tumefactive Demyelination

Cerebrospinal fluid picture in TD is usually guided by the underlying cause of demyelination. In other cases, CSF is usually normal or may show a mild rise in protein or cells. OCBs in CSF can be seen in 50–70% of the patients, and as per our current understanding, do not necessarily indicate underlying pathology to be MS.

It is imperative to rule out aquaporin-4 and MOG antibody disease in TD. Paraneoplastic and autoimmune etiologies also mandate exclusion by relevant investigations.

Treatment of Tumefactive Demyelination

Acute treatment rests on the use of IV steroids for 3–5 days. Steroid refractoriness has been defined as failure of expanded disability status scale (EDSS) improvement by at least one point in 7 days after finishing steroids.[46] Guidelines for escalation to plasmapheresis have been proposed by Weinshenker et al.[50] They suggested plasmapheresis to be considered as a second-line treatment if a minimum duration of the deficit is 21 days from the onset and 14 days from the commencement of IV steroid therapy, or 12 days from the onset if the deficit continues to worsen beyond 5 full days after starting steroid treatment. However, we believe that since the "time is tissue" principle even in cases of demyelination, complementing plasmapheresis along with initial steroids can hasten the recovery, given their differing mechanisms of action. Patients may require decompressive hemicraniectomy in case of larger tumefactive lesions for mass effect amelioration.

In cases of TD occurring in the setup of MS, standard DMTs should be reasonable to use. However, caution exists in the use of natalizumab and fingolimod in TD, as this drug has been implicated in its causation as well.[51] Immune reconstitution therapies have been remotely used in the treatment of TD associated with MS. One patient had a successful outcome with cladribine use.[52] Nevertheless,

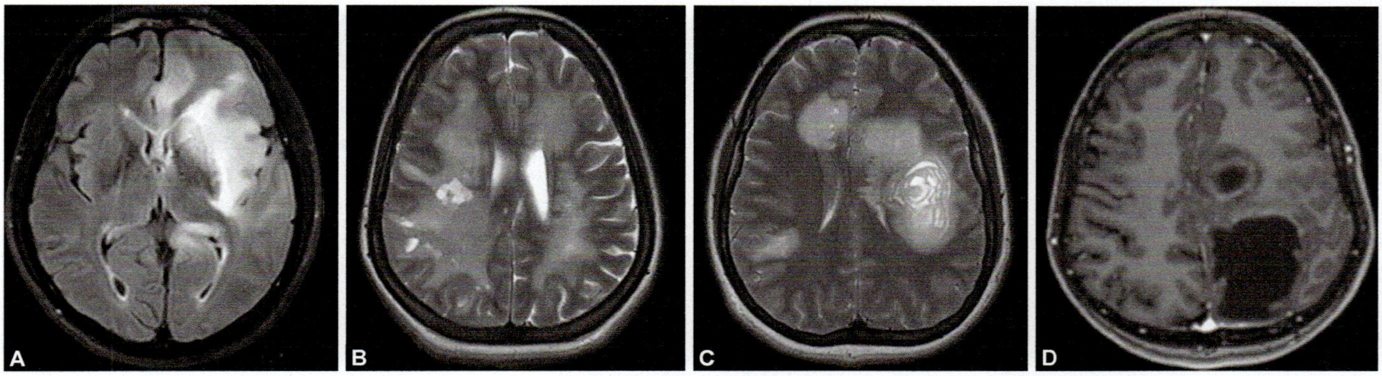

FIGS. 4A TO D: Four patterns of atypical idiopathic inflammatory demyelinating lesions as defined by the MAGNIMS (Magnetic Resonance Imaging in Multiple Sclerosis) group. (A) Infiltrative type; (B) Megacystic type; (C) Balo's like; (D) Ring-like.

TD has been well recognized as a complication of abrupt withdrawal of fingolimod[53] and natalizumab[54] in MS. In such a case, there is a positive role of plasmapheresis, IVIG, and rituximab. Cyclophosphamide also has a role as bridging therapy in case of rebound disease before switching to another DMT.[54] Similarly in cases with underlying aquaporin-4 and MOG antibody pathology, treatment should be guided by the underlying disease. Most authors do not advocate longer immunomodulation in events of isolated TD. However, in case of recurrent TD events, reports of successful use of azathioprine,[45,55] mycophenolate mofetil (MMF),[55] methotrexate,[55] and cyclophosphamide[55] well exist in the literature. Given the robust autoantibody responses involved in immunopathogenesis, there have been reports of positive treatment outcomes with the use of B-cell therapies. Rituximab (anti-CD20 therapy) has been successfully employed and has increasingly found its role in the treatment of TD.[56,57] On the other hand, a case report witnessing the paradoxical appearance of a tumefactive lesion, shortly after rituximab infusion for MS, creates a caution note for its use.[58]

Acute Hemorrhagic Leukoencephalitis

Also known as Hurst's disease, or Weston Hurst's disease,[23] AHL forms an extreme spectrum of ADEM with fulminant progression causing a relentless course to death usually within a week of symptom onset. First described in 1941, it comprises nearly 2% of pediatric ADEM cases;[59] however, recent cases have been reported with the onset of the COVID-19 pandemic as well.[60,61] ADEM though is more common in children; however, AHL may be seen in adults, more so frequently in males. The usual presentation is one of encephalopathy with polyfocal symptomatology. Viral prodrome as a trigger is seen, as commonly as in usual "ADEM." The mortality rate is high, up to the rate of 70% in some case series.[62]

The pathology of AHL mimics that of ADEM with evidence of perivenous demyelination and fibrinoid vascular necrosis resulting in perivenous microhemorrhages. The degree of pathological insult in the form of axonal damage, hemorrhage, and edema is more common in AHL than in ADEM. The inflammation in biopsy specimens is prominent with infiltration by neutrophils, macrophages, and lymphocytes.[63]

Radiology of Acute Hemorrhagic Leukoencephalitis

Computed tomography findings in AHL may mimic hemorrhagic infarcts, infectious encephalitis, mass lesions, or other demyelination. Brain MRI is the diagnostic modality of choice and shows evidence of confluent white matter lesions with significant edema, mass effect, and microhemorrhages. The common locations of lesions are cerebral white matter, brainstem, and cord, though isolated brainstem involvement is also seen.[64] Gray matter involvement is variable, and the contrast enhancement pattern is not specific and inconsistent. The findings on susceptibility-weighted images (SWIs) in AHL cases are quite specific and cannot be underscored.[63] In addition to confluent hemorrhages, SWI has evidence of nondisplaced medullary veins with concomitant petechial hemorrhages, which helps in its differentiation from mass lesions.

Treatment of Acute Hemorrhagic Leukoencephalitis

Treatment of AHL follows the principles of ADEM management; however, given the aggressive nature of the disease and high mortality, it warrants earlier and aggressive immunomodulation. Although cases with a good response to steroids are reported, these are only a handful and represent a minority of cases only.[65,66]

Apart from the use of steroids and plasmapheresis, IVIG has been used in individual cases. Quick escalation to cyclophosphamide has helped in the stabilization of the disease in case reports.[67]

Despite the aggressive use of immunomodulators, it is not uncommon for the disease to have an unfavorable outcome and mortality.[68]

CONCLUSION

The AIIDLs are a separate group of heterogenous disorders that stand out from the common demyelinating syndromes by their clinicoradiological atypicality. Since the MAGNIMS group has radiologically classified these disorders, we believe that the uncommon demyelination should be grouped under this rubric for uniformity and hence, avoid the existing confusion about terminology of these disorders. Identification and categorization into one of the phenotypes can help guide therapeutic decisions as well. Given their rarity and the fact that most of the experience with these disorders is experience-based, we still have a long way to go in defining treatment guidelines for these disorders.

REFERENCES

1. Wallner-Blazek M, Rovira A, Fillipp M, Rocca MA, Miller DH, Schmierer K, et al. Atypical idiopathic inflammatory demyelinating lesions: prognostic implications and relation to multiple sclerosis. J Neurol. 2013;260(8):2016-22.
2. Balo J. Encephalitis periaxialis concentrica. Arch Neurol Psychiatry. 1928;19(2):242.
3. Purohit B, Ganewatte E, Schreiner B, Kollias S. Balo's concentric sclerosis with acute presentation and coexisting multiple sclerosis-typical lesions on MRI. Case Rep Neurol. 2015;7(1):44-50.
4. Bhoi SK, Naik S, Kalita J, Misra UK. Multifocal Balo's concentric sclerosis in children: report of a case and review of literature. J Neurosci Rural Pract. 2017;8(Suppl 1):S136-8.
5. Mowry EM, Woo JH, Ances BM. Baló's concentric sclerosis presenting as a stroke-like syndrome. Nat Clin Pract Neurol. 2007;3(6):349-54.
6. Darke M, Bahador FM, Miller DC, Litofsky NS, Ahsan H. Baló's concentric sclerosis: imaging findings and pathological correlation. J Radiol Case Rep. 2013;7(6):1-8.
7. Amini Harandi A, Esfandani A, Pakdaman H, Abbasi M, Sahraian MA. Balo's concentric sclerosis: an update and comprehensive literature review. Rev Neurosci. 2018;29(8):873-82.
8. Moore GR, Neumann PE, Suzuki K, Lijtmaer HN, Traugott U, Raine CS. Balo's concentric sclerosis: new observations on lesion development. Ann Neurol. 1985;17(6):604-11.
9. Stadelmann C, Ludwin S, Tabira T, Guseo A, Lucchinetti CF, Leel-Ossy L, et al. Tissue preconditioning may explain concentric lesions in Baló's type of multiple sclerosis. Brain J Neurol. 2005;128(Pt 5):979-87.
10. Chitnis T, Hollmann TJ. CADASIL mutation and Balo concentric sclerosis: a link between demyelination and ischemia? Neurology. 2012;78(3):221-3.
11. Kastrup O, Stude P, Limmroth V. Balo's concentric sclerosis. J Neurol. 2002;249(7):811-4.
12. Graber JJ, Kister I, Geyer H, Khaund M, Herbert J. Neuromyelitis optica and concentric rings of Baló in the brainstem. Arch Neurol. 2009;66(2):274-5.
13. Kavanagh EC, Heran MKS, Fenton DM, Lapointe JS, Nugent RA, Graeb DA. Diffusion-weighted imaging findings in Balo concentric sclerosis. Br J Radiol. 2006;79(943):e28-31.
14. Mowry EM, Woo JH, Ances BM. Technology insight: can neuroimaging provide insights into the role of ischemia in Baló's concentric sclerosis? Nat Clin Pract Neurol. 2007;3(6):341-8.
15. Li Y, Xie P, Fan X, Tang H. Balò's concentric sclerosis presenting with benign clinical course and multiple sclerosis-like lesions on magnetic resonance images. Neurol India. 2009;57(1):66-8.
16. Wang C, Zhang KN, Wu XM, Huang G, Xie XF, Qu XH, et al. Balo's disease showing benign clinical course and coexistence with multiple sclerosis-like lesions in Chinese. Mult Scler Houndmills Basingstoke Engl. 2008;14(3):418-24.
17. Behrens JR, Wanner J, Kuchling J, Ostendorf L, Harms L, Ruprecht K, et al. 7 Tesla MRI of Balo's concentric sclerosis versus multiple sclerosis lesions. Ann Clin Transl Neurol. 2018;5(8):900-12.
18. Airas L, Kurki T, Erjanti H, Marttila RJ. Successful pregnancy of a patient with Balo's concentric sclerosis. Mult Scler Houndmills Basingstoke Engl. 2005;11(3):346-8.
19. Kania K, Ambrosius W, Kozubski W, Kalinowska A. Case report: Baló's concentric sclerosis-like lesion in a patient with relapsing-remitting multiple sclerosis treated with dimethyl fumarate. Front Neurol. 2022;13:891113.
20. Stork L, Ellenberger D, Beißbarth T, Friede T, Lucchinetti CF, Brück W, et al. Differences in the responses to apheresis therapy of patients with 3 histopathologically classified immunopathological patterns of multiple sclerosis. JAMA Neurol. 2018;75(4):428-35.
21. Tzanetakos D, Vakrakou AG, Tzartos JS, Velonakis G, Evangelopoulos ME, Anagnostouli M, et al. Heterogeneity of Baló's concentric sclerosis: a study of eight cases with different therapeutic concepts. BMC Neurol. 2020;20(1):400.
22. Hardy TA, Beadnall HN, Sutton IJ, Mohamed A, Jonker BP, Buckland ME, et al. Baló's concentric sclerosis and tumefactive demyelination: a shared immunopathogenesis? J Neurol Sci. 2015;348(1-2):279-81.
23. Hardy TA, Reddel SW, Barnett MH, Palace J, Lucchinetti CF, Weinshenker BG. Atypical inflammatory demyelinating syndromes of the CNS. Lancet Neurol. 2016;15(9):967-81.
24. Capet N, Levraut M, Delourme A, Thomel-Rocchi O, Bourg V, Cabre P, et al. Marburg multiple sclerosis variant: complete remission with very early administration of mitoxantrone—a case report. Neurol Ther. 2021;11(1):507-13.
25. Nagaishi A, Fukudome T, Matsuya N, Masuda-Narita T, Iwano F, Misu T, et al. A long-term survival case of Marburg type multiple sclerosis successfully treated with mitoxantrone: a case report and review of literature. Neuroimmunol Rep. 2021;1:100044.
26. Koska V, Förster M, Brouzou K, Hatami M, Arat E, Aytulun A, et al. Case report: successful stabilization of Marburg variant multiple sclerosis with ocrelizumab following high-dose cyclophosphamide rescue. Front Neurol. 2021;12:696807.
27. Jeffery DR, Lefkowitz DS, Crittenden JP. Treatment of Marburg variant multiple sclerosis with mitoxantrone. J Neuroimaging. 2004;14(1):58-62.
28. Bitsch A, Wegener C, da Costa C, Bunkowski S, Reimers CD, Prange HW, et al. Lesion development in Marburg's type of acute multiple sclerosis: from inflammation to demyelination. Mult Scler Houndmills Basingstoke Engl. 1999;5(3):138-46.
29. Elenein RG, Sharer LR, Cook SD, Pachner AR, Michaels J, Hillen ME. A second case of Marburg's variant of multiple sclerosis with vasculitis and extensive demyelination. Mult Scler J. 2011;17(12):1531-8.
30. Suzuki M, Kawasaki H, Masaki K, Suzuki SO, Terada T, Tsuchida T, et al. An autopsy case of the Marburg variant of multiple sclerosis (acute multiple sclerosis). Intern Med. 2013;52(16):1825-32.

31. Capello E, Mancardi GL. Marburg type and Balò's concentric sclerosis: rare and acute variants of multiple sclerosis. Neurol Sci. 2004;25(Suppl 4):S361-3.
32. Avila-Ornelas J, Labat E, Alfonso G, Serrano C, Fiorito F. An extremely aggressive case of Marburg's disease treated with high dose cyclophosphamide. A case report. Mult Scler Relat Disord. 2019;31:51-3.
33. Sharrack B, Saccardi R, Alexander T, Badoglio M, Burman J, Farge D, et al. Autologous hematopoietic stem cell transplantation and other cellular therapy in multiple sclerosis and immune-mediated neurological diseases: updated guidelines and recommendations from the EBMT Autoimmune Diseases Working Party (ADWP) and the Joint Accreditation Committee of EBMT and ISCT (JACIE). Bone Marrow Transplant. 2020;55(2):283-306.
34. Gobbin F, Marangi A, Orlandi R, Richelli S, Turatti M, Calabrese M, et al. A case of acute fulminant multiple sclerosis treated with alemtuzumab. Mult Scler Relat Disord. 2017;17:9-11.
35. Kurul S, Çakmakçi H, Dirik E, Kovanlikaya A. Schilder's disease: case study with serial neuroimaging. J Child Neurol. 2003;18(1):58-61.
36. Poser CM, Goutières F, Carpentier MA, Aicardi J. Schilder's myelinoclastic diffuse sclerosis. Pediatrics. 1986;77(1):107-12.
37. Bacigaluppi S, Polonara G, Zavanone ML, Campanella R, Branca V, Gaini SM, et al. Schilder's disease: noninvasive diagnosis? Neurol Sci. 2009;30(5):421-30.
38. Rovira Á, Auger C, Rovira A. Other noninfectious inflammatory disorders. Handb Clin Neurol. 2016;135:425-46.
39. Loes DJ, Fatemi A, Melhem ER, Gupte N, Bezman L, Moser HW, et al. Analysis of MRI patterns aids prediction of progression in X-linked adrenoleukodystrophy. Neurology. 2003;61(3):369-74.
40. Pretorius ML, Loock DB, Ravenscroft A, Schoeman JF. Demyelinating disease of Schilder type in three young South African children: dramatic response to corticosteroids. J Child Neurol. 1998;13(5):197-201.
41. Kraus D, Konen O, Straussberg R. Schilder's disease: noninvasive diagnosis and successful treatment with human immunoglobulins. Eur J Paediatr Neurol. 2012;16(2):206-8.
42. Agarwal A, Pinho M, Raj K, Yu FF, Bathla G, Achilleos M, et al. Neurological emergencies associated with COVID-19: stroke and beyond. Emerg Radiol. 2020;27(6):747-54.
43. Netravathi M, Dhamija K, Gupta M, Tamborska A, Nalini A, Holla VV, et al. COVID-19 vaccine associated demyelination and its association with MOG antibody. Mult Scler Relat Disord. 2022;60:103739.
44. Garg RK, Malhotra HS, Kumar N, Pandey S, Patil MR, Uniyal R, et al. Tumefactive demyelinating brain lesion developing after administration of adenovector-based COVID-19 vaccine: a case report. Neurol India. 2022;70(1):409.
45. Wadhwa A, Chatterjee A, Chaudhry N, Laskar S, Chandan S. A case of relapsing-remitting tumefactive demyelination. Ann Indian Acad Neurol. 2019;22(1):124.
46. Jiménez Arango JA, Uribe Uribe CS, Toro González G. Lesser-known myelin-related disorders: focal tumor-like demyelinating lesions. Neurologia. 2015;30(2):97-105.
47. Cianfoni A, Niku S, Imbesi SG. Metabolite findings in tumefactive demyelinating lesions utilizing short echo time proton magnetic resonance spectroscopy. Am J Neuroradiol. 2007;28(2):272-7.
48. Takenaka S, Shinoda J, Asano Y, Aki T, Miwa K, Ito T, et al. Metabolic assessment of monofocal acute inflammatory demyelination using MR spectroscopy and (11)C-methionine-, (11)C-choline-, and (18)F-fluorodeoxyglucose-PET. Brain Tumor Pathol. 2011;28(3):229-38.
49. Seewann A, Enzinger C, Filippi M, Barkhof F, Rovira A, Gass A, et al. MRI characteristics of atypical idiopathic inflammatory demyelinating lesions of the brain. J Neurol. 2008;255(1):1-10.
50. Weinshenker BG, O'Brien PC, Petterson TM, Noseworthy JH, Lucchinetti CF, Dodick DW, et al. A randomized trial of plasma exchange in acute central nervous system inflammatory demyelinating disease. Ann Neurol. 1999;46(6):878-86.
51. Okada K, Hashimoto T, Kobata M, Kakeda S, Takahashi T, Hirato J. Tumefactive demyelination with a transient appearance of oligoclonal bands in MS under fingolimod. Neurol Neuroimmunol Neuroinflammation. 2018;5(5):e484.
52. Inshasi JS, Sarathchandran P, Thakre MC, Al Talai NS, Al Suwaidi R, Al Madani A. Oral cladribine is effective in the treatment of tumefactive demyelination in relapsing remitting multiple sclerosis: a case report. Open Neurol J. 2020;14(1).
53. Barry B, Erwin AA, Stevens J, Tornatore C. Fingolimod rebound: a review of the clinical experience and management considerations. Neurol Ther. 2019;8(2):241-50.
54. Patti F, Leone C, Zappia M. Clinical and radiologic rebound after discontinuation of natalizumab therapy in a highly active multiple sclerosis patient was not halted by dimethyl-fumarate: a case report. BMC Neurol. 2015;15(1):252.
55. Nagappa M, Taly AB, Sinha S, Bharath RD, Mahadevan A, Bindu PS, et al. Tumefactive demyelination: clinical, imaging, and follow-up observations in thirty-nine patients. Acta Neurol Scand. 2013;128(1):39-47.
56. Fan X, Mahta A, De Jager PL, Kesari S. Rituximab for tumefactive inflammatory demyelination: a case report. Clin Neurol Neurosurg. 2012;114(10):1326-8.
57. Sempere AP, Feliu-Rey E, Sanchez-Perez R, Nieto-Navarro J. Rituximab for tumefactive demyelination refractory to corticosteroids and plasma exchange. J Neurol Neurosurg Psychiatry. 2013;84(12):1338-9.
58. Naser Moghadasi A. Tumefactive demyelinating lesions in a patient with multiple sclerosis developed two days after the injection of rituximab. Acta Neurol Taiwanica. 2020;29(4):124-7.
59. Tenembaum S, Chamoles N, Fejerman N. Acute disseminated encephalomyelitis: a long-term follow-up study of 84 pediatric patients. Neurology. 2002;59(8):1224-31.
60. Varadan B, Shankar A, Rajakumar A, Subramanian S, Sathya AC, Hakeem AR, et al. Acute hemorrhagic leukoencephalitis in a COVID-19 patient—a case report with literature review. Neuroradiology. 2021;63(5):653-61.
61. Manzano GS, McEntire CRS, Martinez-Lage M, Mateen FJ, Hutto SK. Acute disseminated encephalomyelitis and acute hemorrhagic leukoencephalitis following COVID-19: systematic review and meta-synthesis. Neurol Neuroimmunol Neuroinflamm. 2021;8(6):e1080.
62. Grzonka P, Scholz MC, De Marchis GM, Tisljar K, Rüegg S, Marsch S, et al. Acute hemorrhagic leukoencephalitis: a case and systematic review of the literature. Front Neurol. 2020;11:899.
63. Kao HW, Alexandru D, Kim R, Yanni D, Hasso AN. Value of susceptibility-weighted imaging in acute hemorrhagic leukoencephalitis. J Clin Neurosci. 2012;19(12):1740-1.
64. Abou Zeid NE, Burns JD, Wijdicks EFM, Giannini C, Keegan BM. Atypical acute hemorrhagic leukoencephalitis (Hurst's disease) presenting with focal hemorrhagic brainstem lesion. Neurocrit Care. 2010;12(1):95-7.
65. Solis WG, Waller SE, Harris AK, Sugo E, Hansen MA, Lechner-Scott J. Favorable outcome in a 33-year-old female with acute hemorrhagic leukoencephalitis. Case Rep Neurol. 2017;9(1):106-13.
66. Payne ET, Rutka JT, Ho TK, Halliday WC, Banwell BL. Treatment leading to dramatic recovery in acute hemorrhagic leukoencephalitis. J Child Neurol. 2007;22(1):109-13.
67. Markus R, Brew BJ, Turner J, Pell M. Successful outcome with aggressive treatment of acute hemorrhagic leukoencephalitis. J Neurol Neurosurg Psychiatry. 1997;63(4):551-2.
68. Martins HM, Teixeira-Jr AL, Lana-Peixoto MA. Acute hemorrhagic leukoencephalitis mimicking herpes simplex encephalitis: case report. Arq Neuropsiquiatr. 2004;62:139-43.

70

CHAPTER

Autoimmune Encephalitis

Jino Vincent, Bijoy Jose, Sudheeran Kannoth, Anandkumar Anandakuttan

INTRODUCTION

Autoimmune encephalitis (AE) is one of the most common forms of encephalitis in current practice. It can be defined as encephalitis caused by inflammation secondary to an autoimmune response to the brain. The classical phenotype of AE, limbic encephalitis (LE) was reported by Corsellis in 1968. The nonparaneoplastic form was described by Lord Brain in 1966 as Hashimoto's encephalitis. Though initially considered rare, with increasing awareness among neurophysicians and the community, with the availability of modern diagnostic facilities like magnetic resonance imaging (MRI) of the brain and neuroimmunology laboratory services, this has emerged as one of the most common forms of encephalitis across the globe. The prevalence of AE is 13.7/100,000, which is not significantly different from that of all infectious encephalitis (11.6/100,00), including the viral subcategory (8.3/100,000). The incidence rates of AE and infectious encephalitis are 0.8/100,000 and 1.0/100,000 person-years respectively.

CLASSIFICATION

Based on the etiology, structures involved and antibody types, AE is classified as shown in **Table 1**.

Paraneoplastic AE can precede or follow a malignancy. It represents an immune reaction against cancer tissue which is cross-reacting with the nervous system. The non-paraneoplastic can be further subclassified as postinfectious, iatrogenic, and idiopathic. There are cases of AE fulfilling the diagnostic criteria, but in which no antibodies are identified. These are called seronegative AE. Many autoimmune illnesses are thought to be postinfectious. Acute disseminated encephalomyelitis (ADEM) is the classical postinfectious AE. Following the coronavirus disease (COVID) pandemic, more cases of postinfectious AE are being reported. Iatrogenic AE is a relatively new consideration. Chemotherapeutic drugs known as immune checkpoint inhibitors (ICIs) are suspected to cause this.

TABLE 1: Classification of autoimmune encephalitis.

Etiology	Structures involved	Type of antibody detected
• Paraneoplastic • Postinfectious • Iatrogenic • Idiopathic	• Limbic encephalitis • Cortical/subcortical • Diencephalon • Basal ganglia/striatal • Rhombencephalon • Brainstem • Cerebellar • Encephalomyelitis • Meningoencephalitis • Combined	• Neuronal cell surface antibodies • Antibodies against intracellular targets • Seronegative in the absence of antibodies

Many named antibodies are frequently associated with AE. Antibodies, on the other hand, are not always the cause of disease in T cell-mediated diseases which typically underlie paraneoplastic encephalitis. Contrary to this, AE is mostly an antibody-mediated autoimmune reaction and the antibodies are located on the neuronal surface. For example, the leucine-rich glioma inactivated 1 (LGI1) antibody attaches to the target molecule and activates complement, causing tissue death. There is no complement activation or tissue death in, for instance, the anti-N-methyl-D-aspartate (NMDA) receptor encephalitis, but rather, there occurs an internalization of the receptors. In cases of seronegative AE, no particular antibodies have been discovered. The etiology in this group could be mediated by T cells or undiscovered antibodies.

Age and Sex Distribution

As with many autoimmune disorders, women are more likely to be affected than men (up to 65%). However, incidence and prevalence rates among men are on the rise and the sex difference is becoming less distinct. AE has been reported in patients as young as 2 months of life to over the ninth decade. Some AE, e.g., anti-NMDAR and anti-gamma-aminobutyric acid receptor (GABAR) are more common in younger age groups, usually presenting with movement disorders and/or seizures. Over the age of 70 years, presentation with seizures may prompt consideration of AMPA (amino-3-hydroxy-5-methyl-4-isoxazolepropionic acid) and voltage-gated potassium channel (VGKC) AE. AE does not appear to have hereditary underpinnings. Some studies suggest that incidence, as especially of glutamic acid decarboxylase 65 (GAD65) antibody encephalitis may be substantially higher among black individuals.

CLINICAL FEATURES

The range of clinical manifestations in AE is rather extremely wide, from altered sensorium to deep coma, focal/generalized seizures to status epilepticus (or epilepsia partialis continua). Behavioral symptoms are common and might lead to diagnostic consideration of psychiatric disorders. Abnormal conduct, psychosis, anxiety, depression, automatism, hallucinations, and delusions are examples of behavioral symptoms. The location and intensity of the inflammation often determine the symptoms. It is not uncommon for the speech and language to be involved. In anti-NMDAR encephalitis, echolalia, mutism and other motor language impairments are frequent. Memory loss and personality shifts are also common. Dementia-like symptoms, mimicking frontotemporal, or Alzheimer's dementia, or even Creutzfeldt–Jakob disease (CJD) have been commonly described. Movement disorders such as myoclonus, chorea, athetosis, tremors, oculogyric crisis, and orofacial dyskinesia may be present. Other symptoms associated with AE include parkinsonism and cerebellar ataxia. Symptoms and signs of autonomic dysfunction are also described and can include bradycardia, tachycardia, cardiac conduction block, diarrhea, constipation, piloerection, bladder dysfunction, erectile dysfunction, paroxysmal sweating, tachycardia, and fluctuating blood pressure **(Tables 2 to 4)**.

TABLE 2: List of antibodies and syndromes.

Name of antibody	Location	Clinical syndrome	Associations
ANNA1 (antineuronal nuclear autoantibody-1/anti-Hu)	Antibodies against intracellular antigens	LE, encephalomyelopathy, subacute sensory neuronopathy	Small-cell lung carcinoma (SCLC)
ANNA-2 (antineuronal nuclear autoantibody-2/anti-Ri)	Antibodies against intracellular antigens	Cerebellar degeneration, opsoclonus, brainstem encephalitis	Breast and gynecological malignancy
ANNA-3 (antineuronal nuclear autoantibody-3)	Antibodies against intracellular antigens	Cerebellar degeneration	SCLC
AGNA-1 (anti-glial nuclear antibody-1/SOX-1)	Antibodies against intracellular antigens	LEMS, cerebellar degeneration, sensory neuronopathy, LE	SCLC
Anti Tr/DNER (delta/notch-like epidermal growth factor-related protein)	Antibodies against intracellular antigens	Cerebellar degeneration, LE	Hodgkin's lymphoma
Anti-amphiphysin	Antibodies against intracellular antigens	Stiff-person syndrome, encephalomyelitis	Breast, SCLC
Anti CRMP5 (collapsin response mediator protein 5)/anti-CV2	Antibodies against intracellular antigens	Encephalomyelitis, chorea, optic nerve, uveitis, peripheral neuropathy	SCLC, thymoma
Anti-Ma2/Ta	Antibodies against intracellular antigens	Excessive daytime sleepiness, vertical ophthalmoparesis, or both associated with LE	Testicular malignancy
Anti-LGI1 (anti-leucine-rich glioma inactivated 1)	Antibodies against ion channels and other cell-surface proteins	Limbic encephalitis, fasciobrachial dystonic seizures	>90% with HLA-DRB1*07:01; hyponatremia common
Anti-CASPR2 (anti-contactin-associated protein-like 2)	Antibodies against ion channels and other cell-surface proteins	Morvan's syndrome or limbic encephalitis	Thymoma (20%)
Anti-NMDAR (anti-N-methyl D-aspartate receptor)	Antibodies against cell surface and synaptic receptors	Anti-NMDA receptor encephalitis	Ovarian teratoma in 60% of adult females
Anti-GlyR (anti-glycine receptor)	Antibodies against cell surface and synaptic receptors	Stiff-person spectrum disorder PERM (progressive encephalopathy with rigidity and myoclonus), limbic encephalitis	Thymoma, lung cancer
Anti-VGCC (anti-voltage-gated calcium channel)	Antibodies against cell surface and synaptic receptors	LEMS, cerebellar degeneration, LE	SCLC
Alpha-3 ganglionic acetylcholine receptor antibody	Antibodies against cell surface and synaptic receptors	Autonomic ganglionopathy, LE	SCLC

Continued

Continued

Name of antibody	Location	Clinical syndrome	Associations
Anti-AMPAR (anti-amino-3-hydroxy-5-methyl-4-isoxazolepropionic acid receptor)	Antibodies against cell surface and synaptic receptors	Limbic encephalitis, subacute psychiatric symptoms	SCLC, thymoma, breast
Anti-GABA-A (anti-gamma aminobutyric acid-A)	Antibodies against synaptic receptors	Encephalitis with prominent seizures and status epilepticus	Thymoma
Anti-GABA-B (anti-gamma aminobutyric acid-B)	Antibodies against synaptic receptors	Limbic encephalitis, seizures	SCLC, neuroendocrine
Anti-DPPX-6 (antibodies against dipeptidyl peptidase-like protein 6)	Antibodies against ion channels and other cell-surface proteins	Encephalitis, myoclonus, hyperekplexia	Diarrhea, cachexia
Anti-IgLON5	Antibodies against cell surface	Sleep disorder (REM and NREM parasomnias, sleep apnea), bulbar syndrome, progressive supranuclear, palsy-like syndrome, cognitive syndrome ± chorea	Strong association with the HLA-DRB1*10:01 allele
Anti-mGluR1 (anti-metabotropic glutamate receptor 1)	Antibodies against synaptic receptors	Cerebellar degeneration, encephalitis	Hematologic malignancy and one patient had a concurrent cutaneous T-cell lymphoma
Anti-mGluR5 (anti-metabotropic glutamate receptor 5)	Antibodies against synaptic receptors	Limbic encephalitis, often including movement disorders, sleep dysfunction, and seizures	Hodgkin's lymphoma (Ophelia syndrome) or SCLC
Anti-GFAP (anti-glial fibrillary acidic protein)	Intermediate protein uniquely found in astrocytes in the CNS, nonmyelinating Schwann cells in the PNS and enteric glial cells	Autoimmune meningoencephalitis or encephalitis, with or without myelitis, optic disc edema and optic papillitis	One-third of the patients had a past or current systemic tumor
Anti-GAD65 (anti-glutamic acid decarboxylase 65)	Antibodies against intracellular antigens	Stiff-person, cerebellar syndrome, limbic encephalitis	Thymoma

(CNS: central nervous system; HLA: human leukocyte antigen; LE: limbic encephalitis; LEMS: Lambert–Eaton myasthenic syndrome; NMDA: N-methyl-D-aspartate; NREM: nonrapid eye movement; PNS: peripheral nervous system; REM: rapid eye movement)

TABLE 3: Clinical presentations with associated antibodies in autoimmune encephalitis (AE).

Neuropsychiatric	Anti-NMDAR, Anti-AMPAR, CASPR2, Anti-CRMP5, Anti-GABA$_A$R, GAD65, ANNA1, Anti-LGI1, Anti-Ma1/2, MOG, AGNA1
Cognitive disorder	Anti-GABA$_B$R, Anti-AMPAR, IgLON5, CASPR2, Anti-NMDAR, LGI1, GAD65, ANNA1, Anti-CRMP5, Ma2, Anti-amphiphysin, Zic-4, ANNA2
Movement disorder	Anti-NMDAR (complex—chorea, stereotypies and dystonia, tremor), anti-DPPX (myoclonus, tremors, hyperekplexia), anti-GlyR (myoclonus, hyperekplexia), IgLON5 (chorea), anti-LGI1 (chorea), anti-CRMP5 (chorea), ANNA1 (chorea), anti-GFAP (dyskinesia)
Tremors	Anti-AMPAR, CASPR2, anti-LGI1, anti-DPPX, anti-GABA$_B$R, anti-GlyR, anti-mGluR1, anti-NMDAR, anti-GFAP
Autonomic dysfunction	Anti-NMDAR, ANNA1, anti-CRMP5, anti-VGCC, anti-GFAP
Central apnea	Anti-NMDAR
Focal seizures	Anti-LGI1 (faciobrachial dystonic seizures, piloerection, paroxysmal dizziness spells), CASPR2
Seizures	Anti-GABA$_A$R/GABA$_B$R (status epilepticus), anti-AMPAR, anti-NMDAR, anti-GlyR (status epilepticus), GAD65, MOG
Peripheral nerve hyperexcitability	CASPR2 (neuromyotonia, fasciculations, cramps and myokymia)
Morvan's syndrome	CASPR2
Diarrhea/weight loss	Anti-DPPX
Stiff person	Anti-GlyR, anti-amphiphysin, GAD65, anti-GABA$_B$R (PERMS)
Optic neuritis	MOG, anti-CRMP5, NMO, anti-GFAP
Myelitis	MOG, NMO, anti-GFAP, anti-amphiphysin, ANNA1, anti-CRMP5

Continued

Continued

Sleep disorder	IgLON5 (parasomnias, sleep apnea), CASPR2, anti-LGI1, NMO, MOG, anti-NMDAR, anti-Ma2, anti-mGluR5
Atypical parkinsonism	IgLON5 (PSP), ANNA2, anti-LGI1, anti-AMPAR, CASPR2, anti-GlyR, anti-Ma2, anti-CRMP5, anti-DPPX
Gait disturbance	CASPR2 (episodic/persistent ataxia), IgLON5 (axial rigidity and gait freezing), anti-CRMP5 (cerebellar ataxia), GAD65 (cerebellar ataxia), anti-GABA$_B$R (ataxia), anti-VGCC, AGNA1, anti-mGluR1 (ataxia)
Rhombencephalitis	Anti-GlyR, NMO, MOG, anti-Ma2, anti-GQ1b, KLHL11, antineurochondrin, ANNA2, Zic-4, ANNA1
Stridor	IgLON5, ANNA2, anti-GlyR
Pain	CASPR2, anti-LGI1, anti-Gly R (allodynia, dysaesthesia and prominent pruritus)
Encephalomyelitis	ANNA1, anti-CRMP5, anti-GlyR, antiamphiphysin, anti-Ma2, ANNA 3, anti-PCA2, MOG, anti-GFAP
Cerebellar encephalitis	ANNA2, ANNA1, GAD65, anti-Ma1/2, AGNA, anti-VGCC, anti-CRMP5, Zic-4, anti-mGluR1, ANNA3, anti-PCA2, anti-GFAP
Hyponatremia	Anti-LGI1 (SIADH)
Uveitis	Anti-CRMP5
Opsoclonus myoclonus	ANNA2, anti-GABA$_B$R, ANNA1, anti-NMDAR, anti-GlyR
Type 1 diabetes mellitus	GAD65
LEMS	Anti-VGCC, anti-CRMP5, AGNA, anti-PCA2
Sensory neuronopathy	ANNA1, anti-CRMP5, antiamphiphysin, ANNA 3
Neuropathy	Antiamphiphysin, anti-VGCC, anti-CRMP5, anti-GFAP, anti-AMPAR, IgLON5

(AGNA1: antiglial nuclear antibody-1; AMPAR: amino-3-hydroxy-5-methyl-4-isoxazolepropionic acid receptor; ANNA: antineuronal nuclear autoantibody; CASPR2: contactin-associated protein-like 2; CRMP5: collapsin response mediator protein 5; DPPX: dipeptidyl peptidase-like protein-6; GABA$_A$R: gamma-aminobutyric acid type A receptor; GAD65: glutamic acid decarboxylase 65; GFAP: glial fibrillary acidic protein; GQ1b: ganglioside antibody; GlyR: glycine receptor; KLHL11: Kelch-like protein 11; LGI1: leucine-rich glioma inactivated 1; mGluR: metabotropic glutamate receptor; MOG: myelin oligodendrocyte glycoprotein; NMDAR: N-methyl-D-aspartate receptor; NMO: neuromyelitis optica; PCA-2: Purkinje cell antibody-2; PERMS: progressive encephalopathy with rigidity and myoclonus syndrome; SIADH: syndrome of inappropriate antidiuretic hormone; VGCC: voltage-gated calcium channel; Zic-4: zinc-finger protein 4)

TABLE 4: Anatomical involvement and associated antibody.

Anatomical location	Associated antibody
Cortical–limbic	ANNA1, GAD65, anti-GABA$_B$R, anti-AMPAR, anti-LGI1, anti-VGCC
Cortical–extra limbic	Anti-NMDAR, anti-VGCC, anti GABA$_A$R
Subcortical–basal ganglia	Anti-CRMP5, anti-NMDAR, anti-D2
Cerebellum	ANNA1, GAD65, anti-VGCC
Brainstem and spinal cord	Anti-Ma, ANNA2, ANNA1, anti-GlyR, GAD65, anti-CRMP5

(AMPAR: amino-3-hydroxy-5-methyl-4-isoxazolepropionic acid receptor; ANNA: antineuronal nuclear autoantibody; CRMP5: collapsin response mediator protein 5; D2: dopamine receptor 2; GABA$_B$R: gamma-aminobutyric acid type B receptor; GAD65: glutamic acid decarboxylase 65; GlyR: glycine receptor; LGI1: leucine-rich glioma inactivated 1; NMDAR: N-methyl-D-aspartate receptor; VGCC: voltage-gated calcium channel)

Diagnosis

A definite diagnosis of AE is only possible by a histopathological examination of the brain tissue, which will demonstrate immune-mediated tissue damage after ruling out other causes. But in actual clinical practice, it is difficult to obtain brain biopsies. In 2016, the diagnostic criteria were proposed by Graus et al. **(Box 1)**.

CLINICAL INSTRUMENTS AND SCALES

Several structured scales have now been proposed and validated to aid diagnosis and assess severity of AE. These include:

- *CASE score (Clinical Assessment Scale for Autoimmune Encephalitis)*: Specific score to assess severity of AE.
- *APE2 score (Antibody Prevalence in Epilepsy and Encephalopathy score)*: To predict seropositivity of neural-specific antibodies and favorable response to an immunotherapy trial among patients with epilepsy; score of ≥4 is a predictor of neuronal antibody positivity (98% sensitivity, 84% specificity).
- NAAs confidence scale (Neuronal Autoantibody confidence scale): The antibody detected is clinically relevant if score ≥2, with an odds ratio of 50.3 [confidence interval (CI) 8.2–309.9, $p < 0.0001$].

APPROACH TO DIAGNOSIS OF AUTOIMMUNE ENCEPHALITIS

Diagnosis of autoimmune encephalitis is possible only with a high level of clinical suspicion. One of the dictums in the diagnosis of AE is that age is no bar. It has been reported from 2.5 months of age to the ninth decade. The long-held adage that autoimmune illnesses does not usually occur in men and old age is now rescinded. Unlike the standard depiction of young females in systemic autoimmunity, male and elderly AEs have now been documented with anti-LGI1, contactin-associated protein-like 2 (CASPR2), anti-dipeptidyl peptidase-like protein-6 (anti-DPPX), and antineuronal nuclear autoantibody-1 (ANNA1) antibodies. History or family history of autoimmunity is an important clue that makes the possibility of AE stronger. One of the

BOX 1 Diagnostic criteria for autoimmune encephalitis.

Diagnostic criteria for possible autoimmune encephalitis

All three of the following:

1. Subacute onset (<3 months) of working memory deficits, altered mental status, or psychiatric symptoms
2. At least one of the following:
   a. New focal CNS findings
   b. Seizures (new onset)
   c. CSF pleocytosis (>5/mm^3)
   d. MRI features suggestive of encephalitis
3. Reasonable exclusion of alternative causes:
   Exclusion of the following:
   a. CNS infection, septic encephalopathy, metabolic encephalopathy
   b. Drug toxicity: Seizures, PRES, serotoninergic syndrome, NMS, drug withdrawal
   c. Cerebrovascular disease, neoplastic disorders, CJD, epileptic disorders
   d. Rheumatologic disorders (lupus, sarcoidosis, others)
   e. Reye's syndrome and mitochondrial diseases, inborn errors of metabolism (children)

Diagnostic criteria for definite autoimmune limbic encephalitis

All four of the following criteria:

1. Subacute onset (<3 months) of working memory deficits, seizures or psychiatric symptoms
2. Bilateral MRI abnormalities restricted to medial temporal lobes
3. At least one of the following:
   a. CSF pleocytosis (>5/mm^3)
   b. EEG with epileptic or slow wave activity in temporal lobes
4. Reasonable exclusion of alternative causes:
   a. Lupus, Sjögren's, Kikuchi, Behçet, glioma, herpes, syphilis, Whipple
   b. If one of the first three criteria is not met, diagnosis of definite LE can be made only by the detection of antibodies against cell surface, synaptic, or onconeural protein

Diagnostic criteria for autoantibody negative probable AE

Diagnosis can be made when all four of the following criteria have been met:

1. Rapid progression (<3 months) of working memory deficits (short-term memory loss), altered mental status, or psychiatric symptoms
2. Exclusion of well-defined syndromes of autoimmune encephalitis (Bickerstaff's, typical LE, ADEM)
3. Absence of well-characterized autoantibodies in serum and CSF, and at least two of the following:
   a. MRI abnormalities suggestive of AE (excluding some mitochondrial or metabolic causes with symmetrical patterns)
   b. CSF pleocytosis, OCB or elevated CSF IgG index, or both
   c. Brain biopsy showing inflammatory infiltrates and excluding other disorders (e.g., tumor)
4. Reasonable exclusion of alternative causes

(ADEM: acute disseminated encephalomyelitis; AE: autoimmune encephalitis; CJD: Creutzfeldt–Jakob disease; CNS: central nervous system; CSF: cerebrospinal fluid; EEG: electroencephalogram; IgG: immunoglobulin G; LE: limbic encephalitis; MRI: magnetic resonance imaging; NMS: neuroleptic malignant syndrome; OCB: oligoclonal band; PRES: posterior reversible encephalopathy syndrome)

Source: Graus F, Titulaer MJ, Balu R, Benseler S, Bien CG, Cellucci T, et al. A clinical approach to diagnosis of autoimmune encephalitis. Lancet Neurol. 2016;15(4):391-404.

most common associations among patients with AE is hypothyroidism. In cases with suspected AE, a history of cancer, either personal or familial, and smoking should be obtained. Physical examination may reveal signs of autoimmunity like vitiligo, arthritis, lichen planus, evidence of thyroid dysfunction, rashes, orogenital ulcers, cachexia, and hyperpigmentation. On laboratory testing, elevated erythrocyte sedimentation rate (ESR), hyponatremia, raised serum globulins, and the presence of other autoimmune markers, such as rheumatoid factor, antinuclear antibody (ANA), and thyroid antibodies, and cancer markers all point to underlying autoimmunity. Inflammatory cerebrospinal fluid (CSF) is a crucial finding in a case of suspected AE. Another significant predictor of AE is mildly elevated protein without pleocytosis. The presence of oligoclonal bands (OCBs) in the CSF as well as an elevated immunoglobulin G (IgG) index should be sought. Findings on the electroencephalogram (EEG), like extreme delta brushes, are also indicative of a diagnosis of AE.

In many instances, especially early in the course of the disease, no imaging abnormalities can be found. The most sensitive imaging modality is MRI with contrast, and positive results can be found in more than half of the cases. The mesial temporal lobes and limbic systems are the most common sites of involvement, with cortical thickness and high T2/fluid-attenuated inversion recovery (FLAIR) signal intensity in these regions. The most prevalent type of involvement is bilateral (60%), whilst asymmetric. The lateral temporal lobe and insula are usually unaffected; however, the basal ganglia can be involved, which helps distinguish it from herpes simplex virus (HSV) encephalitis, which typically spares the basal ganglia **(Flowchart 1)**.

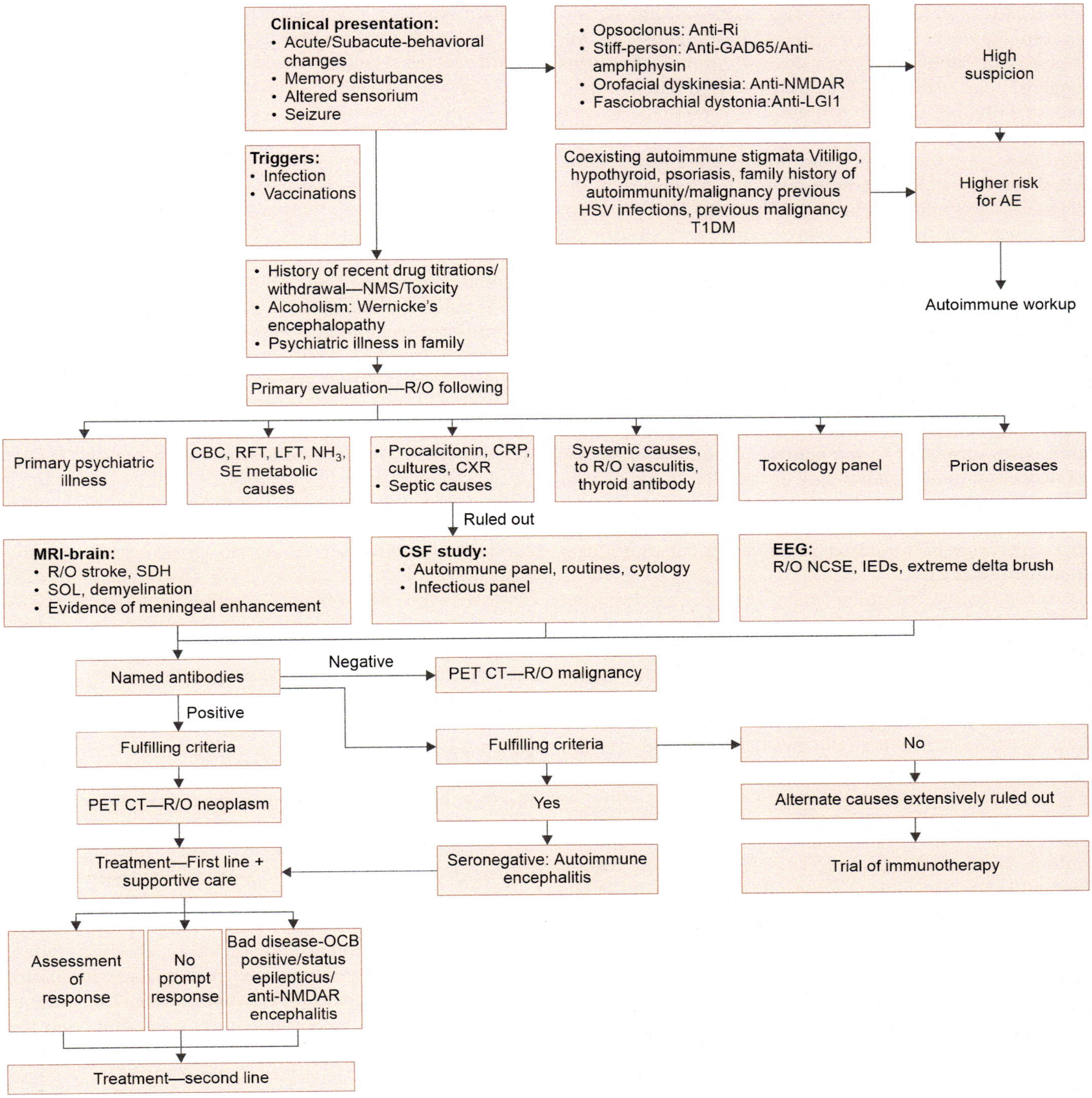

FLOWCHART 1: Algorithm for diagnosis and treatment of autoimmune encephalitis.

(AE: autoimmune encephalitis; CBC: complete blood count; CRP: C-reactive protein; CSF: cerebrospinal fluid; CT: computed tomography; CXR: chest X-ray; EEG: electroencephalogram; GAD65: glutamic acid decarboxylase 65; HSV: herpes simplex virus; IEDs: interictal epileptiform discharges; LFT: liver function test; LGI1: leucine-rich glioma inactivated 1; MRI: magnetic resonance imaging; NCSE: nonconvulsive status epilepticus; NH_3: ammonia; NMDAR: N-methyl D-aspartate receptor; NMS: neuroleptic malignant syndrome; PET: positron emission tomography; RFT: renal function test; R/O: rule out; SDH: sub-dural hematoma; SE: serum electrolytes; SOL: space occupying lesion; T1DM: type 1 diabetes mellitus)

NEUROIMMUNOLOGY LABORATORY EVALUATION

Laboratory evaluation is crucial to the diagnosis of AE. In an epidemiological study from France, 23% of cases were seronegative, which indicates the major role for neuroimmunology laboratory testing in the diagnosis of AE. In the right clinical setting, a positive antibody confirms diagnosis, e.g., in the case of a positive CSF NMDA antibody, even if only one domain symptom is present, a definite diagnosis of anti-NMDA receptor encephalitis can be made. However, absence of such antibodies does not exclude the diagnosis. Paired sample testing is preferred as the diagnosis can sometimes be missed by testing CSF or serum alone. Instead of testing for a single antibody, testing for an entire panel of antibodies is recommended as the clinical features associated with different antibodies may overlap. For example, an encephalomyelitis presentation may be ANNA1-associated as well as anti-amphiphysin-associated AE. LE can be associated with voltage-gated calcium channel (VGCC) antibodies as well as VGKC antibody-like LGI1 or CASPR2. Antibody testing should not, however, replace clinical judgment. Sometimes, testing may reveal antibodies unrelated to the clinical presentation. Hence, all neuroimmunology laboratory test results should only be interpreted in context of the clinical presentation. Testing should be performed with samples before immunotherapy as results may be rendered negative after institution of treatment **(Box 2)**.

Seronegative samples may contain unclassified antibodies. These are newer antibodies that have not yet been elucidated, named, or characterized. Only research labs supervised by competent autoimmune neurologists may recognize and report them. Since all the AEs are not always accompanied by antibodies, such cases are classified as seronegative if they fulfil the seronegative AE criteria and the patient has to be treated with immunosuppression.

Type of Testing

Indirect immunofluorescence (IIF) is the routine testing technique used in neuroimmunology laboratories. Other techniques used are western blot, dot blot, enzyme-linked immunosorbent assay (ELISA), radioimmunoassay (RIA), and electrophoresis. Immunofluorescence is a screening test for many antibodies and is usually confirmed with techniques such as western blot or dot blot. For paraneoplastic antibodies, testing with IIF on tissue followed by western blot or dot blot is the recommended method. For cell surface antibodies, testing with immunofluorescence on transfected cells (cell-based assays) is preferred. RIA or ELISA is used for testing ion channel antibodies.

BOX 2 **Pitfalls in laboratory testing for autoimmune encephalitis.**

- Testing after initiation of immunotherapy can result in false-negative results
- Testing after intravenous immunoglobulin administration may result in false positive results
- Testing unpaired sample, i.e., serum or CSF alone can result in false negative results
- Testing for a single antibody instead of a panel of antibodies can result in false-negative results

(CSF: cerebrospinal fluid)

IMAGING

Many people with AE have normal MRIs. T2 prolongation in many affected brain regions is the most common abnormality. T1 prolongation (LGI1 antibody) and diffusion restriction [LGI1 and glial fibrillary acidic protein (GFAP) antibody] are two other abnormalities. T2 and FLAIR abnormalities, diencephalic T2 hyperintensities in Ma/Ta antibody encephalitis, linear periventricular hyperintensities in GFAP antibody-associated AE, and basal ganglia abnormalities are seen in collapsing response mediator protein 5 (CRMP5) antibody-associated AE and anti-dopamine receptor 2 (D2) antibody AE. Fluorodeoxyglucose positron emission tomography (FDG-PET) scans are used to diagnose AE and to screen for a primary tumor/malignancy in individuals with suspected paraneoplastic encephalitis. Aside from this, the presence of another autoimmune/inflammatory illness elsewhere in the body may indicate a diagnosis of AE. Thyroiditis or arthritis disclosed on whole-body PET-computed tomography (CT), for example, will provide insight into the autoimmune etiology of encephalitis. In FDG-PET-CT of the brain, the most common brain abnormalities are hypermetabolism or hypometabolism in different regions.

ELECTROENCEPHALOGRAM

Electroencephalogram is frequently abnormal in AE. Low background activity is the most common abnormality. EEG suppression, which comprises dampened rapid activity as well as decreased continuity, is generally classified as an acute-stage EEG abnormality. In anti-NMDAR encephalitis, delta brush is seen and alpha-beta rhythms are initially suppressed. This is followed by the disappearance of theta rhythms, leaving only delta waves in the most extreme cases. There are certain signature EEG abnormalities like extreme delta brush named so because of its resemblance to the neonatal EEG pattern known as delta brush.

Two distinct EEG patterns characterize LGI1 encephalitis. The first pattern is frequent subclinical temporal lobe seizures in the absence of interictal epileptiform discharges, while the second is lateralized frontal lobe "direct current (DC) shift" or infraslow activity and associated electrodecremental response. The lateralized infraslow activity serves as an easily identifiable EEG marker of contralateral motor spasms clinically described as faciobrachial dystonic seizures (FBDSs). Hyperventilation-induced focal temporal lobe seizures have also been identified as characteristic of anti-LGI1 encephalitis.[1]

CEREBROSPINAL FLUID EXAMINATION

In many situations, CSF can be normal, but this should not preclude the clinician from suspecting AE. The most common abnormality is an increase in protein without pleocytosis. Even a small increase in protein is significant. In a smaller number of cases, higher concentrations, i.e., >100 mg/dL have been documented. Pleocytosis, elevated proteins, normal or low glucose [e.g., in neuromyelitis optica spectrum disorder (NMOSD), anti-GFAP-related AE], raised IgG index, IgG synthesis rate, and the presence of distinct OCBs are all possible findings. Inflammatory CSF is more often found in anti-NMDAR, anti-$GABA_B$, anti-DPPX, and anti-AMPAR AEs. Anti-LGI1, CASPR2, anti-$GABA_AR$, and glycine receptor antibodies are more frequently related to noninflammatory CSF. Pleocytosis is seen in 50% or more cases of anti-NMDAR, anti-$GABA_A$, anti-DPPX, and anti-AMPAR AE. Though the median cell count in CSF is generally low, counts as high as 950/μL have been reported. Unique OCB is more often reported with anti-GAD, anti-$GABA_BR$, and anti-NMDAR AE.[2]

AUTOIMMUNE ENCEPHALITIS VARIETIES

Limbic Encephalitis

Subacute onset memory impairment, confusion, psychiatric symptoms, and seizures are all indicators of LE. The subacute onset of short-term memory loss is thought to be the disorder's characteristic, yet it can be overlooked due to the presence of other symptoms **(Box 3)**.

BOX 3 Diagnostic criteria of limbic encephalitis.

All the four criteria must be met to make the diagnosis of definite limbic encephalitis:

1. Subacute onset (rapid progression of <3 months) of working memory deficits, seizures, or psychiatric symptoms suggesting involvement of the limbic system
2. Bilateral brain abnormalities on T2-weighted fluid-attenuated inversion recovery MRI highly restricted to the medial temporal lobes
3. At least one of the following:
   a. CSF pleocytosis (white blood cell count of >5 cells/mm^3)
   b. EEG with epileptic or slow-wave activity involving the temporal lobe
4. Exclusion of alternate diagnosis

(CSF: cerebrospinal fluid; EEG: electroencephalogram; MRI: magnetic resonance imaging)

Source: Graus F, Titulaer MJ, Balu R, Benseler S, Bien CG, Cellucci T, et al. A clinical approach to diagnosis of autoimmune encephalitis. Lancet Neurol. 2016;15(4):391-404.

Paraneoplastic Limbic Encephalitis

Limbic encephalitis is considered as a high-risk disorder for paraneoplastic syndrome though there are many cases of non-paraneoplastic syndromes and antibodies described in the last decade. It occurs in <1 in 10,000 patients. Paraneoplastic and nonparaneoplastic LE are clinically indistinguishable. Histopathology shows lymphocytic infiltration of intraparenchymal vessels. There is a T cell-dominant inflammation with neuronal loss and microglial activation. They present with subacute onset cognitive dysfunction, change in personality, seizures (both focal and generalized), irritability, hallucinations, limb weakness, disorientation, short-term amnesia, and altered sensorium. It is rare in children. Carcinoma of lung, breast, and testes are the common neoplasms involved. It precedes cancer in about 60% of the cases. MRI is abnormal in 57% of the cases and neuronal antibody is detected in 60% of the cases. EEG frequently shows sharp and slow waves. Treatment of the tumor is the most important step in the management. Patients with ANNA1 and anti-Ma2/Ta in serum have a poor prognosis. Antibody-negative paraneoplastic LE and anti-$GABA_BR$ positive patients tend to do better.[3,4]

Anti-NMDA Receptor Autoimmune Encephalitis

Antibodies against the NMDA NR-1 glutamate receptor cause this clinically distinct syndrome. Young females are disproportionately affected, with a sex ratio of 4:1. In the age groups of <12 years and >45 years, the female preponderance is less evident. It is linked to ovarian teratoma in women of reproductive age. Six categories of symptoms are present: psychiatric/behavioral symptoms, speech disorders, seizure, movement disorders, decreased state of consciousness, and autonomic dysfunction/central hypoventilation. Seizures and abnormal movements are the most common symptoms in young children. Orofacial dyskinesia, trunk and limb dyskinesia, motor automatism, and oculogyric crises are among the movement disorders. Hemiparesis and hemiataxia are uncommon monosymptomatic manifestations.

Patients with recurrent symptoms after herpes simplex encephalitis must have their CSF tested for the presence of NMDA receptor antibodies. The relapsing form of herpes simplex encephalitis is an autoimmune disorder that can be difficult to distinguish from full-blown anti-NMDA receptor encephalitis. It affects 20% of herpes simplex encephalitis patients and manifests as new-onset choreoathetosis in children or psychiatric symptoms in the elderly a few weeks or months after the viral infection **(Box 4)**.

Bickerstaff's Brainstem Encephalitis

It is characterized by subacute onset progressive ophthalmoplegia with altered consciousness and ataxia. By definition, the duration should be <4 weeks. Usually, post-infectious disease is associated with ganglioside (GQ1b) IgG antibodies. Bilaterally symmetrical ophthalmoplegia,

BOX 4 Diagnostic criteria of anti-NMDAR encephalitis.

Probable anti-NMDA receptor encephalitis

Diagnosis can be made when all three of the following criteria have been met:

1. Rapid-onset (<3 months) of at least four of the six following major groups of symptoms:
   a. Abnormal (psychiatric) behavior or cognitive dysfunction
   b. Speech dysfunction (pressured speech, verbal reduction, mutism)
   c. Seizures
   d. Movement disorder, dyskinesias, or rigidity/abnormal postures
   e. Decreased level of consciousness
   f. Autonomic dysfunction or central hypoventilation
2. At least one of the following laboratory study results:
   a. Abnormal EEG (focal or diffuse slow or disorganized activity, epileptic activity, or extreme delta brush)
   b. CSF with pleocytosis or oligoclonal bands
3. Reasonable exclusion of other disorders

Diagnosis can also be made in the presence of three of the above groups of symptoms accompanied by a systemic teratoma

Definite anti-NMDA receptor encephalitis

Diagnosis can be made in the presence of one or more of the six major groups of symptoms and IgG anti-GluN1 antibodies, after reasonable exclusion of other disorders

(EEG: electroencephalogram; IgG: immunoglobulin G; NMDA: N-methyl-D-aspartate)

Source: Graus F, Titulaer MJ, Balu R, Benseler S, Bien CG, Cellucci T, et al. A clinical approach to diagnosis of autoimmune encephalitis. Lancet Neurol. 2016;15(4):391-404.

pupillary involvement, bulbar palsy, facial palsy, limb weakness, and Babinski signs are common findings. This syndrome shares its spectrum with Miller Fisher syndrome. CSF pleocytosis occurs in 45% of the patients. Brain MRI is usually normal, but brain stem abnormalities on T2-weighted FLAIR imaging are present in 23% of patients. A definitive diagnosis of Bickerstaff's brain stem encephalitis requires demonstration of antibodies but in up to 32% of patients, it is not detectable. Measurement of these antibodies allows confirmation of the diagnosis in patients with incomplete syndromes or atypical symptoms, or when the altered mental status prevents the assessment of ataxia **(Box 5)**.

Anti-LGI1 and CASPR2 Antibody-related Autoimmune Encephalitis

Initially, these two antibodies were classified as voltage-gated potassium channel antibodies, but later their antigenic targets were discovered to be distinct. CASPR2 was first reported as Morvan syndrome, a syndrome of LE and peripheral nerve hyperexcitability, and LGI1 antibody as LE. The median age of onset of anti-LGI AE is 66 years, and range from 17 to 84 years, with a male predominance of 78%. CASPR2 AE has a median age of onset of 66 years with a range from 25 to 77 years, with male predominance as high as 89%. Peripheral nerve hyperexcitability, autonomic instability with profuse sweating, and sleeplessness with encephalopathy are all symptoms of the Morvan syndrome. The expanded spectrum of each of these antibodies was later described. Based on subsequent studies, faciobrachial dystonic seizure (FBDS) appears to be highly specific for anti-LGI1 AE. Both antibodies have an extended spectrum that includes limb encephalitis, dysautonomia, neuromyotonic peripheral nerve hyperexcitability, seizures (focal, piloerection, gelastic), ictal bradycardia, status epilepticus, memory impairment, movement disorders, and discomfort. Dementia-like and psychiatric manifestations are also well-documented. Brief dystonic posturing of the upper limb and face characterizes FBDS. It is thought to be on the borderline of seizure and dystonia. This is explained by the activation of a neuronal network encompassing bilateral frontal, bilateral basal ganglia, and bilateral temporal areas, primarily hippocampi and amygdala, cortical and subcortical structures. The contralateral basal ganglia reveal abnormalities on MRI and PET scans. Antiepileptics are ineffective against FBDS, however, immunosuppressants are effective. The most associated malignancy is thymoma.

BOX 5 Diagnostic criteria of Bickerstaff's encephalitis.

Probable diagnosis can be made when both of the following criteria have been met:

1. Subacute onset (rapid progression of <4 weeks) of all the following symptoms:
   a. Decreased level of consciousness
   b. Bilateral external ophthalmoplegia
   c. Ataxia
2. Reasonable exclusion of alternative causes

Definite Bickerstaff's brainstem encephalitis

The presence of positive IgG anti-GQ1b antibodies is definitive of diagnosis even if bilateral external ophthalmoplegia is not complete or ataxia cannot be assessed, or if recovery has occurred within 12 weeks after onset

(IgG: immunoglobulin G; GQ1b: ganglioside antibody)

Source: Graus F, Titulaer MJ, Balu R, Benseler S, Bien CG, Cellucci T, et al. A clinical approach to diagnosis of autoimmune encephalitis. Lancet Neurol. 2016;15(4):391-404.

Anti-GABA$_B$ Receptor Autoimmune Encephalitis

The common presenting symptoms are seizures, cognitive and behavioral symptoms. Men are more likely to be affected by anti-GABA$_B$R AE (62.8%). Cases involving children have also been documented. The most common presenting symptom is seizures (84%). The most common syndrome is LE, which is followed by rapidly progressing dementia and seizures. Seizures can be focal or generalized. Complex partial seizures and super refractory status are also common. Autonomic dysfunction, movement disorders, cerebellar ataxia, focal neurological deficits, and sleep disorders are less common. CSF pleocytosis is common—76% cases. Unilateral or bilateral temporal lobe hyperintensities in the MRI brain are seen in up to 54.8% of cases. EEG shows temporal lobe seizure, interictal epileptiform abnormalities, or focal temporal slowing in up to 57.6% of cases. Tumor was detected in up to 49.5% of cases, with small-cell carcinoma lung being the most common (91.3%) followed by thymoma, melanoma, carcinoid, and neuroendocrine tumors. Treatment response to immunotherapy or immunotherapy with cancer therapy yielded partial or complete remission in 86.3% of cases.[5]

Anti-AMPA Receptor Autoimmune Encephalitis

Confusion, cognitive impairment, LE, seizures, and psychiatric problems are among the symptoms of AMPAR antibody-mediated AE. Young people frequently experience psychiatric issues. LE affects more women than males. Focal weakness, dysautonomia, cerebellar ataxia, apraxia, upper motor neuron (UMN) signs, aphasia, involuntary movements, and sensory abnormalities are less prevalent symptoms. Mean age of onset is 53.1 years (range 14–92 years), while females account for 65.5% of cases. Neoplasms are found in 66.7% of the patients. The thymus and lung are the most prevalent related neoplasms, followed by breast and ovary. Psychiatric symptoms are linked to the existence of a tumor. In 86.2% of patients, an MRI of the brain can be abnormal. In 44.8% of instances, the EEG is abnormal, with most of the slowing being nonspecific. In 66.7% of cases, routine CSF tests yield abnormal results. The treatment response is excellent, with an 84% survival rate. In the long run, psychiatric presentation is associated with a poor prognosis.[6]

Anti-glycine Receptor Autoimmune Encephalitis

A progressive encephalopathy with rigidity and myoclonus (PERM) syndrome has been described. Apart from that, patients may also present with seizures. The age of presentation ranges from 1 to 75 years. The epilepsy group has a younger mean age than the PERM group (27.15 vs. 43.18 years). In the PERM group, men are more involved, while in the epilepsy group, women are more. Autoimmune disorders have been linked to 25% of the cases. The most typical presentation is subacute, but it can also be acute or chronic. Muscle spasms in the limbs, trunk, and neck, and also myoclonus associated with walking difficulties and falls, are the most common symptoms (69%). The second most prevalent symptom is excessive startle. Diplopia, nystagmus, ptosis, and slow/jerky eye movements affect 42% of people, whereas trismus and swallowing issues, facial numbness, and speech difficulty affect 40% of people. 13% can have seizures and 29% cognitive problems. Pyramidal signs, cerebellar ataxia, autonomic dysfunction, and laryngospasm, respiratory failure necessitating ventilation are among the other symptoms. In PERM, the MRI brain is usually normal. Malignancy is found in 16% of the patients. Thymoma, lymphoma, breast cancer, Hodgkin's disease, and small-cell carcinoma are the most frequent cancers. A good response to immunotherapy is seen in 46% of cases, whereas a partial response is seen in 38% of cases.[6]

Anti-DPPX Autoimmune Encephalitis

Central nervous system (CNS) hyperexcitability, cognitive impairment, and gastrointestinal (GI) problems are all signs of this illness. Myoclonus, tremor, seizures, and hyperekplexia are indications of CNS hyperexcitability. The median age of presentation is 52 years (13–76 years), with a male predominance of 69%. In 77% of cases, weight loss, diarrhea and significant GI symptoms are present. In 77% of patients, there are indications of CNS hyperexcitability. In 8% of cases, PERM is observed. In 92% of cases, cognitive decline, memory impairment, and changed mental status are present. In 67% of cases, the triad of prodromal weight loss/GI symptoms, cognitive dysfunction/altered mental status, and CNS hyperexcitability are seen. Up to 7.6% of the patients has a B-cell neoplasm such as mantle cell lymphoma, B-cell lymphoma, or B-cell chronic lymphocytic leukemia (CLL). The hippocampus, amygdala, cingulum, and tempero-occipital cortex has the most inflammatory infiltrate, with the pons, cerebellum, and medulla showing lesser involvement. 46% respond well to immunotherapy, 14% improve moderately, and death occurs in 17%. Relapse occurs in 23% of patients, primarily after treatment is stopped.[7]

Anti-GFAP Autoimmune Encephalitis

Subacute onset (<8 weeks) encephalopathy (57%), seizures (19%), psychiatric symptoms (29%), tremor (41%), headache (39%), and vomiting are all common clinical presentations of GFAP antibody-related meningoencephalitis Meningeal signs, sensory, and mild motor symptoms of myelopathy (24%) and visual blurring due to optic disc edema (32%), ataxia (29%), and irregular eye movement (16%) are also seen. Dementia, cranial neuropathy, peripheral neuropathy, dysautonomia and epilepsy are some of the other symptoms. The average age of presentation is 44 years (with a range of 8–103 years), with women accounting for 54% of cases. Inflammation of the meninges, brain, or spine, or both, is found in 81% of cases. In 54% of cases, perivascular MRI brain enhancement is evident, and in 66% of cases, gadolinium-enhancing lesions are seen. Punctate and cerebellar enhancement, serpentine enhancement, ependymal enhancement, and leptomeningeal enhancement are all common findings. Spine MRI shows longitudinally extensive lesions in 75% cases. Normal MRI is reported in 18% cases. Neoplasm is reported in 22% cases, CSF shows pleocytosis in 88% (with a median of 78/μL and range 13–550/μL). In 83% of patients, there is an increase in protein (median 80 mg/dL, range 44–205 mg/dL), and in 54% percent of cases, there are unique OCBs in the CSF. Histopathology demonstrates chronic inflammation with abundant microglia but no vasculitis. 21% percent of the patients have other autoimmune illnesses. Neoplasms are found in 34% of the cases, with 66% of them developing a tumor 2 years following the onset of neurological symptoms. The most prevalent tumor is ovarian teratoma, which is followed by adenocarcinoma, lymphoma, and glioma. Prodromal flu symptoms are reported in 29% of the cases. The most prevalent coexisting antibody is NMDA IgG, followed by aquaporin-4 (AQP4) IgG. Almost 87.5% cases respond well to corticosteroids.[8]

IgLON5 Autoimmune Encephalitis

Affects men and women equally. The median age of presentation is 62 years (45–79 years). 10% cases have associated autoimmune diseases. 11% have associated malignancy. CSF protein is elevated in 48.8% cases, pleocytosis in 24.4% cases, OCB in 10.3% cases, tau in 16.7% and phosphorylated tau in 28.6% cases in CSF; IGLON5 is detected in 100% of serum and 94.9% of CSF. Histopathology shows neuronal loss and hyperphosphorylated tau accumulation, which is maximum in the hypothalamus and tegmentum, reducing as moving towards the hippocampus, periaqueductal gray matter, medulla oblongata, and upper cervical cord. Substantia nigra, basal ganglia, thalamus, cortex, and cerebellum are unaffected or mildly affected, unlike primary tauopathies. A definite IgLON5 diagnosis can be made with the characteristic neuropathological finding with antibody detection in serum or CSF. A probable IGLON5 diagnosis can be made if neuropathological findings are present with a clinical history or correlation with human leukocyte antigen (HLA) (HLA-DRB1*1001 and HLA-DQB1*0501) with unknown antibody status, and possible when pathological findings are present without immunological or clinical information. Patients present with insidious onset progressive sleep and brainstem disorders initially. Neuropsychiatric disorders such as cognitive decline, memory deficit, and hallucinations, dysautonomia, urinary incontinence, urgency, constipation, anhidrosis, and hyperexcitability appear later. Hyperexcitability includes myoclonus, exaggerated startle, and cramps. Sleep disorders include rapid eye movement (REM) and non-rapid eye movement (NREM) parasomnia, sleep-disordered breathing with stridor, and obstructive sleep apnea (OSA). Polysomnography is abnormal in 95% of cases. Brainstem dysfunction includes dysarthria (38%), dysphagia (67%), oculomotor abnormalities (43%)—vertical and horizontal gaze palsy, nystagmus, ptosis, and hypermetric saccades, gait instability, movement disorders including chorea, parkinsonism, and dystonia. According to the predominant symptoms at presentation, the disease is classified as: (1) sleep disorder with parasomnias with sleep breathing disorder; (2) bulbar syndrome with dysphagia, sialorrhea, stridor or acute respiratory insufficiency; (3) progressive supranuclear palsy-like syndrome; (4) cognitive decline with or without chorea. MRI is abnormal in 19.3% of cases-predominantly brainstem atrophy and cerebellar atrophy Peripheral nervous system involvement with fasciculations, muscle cramps, and peripheral neuropathy is seen in 32% of the cases. Mortality is around 34%. Monoimmunotherapy showed a response in 31.8%, while combination therapy showed a response in 66.7%.[9]

GAD-associated Autoimmune Encephalitis

Glutamic acid decarboxylase 65 is required for the conversion of glutamic acid to GABA. GABA is the inhibitory neurotransmitter of the CNS. Hence, an imbalance is likely to be caused by these antibodies resulting in hyperexcitability of neurons. GAD65 antibodies target intracellular antigens. A wide spectrum of disorders is associated with GAD65 autoimmunity such as type 1 diabetes mellitus (T1DM), stiff-person syndrome, treatment-refractory epilepsy, cerebellar ataxia, and progressive encephalomyelitis with rigidity and myoclonus. LE presentation of GAD65 positive cases range from 1 to 70 years. The median age among pediatric cases was 10 years (range 1–17 years), and for adults, it was 39.5 (19–70 years). Adult cases are primarily young women (59%) while pediatric cases are largely males (57%). Systemic autoimmune disorders are found in 48% of cases (T1DM common). Cancer association is found in 10% of cases. Small-cell carcinoma and thymoma are frequent. Symptom at onset is seizure in 97% cases (upto 24% can be refractory status epilepticus). Epilepsia partialis continua is also reported in a few. Up to 59% cases can have memory impairment and impairment of other cognitive domains is seen in 40% of cases (impairment of orientation, execution, and language). Psychiatric symptoms are the third most common symptom, affecting 28% of patients (depression, behavior, and personality changes). Other rarer associated manifestations include myoclonus, facial cramps, stiff-person syndrome, cerebellar ataxia, hyperphagia, gaze-evoked nystagmus, and tinnitus. MRI brain is abnormal in 78% of the cases (temporal lobe in 59% cases, multifocal abnormalities in 16% cases). EEG shows epileptiform abnormalities in 77% of the cases—temporal lobe in 70%, multifocal in 22%, and generalized in 7% cases. CSF shows pleocytosis in 27% of cases (7–114 cells/mm^3), OCB is positive in 51.2% of cases. Hyponatremia is rare, unlike other LE. Other antibodies can be positive in 19% of cases (anti-$GABA_A$, anti-$GABA_B$, and anti-VGKC). Approximately 55% of patients benefit from immunotherapy.[10]

Anti-$GABA_A$ Receptor Autoimmune Encephalitis

Gamma-aminobutyric acid type A receptors modulate the fast inhibitory actions of GABA. $GABA_A$ antibody binding causes internalization of the receptors with neuronal hyperexcitability. Median age of onset is 47 years (2.5 months to 88 years). Adults make up 64% of the cases, and children make up 36%. Females are more affected than males in adults. The presentation includes seizures, both focal and generalized, encephalopathy presenting with cognitive impairment, impaired sensorium, and behavioral changes, and both seizure and encephalopathy in 58% of cases. Status epilepticus can be seen in upto 41% of individuals who present with a seizure.

Psychiatric symptoms may be the presentation in 36% of cases, including behavioral changes, personality changes, depression, anxiety, hallucinations, and catatonia. Movement disorders occur in 14% of cases, chorea/

choreoathetosis, ataxia, orofacial dyskinesia, and other involuntary movements are described. In 8% of cases, dysautonomia is noted. Thymoma is the most common neoplasm, accounting for 64% of cases, followed by Hodgkin's disease, non-Hodgkin's lymphoma (NHL), rectal carcinoma, multiple myeloma, and small-cell carcinoma. In 28% of the cases, there is a preceding infection or fever. Other autoantibodies are found in 36% of the cases, and other autoimmune disorders are found in 18%. There is a higher degree of sensitivity in serum antibody testing than in CSF. The most frequent lesion in MRI is cortical and subcortical multifocal FLAIR/T2 abnormalities, which are seen in 83% of the patients. Gadolinium-enhancing lesions are seen in 8% of the cases, while diffusion restriction is seen in 4%. Cerebellar, basal ganglia, brainstem, and leptomeningeal enhancement are uncommon observations. In 94% of cases, the EEG is abnormal, with epileptiform abnormalities in 77%, focal and generalized slowness in 47%, and both in 27% of abnormal EEGs. CSF is abnormal in 57% of the cases, with lymphocytic pleocytosis (range 7–154/mm^3) seen in nearly half of them, increased protein in 32%, and OCB in 14%. Among those who undergo immunotherapy, 36% achieve a complete recovery, 44% have a partial recovery, and 20% have a poor recovery.[11]

Neuromyelitis Optica Spectrum Disorder Autoimmune Encephalitis

Myelin oligodendrocyte glycoprotein (MOG) IgG antibody associated disease has a wide range of presentations, including optic neuritis, transverse myelitis, and ADEM. Encephalitis presentation is rare, and LE presentation is even rarer. FLAMES (FLAIR hyperintense cortical lesions in MOG-associated encephalitis with seizures) is a novel subentity of MOG-associated disease characterized by unilateral or bilateral cortical encephalitis with possible meningeal inflammation. FLAMES show male predominance (60%), with a mean age of 29 years (11–46 years). Clinical presentation include seizures (85%), headache (70%), and fever (65%). CSF may show pleocytosis (29–311/mm^3). Unlike MOG IgG, AQP4 IgG is associated with brainstem encephalitis.[12]

Hashimoto's Encephalitis

It has been reported from the first to eighth decades of life, women are disproportionately affected. Usually, overt or subclinical thyroid illness, mainly hypothyroidism, is present. With normal or nonspecific CSF and brain MRI abnormalities, patients develop encephalopathy, which can be accompanied by seizures, myoclonus, hallucinations, and stroke-like events. Most patients who are treated with corticosteroids have good outcomes, hence renamed steroid-responsive encephalopathy with autoimmune thyroiditis. Hashimoto's encephalopathy has been currently classified as probable autoimmune encephalitis **(Box 6)**.

BOX 6 Diagnostic criteria of Hashimoto's encephalitis.

When all six of the following criteria have been met:

1. Encephalopathy with seizures, myoclonus, hallucinations, or stroke-like episodes
2. Subclinical or mild overt thyroid disease (usually hypothyroidism)
3. Brain MRI normal or with nonspecific abnormalities
4. Presence of serum thyroid (thyroid peroxidase, thyroglobulin) antibodies
5. Absence of well-characterized neuronal antibodies in serum and CSF
6. Reasonable exclusions of alternative causes

(CSF: cerebrospinal fluid; MRI: magnetic resonance imaging)

Source: Graus F, Titulaer MJ, Balu R, Benseler S, Bien CG, Cellucci T, et al. A clinical approach to diagnosis of autoimmune encephalitis. Lancet Neurol. 2016;15(4):391-404.

PEDIATRIC AUTOIMMUNE ENCEPHALITIS

Children present with rapid-onset symptoms, unlike adults. Prodromal symptoms are reported in >50% of the cases. Seizure is the most common symptom in pediatric AE. One-third of them present with abnormal movements such as ataxia, chorea, dystonia, and tremor. Cognitive dysfunction is one of the cardinal symptoms. Development and language regression may be the presenting feature in pediatric AE. Assessing memory impairment is challenging in the pediatric age group. Behavioral changes such as stereotypy, irritability, hyperactivity, hypersexuality, insomnia, and anger outbursts are common. Psychiatry symptoms occur in 50% of cases ranging from personality changes to frank psychosis. New-onset psychosis in children should warn of an AE. The difference in presentation from adults can be accounted for by the developing brain in children, where neuronal circuitry, neurotransmitter density, and myelination are different. Children with AE present with multifocal neuropsychiatric symptoms than isolated clinical syndrome. Tumors are less often associated with pediatric AE than adults **(Box 7)**.[13]

DIFFERENTIAL DIAGNOSIS

Infectious meningoencephalitis is the most likely differential diagnosis as clinically, they are indistinguishable. As a result, CSF analysis is used to differentiate the conditions. Except in the very early stages of the disease, pleocytosis is usually the rule in infectious meningoencephalitis, whereas the absence of pleocytosis indicates an AE/metabolic encephalopathy. Even if pleocytosis occurs in AE, it is generally moderate and lymphocytic. In AE, CSF glucose levels will be normal (except in rare cases of NMOSD and GFAP-related meningoencephalitis), while in viral encephalitis it will be normal and in bacterial meningoencephalitis it will be low. Bacterial meningoencephalitis causes neutrophilic leukocytosis, and is characterized by low glucose and high protein levels. One of the most prevalent abnormalities in AE is mildly elevated CSF protein with no pleocytosis and

BOX 7 Diagnostic criteria for pediatric AE.

1. Acute or subacute onset of neurologic and or psychiatric symptoms of <3 months duration in a previously healthy child
2. Clinical evidence of neurologic dysfunction:
   a. Altered mental status/consciousness level or EEG with sowing or epileptiform abnormalities
   b. Focal neurologic deficit
   c. Cognitive difficulties
   d. Acute developmental regression
   e. Movement disorders other than tics
   f. Psychiatric symptoms
   g. Unexplained seizures
3. Evidence for neuroinflammation:
   a. CNS inflammatory changes
   b. MRI features of encephalitis
   c. Brain biopsy showing inflammatory infiltrates excluding other causes
4. Presence of well-characterized antibodies in serum and or CSF
5. Exclusion of alternative causes including other causes of CNS inflammation

Definite antibody-positive diagnosis—criteria 1+ more than one feature from criteria 2, one or more feature from criteria 3, and both criteria 4 and 5 fulfilled

Probable antibody-negative AE—criteria 1+ more than one feature from criteria 2, one or more features from criteria 3, and criteria 5 fulfilled but criteria 4 not met

Possible AE—criteria 1+ more than one feature from criteria 2, criteria 5 fulfilled, but features from criteria 3 and 4 are not available

(AE: autoimmune encephalitis; CNS: central nervous system; CSF: cerebrospinal fluid; EEG: electroencephalogram; MRI: magnetic resonance imaging)

Source: With permission from Cellucci, et al (2020).[13]

normal glucose. Differentiating AE from infectious causes such as bacteria, viruses, and fungi relies heavily on CSF analysis. To rule out infectious causes, routine CSF analysis, cytology, microorganism staining, culture, and a molecular testing panel for DNA/RNA of the infective organism are required.

Metabolic encephalopathy is the other closest differential diagnosis. Hepatic encephalopathy, uremic encephalopathy, hypo/hypernatremia, hypo/hyperthyroidism, hypo/hypercalcemia, hypo/hyperphosphatemia, hypo/hypermagnesemia, and hyperammonemia can exactly mimic AE, and full metabolic profile should be done to rule out metabolic encephalopathy. Septic encephalopathy, drug toxicity, other toxicities, cerebrovascular diseases, neoplastic diseases, CJD, primary and secondary CNS vasculitis, epileptic disorders and encephalopathy, systemic autoimmune diseases with CNS involvement such as systemic lupus erythematosus, sarcoidosis, Kleine-Levin syndrome, Reye's syndrome and inborn errors of metabolism in children, Rasmussen encephalitis, febrile infection-related epilepsy syndrome (FIRES), idiopathic hemiconvulsion hemiplegia and epilepsy syndrome (IHHE), acute encephalitis with refractory repetitive partial seizures (AERRPS) can be considered as differentials for AE.

MANAGEMENT

The most crucial part of AE management is immunotherapy. In cases of paraneoplastic AE, treatment of the neoplasm is the most important step. But symptomatic management and supportive care should not be neglected. Comprehensive management is essential for treatment success, and there are multiple domains of symptoms involving different parts of the neuroaxis such as psychiatry, critical care, and infectious disease. With AE syndromes recently recognized and significant heterogeneity within syndromes, the treatment recommendations are not purely based on randomized controlled trials. Currently, little data is available, fulfilling evidence-based medicine.

- Patients treated with immunotherapy do better and have lesser relapses than those who are not treated
- Early treatment has better results.
- Those with failed first-line treatment improve with second-line treatment and have fewer relapses.

Worldwide, high-dose steroids are usually recommended for first-line immunotherapy. Methylprednisolone 1 g infusion intravenously daily for 3–7 days is the standard regime. Plasma exchange (PLEX)/Intravenous immunoglobulin (IVIgG) is preferred when steroids are contraindicated. If there is no significant improvement at the end of the initial therapy, consider intravenous immunoglobulin G (IVIgG) or PLEX. IVIgG is preferred in the case of agitated patients, those with dysautonomia, bleeding disorders, and hemodynamic instability. The dose of IVIgG is 2 g/kg of body weight and is given over 2–5 days. PLEX is preferred in those with severe hyponatremia and thrombotic risk and those with associated brain and spinal cord demyelination. PLEX is typically 5–10 exchanges every other day. Consider adding PLEX/IVIgG and steroids from the beginning of treatment if the disease is severe, like anti-NMDAR AE, status epilepticus, or severe dysautonomia. If there is no improvement in 2–4 weeks after a combined therapy, consider adding second-line therapy. Rituximab is preferred in confirmed or suspected antibody-mediated disease and cyclophosphamide in AE with cell-mediated autoimmunity like paraneoplastic AE. The dose of rituximab is 375 mg/m^2 weekly for 4 weeks or 1 g doses 2 weeks apart (total of 2 g). Dose of cyclophosphamide is 600–1,000 mg/m^2.

How long to treat is an unanswered question. Some experts prefer a short course of treatment, like 6 months, and others prefer 2–3 years of treatment. If there is no response to second-line therapy, consider tocilizumab or bortezomib. The dose of bortezomib is 1.3 mg/m^2 on day 1, 4, 8, and 11, given subcutaneously. Tocilizumab is administered at 8 mg/kg intravenous once a month. Abrupt discontinuation of immunotherapy is to be avoided to prevent relapse. Bridging immunotherapy has to be started before discharge. Usually, patients are started on oral prednisolone 1–2 mg/kg after completing the acute therapy and tapered over weeks to months, depending on the clinical response. If needed, long-term immunotherapy should be initiated. It is better to continue on long-term immunosuppression in neuronal surface antibody-positive cases as the risk of relapses is high. In long-term immunosuppression, azathioprine and mycophenolate mofetil are used. Rituximab is also an effective alternative to these drugs. The dose of azathioprine is 2–3 mg/kg/day, and mycophenolate mofetil 2,000 mg/day and can be hiked to 3,000 mg/day if there is no response.

In paraneoplastic syndrome, tumor treatment is more beneficial as T cell-mediated diseases are resistant to immunotherapy in most cases. In inoperable cases, debulking of tumor with surgery, radiation, or chemotherapy can help to improve the neurological condition by reducing the immunological drive. Low Karnofsky Performance Status scales may be due to paraneoplastic neurologic syndrome rather than cancer and should not prevent aggressive cancer therapy. Although cancer treatment improves paraneoplastic neurologic syndrome, the introduction of ICIs can worsen existing paraneoplastic syndrome or trigger a new one due to uninhibited immune reaction against tumor antigens. Paraneoplastic AE in the setting of ICI is usually well responsive to steroids. According to the European Society of Medical Oncology, starting steroids and interrupting ICI is recommended if a moderate-intensity side effect occurs and altogether discontinuing if a severe side effect occurs. Moderate-to-severe adverse effects include meningitis and encephalitis. If no other alternatives are available, a rechallenge of ICI can be considered if the patient agrees, considering the risks and benefits after a sufficient course of steroid treatment.[14]

SUPPORTIVE MANAGEMENT

Benzodiazepines such as diazepam and clonazepam, antipsychotics like quetiapine, and mood stabilizers like valproate are used in managing psychiatric symptoms. The clinician should be cautious to avoid oversedation and polypharmacy, avoid drugs lowering seizure threshold like olanzapine, and avoid medication that prolongs QT interval like haloperidol in susceptible patients. Regarding management of seizures, sodium channel blockers such as carbamazepine and lacosamide may be preferred in anti-LGI1 AE. Thiopentone, ketamine, and propofol are used in refractory status epilepticus. In the case of movement disorders, benzodiazepines are useful in the management of myoclonus, stiff-person syndrome, PERM, catatonia, dystonia, and stereotypy. Anticholinergics are useful in the management of dystonia. Baclofen and tizanidine are also used in management of dystonia and spasticity.

Dopamine blockers like risperidone and depleters like tetrabenazine are used to manage tic, hemiballismus, chorea, athetosis, and hyperkinesia. Levodopa and dopamine agonists are used for parkinsonism, rigidity, and akinetic mutism. In the case of antipsychotic use, the clinician should be aware of the paradoxical worsening and development of neuroleptic malignant syndrome. In dysautonomia and psychosis, caution should be exercised when administering anticholinergics. The same can be said for dopaminergic medications in psychosis. In dysautonomia, alpha blockers, beta blockers, and/or acetylcholinesterase inhibitors are used for patients with an increased sympathetic drive.

In postural hypotension, midodrine and fludrocortisone are used. Temporary pacemakers are used for cardiac block and severe arrhythmia, total parenteral nutrition for severe gastric dysmotility, and antimuscarinics for urinary incontinence. Sleep hygiene should be encouraged, and melatonin can be added to optimize the sleep–wake cycle. In addition, benzodiazepines, zolpidem, and nonbenzodiazepine hypnotics can be used to treat insomnia. Patients with spasticity, ataxia, and mobility issue will benefit from physiotherapy. Patients with cognitive deficits should undergo neuropsychology evaluation and cognitive rehabilitation.

FOLLOW-UP SCREENING

If onconeural antibodies are positive but no cancer is detected, continue cancer screening for 4 years. Treat neurologic relapses with intravenous methylprednisolone (IVMP)/cyclophosphamide as necessary but avoid long-term immunosuppression. If a neuronal surface antibody is found to be positive with high clinical significance and a typical clinical picture, cancer surveillance for 2–4 years is indicated. The frequency of cancer screening is determined by the antibody type; for example, anti-AMPAR/$GABA_BR$ requires regular screening, but anti-LGI1 requires less frequent screening. Patients with severe disease or other risk factors, including CSF OCBs or relapses, are placed on long-term immunosuppression.

INDIAN PERSPECTIVE

Most AE literature originates from Western countries. Asian countries, like South Korea, have reported AE and in contrast to western countries, have reported more seronegative AE. In 2013, we established the country's first dedicated neuroimmunology laboratory for diagnosing AE at AIMS, Kochi. The large number of cases we have studied indicates that seronegative cases are more common. Seropositive people are more likely to have NMDA AE, followed by GAD65, anti-LGI1, and CASPR2. Even though MOG IgG is more frequently positive, AE presentation is uncommon. GAD65 antibody levels are low in Indian patients based on our cohort; the highest value at this time is <5,000 IU/mL. In our experience, onconeural antibody positivity is also rare.

In terms of treatment, we have observed that early aggressive immunotherapy provides better results. We use a combination of IVMP with IVIgG/PLEX for severe AE, like those who present with status epilepticus, have a long duration of disease prior to hospitalization, and seropositive cases who do not respond to IVMP within a few days. This is usually followed by rituximab treatment.

CONCLUSION

Autoimmune encephalitis is evolving into one of the most common causes of encephalitis now. Understanding of the clinical phenotype of this syndrome is very important for making an early diagnosis. Early diagnosis leads to early treatment and better outcomes. Clinical evaluation and neuroimmunology laboratory evaluation are important for making the diagnosis of AE. There is a significant difference in phenotype and antibody positivity pattern in the Indian population compared to the Western population.

REFERENCES

1. Hébert J, Muccilli A, Wennberg RA, Tang-Wai DF. Autoimmune Encephalitis and Autoantibodies: A Review of Clinical Implications. J Appl Lab Med. 2022;7(1):81-98.
2. Blinder T, Jan Lewerenz J. Cerebrospinal Fluid Findings in Patients with Autoimmune Encephalitis—A Systematic Analysis. Front Neurol. 2019;10:804.
3. Altabakhi IW, Babiker HM. Paraneoplastic Limbic Encephalitis. In: StatPearls [Internet]. Treasure Island (FL): StatPearls Publishing; 2023.
4. Gultekin SH, Rosenfeld MR, Voltz R, Eichen J, Posner JB, Dalmau J. Paraneoplastic limbic encephalitis: neurological symptoms, immunological findings and tumour association in 50 patients. Brain. 2000;123(7):1481-94.
5. van Coevorden-Hameete MH, de Bruijn MAAM, de Graaff E, Bastiaansen DAEM, Schreurs MWJ, Demmers JAA, et al. The expanded clinical spectrum of anti-$GABA_BR$ encephalitis and added value of KCTD16 autoantibodies. Brain. 2019;142(6):1631-43.
6. Swayne A, Tjoa L, Broadley S, Dionisio S, Gillis D, Jacobson L, et al. Antiglycine receptor antibody related disease: a case series and literature review. Eur J Neurol. 2018;25(10):1290-8.
7. Hara M, Ariño H, Petit-Pedrol M, Sabater L, Titulaer MJ, Martinez-Hernandez E, et al. DPPX antibody-associated encephalitis: Main syndrome and antibody effects. Neurology. 2017;88(14):1340-8.
8. Flanagan EP, Hinson SR, Lennon VA, Fang B, Aksamit AJ, Morris PP, et al. Glial fibrillary acidic protein immunoglobulin G as biomarker of autoimmune astrocytopathy: Analysis of 102 patients. Ann Neurol. 2017;81(2):298-309.
9. Nissen MS, Blaabjerg M. Anti-IgLON5 Disease: A Case with 11-year Clinical Course and Review of the Literature. Front Neurol. 2019;10:1056.
10. Gagnon M, Savard M. Limbic Encephalitis Associated with GAD65 Antibodies: Brief Review of the Relevant literature. Can J Neurol Sci. 2016;43(4):486-93.
11. Guo CY, Gelfand JM, Geschwind MD. Anti-gamma-aminobutyric acid receptor type A encephalitis: a review. Curr Opin Neurol. 2020;33(3):372-80.
12. Budhram A, Mirian A, Le C, Hosseini-Moghaddam SM, Sharma M, Nicolle MW. Unilateral cortical FLAIR-hyperintense Lesions in Anti-MOG-associated Encephalitis with Seizures (FLAMES): characterization of a distinct clinico-radiographic syndrome. J Neurol. 2019;266(10):2481-7.
13. Cellucci T, Van Mater H, Graus F, Muscal E, Gallentine W, Klein-Gitelman MS, et al. Clinical approach to the diagnosis of autoimmune encephalitis in the pediatric patient. Neurol Neuroimmunol Neuroinflamm. 2020;7(2):e663.
14. Abboud H, Probasco J, Irani SR, Ances B, Benavides DR, Bradshaw M, et al; Autoimmune Encephalitis Alliance Clinicians Network. Autoimmune encephalitis: proposed recommendations for symptomatic and long-term management. J Neurol Neurosurg Psychiatry. 2021;92(8): 897-907.

Part 4E: Movement Disorders

71

CHAPTER

Parkinson's Disease

Shweta Prasad, Vikram V Holla, Pramod Kumar Pal

INTRODUCTION

Parkinson's disease (PD) is a chronic, progressive, and neurodegenerative disorder that was first described in 1817 by James Parkinson, a 19th-century English physician in "An essay on the Shaking Palsy" wherein it was referred to as the "shaking palsy" or the Latin term "paralysis agitans".[1] In 1897, Charcot argued against the term "paralysis agitans" and recommended the disorder be named after Parkinson. PD is the second most prevalent neurodegenerative disorder Alzheimer's dementia and has been observed to affect 1% of the population over 65 years of age.[2] PD is seldom observed before 50 years of age and shows a fivefold to tenfold increase beyond the 6th decade.[3] Owing to this, PD has frequently been considered a geriatric disease with an average age at onset (AAO) of 55–60 years. However, approximately 5–10% of patients develop symptoms before the age of 50 years and are referred to as early onset PD.[4]

It is clinically characterized by the *sine qua non* of bradykinesia, rigidity, and rest tremor,[5] while from a pathological perspective, PD is characterized by the loss of dopaminergic neurons in the substantia nigra pars compacta (SNpc) and widespread α-synuclein accumulation.[6] Apart from the classical motor symptoms, PD is associated with a wide gamut of nonmotor symptoms (NMS) encompassing the domains of neuropsychiatric symptoms, cognitive dysfunction, sleep dysfunction, autonomic dysfunction, and sensory dysfunction.[7] The discovery of dopamine deficiency in PD in the 1960s and the subsequent introduction of levodopa have significantly contributed to the improvement of quality of life and life expectancy. However, the treatment of NMS and slowing of disease progression remain important unmet needs. Furthermore, patients tend to develop motor complications and reduced efficacy of levodopa as the disease progresses owing to which surgical intervention in the form of deep brain stimulation (DBS) is often necessary. This chapter aims to provide a comprehensive overview of PD by primarily discussing the epidemiology, clinical features, diagnosis, investigations, and management.

EPIDEMIOLOGY

The prevalence rate of PD is highly variable and ranges between 18 and 418 per 100,000 worldwide with a reduction to 102–190 per 100,000 when adjusted for multiple factors.[8] An incidence rate of 37.55 per 100,000 women and 61.21 per 100,000 men above the age of 40 years has been reported. The incidence rates are suggested to steadily increase over time, from 3.26 per 100,000 at age 40–49 to 103.48 over the age of 80.[9] In India, the prevalence of PD is highly variable. In Northern India (Kashmir), the prevalence rate is 14.1 per 100,000,[10] whereas in South India (Bengaluru), the prevalence rate has been reported as 8 per 100,000.[11] In Eastern India (West Bengal), the prevalence rate ranges from 16 per 100,000 in rural areas[12] to 80 per 100,000 in urban areas,[13] while in an urban Parsi community in Western India (Mumbai), the prevalence rate was reported as 328.3 per 100,000.[14] These differences in prevalence rates may either reflect variability in methodology or may represent actual differences in etiology based on genetic background or environmental exposure. Epidemiological studies in the western population have reported an AAO of 59.6 ± 10 years.[15] Similarly, the AAO in Asia has been reported to range from 60 to 69 years.[16] The average AAO of PD in the Indian population has been reported to be 51.1 ± 11.8 years, which is earlier in comparison to reports from other countries.[17]

Gender-based prevalence of PD is uncertain with conflicting results across studies. A marginal male predominance has been reported by several clinic-based studies; however, this result has not been replicated by door-to-door studies. A higher prevalence in men may be attributable to an increased X-linked genetic predisposition, the influence of sex hormones, or increased exposure to probably causative environmental factors. Over the past generation, the global burden of PD has more than doubled as a result of increasing numbers of older people, with potential contributions from longer disease duration and environmental factors.[18]

Genetic factors are suggested to play a strong role in the etiology of PD and family history is associated with an increased risk of PD.[19] It is uncertain if this increased risk is suggestive of increased genetic susceptibility, actual genetic inheritance, common exposure, or a recall bias. A large number of factors have been associated with either an increased or decreased risk of developing PD.[20] However, establishing these associations is difficult owing to recall bias, latency between exposure and onset of PD, etc. **Box 1** lists the factors linked with either an increased or decreased risk of PD.

PATHOLOGY AND PATHOPHYSIOLOGY

Parkinson's disease is characterized by two major pathological processes—firstly, a premature selective loss of dopamine neurons, and secondly, accumulation of Lewy bodies which are composed of misfolded α-synuclein. A stepwise degeneration of neurons has been observed, with each affected site corresponding to specific symptomatology[6] **(Fig. 1)**. α-synuclein may spread transcellularly by a prion-like process, and this may contribute to the progression of PD pathology.[21] An approximate 30–70% cell loss in the SNpc has been associated with motor symptoms.[22]

BOX 1 **Factors associated with increased or decreased risk of Parkinson's disease.**

Increased risk of PD:
- *Demographic factors*: Elderly white male
- *Genetic factors*: Family history of PD or essential tremor; early onset of PD
- *Environmental factors*: Well-water, MPTP; MPTP-like compounds; pesticide exposure—insecticide, herbicide, rodenticide, fumigants, fungicides; metal exposure—manganese, lead, mercury, copper, and lead

Decreased risk of PD:
- *Antioxidants*: Vitamin A, vitamin C, vitamin E, and β-carotene
- *Diet*: Coffee, tea, and niacin-containing foods
- *Miscellaneous*: Cigarette smoking and consumption of alcohol

(MPTP: 1-methyl-4-phenyl-1,2,3,6-tetrahydropyridine; PD: Parkinson's disease)

While the symptoms of bradykinesia and rigidity can be attributed to dopamine deficiency in the basal ganglia and its effect on the direct and indirect pathways, the pathophysiology of tremor may have a distinct basis as it does not always respond to levodopa treatment and may involve a cerebellar circuit which is triggered by the basal ganglia.[23,24] In recent years, converging evidence from neuroimaging and neurophysiological techniques has successfully demonstrated an imbalance of neurotransmitters to underlie the motor and NMS of PD. The predominant neurotransmitter changes in the basal ganglia structures include a decrease in dopamine, γ-aminobutyric acid (GABA), and adenosine and an increase in glutamate and acetylcholine at different levels of striatal connections.[25]

A genetic basis for PD is now well established, wherein, familial PD is defined as the familial clustering of affected individuals or evidence of Mendelian inheritance of the disease trait.[26] The first mutation known to cause parkinsonism, i.e., a mutation in the α-synuclein (*SNCA*) gene was reported in 1997.[27] Genetic research has led to the identification of several monogenic forms of PD and numerous genetic risk factors. Monogenic forms account for about 30% of familial and 3–5% of sporadic cases.[19] Non-Mendelian forms of PD have also been reported and

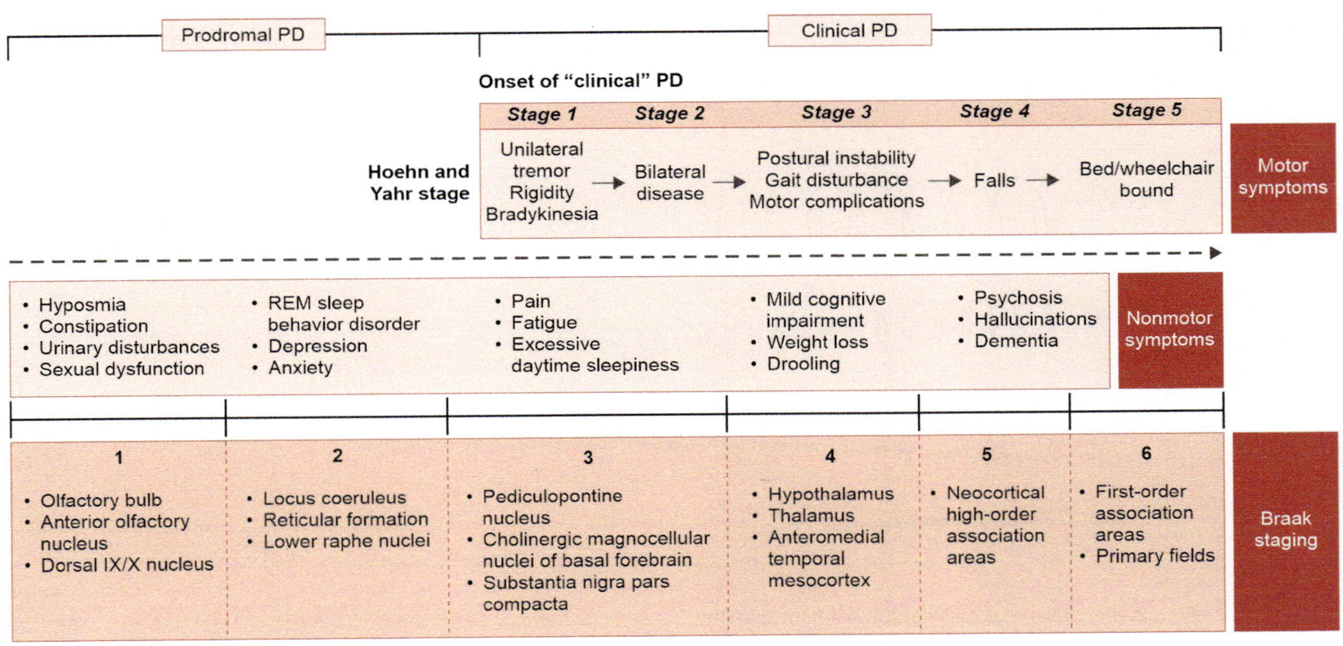

FIG. 1: Natural history of Parkinson's disease.
(REM: rapid eye movement)

this indicates that PD is genetically heterogeneous. The identification of epidemiological risk factors such as heavy metals, pesticides, etc. implies that the etiology of PD is complex. The etiology of PD is multifactorial and may result from an elaborate complex interplay of genes, modifying effects by susceptibility alleles, environmental exposures, gene–environment interactions, unknown factors, and the possible direct impact on the brain.[19]

CLINICAL FEATURES

The core motor clinical features of PD are bradykinesia, rest tremor, rigidity, and postural instability. MDS-PD criteria do not consider postural instability as the core clinical feature.[5] Three stages have been suggested based on the motor symptoms **(Fig. 1)**:[28]

1. *Preclinical PD*: Asymptomatic patient with neurodegeneration-related PD.
2. *Prodromal PD*: The patient has clinical signs or symptoms suggestive of neurodegeneration but not amounting to a diagnosis of clinical PD as per diagnostic criteria.
3. *Clinical PD*: The patient has bradykinesia with either rest tremor, rigidity, or both.

Besides the motor symptoms, patients with PD develop a variety of NMS, a few of which may antedate the motor symptoms by several years. NMS has been established as part of the disease process and has been established as prodromal markers.[29] A holistic approach incorporating both the motor symptoms and NMS is vital to arrive at a definitive diagnosis of PD. Early PD may go undiagnosed due to a multitude of vague and nonspecific symptoms. With the advancing PD, patients tend to develop motor complications in the form of either motor fluctuations, dyskinesia, or freezing of gait (FOG). Identifying these symptoms is crucial to make appropriate adjustments to medication.

Motor Symptoms

Bradykinesia

Bradykinesia is a general term used to describe an overall slowness and poverty of body and limb movements and is the most disabling and consistent component of PD. Along with slowness, there should be a progressive reduction in amplitude of movement (hypokinesia) to qualify as bradykinesia **(Video 1)**. Bradykinesia may be subtle to begin with and noticed as micrographia **(Fig. 2)**, reduced arm swing **(Video 1)**, reduced blink or facial expression. Later, with disease progression, it may be more evident with slowness in daily activities and gait. Bradyphrenia, a slowing of the thought process, may often be misinterpreted as dementia, especially in older patients. Generalized bradykinesia observed in older patients may be attributable to comorbidities or normal age-related slowing. The slowness of movements can also occur with apathy, depression, and pyramidal and cerebellar disorders, but the absence of a progressive reduction in amplitude of the movements differentiates these from parkinsonian slowness.

Tremor

Tremor is a presenting symptom in up to 70% of patients with PD. Classically, the tremor starts at rest and is asymmetrical at the onset with a frequency of 4–6 Hz. In the early stages, the tremor may be intermittent, restricted to only the thumb, and only appear during periods of stress. On occasion, the tremor may also be an action tremor which is observed while a limb is held against gravity or while executing voluntary movements. There may be a re-emergent component of postural tremor with varying latency. An isolated head, jaw, or trunk tremor is unlikely in the early stages of PD and an alternate diagnosis should be considered in such a situation. A subsection of patients can

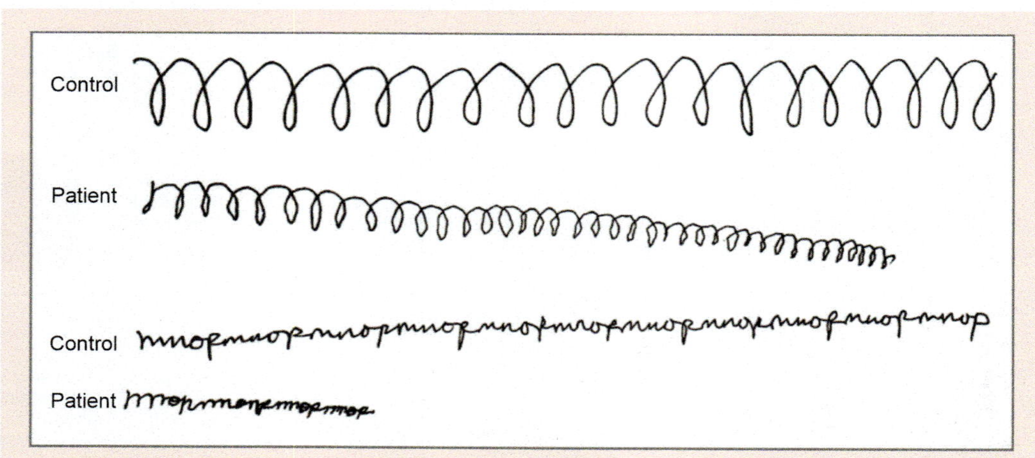

FIG. 2: Illustration of micrographia. In comparison to controls, the size of loops and letters drawn by the patient show a gradual diminution in size.

demonstrate a tremor-predominant phenotype wherein the severity of tremor is more than the rigidity and bradykinesia **(Video 2)**. Additionally, the rate of progression and underlying pathophysiology in this subsection is considered to be slightly different.

Rigidity

Rigidity is reported by patients as muscle stiffness and contributes to muscle pain, aches, fatigue, and clumsiness of hands. It is assessed as the degree of resistance to passive movement of limbs in both directions. Isolated cogwheel rigidity without lead pipe rigidity does not qualify as a core feature. In the early stages of PD, the rigidity is often asymmetric, and subtle, predominantly affecting appendicular musculature. Mild rigidity may be detectable by voluntary movement of the contralateral limb during examination (Froment's maneuver). Bradykinesia and rigidity frequently affect the same limb. As the disease progresses, several other regions and other joints get involved, which results in a stooped posture. Pre-existing joint problems must be ruled out before evaluation, since joint pain secondary to arthritis may also lead to an increase in tone which may be misinterpreted as rigidity. Rigidity and bradykinesia can also lead to reduced joint mobility and often patients may present with frozen shoulder to the orthopedician. Similar to the presence of a tremor-dominant phenotype, another motor phenotype of PD is the akinetic-rigid variant where rigidity and bradykinesia are the dominating symptoms. This subgroup is considered to be associated with the involvement of frontal networks and tends to demonstrate a higher occurrence of cognitive impairment.

Postural Instability and Gait Disturbance

Impairment of gait and balance is common in advanced PD and seldom observed in early PD. For this reason, it is no more considered an essential feature in MDS-PD diagnostic criteria. In the early stages, patients have discreet signs in the form of a slowing of gait and shortening of stride length, a tendency to trip after walking for a while, and difficulty maneuvering narrow lanes. Patients may also have slight flexion of the trunk to one side. Significant impairment in the early stages is usually indicative of different pathology. In the later stages of PD, these abnormalities are obvious and significantly contribute to morbidity. Patients may have difficulty with gait initiation and turning, and may develop festination, retropulsion, and freezing. Impairment of postural reflexes in the advanced stage leads to falls while standing or walking. Other causes for postural instability and gait disturbances should be evaluated and ruled out, especially in older patients.

Nonmotor Symptoms

Nonmotor symptom often predates the onset of motor symptoms and can add a significant burden to the patient's quality of life.[7] NMS has been shown to correlate with the pathological process described by Braak,[6] and NMS reported by patients may vary based on the stage and subtype of PD.

Nonmotor symptoms can be grouped into sensory symptoms (anosmia/hyposmia, pain, and excessive sweating), neuropsychiatric (depression, anxiety, apathy, psychosis, and impulse control disorders), cognitive, autonomic (orthostatic hypotension, urinary, sexual, and gastrointestinal), sleep-related (insomnia, rapid eye movement sleep behavior disorder, excessive daytime sleepiness, restless leg, periodic limb movements, and snoring), and others (weight loss, physically or mentally tired).[30] Of these, certain NMS such as hyposmia, depression, anxiety, sleep abnormalities, and constipation may antedate the motor onset, whereas cognitive abnormality, orthostatic hypotension, and urinary and sexual dysfunctions occur with advanced PD and are a red flag if occur in the early stage.

Motor Complications

With the progression of the disease and continued levodopa intake for around 3–5 years, motor complications can start to appear in the form of motor fluctuations, levodopa-induced dyskinesia, and gait disturbances.[31]

Motor Fluctuations

These include wearing OFF (gradual loss of efficacy of dopaminergic medication before the next dose of medication), OFF state (complete loss of levodopa effect before the next dose), delayed ON (onset of levodopa effect prolonged than usual), dose failure (no levodopa effect of the dose warranting additional dose), and sudden OFFs (unpredictable and sudden OFF state).

Dyskinesias

Commonly observed levodopa-induced dyskinesia is peak dose dyskinesia which is often choreiform **(Video 3)** and occurs during the peak effect of levodopa. It can also be dystonic or rarely myoclonic. The second type of dose-related dyskinesia is biphasic dyskinesia which tends to occur during the onset and wearing off of the levodopa effect and is characteristically short-lasting lower limb-predominant dystonia. Patients can also have early morning OFF state dystonia due to a lack of levodopa effect in the early morning.

Freezing of Gait

Freezing of gait and postural instability occur in the advanced stage of the disease. Freezing can occur with the initiation of gait (gait initiation or ignition failure) while turning (turn hesitancy), with narrow passages and obstacles or during dual tasking. Freezing in PD often improves with visual or auditory cues **(Video 4)**.[32]

DIAGNOSIS

The diagnosis of PD remains essentially clinical and only partly aided by supportive ancillary imaging and investigations. The diagnostic approach when evaluating a case of suspected PD is to look for essential features of PD, supportive features to increase the certainty of diagnosis, red flag signs that suggest a possibility of an alternative diagnosis, and clinical features that are inconsistent and exclude the diagnosis of PD. Till the late 1980s, formal diagnostic criteria for PD were not available and the diagnostic accuracy was around 75%.[33]

The United Kingdom Parkinson Disease Society Brain Bank Criteria

The first and most widely used formal diagnostic criteria are the United Kingdom Parkinson's Disease Society Brain Bank (UKPDSBB) clinical diagnostic criteria.[34] As the first step, it requires the presence of bradykinesia with at least one of the three cardinal signs of parkinsonism, i.e., muscular rigidity, 4–6 Hz rest tremor, and postural instability. Once parkinsonism is established, the second step is to exclude alternative causes in the absence of exclusion criteria. Finally, the definitive diagnosis of PD is made by the third step, which requires the presence of three or more supportive criteria.[34] Based on clinicopathological studies, the diagnostic accuracy of UKPDSBB was >80%.[5]

Over the next decade, few other criteria were put forth with different levels of diagnostic certainty of possible, probable, or definite PD incorporating various investigations and pathological confirmation by autopsy.[35–37] However, none of these achieved the wide clinical and research utility as that of UKPDSBB criteria. With the routine use of these criteria, a few limitations were noted. Positive family history is an exclusion criterion according to the UKPDSBB which is counterintuitive to our recent understanding of genetic PD. Furthermore, none of these criteria considered nonmotor features despite these symptoms being very prevalent and significant in patients with PD. In the Gelb criteria, bradykinesia is not considered an essential feature for the diagnosis of PD despite being the most important finding in patients with PD.

International Parkinson and Movement Disorder Society PD Criteria

Recently, the International Parkinson and Movement Disorders Society (MDS) proposed a new diagnostic criterion (MDS-PD) specifically for use in research. However, this can also be used as a general guide for clinical diagnosis.[38] The MDS-PD criterion is a three-step process with the first step establishing parkinsonism by the presence of bradykinesia with rest tremor or rigidity **(Box 2; Flowchart 1)**. Once the parkinsonism is established, the next step is to attribute it to PD when none of the exclusion criteria are present and the supportive criteria are counterbalanced by red flag signs. Based on the number of supportive criteria and red flags, two levels of diagnostic certainty have been proposed as clinical established and clinically probable. The new criteria incorporate NMS as well in the supportive criteria, compared to earlier criteria where postural instability was not a part of essential criteria, dementia is not an exclusion criterion and an expert physician evaluating the patient can exclude the diagnosis of PD if the physician feels that an alternative diagnosis is more likely than PD.[38]

Prodromal PD

Acknowledging the well-established stage of prodromal PD, the MDS has proposed a criterion of prodromal PD to aid in the diagnosis of those patients who have early symptoms or signs of PD neurodegeneration but are not sufficient enough to establish the clinical diagnosis based on the motor parkinsonism, i.e., those not satisfying essential criteria. However, in the absence of clear neuroprotective/disease-modifying therapy for prodromal PD, the criterion is developed only for research purposes and has no definitive role in clinical practice.

Overall, the clinical diagnostic criteria have a similar diagnostic accuracy of around 80%.[39] Even though these criteria have helped in maintaining uniformity, improving inter-rater reproducibility in research, and aiding in diagnosis by clinicians with less expertise in PD, the diagnostic accuracy of an experienced clinician is at par with UKPDSBB criteria and has higher specificity (83.5% *vs.* 34%) with a mild reduction in sensitivity (81.3% *vs.* 90.8%).[33,38] For these reasons, clinical expert opinion will remain the gold standard diagnostic technique till definitive validated diagnostic markers are available. This is acknowledged in the MDS-PD criteria as well with the clinical expert opinion of the most likely possibility of an alternative diagnosis other than PD as one of the absolute exclusion criteria. However, the definition of a clinical expert is not defined.

DIFFERENTIAL DIAGNOSIS

Owing to the lack of a definitive diagnostic test for PD, misdiagnosis is quite common. In the earlier stages of PD, it can be challenging to differentiate from other causes of parkinsonism. While evaluating a patient with suspected PD, both the clinical assessment and diagnostic criteria focus on red flags that hint at a possibility of alternative diagnosis and exclusion criteria which essentially rule out the possibility of PD. Atypical parkinsonian syndromes or Parkinson-plus syndromes are the most common PD mimics one can encounter in clinical practice. In addition, a few other etiologies that need to be considered are normal aging in very late-onset PD, essential tremor (ET) in tremor-dominant PD, and structural cause in persistently unilateral parkinsonism.[40–52]

BOX 2 International Parkinson and Movement Disorder Society Parkinson's disease (MDS-PD) clinical diagnostic criteria.

Essential criteria:

- Parkinsonism defined as bradykinesia, in combination with at least 1 of rest tremor or rigidity

Supportive criteria:

- Clear and dramatic beneficial response to dopaminergic therapy. During initial treatment, patient returned to normal or near-normal level of function. In the absence of clear documentation of initial response, a dramatic response can be classified as:
  a. Marked improvement with dose increases or marked worsening with dose decreases. Mild changes do not qualify. Document this either objectively (>30% in UPDRS III with change in treatment), or subjectively (clearly documented history of marked changes from a reliable patient or caregiver)
  b. Unequivocal and marked ON/OFF fluctuations, which must have at some point included predictable end-of-dose wearing off
- Presence of levodopa-induced dyskinesia
- Rest tremor of a limb, documented on clinical examination (in past, or on current examination)
- The presence of either olfactory loss or cardiac sympathetic denervation on MIBG scintigraphy

Absolute exclusion criteria:

- Unequivocal cerebellar abnormalities, such as cerebellar gait, limb ataxia, or cerebellar oculomotor abnormalities (e.g., sustained gaze evoked nystagmus, macro square wave jerks, hypermetric saccades)
- Downward vertical supranuclear gaze palsy, or selective slowing of downward vertical saccades
- Diagnosis of probable behavioral variant frontotemporal dementia or primary progressive aphasia, defined according to consensus criteria within the first 5 years of disease
- Parkinsonian features restricted to the lower limbs for >3 years
- Treatment with a dopamine receptor blocker or a dopamine-depleting agent in a dose and time-course consistent with drug-induced parkinsonism
- Absence of observable response to high-dose levodopa despite at least moderate severity of disease
- Unequivocal cortical sensory loss (i.e., graphesthesia, stereognosis with intact primary sensory modalities), clear limb ideomotor apraxia, or progressive aphasia
- Normal functional neuroimaging of the presynaptic dopaminergic system
- Documentation of an alternative condition known to produce parkinsonism and plausibly connected to the patient's symptoms, or, the expert evaluating physician, based on the full diagnostic assessment, feels that an alternative syndrome is more likely than PD

Red flags:

- Rapid progression of gait impairment requiring regular use of wheelchair within 5 years of onset
- A complete absence of progression of motor symptoms or signs over 5 or more years unless stability is related to treatment
- *Early bulbar dysfunction*: Severe dysphonia or dysarthria (speech unintelligible most of the time) or severe dysphagia (requiring soft food, NG tube, or gastrostomy feeding) within first 5 years
- *Inspiratory respiratory dysfunction*: Either diurnal or nocturnal inspiratory stridor or frequent inspiratory sighs
- Severe autonomic failure in the first 5 years of disease. This can include:
  - *Orthostatic hypotension*—orthostatic decrease of blood pressure within 3 minutes of standing by at least 30 mm Hg systolic or 15 mm Hg diastolic, in the absence of dehydration, medication, or other diseases that could plausibly explain autonomic dysfunction, or
  - Severe urinary retention or urinary incontinence in the first 5 years of disease (excluding long-standing or small amount stress incontinence in women) that is not simply functional incontinence. In men, urinary retention must not be attributable to prostate disease, and must be associated with erectile dysfunction
- Recurrent (>1/year) falls because of impaired balance within 3 years of onset
- Disproportionate anterocollis (dystonic) or contractures of hand or feet within the first 10 years
- Absence of any of the common nonmotor features of disease despite 5 years disease duration. These include sleep dysfunction (sleep-maintenance insomnia, excessive daytime somnolence, symptoms of REM sleep behavior disorder), autonomic dysfunction (constipation, daytime urinary urgency, and symptomatic orthostasis), hyposmia, or psychiatric dysfunction (depression, anxiety, or hallucinations)
- Otherwise-unexplained pyramidal tract signs, defined as pyramidal weakness or clear pathologic hyperreflexia (excluding mild reflex asymmetry and isolated extensor plantar response)
- *Bilateral symmetric parkinsonism*: The patient or caregiver reports bilateral symptom onset with no side predominance, and no side predominance is observed on objective examination

(MIBG: metaiodobenzylguanidine; NG: nasogastric; PD: Parkinson's disease; REM: rapid eye movement; UPDRS: unified Parkinson's disease rating scale)

Source: Adapted from Postuma et al., 2015.[38]

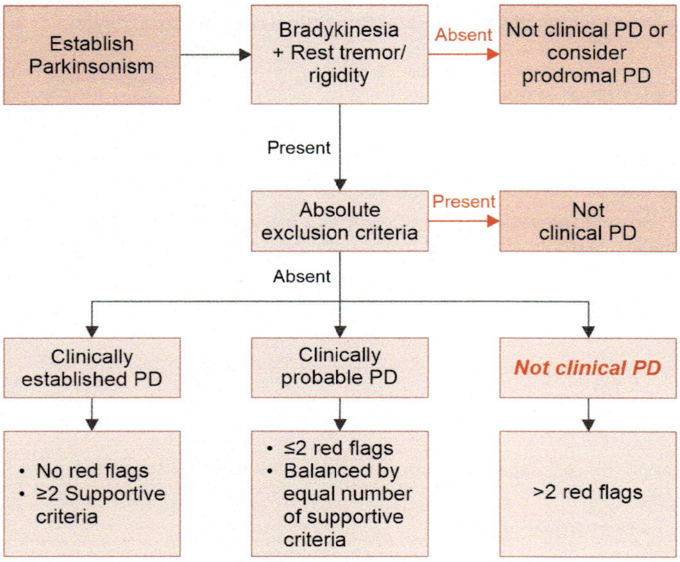

FLOWCHART 1: MDS-PD diagnostic criteria.

(MDS: International Parkinson and Movement Disorders Society; PD: Parkinson's disease)

Parkinson-plus Syndromes

The most common syndrome one has to differentiate from PD is atypical parkinsonism or Parkinson-plus syndromes, which constitutes multiple system atrophy (MSA), progressive supranuclear palsy (PSP), corticobasal ganglia degeneration, and dementia with Lewy body. In addition, vascular parkinsonism (VP) and normal pressure hydrocephalus (NPH) also pose a diagnostic challenge while differentiating from PD.

Multiple System Atrophy

Among the parkinsonian and cerebellar subtypes of MSA, MSA-Parkinson type (MSA-P) bears a very close resemblance to PD as it can have asymmetrical onset parkinsonism with tremor, rapid eye movement behavioral disorder (RBD), and in a few cases can be levodopa responsive as well.[53] However, unlike PD, the tremor is often postural and jerky with a very rare occurrence of classical pill-rolling rest tremor; the other classical NMS such as hyposmia is rare, and the levodopa responsiveness is suboptimal and ill-sustained. In addition, patients tend to have early and prominent levodopa-induced craniofacial dystonia in contrast to appendicular dyskinesia in PD. The key differences lie in the early and prominent autonomic failure, which is paramount for the diagnosis of MSA-P.[42] Furthermore, patients with MSA-P develop postural instability and dysphagia early in the disease course and are often disabling. Imaging evidence of asymmetrical posterior putaminal predominant, middle cerebellar peduncle, pontine and cerebellar atrophy, and hot cross bun sign can aid in the diagnosis.

Progressive Supranuclear Palsy

The recent PSP classification has various subtypes. Of these, probable PSP with predominant parkinsonism (PSP-P) subtype in the early stages can mimic PD with asymmetrical and limb onset parkinsonism with or without tremor and/or levodopa responsiveness.[54] Classical midbrain atrophy on magnetic resonance imaging (MRI) may be absent in the early stages and dopamine uptake imaging may also mimic PD compounding the diagnostic difficulty. However, the presence of or eventual occurrence of vertical gaze or saccadic impairment, square wave jerks, lid opening apraxia, photophobia, early dysphagia or dysarthria, and/or early falls point toward an underlying PSP pathology. Features distinguishing PSP-P from PD include supranuclear vertical gaze palsy, early postural instability with backward falls, prominent axial rigidity, dysarthria, dysphagia, and subcortical dementia.[44]

Corticobasal Syndrome

Similar to PD, corticobasal syndrome (CBS) classically presents with asymmetric parkinsonism. However, unlike PD, CBS has additional features of stimulus-sensitive myoclonus, apraxia, cortical sensory impairment, and cognitive decline that excludes the diagnosis of PD. In addition, CBS is rarely levodopa responsive and even when responsive, it is suboptimal and transient. Imaging findings of asymmetrical parietal atrophy in CBS may aid in the differentiation.[46]

Vascular Parkinsonism

Patients with VP usually have a lower body-predominant symmetrical parkinsonism with short-stepping gait and early cognitive and urinary disturbance which are red flags against a diagnosis of PD. However, in selected cases, the presentation may mimic that of PD with asymmetrical and upper limb presentations, especially with strategic infarcts involving the basal ganglia circuits. Levodopa responsiveness has also been observed in some of these cases. The presence of vascular risk factors, step-wise progression of cumulative vascular insults, the imaging evidence of the infarct responsible for the findings, and the additional signs and symptoms related to these lesions should suggest a diagnosis of VP instead of PD.[49]

Normal Pressure Hydrocephalus

Owing to the lower body-predominant symmetrical parkinsonism with early cognitive impairment, urinary disturbance, and poor levodopa responsiveness, the common diagnostic confusion is with VP rather than PD. However, in rare instances, there may be tremor and upper limb involvement which may raise the possibility of PD. The tremor is often postural or kinetic instead of the classical rest tremor of PD. Imaging findings play a significant role in confirming a diagnosis of NPH.[48]

Other Differential Diagnoses

Normal Aging

Commonly observed normal findings in the elderly such as a stooped posture, stiffness, slowness of movement, and postural instability can often be misdiagnosed as PD leading to unwarranted medication intake.[40] Additionally, it is not uncommon to find kinetic or postural tremor or a false positive Froment's maneuver in a normal elderly person compounding the diagnostic difficulty. However, the subtle and symmetrical nature of these findings, with relatively normal arm swing and heel strike, and the nonresponsiveness to levodopa should suggest normal aging instead of PD.

Essential Tremor

Essential tremor and tremor-dominant PD are very similar in presentation and, at times, are difficult to differentiate. In addition, assessment of bradykinesia can be difficult due to superimposed tremors adding to the difficulty. Furthermore, ET may be asymmetric at onset; rest tremor may be present at later stages and the Froment's maneuver can also be positive although often cogwheeling rather than lead pipe rigidity seen in PD. Levodopa responsiveness of PD, which is very helpful in differentiating PD from other parkinsonian syndromes, may not be of much help in differentiating from ET as it is well known that PD tremor may not be levodopa responsive. ET and PD can coexist in a single patient. However, positive family history, head and voice tremor, absence of significant rigidity, and bradykinesia can aid in differentiating ET from PD.[41] When in doubt even after clinical evaluation, dopamine uptake imaging can help in differentiating between the two.

Drug-induced Parkinsonism

Drug-induced Parkinsonism (DIP) is a common cause of secondary parkinsonism that usually has symmetric onset with a postural tremor but may present with asymmetric parkinsonism and rest tremor mimicking PD.[51] The presence of the classical NMS of PD such as anosmia/hyposmia, RBD, etc. may suggest a possibility of PD rather than DIP. Proper drug history is important as symptoms usually develop during treatment with medications such as dopamine-depleting agents, dopamine antagonists, and antipsychotics. Recovery often ensues within 6 months of the drug withdrawal.[52] In selected cases, dopamine uptake imaging may help in confirming the diagnosis.

Systemic Disorders

Rarely, symptoms of systemic illnesses may mimic PD and should be considered while evaluating a case of parkinsonism. These include: (1) metabolic disorders—hypoparathyroidism, hypothyroidism, and acquired hepatocerebral degeneration, (2) infectious diseases, (3) autoimmune diseases, (4) paraneoplastic disorder, (5) space-occupying brain lesions, (6) trauma, and (7) some of the genetic disorders such as juvenile Huntington's disease, Wilson's disease, spinocerebellar ataxia types 2 and 3, and neurodegeneration with brain iron accumulation.[50] Relevant investigations such as blood biochemical parameters, imaging, and appropriate genetic testing would help in identifying the underlying alternative diagnosis.

INVESTIGATIONS

Parkinson's disease is essentially a clinical diagnosis and investigations are sparingly needed and are primarily performed to rule out the possibility of alternate diagnosis in the presence of red flags or atypical features. In some instances, investigations are performed to estimate the severity of NMS as in autonomic function testing or sleep studies. In rare instances, investigations are performed primarily to confirm the diagnosis of PD. This is relevant in the setting of early PD wherein symptoms may be subtle or confounded by comorbidities.

Imaging

MRI Brain

The MRI brain in early PD often helps to rule out structural causes of parkinsonism and is usually performed to look for imaging patterns suggestive of atypical parkinsonism such as PSP, MSA, VP, or NPH. Routine sequences of MRI brain in PD are essentially normal. Special MRI sequences such as iron-specific sequences show the degeneration of nigrosome-1 (dorsal nigral hyperintensity), and neuromelanin-sensitive sequences display reduced signal intensity, size, and volume of SN. However, these findings do not add significantly to the clinical opinion and are neither sensitive nor specific to PD as they may be seen in several parkinsonian syndromes; hence, limiting their utility.[55–57]

Molecular Imaging

Dopaminergic imaging is either presynaptic such as Dopamine transporter scan (DaTscan) single-photon emission computerized tomography (SPECT) utilizing ^{123}I-ioflupane tracer or positron emission tomography (PET) utilizing 18-fluorodopa (fluorodopa-PET) or postsynaptic dopaminergic imaging such as those utilizing postsynaptic D2 receptors. Presynaptic dopaminergic imaging is commonly used in clinical practice and research rather than postsynaptic dopaminergic imaging.[58–60] Striatal dopamine depletion can be visualized using the DaTscan or fluorodopa-PET.

These modalities can improve the diagnostic accuracies in certain selected situations. Dopaminergic imaging is very useful in differentiating tremor-dominant PD from ET syndromes with high sensitivity (87–98%) and specificity (80–100%).[61] It is also useful and indicated in differentiating PD from DIP or functional parkinsonism. Another situation is for differentiating PD from healthy controls as in those cases with normal aging-related slowing. However, these imaging modalities are not useful in differentiating PD from other neurodegenerative parkinsonism and should not be used for such cases.

Occasionally, patients with suspected clinical PD may have scans without evidence of dopaminergic deficit (SWEDD).[62] Controversy exists regarding the implications of SWEDD; whether these patients are a benign subtype of PD or PD mimics. A recent systematic review found that although most cases of SWEDD were a misdiagnosis of PD, a small group were irrefutably clinically PD.[59] This raises doubts about the fixed relationship between the diagnosis of nigrostriatal parkinsonism and dopaminergic tracer binding. According to the MDS-PD criteria, SWEDD, i.e., normal functioning neuroimaging of the presynaptic dopaminergic system is an exclusion criterion and is not consistent with the diagnosis of clinical PD.

Other Imaging Modalities

Transcranial brain parenchyma sonography shows nigral hyperechogenicity in the early stages of PD and is an imaging biomarker for PD.[63] However, in a significant percentage, the adequate window for sonography cannot be achieved and also the sensitivity and specificity are inadequate for routine clinical use.

Metaiodobenzylguanidine (MIBG) scintigraphy is useful to detect myocardial sympathetic denervation, a feature common in PD but rarely seen in atypical PD or PD mimics.[64] For this reason, abnormal cardiac MIBG scintigraphy is one of the four supportive criteria in MDS-PD diagnostic criteria. However, MIBG scintigraphy is not as widely available compared to MRI or dopaminergic molecular imaging.

Ancillary Diagnostic Tests

Several modalities of testing exist that complement and strengthen a clinical diagnosis **(Box 3)**. Currently, no clinically useful diagnostic biomarkers exist. However, several have been associated with an increased risk of PD and may be indicative of disease progression.[65,66] A definitive diagnosis of PD requires an autopsy, however, recent evidence indicates that a peripheral tissue biopsy also may serve the purpose.[67,68] Olfactory dysfunction is present in a vast majority of patients with early PD. It aids in diagnosis and is simple to test.[29,69,70]

Genetic Testing

Genetic testing is an important diagnostic modality when evaluating a patient with PD, especially in the setting of juvenile or young-onset PD, family history of PD or with a history of consanguinity in parents where genetic causes constitute around 20–40% of the cohort. With the increasing availability of next-generation sequencing and its reducing cost, genetic variants of PD are being frequently identified. However, it is imperative to not all genetic variants are directly causative, rather they may increase susceptibility for sporadic PD.

In several cases, certain clinical features are often strongly suggestive of a genetic etiology of PD rather than idiopathic PD. These features include lower limb onset of symptoms, predominant dystonia, early levodopa-induced dyskinesia and dyskinesia to a very low dose of levodopa, etc. A summary of these features for the common monogenic variants of PD is listed in **Tables 1 and 2**.[71,72]

BOX 3 Ancillary diagnostic tests for Parkinson's disease (PD).

1. *Biomarkers*:
    - No clinically useful diagnostic biomarkers in blood/cerebrospinal fluid at present
    - *Early PD*:
        - Reduced serum brain-derived neurotrophic factor
        - Altered fecal microbiota
2. *Tissue diagnosis*:
    - Alpha-synuclein deposits in gastrointestinal and submandibular gland biopsy specimens in prodromal and clinical PD
3. *Olfactory testing*:
    - Easy to test
    - *Tests*: Indian Smell Identification Test (INSIT), University of Pennsylvania Smell Identification test (UPSIT), Sniffin' sticks
    - Olfactory dysfunction and abnormal DaTscan favors a diagnosis of PD
4. *Genetic testing*:
    - Limited to situations where a specific genetic cause is suspected
        - Juvenile onset PD with no family history
        - Patients in the premotor stage with significant family history
    - Presymptomatic testing in the background of family history is not advocated

TABLE 1: Autosomal dominant genetic variants of Parkinson's disease with key clinical features.

Locus	Gene	Clinical features
PARK1	*SNCA* (Alpha-synuclein)	• Early or late onset • Parkinsonism, dementia, and visual hallucinations • Less tremor • Faster clinical deterioration • Myoclonus • Hyperventilation
PARK3	Unknown	• Late onset • Dementia may be present • Good response to dopaminergic drugs • Penetrance <40%
PARK4	*SNCA* (Alpha-synuclein triplication)	• Early onset • Rapid progression • Postural tremor • Asymmetric limb "heaviness" and rigidity • *Atypical features*: Autonomic dysfunction, dementia, early weight loss, myoclonus, and seizures
PARK5	*UCHL1*	• Late onset • Similar to typical PD
PARK8	*LRRK2*	• Late onset • Resembles typical sporadic PD • Good response to levodopa • Psychiatric symptoms

(PD: Parkinson's disease)

TABLE 2: Autosomal recessive genetic variants of Parkinson's disease with key clinical features.

Locus	Gene	Clinical features
PARK2	*PRKN*	• Juvenile onset • Slow progression • High incidence of focal dystonia • Good response to dopaminergic therapy • Symmetric presentation • Levodopa-induced dyskinesia and motor fluctuations common • Hyperreflexia
PARK6	*PINK1*	• Early onset • Slow progression • Good and long-lasting response to levodopa
PARK7	*PARK7 (DJ1)*	• Early onset • Slow progression • Variable clinical severity • Sustained response to levodopa • Psychiatric symptoms
PARK9	*ATP13A2* (Kufor–Rakeb syndrome)	• Juvenile onset • Atypical features such as spasticity, dementia supranuclear gaze palsy • Facial and finger minimyoclonus • Good response to levodopa
PARK14	*PLA2G6*	• Early onset • Dystonia parkinsonism

MANAGEMENT

The treatment of PD is primarily symptomatic and the approach has to be individualized based on the stage of illness, age of the patient, and side effect profile. Although the primary aim of treatment is the reduction of motor disability, NMS, if present, should also be addressed.

Assessment of Disease Severity

Before starting treatment and during treatment, disease severity should be quantified and staged using validated scales and questionnaires. The commonly used scales are:

- *Modified Hoehn and Yahr (HY) scale*: The HY scale is frequently used to describe the symptom progression in PD and has five stages ranging from 0 to 5 **(Fig. 1)**.[73]
- *Unified Parkinson's disease rating scale (UPDRS)*: This is the most widely used clinical rating scale for PD.[74] Section III of the UPDRS—motor examination—should be routinely used to quantify the motor symptoms of PD.
- *MDS-UPDRS*: A new version of UPDRS was proposed by the MDS by retaining the strengths of UPDRS, resolving the identified problems and incorporating several clinically pertinent PD-related questions which were inadequately captured in the original version. The basic pattern was maintained with section III assessing the motor manifestation of PD.[75]

BOX 4 Guidelines for management of PD.

1. Determine the need for treatment
2. Significant variations exist in the impact of symptoms on a patient's quality of life
3. The type of symptom, patient's occupation, and the benefit to adverse effect ratio of medication must be considered for initiation of treatment
4. A flexible and practical approach has to be employed, and decision making must involve the patient and caregiver
5. The possibility of day-to-day fluctuations in symptoms has to be explained to the patient
6. Patients should be permitted to modify dosing based on the response obtained
7. Due credence must be given to reports of adverse effects, and appropriate changes should be made
8. The significance of regular medication and follow-up must be emphasized

(PD: Parkinson's disease)

- *NMS questionnaire (NMSQuest)*: As NMS plays a crucial role in the symptom complex of PD, adequate documentation and quantification are necessary. The NMSQuest is a comprehensive questionnaire that assesses the presence or absence of 10 domains of NMS and can either be administered by the physician or provided to a patient for self-completion.[76]
- *MDS-NMS questionnaire*: In contrast to NMSQuest, MDS-NMS quantifies the severity of the NMS as well so that it can be used to assess the response to various medications and monitor the progression of these symptoms.[30]
- *Nonmotor fluctuation assessment (NoMoFA) questionnaire*: This questionnaire, in addition to quantifying the NMS, also captures the medication-related NMS ON–OFF fluctuation akin to motor fluctuations.[77]

Pharmacological Management of Motor Symptoms

Several factors, which govern the choice of treatment, are listed in **Box 4. Flowchart 2** shows a possible approach to the treatment of PD. The choice of the drug has to be based on the age of the patient, symptom causing the greatest disability, and coexisting NMS. Drugs commonly used in the treatment of PD are summarized in **Table 3.**

Levodopa

Levodopa is the gold standard drug for the treatment of PD and no other drug has been shown to match up to the benefits obtained. Levodopa is a precursor of dopamine and is absorbed in the gastrointestinal tract at the level of the small intestine. Levodopa is metabolized to dopamine by aromatic acid decarboxylase, and to 3-O-methyldopa by catechol-O-methyltransferase (COMT) in the peripheral tissue. This peripheral conversion of levodopa significantly reduces the

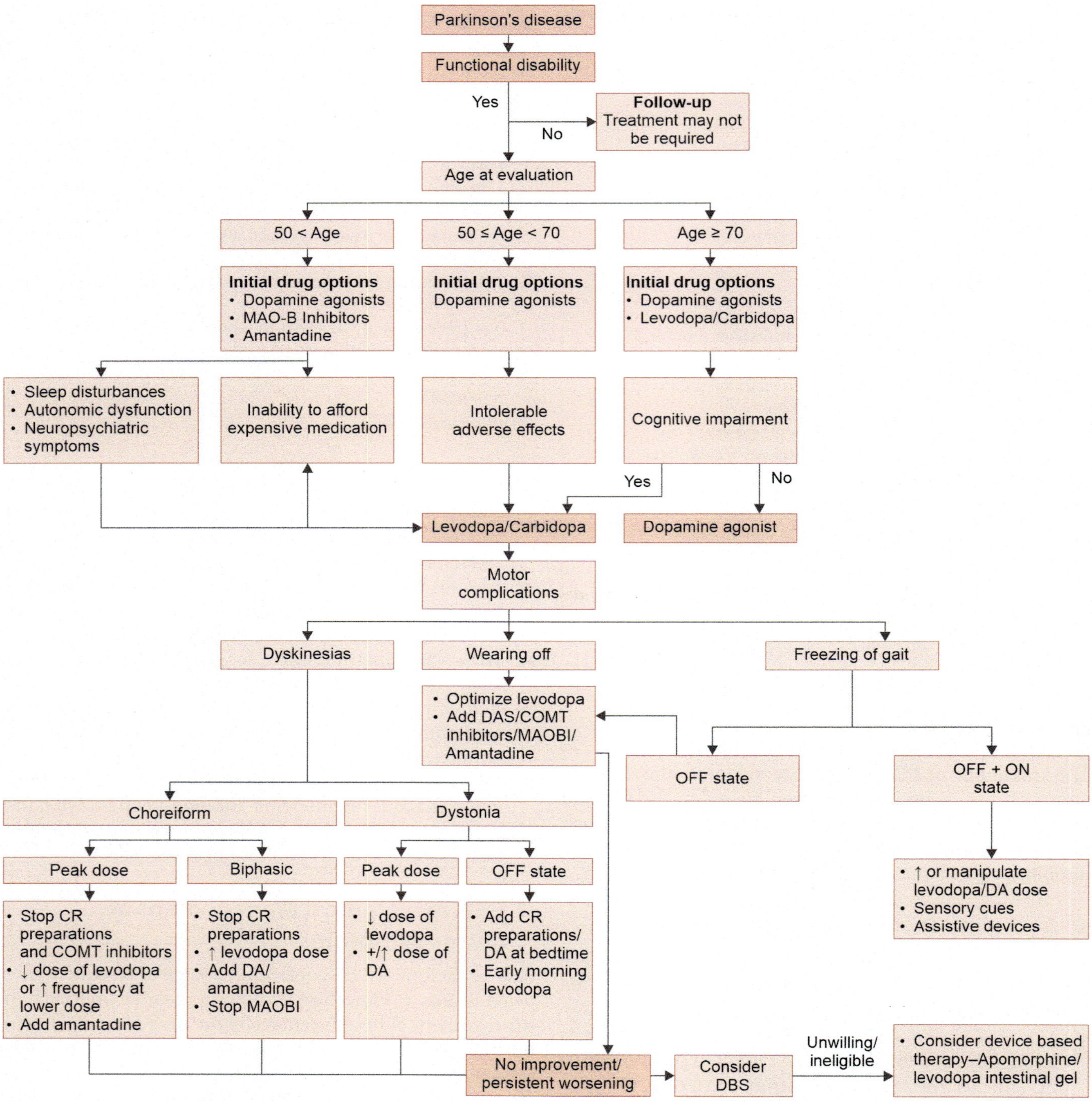

FLOWCHART 2: Treatment of Parkinson's disease.
(DBS: deep brain stimulation; MAO-B: monoamine oxidase type B)

availability of levodopa in the brain. To reduce this peripheral conversion, levodopa is administered in combination with decarboxylase inhibitors such as carbidopa or benserazide. The most commonly used preparations in India are levodopa + carbidopa available as regular and controlled release (CR) preparations, and less often levodopa + benserazide.

The treatment may be initiated with either a regular or CR preparation and should follow a "start slow" and "go slow" regimen, i.e., start with a low dose and slowly titrate upward based on the clinical response and to reduce the occurrence of adverse effects. For better intestinal absorption, levodopa should ideally be consumed either half hour before, or one

TABLE 3: Drugs commonly used in the treatment of Parkinson's disease.

Drug	Starting dose	Maintenance dose	Side effects
Levodopa	½ tablet 100/25 mg or 100/10 mg of levodopa/carbidopa	800 mg/day	Nausea, postural giddiness
Dopamine agonists:			
Pramipexole	0.125 mg TID	0.75–3 mg/day	Daytime somnolence, leg edema, and ICD
Ropinirole	0.25 mg TID	9–24 mg/day	Daytime somnolence, leg edema, and ICD
MAO-B inhibitors:			
Rasagiline	0.5 mg OD	1 mg/day	Worsen dopaminergic adverse effects, increase dyskinesia, confusion, hallucinations, and serotonin syndrome
Selegiline	5 mg OD	5–10 mg/day	Worsen dopaminergic adverse effects, increase dyskinesia, confusion, hallucinations, and serotonin syndrome
Safinamide	50 mg OD	100 mg/day (OD)	Nausea, insomnia, and hypertension
COMT inhibitor:			
Entacapone	200 mg with every dose of levodopa	1,600 mg/day	Peak dose dyskinesia
NMDA receptor blocker:			
Amantadine	100 mg OD	200 mg/day	Hallucinations, confusion, nightmares, ankle edema, livedo reticularis, dry mouth, hyponatremia
Anticholinergics:			
THP	2 mg OD	6 mg/day	Dry mouth, postural giddiness, blurred vision, urinary retention, constipation, and confusion
Benztropine	0.5 mg OD	6 mg/day	Dry mouth, postural giddiness, blurred vision, urinary retention, constipation, and confusion

(COMT: catechol-O-methyltransferase; ICD: impulse control disorder; MAO-B: monoamine oxidase type B; NMDA: N-methyl-D-aspartate; OD: once daily; THP: trihexyphenidyl)

and a half hours after meals. For those who cannot tolerate levodopa without meals, it can be taken with light snacks not rich in protein, as protein can reduce the intestinal absorption of levodopa. The most common side effects of levodopa after initiation of treatment include nausea and postural giddiness. Domperidone may be prescribed half hour prior to each dose for a few days to weeks till the patient can tolerate levodopa.

Controlled release preparations are beneficial as they have a prolonged half-life and a slower decline in plasma levels and clinical effects. It is helpful for the reduction of motor fluctuations and may be used at bedtime to improve mobility during the night. However, CR preparations have a delayed onset of action and need a higher dose in comparison to regular preparations of levodopa. CR preparations should be avoided or discontinued in patients with advanced PD who may have gastrointestinal dysmotility that may lead to erratic and unpredictable absorption of levodopa and may worsen peak dose dyskinesia.

Other newer preparations of levodopa are approved for clinical use. Levodopa-carbidopa intestinal gel (LCIG) that is administered directly to the jejunum through percutaneous jejunal tube aids in steady delivery and absorption of levodopa preventing motor fluctuation and improving levodopa-induced dyskinesia in advanced PD. Inhalational levodopa, which is absorbed by the pulmonary system bypassing the gastrointestinal system, helps in rapid levodopa absorption and prolonged clinical benefit.[78] Inhalational levodopa can be utilized as rescue therapy and also to improve wearing OFF states. However, these preparations are not available in India.

Prolonged treatment with levodopa will invariably lead to the production of dyskinesias. It has been observed that after 5 years of treatment, 50% of patients develop motor fluctuations including dyskinesias and about 80% of patients develop these complications after 10 years of treatment.[79] A daily dose of <600 mg has been suggested to aid in delaying the onset of motor complications.[80] Additional agents such as dopamine agonists (DAs) or monoamine oxidase type B (MAO-B) inhibitors should be considered if a higher dose of levodopa is required.

Dopamine Agonists

Dopamine agonists may either be used as a monotherapy in early PD or adjunct treatment in advanced PD. These are especially useful when patients on prolonged levodopa treatment start to develop motor complications. DAs can either be ergot derivatives—bromocriptine, lisuride, pergolide, and cabergoline or nonergot derivatives—pramipexole, ropinirole, rotigotine, and apomorphine. Nonergot DAs are preferable owing to the side effect profile of the ergot group. DAs are preferred in younger-onset PD as it delays the occurrence of levodopa-induced dyskinesia and younger patients can better tolerate DAs compared to elderlies.

Dopamine agonists must be started at a very low dose with a slow increase in the dose, e.g., pramipexole should be started at 0.125 mg TID for a week and gradually increased at 0.125 mg per week to a dose of 0.5 mg TID. Rotigotine is a unique DA since it can be administered as a transdermal patch and provides continuous drug delivery. DAs have a troublesome adverse effect profile of daytime somnolence, orthostatic hypotension, leg edema, cognitive and behavioral side effects, and impulse control disorders.[81] Hence, DAs should be avoided in patients with symptomatic postural hypotension or psychosis and used with caution in those working as heavy machinery operators, drivers, etc.

Monoamine Oxidase Type B Inhibitors

The MAO-B inhibitors are frequently utilized as first-line therapy, especially in patients with mild symptoms. Rasagiline can be used as monotherapy at 1 mg/day in early PD and has recently gained popularity owing to its neuroprotective properties and possible utility as a disease-modifying agent.[82] However, because of the confounding symptomatic effect and lack of long-term benefits of early start rasagiline, this drug is no longer recommended as a disease-modifying treatment. Selegiline has been shown to significantly delay the need for initiation of levodopa treatment.[83] Safinamide is a reversible MAO-B inhibitor that has been recently introduced and has been shown to prolong ON time without significant dyskinesia. It is used only as an add-on to levodopa in mid- to late-stage PD.[84] It is started at a dose of 50 mg/day and increased to 100 mg/day over 1–2 weeks.

Catechol-O-methyltransferase Inhibitors

Catechol-O-methyltransferase inhibitors act by reducing the peripheral and central degradation of levodopa, hence, increasing its availability and prolonging the effect of levodopa. Thus, COMT inhibitors are often started with the onset of wearing OFFs with levodopa. They do not have an inherent dopaminergic effect and hence are not effective without levodopa. Entacapone is a frequently used reversible peripheral COMT inhibitor and 200 mg should be given along with every dose of levodopa. The maximum dose of entacapone is 1,600 mg/day, i.e., 8 tablets. Tolcapone, another central and peripheral COMT inhibitor, is no longer used due to hepatotoxicity. Entacapone can induce or worsen peak-dose dyskinesia and hence is often discontinued with the onset of disabling peak-dose dyskinesia that cannot be mitigated by reducing the levodopa dose.

N-Methyl-D-Aspartate Receptor Blockers

Amantadine is widely used for its antidyskinetic effect in the late stages of PD. It is also used as monotherapy or adjunct therapy in early PD. The usual dose of amantadine is 200–400 mg per day divided into 2–3 doses/day. Recently extended-release preparation is available that can be administered once a day. Amantadine should be cautiously used in the elderly owing to the wide side effect profile, which includes hallucinations, confusion, nightmares, ankle edema, livedo reticularis, dry mouth, and hyponatremia.

Anticholinergics

Trihexyphenidyl and benztropine are inexpensive and low-risk monotherapy options for young patients with tremor-dominant PD. However, levodopa is superior to them for both tremor and bradykinesia improvement.[85] Trihexyphenidyl can be started at 2 mg once daily and gradually increased to 2 mg TID. Benztropine should be started at 0.5 mg once daily and gradually increased to 2 mg TID. They should be avoided in elderly patients due to common adverse effects such as dry mouth, postural giddiness, blurred vision due to angle-closure glaucoma, urinary retention, constipation, and confusion.

Newer Drugs

Istradefylline, a novel adenosine A2A receptor antagonist, antagonizes adenosine in the indirect pathway tipping the balance toward increased dopaminergic activity thereby improving the levodopa effect, reducing dyskinesia, and decreasing OFF periods.[86] It is given in once a dose with starting dose of 20 mg/day that can be increased to 40 mg/day. Several new drugs such as Pardoprunox (SLV-308) and Rytary (IPX066) are in the trial stages and are being explored as possible monotherapies.[87] Newer drugs with novel mechanisms of action such as immunotherapies to prevent α-synuclein aggregation and deposition, increased clearance by ambroxol, viral vector-mediated gene therapies, and stem cell therapies are in the experimental stage.

Pharmacological Management of NMS

Nonmotor symptoms are one of the major parts of PD symptomatology which can be more pronounced and troublesome in advanced PD. Appropriate therapy targeted toward these NMS helps in improving the quality of life of patients with PD over and above that offered by levodopa. Treatment of common NMS is provided in **Box 5**.[88–90]

Management of Advanced PD

Pharmacological Treatment of Motor Fluctuations

As the disease advances, a significant number of patients will be on multiple PD-related medications which need to be adjusted to obtain a good quality ON state without dyskinesia and reduce the overall OFF states. To adequately manage the motor fluctuations and levodopa-related dyskinesias, it is important to understand the interaction between the timing of the medications and the occurrence of different motor fluctuations. For example, wearing off and OFF states can be managed by prolonging the dopaminergic effect either by increasing levodopa, prolonging the levodopa effect either by taking long-acting preparation or by adding MAO-B or COMT inhibitors. Likewise, levodopa-induced

BOX 5 Pharmacological treatment of nonmotor symptoms.

1. *Neuropsychiatric symptoms*:
   - *Depression*: Selective serotonin reuptake inhibitors and selective norepinephrine reuptake inhibitors. Tricyclic antidepressants should be used with caution in old patients
   - *Psychosis*: Quetiapine, olanzapine, or clozapine
   - *Dementia*: Rivastigmine
2. *Sleep symptoms*:
   - *REM behavior disorder*: Clonazepam and melatonin
   - *Excessive daytime sleepiness*: Modafinil
   - *Restless leg syndrome*: Clonazepam
3. *Autonomic symptoms*:
   - *Urinary dysfunction*: Anticholinergic drugs—oxybutynin, alpha-1 agonists, and antispasmodics
   - *Erectile dysfunction*: Sildenafil
   - **Orthostatic hypotension*: Fludrocortisone, midodrine
4. *Gastrointestinal symptoms*:
   - *Constipation*: High-fiber diet and lactulose
   - *Drooling*: Anticholinergics (caution in elderly, bladder disturbances, and psychosis), intraparotid botulinum toxin injection
   - *Gastroparesis*: Domperidone, tegaserod, and mosapride
5. *Other symptoms*:
   - Pain usually responds to the optimization of dopaminergic treatment

*Nonpharmacological methods such as the use of elastic stockings, an increase in salt and water intake, and gradual change of posture should be tried in orthostatic hypotension before starting medication.

(REM: rapid eye movement)

peak-dose dyskinesias can be managed by either giving a lower but frequent dose of levodopa, the addition of DAs with a reduction of levodopa dose, or by adding amantadine. Management of various types of motor fluctuations is given in **Flowchart 2**.

Surgical and Other Device-aided Therapies in Advanced PD

With the progression of the disease, medication adjustment alone cannot satisfactorily improve the dyskinesia-free ON state without worsening the OFF periods. In addition, with advanced PD, the patient may not tolerate the combination of drugs reducing the options of medications that can be used. At this juncture, surgical and other device-aided therapies help in providing a good quality of life for a patient with advanced PD. Surgical intervention in the management of PD is typically restricted to advanced stages of PD and consists of either DBS or lesioning procedures. Magnetic resonance-guided focused ultrasound (MRgFUS) is a novel noninvasive lesioning therapy.[91] Other device-aided therapies are LCIG and continuous subcutaneous apomorphine pump (CSAP).[92] DBS, LCIG, and CSAP provide similar benefit in the control of motor fluctuation including dyskinesia and also improve certain NMS. They differ in the side effect profile and the choice should be individualized.

BOX 6 Indications and contraindications for DBS.

Indications for DBS:
- Levodopa-responsive PD
- Presence of motor fluctuations/dyskinesias
- Adequate trial of dopaminergic medications given
- Good family support
- Ability to come for programming

Contraindications:
- Atypical Parkinsonism
- Dementia
- Severe psychosis/depression
- Severe autonomic dysfunction/postural instability
- Severe systemic illness

Symptoms which may not improve after DBS:
- Levodopa nonresponsive symptoms of PD such as speech and swallowing disturbances, freezing, and postural instability
- Unpredictable OFF periods
- Cognitive impairment

Symptoms that may worsen or appear after DBS:
- Gait disturbances
- Dysarthria
- Mood/behavior disturbances
- Impulse control disorders

(DBS: deep brain stimulation; PD: Parkinson's disease)

Deep Brain Stimulation

Deep brain stimulation targeting either the subthalamic nucleus (STN) or globus pallidus interna (GPi) is widely accepted for advanced PD with inadequately controlled symptoms with medications **(Video 5)**. The common indications of DBS are to improve OFF state disability, peak-dose dyskinesia, and tremor **(Box 6)**. In addition, STN DBS will also result in a reduction in medications. Good response of motor symptoms to levodopa is a mandatory criterion for consideration of DBS.[93] However, patients of PD with tremors, even if not adequately responding to levodopa, can be subjected to DBS. Cognitive impairment, psychosis, autonomic dysfunction, severe psychiatric comorbidity or systemic illness, and advanced age in the patients are relative contraindications to DBS.[94] Unpredictable OFF states, severe freezing, gait and balance problems, and severe hypophonia unresponsive to levodopa may not improve with DBS. Appropriate patient selection is a critical step for a successful outcome after DBS. The ability of a patient to afford DBS and the recurring costs involved should also be considered before suggesting DBS. It is imperative to explain realistic outcomes of DBS to patients since several symptoms of PD do not improve after DBS.

Lesioning Procedures

The advent of DBS has significantly reduced the utility of lesioning procedures in PD, which were frequently performed in the past. The thalamus (ventral intermediate nucleus), GPi, and STN are the commonly used sites in PD. Although this procedure has been shown to produce improvement in some symptoms such as tremors, bilateral lesioning can lead to significant speech and bulbar side effects reducing the utility of lesioning in PD. At present, the use of lesioning in PD may be limited to thalamic lesioning in patients with treatment-resistant tremor-dominant PD especially when the tremor is significantly asymmetrical and predominantly affects the dominant hand.[95] Unilateral pallidotomy may be performed in cases with severe dyskinesia. STN lesioning is avoided due to severe adverse effects such as hemiballismus.

Other Device-aided Therapies

These therapies are often employed in patients either ineligible for DBS or those who are unwilling for surgical intervention. These are easily reversible if the patient decides to discontinue the therapy and hence can also be used as a bridge for eventual DBS surgery.[92]

Levodopa–carbidopa intestinal gel is administered by an endoscopically placed percutaneous gastrostomy tube extending to the upper jejunum. It can aid in the steady delivery of levodopa and can be maintained as monotherapy. Significant improvement in OFF states and dyskinesia is noted. However, device-related side effects such as abdominal pain are the most common side effect. In addition, patients may develop significant neuropathy with long-term use of pump. A CSAP, similar to LCIG, aims toward steady-state dopaminergic stimulation to improve OFF states without significant dyskinesias. The apomorphine is delivered by an external subcutaneous pump that can be carried around the neck or waist. The common side effects are local pain, subcutaneous nodules, and apomorphine-related cognitive and behavioral side effects. Both these modalities have the disadvantage of having an external device that needs to be carried around in contrast to a completely internalized device in DBS.

Nonpharmacological Treatment for PD

Despite optimal medical management, patients persist to experience a wide range of symptoms that significantly affect their quality of life. Several nonpharmacological managements such as physiotherapy, yoga, Tai chi, cognitive and behavior training, and dance intervention have been shown to produce symptomatic relief.[96,97] FOG, which is a troublesome motor complication, has been shown to respond to visual or auditory external cues. Visual cues in the form of striped floors have frequently been reported to aid in alleviating FOG.[98,99]

CONCLUSION

Parkinson's disease is a chronic, neurodegenerative disorder that shows significant variability in signs and symptoms based on the stage of illness. Diagnosis of PD in the early stages may be challenging and other diagnoses must be ruled out. NMS often overshadows the motor symptoms and due consideration must be given while planning treatment.

VIDEO LEGENDS

Video 1: Bradykinesia: Video demonstrates bradykinesia in the form of an asymmetric reduction (right>left) in amplitude of finger tapping, hand movement, rapid alternating movement and leg agility. The patient also has a stooped posture with reduced arm swing while walking, slowness of gait with freezing and a positive pull test.

Video 2: Tremor dominant Parkinson's disease (PD): Video demonstrates the tremor dominant phenotype of PD wherein the patient has a severe rest and action tremor of bilateral upper and lower limbs (left>right).

Video 3: Choreiform peak dose dyskinesia occurring post comsumption of dopaminergic medication (levodopa–carbidopa). Segment 1: Mild choreiform dyskinesia. Segment 2: Severe choreiform dyskinesia.

Video 4: Freezing of gait: The patient has significant gait freezing with improves significantly with visual cues.

Video 5: Effect of bilateral STN DBS in a patient with akinetic rigid variant of PD: In the Pre DBS, OFF state, the patient has significant bradykinesia and freezing of gait. In the post DBS. OFF state, the patient has no evident bradykinesia and gait is normal.

(DBS: deep brain stimulation; PD: Parkinson's disease; STN: subthalamic nucleus)

REFERENCES

1. Goetz CG. The history of Parkinson's disease: early clinical descriptions and neurological therapies. Cold Spring Harb Perspect Med. 2011;1(1):a008862.
2. de Lau LM, Breteler MM. Epidemiology of Parkinson's disease. Lancet Neurol. 2006;5(6):525-35.
3. Twelves D, Perkins KS, Counsell C. Systematic review of incidence studies of Parkinson's disease. Mov Disord. 2003;18(1):19-31.
4. Spica V, Pekmezovic T, Svetel M, Kostic VS. Prevalence of non-motor symptoms in young-onset versus late-onset Parkinson's disease. J Neurol. 2013;260(1):131-7.
5. Hughes AJ, Daniel SE, Kilford L, Lees AJ. Accuracy of clinical diagnosis of idiopathic Parkinson's disease: a clinicopathological study of 100 cases. J Neurol Neurosurg Psychiatry. 1992;55(3):181-4.
6. Braak H, Del Tredici K, Rub U, de Vos RA, Jansen Steur EN, Braak E. Staging of brain pathology related to sporadic Parkinson's disease. Neurobiol Aging. 2003;24(2):197-211.
7. Chaudhuri KR, Healy DG, Schapira AH, National Institute for Clinical E. Non-motor symptoms of Parkinson's disease: diagnosis and management. Lancet Neurol. 2006;5(3):235-45.
8. Zhang Z-X, Román GC. Worldwide occurrence of Parkinson's disease: an updated review. Neuroepidemiology. 1993;12(4): 195-208.
9. Hirsch L, Jette N, Frolkis A, Steeves T, Pringsheim T. The Incidence of Parkinson's Disease: A Systematic Review and Meta-Analysis. Neuroepidemiology. 2016;46(4):292-300.

10. Razdan S, Kaul RL, Motta A, Kaul S, Bhatt RK. Prevalence and pattern of major neurological disorders in rural Kashmir (India) in 1986. Neuroepidemiology. 1994;13(3):113-9.
11. Gourie-Devi M. Epidemiology of neurological disorders in India: review of background, prevalence and incidence of epilepsy, stroke, Parkinson's disease and tremors. Neurol India. 2014;62(6):588-98.
12. Das S, Sanyal K. Neuroepidemiology of major neurological disorders in rural Bengal. Neurol India. 1996;44(2):47-58.
13. Das S, Sanyal K, Moitra A. A pilot study on neuroepidemiology in urban Bengal. Indian J Public Health. 1998;42(2):34-36, 41.
14. Bharucha NE, Bharucha EP, Bharucha AE, Bhise AV, Schoenberg BS. Prevalence of Parkinson's disease in the Parsi community of Bombay, India. Arch Neurol. 1988;45(12):1321-3.
15. Simuni T, Caspell-Garcia C, Coffey CS, Weintraub D, Mollenhauer B, Lasch S, et al. Baseline prevalence and longitudinal evolution of non-motor symptoms in early Parkinson's disease: the PPMI cohort. J Neurol Neurosurg Psychiatry. 2018;89(1):78-88.
16. Muangpaisan W, Hori H, Brayne C. Systematic review of the prevalence and incidence of Parkinson's disease in Asia. J Epidemiol. 2009;19(6):281-93.
17. Surathi P, Kamble N, Bhalsing KS, Yadav R, Pal PK. Prescribing pattern for Parkinson's disease in Indian community before referral to tertiary center. Can J Neurol Sci. 2017;44:705-10.
18. Dorsey ER, Elbaz A, Nichols E, GBD 2016 Parkinson's Disease Collaborators. Global, regional, and national burden of Parkinson's disease, 1990–2016: a systematic analysis for the Global Burden of Disease Study 2016. Lancet Neurol. 2018;17(11):939-53.
19. Klein C, Westenberger A. Genetics of Parkinson's disease. Cold Spring Harb Perspect Med. 2012;2(1):a008888.
20. Chen H, Ritz B. The search for environmental causes of Parkinson's disease: Moving forward. J Parkinsons Dis. 2018;8(s1):S9-S17.
21. Visanji NP, Brooks PL, Hazrati LN, Lang AE. The prion hypothesis in Parkinson's disease: Braak to the future. Acta Neuropathol Commun. 2013;1(1):1-12.
22. Jankovic J. Progression of Parkinson disease: are we making progress in charting the course? Arch Neurol. 2005;62(3):351-2.
23. Helmich RC, Hallett M, Deuschl G, Toni I, Bloem BR. Cerebral causes and consequences of parkinsonian resting tremor: a tale of two circuits? Brain. 2012;135(Pt 11):3206-26.
24. Dirkx MF, den Ouden HE, Aarts E, Timmer MH, Bloem BR, Toni I, et al. Dopamine controls Parkinson's tremor by inhibiting the cerebellar thalamus. Brain. 2017;140(3):721-34.
25. van Nuland AJ, den Ouden HE, Zach H, Dirkx MFM, van Asten JJA, Scheenen TWJ, et al. GABAergic changes in the thalamocortical circuit in Parkinson's disease. Hum Brain Mapp. 2020;41(4):1017-29.
26. Schiesling C, Kieper N, Seidel K, Krüger R. Familial Parkinson's disease–genetics, clinical phenotype and neuropathology in relation to the common sporadic form of the disease. Neuropathol Applied Neurobiol. 2008;34(3):255-71.
27. Polymeropoulos MH, Lavedan C, Leroy E, Ide SE, Dehejia A, Dutra A, et al. Mutation in the α-synuclein gene identified in families with Parkinson's disease. Science. 1997;276(5321):2045-7.
28. Berg D, Postuma RB, Bloem B, Chan P, Dubois B, Gasser T, et al. Time to redefine PD? Introductory statement of the MDS Task Force on the definition of Parkinson's disease. Mov Disord. 2014;29(4):454-62.
29. Postuma RB, Berg D. Advances in markers of prodromal Parkinson disease. Nat Rev Neurol. 2016;12(11):622-34.
30. Chaudhuri KR, Schrag A, Weintraub D, Rizos A, Rodriguez-Blazquez C, Mamikonyan E, et al. The movement disorder society nonmotor rating scale: Initial validation study. Mov Disord. 2020;35(1):116-33.
31. Ondo WG. Motor complications in Parkinson's disease. Int J Neurosci. 2011;121 Suppl 2:37-44.
32. Giladi N, Treves TA, Simon ES, Shabtai H, Orlov Y, Kandinov B, et al. Freezing of gait in patients with advanced Parkinson's disease. J Neural Transm (Vienna). 2001;108(1):53-61.
33. Rizzo G, Copetti M, Arcuti S, Martino D, Fontana A, Logroscino G. Accuracy of clinical diagnosis of Parkinson disease. Neurology. 2016;86(6):566.
34. Gibb WR, Lees AJ. The relevance of the Lewy body to the pathogenesis of idiopathic Parkinson's disease. J Neurol Neurosurg Psychiatry. 1988;51(6):745-52.
35. Gelb DJ, Oliver E, Gilman S. Diagnostic criteria for Parkinson disease. Arch Neurol. 1999;56(1):33-9.
36. Larsen JP, Dupont E, Tandberg E. Clinical diagnosis of Parkinson's disease. Proposal of diagnostic subgroups classified at different levels of confidence. Acta Neurol Scand. 1994;89(4):242-51.
37. Calne D, Snow B, Lee C. Criteria for diagnosing Parkinson's disease. Ann Neurol. 1992;32(S1):S125-7.
38. Postuma RB, Berg D, Stern M, Poewe W, Olanow CW, Oertel W, et al. MDS clinical diagnostic criteria for Parkinson's disease. Move Disord. 2015;30(12):1591-601.
39. Marsili L, Rizzo G, Colosimo C. Diagnostic criteria for Parkinson's disease: from James Parkinson to the concept of prodromal disease. Front Neurol. 2018;9:156.
40. Bennett DA, Beckett LA, Murray AM, Shannon KM, Goetz CG, Pilgrim DM, et al. Prevalence of parkinsonian signs and associated mortality in a community population of older people. N Engl J Med. 1996;334(2):71-6.
41. Jankovic J. Essential tremor: clinical characteristics. Neurology. 2000;54(11 Suppl 4):S21-5.
42. Gilman S, Wenning GK, Low PA, Brooks DJ, Mathias CJ, Trojanowski JQ, et al. Second consensus statement on the diagnosis of multiple system atrophy. Neurology. 2008;71(9):670-6.
43. Williams DR, de Silva R, Paviour DC, Pittman A, Watt HC, Kilford L, et al. Characteristics of two distinct clinical phenotypes in pathologically proven progressive supranuclear palsy: Richardson's syndrome and PSP-parkinsonism. Brain. 2005;128(Pt 6):1247-58.
44. Litvan I, Mangone CA, McKee A, Verny M, Parsa A, Jellinger K, et al. Natural history of progressive supranuclear palsy (Steele-Richardson-Olszewski syndrome) and clinical predictors of survival: a clinicopathological study. J Neurol Neurosurg Psychiatry. 1996;60(6):615-20.
45. Stamelou M, Alonso-Canovas A, Bhatia KP. Dystonia in corticobasal degeneration: a review of the literature on 404 pathologically proven cases. Mov Disord. 2012;27(6):696-702.
46. Armstrong MJ, Litvan I, Lang AE, Bak TH, Bhatia KP, Borroni B, et al. Criteria for the diagnosis of corticobasal degeneration. Neurology. 2013;80(5):496-503.
47. Morishita T, Foote KD, Okun MS. INPH and Parkinson disease: differentiation by levodopa response. Nat Rev Neurol. 2010;6(1):52-6.
48. Ali K, Morris HR. Parkinson's disease: chameleons and mimics. Pract Neurol. 2015;15(1):14-25.
49. Gupta D, Kuruvilla A. Vascular parkinsonism: what makes it different? Postgrad Med J. 2011;87(1034):829-36.
50. Lehosit JB, Cloud LJ. (2015) Early Parkinsonism: Distinguishing Idiopathic Parkinson's disease from other syndromes. [online] Available from https://www.mdedge.com/jcomjournal/article/146588/neurology/early-parkinsonism-distinguishing-idiopathic-parkinsons-disease. [Last accessed April, 2023]
51. Shin HW, Chung SJ. Drug-induced parkinsonism. J Clin Neurol. 2012;8(1):15-21.
52. Brigo F, Erro R, Marangi A, Bhatia K, Tinazzi M. Differentiating drug-induced parkinsonism from Parkinson's disease: an update on non-motor symptoms and investigations. Parkinsonism Relat Disord. 2014;20(8):808-14.
53. Wenning GK, Stankovic I, Vignatelli L, Fanciulli A, Calandra-Buonaura G, Seppi K, et al. The movement disorder society criteria for the diagnosis of multiple system atrophy. Mov Disord. 2022;37(6):1131-48.
54. Höglinger GU, Respondek G, Stamelou M, Kurz C, Josephs KA, Lang AE, et al. Clinical diagnosis of progressive supranuclear palsy: the movement disorder society criteria. Mov Disord. 2017;32(6):853-64.
55. Mahlknecht P, Hotter A, Hussl A, Esterhammer R, Schocke M, Seppi K. Significance of MRI in diagnosis and differential diagnosis of Parkinson's disease. Neurodegener Dis. 2010;7(5):300-18.

56. Scherfler C, Gobel G, Muller C, Nocker M, Wenning GK, Schocke M, et al. Diagnostic potential of automated subcortical volume segmentation in atypical parkinsonism. Neurology. 2016;86(13): 1242-9.
57. Tuite P. Magnetic resonance imaging as a potential biomarker for Parkinson's disease. Transl Res. 2016;175:4-16.
58. Saeed U, Compagnone J, Aviv RI, Strafella AP, Black SE, Lang AE, et al. Imaging biomarkers in Parkinson's disease and Parkinsonian syndromes: current and emerging concepts. Transl Neurodegener. 2017;6:8.
59. Erro R, Schneider SA, Stamelou M, Quinn NP, Bhatia KP. What do patients with scans without evidence of dopaminergic deficit (SWEDD) have? New evidence and continuing controversies. J Neurol Neurosurg Psychiatry. 2016;87(3):319-23.
60. Papathanasiou ND, Boutsiadis A, Dickson J, Bomanji JB. Diagnostic accuracy of (1)(2)(3)I-FP-CIT (DaTSCAN) in dementia with Lewy bodies: a meta-analysis of published studies. Parkinsonism Relat Disord. 2012;18(3):225-9.
61. Morbelli S, Esposito G, Arbizu J, Barthel H, Boellaard R, Bohnen NI, et al. EANM practice guideline/SNMMI procedure standard for dopaminergic imaging in Parkinsonian syndromes 1.0. Eur J Nucl Med Mol Imag. 2020;47(8):1885-912.
62. Marek K, Jennings D, Seibyl J. Imaging the dopamine system to assess disease-modifying drugs: studies comparing dopamine agonists and levodopa. Neurology. 2003;61(6 Suppl 3):S43-48.
63. Li DH, He YC, Liu J, Chen SD. Diagnostic accuracy of transcranial sonography of the substantia nigra in Parkinson's disease: A systematic review and meta-analysis. Sci Rep. 2016;6:20863.
64. Treglia G, Cason E, Stefanelli A, Cocciolillo F, Di Giuda D, Fagioli G, et al. MIBG scintigraphy in differential diagnosis of Parkinsonism: a meta-analysis. Clin Auton Res. 2012;22(1):43-55.
65. Poewe W, Seppi K, Tanner CM, Halliday GM, Brundin P, Volkmann J, et al. Parkinson disease. Nat Rev Dis Primers. 2017;3:17013.
66. Scheperjans F. Can microbiota research change our understanding of neurodegenerative diseases? Neurodegener Dis Manag. 2016;6(2):81-5.
67. Stokholm MG, Danielsen EH, Hamilton-Dutoit SJ, Borghammer P. Pathological alpha-synuclein in gastrointestinal tissues from prodromal Parkinson disease patients. Ann Neurol. 2016;79(6):940-9.
68. Vilas D, Iranzo A, Tolosa E, Aldecoa I, Berenguer J, Vilaseca I, et al. Assessment of alpha-synuclein in submandibular glands of patients with idiopathic rapid-eye-movement sleep behaviour disorder: a case-control study. Lancet Neurol. 2016;15(7):708-18.
69. George J, Jose T, Behari M. Use of Indian smell identification test for evaluating olfaction in idiopathic Parkinson's disease patients in India. Neurol India. 2013;61(4):365-70.
70. Haehner A, Hummel T, Reichmann H. Olfactory loss in Parkinson's disease. Parkinsons Dis. 2011;2011:450939.
71. Tan EK, Jankovic J. Genetic testing in Parkinson disease: promises and pitfalls. Arch Neurol. 2006;63(9):1232-7.
72. McInerney-Leo A, Hadley DW, Gwinn-Hardy K, Hardy J. Genetic testing in Parkinson's disease. Mov Disord. 2005;20(1):1-10.
73. Goetz CG, Poewe W, Rascol O, Sampaio C, Stebbins GT, Counsell C, et al. Movement Disorder Society Task Force report on the Hoehn and Yahr staging scale: status and recommendations. Mov Disord. 2004;19(9):1020-8.
74. Ramaker C, Marinus J, Stiggelbout AM, Van Hilten BJ. Systematic evaluation of rating scales for impairment and disability in Parkinson's disease. Mov Disord. 2002;17(5):867-76.
75. Goetz CG, Tilley BC, Shaftman SR, Stebbins GT, Fahn S, Martinez-Martin P, et al. Movement Disorder Society-sponsored revision of the Unified Parkinson's Disease Rating Scale (MDS-UPDRS): scale presentation and clinimetric testing results. Mov Disord. 2008;23(15):2129-70.
76. Chaudhuri KR, Martinez-Martin P, Schapira AH, Stocchi F, Sethi K, Odin P, et al. International multicenter pilot study of the first comprehensive self-completed nonmotor symptoms questionnaire for Parkinson's disease: the NMSQuest study. Mov Disord. 2006;21(7):916-23.
77. Kleiner G, Fernandez HH, Chou KL, Fasano A, Duque KR, Hengartner D, et al. Non-motor fluctuations in Parkinson's disease: Validation of the non-motor fluctuation assessment questionnaire. Mov Disord. 2021;36(6):1392-400.
78. Glenardi G, Handayani T, Barus J, Mangkuliguna G. Inhaled Levodopa (CVT-301) for the Treatment of Parkinson Disease. Neurol Clin Pract. 2022;12(2):139.
79. DeMaagd G, Philip A. Parkinson's Disease and Its Management: Part 4: Treatment of Motor Complications. P T. 2015;40(11):747-73.
80. Group PS. Levodopa and the progression of Parkinson's disease. N Engl J Med. 2004;2004(351):2498-508.
81. Antonini A, Tolosa E, Mizuno Y, Yamamoto M, Poewe WH. A reassessment of risks and benefits of dopamine agonists in Parkinson's disease. Lancet Neurol. 2009;8(10):929-37.
82. Olanow CW, Rascol O, Hauser R, Feigin PD, Jankovic J, Lang A, et al. A double-blind, delayed-start trial of rasagiline in Parkinson's disease. N Engl J Med. 2009;361(13):1268-78.
83. Parkinson Study Group. Datatop: A multicenter controlled clinical trial in early parkinson's disease. Parkinson study group. Arch Neurol. 1989;46(10):1052-60.
84. Borgohain R, Szasz J, Stanzione P, Meshram C, Bhatt MH, Chirilineau D, et al. Two-year, randomized, controlled study of safinamide as add-on to levodopa in mid to late Parkinson's disease. Mov Disord. 2014;29(10):1273-80.
85. Sahoo LK, Holla VV, Batra D, Prasad S, Bhattacharya A, Kamble N, et al. Comparison of effectiveness of trihexyphenidyl and levodopa on motor symptoms in Parkinson's disease. J Neural Transm (Vienna). 2020;127(12):1599-606.
86. Berger AA, Winnick A, Welschmeyer A, Kaneb A, Berardino K, Cornett EM, et al. Istradefylline to Treat Patients with Parkinson's Disease Experiencing "Off" Episodes: A Comprehensive Review. Neurol Int. 2020;12(3):109-29.
87. Pahwa R, Lyons KE. Treatment of early Parkinson's disease. Curr Opin Neurol. 2014;27(4):442-9.
88. Muzerengi S, Contrafatto D, Chaudhuri KR. Non-motor symptoms: identification and management. Parkinsonism Relat Disord. 2007;13 Suppl 3:S450-6.
89. Sprenger F, Poewe W. Management of motor and non-motor symptoms in Parkinson's disease. CNS Drugs. 2013;27(4):259-72.
90. Aurora RN, Zak RS, Maganti RK, Auerbach SH, Casey KR, Chowdhuri S, et al. Best practice guide for the treatment of REM sleep behavior disorder (RBD). J Clin Sleep Med. 2010;6(1):85-95.
91. Schlesinger I, Sinai A, Zaaroor M. MRI-guided focused ultrasound in Parkinson's disease: A Review. Parkinsons Dis. 2017;2017:8124624.
92. Timpka J, Nitu B, Datieva V, Odin P, Antonini A. Device-aided treatment strategies in advanced Parkinson's disease. Int Rev Neurobiol. 2017;132:453-74.
93. Defer GL, Widner H, Marié RM, Rémy P, Levivier M. Core assessment program for surgical interventional therapies in Parkinson's disease (CAPSIT-PD). Mov Disord. 1999;14(4):572-84.
94. Lang AE, Widner H. Deep brain stimulation for Parkinson's disease: patient selection and evaluation. Mov Disord. 2002;17 Suppl 3: S94-101.
95. Okun MS, Vitek JL. Lesion therapy for Parkinson's disease and other movement disorders: update and controversies. Mov Disord. 2004;19(4):375-89.
96. Bloem BR, de Vries NM, Ebersbach G. Nonpharmacological treatments for patients with Parkinson's disease. Mov Disord. 2015;30(11):1504-20.
97. Li S, Dong J, Cheng C, Le W. Therapies for Parkinson's diseases: alternatives to current pharmacological interventions. J Neural Transm (Vienna). 2016;123(11):1279-99.
98. Okuma Y. Practical approach to freezing of gait in Parkinson's disease. Pract Neurol. 2014;14(4):222-30.
99. Ginis P, Nackaerts E, Nieuwboer A, Heremans E. Cueing for people with Parkinson's disease with freezing of gait: A narrative review of the state-of-the-art and novel perspectives. Ann Phys Rehabil Med. 2018;61(6):407-13.

72

CHAPTER

Parkinson Plus Syndromes

Divyani Garg, Vinay Goyal

INTRODUCTION

Parkinson-plus syndrome is an overarching term denoting a group of neurodegenerative conditions, in which patients demonstrate features of dopaminergic deficiency, such as hypomimia, rigidity, bradykinesia, tremor, and loss of postural reflexes.[1] However, unlike typical Parkinson's disease, the response to levodopa is poor and ill-sustained, loss of ambulation is early, and progression is more debilitating.[2] The conditions included within this broad term include progressive supranuclear palsy (PSP), multiple system atrophy (MSA), and corticobasal degeneration (CBD). Dementia with Lewy bodies (DLB) is also considered to be a part of this syndrome, although it is now believed to fall in the spectrum of Lewy Body dementia, along with Parkinson's disease with dementia (PDD). These four disorders are also popularly referred to as "atypical parkinsonism".[3]

Parkinson's plus syndrome includes both tauopathy [PSP and corticobasal syndrome (CBS)] and synucleinopathy (MSA and DLB). Some features of tauopathy include the presence of cognitive impairment, early falls, the presence of supranuclear gaze palsy, apraxia, myoclonus, dystonia, etc. Synucleinopathies like MSA have a prominence of autonomic dysfunction, manifesting as urinary urgency and urge incontinence, significant postvoid residue, frequency, erectile dysfunction, and orthostatic hypotension. These features combine with features of parkinsonism (bradykinesia, tremor, and rigidity) to varying extents. Apart from the common syndromes mentioned above, less common Parkinson-plus syndromes include frontotemporal dementia with chromosome 17 (FTDP-17), parkinsonism-dementia complex of Guam, pallidonigral degeneration, Wilson's disease, and Huntington's disease.[4]

It is important to recognize clinical features which are considered red flags for Parkinson-plus syndromes, as these syndromes usually indicate a poorer prognosis, greater morbidity, and earlier mortality in comparison to Parkinson's disease.

EPIDEMIOLOGY

The prevalence of PSP ranges from 5 to 10 per 100,000 individuals, while MSA is 5 per 100,000 individuals. For CBD, it is estimated to be 1 per 100,000 individuals. The prevalence of DLB in individuals above the age of 65 years is 0.4%.[3]

These are progressive disorders, with a median life span ranging between 5 and 7 years, although overall the range may be longer.

PROGRESSIVE SUPRANUCLEAR PALSY

Progressive supranuclear palsy was originally described by Steele, Richardson, and Olszewski in 1964, among patients who manifested with supranuclear gaze palsy, postural instability (PI), cognitive impairment, and dystonia.[5] They also described the presence of argyrophilic globose and flame-shaped inclusions throughout the brainstem and cortical and subcortical structures, which eventually were determined to be tau inclusions. PSP is a 4-repeat (4R) tauopathy, with tau filaments being arranged as straight filaments.[6] The usual age at onset is in the seventh decade. It is the most common Parkinson-plus syndrome.

Pathology

Extensive atrophy is observed, particularly involving the midbrain tectum, superior cerebellar peduncle (SCP), subthalamic nucleus, and frontal cortices.[7] Tufted astrocytes are pathognomonic for PSP. 4R globose neurofibrillary tangles, coiled bodies, and threads are also seen.

Clinical Phenotypes

- Although 10 subtypes of PSP have now been described, certain features are classical, as seen in PSP-Richardson syndrome (PSP-RS).
- *Face*: Staring look with decreased blinking, procerus dystonia (referred to as the "procerus sign" or "omega sign"), prominent nasolabial folds, furrowed brow—giving rise to an "angry" look
- *Speech*: Hypophonic, growling
- *Gait*: Broad based, slightly ataxic, arms extended, referred to as the "gunslinger" gait. "Drunken sailor" gait refers to difficulty in pivoting while turning, leading to an unstable gait.
- *Rocket sign*: Tendency to suddenly get up from a chair, due to loss of insight.
- *Applause sign*: Frontal dysfunction, in which the patient perseveres in clapping despite being instructed to clap only thrice.
- *Eyes*: Multiple eye signs are seen in PSP. These include:
  - Square wave jerks
  - Loss of vertical optokinetic nystagmus
  - Slow vertical saccades
  - Round-the-houses sign
  - Zig-zag sign[8]
  - Vertical supranuclear gaze palsy
  - Blepharospasm, apraxia of eyelid opening

The other rarer variants of PSP include:[9]

- *PSP-parkinsonism (PSP-P)*: These patients have levodopa-responsive, asymmetric parkinsonism with rest tremors. The levodopa response is soon lost. The patients go on to develop the classic signs of PSP. This is the second most common type after PSP-RS.[10]
- *PSP-pure gait freezing (PSP-PGF)*: These patients develop early gait freezing, loss of balance.
- *PSP-speech/language disorder (PSP-SL)*: Nonfluent primary progressive aphasia or progressive apraxia of speech
- *PSP-CBS* : Associated with the corticobasal syndrome
- *PSP-ocular motor dysfunction (PSP-OM)*: Initial symptoms with oculomotor features
- *PSP-predominant frontal presentation (PSP-F)*: Initial frontal features, including behavior and personality changes
- *PSP-cerebellar ataxia (PSP-C)*: Ataxia is an initial feature
- *PSP-primary lateral sclerosis (PSP-PLS)*: Begins with spasticity, similar to *PLS*
- PSP-Pi

  These are summarized in **Table 1**.

TABLE 1: Some variants of PSP with main clinical features.

PSP variant	Chief clinical features
PSP-RS	Classical phenotype, most common. Characterized by early falls, bradykinesia, eye signs, and frontal lobe dysfunction
PSP-P	• May be misdiagnosed as PD • Characterized by asymmetrical parkinsonism, limb rigidity, early rapid progression, axial rigidity, and eye signs may be absent in the early stages
PSP-PAGF	Gait initiation failure, axial rigidity, and postural instability; parkinsonian features are usually lacking
PSP-PNFA	Language dysfunction and apraxia of speech
PSP-CBS	Combination of PSP with cortical sensory loss, dystonia, myoclonus, and alien limb phenomenon
PSP-F	Behavioral disturbances, social disinhibition, and emotional outbursts
PSP-C	Rare, cerebellar signs seen

(CBS: corticobasal syndrome; PD: Parkinson's disease; PAGF: pure akinesia with gait freezing; PNFA: progressive nonfluent aphasia; PSP-C: progressive supranuclear palsy-cerebellar ataxia; PSP-F: progressive supranuclear palsy-frontal; PSP-P: progressive supranuclear palsy-parkinsonism)

Radiological Features

Many radiological features have been described in PSP, based on the differential atrophy of the midbrain compared to pons.[11]

Magnetic Resonance Imaging

- *Hummingbird sign*: Midbrain atrophy on the sagittal plane, with the concavity of the upper border, resembling the head and bill of a hummingbird. The body of the bird is formed by the preserved pons.
- *Mickey Mouse sign*: Rounded appearance of the cerebral peduncles at the midbrain level on the axial section.
- *Morning glory sign*: Concavity of the margins of the tegmentum of the midbrain in the axial section
- *MR Parkinsonism index (MRPI)*: MRPI is a ratio of the pons: midbrain area viz-a-viz area of the middle cerebellar peduncle (MCP) compared to SCP [MRPI = (P/M)*(MCP/SCP)]. MRPI above 13.55 may help to distinguish PSP-RS from MSA-P and PD.[12]
- *Midbrain to pons area ratio*: The normal ratio is 0.24. A ratio of below 0.12 indicates significant midbrain atrophy in PSP.
- *Midbrain anterior-to-posterior diameter*: Reduction of the midbrain anteroposterior diameter below 12 mm from the interpeduncular groove.

Positron Emission Tomography

Hypometabolism involving the frontal cortex, midbrain, cingulate cortex, caudate, and thalamus may be seen.

Single-photon Emission Computed Tomography

Hypoperfusion involves the same regions as on positron emission tomography (PET).

Dopamine Active Transporter Scan

Decreased dopamine binding in the putamen and caudate nucleus is seen in PSP.

Diagnosis

The clinical diagnosis of PSP is based on the Movement Disorders Society criteria, published in 2017.[13] Patients have to meet basic criteria, that is, mandatory inclusion and exclusion criteria. There are also four core features (ocular motor dysfunction, PI, akinesia, and cognitive dysfunction), with three levels of certainty: level 1 (higher certainty) to level 3 (lower certainty). Certain clinical clues and imaging findings constitute supportive criteria. Clinical clues include levodopa resistance, hypokinetic-spastic dysarthria, dysphagia, and photophobia. Imaging clues include predominantly midbrain atrophy/hypometabolism, and postsynaptic dopamine dysfunction of the striatum.

Treatment

Although there is no curative therapy, there are many symptoms in PSP that can be addressed.[14]

Motor symptoms of parkinsonism—a trial of levodopa should be considered for all patients with PSP. Levodopa can be incremented every 2 weeks, which is a faster rate compared to patients with PD and built up to 1,000 mg/day. If there is no response, levodopa should be tapered off and stopped over 6–8 weeks. Dopaminergic agents may also be used.

Amantadine may also assist in improving energy, reducing fatigue and improving axial rigidity.

In PSP-PGF, cholinesterase inhibitors (ChEIs) such as donepezil may lead to improvement.

Botulinum toxin may help in the management of disabling dystonia. Pseudobulbar affect may respond to selective serotonin reuptake inhibitors like sertraline or citalopram.

CORTICOBASAL DEGENERATION

Corticobasal degeneration is a 4R tauopathy. The terms "CBD" and "CBS" are often used interchangeably. The former term refers to a neuropathological entity, whereas the latter term refers to a phenotypic syndrome. In 2002, pathological criteria were established.[15] In 2013, clinical diagnostic criteria were established.[16] CBD can present in diverse manners, including the classical CBS phenotype, PSP, Alzheimer's disease, and FTD with TDP-43.[17] The usual age of onset is in the mid-sixties. The median survival is 5.5–8 years. **Figure 1** represents the CBS-CBD overlap.

Pathology

Corticobasal degeneration is a tauopathy and is characterized by the presence of hyperphosphorylated tau protein. Astrocytic plaques are a hallmark.[18] Ballooned/achromatic neurons are pathognomonic for CBD.[19] Another important pathological feature is the presence of astrocytic plaques in CBD, unlike tufted astrocytes seen in PSP. CBD is considered to be a network disorder. In the earlier stages, the dorsolateral prefrontal cortex and basal ganglia are chiefly affected. In the more advanced stages, posterior areas also become involved.

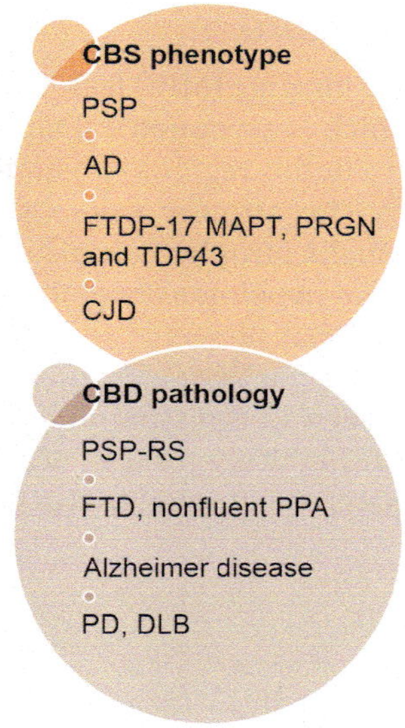

FIG. 1: Overlap of corticobasal degeneration pathology with corticobasal phenotype.

(AD: Alzheimer's disease; CBD: corticobasal degeneration; CBS: corticobasal syndrome; CJD: Creutzfeldt–Jakob disease; DLB: dementia with Lewy bodies; FTDP-17: frontotemporal dementia with chromosome 17; MAPT: microtubule-associated protein tau; PD: Parkinson disease; PPA: primary progressive aphasia; PRGN: progranulin; PSP: progressive supranuclear palsy; RS: Richardson's syndrome)

Clinical Features

A hallmark feature of CBD is striking asymmetry or even unilaterality.[20] CBD features a combination of cortical and extrapyramidal dysfunction. Features of cortical dysfunction include cortical sensory deficits, alien limb phenomenon, and apraxia. Features of extrapyramidal dysfunction include parkinsonism, dystonia, and myoclonus.

Alien limb phenomenon, seen in up to 50% of patients, may be of the posterior or sensory type, which is associated with hemi-neglect.[21] It may be stimulus-induced and position dependent. The patient perceives that the limb is alien or not part of his body. Alien limb phenomenon may also be of the anterior or frontal type. It affects the dominant hand and is characterized by inter manual conflict. In inter manual conflict, the affected hand interferes with the activities of the opposite hand. Other frontal release signs may be associated.

Dystonia and myoclonus are also seen. The myoclonus is of the cortical type and affects the distal limb. Parkinsonism is highly asymmetrical. Apraxia is a hallmark feature of CBS and is severe.

Radiological Features

Magnetic resonance imaging (MRI) features of CBD include cortical atrophy which is asymmetrical and predominantly involves the perirolandic regions, posterior frontal, and parietal regions.[22] The atrophy worsens as the disease advances. Basal ganglia atrophy may also be seen. Corpus callosum atrophy and hypointensity of the basal ganglia on T2-weighted imaging may be seen.

On the dopamine active transporter (DAT) scan, reduced uptake is seen in the striatum and asymmetrical uptake involving the hemispheres. PET scan may also show decreased metabolism over the perisylvian region, thalamus, and striatum.

Diagnosis

The diagnostic criteria by Armstrong et al. are used to diagnose CBD.[16] Probable CBD requires the presence of asymmetric features of insidious onset and gradual progression. At least two cortical features must be present out of orobuccal or limb apraxia, cortical sensory loss, and alien limb phenomenon more than simple levitation. At least two extrapyramidal features must be present out of limb rigidity/akinesia, limb dystonia, and limb myoclonus.

Corticobasal Degeneration Phenotypes

These include:

- CBS (probable/possible)
- Frontal behavioral spatial syndrome
- Nonfluent/agrammatic variant of primary progressive aphasia
- PSP syndrome

Treatment

There is currently no disease modifying therapy for CBD. Treatment is symptomatic. Parkinsonism may demonstrate mild-to-moderate response to levodopa therapy, although the response is transitory. Myoclonus is treated with clonazepam. Dystonia may need botulinum neurotoxin therapy or baclofen. Tremor may be managed using topiramate, propranolol, primidone, or clonazepam. Depression may necessitate serotonin reuptake inhibitors.

MULTIPLE SYSTEM ATROPHY

Multiple system atrophy is a sporadic, adult-onset, and neurodegenerative condition characterized by prominent autonomic failure, in varying combinations with parkinsonism and cerebellar dysfunction.[23] Based on selective neuronal loss in either the striatonigral pathways or the olivopontocerebellar pathways, it is subtyped into MSA-parkinsonism type (MSA-P) or MSA-cerebellar type (MSA-C). The disease is inexorably progressive, with a mean survival of 7–9 years.

Pathology

In MSA-C, there may be marked atrophy of the pons and MCPs, substantia nigra, locus coeruleus, striatum, and Onuf's nucleus in the sacral spinal cord.[24] Loss of neurons in the intermediolateral column of the spinal cord leads to autonomic dysfunction. Lewy bodies are not seen. Glial cytoplasmic inclusions (GCI) are considered to be the hallmark of MSA, and are present in the motor and premotor cortices, striatal, cerebellar, and autonomic nervous systems. GCIs contain alpha-synuclein.

Clinical Features

Although MSA is defined as occurring above the age of 30 years, the usual age at onset is in the sixth decade. Young onset MSA is defined as onset between the ages of 30 and 40 years.[25] A prodromal premotor phase is known, characterized by urinary or sexual dysfunction, rapid eye movement sleep behavior disorder (RBD), stridor, etc.

Autonomic failure is usually an early feature. Features of autonomic dysfunction include lower urinary tract symptoms, and features of cardiovascular autonomic dysfunction. Urinary dysfunction includes urinary frequency, urgency, and significant urinary retention, in the absence of other extenuating causes, such as benign prostatic hyperplasia in men and pelvic floor prolapse in women, etc. In comparison to autonomic dysfunction in PD, where the pathology is postganglionic, in MSA, autonomic dysfunction is preganglionic.

Features of cardiovascular autonomic dysfunction include orthostatic hypotension, which may present as presyncope, dizziness, nausea or fatigue on standing, or coat hanger pain. Objectively, orthostatic hypotension is defined as a fall in systolic BP by 20 mm Hg or diastolic BP by 10 mm Hg at three minutes of standing. In the new diagnostic criteria, this time may be extended up to 10 minutes of standing, to satisfy the criteria for probable MSA.[26]

Patients with MSA-P demonstrate the predominance of parkinsonian features, although some features of cerebellar ataxia are also usually present. Similarly, patients with MSA-C demonstrate predominant cerebellar features with variable degrees of parkinsonism. MSA patients infrequently demonstrate the typical "pill-rolling" tremor associated with PD. Myoclonic tremor or polyminimyoclonus may be observed. Other features of MSA include postural abnormalities (disproportionate anterocollis, camptocormia, and Pisa syndrome), orofacial dyskinesias involving the lower face, contractures of the hands and feet, cold hands and feet, and other features. "Wheelchair sign" refers to the early loss of ambulation in these patients within 5 years of onset of motor symptoms.

Nonmotor features include inspiratory stridor, snoring, pathological laughter, and crying. Inspiratory stridor may occur in advanced stages of the disease, due to atrophy of the posterior cricoarytenoid muscles. Sleep-related disorders include obstructive sleep apnea (OSA) and RBD.

Radiological Features

Magnetic Resonance Imaging

- *Putaminal rim/slit sign*: Hyperintense signal change along the posterolateral putamen in MSA-P, due to neuronal loss and gliosis.
- *Hot-cross bun sign*: Atrophy of the median raphe and transverse pontine fibers on the axial section, giving rise to a cruciform appearance. The pontine tegmentum and corticospinal tracts remain preserved.
- Atrophy and signal change in the MCPs. The normal width of the MCP is 9.8 ± 0.66 mm, which is significantly reduced in MSA.
- Cerebellar and pontine atrophy

Fluorodeoxyglucose-positron Emission Tomography Scan

Decreased striatal metabolism is seen in MSA. In MSA-C, cerebellar and pontine hypometabolism may be seen additionally, whereas striatal hypometabolism is prominent in MSA-P.

Dopaminergic Imaging

^{18}F dopa-PET shows reduced uptake in the posterior putamen, with an anteroposterior gradient, as well as reduced caudate uptake. Single-photon emission computed tomography (SPECT) and DAT show decreased striatal binding, which is usually symmetrical.

Metaiodobenzylguanidine Scintigraphy

Due to the postganglionic nature of sympathetic dysfunction, PD patients show reduced innervation on cardiac metaiodobenzylguanidine (MIBG) scan, which is normal among patients with MSA.[27]

Diagnosis

Diagnosis is based on the recently published diagnostic criteria, published by the Movement Disorders society.[28] Four levels of diagnostic certainty have been established—(1) neuropathologically established MSA, (2) clinically established MSA, (3) clinically probable MSA, (4) and possible prodromal MSA. The hallmark is autonomic dysfunction, which is defined based on the presence of any one of unexplained urinary urge incontinence, unexplained voiding difficulties with postvoid residue >100 mL, or neurogenic orthostatic hypotension at 3 minutes standing [drop in systolic blood pressure (BP) of at least 20 mm Hg and diastolic BP of at least 10 mm Hg].

Additionally, patients should have either poorly levodopa-responsive parkinsonism or cerebellar syndrome. In addition, patients should demonstrate at least two supportive features and one MRI feature to fulfill the diagnosis of clinically established MSA. Supportive features include rapid progression within 3 years of onset of motor symptoms, significant PI within 3 years of onset of motor symptoms, and levodopa-induced craniocervical dystonia[29] in the absence of limb dystonia, severe dysphagia/dysarthria within 3 years of motor onset, and unexplained Babinski sign.

Treatment

For the treatment of parkinsonism, levodopa therapy may yield some response in 30% of the cases, although it is poorly sustained. Patients should be given a trial of 1,000 mg of levodopa for at least 1 month before labeling to have levodopa nonresponsiveness. Levodopa may induce craniocervical dystonias without limb dyskinesias. No specific treatment is available for ataxia. Dystonia may require treatment with botulinum toxin injection.

Management of autonomic dysfunction is paramount.[30] Several nonpharmacological measures may be of benefit for orthostatic hypotension, such as frequent, smaller meals, increased fluid intake, several physical maneuvers while standing, and the use of elastic stockings and abdominal binders. Pharmacological measures include fludrocortisone, midodrine, pyridostigmine, and ephedrine. Urinary urgency and urge incontinence may be managed using oxybutynin, and trospium chloride. For significant postvoid residue, clean intermittent catheterization may be of benefit.

DEMENTIA WITH LEWY BODIES

The term Lewy body dementias refer to DLB and PDD.[31] Both DLB and PDD are characterized by the presence of cortical Lewy bodies. Lewy body dementias are characterized by the presence of dementia, visual hallucinations, fluctuations, RBD, and visuospatial abnormalities. In DLB, dementia usually occurs early in the course of the disease, preceding parkinsonism. In PDD, dementia occurs in the setting of well-established PD.[32]

Pathology

Neuropathology of both DLB and PDD demonstrates limbic and cortical Lewy bodies and Lewy neurites, which are aggregates of alpha-synuclein. There is a loss of dopaminergic neurons in the midbrain and cholinergic neurons in the ventral forebrain neurons. Neuritic plaques containing amyloid and neurofibrillary tangles are also seen.

Clinical Features

Dementia

Cognitive impairment is an early feature of DLB and sets in before the advent of extrapyramidal features.[33] Visual hallucinations, disorders of attention and executive function, and short-term memory impairment which improves with cueing (retrieval deficit) are prominent features.

Neuropsychiatric Features

Visual hallucinations occur, which are usually animate and vivid. Visual hallucinations are present in 54–70% of patients with DLB.[34] Although visual hallucinations are usually simple, complex hallucinations can also occur. The patient may see small animals, children, or deceased relatives.[35] Initially, these delusions do not provoke emotion or fear. Visual illusions may also occur, particularly in the dark, in which objects may be mistaken for a person. Delusions of persecution, paranoia, and theft may also occur. The patient may mistake their partner for an imposter, referred to as Capgras syndrome.

Parkinsonism

Extrapyramidal features are usually sent in after the onset of dementia. Parkinsonism is usually symmetric, although an asymmetrical pill-rolling rest tremor may be present. Unlike PD, the response to levodopa is poor and ill-sustained.

Fluctuations

These are variations in alertness and attention that fluctuate throughout the day. The patient may lose the train of thought, appear to daydream, stare into space, have episodes of disorganized speech, or sleep more than usual during the day, despite adequate sleep the previous night.[36]

Other Features

Neuroleptic sensitivity is an important feature of DLB.[37] Patients with DLB may experience significant worsening of parkinsonism on exposure to neuroleptic drugs, as well as cognitive deterioration and impaired alertness and attention. They are also predisposed to the neuroleptic malignant syndrome. Other features of DLB include RBD, autonomic dysfunction, and repeated, early falls.

Radiological Features

Magnetic Resonance Imaging

Atrophy in the posterior parietal cortices is seen, with relative preservation of the mesial temporal structures, which are affected by Alzheimer disease.[38]

Single-photon Emission Computed Tomography/Positron Emission Tomography Imaging

Generalized low uptake on SPECT/PET with reduced occipital activity is seen. "Cingulate island sign" may also be seen. In the "cingulate island sign", a higher metabolism is seen in the posterior cingulate region compared to the cuneus and precuneus region.[39]

Dopamine Active Transporter Imaging

Reduced striatal binding is seen in DLB, but not in Alzheimer's disease.

Diagnosis

The diagnostic criteria for DLB were revised in 2017 by the fourth consensus statement of the DLB Consortium.[40] The diagnostic categories include probable and possible DLB. Essential criteria are required for diagnosis, which includes the presence of cognitive impairment, which interferes with social or occupational function or activities of daily living. The initial deficits involve attention, visuospatial function, and executive function, but may evolve to involve short-term memory retrieval. Core clinical features include fluctuations in attention/alertness, visual hallucinations, RBD, and parkinsonism. Supportive clinical features include neuroleptic sensitivity, falls, syncope, autonomic dysfunction, nonvisual hallucinations, hyposmia, hypersomnia, delusions, mood changes, and apathy.

Supportive biomarkers include relative preservation of mesial temporal lobes on CT/MRI, decreased uptake on PET/SPECT with reduced activity in the occipital regions with cingulate island sign, posterior slowing on EEG.[32]

Treatment

For cognitive symptoms, ChEIs including donepezil and rivastigmine are used.[41] Memantine may also have some benefits for cognitive symptoms. ChEIs also improve apathy and hallucinations and delusions. Antipsychotics are usually avoided due to neuroleptic sensitivity. Low-dose quetiapine and clozapine on pimavanserin may be of some benefit. For depression, selective serotonin reuptake inhibitors, serotonin-norepinephrine reuptake inhibitors, and mirtazapine may be of use. For parkinsonism, levodopa therapy may be tried at the minimum dose that does not worsen psychotic features **(Table 2)**.[42]

TABLE 2: Treatment options for dementia with Lewy bodies.

Domain	Treatment
Cognitive dysfunction	Cholinesterase inhibitors, NMDA antagonists
Extrapyramidal features	Levodopa
Mood symptoms	Antidepressants (SSRIs, SNRIs)
Sleep related issues	Benzodiazepines, melatonin
Orthostatic hypotension	Fludrocortisone, midodrine

(NMDA: N-methyl-D-aspartate; SNRI: selective norepinephrine reuptake inhibitor; SSRI: selective serotonin reuptake inhibitor)

CONCLUSION

Parkinsonism-plus syndromes include various forms of atypical parkinsonism, including PSP, MSA, CBD, and DLB. These syndromes are characterized by distinct clinical and neuropathological features, but share certain common features, including a lack of sustained response to levodopa therapy, more rapid progression and poorer prognosis compared to Parkinson's disease. These syndromes include both tauopathies (PSP and CBD) and synucleinopathies (MSA and DLB). Diagnostic criteria have evolved, to increase diagnostic certainty. In the absence of definitive disease modifying therapy, treatment remains largely symptomatic.

REFERENCES

1. Olfati N, Shoeibi A, Litvan I. Progress in the treatment of Parkinson-Plus syndromes. Parkinsonism Relat Dis. 2019;59:101-10.
2. McFarland NR. Diagnostic Approach to Atypical Parkinsonian Syndromes. Continuum (Minneap Minn). 2016;22(4 Movement Disorders):1117-42.
3. Levin J, Kurz A, Arzberger T, Giese A, Höglinger GU. The Differential Diagnosis and Treatment of Atypical Parkinsonism. Dtsch Arztebl Int. 2016;113(5):61-9.
4. Mitra K, Gangopadhaya PK, Das SK. Parkinsonism plus syndrome—a review. Neurol India. 2003;51(2):183-8.
5. Steele JC, Richardson JC, Olszewski J. Progressive supranuclear palsy. a heterogeneous degeneration involving the brain stem, basal ganglia and cerebellum with vertical gaze and pseudobulbar palsy, nuchal dystonia and dementia. Arch Neurol. 1964;10:333-59.
6. Arai T, Ikeda K, Akiyama H, Shikamoto Y, Tsuchiya K, Yagishita S, et al. Distinct isoforms of tau aggregated in neurons and glial cells in brains of patients with Pick's disease, corticobasal degeneration and progressive supranuclear palsy. Acta Neuropathol. 2001;101(2):167-73.
7. Dickson DW, Rademakers R, Hutton ML. Progressive supranuclear palsy: pathology and genetics. Brain Pathol. 2007;17(1):74-82.
8. Abate F, Picillo M, Della Rocca G, Barone P, Erro R. The "zig-zag" sign in progressive supranuclear palsy. Parkinsonism Relat Disord. 2020;79:86-7.
9. Krzosek P, Madetko N, Migda A, Migda B, Jaguś D, Alster P. Differential diagnosis of rare subtypes of progressive supranuclear palsy and PSP-like syndromes—infrequent manifestations of the most common form of atypical parkinsonism. Front Aging Neurosci. 2022;14:804385.
10. Ling H. Clinical approach to progressive supranuclear palsy. J Mov Disord. 2016;9(1):3-13.
11. Whitwell JL, Höglinger GU, Antonini A, Bordelon Y, Boxer AL, Colosimo C, et al. Radiological biomarkers for diagnosis in PSP: Where are we and where do we need to be? Mov Disord. 2017;32(7): 955-71.
12. Nigro S, Antonini A, Vaillancourt DE, Seppi K, Ceravolo R, Strafella AP, et al. Automated MRI Classification in Progressive Supranuclear Palsy: A Large International Cohort Study. Mov Disord. 2020;35(6):976-83.
13. Hoglinger GU, Respondek G, Stamelou M, Kurz C, Josephs KA, Lang AE, et al. Clinical diagnosis of progressive supranuclear palsy: The movement disorder society criteria. Mov Disord. 2017;32(6): 853-64.
14. Rowe JB, Holland N, Rittman T. Progressive supranuclear palsy: Diagnosis and management. Pract Neurol. 2021;21(5):376-83.
15. Dickson DW, Bergeron C, Chin SS, Duyckaerts C, Horoupian D, Ikeda K, et al. Office of rare diseases neuropathologic criteria for corticobasal degeneration. J Neuropathol Exp Neurol. 2002;61(11): 935-46.
16. Armstrong MJ, Litvan I, Lang AE, Bak TH, Bhatia KP, Borroni B, et al. Criteria for the diagnosis of corticobasal degeneration. Neurology. 2013;80(5):496-503.
17. Ling H, O'Sullivan SS, Holton JL, Revesz T, Massey LA, Williams DR, et al. Does corticobasal degeneration exist? A clinicopathological re-evaluation. Brain. 2010;133(Pt 7):2045-57.
18. Parmera JB, Rodriguez RD, Studart Neto A, Nitrini R, Brucki SMD. Corticobasal syndrome: A diagnostic conundrum. Dement Neuropsychol. 2016;10(4):267-75.
19. Rebeiz JJ, Kolodny EH, Richardson EP. Corticodentatonigral degeneration with neuronal achromasia: a progressive disorder of late adult life. Trans Am Neurol Assoc. 1967;92:23-26.
20. Constantinides VC, Paraskevas GP, Paraskevas PG, Stefanis L, Kapaki E. Corticobasal degeneration and corticobasal syndrome: A review. Clin Parkinsonism Relat Disord. 2019;1:66-71.
21. Graff-Radford J, Rubin MN, Jones DT, Aksamit AJ, Ahlskog JE, Knopman DS, et al. The alien limb phenomenon. J Neurol. 2013; 260(7):1880-8.
22. Koyama M, Yagishita A, Nakata Y, Hayashi M, Bandoh M, Mizutani T. Imaging of corticobasal degeneration syndrome. Neuroradiology. 2007;49(11):905-12.
23. Fanciulli A, Stankovic I, Krismer F, Seppi K, Levin J, Wenning GK. Multiple system atrophy. Int Rev Neurobiol. 2019;149:137-92.
24. Koga S, Dickson DW. Recent advances in neuropathology, biomarkers and therapeutic approach of multiple system atrophy. J Neurol Neurosurg Psychiatry. 2018;89(2):175-84.
25. Batla A, De Pablo-Fernandez E, Erro R, Reich M, Calandra-Buonaura G, Barbosa P, et al. Young-onset multiple system atrophy: Clinical and pathological features. Mov Disord. 2018;33(7):1099-107.
26. Sun Z, Jia D, Shi Y, Hou X, Yang X, Guo J, et al. Prediction of orthostatic hypotension in multiple system atrophy and Parkinson disease. Sci Rep. 2016;6:21649.
27. Skowronek C, Zange L, Lipp A. Cardiac 123I-MIBG Scintigraphy in Neurodegenerative Parkinson Syndromes: Performance and Pitfalls in Clinical Practice. Front Neurol. 2019;10:152.
28. Wenning GK, Stankovic I, Vignatelli L, Fanciulli A, Calandra-Buonaura G, Seppi K, et al. The movement disorder society criteria for the diagnosis of multiple system atrophy. Mov Disord. 2022;37(6):1131-48.
29. Boesch S, Wenning G, Ransmayr G, Poewe W. Dystonia in multiple system atrophy. J Neurol Neurosurg Psychiatry. 2002;72(3):300-3.
30. Burns MR, McFarland NR. Current management and emerging therapies in multiple system atrophy. Neurotherapeutics. 2020;17(4):1582-602.
31. Gomperts SN. Lewy Body Dementias: Dementia with Lewy bodies and Parkinson disease dementia. Continuum (Minneap Minn). 2016;22(2, Dementia):435-63.
32. Armstrong MJ. Advances in dementia with Lewy bodies. Ther Adv Neurol Disord. 2021;14:17562864211057666.
33. Goldman JG, Williams-Gray C, Barker RA, Duda JE, Galvin JE. The spectrum of cognitive impairment in Lewy body diseases. Mov Disord. 2014;29(5):608-21.
34. Heitz C, Noblet V, Cretin B, Philippi N, Kremer L, Stackfleth M, et al. Neural correlates of visual hallucinations in dementia with Lewy bodies. Alzheimers Res Ther. 2015;7(1):6.

35. Cagnin A, Gnoato F, Jelcic N, Favaretto S, Zarantonello G, Ermani M, et al. Clinical and cognitive correlates of visual hallucinations in dementia with Lewy bodies. J Neurol Neurosurg Psychiatry. 2013;84(5):505-10.
36. Ferman TJ, Smith GE, Boeve BF, Ivnik RJ, Petersen RC, Knopman D, et al. DLB fluctuations: Specific features that reliably differentiate DLB from AD and normal aging. Neurology. 2004;62(2):181-7.
37. Baskys A. Lewy body dementia: the litmus test for neuroleptic sensitivity and extrapyramidal symptoms. J Clin Psychiatry. 2004;65(Suppl 11):16-22.
38. Scamarcia PG, Agosta F, Caso F, Filippi M. Update on neuroimaging in non-Alzheimer's disease dementia: a focus on the Lewy body disease spectrum. Curr Opin Neurol. 2021;34(4):532-8.
39. Graff-Radford J, Murray ME, Lowe VJ, Boeve BF, Ferman TJ, Przybelski SA, et al. Dementia with Lewy bodies: basis of cingulate island sign. Neurology. 2014;83(9):801-9.
40. McKeith IG, Boeve BF, Dickson DW, Halliday G, Taylor JP, Weintraub D, et al. Diagnosis and management of dementia with Lewy bodies: Fourth consensus report of the DLB consortium. Neurology. 2017;89(1):88-100.
41. Boot BP, McDade EM, McGinnis SM, Boeve BF. Treatment of Dementia with Lewy Bodies. Curr Treat Options Neurol. 2013;15(6):738-64.
42. Molloy S, McKeith IG, O'Brien JT, Burn DJ. The role of levodopa in the management of dementia with Lewy bodies. J Neurol Neurosurg Psychiatry. 2005;76(9):1200-3.

73 CHAPTER

Hyperkinetic Movement Disorders

Mrinal Acharya, Kalyan B Bhattacharyya

INTRODUCTION

C David Marsden and Stanley Fahn defined movement disorders as those conditions where there is either a paucity of normal physiological movements or an excess of abnormal involuntary movements. Movement disorders are of two types—*(1) hyperkinetic* and *(2) hypokinetic*. Hyperkinetic disorders are also known as dyskinesias.[1] Dyskinesias encompass five patterns—*(1) tremors, (2) myoclonus, (3) tics, (4) chorea,* and *(5) dystonia*. Hypokinetic movement disorders comprise parkinsonian syndromes. Some rare patients present with a mixed movement disorder. Different etiological conditions can present with similar clinical syndromes; thus, a syndromic approach is often complex and confusing. However, recognizing the phenomenology of different movement disorders is an essential first step, followed by a step-by-step approach that will eventually lead to a list of differential diagnoses. Basic steps such as history and examination are vital in evaluating movement disorder patients like any other neurological disorder. However, certain aspects need extra emphasis in movement disorder patients. Concerning history, drug, and family history are important as several movement disorders are drug-induced or inherited. Regarding the neurological examination, special attention is to be paid to the gait, postural reflexes, and eye movements, and tests for bradykinesia and rigidity are indicated as these are usually not included within the routine neurological examination and often concentrate on the pyramidal system.

GENERAL APPROACH

Because of the exhaustive list of etiological causes of movement disorders and diverse clinical presentation, it is vital to use a step-by-step organized approach in a movement disorder patient. A three-step approach is suggested by experts when evaluating a movement disorders patient.

The *first step* is identifying whether the patient has hypo- or hyperkinetic movement disorder. Regarding hyperkinetic movement disorders, it is vital to classify the presenting abnormal movement best fits into which pattern of dyskinesia. Is it a rhythmic (tremor), or one of the three forms of jerks (chorea, tics, or myoclonus), or sustained posturing (dystonia)? Typical features of forms of dyskinesias help to classify them. For example, although both myoclonus and tics are jerky movements, tics are suppressible while myoclonus is not. Also, tic patients sometimes describe a rising inner tension when suppressing tics. Chorea is typified by jerky movements flitting from one body part to another, in contrast to tics which are stereotyped. Quasi-purposive movements, where the patient seemingly uses a part of the involuntary movement to do a task to hide the abnormal movement, are also typical of chorea. Dystonia is characterized by sustained postures. The presence of a sensory trick is generally seen in dystonia but not in other dyskinesia.

The *second step* is to note the anatomical distribution of the movement disorder, whether it is focal, multifocal, generalized, or unilateral. A particular predilection for a specific body part or a definite pattern often points toward a definitive diagnosis. The age of the patient and associated neurological (cognitive decline, epilepsy, and spasticity) and non-neurological (organ failure, blood investigations) involvement, apart from the movement disorder, are also important.

The *third step* is needed to integrate the above findings to synthesize a list of differential diagnoses and order appropriate investigations to come to a definitive diagnosis.

In this regard, when attempting to form a list of possible etiology for the movement disorder in a particular patient, it is helpful to remember that, in general, causes of movement disorders fall into four main categories:

1. *Primary or idiopathic*: These tend to be pure movement disorders (no other neurological or systemic features) that are nonprogressive. These disorders are often inherited and without any identifiable structural brain damage.

2. *Secondary*: These movement disorders are caused by identifiable secondary causes such as brain injury, infection, or drug use. Other systems may be involved, and other neurological signs may occur. The defining feature of these conditions is the presence of a precipitating factor, and sometimes a disorder may be delayed after the precipitating event (i.e., tardive movement disorders). Secondary movement disorders are usually static and do not progress if the precipitating factor is no longer active.
3. *Heredodegenerative*: These are movement disorders that occur as part of a generalized degenerative process affecting the nervous system. These disorders usually have a progressive course. Clinical presentation is variable, often presenting with mixed movement disorders and other neurological involvement. Movement disorder is sometimes a minor part of the overall neurological systemic dysfunction.
4. *Psychogenic*: Usually have a diverse presentation coupled with other unusual clinical manifestations and often (but not necessarily) the presence of psychological disturbance.

PLANNING INVESTIGATIONS

It is important to exclude treatable causes of movement disorders. Treatable movement disorders such as Wilson's disease or dopa-responsive dystonia are rare, but there should be a high index of suspicion for these. The differential diagnosis of heredodegenerative movement disorders is usually very long, and investigating the different possibilities is difficult and expensive. Other neurological involvements and systemic manifestations are often helpful in narrowing down the differential diagnosis. A patient presenting with peripheral neuropathy associated with generalized dystonia or dystonia associated with deafness has a much shorter list of differential diagnosis than of heredodegenerative dystonia in general. Investigations can be narrowed down by using syndromic associations.

Tremor

A tremor is a regular, hyperkinetic movement in which a body part oscillates around an axis. Tremor occurs when alternating and synchronous contractions of reciprocally innervated agonistic and antagonistic muscles cause a symmetrical displacement about the midpoint in both directions.[2]

Using a series of three questions focusing on history and phenomenology, we demonstrate a practical approach to patients with a tremor in the outpatient setting.

1. *Is the movement disorder a tremor?*
2. *Is the tremor isolated, or are there accompanying neurologic abnormalities?*
3. *What are the phenomenological features of the tremor?*

Although tremors are classified in several ways, the most crucial parameter used to describe tremors is about the movement or position of a body part. Based on this, they are classified as rest or action tremors. Action tremor is further subdivided into a postural or kinetic tremor. When the tremor worsens on approaching a target, it is termed intention tremor, which is a type of kinetic tremor. This classification helps in identifying underlying pathophysiology and etiology, which in turn aids in the management. Tremors can also be classified based on frequency, amplitude, anatomical distribution, exacerbating or alleviating factors, and associated neurological signs.[3,4]

Rest tremor is characteristically present when the involved extremity is supported against gravity. Rest tremors subside with the limb movement. The most common cause of rest tremors is Parkinson's disease (PD). The typical tremor of PD is a 4–6 Hz rest tremor. It is characteristically unilateral at onset and involves the distal upper extremity initially. The classical "pill-rolling" tremor consists of movement at the thumb and forefinger. Rest tremors could also be in the form of flexion-extension of the wrist, pronation-supination at the forearm, and abduction-adduction of the leg. Rest tremor in PD not only involves hands but also involves lips, chin, jaw, and legs, and rarely neck and head. The "re-emergent" tremor appears after an interval of a few seconds of maintaining the arm in front, and it has a similar frequency as that of a rest tremor.[5]

Certain patients develop only a rest tremor, which persists beyond 2 years without manifesting other cardinal signs of PD. The term "*monosymptomatic rest tremor*" has been used to describe these patients. Many of these patients are diagnosed with PD by functional imaging. However, sometimes presynaptic dopaminergic deficit cannot be detected, leading to a diagnosis of scans without evidence of dopaminergic deficits (SWEDDs).[6,7] Parkinsonian syndromes other than PD, such as multiple system atrophy (MSA), progressive supranuclear palsy (PSP), and corticobasal degeneration (CBD), are also important causes of rest tremors. Certain drugs [antipsychotics, antiemetics (metoclopramide), and antivertigo medications (prochlorperazine)] with dopamine receptor-blocking properties can also produce rest tremors.

Action tremor occurs when a limb is voluntarily contracting. It is subdivided into a postural, kinetic, and isometric tremor. Action tremors are the largest group of tremors. Essential tremor (ET) is the most common neurological cause of action tremor. Three important tremor syndromes included under this category are enhanced physiological tremor, ET, and cerebellar and psychogenic tremor (PT). Specific uncommon tremor syndromes such as orthostatic tremor, task-specific tremor, and Holmes tremor (HT) also present with action tremor.

Essential tremor is a symmetrical postural tremor with or without kinetic component that involves hands and forearms, lasting for >3 years and having a gradual onset. The amplitude of the kinetic tremor is more than that of the postural component, and the kinetic tremor typically increases in amplitude as the target is approached (intention tremor). The tremor in ET may involve other body parts such as voice, head, neck, and legs but not in isolation without the involvement of hands. Head, voice, and jaw tremors tend to become more prevalent with longer disease duration. Red flags for the diagnosis of ET are the presence of a unilateral tremor, tremor predominantly in the legs, tremor in a hemi distribution, isolated head tremor with posturing, isolated voice tremor, lip tremor, and predominant rest tremor. ET usually is a monosymptomatic disorder, with tremors as its sole feature.[8-14]

Cerebellar tremor[15-17] is classically defined as an intention tremor, i.e., the tremor that worsens/occurs only on approaching a target. Cerebellar tremors are usually associated with other cerebellar signs. *Dystonic tremor* (DT) syndromes are divided into DT, tremor associated with dystonia (TAWD), and dystonia-gene-associated tremor. The tremor in dystonia involves most commonly the head or arm, followed by the jaw, facial, or voice tremor and at least the legs. In DT, dystonia, as well as tremor (postural/kinetic), is simultaneously present in the same body part, for example, dystonic head tremor. This tremor is position specific. Dystonic head tremor differs from essential head tremor by being jerky, more pronounced when the head is turned to one side, and persistent while lying down. It also shows the null point phenomenon, i.e., tremor decreases when placed in the direction of pull. Sensory tricks, neck pain, and hypertrophy of neck muscles are all seen in dystonic head tremors. Features that favor a dystonic rather than Parkinsonian tremor are task- or position-specific tremor, presence of head tremor, and dystonic voice.[18] Tremor with thumb extension favors DT more than PD rest tremor. Dystonic voice tremor can be differentiated from essential voice tremor by the presence of "geste maneuvers" such as cessation of tremor on changing pitch or singing. *TAWD* is characterized by tremors in one body part and dystonia in another, for example, postural tremors in hands with cervical dystonia. The third type, i.e., *dystonia-gene-associated tremor*, is the presence of tremor in a patient with a family history of dystonia.[19-22]

Task-specific tremor occurs during executing a specific and skilled task that is not associated with abnormal posturing. *Primary writing tremor* is the most common among task-specific tremors. It can be associated with postural and intention tremors. The tremor is a pronation/supination movement at the wrist joint.[23-25] Other examples of task-specific tremors are voice tremors, golfer's tremors, laughing tremors, tremors in musicians, and other trained professionals.

Physiological tremor occurs in all healthy people when muscles are actively used. Physiological tremor is not usually visible to the naked eye because of its low amplitude. It is called an *enhanced physiological tremor* when this tremor becomes visible due to increased sympathetic activity.[26] Enhanced physiological tremor is the most common cause of postural tremor. Certain diseases or drugs can bring about this increased sympathetic activity. The tremor is typically a fine postural or kinetic tremor in the hands and fingers. It is symmetrical and has low amplitude and high frequency. Patients usually give a history of the tremor surfaces only under certain conditions such as stress, fatigue, anxiety, medication use, or caffeine intake. Moreover, such patients do not require further investigation. They improve by the removal of the offending agent.

Orthostatic tremor[27] is a rare, high-frequency symmetrical tremor of 13–16 Hz involving the legs and trunk. It occurs more commonly in women and is typically seen in the sixth to seventh decade. It presents exclusively on standing, decreases on walking, and altogether disappears on sitting or lying down. Patients may only complain of having poor balance while standing and assuming a broad base, which gets relieved on walking. Although classically described in the legs and trunk, it may also be seen in the arms, especially in weight bearing. This tremor may be visible as a fine ripple or palpable or could be heard via a stethoscope placed over the thigh or calf muscles, which produces a thumping sound resembling the sound of a helicopter.

Holmes tremor[28,29] is a rare tremor affecting the proximal parts of the limbs. It is also known as rubral and midbrain tremors. This tremor is typically present at rest and worsens with posture and movement. It has a low frequency (2–5 Hz) and high amplitude. A lesion in the thalamus, upper brainstem, or cerebellum can cause HT. It is essential to differentiate the rest tremor of HT from that of PD. In HT, the rest tremor has a frequency of <4 Hz and involves the proximal part of the limbs, whereas PD causes the classic pill-rolling tremor of 4–6 Hz involving the limbs distally.

Psychogenic tremor is characterized by the presence of rest, postural, or kinetic tremor, but most often, all three types are seen in unison. The tremor characteristically starts in both arms spreading to involve the head and legs. Diagnosis of PT relies on history and clinical examination. A tremor of abrupt onset, with variable characteristics, is suggestive of PT. Excluding other organic tremors to reach a diagnosis of PT is insufficient. Demonstrating reliable signs which are compatible with PT is essential.[30-32]

Drug-induced tremors can present as rest or action tremors. The most common form is the enhanced physiological tremor due to drugs. The elderly population and polypharmacy are substantial risk factors. Drug-induced postural tremor is symmetrical. Tardive tremor most commonly presents as a postural tremor can rarely be present at rest, and is of high amplitude. It typically occurs on exposure to neuroleptic (dopamine receptor-blocking agents) drugs and can resemble a Parkinsonian rest tremor. However, it tends to be more symmetrical than Parkinsonian rest tremors. Usually, this tremor is nonprogressive and responds to drug withdrawal or reduction in dose.[33,34]

Dystonia

Dystonia involves sustained or intermittent muscle contractions, often resulting in twisting and repetitive patterned movements and abnormal postures related to the co-contraction of agonist and antagonist muscles. Core features of dystonia include influence by voluntary action, overflow dystonia (unintentional muscle contraction distinct anatomically from the primary movement), mirror dystonia (unilateral abnormal posturing elicited by contralateral movements),[35] and, in some cases, DT (movements are oscillatory but not strictly rhythmic, jerky, and patterned).[36] Dystonia and DT may also have a directional nature, with movements worse in certain positions and improved in others (a "null point"). Another feature is alleviating maneuvers (sensory tricks or geste antagoniste),[37,38] typically involving simple movements but not forceful opposition to the dystonic movement. Fatigue, anxiety, stress, or heightened emotions can exacerbate dystonia; dystonia decreases with relaxation, generally resolving during sleep.[39-46]

The 2013 consensus classification of dystonia involves two distinct axes: Axis I (clinical characteristics) involves (1) age of onset, (2) body distribution, (3) temporal pattern, and (4) associated clinical features. Axis II (etiology) addresses two complementary characteristics—(1) underlying nervous system pathology (imaging/diagnostic testing) and (2) whether the disorder is inherited, acquired, or idiopathic.[40]

Age of onset and body distribution can clinically differentiate dystonia. Focal dystonia involves a single body region.[47-49] Segmental dystonia involves two or more adjacent body segments, including the involvement of both arms or both legs. Multifocal dystonia involves at least two noncontiguous or more (contiguous/noncontiguous) body regions. Generalized dystonia has truncal involvement and at least two other distant sites. Hemidystonia involves multiple body regions restricted to a single side.[50,51,48]

The temporal pattern of dystonia is subdivided into four distinct types. In a persistent pattern, dystonia presence and severity are roughly similar throughout the day. Action-specific/task-specific dystonia[52] only occurs during a particular activity, such as writing, typing, playing an instrument,[51] or singing. Paroxysmal dystonia involves sudden, discrete episodes of dystonia, with a return to the neurologic baseline.[53,54] Dopa-responsive dystonia classically shows a diurnal variation (mild awakening symptoms and worsening as the day progresses).[55,56]

Dystonia can either be isolated or combined with another movement disorder. In isolated dystonia, dystonia is the only clinical motor feature other than tremors. Dystonia is frequently associated with neuropsychiatric symptoms, whereas cognitive decline generally only occurs in degenerative/progressive dystonias. The rate of symptomatic progression can differentiate dystonia. Focal dystonias generally follow a subacute or slow worsening of symptoms, followed by a plateau, at least initially. Subsequent spread to segmental/multifocal distributions may occur but generally plateaus.[52,57-59]

ETIOLOGIC CLASSIFICATION OF DYSTONIA

Identifiable anatomic changes and patterns of inheritance can differentiate the etiology of dystonia. In most cases of dystonia, brain degeneration or structural brain lesions are absent. Significant changes have occurred in the nomenclature of genetic dystonias and other movement disorders. According to the new nomenclature, only isolated genetic dystonias (dystonia as the primary feature) were designated "DYT" followed by the gene name (e.g., DYT-*TOR1A*, formerly DYT1). In contrast, combined dystonias have a double prefix, including both movement phenotypes (e.g., DYT/PARK-*TAF1*, formerly DYT3). Paroxysmal dyskinesias/dystonias have the prefix PxMD, while those without a consistent core phenotype are designated as mixed movement disorders (MxMD).[53,60,61]

LABORATORY INVESTIGATIONS

Each of the four clinical dimensions described above is important for describing a syndromic pattern, which helps to guide laboratory investigations to delineate etiology, which falls in axis two. Universal algorithms for laboratory investigations in dystonias are challenging because of the remarkable heterogeneity of clinical manifestations and causes. Although there are several diagnostic algorithms, none is comprehensive.

Laboratory investigations depend on body distribution, whether additional neurologic features are present and temporal aspects for dystonias. Diagnostic testing is usually unrevealing for the most common adult-onset focal or segmental dystonias, such as cervical dystonia or blepharospasm. Laryngoscopy is recommended in laryngeal dystonia to rule out structural defects of the vocal apparatus. For the less common adult-onset cases with hemidystonia or generalized dystonia, neuroimaging can help reveal a structural cause. Neuroimaging is also valuable for patients with adult-onset dystonia with the rapid or severe progression of symptoms or if the dystonia coexists with other neurologic features, such as parkinsonism or ataxia. Genetic testing is usually not indicated unless multiple family members are affected, or a specific syndromic pattern leads to suspicion of an inherited disorder. EEG is indicated in patients with paroxysmal attacks of dystonia. EMG is indicated when a neuromuscular disorder (like myotonia or stiff person syndrome) that may resemble dystonia is suspected.

Some laboratory investigations are almost always valuable for dystonias that first emerge at an earlier age (in patients younger than 40 years). Neuroimaging can provide clues to guide diagnostic testing. Beyond this step, strategies vary. A "red flag" approach, in which the identification of characteristic features from the medical history, clinical examination, or neuroimaging guides diagnostic testing, is recommended. Examples include the corneal Kayser–Fleischer ring of Wilson disease[62] or the "eye of the tiger" sign on magnetic resonance imaging (MRI) for neurodegeneration with brain iron accumulation.[63] Although this strategy can be helpful sometimes, it does not provide a comprehensive approach in all cases.[64]

A related strategy is delineating a group of clinical abnormalities that form a recognizable syndromic pattern to guide diagnostic testing. An example is a Lesch–Nyhan disease, where patients present with early-onset generalized dystonia, intellectual disability, tendencies toward self-harm, and elevations of serum uric acid. This syndrome is unique; it is associated only with the *HPRT1* gene, so single gene or enzyme testing is efficient. However, many other disorders present with overlapping syndromes with many causes. It can be challenging even for experts to remember all syndromes, and partial syndromes are hard to recognize. For almost all of the classic phenotypes described for inherited disorders of children, adult-onset variant forms with partial syndromes may occur.[65]

Furthermore, syndromic patterns sometimes need to be more accurate. An example involves the *ATM* gene, which is classically associated with ataxia-telangiectasia in children. However, mutations in this gene can sometimes cause isolated focal or generalized dystonia, sometimes in adults and sometimes without telangiectasias. In the era of shotgun genetic testing that may involve whole exome sequencing or large multigene panels, unexpected results are typical.[66]

A third strategy sometimes recommended is focusing laboratory investigations specifically on disorders for which specific treatments exist. According to this strategy, laboratory testing should focus only on a smaller number of treatable disorders, such as Wilson disease, for which specific treatments are available. This strategy is unwise. Even when the cause does not have a specific treatment, many patients and families find that obtaining a definitive etiologic diagnosis helps to end a long diagnostic process. The information also provides valuable information for counseling regarding the prognosis for the individual affected and the potential risk for family members. Also, the list of treatable disorders has been growing each year, making it challenging to know what disorders should be investigated.[67,68]

Because of the limitations of traditional strategies for laboratory investigations, there is a growing trend toward the greater use of broad dystonia gene panels or whole exome sequencing. The red flags and syndromic strategies are helpful only when the clinical clues point specifically to a single or small number of potential diagnoses to target. Serial genetic testing, starting with the most likely genes, should be avoided because it is frustrating and more expensive than ordering a larger panel. Gene panels are not standardized across testing laboratories.[69]

Even when an etiologic diagnosis is not possible, it is important to follow patients because new problems may arise that point to the cause. For example, some patients may present with isolated focal dystonia of the hand or foot. However, with time, signs of parkinsonism may develop, pointing toward an atypical parkinsonian syndrome. In a child or young adult, this evolution may point to one of many inherited metabolic or degenerative disorders.[70]

Chorea

Chorea[71] refers to involuntary random, irregular, purposeless movements that flow from one body part to another. Randomness is the crucial phenomenological feature in chorea. The movements typically flit from one body region to another in an unpredictable fashion. In addition to randomness and flowing quality, patients with chorea often blend or incorporate the chorea into their regular movements, as if attempting to hide it. This phenomenon is known as *parakinesia*. For example, when chorea is present in the arm, the patient may try to blend chorea by lifting or moving the arm to a target in the same direction as the choreic movements. Another feature of chorea is motor impersistence, an inability to perform sustained motor activities. Tongue protrusion cannot be maintained, and the tongue retracts back into the mouth after several seconds. There is waxing-and-waning grip strength (called *milkmaid's grip*) when the patient attempts to squeeze an examiner's fingers during handgrip.[72,73]

Ballism is a chorea variant characterized by large-amplitude flinging movements involving proximal extremities. Athetosis is characterized by slow writhing movements typically involving distal extremities, although other body parts, such as the face, can be involved. When dystonia, such as dystonic hand posturing, coexists with flowing movements, it is sometimes challenging to separate athetosis from dystonia, resulting in the so-called dystonia-choreoathetosis movements seen in cerebral palsy. The velocity of the chorea can vary. The flowing component of chorea is usually faster than dystonia's but not as fast as the jerking component of myoclonus. However, when chorea has a quick velocity and low amplitude, it may appear quite jerky and can be mistaken for myoclonic jerks. Chorea has a wide variation of severity; patients with a mild degree can appear fidgety, and thus chorea may be overlooked.[74-76]

Chorea can present as an isolated symptom or a mixed movement disorder and can be associated with behavioral and cognitive symptoms, seizures, or symptoms suggestive of polyneuropathy.[77] The different symptom complexes identified with a clinical interview can give the first clues for a diagnosis and prioritization of investigations. Chorea is frequently noticed first by a third person and not by the patient; consequently, the information provided by a caregiver or family member is crucial for a more rigorous history of chorea. As with other neurologic symptoms, the age of onset (adult versus elderly), the acute versus progressive mode of onset, and the type of disease course (remitting, paroxysmal, or continuous) can favor a specific syndrome. Senile chorea is a sporadic idiopathic form of chorea with onset in the elderly without dementia and a benign course.[78,79]

A relatively acute onset of chorea can be the manifestation of stroke.[80] It can also be due to nonketotic hyperglycemia, chorea gravidarum, or drug-induced chorea.[81,82] A subacute course (over a few days or weeks) can be due to an infectious process or autoimmune etiology,[83] including a paraneoplastic syndrome.[84-87] Metabolic etiology may also manifest in a subacute manner. Some cases of drug-induced chorea[88] may have a gradual onset, as in levodopa-induced dyskinesia in PD or neuroleptic-induced dyskinesia.[89,90] A more protracted course of months to years is usually associated with a neurodegenerative condition.[91-93]

Regarding the time course, vascular chorea secondary to a stroke[94] or nonketotic hyperglycemia may have a slowly remitting course. The case of paroxysmal recurrent chorea suggests a different set of differential diagnoses.[54] Three classic forms are described—(1) paroxysmal kinesigenic dyskinesia, (2) paroxysmal nonkinesigenic dyskinesia, and (3) paroxysmal exertion-induced (or exercise-induced) dyskinesia. Although chorea can present in isolation, paroxysmal dyskinesias manifest most commonly with dystonia and chorea. These conditions are classified based on clinical manifestations, mainly concerning the trigger of the episodes. The age of onset, duration, frequency of episodes, and response to treatment have further classified them. Recurrent chorea can also occur in patients with a history of chorea gravidarum or Sydenham chorea who develop chorea when exposed to drugs such as oral contraceptives or phenytoin. However, these cases can assume a distinctive pattern of longer-lasting episodes separated, at times, by years. The presence of chorea in specific body regions also provides important clues for the differential diagnosis. Orofacial chorea frequently associated with dystonia is suggestive of a classic neuroacanthocytosis syndrome (i.e., chorea-acanthocytosis and, less commonly, McLeod syndrome).[95] Orofacial chorea can also be an early feature of neuroferritinopathy.[96]

Chorea-acanthocytosis classically shows the dystonic protrusion of the tongue with an associated difficulty maintaining ingested food in the mouth (feeding dystonia). However, McLeod syndrome, tardive dyskinesia, pantothenate-kinase-associated neurodegeneration,[63,97] and Lesch–Nyhan syndrome can also manifest feeding dystonia.[98] In addition, advanced chorea-acanthocytosis distinctively manifests head drops and truncal/cervical extension. The presence of tics can be found in Huntington's disease (HD) and in classic neuroacanthocytosis syndromes, particularly in chorea-acanthocytosis. Significant behavioral symptoms and cognitive deterioration strongly suggest a neurodegenerative choreic syndrome, HD. Behavioral symptoms[99] often precede the onset of motor symptoms, and formal testing can elicit deficits in cognitive function at the time of a diagnosis based on motor features.[100-102]

Huntington's disease phenocopies[103,104] in which behavioral or cognitive symptoms are part of the clinical presentation include SCA17,[105] HDL2, chorea-acanthocytosis,[106] and dentatorubral-pallidoluysian atrophy (DRPLA). In McLeod syndrome, behavioral problems are more common, and cognitive difficulties are mild. Self-mutilation of the lip and tongue is a clinical manifestation of chorea-acanthocytosis but is uncommon in McLeod syndrome. Lesch–Nyhan syndrome[98] is an X-linked genetic condition in which patients can have self-mutilating behaviors, but the onset occurs in childhood. Chorea gravidarum, antiphospholipid syndrome, or systemic lupus erythematosus is among nondegenerative causes of chorea that can present with concomitant behavioral symptoms, including personality changes, depression, psychotic symptoms, and cognitive impairment. Seizures can be a distinguishing feature of some HD phenotypes, such as chorea-acanthocytosis (30% as presenting feature) and McLeod syndrome, as well as in DRPLA and Huntington's disease-like 1 (HDL1). In DRPLA,[107] it is helpful to recognize that when the age of onset overlaps the mean age of onset of the adult form of HD, seizures rarely occur, and more common presenting features are chorea, in addition to dystonia, parkinsonism, and psychosis.

Myoclonus

Myoclonus refers to a sudden, brief, lightning like muscle contraction. Myoclonus may occur from increased contraction activity (positive myoclonus) or inhibition of contraction activity (negative myoclonus). Dystonic spasms or dyskinetic jerks may be sudden, but they are not lightning brief. A tremor discharge may be brief but does not result in a jerk or sudden movement. Indeed, the myoclonus phenotype is both a jerk (sudden) and the most transient (brief) compared with any other movement disorder phenotype.[108-110]

Myoclonus has many possible etiologies, anatomic sources, and pathophysiologic features.[111] Myoclonus is most often secondary to another disorder. There is an efficient and pragmatic strategy to define the physiology and diagnostic and therapeutic approach for a specific myoclonus case.[112] Myoclonus has popular classification schemes based on clinical presentation and etiology and a separate scheme based on physiology. The classification scheme of Marsden and colleagues organizes the numerous etiologies of myoclonus into four major categories—(1) physiologic, (2) essential, (3) epileptic, and (4) symptomatic. Each clinical category contains myoclonus arising from various etiologies and pathophysiologic mechanisms.[113] Thus, differentiation by clinical-etiologic category is only sometimes pure. In addition, a single etiology can produce different types of myoclonus, and occasionally patients may demonstrate more than one type of myoclonus.[112,114]

Physiologic myoclonus refers to myoclonic jerks that occur as everyday phenomena in almost all people with different frequencies. Concerned observers, such as spouses or close relatives, first notice them. Jerks occurring in sleep or sleep transition are common examples.[115] Normal startle response and hiccups are also physiologic myoclonus. However, some physiologic myoclonus phenotypes may be part of a clinical syndrome or disorder. Hyperekplexia is a pathological condition where an otherwise normal startle response is non-fatigable and symptomatic.

Essential myoclonus is a chronic and relatively stable course in which myoclonus is a prominent or the only symptom.[116]

Epileptic myoclonus occurs in syndromes presenting as chronic seizure disorder (epilepsy). In most instances, the myoclonus is the seizure itself and is called a *myoclonic seizure*. Less commonly, the myoclonus is just one component of the whole seizure manifestation and is a *fragment* of the seizure or epileptic syndrome (eyelid myoclonus with absence seizure).[117] As phenomena related to seizures, these myoclonic jerking episodes are often paroxysmal and unpredictable.[113,118-121]

Symptomatic myoclonus is the most common clinical presentation among myoclonic syndromes. Myoclonus is secondary to a medical or neurologic illness. Seizures may be a significant part of the patient's illness, but seizures are not the primary myoclonus phenotype as in epileptic myoclonus. Other neurologic systems are typically affected and may involve cognition, parkinsonism, ataxia, sleep dysfunction, autonomic symptoms, upper motor neuron findings, and peripheral nerve dysfunction. Almost all the major medical pathophysiologic processes can include myoclonus as a symptom, including metabolic, degenerative,[122] toxic, structural lesion, infectious, and inflammatory.

Clinically, the evaluation of myoclonus is organized into three steps:

1. *Step one:* History and examination with clinical presentation classification
2. *Step two:* Basic ancillary testing
3. *Step three:* Comprehensive testing if indicated

PHYSIOLOGIC CLASSIFICATION

In addition to the clinical and etiologic classification as discussed, the localization of the physiologic mechanism that generates it also classifies myoclonus. The categories are cortical, cortical-subcortical, subcortical-nonsegmental, segmental, and peripheral. This classification paradigm can help with the localization of the underlying lesion, aid in diagnosing certain disorders with characteristic myoclonus physiology, and guide treatment options that may be useful for some physiologic types of myoclonus.

Cortical myoclonus originates with a focal discharge from the primary sensorimotor cortex, which causes a myoclonic jerk after a time interval required for corticospinal transmission. Cortical myoclonus may occur with reflex sensory stimulation (cortical reflex myoclonus), with muscle activation (cortical action myoclonus), with rest (e.g., focal motor seizure), or with any combination of the above. In cortical reflex myoclonus, an exaggerated cortical response to somatosensory stimuli produces the jerk, but subsequently, the whole sensorimotor cortex generates giant somatosensory evoked cortical potentials (SEPs) and reflex myoclonus. Rhythmic or semirhythmic discharges from the sensorimotor cortex can produce a repetitive movement that resembles a tremor.[123-129]

Cortical-subcortical myoclonus is the principal mechanism for myoclonic seizures that occur in primary generalized epileptic syndromes [e.g., juvenile myoclonic epilepsy (JME)] and in some other instances (e.g., minipolymyoclonus). Generalized spike-and-wave discharges on EEG that correlate with the myoclonus confirm this category of physiology. Because this excitation over the sensorimotor cortex is simultaneously widespread, the myoclonus is commonly generalized.[130]

Subcortical-nonsegmental myoclonus is generated from a subcortical site, but the crucial feature is that the myoclonus manifests far beyond the segments near the originating site. The best-characterized types of subcortical-nonsegmental physiologies are reticular-reflex myoclonus[131] and propriospinal myoclonus.[132,133] In both examples, the abnormal activity begins in a focal area of the neuroaxis. Then it spreads in rostral and caudal directions, producing generalized myoclonus due to the bilateral pathways involved.

Segmental myoclonus is generated at a particular segment or contiguous segments of the brainstem or spinal cord. The pathologic motor oscillations in this type of myoclonus occur at a lower frequency than tremors. Segmental myoclonus manifests at, or close to, that particular segment or contiguous body segments (e.g., palatal myoclonus[134] and spinal segmental myoclonus).[135]

Peripheral myoclonus arises due to a peripheral nervous system lesion producing hyperactive motor discharges to its muscle (e.g., hemifacial spasm).[136] The possible role of central reorganization needs to be better defined.[137]

Tics

Tics[138] are intermittent, repeated, and stereotyped movements or sounds.[139] Tics may be rhythmic or nonrhythmic, involve tonic postures or brief jerking movements, and involve a single movement or sequence of movements and sounds, associated with a premonitory urge.[140] Tics have a distinct onset and ending and are usually repeated at unpredictable intervals many times per day. Tics can involve movements or vocalizations and, in some cases, purely sensations.[141,142]

There are two types of tics—motor and phonic—subdivided into the simple and complex grouping. Brief, rapid, abrupt jerk like, nonrhythmic movements that involve only a single muscle or localized group are considered simple (eye blink, head jerk, and shoulder shrug). In contrast, complex tics involve a cluster of simple actions or a more coordinated pattern of movements. Complex motor tics can be nonpurposeful (facial or body contortions) or appear purposeful but serve no purpose [touching, hitting, smelling, jumping, bending, imitating observed movements (echopraxia), and making obscene gestures (copropraxia)]. They may have a dystonic quality (oculogyric movements, sustained mouth opening, body posturing, and torticollis) or tonic character (prolonged tensing of abdominal muscles, immobility, and staring), labeled as *blocking tics*. In some patients (4–5)%, self-injurious (malignant) tics can cause myelopathies, ocular damage, or body injuries. Simple vocal tics include various sounds and noises (grunts, barks, hoots, hollers, moans, groans, sniffs, and throat clearing). Complex vocalizations involve linguistically meaningful vocalizations and utterances; the repetition of words, syllables, or phrases; echolalia (repeating other people's words); palilalia (repeating one's own words); or coprolalia (obscene words or profanity). Although coprolalia is commonly associated with Tourette syndrome, only a minority (10–19%) of individuals with Tourette syndrome have this symptom.[143,144] Vocal alterations can also include pauses and hesitations in speech, word interjections, changes in tone/pitch, and prolongations of words.[145-148]

Some vocalizations can be secondary to a nasal, pharyngeal, chest, or abdominal motor tic. A rapid chest or abdomen contraction can lead to air expulsion and the production of a simple vocalization. Tics can mimic almost any movement or sound. Uncommon tics may include anterior-posterior movements of the external ear, sign language tics, palatal movements, air swallowing, vomiting, and retching.[149]

Unlike other movement disorders such as chorea, the stereotyped nature of tics makes them easily recognizable. It is usually possible to enumerate a small number of distinct tics a child has at any time. Parents of children with tics are often able to list the particular set of movements that the child currently has, as well as a history of which movements were present at a given time.[150] This characteristic, recognizable, and repetitive nature helps to distinguish tics from other movement disorders. In particular, they are easily distinguished from tremors, myoclonus, stereotypies, and other disorders by a discrete beginning and end.[151,152]

Similarly, they are usually easily distinguished from dystonia by the absence of sensory tricks. In tic disorders, the movement usually remains under the child's voluntary control. However, in some cases of rapid sequences of tics, or tics with prolonged abnormal postures, it may be difficult for an observer to distinguish between a tic disorder and chorea, myoclonus, stereotypies, or dystonia.[153,154]

Tics must be differentiated from drug-induced movements (akathisia, dystonia, and parkinsonism), obsessive-compulsive behaviors, hyperactivity, antisocial behaviors, and stereotypies.[155] In contrast to tics, commonly associated with a premonitory urge,[156] compulsions are complex activities performed to prevent or relieve anxiety, are executed in a rigid pattern, and are usually done in response to an obsession.[157] Motor stereotypies typically have an earlier onset, fixed pattern, rhythmic quality, prolonged duration, and lack of a premonitory urge and stop abruptly with distraction. Individuals with stuttering may also have an array of nonspeech motor tic-like behaviors, including eye blinking, ocular deviation, head jerks, and limb and trunk movements. In practice, repetitive sniffing, throat clearing, and coughing tics are often mistakenly attributed to allergies, sinusitis, or pulmonary issues; eye blinking tics are often misdiagnosed as blepharospasm, and ocular tics are confused with opsoclonus. Psychogenic disorders that present with tic-like movements can arise in childhood but are more common in adults;[158] they are also more common in females than in males. Nevertheless, it may be difficult, at times, to distinguish a functional movement in an individual with preexisting typical tics. Predisposing factors, the lack of a premonitory sense, the inability to suppress the tics and other functional movements briefly, and the lack of response to otherwise effective therapies usually help to identify psychogenic movement disorders.[159,160]

Specific tic syndromes have been classified into five tic categories:[161]

1. *Provisional tic disorder*: Tics (motor or vocal) have been present for <1 year since the first tic onset, and onset is before age 18 years. The disturbance cannot be attributable to the psychological effects of a substance or other medical conditions.
2. *Chronic motor or vocal tic disorder* indicates the presence of either motor or vocal tics, but not both, for longer than 1 year, without regard for tic frequency with onset before 18 years of age.
3. *Tourette disorder (Tourette syndrome)*: Presence of multiple motor tics and at least one vocal tic, a waxing and waning course, a duration of longer than 1 year, with onset before 18 years of age (for Tourette syndrome was before 21 years of age).
4. The last two categories (*other specified tic disorder* and *unspecified tic disorder*) apply to those tic disorders that cause clinical distress/impairment but do not meet the criteria for either of the three tic disorders as mentioned earlier or any neurodevelopmental disorder.[162,163]

Abnormal Movements in Sleep

Abnormal movements and behaviors during sleep are part of a larger group of nocturnal events that may occur during sleep, wake, or transition into or out of sleep.[164] These events are usually common in the early phase of life. They are usually classified according to the type of movement (i.e., simple or complex) and the underlying sleep physiology, i.e., whether movements are associated with transitions of sleep and wake, nonrapid eye movement (NREM), or rapid eye movement (REM) sleep. Nocturnal events are categorized into simple (e.g., single movements, repetitive or periodic movements, and rhythmical movements) and complex (e.g., sleep talking, sleepwalking, sleep terrors, and dream enactment). A detailed history from the patient and, ideally, a bed partner or caregiver witness is the cornerstone of establishing clues about the underlying etiology. The challenge for the clinician is to recognize when certain nocturnal events signal an underlying treatable disorder, an emerging neurological abnormality, or a benign age-appropriate episode.[165,166]

Most simple movements occur during the transition from wake to sleep, sleep to wake, or during light, NREM sleep. Complex behaviors can result from disrupting the control mechanisms of the three ordinary states of being—(1) wake, (2) NREM sleep, and (3) REM sleep.[167,168]

Occasionally, simple, or complex motor patterns during sleep are a manifestation of seizures, dissociative psychiatric events, or even physiological states such as hypoglycemia. Therefore, clinicians should be aware that nocturnal events may be a manifestation of specific neurologic, medical, psychiatric, or sleep disorders. On the other hand, some of these behaviors, specifically arousal disorders and nightmares, may be normal in childhood.[169]

Simple movements during sleep are typically quick, single movements involving only one body area. They tend to occur in the transition periods between sleep and wakefulness. Periodic or rhythmic movements in or around sleep include body or head rocking or banging, hypnagogic foot tremor, and periodic limb movements of sleep.[170]

Complex movements and behaviors during sleep, or parasomnias, encompass common or bizarre behaviors[171] and seemingly purposeful movements, perceptions, dreaming, and autonomic output during sleep or sleep transitions. While the simple movements described above tend to occur during the transition between sleep and wakefulness, more complex behaviors may occur in various sleep states.[172,173]

Parasomnias are classified into three major groups—(1) events associated with NREM sleep, (2) events associated with REM sleep, and (3) other parasomnias. Events associated with NREM sleep include disorders of arousal (e.g., sleepwalking, sleep terrors, and confusional arousals) and a sleep-related eating disorder. REM sleep-related parasomnias include recurrent isolated sleep paralysis, nightmares, and REM sleep behavior disorder (RBD).[174,175]

CONCLUSION

Although an expert clinician can quickly identify the features of hyperkinetic disorders, a thorough documentation of the observed features should be done to avoid mistakes and allow review and comparison of the phenotype. Evaluation of patients presenting with hyperkinetic movement disorder must include a complete neurological examination and an appraisal of the effect of the movement disorder on overall motor function and quality of life. Observation of the disorder itself should include the phenomenology of the disorder, the time course, the evolution of symptoms, triggers and suppressibility, and the anatomic distribution. The description of the phenomenology should include duration, speed, amplitude, jerkiness, repeatability, stereotyped quality, and the number of different identifiable movements or postures. The time course should be described in terms of rhythmicity, whether it is intermittent with intervening more normal movement, whether movements are sustained or ongoing, and whether there are discrete submovements or movement fragments or whether the movement appears to be continuously flowing. Possible triggers should be assessed from the history and examination, including attempted movement, posture, rest, and emotional state. Suppressibility can be tested in the clinic or assessed from the history. The presence of inner restlessness or urge to move should be questioned. Distractibility evaluates whether unrelated mental or physical tasks (as opposed to asking the patient to suppress voluntarily) result in movement suppression. Distractibility can be seen in tics, stereotypies, and psychogenic movements.[176] Taking a video of the clinical interview and medical examination is valuable if the patient approves. This allows the examiner to review the phenomenology of the hyperkinetic disorder, seek expert consultation, and visually compare phenomenology changes during the natural course of the condition. A well-constructed video recording can convey more accurate information than standard clinical notes. The approach to history taking and examination of the hyperkinetic movement disorder patient is an art that should be practiced during clinical evaluation. Over-reliance upon unfocused investigations can sometimes be dangerous, which runs the risk of giving false-positive outcomes, prolonged diagnostic pathways, and increased financial burden.

REFERENCES

1. Caviness JN. Segmental Myoclonus. In: Albanese A, Jankovic J (Eds). Hyperkinetic Movement Disorders. West Sussex, United Kingdom: Wiley-Blackwell; 2012. pp. 221-36.
2. Louis ED. Essential tremor. Arch Neurol. 2000;57:1522-24.
3. Bhatia KP, Bain P, Bajaj N, Elble RJ, Hallett M, Louis ED, et al. Consensus Statement on the classification of tremors. From the task force on tremor of the International Parkinson and Movement Disorder Society. Mov Disord. 2018;33(1):75-87.
4. Louis ED. Tremor. Continuum (Minneap Minn). 2019;25(4):959-75.
5. Jankovic J, Schwartz KS, Ondo W. Re-emergent tremor of Parkinson's disease. J Neurol Neurosurg Psychiatry. 1999;67(5): 646-50.
6. Oravivattanakul S, Benchaya L, Wu G, Ahmed A, Itin I, Cooper S, et al. Dopamine transporter (DaT) scan utilization in a movement disorder center. Mov Disord Clin Pract. 2015;3(1):31-5.
7. Waln O, Wu Y, Perlman R, Wendt J, Van AK, Jankovic J. Dopamine transporter imaging in essential tremor with and without parkinsonian features. J Neural Transm (Vienna). 2015; 122(11):1515-21.
8. Phibbs F, Fang JY, Cooper MK, Charles DP, Davis TL, Hedera P. Prevalence of unilateral tremor in autosomal dominant essential tremor. Mov Disord. 2009;24(1):108-11.
9. Louis ED. The primary type of tremor in essential tremor is kinetic rather than postural: cross-sectional observation of tremor phenomenology in 369 cases. Eur J Neurol. 2013;20(4):725-7.
10. Sternberg EJ, Alcalay RN, Levy OA, Louis ED. Postural and intention tremors: a detailed clinical study of essential tremor vs. Parkinson's disease. Front Neurol. 2013;4:51.
11. Rao AK, Gilman A, Louis ED. Balance confidence and falls in nondemented essential tremor patients: the role of cognition. Arch Phys Med Rehabil. 2014;95(10):1832-7.
12. Hardesty DE, Maraganore DM, Matsumoto JY, Louis ED. Increased risk of head tremor in women with essential tremor: longitudinal data from the Rochester Epidemiology Project. Mov Disord. 2004;19(5):529-33.
13. Robakis D, Louis ED. Head tremor in essential tremor: "yes-yes", "no-no", or "round and round"? Parkinsonism Relat Disord. 2016;22:98-101.
14. Jain S, Lo SE, Louis ED. Common misdiagnosis of a common neurological disorder: how are we misdiagnosing essential tremor? Arch Neurol. 2006;63(8):1100-4.
15. Bodranghien F, Bastian A, Casali C, Hallett M, Louis ED, Manto M, et al. Consensus paper: revisiting the symptoms and signs of cerebellar syndrome. Cerebellum 2016;15(3):369-91.
16. Lenka A, Louis ED. Revisiting the clinical phenomenology of "cerebellar tremor": beyond the intention tremor. Cerebellum. 2019;18(3):565-74.
17. Holmes G. The Croonian lectures on the clinical symptoms of cerebellar disease and their interpretation. Lecture I. 1922. Cerebellum. 2007;6(2):142-7.
18. Postuma RB, Berg D, Stern M, Poewe W, Olanow CW, Oertel W, et al. MDS clinical diagnostic criteria for Parkinson's disease. Mov Disord. 2015;30(12):1591-601.
19. Defazio G, Conte A, Gigante AF, Fabbrini G, Berardelli A. Is tremor in dystonia a phenotypic feature of dystonia? Neurology. 2015; 84:1053-9.
20. Defazio G, Gigante AF, Abbruzzese G, Bentivoglio AR, Colosimo C, Esposito M, et al. Tremor in primary adult-onset dystonia: prevalence and associated clinical features. J Neurol Neurosurg Psychiatry. 2013;84(10):404-8.
21. Pandey S, Sarma N. Tremor in dystonia. Parkinsonism Relat Disord. 2016;29:3-9.
22. Agnew A, Frucht SJ, Louis ED. Supine head tremor: a clinical comparison of essential tremor and spasmodic torticollis patients. J Neurol Neurosurg Psychiatry. 2012;83(2):179-81.
23. Rana AQ, Vaid HM. A review of primary writing tremor. Int J Neurosci. 2012;122(3):114-8.
24. Hai C, Yu-ping W, Hua W, Ying S. Advances in primary writing tremor. Parkinsonism Relat Disord. 2010;16(9):561-5.
25. Papapetropoulos S, Singer C. Treatment of primary writing tremor with botulinum toxin type A injections: report of a case series. Clin Neuropharmacol. 2006;29(6):364-7.
26. Elble RJ, Higgins C, Elble S. Electrophysiologic transition from physiologic tremor to essential tremor. Mov Disord. 2005;20(8): 1038-42.
27. Benito-León J, Domingo-Santos Á. Orthostatic tremor: An update on a rare entity. Tremor Other Hyperkinet Mov (N Y) 2016;6:411.
28. Raina GB, Cersosimo MG, Folgar SS, Giugni JC, Calandra C, Paviolo JP, et al. Holmes tremor: clinical description, lesion localization, and treatment in a series of 29 cases. Neurology 2016;86(10): 931-8.
29. Tan H, Turanli G, Ay H, Saatçi I. Rubral tremor after thalamic infarction in childhood. Pediatr Neurol. 2001;25(5):409-12.
30. Schwingenschuh P, Deuschl G. Functional tremor. Handb Clin Neurol 2016;139:229-33.
31. Thenganatt MA, Jankovic J. Psychogenic tremor: a video guide to its distinguishing features. Tremor Other Hyperkinet Mov (N Y). 2014;4:253.
32. Schwingenschuh P, Katschnig P, Seiler S, Saifee TA, Aguirre-gomozcorta M, Cordivari C, et al. Moving toward "laboratory-supported" criteria for psychogenic tremor. Mov Disord. 2011; 26(14):2509-15.
33. Sethi KD, Zamrini EY. Asymmetry in clinical features of drug-induced parkinsonism. J Neuropsychiatry Clin Neurosci. 1990;2(1): 64-6.
34. Quinn NP, Schneider SA, Schwingenschuh P, Bhatia KP. Tremor—some controversial aspects. Mov Disord. 2011;26(1):18-23.
35. Sitburana O, Wu LJ, Sheffield JK, Davidson A, Jankovic J. Motor overflow and mirror dystonia. Parkinsonism Relat Disord. 2009;15(10):758-61.
36. Grütz K, Klein C. Dystonia updates: definition, nomenclature, clinical classification, and etiology. J Neural Transm (Vienna). 2021;128(4):395-404.
37. Munhoz RP, Lang AE. Gestes antagonistes in psychogenic dystonia. Mov Disord. 2004;19(3):331-2.
38. Baizabal-Carvallo JF, Jankovic J. Examiner manoeuvres "sensory tricks" in functional (psychogenic) movement disorders. J Neurol Neurosurg Psychiatry. 2017;88(5):453-5.
39. Burkhard PR. Acute and subacute drug-induced movement disorders. Parkinsonism Relat Disord. 2014;20(suppl 1):S108-12.
40. Albanese A, Bhatia K, Bressman SB, Delong MR, Fahn S, Fung VSC, et al. Phenomenology and classification of dystonia: a consensus update. Mov Disord. 2013;28(7):863-73.
41. Balint B, Mencacci NE, Valente EM, Pisani A, Rothwell J, Jankovic J, et al. Dystonia. Nat Rev Dis Primers. 2018;4(1):25.
42. Albanese A, Lalli S. Is this dystonia? Mov Disord. 2009;24(12): 1725-31.
43. Morales-Briceno H, Fung VSC, Bhatia KP, Balint B. Parkinsonism and dystonia: Clinical spectrum and diagnostic clues. J Neurol Sci. 2022;433:120016.
44. Stephen CD, Perez DL, Chibnik LB, Sharma N. Functional dystonia: a case-control study and risk prediction algorithm. Ann Clin Transl Neurol. 2021;8(4):732-48.
45. Dressler D. Nonprimary dystonias. Handb Clin Neurol. 2011;100: 513-38.

46. Berlot R, Bhatia KP, Kojović M. Pseudodystonia: a new perspective on an old phenomenon. Parkinsonism Relat Disord. 2019;62: 44-50.
47. Tolosa E, Martí MJ. Blepharospasm-oromandibular dystonia syndrome (Meige's syndrome): Clinical aspects. Adv Neurol. 1988; 49:73-84.
48. Conti AM, Pullman S, Frucht SJ. The hand that has forgotten its cunning—lessons from musicians' hand dystonia. Mov Disord. 2008;23(10):1398-406.
49. Comella C, Bhatia K. An international survey of patients with cervical dystonia. J Neurol. 2015;262(4):837-48.
50. Battistella G, Termsarasab P, Ramdhani RA, Fuertinger S, Simonyan K. Isolated focal dystonia as a disorder of large-scale functional networks. Cereb Cortex. 2017;27(2):1203-15.
51. Lalli S, Albanese A. The diagnostic challenge of primary dystonia: evidence from misdiagnosis. Mov Disord. 2010;25(11):1619-26.
52. Stahl CM, Frucht SJ. Focal task specific dystonia: a review and update. J Neurol. 2017;264(7):1536-41.
53. Erro R, Sheerin UM, Bhatia KP. Paroxysmal dyskinesias revisited: a review of 500 genetically proven cases and a new classification. Mov Disord. 2014;29(9):1108-16.
54. Gardiner AR, Jaffer F, Dale RC, Labrum R, Erro R, Meyer E, et al. The clinical and genetic heterogeneity of paroxysmal dyskinesias. Brain. 2015;138(Pt 12):3567-80.
55. Wijemanne S, Jankovic J. Dopa-responsive dystonia—clinical and genetic heterogeneity. Nat Rev Neurol. 2015;11(7):414-24.
56. Segawa M. Dopa-responsive dystonia. Handb Clin Neurol. 2011; 100:539-57.
57. Evatt ML, Freeman A, Factor S. Adult-onset dystonia. Handb Clin Neurol 2011;100:481-511.
58. Frucht L, Perez DL, Callahan J, MacLean J, Song PC, Sharma N, et al. Functional dystonia: differentiation from primary dystonia and multidisciplinary treatments. Front Neurol. 2020;11:605262.
59. Klein C, Münchau A. Progressive dystonia. Handb Clin Neurol. 2013;113:1889-97.
60. Klein C, Lohmann K, Marras C. Hereditary dystonia overview. In: Adam MP, Ardinger HH, Pagon RA (Eds). GeneReviews. Seattle (WA): University of Washington; 1993-2022.
61. Marras C, Lang A, van de Warrenburg BP, Sue CM, Tabrizi SJ, Bertram L, et al. Nomenclature of genetic movement disorders: Recommendations of the international Parkinson and movement disorder society task force. Mov Disord. 2016;31(4):436-57.
62. Brooker S, Mishra S, Bega D. Wilson disease. Pract Neurol. 2021;9:36-9.
63. Hayflick SJ, Kurian MA, Hogarth P. Neurodegeneration with brain iron accumulation. Handb Clin Neurol. 2018;147:293-305.
64. Donzuso G, Mostile G, Nicoletti A, Zappia M. Basal ganglia calcifications (Fahr's syndrome): related conditions and clinical features. Neurol Sci. 2019;40(11):2251-63.
65. Lange LM, Junker J, Loens S, Baumann H, Olschewski L, Schaake S, et al. Genotype-phenotype relations for isolated dystonia genes: MDSGene systematic review. Mov Disord. 2021;36(5):1086-103.
66. Di Fonzo A, Monfrini E, Erro R. Genetics of movement disorders and the practicing clinician; who and what to test for? Curr Neurol Neurosci Rep. 2018;18(7):37.
67. Chopra M, Gable DL, Love-Nichols J, Tsao A, Rockowitz S, Sliz P, et al. Mendelian etiologies identified with whole exome sequencing in cerebral palsy. Ann Clin Transl Neurol. 2022;9(2):193-205.
68. Steeves TD, Day L, Dykeman J, Jette N, Pringsheim T. The prevalence of primary dystonia: a systematic review and meta-analysis. Mov Disord. 2012;27(14):1789-96.
69. Donohue KE, Gooch C, Katz A, Wakelee J, Slavotinek A, Korf BR, et al. Pitfalls and challenges in genetic test interpretation: an exploration of genetic professionals experience with interpretation of results. Clin Genet. 2021;99(5):638-49.
70. Jinnah HA, Albanese A, Bhatia KP, Cardoso F, Prat GD, de Koning TJ, et al. Treatable inherited rare movement disorders. Mov Disord. 2018;33(1):21-35.
71. Vale TC, Cardoso F. Chorea: a journey through history. Tremor Other Hyperkinet Mov (N Y). 2015;5:tre-5-296.
72. Walker RH. Chorea. Continuum (Minneap Minn). 2013;19(5, Movement Disorders):1242-63.
73. Walker RH. Thoughts on selected movement disorder terminology and a plea for clarity. Tremor Other Hyperkinet Mov (N Y). 2013; 3:tre-03-203-4656-2.
74. Sanger TD, Chen D, Fehlings DL, Hallett M, Lang AE, Mink JW, et al. Definition and classification of hyperkinetic movements in childhood. Mov Disord. 2010;25(11):1538-49.
75. Mestre TA. Chorea. Continuum (Minneap Minn). 2016;22 (4 Movement Disorders):1186-207.
76. Termsarasab P. Chorea. Continuum (Minneap Minn). 2019; 25(4):1001-35.
77. Jankovic J, Roos RA. Chorea associated with Huntington's disease: to treat or not to treat? Mov Disord. 2014;29(11):1414-8.
78. Macerollo A, Martino D. What is new in tics, dystonia and chorea? Clin Med (Lond). 2016;16(4):383-9.
79. Wild EJ, Tabrizi SJ. The differential diagnosis of chorea. Pract Neurol. 2007;7(6):360-73.
80. Caproni S, Colosimo C. Movement disorders and cerebrovascular diseases: from pathophysiology to treatment. Expert Rev Neurother. 2017;17(5):509-19.
81. Silva GD, Parmera JB, Haddad MS. Acute chorea: case series from the emergency room of a Brazilian tertiary-level center. Arq Neuropsiquiatr. 2021;79(3):233-7.
82. Zesiewicz TA, Sullivan KL. Drug-induced hyperkinetic movement disorders by nonneuroleptic agents. Handb Clin Neurol. 2011;100:347-63.
83. Honorat JA, McKeon A. Autoimmune movement disorders: A clinical and laboratory approach. Curr Neurol Neurosci Rep. 2017; 17(1):4.
84. Cardoso F, Seppi K, Mair KJ, Wenning GK, Poewe W. Seminar on choreas. Lancet Neurol. 2006;5(7):589-602.
85. Marvi MM, Lew MF. Polycythemia and chorea. Handb Clin Neurol. 2011;100:271-6.
86. Vigliani MC, Honnorat J, Antoine JC, Vitaliani R, Giometto B, Psimaras D, et al. Chorea and related movement disorders of paraneoplastic origin: the PNS EuroNetwork experience. J Neurol. 2011;258(11):2058-68.
87. Popławska-Domaszewicz K, Florczak-Wyspiańska J, Kozubski W, Michalak S. Paraneoplastic movement disorders. Rev Neurosci. 2018;29(7):745-55.
88. Feinstein E, Walker R. An update on the treatment of chorea. Curr Treat Options Neurol. 2018;20(10):44.
89. Tran TN, Vo TNN, Frei K, Truong DD. Levodopa-induced dyskinesia: clinical features, incidence, and risk factors. J Neural Transm (Vienna). 2018;125(8):1109-17.
90. Espay AJ, Morgante F, Merola A, Fasano A, Marsili L, Fox SH, et al. Levodopa-induced dyskinesia in Parkinson disease: Current and evolving concepts. Ann Neurol. 2018;84(6):797-811.
91. de Gusmao CM, Waugh JL. Inherited and acquired choreas. Semin Pediatr Neurol. 2018;25:42-53.
92. Martinez-Ramirez D, Walker RH, Rodríguez-Violante M, Gatto EM. Review of hereditary and acquired rare choreas. Tremor Other Hyperkinet Mov (N Y). 2020;10:24.
93. Peall KJ, Kurian MA. Benign hereditary chorea: an update. Tremor Other Hyperkinet Mov (N Y). 2015;5:314.
94. Mehanna R, Jankovic J. Movement disorders in cerebrovascular disease. Lancet Neurol. 2013;12(6):597-608.
95. Walker RH, Jung HH, Danek A. Neuroacanthocytosis. Handb Clin Neurol. 2011;100:141-51.

96. Marshall RD, Collins A, Escolar ML, Jinnah HA, Klopstock T, Kruer MC, et al. Diagnostic and clinical experience of patients with pantothenate kinase-associated neurodegeneration. Orphanet J Rare Dis. 2019;14(1):174.
97. Di Meo I, Tiranti V. Classification and molecular pathogenesis of NBIA syndromes. Eur J Paediatr Neurol. 2018;22(2):272-84.
98. Jinnah HA, Visser JE, Harris JC, Verdu A, Larovere L, Ceballos-Picot I, et al. Delineation of the motor disorder of Lesch-Nyhan disease. Brain. 2006;129(Pt 5):1201-17.
99. Teixeira AL, de Souza LC, Rocha NP, Furr Stimming E, Lauterbach EC. Revisiting the neuropsychiatry of Huntington's disease. Dement Neuropsychol. 2016;10(4):261-6.
100. Stoker TB, Mason SL, Greenland JC, Holden ST, Santini H, Barker RA. Huntington's disease: diagnosis and management. Pract Neurol. 2022;22(1):32-41.
101. Reilmann R, Leavitt BR, Ross CA. Diagnostic criteria for Huntington's disease based on natural history. Mov Disord. 2014;29(11): 1335-41.
102. Ross CA, Reilmann R, Cardoso F, McCusker EA, Testa CM, Stout JC, et al. Movement Disorder Society Task Force Viewpoint: Huntington's disease diagnostic categories. Mov Disord Clin Pract. 2019;6(7):541-6.
103. Schneider SA, Bird T. Huntington's disease, Huntington's disease look-alikes, and benign hereditary chorea: what's new? Mov Disord Clin Pract. 2016;3(4):342-54.
104. Schneider SA, Bhatia KP. Huntington's disease look-alikes. Handb Clin Neurol. 2011;100:101-12.
105. Toyoshima Y, Takahashi H. Spinocerebellar ataxia type 17 (SCA17). Adv Exp Med Biol. 2018;1049:219-31.
106. Feriante J, Gupta V. Neuroacanthocytosis. In: StatPearls. Treasure Island: StatPearls Publishing; 2021.
107. Burke JR, Wingfield MS, Lewis KE, Roses AD, Lee JE, Hulette C, et al. The Haw River syndrome: Dentatorubropallidoluysian atrophy (DRPLA) in an African-American family. Nat Genet. 1994; 7(4):521-4.
108. Caviness JN. Myoclonus. Continuum (Minneap Minn). 2019;25(4): 1055-80.
109. Caviness JN. Primary care guide to myoclonus and chorea. Characteristics, causes, and clinical options. Postgrad Med. 2000;108(5):163-6.
110. Nardocci N. Myoclonus-dystonia syndrome. Handb Clin Neurol. 2011;100:563-75.
111. Marsden CD, Hallett M, Fahn S. The nosology and pathophysiology of myoclonus. In: Marsden CD, Fahn S (Eds). Movement disorders. London, United Kingdom: Butterworths; 1982. pp. 196-248.
112. Caviness JN. Clinical neurophysiology of myoclonus. In: Hallett M (Ed). Movement disorders. Handbook of Clinical Neurophysiology. Vol 1. Amsterdam, the Netherlands: Elsevier; 2003. pp. 521-48.
113. Avanzini G, Shibasaki H, Rubboli G, Canafoglia L, Panzica F, Franceschetti S, et al. Neurophysiology of myoclonus and progressive myoclonus epilepsies. Epileptic Disord. 2016;18(S2): 11-27.
114. Caviness JN, Brown P. Myoclonus: current concepts and recent advances. Lancet Neurol. 2004;3(10):598-607.
115. Frauscher B, Gabella D, Mitterling T, Biermayr M, Bregler D, Ehrmann L, et al. Motor events during healthy sleep: A quantitative polysomnographic study. Sleep. 2014;37(4):763-73.
116. Chokroverty S, Manocha MK, Duvoisin RC. A physiologic and pharmacologic study in anticholinergic-responsive essential myoclonus. Neurology. 1987;37(4):608-15.
117. Wilkins DE, Hallett M, Erba G. Primary generalized epileptic myoclonus: a frequent manifestation of minipolymyoclonus of central origin. J Neurol Neurosurg Psychiatry. 1985;48(6): 506-16.
118. Caviness JN. Epileptic myoclonus. In: Sirven JI, Stern JM (Eds). Atlas of video-EEG monitoring. New York, NY: McGraw-Hill Medical; 2011. pp. 309-28.
119. Genton P, Thomas P, Kasteleijn-Noist Trenité DG, Medina MT, Salas-Puig J. Clinical aspects of juvenile myoclonic epilepsy. Epilepsy Behav. 2013;28(suppl 1):S8-S14.
120. Tan KM, Lennon VA, Klein CJ, Boeve BF, Pittock SJ, et al. Clinical spectrum of voltage-gated potassium channel autoimmunity. Neurology. 2008;70(20):1883-90.
121. Michelucci R, Pasini E, Riguzzi P, Andermann E, Kälviäinen R, Genton P. Myoclonus and seizures in progressive myoclonus epilepsies: pharmacology and therapeutic trials. Epileptic Disord. 2016;18(2):145-53.
122. Marsden CD, Harding QE, Obeso JA, Lu CS. Progressive myoclonic ataxia (the Ramsay Hunt syndrome). Arch Neurol. 1990;47(10): 1121-5.
123. Caviness JN, Adler CH, Beach T. Myoclonus in Lewy body disorders. In: Fahn S, Frucht SJ, Hallett M, Truong D (Eds). Myoclonus and Paroxysmal Dyskinesias. Advances in neurology, Volume 89. New York, NY: Lippincott Williams & Wilkins; 2002. pp. 23-30.
124. Sifoglu A, Gunduz A, Kiziltan G. Dopaminergic medication unrelated myoclonus is less related to tremor in idiopathic Parkinson's disease. Neurol Sci. 2017;38(4):679-82.
125. Beagle AJ, Darwish SM, Ranasinghe KG, La AL, Karageorgiou E, Vossel KA. Relative incidence of seizures and myoclonus in Alzheimer's disease, dementia with Lewy bodies, and fronto-temporal dementia. J Alzheimers Dis. 2017;60(1):211-23.
126. Okuma Y, Fujishima K, Miwa H, Mori H, Mizuno Y. Myoclonic tremulous movements in multiple system atrophy are a form of cortical myoclonus. Mov Disord. 2005;20(4);451-6.
127. Grijalvo-Perez AM, Litvan I. Corticobasal degeneration. Semin Neurol. 2014;34(2):160-73.
128. Iwasaki Y. Creutzfeldt-Jakob disease. Neuropathology. 2017;37(2): 174-88.
129. Alvarez M, Caviness JN. Primary progressive myoclonus of aging. Mov Disord. 2008;23(12):1658-64.
130. Gupta HV, Caviness JN. Post-hypoxic myoclonus: current concepts, neurophysiology, and treatment. Tremor Other Hyperkinet Mov (NY). 2016;6:409.
131. Ong MT, Sarrigiannis PG, Baxter PS. Post-anoxic reticular reflex myoclonus in a child and proposed classification of post-anoxic myoclonus. Pediatr Neurol. 2017;68:68-72.
132. Brown P, Thompson PD, Rothwell JC, Day BL, Marsden CD, et al. Axial myoclonus of propriospinal origin. Brain. 1991;114 (pt 1A):197-214.
133. Antelmi E, Provini F. Propriospinal myoclonus: The spectrum of clinical and neuro physiological phenotypes. Sleep Med Rev. 2015;22:54-63.
134. Deuschl G, Mischke G, Schenck E, Schulte-Mönting J, Lücking CH, et al. Symptomatic and essential rhythmic palatal myoclonus. Brain. 1990;113(pt 6):1645-72.
135. Deuschl G, Wilms H. Palatal tremor: the clinical spectrum and physiology of a rhythmic movement disorder. In: Fahn S, Frucht SJ, Hallett M, Truong D (Eds). Myoclonus and Paroxysmal Dyskinesias. Advances in Neurology, Volume 89. New York, NY: Lippincott Williams and Wilkins; 2002. pp. 115-30.
136. Chaudhry N, Srivastava A, Joshi L. Hemifacial spasm: the past, present and future. J Neurol Sci. 2015;356(1–2):27-31.
137. Shin HW, Ye BS, Kim J, Kim SM, Sohn YH. The contribution of a spinal mechanism in developing peripheral myoclonus: A case report. Mov Disord. 2007;22(9):1350-1.
138. Singer HS. Tics and Tourette syndrome. Continuum (Minneap Minn). 2019;25(4):936-58.
139. Knight T, Steeves T, Day L, Lowerison M, Jette N, Pringsheim T. Prevalence of tic disorders: A systematic review and meta-analysis. Pediatr Neurol. 2012;47(2):77-90.
140. Woods DW, Piacentini J, Himle MB, Chang S. Premonitory Urge for Tics Scale (PUTS): Initial psychometric results and examination of the premonitory urge phenomenon in youths with tic disorders. J Dev Behav Pediatr. 2005;26(6):397-403.

141. Singer HS. Tics and Tourette Syndrome. In: Singer HS, Mink J, Gilbert DL, Jankovic J (Eds). Movement Disorders in Childhood, 2nd edition. London, UK: Elsevier; 2016. pp. 81-109.
142. Robertson MM, Eapen V, Singer HS, Martino D, Scharf JM, Paschou P, et al. Gilles de la Tourette syndrome. Nat Rev Dis Primers. 2017;3:16097.
143. Comings DE, Comings BG. A controlled study of Tourette syndrome. I. Attention-deficit disorder, learning disorders, and school problems. Am J Hum Genet. 1987;41(5):701-41.
144. Fernandez TV, State MW, Pittenger C. Tourette Disorder and Other Tic Disorders. In: Geschwind DH, Paulson HL, Klein C (Eds). Handbook of Clinical Neurology. Amsterdam, the Netherlands: Elsevier; 2018. pp. 343-54.
145. Cavanna AE, Robertson MM, Critchley HD. Catatonic signs in Gilles de la Tourette syndrome. Cogn Behav Neurol. 2008;21(1):34-7.
146. Robertson MM, Trimble MR, Lees AJ. Self-injurious behaviour and the Gilles de la Tourette syndrome: a clinical study and review of the literature. Psychol Med. 1989;19(3):611-25.
147. Lin H, Katsovich L, Ghebremichael M, Findley DB, Grantz H, Lombroso PJ, et al. Psychosocial stress predicts future symptom severities in children and adolescents with Tourette syndrome and/or obsessive-compulsive disorder. J Child Psychol Psychiatry. 2007;48(2):157-66.
148. Mahone EM, Bridges D, Prahme C, Singer HS. Repetitive arm and hand movements (complex motor stereotypies) in children. J Pediatr. 2004;145(3):391-5.
149. Kompoliti K, Goetz CG. Hyperkinetic movement disorders misdiagnosed as tics in Gilles de la Tourette syndrome. Mov Disord. 1998;13(3):477-80.
150. Gaze C, Kepley HO, Walkup JT. Co-occurring psychiatric disorders in children and adolescents with Tourette syndrome. J Child Neurol. 2006;21(8):657-64.
151. Shprecher DR, Gannon K, Agarwal N, Shi X, Anderson JS. Elucidating the nature and mechanism of tic improvement in tourette syndrome: A pilot study. Tremor Other Hyperkinet Mov (NY). 2014;4:217.
152. Eapen V, Lees AJ, Lakke JP, Trimble MR, Robertson MM. Adult-onset tic disorders. Mov Disord. 2002;17(4):735-40.
153. Erenberg G, Cruse RP, Rothner AD. The natural history of Tourette syndrome: a follow-up study. Ann Neurol. 1987;22(3):383-5.
154. Pappert EJ, Goetz CG, Louis ED, Blasucci L, Leurgans S. Objective assessments of longitudinal outcome in Gilles de la Tourette's syndrome. Neurology. 2003;61(7):936-40.
155. Vijayakumar D, Jankovic J. Drug-induced dyskinesia, part 2: Treatment of tardive dyskinesia. Drugs. 2016;76(7):779-87.
156. Kwak C, Dat Vuong K, Jankovic J. Premonitory sensory phenomenon in Tourette's syndrome. Mov Disord. 2003;18(12):1530-3.
157. Banaschewski T, Woerner W, Rothenberger A. Premonitory sensory phenomena and suppressibility of tics in Tourette syndrome: Developmental aspects in children and adolescents. Dev Med Child Neurol. 2003;45(10):700-3.
158. Soman T, Lang AE. Movement disorders. Continuum (Minneap Minn). 2009;15(6, Childhood Neurologic Disorders in Adulthood): 167-90.
159. Baizabal-Carvallo JF, Jankovic J. The clinical features of psychogenic movement disorders resembling tics. J Neurol Neurosurg Psychiatry. 2014;85(5):573-5.
160. Jankovic J, Mejia NI. Tics associated with other disorders. Adv Neurol. 2006;99:61-8.
161. Definitions and classification of tic disorders. The Tourette Syndrome Classification Study Group. Arch Neurol. 1993;50(10): 1013-6.
162. American Psychiatric Association. Diagnostic and statistical manual of mental disorders, 5th edition (DSM-5). Washington, DC: American Psychiatric Association; 2013.
163. Martino D, Ganos C, Pringsheim TM. Tourette syndrome and chronic tic disorders: the clinical spectrum beyond tics. Int Rev Neurobiol. 2017;134:1461-90.
164. International Classification of Sleep Disorders, 3rd edition. Darien, IL: American Academy of Sleep Medicine; 2014.
165. Ohayon MM, Guilleminault C, Priest RG. Night terrors, sleepwalking, and confusional arousals in the general population: their frequency and relationship to other sleep and mental disorders. J Clin Psychiatry. 1999; 60:268.
166. Vaughn BV, Ali I. Sleep and epilepsy: opportunities for diagnosis and treatment. Neurol Clin. 2012;30:1249.
167. Laganière C, Pennestri MH, Rassu AL, Barateau L, Chenini S, Evangelista E, et al. Disturbed nighttime sleep in children and adults with rhythmic movement disorder. Sleep. 2020;43: zsaa105.
168. Wichniak A, Tracik F, Geisler P, Ebersbach G, Morrissey SP, Zulley J. Rhythmic feet movements while falling asleep. Mov Disord. 2001;16:1164.
169. D'Cruz OF, Vaughn BV. Nocturnal seizures mimic REM behavior disorder. Am J Electroneurodiagnostic Technol. 1997;37:258.
170. Dyken ME, Afifi AK, Lin-Dyken DC. Sleep-related problems in neurologic diseases. Chest. 2012;141:528.
171. Rice E, Fisher C. Fugue states in sleep and wakefulness: A psychophysiological study. J Nerv Ment Dis. 1976;163:79.
172. Tinuper P, Bisulli F, Cross JH, Hesdorffer D, Kahane P, Nobili L, et al. Definition and diagnostic criteria of sleep-related hypermotor epilepsy. Neurology. 2016;86:1834.
173. Foldvary-Schaefer N, Alsheikhtaha Z. Complex nocturnal behaviors: nocturnal seizures and parasomnias. Continuum (Minneap Minn). 2013;19:104.
174. Schenck CH, Milner DM, Hurwitz TD, Bundlie SR, Mahowald MW. A polysomnographic and clinical report on sleep-related injury in 100 adult patients. Am J Psychiatry. 1989;146:1166.
175. Schenck CH, Mahowald MW. REM sleep behavior disorder: clinical, developmental, and neuroscience perspectives 16 years after its formal identification in SLEEP. Sleep. 2002;25:120.
176. van der Salm SM, de Haan RJ, Cath DC, Rootselaar AF, Tijssen MAJ. The eye of the beholder: Inter-rater agreement among experts on psychogenic jerky movement disorders. J Neurol Neurosurg Psychiatry. 2013;84(7):742-7.

74

CHAPTER

Wilson's Disease

DV Seshagiri, Sanjib Sinha

INTRODUCTION

Wilson's disease (WD) is an inborn error of copper metabolism resulting in excess accumulation of copper in the various parts of the human body, most commonly involving the liver and brain. The first clinical description of WD was done by Wilson SAK (1911), where he described four patients with the title progressive lenticular degeneration, a familial nervous system disease associated with liver cirrhosis. He gave a detailed clinical description of these patients and autopsy findings. The association of the Kayser–Fleischer (KF) ring with the sunflower cataract was described by Siemerling and Oloff (1922). The autosomal recessive pattern of inheritance was documented in 30 families by Bearn (1960). Excessive copper deposition in the liver, in a patient dying with WD, was initially reported by Austrian pathologist Rumpel (1913). The discovery of penicillamine therapy (1960), improving this fatal disease, revolutionized the management aspect of WD. Till today penicillamine is the most commonly used medication for WD in the world.[1] With early recognition of this fatal disease and initiation of appropriate treatment, these patients can have a normal life expectancy. With the advancement in science over the last 3–4 decades, WD can be diagnosed easily with currently available tests; however, the clinician needs knowledge about the disease and a high index of suspicion to pick up early, thereby preventing morbidity and mortality.

EPIDEMIOLOGY

The incidence and prevalence of WD vary widely depending on the screening method used to estimate. The first epidemiological studies on WD done by Sternlieb (1968) quoted the incidence to be at 5 per million, subsequently in East Germany between 1949 and 1977 Bachman (1979) found it to be 29 per million. The clinical prevalence studies underestimate the true prevalence, as there can be many asymptomatic WD patients in the community. It is also important to recognize the asymptomatic WD patients due to the high therapeutic potential advantage. Screening of newborns for the WD with dried blood spot (using holo-ceruloplasmin assay) method was disappointing. However, the study using older children 6 months to 9 years yielded a prevalence of 124 per million in the UK. The authors suggested 3 years as the appropriate age for screening for WD. In Korean children between 3 months and 15 years old, the dried blood spot method found a higher prevalence of 717 per million. H1069Q was the most common mutation observed in the European population. In Japanese R778L and Spanish M645R mutations were common. There exist population isolates where WD had a very high prevalence of 370 per million births in the Sardinian population. Rucar from Romania showed the highest prevalence in the world with 885 per million genetically confirmed study.[2] The genetic prevalence may be four times higher compared to the clinical prevalence. The global prevalence of WD estimated by WHO was 1 per 10,000–30,000. There were no Indian studies estimating the prevalence of WD, however, in the pediatric liver disease population, WD accounts for 7.6–19.7% in tertiary hepatobiliary centers, and about 15–20 new WD patients were diagnosed annually in a neurology referral center.[3]

PATHOLOGY AND PATHOPHYSIOLOGY

Wilson's disease is an autosomal recessive disorder with a genetic defect in the membrane protein called ATP7B, which plays a vital role in the copper transportation mechanisms. ATP7B is expressed abundantly in the liver and to a lesser extent in the brain, kidney, heart, and lung. The impaired function in the ATP7B in patients with WD causes abnormal copper homeostatic mechanisms resulting in excessive accumulation of copper predominantly in the liver, brain, and other systems. The ATP7B transporter protein facilitates the expulse of copper from the liver through biliary secretions. Excess copper in the liver stimulates the trafficking of ATP7B protein by trans-Golgi apparatus, in the hepatocyte close to the apical membrane of the biliary canaliculus, where copper is incorporated into the nascent ceruloplasmin. This excess copper removal mechanism is being affected, resulting in an abnormally high amount of copper accumulation in the liver. Ceruloplasmin is the major copper-carrying protein, almost 90% of the copper, circulates bounding to ceruloplasmin. ATP7B dysfunction resulting in failure to incorporate copper into the nascent ceruloplasmin may lead to unstable compound and early destruction resulting in low serum ceruloplasmin. Though there is excess copper accumulation in the various organs in the body, total serum copper will be low, as there is low ceruloplasmin-bound copper. However, serum free copper is always high, which is difficult to measure in the routine laboratory. The amount of free copper is responsible for the various toxic effects found in the WD. The exact mechanism by which free copper causes liver, brain, and other organ injury is not clear, and the possible mechanism is copper-induced oxidative stress. Intracellular copper-induced oxidative stress generates hydroxyl radicals, glutathione, and reduced superoxide dismutase, which can cause membrane damage leading to apoptosis and cell death.[3,4]

CLINICAL PRESENTATION

Though WD is a multisystem disease, the predominant organs involved are the liver and brain. The liver is the earliest organ involved in the disease process, and the liver symptoms manifest at an early age in the first decade of life. WD rarely manifests before 3–5 years. Only a few cases were reported in those below 3 years of age. Hepatic presentation occurs in 83% present before 10 years, 52% between 10 and 18 years, and 24% >18 years. Neurological presentation occurs 17% before 10 years, 48% between 10 and 18 years, and 74% >18 years. Studies showed symptom onset to diagnosis was shorter with hepatic presentation (6 months) than neuropsychiatric presentation (18 months). The frequency of hepatic and neurological presentation depends on the pattern of patients visiting the reporting institute, viz., neurological and hepatic institutes, with respective authors, might report higher frequencies in their respective specialities.[3,5]

Hepatic Presentations[3,6]

Wilson's disease presents with wide varied type of presentations from asymptomatic stage to acute liver failure (ALF).

- *Asymptomatic liver disease*: The regular practice of family screening for the WD showed asymptomatic liver abnormalities; there can be a mild elevation of liver enzymes alone (18–23%). Some of them may have mild hepatomegaly or splenomegaly on physical examinations; it is not uncommon to find liver cirrhosis in asymptomatic patients with WD while screening siblings.
- *Symptomatic liver disease*: Patient manifest with mild liver disease to liver cell failure requiring liver transplantation (LT). The most common symptoms are nausea, jaundice, vomiting, and anorexia (37–44%), then ascites (23–26%) with either splenomegaly, hepatomegaly, or both (16–29%).
- *Acute hepatitis*: Patients often present with anorexia, nausea, jaundice, and elevation of transaminases, conjugated hyperbilirubinemia. It accounts for 10–25%. The presentation needs to be distinguished from acute viral hepatitis, drug-induced hepatitis, and autoimmune hepatitis. One needs to consider WD as one of the differentials during evaluating children and adolescents with acute hepatitis, particularly if the virus serology is negative.
- *Acute liver cell failure*: It usually starts with the acute hepatitis-like presentation but might rapidly progress to deep jaundice, coagulation failure, ascites, encephalopathy, hemolysis, coagulopathy, and renal failure. The reported frequency is around 8–20% and observed more commonly in patients with WD, who stops chelating agents abruptly.
- *Acute on chronic liver failure*: Sometimes, acute viral hepatitis may unmask the preexisting chronic liver disease related to WD. In 42–43% of patients, the cause for underlying chronic liver disease was WD in this type of presentation.
- *Chronic liver disease*: Patients usually present with nonspecific symptoms such as anorexia, malaise, nausea, and jaundice. They can also have amenorrhea, delayed puberty, and polyarthralgia. It is often seen in adolescents and accounts for 10–30% of hepatic presentations.
- *Cirrhosis*: Liver cirrhosis can be incidentally detected in neurological WD. It is not surprising to observe liver cirrhosis while screening the siblings. Cirrhosis is often detected when they present with complications like variceal bleeding related to portal hypertension, hepatorenal syndrome, ascites, and sometimes with spontaneous bacterial presentations. About 35–60% of them present with complications related to cirrhosis.
- *Fatty liver*: The presence of nonalcoholic fatty liver in a child should raise the suspiciousness of WD. The frequency of fatty liver in various studies ranges between 28 and 35.7%.
- *Malignancies*: The occurrence of hepatocellular carcinoma (HCC) in WD is less; uncommonly noted in patients with cirrhosis. However, rare reports showing the occurrence of HCC in noncirrhotic hepatic WD have been documented. Though the risk of HCC is low, some clinicians recommend screening for HCC in patients with hepatic WD, as early recognition of HCC has potential treatment options.

Neurological Features[5,7-9]

Patients with neurological WD usually present in the second decade and after. However, an occurrence at the young age of 6 years and 72 years was reported. The later presentation of neurological WD, may be explained that, after the initial involvement of the liver, over-spillage of copper from the liver may affect other organs like the brain. The liver is almost always involved in neurological WD, though it may be asymptomatic many times. The presenting neurological symptoms may vary considerably, including parkinsonism, tremor, ataxia, myoclonus, athetosis, dystonia, dysphagia, dysarthria, drooling, chorea, tic disorder, seizures, and cognitive impairment.

- *Parkinsonism*: Parkinsonism features such as hypomimia, bradykinesia, rest tremor, slow shuffling gait, and occasional postural imbalance have been reported in 16–62% of the WD presenting with neurological manifestations.
- *Tremor*: Wilson's disease can present with many types of tremors, and they may change in character as the disease evolves (dynamic tremor) and improves with decoppering treatment. Tremors can resemble essential tremor (ET), dystonic tremor, parkinsonian rest tremor, and rubral tremor. The characteristic wing beating tremor (the tremor appears after a few seconds, after assuming wing beating position of the upper limbs—the extension of shoulders, flexion of elbows, and palms facing down) found in WD is a low frequency, high amplitude, and sometimes disabling. Tremor is commonly bilateral, asymmetrical/symmetrical, and can have unilateral also.
- *Dystonia*: It can be the initial presentation in 11–65% of the patients, and during the course of the illness, dystonia can be found in 38–65% of patients with neurological WD. Patients can manifest with focal, segmental, and generalized dystonia with varying severity. The facial muscles dystonia with hypomimia produces characteristic facies, which is the common focal dystonia in WD. Dystonic dropped jaw with parkinsonian face produces open mouth, sometimes labeled as "vacuous smile", risorius, and zygomaticus muscles spasmodic contraction may result in fixed forced smile referred as "risus sardonicus". A vacuous smile and risus sardonicus give rise to the characteristic facial appearance in WD. Other focal dystonias include cervical dystonia, writer's cramps, and blepharospasm; and these can be a part of generalized dystonia. Drooling, dysarthria, and dysphagia, commonly found in WD may be the result of dystonia involving facial muscles, pharyngeal muscles, tongue, and vocal cords.
- *Ataxia*: The reported frequency of ataxia in WD is around 30%. Intentional tremors, dysarthria, and broad-based gait are commonly seen associated with other movement disorders such as tremor and dystonia. However, isolated cerebellar ataxia and nystagmus suggestive of cerebellar damage are not usually found in WD.
- *Chorea*: Less frequently observed movement disorder in WD, about 6–16% in the neurological presentation was reported. Involuntary irregular, unpredictable movements interfering with normal activities involving the face, head, neck, trunk, and extremities are called chorea. Chorea, when associated with slow writhing movements of the face, head, and extremities called choreoathetosis, and confluent choreiform movements may result in ballistic movements.
- *Epilepsy*: The reported frequency of WD is about 6.2 and 8.3% in two larger studies involving 200 and 490 patients, respectively. Various causes for seizures were proposed including, atrophy and lesions of the cortical white matter involving in the frontal lobes predominantly, less frequently involving parietal, and occipital lobes.[7,10]
- *Other neurological symptoms*: Few studies/case reports suggest the involvement of peripheral nerves and autonomic nervous system in WD. Liver disease, excess copper, copper deficiency resulting from zinc therapy, and D-penicillamine (DP) therapy can be proposed to be the cause of neuropathy in WD. However, it is difficult to conclude the etiology of neuropathic illness. The clinician treating WD needs to keep a careful watch on neuropathic symptoms like sensory ataxic myeloneuropathy, which can be a sign of copper deficiency indicating excessive decoppering therapy. Autonomic dysfunction and small fiber neuropathy were reported, but not orthostatic hypotension. Olfactory disturbances, proportional to the severity of neurological involvement; pyramidal signs, myoclonus, tics, painful legs, headache, sleep disturbances, and taste disturbances can also be observed in WD.

Psychiatric Presentation[9,11]

Wilson's disease can present like a pure psychiatric disease or psychiatric symptoms develop during the disease course and can be associated with both neurological and hepatic WD. Diagnosis of WD is often delayed with a pure psychiatric presentation of WD, as it requires a high index of suspicion in the routine psychiatry practice. The median delay was around 2.5 years. All kinds of psychiatric presentations can be found in WD.

Depression is one of the common manifestations. Major depressive disorder can be found between 4 and 47.8%, depending upon the study center and assessment tools used for the diagnosis of WD. Bipolar disorder was found in 18–30%, while mania and hypomania were noted in 39% in one study. Significant anxiety symptoms were reported in up to 20–62% of patients and panic disorder in 8.7% of patients. Psychotic symptoms can be the initial presenting symptoms in 4.2% of patients. Schizophrenia was diagnosed in 11% of patients with WD. During the course of the illness, studies have reported psychotic symptoms up to 40%. Patients with WD have increased sensitivity to neuroleptic medications. It is not uncommon that, the diagnosis of WD would be established, when these patients develop involuntary movements after initiation of antipsychotic medications and a neurologist evaluate the patient.

Ophthalmologic Manifestations

The Kayser–Fleischer (KF) ring **(Fig. 1)**, once considered a pathognomonic feature of WD, is present in almost all patients with neurological WD, 50% hepatic WD, 20–30% of presymptomatic WD. KF ring usually appears as a bilateral peripheral corneal ring with brownish, greenish, and yellowish discoloration resulting from the deposition of copper pigments in the Descemet membrane. The KF ring usually starts appearing from the superior margin, then the inferior margin, and medial and lateral margins of the cornea. With adequate treatment of WD, the KF ring fades away in the opposite direction; the superior margin ring disappears last. This pattern of formation and fading of the KF ring was thought to be related to the vertical flow of aqueous fluid in the anterior chamber of the eye. KF ring was once thought to be specific for WD. However, similar rings were found in other disorders like primary biliary cirrhosis, chronic cholestasis associated with serum bilirubin >20 mg/dL, multiple myeloma, monoclonal gammopathies, and arcus senilis. These rings may be the result of excessive deposition of copper, other metals, or bilirubin. The clinician needs to be careful when evaluating hepatic disease with a KF ring as there is a possibility of false positive and false negative KF ring.[7]

Sunflower cataract was once thought to be a pathognomonic manifestation of WD. However, subsequent studies found that sunflower cataract is a rare manifestation of the WD. The cataract is characterized by the deposition of the copper pigments in the capsule of the lens resembling a sunflower (central disk with radiating petal-like fronds). Sunflower cataract usually does not cause visual impairment.[7]

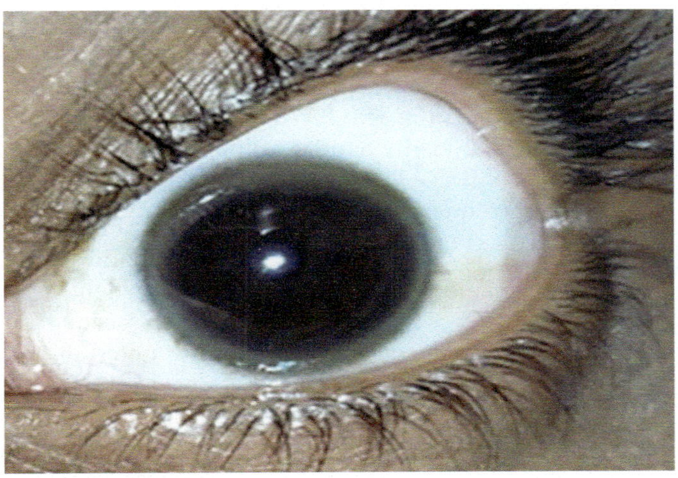

FIG. 1: Showing brown color ring at the corneal limbus suggestive of Kayser–Fleischer (KF) ring.

DIAGNOSIS OF WILSON'S DISEASE

The clinical presentation of WD is widely varied. The clinicians should be familiar with various forms of the presentation of this fatal, treatable genetic disorder. Once there is a high index of suspiciousness, the diagnosis of WD is not difficult, particularly in the neurological WD. The presence of low serum ceruloplasmin/copper, neurological syndrome, corneal KF ring, and MRI changes clinches the diagnosis of WD. However, hepatic presentations such as acute liver cell failure and intravascular hemolytic presentations sometimes pose a significant diagnostic challenge.

- *Serum ceruloplasmin*: Ceruloplasmin synthesized in hepatic microsomes as an inactive apoceruloplasmin. Adding six copper atoms results in holoceruloplasmin (active). The holoceruloplasmin carries 90% of serum copper. The genetic defect in the *ATP7B* gene causes failure to incorporate copper, resulting in a decrease in the active ceruloplasmin. The active ceruloplasmin decreased in WD. However, the currently available laboratory tests measures both ceruloplasmins (total) together. Though the total ceruloplasmin decreased in WD, there can be false positive and false negative results. Ceruloplasmin is acute phase reactant elevated in tissue damage, infection/inflammation.[3,12,13]
- *Serum copper*: As there is a significantly low level of copper carrying protein (serum ceruloplasmin) in the plasma, the total serum copper is low in WD in proportion to the low ceruloplasmin. However, free serum copper is elevated in WD, which is difficult to measure. In the presence of low ceruloplasmin, normal or elevated copper indicates an increase in unbound copper. Total unbound copper can be estimated by a formula:

  $$\text{Unbound serum copper } \mu g/L = \text{Total serum copper} - 3.15 \times [\text{serum ceruloplasmin (mg/L)}]$$

  The problem with this formula is that it depends on the accuracy of the method used to estimate ceruloplasmin and copper and is not useful as a diagnostic marker.[3,12,13]
- *24 hours urinary copper*: Measurement of 24 hours urinary copper may roughly reflect the free copper in the blood; however, the diagnostic value depends upon the normal kidney function. The chances of contamination of urinary samples are high, resulting in false high values. One should be reminded of the practical difficulty in collecting complete 24 hours urinary samples in children and neurological patients. Children with asymptomatic siblings can have lower urinary copper. Hence, the lower cut-off value of urinary copper may be more sensitive.[3,12,13]
- *Relative exchangeable copper (REC)*: Ultrafiltrable copper and copper that is loosely bound to albumin and

amino acids constitute the free serum copper which is not bound to the ceruloplasmin. The percentage of free copper to the total copper (unbound + ceruloplasmin bound copper) is called REC. A cut-off above 18.5% was found to be diagnostic of WD with 100% sensitivity and specificity. REC can also be used to discriminate heterozygous carriers, WD patients, and normal subjects; hence can also be used for family screening. This is a research tool, not widely used, and has significant potential for a promising role in the diagnosis and monitoring of WD.[3,13]

- *Hepatic copper estimation*: Accumulation of copper in the liver is one of the important features of WD. However, histological evaluation with rhodamine stains shows the only focal accumulation of copper in 10% of patients. Estimation of copper in the dry hepatic tissue is the method of choice. A recent study with a 691-sample size showed a cut-off of 209 mg/g of dry weight of liver, having a sensitivity of 99.4% and specificity was around 96.1%. However, sampling errors and nonhomogenous distribution of copper in the liver may significantly affect the results.[3,12,13]
- *Liver biopsy*: Usually, liver histology/biopsy is not done for routine diagnosis of WD. For the evaluation of alternate causes and inconclusive noninvasive tests, a liver biopsy may be done. In the early stages of the WD, histology shows microvascular and macrovascular mild steatosis and focal hepatocellular necrosis, and these findings usually mislead the diagnosis of nonalcoholic fatty liver. Features of chronic hepatitis mimic autoimmune hepatitis, and advanced disease may show markers of fibrosis. The ultrastructural analysis finding may help in the diagnosis of WD in the early steatosis phase of the disease.[3,12,13]
- *Brain imaging*: Imaging the brain with MRI in patients with WD contributed to a significant understanding of pathoanatomy of the WD. MRI brain is one of the most sensitive diagnostic tools for the diagnosis of neurological WD. At least one regional brain abnormality can be found in all the symptomatic untreated neurological WD. The imaging findings are almost diagnostic in the presence of the appropriate clinical settings. The imaging abnormalities improve significantly with adequate decoppering therapy and are useful for disease monitoring. The most prominent feature in the brain MRI is T2W and fluid-attenuated inversion recovery (FLAIR) hyperintensities involving bilateral basal ganglia, thalamus, pontine, and mesencephalic white matter. The characteristic imaging signs found in WD are "face of the giant panda" in the midbrain, "miniature panda" in the pons, and "central pontine myelinolysis"—like presentations.[12,14-16] The frequencies of various parts of the brain involvement are described in the **Table 1** and signs are described in the **Figure 2**.
- *Genetic testing*: It is usually not required in presence of typical biochemical, clinical, and imaging abnormalities associated with WD. However, Sanger sequencing of ATP7B usually establishes the genetic diagnosis of WD. Demonstration of biallelic, two known pathogenic mutations in the *ATP7B* gene, establishes the genetic diagnosis of the WD. Around 907 deleterious variants are identified. The genetic tests could not identify the pathogenic variant in 1–27% of affected patients. Some part of this could be partially explained by incomplete genetic analysis. However, even in complete genetic analysis, the detection rate for the pathogenic variant was 77–98%. The additional genetic mechanisms like uniparental disomy and complex structural genomic variants involved in the pathogenesis of the disease might be the reason for the missing of the pathogenic variants. The proposed flow chart for genetic testing in WD is 1st step—Sanger sequencing of *ATP7B* gene (archives molecular diagnosis most of the times)—if negative then 2nd step—multiplex ligation-dependent probe amplification (MLPA) for large deletions and promotor analysis by Sanger sequencing—if negative 3rd step—entire ATP7B sequence analysis by next-generation sequencing (NGS), including untranslated regions (UTRs) and intron, if negative, the clinician needs to be asked to review the diagnosis and whole exome/genome sequencing may be done to look for the disease mimics.[17]
- *Family screening*: Screening for WD is important to detect this fatal disease in the presymptomatic phase and initiate appropriate treatment, which may prevent the occurrence of the disease. There are 25% chances of affecting siblings and 0.5% chances in the offspring of the index patient from a nonconsanguineous parentage.

TABLE 1: Topographic distribution of MRI brain lesions in patients with Wilson's disease.

Site of brain pathology	MRI brain abnormalities (%)	
	Sinha S et al. (*n* = 100)	**Yu XE et al. (*n* = 364)**
Putamen	72%	81.0%
Globus pallidus	40%	15.4%
Caudate nucleus	61%	34.3%
Thalamus	58%	36.0%
Pons	20%	46.4%
Midbrain	49%	33.5%
Frontal lobe	6%	3.2%
Parietal lobe	0%	3.3%
Temporal lobe	3%	3.3%
Cerebellum	10%	2.2%
Corpus callosum	0%	2.2%
Occipital lobe	0%	0%
Medulla oblongata	12%	0%

(MRI: magnetic resonance imaging)

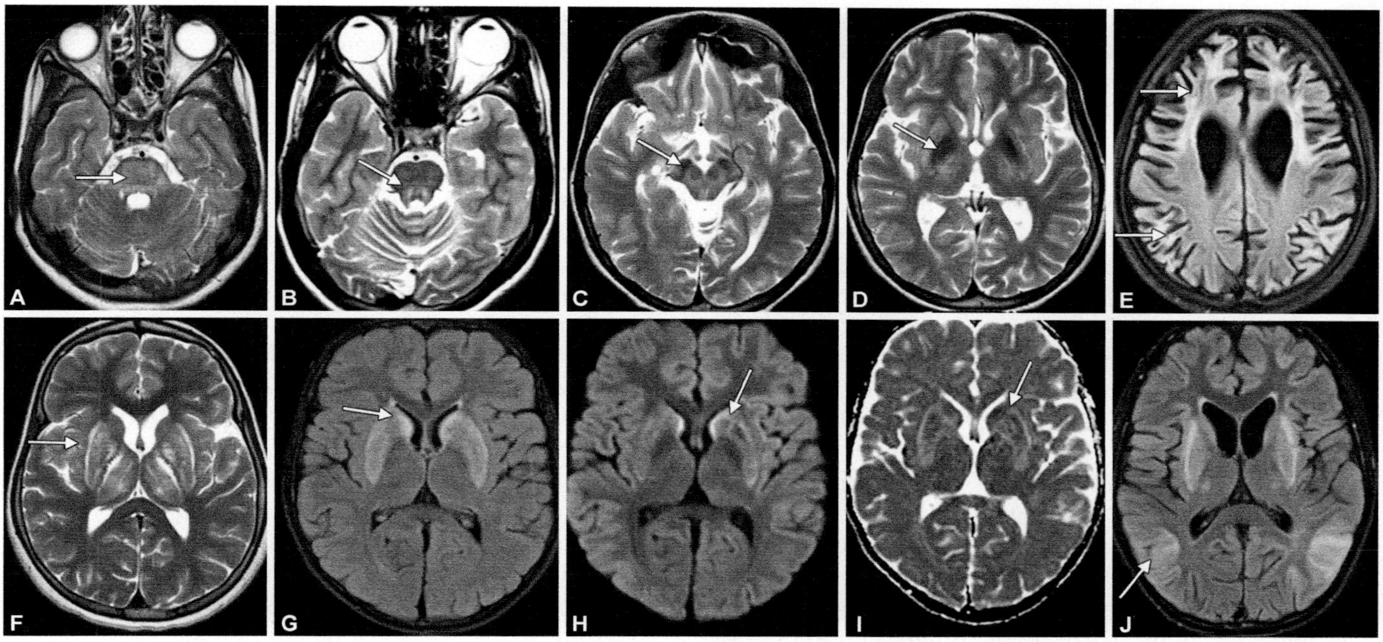

FIGS. 2A TO J: Spectrum of magnetic resonance imaging (MRI) findings in patients with Wilson's disease (WD). Figures A, B, C, D, and F are T2-weighted (T2W) MRI brain images. (A) Central pontine myelinolysis like picture (white arrow); (B) Characteristic miniature panda sign (white arrow); (C) Giant panda sign (white arrow); (D) Hypointensity in the globus pallidus; (E) T2 FLAIR image showing atrophy in frontal and parietal lobes (white arrows); (F) Bright claustrum sign (white arrow); (G) T2 FLAIR image showing involvement of caudate and putamen; (H) Diffusion-weighted imaging (DWI) and (I) Apparent diffusion coefficient (ADC) map showing diffusion restriction in the caudate suggestive acute illness (white arrow); (J) Parietal cortex involvement (white arrow) along with putamen.

Screening is recommended for siblings, parents, and offspring. WD is rarely symptomatic before 3 years of age. Screening can be done after 3 years with serum ceruloplasmin, 24 hours urinary copper, KF ring, and ultrasound abdomen for liver pathology. The negative results of these screening tests do not exclude the presymptomatic disease and need to be repeated for better sensitivity. Mutation analysis of the index patient in the sibling may be the most reliable way of screening, which can be done once, even at an early age.[12]

- *Leipzig and modified Leipzig scoring system*: There is no single test to diagnose WD confidently. At the 8th International Meeting on WD, Leipzig 2001 developed a scoring system that provides good diagnostic accuracy. The Leipzig score was modified by a consortium of Indian researchers who developed clinical practice guidelines for the WD. A modified Leipzig score of 4 or more establishes the diagnosis of WD. The scoring system helps to understand the diagnostic value of each test. The higher the abnormality of a test, there is more likely to establish the diagnosis. The scorings in bracket () are as follows. KF ring present (2), absent (0); serum ceruloplasmin 0–5 mg/dL (3), 6–10 mg/dL (2), 11–20 mg/dL (1), >20 mg/dL (0); 24 hours urinary copper (in the absence of acute hepatitis) <40 µg (0), 40–100 µg (1), and >100 µg (2); Coombs-negative hemolytic anemia with liver disease absent (0), present (1); both chromosomes mutation detected (4), detected on single chromosome (1); Orcein- or rhodanine-positive granules on liver biopsy (1); neurobehavioral symptoms present (2), absent (0); typical features on MRI brain absent (0), present (1); history of WD in the family absent (1), present (2).[3,12]

MANAGEMENT OF WILSON'S DISEASE

Decoppering therapy is the mainstay of the treatment for WD. The decoppering therapy can reverse some of the pathological changes and clinical symptoms. Presymptomatic patients can prevent the occurrence of the disease. There are no randomized studies regarding the effectiveness of decoppering medications in WD.

- *Dimercaprol*: It is also called British anti-Lewisite (BAL), it was the first chelating used to treat WD. Earlier studies had demonstrated good improvement with BAL. However, due to significant side effects, and frequent intramuscular injections, it is not used currently for WD management.
- *D-penicillamine (DP)*: It is the most used chelating agent for WD in the world. DP makes disulfide bonds with copper and is excreted in the urine. DP binds with free copper, which is not bound to ceruloplasmin and is the principal mechanism of action. DP also chelates copper from the tissue-resident complexes due to its high affinity.

One gram of DP can combine with 200 mg of copper based on the chemical mechanism; however, in vivo, 1 g of DP can chelate only 2 mg of copper. The recommended dose of DP is 1,000–1,500 mg/day in 2–3 divided doses. In children, the dose is 20 mg/kg/day up to a maximum of 1,500 mg/day. DP is incompletely absorbed from the gastrointestinal tract. It needs to be taken 1 hour before or 2 hours after food. Antacids, iron, zinc, and food decrease the absorption of DP. While treating neurological WD with DP, it is preferable to "start low go slow" as there is a chance of DP-induced neurological worsening in a subset of patients. DP-induced neurological worsening was hypothesized, related to excessive generation of free copper by the DP. However, such DP-induced worsening is sometimes difficult to differentiate from the natural disease progression/ noncompliant with medication. The maintenance dose of DP is 1,000 mg/day. DP at recommended doses can cause significant side effects in up to 30% of patients leading to discontinuation in some patients. Early adverse reactions, which occur usually within 3 weeks, most of them are related to hypersensitivity reactions, including fever, generalized pruritus, lymphadenopathy, urticarial eruptions, exfoliative dermatitis, arthralgia, leukopenia, and thrombocytopenia. The late reactions usually occur from 3 weeks to a few years after initiation of DP, renal impairment, Good–Pasture syndrome, drug-induced myasthenia, lupus-like syndrome, hypogeusia, hair loss, and bone marrow suppression.[18,19]

- *Trientine (triethylenetetramine)*: Trientine was first introduced in 1969 to overcome the side effects of DP. Trientine has a different structure compared to DP, lacking sulfhydryl; however, the mechanism of action is similar. It combines with nonceruloplasmin-bound copper and facilitates the excretion of copper from the kidney, similar to DP. It is given orally and is poorly absorbed through the gastrointestinal tract compared to DP. The compound is unstable at higher temperatures and needs to be stored at 2–80°C. Trientine is usually prescribed at 750 mg–1,500 mg/day initially, and the maintenance dose is around 750–1,000 mg/day. Given at 2–3 divided doses 1 hour before or 2 hours after food. It has similar chelating potency when compared with DP. However, controversial data regarding efficacy when compared with DP exists. The side effects are four times less compared to DP. The side effects include lupus-like reactions, chelation of iron resulting in sideroblastic anemia, skin rashes, hemorrhagic gastritis, and loss of taste. Neurological deterioration can occur similar to DP. Hence, "start low, go slow" strategy applies to trientine also. Trientine can be used as monotherapy for WD in view of a good safety profile. However, high cost, strict temperature control for storage, and not being widely available make the trientine less frequently used medication for WD compared to DP. Trientine recently launched in the Indian market.[18-20]
- *Zinc salts*: It predominantly act by interfering with the absorption of copper from the gastrointestinal tract creating a negative copper balance. Zinc acetate, zinc sulfate, and zinc gluconate are the salts used for the treatment of WD. Zinc induces metallothionein synthesis about 25-folds in the enterocytes. Metallothioneins have a high affinity to bind some metals, and copper has more affinity compared to zinc. Hence, copper replaces zinc. The copper absorbed in the enterocytes by metallothioneins is prevented from entering the bloodstream and passes into stools when they shred during the normal cell turnover process. The usual zinc dose in adults is 150–300 mg of elemental zinc, which needs to be taken 30–60 minutes before food in 2–3 divided doses. Once daily dosage of zinc is not effective. Zinc is less potent as a decoppering agent compared to currently used chelating agents. It is commonly used as maintenance therapy in presymptomatic patients. Because of lesser adverse effects, low cost, and wide availability, some clinicians started using zinc for maintenance therapy for symptomatic WD, as well as for the initial treatment, particularly for the neurological form of WD. However, deterioration of liver disease has been reported during zinc therapy. Zinc requires around 3 weeks for full activation of metallothioneins, which results in the slow onset of action. Zinc is tolerated well, and the most common side effects are nausea and vomiting. Zinc causes gastric irritation and ulcers and asymptomatic elevation of pancreatic enzymes mimicking pancreatitis. Zinc sulfate form is commonly attributed to the dyspepsia symptoms. Zinc is also reported to cause neurological worsening in 7.3%, though this neurological worsening could be part of natural disease progression. Zinc therapy can rarely cause a copper deficiency in WD as well as non-WD, which manifest as anemia, leukopenia, neutropenia, sensory ataxia, and myelopathy. The symptoms improve with stopping/reducing the dose of zinc.[18,19,21]
- *Tetrathiomolybdate (TTM)*: Currently available decoppering agents do not cross the blood–brain barrier (BBB), and there is a risk of excessive generation of free copper, which can be responsible for the initial progression of the illness, requires frequent dosing in the fasting state and needs to be taken apart from the meal. Though TTM was in clinical studies since 1986 in the form of ammonium TTM, it was not approved for clinical use as it was an unstable compound. The new form, bis-choline TTM (WTX101), completed phase II clinical trials, and phase III trials are ongoing. Though not completely understood, this chelating agent works by a different mechanism of action, forms tripartite complexes along with free copper and albumin, thereby avoiding free copper-induced worsening, removes intracellular copper, increases the biliary secretion of copper, and crosses BBB. In the phase II trial, there was

no neurological deterioration. Hence, this bis-choline TTM is expected to be a more efficient chelating agent that may prevent the disease progression, particularly in the neurological form of WD. The medication has the advantage of a once-daily dose, which is well tolerated but can cause elevation of liver transaminases, which can be reversible after stopping/reducing the dose.[18,19,22,23]

- *Liver transplantation (LT)*: Curative treatment for the WD is LT. However, LT has its limitations related to donor availability, surgical complications in both donor and patient, the requirement of long-term immunosuppression, and graft rejection. The indication for LT is ALF (acute liver failure), where patients present with coagulation defects and encephalopathy. The ALF presentation is most often fatal. However, emergency LT may have a good prognosis. Patients with acute on chronic liver disease and end-stage liver disease may be offered LT if they are deteriorating even with standard medical therapy.

To conclude, a failure of medical therapy in neurological WD is difficult, as neurological symptoms improve up to 3 years, and the reversibility of neurological symptoms after a long interval is difficult to predict either related to medication/related to LT. Hence, it is difficult to establish the indications for LT in neurological WD. In a recent study that included 18 patients with neurological WD for LT, only 8% had a major improvement in the neurological disability, 22.2% died due to complications, and there was no comparison with best medical management. There is no obvious evidence/indication for LT for neurological WD. The outcome of LT is excellent in ALF, as there is no disease recurrence. The LT reverses the basic pathology. Serum copper, ceruloplasmin, 24 hours urinary copper may also become normalized in a few months. Most of these patients do not require decoppering therapy post LT.[24]

- *Diet*: Copper-restricted diet, considered for the long-time as a part of managing WD. However, evidence for this is lacking. Low copper diet increases, high copper diet reduces the absorption of copper. However, retention of copper was higher with a high copper diet. Experts advise during the acute phase of the illness, a low copper diet, after 1 year during the maintenance phase of illness, a diet with very high copper content such as starfish and liver needs to be avoided.[18]
- *Symptomatic therapy*: It is required for various hepatic and neurological manifestations. Various degenerative movement disorders are being treated with symptomatic treatment to improve the quality of life. However, the literature regarding symptomatic therapy for neurological manifestation in the WD is lacking. For tremors, one could prefer propranolol, as this can also be used for portal hypertension; primidone/clonazepam is another option. Thalamotomy or thalamic deep brain stimulation (DBS) can be tried in drug refractory and disabling patients. Dystonia can be treated with clonazepam, anticholinergics, botulinum toxin, baclofen, dopaminergic agonists, oxcarbazepine, gabapentin, and GPi-DBS. Parkinsonism might be treated with levodopa, apomorphine, and amantadine. Chorea might be treated with tetrabenazine, and drooling with anticholinergics and in extreme cases, botulinum toxin in salivary glands. The benefit of symptomatic therapy is minimal and often difficult to differentiate from gradual recovery resulting from decoppering therapy.[8,25,26]

Pregnancy

Pregnancy needs to be avoided during the acute phase of WD, as abnormal brain and liver functions can have an adverse pregnancy outcome. One needs to continue the decoppering therapy during pregnancy as there are chances of disease reactivation and the possibility of ALF. The pregnancy category of DP, trientine, and zinc are D, C, and A, respectively. However, in a small series of patients, no significant teratogenicity of decoppering agents in the pregnancy was found. It is recommended to reduce the dose of DP and trientine up to 50% during the pregnancy. No change in the medication required for zinc.[8,25,27]

Assessment Scales

It is important to quantify the improvement to ensure the adequacy of decoppering therapy and the compliance of therapy. Objective quantification of the disease burden helps to understand the dynamic nature of the disease and appropriate therapy can be guided. Model for end-stage liver disease (MELD), and Child-Pugh are used for liver disease, Global Assessment Scale for Wilson's disease (GAS for WD), and Unified Wilson's Disease Rating Scale (UWDRS) are used for neurological disease severity assessment.[3]

SPECIAL FEATURES IN THE INDIAN CONTEXT

Since Dastur and Wadia's initial description of WD from India in 1963, there has been a significant contribution from Indian researchers, describing the clinical, imaging, management, genetic, and other aspects of WD. There is a significant male preponderance of WD prevalence in the Indian literature; the age of onset is lower in Indian WD compared to European WD. About 50% of patients in western countries have H1069Q mutations in patients with WD. Though there is a high prevalence of consanguineous parentage in the Indian settings, the mutation pattern was widely distributed; this phenomenon was called "Indian paradox" by some authors. Thirty-six mutations were reported by a south Indian study from 102 families recently, of which 13 were novel mutations. The most common mutation in India was p.C271*, as it was found in various studies with allelic frequency in the western (20.2%), sothern (10%), and eastern (16%) parts of India. WD involves management by multiple specialties; there was a felt need to develop clinical practice guidelines for this preventable, treatable, and fatal disease suitable for the Indian settings. The Indian national societies, related to three specialties, (hepatology, pediatric hepatology, and neurology) got together and formed the clinical practice guidelines in 2018. These guidelines give the clinical presentation, diagnostic aspect, management, and monitoring of the patients with WD. Modified Leipzig score developed by this Indian consortium helps to diagnose the patients with WD easily in the Indian scenario.[28-30]

CONCLUSION

Wilson disease can mimic common hepatological neurological, and psychiatric disorders. It is worth screening for WD in most of these presentations to recognize and treat it early otherwise, this is a fatal disease. The diagnosis of WD is not difficult most of the times if there is a high index of suspicion. The diagnosis should be accurate, as WD requires lifelong treatment, and the available medications are relatively safe though periodic monitoring is required. Compliance of the medications is of utmost importance, which needs to be stressed at the diagnosis and follow-up visits. The life expectancy for patients with WD can be estimated to be equal to the normal population, with early diagnosis, regular compliance with the medications, and monitoring.

REFERENCES

1. Walshe JM. History of Wilson disease: a personal account. Handb Clin Neurol. 2017;142:1-5.
2. Lo C, Bandmann O. Epidemiology and introduction to the clinical presentation of Wilson disease. Handb Clin Neurol. 2017;142:7-17.
3. Nagral A, Sarma MS, Matthai J, Kukkle PL, Devarbhavi H, Sinha S, et al. Wilson's Disease: Clinical Practice Guidelines of the Indian National Association for Study of the Liver, the Indian Society of Pediatric Gastroenterology, Hepatology and Nutrition, and the Movement Disorders Society of India. J Clin Exp Hepatol. 2019;9(1):74-98.
4. Scheiber IF, Brůha R, Dušek P. Pathogenesis of Wilson disease. Handb Clin Neurol. 2017;142:43-55.
5. Taly AB, Meenakshi-Sundaram S, Sinha S, et al. Wilson disease: description of 282 patients evaluated over 3 decades. Medicine (Baltimore). 2007;86(2):112-21.
6. Boga S, Ala A, Schilsky ML. Hepatic features of Wilson disease. Handb Clin Neurol. 2017;142:91-9.
7. Członkowska A, Litwin T, Chabik G. Wilson disease: neurologic features. Handb Clin Neurol. 2017;142:101-19.
8. Dusek P, Litwin T, Członkowska A. Neurologic impairment in Wilson disease. Ann Transl Med. 2019;7(Suppl 2):S64.
9. Lorincz MT. Neurologic Wilson's disease. Ann N Y Acad Sci. 2010;1184:173-87.
10. Prashanth LK, Sinha S, Taly AB, A Mahadevan, Vasudev MK, Shankar SK. Spectrum of epilepsy in Wilson's disease with electroencephalographic, MR imaging and pathological correlates. J Neurol Sci. 2010;291(1-2):44-51.
11. Zimbrean P, Seniów J. Cognitive and psychiatric symptoms in Wilson disease. Handb Clin Neurol. 2017;142:121-40.
12. Ferenci P. Diagnosis of Wilson disease. Handb Clin Neurol. 2017;142:171-80.
13. Woimant F, Djebrani-Oussedik N, Poujois A. New tools for Wilson's disease diagnosis: exchangeable copper fraction. Ann Transl Med. 2019;7(Suppl 2):S70.
14. Sinha S, Taly AB, Ravishankar S, Prashanth LK, Venugopal KS, Arunodaya GR, et al. Wilson's disease: cranial MRI observations and clinical correlation. Neuroradiology. 2006;48(9):613-21.
15. Sinha S, Taly AB, Prashanth LK, Ravishankar S, Arunodaya GR, Vasudev MK. Sequential MRI changes in Wilson's disease with de-coppering therapy: a study of 50 patients. Br J Radiol. 2007;80(957):744-9.
16. Yu XE, Gao S, Yang RM, Han YZ. MR Imaging of the Brain in Neurologic Wilson Disease. AJNR Am J Neuroradiol. 2019;40(1):178-83.
17. Espinós C, Ferenci P. Are the new genetic tools for diagnosis of Wilson disease helpful in clinical practice? JHEP Rep. 2020;2(4):100114.
18. Członkowska A, Litwin T. Wilson disease—currently used anticopper therapy. Handb Clin Neurol. 2017;142:181-91.
19. Litwin T, Dzieżyc K, Członkowska A. Wilson disease-treatment perspectives. Ann Transl Med. 2019;7(Suppl 2):S68.
20. Rupp C, Weiss KH. Oral chelator treatment of Wilson disease: trientine. In: Kerkar N, Roberts EA (Eds). Clinical and Translational Perspectives on Wilson disease. London: Academic Press; 2019. pp. 365-72.
21. Sinha S, Taly AB. Withdrawal of penicillamine from zinc sulphate-penicillamine maintenance therapy in Wilson's disease: promising, safe and cheap. J Neurol Sci. 2008;264(1-2):129-32.
22. Rupp C, Weiss KH. Tetrathiomolybdate (TTM). In: Weiss KH, Schilsky M (Eds). Wilson Disease. Academic Press, London: 2019. pp. 197-201.
23. Weiss KH, Askari FK, Czlonkowska A, Ferenci P, Bronstein JM, Bega D, et al. Bis-choline tetrathiomolybdate in patients with Wilson's disease: an open-label, multicentre, phase 2 study. Lancet Gastroenterol Hepatol. 2017;2(12):869-76.
24. Poujois A, Sobesky R, Meissner WG, Brunet AS, Broussolle E, Laurencin C, et al. Liver transplantation as a rescue therapy for severe neurologic forms of Wilson disease. Neurology. 2020;94(21):e2189-e2202.
25. Litwin T, Dušek P, Członkowska A. Symptomatic treatment of neurologic symptoms in Wilson disease. Handb Clin Neurol. 2017;142:211-23.
26. Hedera P. Treatment of Wilson's disease motor complications with deep brain stimulation. Ann N Y Acad Sci. 2014;1315:16-23.
27. Sinha S, Taly AB, Prashanth LK, Arunodaya GR, Swamy HS. Successful pregnancies and abortions in symptomatic and asymptomatic Wilson's disease. J Neurol Sci. 2004;217(1):37-40.
28. Kumar N, Prashant LK, Goyal V. Wilson's Disease Update: An Indian Perspective. Ann Indian Acad Neurol. 2021;24(5):652-63.
29. Kumar SS, Kurian G, Eapen CE, Roberts EA. Genetics of Wilson's disease: a clinical perspective. Indian J Gastroenterol. 2012;31(6):285-93.
30. Aggarwal A, Chandhok G, Todorov T, Parekh S, Tilve S, Zibert A, et al. Wilson disease mutation pattern with genotype-phenotype correlations from Western India: confirmation of p.C271* as a common Indian mutation and identification of 14 novel mutations. Ann Hum Genet. 2013;77(4):299-307.

75

CHAPTER

Deep Brain Stimulation

Milind Deogaonkar

INTRODUCTION

Deep brain stimulation (DBS) has now become an established therapeutic option in the treatment of movement disorders,[1] psychiatric disorders,[2] and chronic pain.[3] It is also being explored for a variety of other indications such as addiction, obesity, stroke, and cognitive disabilities. Functional modulation of various circuits of the brain by placing electrodes at various nuclei in the circuit has resulted in the treatment of previously untreatable neurological and psychiatric disorders. For the purpose of this chapter, we will discuss DBS in relation to movement disorders.

HISTORICAL PERSPECTIVE

Neuromodulation using electrical impulses was identified in 1809 by Rolando.[4] Modern use of stimulation was first reported by Hassler during stereotactic surgeries for ablation of the pallidum.[5] Chronic electrical stimulation using implanted devices came much later. Bechtereva and colleagues in Russia[6] did the first implanted DBS. They did report benefits with chronic DBS of the thalamus, striatum, and pallidum. After Brice and Mcllelan,[7] Siegfried,[8,9] Benabid[10,11] published reports of the use of chronic electrical stimulation or DBS for the treatment of movement disorders, the procedure became a clinical alternative. Due to the reversibility and adjustability, DBS has become the neurosurgical standard of care for movement disorders such as PD, dystonia, and essential tremor over the past few decades.[12-34] It is also being increasingly used in conditions such as Tourette's syndrome,[35-42] chronic pain,[43-48] and psychiatric disorders such as depression[49-53] and obsessive-compulsive disorder (OCD).[54-59]

MECHANISM OF ACTION OF DEEP BRAIN STIMULATION

Deep brain stimulation creates a reversible electrical field on the surrounding nervous tissue causing inhibition of neurons and activation of axons. There appears to be a combination of inhibition of neurons, modulation of abnormal patterns of activity, and activation of axons.[1] Initial observations suggested that high-frequency stimulation (HFS) caused inhibition of the cellular activity in the nucleus thereby mimicking a transient lesion-like effect.[1] DBS lead is shown to disrupt local synaptic function and neuronal firing thereby leading to a "functional deafferentation" and/or "functional inactivation". Studies have shown that DBS can induce inhibition of cellular activity or of neural network functions by direct inhibition of membrane action potentials, by retrograde activation of upstream neuronal structures, or by a shutdown of neurotransmitter release in the subthalamic nucleus (STN).[60] Though, there is complexity in the understanding the exact mechanism of DBS action, various hypotheses postulate inhibition at the neuronal level, activation at the axonal level, as well as interruption of excessive and abnormally patterned neuronal activity in the neural networks.[61-67]

DEEP BRAIN STIMULATION SURGERY

The Team

Deep brain stimulation is always an undertaking of a multidisciplinary team. The team should include a movement disorder neurologist, neuropsychologist, neurophysiologist, psychiatrist, neuroradiologist, and neurosurgeon. The movement disorder neurologist can help confirm the accurate diagnosis. Neuropsychologist helps in preoperative as well as postoperative cognitive assessments. Neurophysiologist helps in the intraoperative mapping **(Fig. 1)**. The psychiatrist plays the same role as a neurologist in DBS for psychiatric disorders. Neuroradiologist helps in selection of patients and rules out patients with structural problems that may cause problems in surgical access or trajectory. The DBS programming can be performed by the neurosurgeon or neurologist. A rehabilitation team (e.g.,

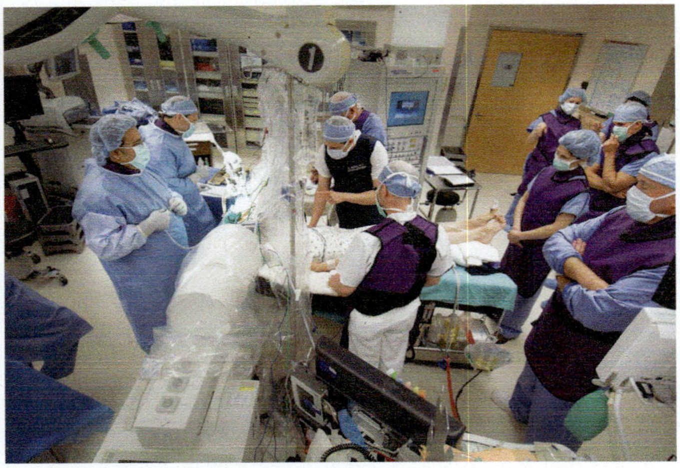

FIG. 1: A view of DBS operating room showing the team at work including neurologist, neurosurgeon, and neurophysiologist.

physical and occupational therapy) can also help optimize motor outcomes after surgery.

Surgical Patient Selection Criteria

- *General criteria*:
  - Patients must be able to tolerate the various components of surgery.
  - Social support structure to comply with the demands of surgery and postoperative care.
  - The procedure, outcomes, risks benefits, and alternatives as well as which symptoms will improve and which will not, need to be explained to patient and family.
  - DBS is not a one-step procedure. It is continuous postoperative programming that the patient needs to be able to come for.
  - Medical comorbidities need to be optimized, etc.
- *Neuropsychological criteria*:
  - Cognitive problems, neuropsychological problems, and psychiatric problems can preclude DBS candidacy.
  - Patients with mild cognitive impairment (MCI) can be the candidates for surgery but with a sound understanding of the risk of postoperative decline in cognitive status.
  - Psychiatric conditions such as anxiety and depression must be medically optimized preoperatively and may need an intraoperative anxiety counselor who is generally provided by neuropsychology and stands by the side of the patient and talks to them to reduce anxiety.
  - Patients with delusional psychosis or severe personality disorder, such as borderline personality disorder are not candidates.
- *Disease-specific selection criteria*:
  - *Parkinson's disease (PD)*:
    - Idiopathic PD with a good response to levodopa.
    - Tremor, rigidity, bradykinesia, dystonia, motor fluctuations, and drug-induced dyskinesia are the symptoms that will most benefit with a DBS.
    - Midline symptoms such as balance speech and swallowing do not respond as well to DBS.
    - Levodopa ON and OFF testing is the best indicator of DBS response.
    - More than 30% improvement in ON and OFF testing is needed unless the patient is tremor dominant.
    - Magnetic resonance imaging (MRI) with no structural abnormality that could preclude the access to deeper brain areas.
  - *Tremor*:
    - DBS helps the most with essential tremor and PD tremor.
    - Rubral or cerebellar outflow tremors do not respond as well, but DBS can be offered as a limited benefit procedure.
    - Proximal limb, head, or truncal tremors respond less than distal tremors.
    - Midline tremors need bilateral DBS.
  - *Dystonia*:
    - Primary generalized dystonias (PGDs) are the best candidates for DBS.[18,68,69] Tardive dystonia is one of the secondary dystonias that responds well to DBS.[70-72]
    - Primary generalized dystonia can show improvements in rating scales from 50 to 80%.
    - Cervical dystonia (CD) also responds well to DBS[73] and so do focal dystonias[74] and so do task-specific dystonias.
    - DYT1+ (mutation on chromosome 9q) dystonias have better response amongst the PGDs. Medication refractory juvenile-onset PGDs with DYT1+ are by and far the best candidates.[13,75]

Surgical Targets for Deep Brain Stimulation

The three most common targets for movement disorder DBS are the STN, globus pallidus internus (GPi), and the ventral intermediate nucleus (VIM) of the thalamus. GPi and STN DBS both are good targets for PD and improve all the major symptoms of PD. STN DBS also helps reduce the PD medications.[76-78] STN is used most often for PD and GPI for dystonia.[12,13,18,70,72,79-85] VIM is primarily used for ET and dystonic tremors.[29,86] Details of individual targets are as follows:

- *The subthalamic nucleus*:
  - STN (also called Corpus Luysi) plays a pivotal role in motor control, is a nodal point in the basal ganglia

thalamocortical "motor" circuit, and alteration in neuronal activity in this structure has been implicated in the underlying pathophysiology of multiple movement disorders, i.e., PD, hemiballismus, and drug-induced dyskinesia.
  - Though STN is most often used for PD, GPi too provides similar benefits in properly selected subsets of PD patients.[87]
  - STN DBS helps reduce tremor, bradykinesia, and rigidity.
  - It also improves motor fluctuations and drug-induced dyskinesias.
  - Antiparkinsonian medication must be reduced following STN DBS in the majority of cases as dyskinesia may worsen with STN DBS if reductions in anti-PD medication are not made.
  - Risk of cognitive issues is higher with STN than GPi.
  - More recently STN DBS has been explored for the treatment of primary dystonia with early reports suggesting it is an effective target site for this disorder as well as for PD and may require lower voltages to produce a similar therapeutic benefit.[88,89] At this time, however, GPi remains the primary target for dystonia DBS.
- *Globus pallidus internus*:
  - GPi is a good target for PD as well as dystonia.[90]
  - It is as effective as STN in PD patients.
  - The target within the GPi is the posterolateral "sensorimotor" portion of GPi.
  - GPi DBS, similar to STN DBS effectively treats the cardinal motor signs of PD including tremor, rigidity, bradykinesia, as well as gait and balance disorders provided these axial symptoms respond to antiparkinsonian medication.
  - GPi DBS also significantly reduces motor fluctuations and dyskinesias, which are directly reduced by GPi DBS regardless of whether antiparkinsonian medications are reduced.
  - Patients with severe ON and OFF dystonia or in whom dyskinesia is a severe and disabling symptom may do better with GPi DBS given STN DBS may induce dyskinesia or ON dystonia.
  - GPi DBS also reduces the need for dopaminergic medication. There remains debate over whether GPi DBS allows as much of a reduction as STN with studies suggesting STN DBS may allow a greater reduction, while others report a similar reduction with both sites.
  - It is suggested that GPi DBS is less likely to cause neurocognitive disturbances than STN DBS. As such it may be a safer target site for patients who are showing early indications of cognitive dysfunction.
- *Ventral intermediate nucleus of the thalamus*:
  - VIM is used for the treatment of all tremor types including essential, PD tremor, or tremor that is secondary to disruption of cerebellothalamic outflow as in multiple sclerosis, post-traumatic tremor, or stroke.
  - The somatotopy of the VIM nucleus is well demarcated and serves as a guide for placing the DBS lead. Somatotopically, the face is represented medially in VIM and as one moves lateral in the structure one encounters the arm and then most laterally the leg.
  - VIM DBS is very effective in ET.
  - VIM DBS also helps in dystonic tremors, rubral tremors, and PD tremors.
  - Cerebellar intention tremor is difficult to treat with DBS and only about one-third of patients receive the good functional benefit. Some have argued for placing two leads to cover a greater volume of the motor thalamus since intention tremor generally involves more proximal body parts, which are represented over a greater volume of the motor thalamus.[91]

DEEP BRAIN STIMULATION SURGICAL TECHNIQUE

Though general principles of DBS surgery remain the same, there is some variance in the protocols for the placement of DBS leads.[1,92-95]

The surgical technique has its foundation in stereotaxis principles. It has evolved from a strong reliance on stereotactic atlases, incorporating advances in imaging, and neurophysiological mapping techniques. Currently, most centers performing DBS utilize a variety of these approaches to localize the target of interest. These variations are due to training patterns, surgeon preference, and the logistics of surgical practice. There is no single, right approach as long as the outcomes are good and complications are kept to a minimum. The lack of randomized prospective studies comparing one approach versus another is also a major barrier in this field for advancement and standardization.

Deep brain stimulation surgery primarily involves planning of target and trajectory, placement of stereotactic frame placement, microelectrode recording (MER), lead placement, and implantable pulse generator (IPG) placement.

Presurgical Planning: Indirect and Direct Targeting

The stereotactic targets (STN, GPi, and VIM) are hard to locate on routine structural imaging.[96] High resolution, specialized sequences like T2 fast-spin echo, susceptibility weighted imaging (SWI), and proton density weighted images are better for target visualization.[97-101] All these sequences though do have magnetic warping effects and artifacts[102] so a combination of computed tomography (CT), MRI, and atlas is used to improve the accuracy on Stealth workstation (Framelink Medtronic Inc., Minneapolis, USA) **(Fig. 2)**.

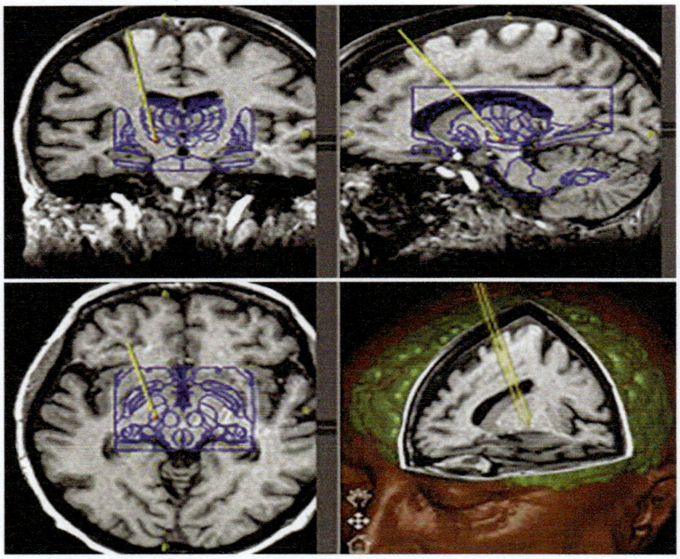

FIG. 2: Planning station view of preprocessed (coregistered, aligned to AC-PC plane) images with overlay of atlas using stealth workstation and processed with stereotactic planning software (Framelink Medtronic Inc., Minneapolis, USA).

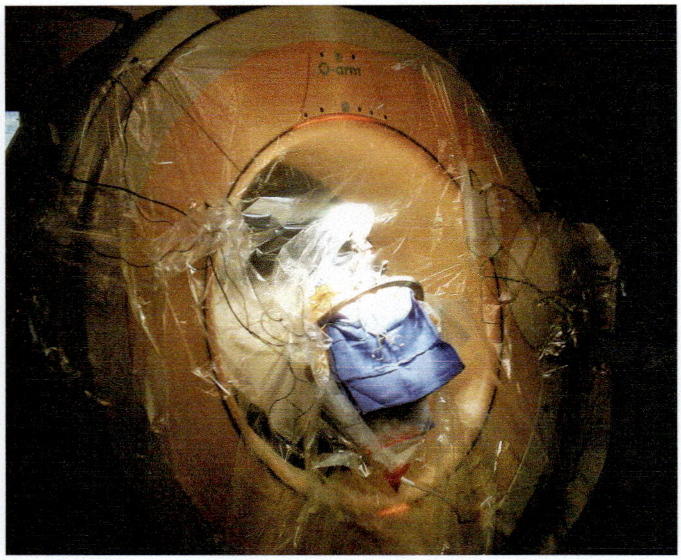

FIG. 3: Asleep DBS using intraoperative CT scan guidance.
(CT: computed tomography; DBS: deep brain stimulation)

Targeting methods differ across centers.[103] In general, the coordinates used for initial target selection are: STN—X = 10–12 mm, Y = 2–5 mm posterior to mid-commissural point or corresponding with the anterior border of red nucleus, Z = 3–5 mm below the intercommissural plane; GPi—X = 19–21 mm, Y = 0–3 mm anterior to mid-commissural point, Z = superior border of optic tract; and VIM—X = 10–14 mm or 11 mm lateral to the wall of the third ventricle, Y = 5–7 mm anterior commissure (AC) to posterior commissure (PC), Z = at the intercommissural plane. The targets are then refined based on direct visualization of the target nucleus borders. Electronic brain atlases are also available to guide stereotactic targeting[104] including deformable brain atlases[105] It is important to note that both the formulaic[106] and atlas-based[107] targeting have limitations in entirely capturing the variability in individual anatomy. Therefore most surgeons use MER and stimulation for intraoperative confirmation.[108] Novel functional stereotactic atlases are being developed to incorporate these intraoperative findings to create probabilistic maps of physiological and functional information.[109]

Trajectory Planning

Trajectories are planned so as to avoid eloquent areas, sulci, vascular structures, and ventricles.

Frame Placement

Placement of the head-frame is generally done under local anesthesia in adults. The frame should be placed parallel to a line extending from the lateral canthus to the tragus, in order to approximately parallel the AC–PC line. Though the frame is the gold standard of stereotaxic targeting, frameless systems are often used as they are supposed to provide more patient comfort.

Surgical Procedure: Awake and Asleep Deep Brain Stimulation

Deep brain stimulation is performed under monitored anesthesia that involves local anesthesia and sedation during parts of the procedure.[110] MER and intraoperative testing are done with patient awake. MER involves obtaining the standard firing pattern of the nucleus, getting movement response to active and passive movements (driving), and defining the borders of the nucleus. Intraoperative testing involves stimulating from the macroelectrode and records the therapeutic response as well as the side effects.

Due the recent improvements in the imaging resolution[111] **(Fig. 3)** nowadays image-guided DBS can be done as effectively as the MER guidance.[112] Image guidance is almost as accurate as MER in placement of DBS.[113,114] Some patients have anxiety in regards to being awake for neurosurgery and asleep DBS has been reported to improve patient comfort and satisfaction.[115] Overall the accuracy of targeting is critical for good clinical outcomes.[116] The following steps are typically taken to minimize targeting error:

- Head positioning to avoid significant brain sag and pneumocephalus.
- Minimizing the egress of cerebrospinal fluid.
- Minimum manipulation once the recording system is in situ.
- Intraoperative imaging with either 2D X-rays[117] or O-Arm (Medtronic, Inc.)[118] **(Fig. 3)**, or intraoperative CT.[119]

Microelectrode Recording

Microelectrode recording is done with microelectrodes with high impedances (typically >0.4 m Ohms) with a tip diameter in the range of 2–4 µm.[120-122] Single cell, extracellular recordings are obtained, filtered, and amplified so as to see and hear the firing patterns of the nucleus using a microdrive that advances in submilimetric steps.[1] Commercially available microelectrodes are made of tungsten or platinum/iridium.

Methods of doing MER differ from center to center, ranging from one track, one electrode, two multiple tracks to multiple electrodes **(Fig. 4)**.[110] Ondo,[123] in a survey of high output centers doing DBS, found 97% of centers use MER. Average number of tracks was 2.3 per electrode and ranged from 1 to 18. Macrostimulation was commonly used to assess the final clinical response in this survey. Multiple electrodes advance strategies are seen less often.[124,125] Use of microelectrode for intraoperative response is uncommonly used and is less reliable.[120,126]

Use of MER is still debated by some. It is argued that accuracy of electrode placement is not enhanced by MER but it adds to risks of complications.[127] Some centers also use semimicroelectrodes for generating the physiological data.[128,129]

Macroelectrode and Intraoperative Responses

Macrostimulation is done to observe therapeutic responses and side effects using either a macroelectrode or a DBS electrode itself.[123] If macrostimulation is done using DBS lead, then the results are more reproducible in postoperative programming. The caveat here is that the macroelectrode stimulation during surgery using the stimulator screening box can be done only in bipolar mode. Macrostimulation still is an important step for lead placement accuracy.

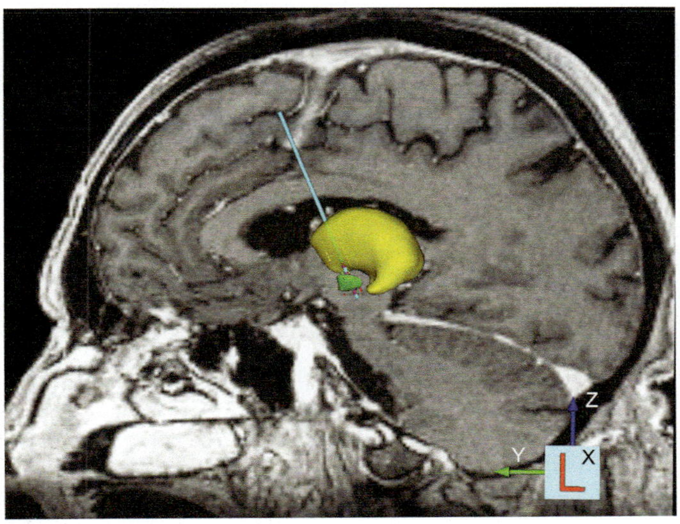

FIG. 4: Multiple tracks during STN mapping and location of final DBS lead in STN (green) seen below thalamus (yellow).
(DBS: deep brain stimulation; STN: subthalamic nucleus)

Deep Brain Stimulation Lead Placement

The most important point during lead placement is to remember that the target (bottom of lead) may not be the point of stimulation.[130,131]

The Medtronic (Medtronic, Minneapolis, MN) electrodes, which are commercially available have four contacts of 1.5 mm in height and 1.27 mm in diameter and differ only in the spacing between contacts: 1.5 mm in the 3387 model and 0.5 mm in the 3389 model. Fluoroscopy is always used to confirm the lead placement and to check for lead displacement during anchoring. Most of the patients will have a transient improvement after lead placement due to microsubthalamotomy which will last 3-7 days.

The intraoperative macrostimulation is done using standard parameters like 1-5 V, 60 microseconds PW, 130 Hz frequency. The therapeutic window that means the difference in amplitude between therapeutic benefits and side effects is assessed.

Implanted DBS is then secured using the burr hole cap under continuous radiological monitoring to prevent lead displacement **(Fig. 5)**. Leads are variously anchored using burr hole ring and cap, and the Medtronic Stimloc anchoring device (Medtronic, Minneapolis, MN), dental cement, miniplates, and screws. The distal DBS lead tip is then covered by cap and tunneled to posterior parietal area. The excess lead is coiled in the subgaleal space.

Placement of the Implantable Pulse Generator

Subsequent step of DBS surgery is to place the IPG in subclavicular region and connect it with the DBS lead with an extension wire. There are various types of available IPG but broadly they can be single channel (Medtronic Soletra) for one DBS lead and dual channel (Medtronic Kinetra) for two leads. This part of surgery is performed under GA, either on the same or subsequent days.

In this, the patient is placed with slight neck extension. The clavicle and subclavicular area is cleaned. A subfascial pocket is made. The extension is tunneled from the posterior parietal incision to the subclavicular pocket. The extension wire is connected to lead and then to the IPG **(Fig. 6)**. Though subclavicular location is the commonest, sometimes it can be placed in subcostal location or over the abdominal wall.

Risks and Complications

Serious complications are few and uncommon.[132] Complications include brain hemorrhage, infection, hardware malfunction, erosion, stimulation-induced complications, and misplaced leads.[133,134]

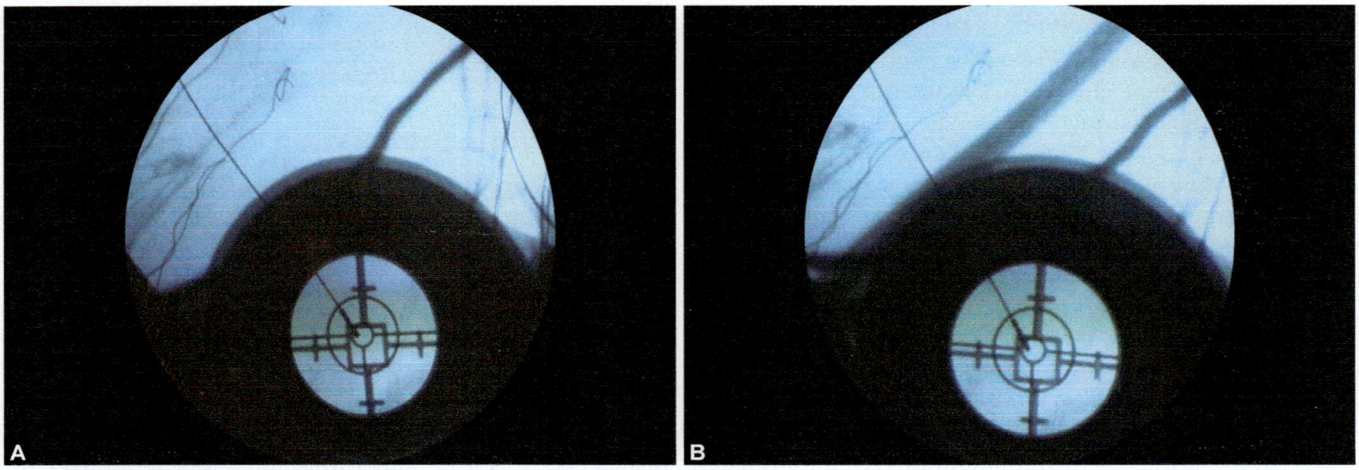

FIGS. 5A AND B: Final DBS lead in place and is under constant fluoroscopic control till it is secured.
(DBS: deep brain stimulation)

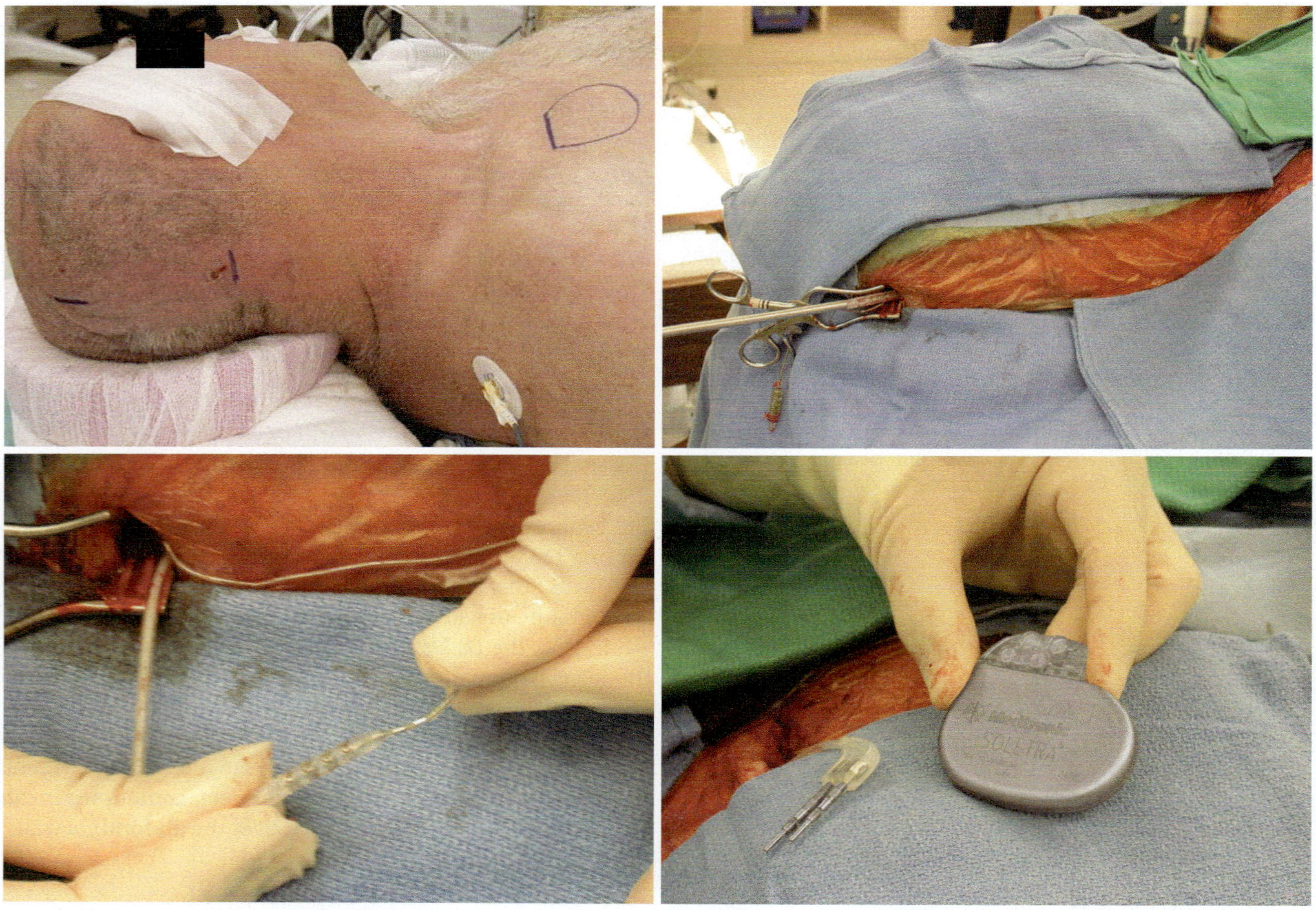

FIG. 6: IPG placement surgery with multiple steps of planning, tunneling, and connection to IPG.
(IPG: implantable pulse generator)

Deep Brain Stimulation Programming

Initial programming is done a month after surgery.[135,136] Initial programming includes monopolar review and determining the optimum monopolar or bipolar setting for improvement in tremors, bradykinesia, and rigidity.[137] The other goal of initial programming is to observe thresholds for side effects that could be capsular stimulation, behavioral issues or sensory symptoms such as parasthesia.[138] Good contacts are those that give the best benefits at lowest amplitudes and have higher thresholds for side effects.

Stimulation-induced Side Effects of DBS

Stimulation-induced capsular stimulation could cause speech impairments including slurring, spastic, or hypovolemic speech.[139] Tripolitie et al. found that Anteromedially placed leads at higher voltage will cause significant speech impairments. Speech is affected less often with GPi leads.[140]

Stimulation can also evoke dyskinesias which are supposed to a sign of accurate lead placement.[138,141] They can be prevented or lessened by slow increase in voltage.[142] GPi DBS does not generally evoke dyskinesias.[138,142]

Though axial symptoms like gait do not get worse with stimulation (unless the bottom contact is used or there is capsular stimulation) they also do not show sustained improvement.[143]

The most common neuropsychiatric side effect in the immediate postoperative period following DBS is transient confusion with an incidence between 1 and 36%.[144] Evidence of greater neuropsychological deficits before surgery is significantly associated with increased confusion and cognitive complications following surgery.[145]

OUTCOMES OF DEEP BRAIN STIMULATION FOR MOVEMENT DISORDERS

Many studies have reported on the outcomes of GPi and STN DBS for the cardinal symptoms of PD. Both targets have been shown to be beneficial.[146,147]

Globus pallidus internus, STN DBS, or both show sustained and significant improvement in PD symptoms.

Ventral intermediate nucleus stimulation has excellent effects on controlling the essential and dystonic tremors with minimal side effects.

Globus pallidus internus stimulation in treatment resistant, primary, generalized genetic dystonias has best outcomes closely followed by tardive dyskinesias and cervical and focal dystonias.

CONCLUSION

Deep brain stimulation is a safe and effective treatment for medically intractable movement disorders. Research for expanding the indications in psychiatric disorders, pain and other areas is ongoing. This can be used in the future for many more medically intractable disorders.

REFERENCES

1. Rezai AR, Machado AG, Deogaonkar M, Azmi H, Kubu C, Boulis NM. Surgery for movement disorders. Neurosurgery. 2008;62 (Suppl 2): 809-38.
2. Zibly Z, Shaw A, Harnof S, Sharma M, Graves C, Deogaonkar M, et al. Modulation of mind: Therapeutic neuromodulation for cognitive disability. J Clin Neurosci. 2014;21(9):1473-7.
3. Sharma M, Shaw A, Deogaonkar M. Surgical options for complex craniofacial pain. Neurosurg Clin N Am. 2014;25(4):763-75.
4. Finger S. Origins of Neuroscience. New York: Oxford Press; 1994.
5. Hassler R, Riechert T, Mundinger F, Umbach W, Ganglberger JA. Physiological observations in stereotaxic operations in extrapyramidal motor disturbances. Brain. 1960;83:337-50.
6. Bechtereva NP, Bondartchuk AN, Smirnov VM, Meliutcheva LA, Shandurina AN. Method of electrostimulation of the deep brain structures in treatment of some chronic diseases. Confin Neurol. 1975;37(1-3):136-40.
7. Brice J, McLellan L. Suppression of intention tremor by contingent deep-brain stimulation. Lancet. 1980;1(8180):1221-2.
8. Blond S, Siegfried J. Thalamic stimulation for the treatment of tremor and other movement disorders. Acta Neurochir Suppl (Wien). 1991;52:109-11.
9. Siegfried J, Shulman J. Deep brain stimulation. Pacing Clin Electrophysiol. 1987;10(1 Pt 2):271-2.
10. Benabid AL, Pollak P, Louveau A, Henry S, de Rougemont J. Combined (thalamotomy and stimulation) stereotactic surgery of the VIM thalamic nucleus for bilateral Parkinson disease. Appl Neurophysiol. 1987;50(1-6):344-6.
11. Benabid AL, Pollak P, Gross C, Hoffmann D, Benazzouz A, Gao DM, et al. Acute and long-term effects of subthalamic nucleus stimulation in Parkinson's disease. Stereotact Funct Neurosurg. 1994;62(1-4):76-84.
12. Tisch S, Zrinzo L, Limousin P, Bhatia KP, Quinn N, Ashkan K, et al. The effect of electrode contact location on clinical efficacy of pallidal deep brain stimulation in primary generalised dystonia. J Neurol Neurosurg Psychiatry. 2007;78(12):1314-9.
13. Parr JR, Green AL, Joint C, Andrew M, Gregory RP, Scott RB, et al. Deep brain stimulation in childhood: An effective treatment for early onset generalised idiopathic dystonia. Arch Dis Child. 2007;92(8):708-11.
14. Cohen OS, Hassin-Baer S, Spiegelmann R. Deep brain stimulation of the internal globus pallidus for refractory tardive dystonia. Parkinsonism Relat Disord. 2007;13(8):541-4.
15. Alterman RL, Shils JL, Miravite J, Tagliati M. Lower stimulation frequency can enhance tolerability and efficacy of pallidal deep brain stimulation for dystonia. Mov Disord. 2007;22(3):366-8.

16. Zhang JG, Zhang K, Ma Y, Hu WH, Yang AC, Chu JS, et al. Follow-up of bilateral subthalamic deep brain stimulation for Parkinson's disease. Acta Neurochir Suppl. 2006;99:43-7.
17. Krauss JK, Yianni J, Loher TJ, Aziz TZ. Deep brain stimulation for dystonia. J Clin Neurophysiol. 2004;21(1):18-30.
18. Lee JY, Deogaonkar M, Rezai A. Deep brain stimulation of globus pallidus internus for dystonia. Parkinsonism Relat Disord. 2007;13(5):261-5.
19. Pahwa R, Lyons KE, Wilkinson SB, Simpson Jr RK, Ondo WG, Tarsy D, et al. Long-term evaluation of deep brain stimulation of the thalamus. J Neurosurg. 2006;104(4):506-12.
20. Ondo WG. Essential tremor: treatment options. Curr Treat Options Neurol. 2006;8(3):256-67.
21. Lee JY, Kondziolka D. Thalamic deep brain stimulation for management of essential tremor. J Neurosurg. 2005;103(3):400-3.
22. Putzke JD, Uitti R, Obwegeser A, Wszolek Z, Wharen R. Bilateral thalamic deep brain stimulation: midline tremor control. J Neurol Neurosurg Psychiatry. 2005;76(5):684-90.
23. Foote KD, Okun MS. Ventralis intermedius plus ventralis oralis anterior and posterior deep brain stimulation for posttraumatic Holmes tremor: two leads may be better than one: technical note. Neurosurgery. 2005;56(2 Suppl):E445.
24. Ushe M, Mink JW, Revilla FJ, Wernle A, Gibson PS, McGee-Minnich L, et al. Effect of stimulation frequency on tremor suppression in essential tremor. Mov Disord. 2004;19(10):1163-8.
25. Putzke JD, Wharen Jr RE, Obwegeser AA, Wszolek ZK, Lucas JA, Turk MF, et al. Thalamic deep brain stimulation for essential tremor: recommendations for long-term outcome analysis. Can J Neurol Sci. 2004;31(3):333-42.
26. Lyons KE, Pahwa R. Deep brain stimulation in Parkinson's disease. Curr Neurol Neurosci Rep. 2004;4(4):290-5.
27. Kumar R, Lozano AM, Sime E, Lang AE. Long-term follow-up of thalamic deep brain stimulation for essential and Parkinsonian tremor. Neurology. 2003;61(11):1601-4.
28. Murata J, Kitagawa M, Uesugi H, Saito H, Iwasaki Y, Kikuchi S, et al. Electrical stimulation of the posterior subthalamic area for the treatment of intractable proximal tremor. J Neurosurg. 2003;99(4):708-15.
29. Tasker RR, Munz M, Junn FS, Kiss ZH, Davis K, Dostrovsky JO, et al. Deep brain stimulation and thalamotomy for tremor compared. Acta Neurochir Suppl. 1997;68:49-53.
30. Benabid AL, Benazzouz A, Hoffmann D, Limousin P, Krack P, Pollak P. Long-term electrical inhibition of deep brain targets in movement disorders. Mov Disord. 1998;13 (Suppl 3):119-25.
31. Benabid AL, Pollak P, Gao D, Hoffmann D, Limousin P, Gay E, et al. Chronic electrical stimulation of the ventralis intermedius nucleus of the thalamus as a treatment of movement disorders. J Neurosurg. 1996;84(2):203-14.
32. Alesch F, Pinter MM, Helscher RJ, Fertl L, Benabid AL, Koos WT. Stimulation of the ventral intermediate thalamic nucleus in tremor dominated Parkinson's disease and essential tremor. Acta Neurochir (Wien). 1995;136(1-2):75-81.
33. Benabid AL, Pollak P, Seigneuret E, Hoffmann D, Gay E, Perret J. Chronic VIM thalamic stimulation in Parkinson's disease, essential tremor and extra-pyramidal dyskinesias. Acta Neurochir Suppl (Wien). 1993;58:39-44.
34. Benabid AL, Pollak P, Gervason C, Hoffmann D, Gao DM, Hommel M, et al. Long-term suppression of tremor by chronic stimulation of the ventral intermediate thalamic nucleus. Lancet. 1991;337(8738):403-6.
35. Diallo R, Welter ML, Mallet L. Therapeutic management of tics in Tourette's syndrome. Rev Neurol (Paris). 2007;163(3):375-86.
36. Okun MS, Rodriguez RL, Mikos A, Miller K, Kellison I, Kirsch-Darrow L, et al. Deep brain stimulation and the role of the neuropsychologist. Clin Neuropsychol. 2007;21(1):162-89.
37. Mink JW, Walkup J, Frey KA, Como P, Cath D, Delong MR, et al. Patient selection and assessment recommendations for deep brain stimulation in Tourette syndrome. Mov Disord. 2006;21(11):1831-8.
38. Anderson TR, Hu B, Iremonger K, Kiss ZHT. Selective attenuation of afferent synaptic transmission as a mechanism of thalamic deep brain stimulation-induced tremor arrest. J Neurosci. 2006;26(3):841-50.
39. Skidmore FM, Rodriguez RL, Fernandez HH, Goodman WK, Foote KD, Okun MS. Lessons learned in deep brain stimulation for movement and neuropsychiatric disorders. CNS Spectr. 2006;11(7):521-36.
40. Visser-Vandewalle V, Ackermans L, van der Linden C, Temel Y, Tijssen MA, Schruers KRJ, et al. Deep brain stimulation in Gilles de la Tourette's syndrome. Neurosurgery. 2006;58(3):E590.
41. Houeto JL, Karachi C, Mallet L, Pillon B, Yelnik J, Mesnage V, et al. Tourette's syndrome and deep brain stimulation. J Neurol Neurosurg Psychiatry. 2005;76(7):992-5.
42. Gilbert DL, Lipps TD. Tourette's Syndrome. Curr Treat Options Neurol. 2005;7(3):211-9.
43. Kringelbach ML, Jenkinson N, Green AL, Owen SLF, Hansen PC, Cornelissen PL, et al. Deep brain stimulation for chronic pain investigated with magnetoencephalography. Neuroreport. 2007;18(3):223-8.
44. Rasche D, Rinaldi PC, Young RF, Tronnier VM. Deep brain stimulation for the treatment of various chronic pain syndromes. Neurosurg Focus. 2006;21(6):E8.
45. Coffey RJ, Lozano AM. Neurostimulation for chronic noncancer pain: An evaluation of the clinical evidence and recommendations for future trial designs. J Neurosurg. 2006;105(2):175-89.
46. Green AL, Nandi D, Armstrong G, Carter H, Aziz T. Post-herpetic trigeminal neuralgia treated with deep brain stimulation. J Clin Neurosci. 2003;10(4):512-4.
47. Levy RM. Deep brain stimulation for the treatment of intractable pain. Neurosurg Clin N Am. 2003;14(3):389-99.
48. Bittar RG, Kar-Purkayastha I, Owen SL, Bear RE, Green A, Wang S, et al. Deep brain stimulation for pain relief: a meta-analysis. J Clin Neurosci. 2005;12(5):515-9.
49. Sartorius A, Henn FA. Deep brain stimulation of the lateral habenula in treatment resistant major depression. Med Hypotheses. 2007;69(6):1305-8.
50. Schlaepfer TE, Cohen MX, Frick C, Kosel M, Brodesser D, Axmacher N, et al. Deep Brain Stimulation to Reward Circuitry Alleviates Anhedonia in Refractory Major Depression. Neuropsychopharmacology. 2008;33(2):368-77.
51. George MS, Nahas Z, Borckardt JJ, Anderson B, Foust MJ, Burns C, et al. Brain stimulation for the treatment of psychiatric disorders. Curr Opin Psychiatry. 2007;20(3):250-4.
52. Carpenter LL. Neurostimulation in resistant depression. J Psychopharmacol. 2006;20(3 Suppl):35-40.
53. Mayberg HS, Lozano AM, Voon V, McNeely HE, Seminowicz D, Hamani C, et al. Deep brain stimulation for treatment-resistant depression. Neuron. 2005;45(5):651-60.
54. Greenberg BD, Malone DA, Friehs GM, Rezai AR, Kubu CS, Malloy PF, et al. Three-year outcomes in deep brain stimulation for highly resistant obsessive-compulsive disorder. Neuropsychopharmacology. 2006;31(11):2384-93.
55. Greenberg BD, Rezai AR. Mechanisms and the current state of deep brain stimulation in neuropsychiatry. CNS Spectr. 2003;8(7):522-6.
56. Cosyns P, Gabriels L, Nuttin B. Deep brain stimulation in treatment refractory obsessive compulsive disorder. Verh K Acad Geneeskd Belg. 2003;65(6):385-99.
57. Millet B, Jaafari N. Treatment of obsessive-compulsive disorder. Rev Prat. 2007;57(1):53-7.
58. Kuhn J, Gründler TOJ, Lenartz D, Sturm V, Klosterkötter J, Huff W. Deep brain stimulation for psychiatric disorders. F Dtsch Arztebl Int. 2010;107(7):105-13.
59. Wichmann T, Delong MR. Deep brain stimulation for neurologic and neuropsychiatric disorders. Neuron. 2006;52(1):197-204.

60. Benabid AL, Wallace B, Mitrofanis J, Xia R, Piallat B, Chabardes S, et al. A putative generalized model of the effects and mechanism of action of high frequency electrical stimulation of the central nervous system. Acta Neurol Belg. 2005;105(3):149-57.
61. Santens P, Boon P, Roost DV, Caemaert J. The pathophysiology of motor symptoms in Parkinson's disease. Acta Neurol Belg. 2003;103(3):129-34.
62. Wichmann T, DeLong MR. Pathophysiology of Parkinson's disease: the MPTP primate model of the human disorder. Ann N Y Acad Sci. 2003;991:199-213.
63. Obeso JA, Rodríguez MC, Gorospe A, Guridi J, Alvarez L, Macias R. Surgical treatment of Parkinson's disease. Baillieres Clin Neurol. 1997;6(1):125-45.
64. Benazzouz A, Hallett M. Mechanism of action of deep brain stimulation. Neurology. 2000;55(12 Suppl 6):S13-6.
65. Hamani C, Saint-Cyr JA, Fraser J, Kaplitt M, Lozano AM. The subthalamic nucleus in the context of movement disorders. Brain. 2004;127(Pt 1):4-20.
66. Hamani C, Lozano AM. Physiology and pathophysiology of Parkinson's disease. Ann N Y Acad Sci. 2003;991:15-21.
67. Baev KV, Greene KA, Marciano FF, Samanta JES, Shetter AG, Smith KA, et al. Physiology and pathophysiology of cortico-basal ganglia-thalamocortical loops: theoretical and practical aspects. Prog Neuropsychopharmacol Biol Psychiatry. 2002;26(4):771-804.
68. Krause M, Fogel W, Kloss M, Rasche D, Volkmann J, Tronnier V. Pallidal stimulation for dystonia. Neurosurgery. 2004;55(6):1361-8.
69. Kupsch A, Klaffke S, Kühn AA, Meissner W, Arnold G, Schneider GH, et al. The effects of frequency in pallidal deep brain stimulation for primary dystonia. J Neurol. 2003;250(10):1201-5.
70. Zhang JG, Zhang K, Wang ZC, Ge M, Ma Y. Deep brain stimulation in the treatment of secondary dystonia. Chin Med J (Engl). 2006;119(24):2069-74.
71. Eltahawy HA, Saint-Cyr J, Giladi N, Lang AE, Lozano AM. Primary dystonia is more responsive than secondary dystonia to pallidal interventions: outcome after pallidotomy or pallidal deep brain stimulation. Neurosurgery. 2004;54(3):613-9.
72. Starr PA, Turner RS, Rau G, Lindsey N, Heath S, Volz M, et al. Microelectrode-guided implantation of deep brain stimulators into the globus pallidus internus for dystonia: techniques, electrode locations, and outcomes. J Neurosurg. 2006;104(4):488-501.
73. Vidailhet M, Vercueil L, Houeto JL, Krystkowiak P, Benabid AL, Cornu P, et al. Bilateral deep-brain stimulation of the globus pallidus in primary generalized dystonia. N Engl J Med. 2005;352(5):459-67.
74. Mehrkens JH, Bötzel K, Steude U, Zeitler K, Schnitzler A, Sturm V, et al. Long-term efficacy and safety of chronic globus pallidus internus stimulation in different types of primary dystonia. Stereotact Funct Neurosurg. 2009;87(1):8-17.
75. Starr PA, Turner RS, Rau G, Lindsey N, Heath S, Volz M, et al. Microelectrode-guided implantation of deep brain stimulators into the globus pallidus internus for dystonia: techniques, electrode locations, and outcomes. Neurosurg Focus. 2004;17(1):E4.
76. Vitek JL. Deep brain stimulation for Parkinson's disease. A critical re-evaluation of STN versus GPi DBS. Stereotact Funct Neurosurg. 2002;78(3-4):119-31.
77. Burchiel KJ, Anderson VC, Favre J, Hammerstad JP. Comparison of pallidal and subthalamic nucleus deep brain stimulation for advanced Parkinson's disease: results of a randomized, blinded pilot study. Neurosurgery. 1999;45(6):1375-82.
78. Deep-Brain Stimulation for Parkinson's Disease Study Group; Obeso JA, Olanow CW, Rodriguez-Oroz MC, Krack P, Kumar R, Lang AE. Deep-brain stimulation of the subthalamic nucleus or the pars interna of the globus pallidus in Parkinson's disease. N Engl J Med. 2001;345(13):956-63.
79. Tisch S, Rothwell JC, Bhatia KP, Quinn N, Zrinzo L, Jahanshahi M, et al. Pallidal stimulation modifies after-effects of paired associative stimulation on motor cortex excitability in primary generalised dystonia. Exp Neurol. 2007;206(1):80-5.
80. Uc EY, Follett KA. Deep brain stimulation in movement disorders. Semin Neurol. 2007;27(2):170-82.
81. Schadt CR, Charles PD, Davis TL, Konrad PE. Thalamotomy, DBS-Vim, and DBS-GPi for generalized dystonia: a case report. Tenn Med. 2007;100(2):38-9.
82. Hung SW, Hamani C, Lozano AM, Poon YYW, Piboolnurak P, Miyasaki JM, et al., Long-term outcome of bilateral pallidal deep brain stimulation for primary cervical dystonia. Neurology. 2007;68(6):457-9.
83. Foncke EM, Bour LJ, Speelman JD, Koelman JHT, Tijssen MAJ. Local field potentials and oscillatory activity of the internal globus pallidus in myoclonus-dystonia. Mov Disord. 2007;22(3):369-76.
84. Krause M, Fogel W, Tronnier V, Pohle S, Hörtnagel K, Thyen U, et al. Long-term benefit to pallidal deep brain stimulation in a case of dystonia secondary to pantothenate kinase-associated neurodegeneration. Mov Disord. 2006;21(12):2255-7.
85. Chen CC, Kühn AA, Trottenberg T, Kupsch A, Schneider GH, Brown P. Neuronal activity in globus pallidus interna can be synchronized to local field potential activity over 3–12 Hz in patients with dystonia. Exp Neurol. 2006;202(2):480-6.
86. Tasker RR. Tremor of parkinsonism and stereotactic thalamotomy. Mayo Clin Proc. 1987;62(8):736-9.
87. Anderson VC, Burchiel KJ, Hogarth P, Favre J, Hammerstad JP. Pallidal vs subthalamic nucleus deep brain stimulation in Parkinson disease. Arch Neurol. 2005;62(4):554-60.
88. Kleiner-Fisman G, Liang GSL, Moberg PJ, Ruocco AC, Hurtig HI, Baltuch GH, et al. Subthalamic nucleus deep brain stimulation for severe idiopathic dystonia: impact on severity, neuropsychological status, and quality of life. J Neurosurg. 2007;107(1):29-36.
89. Sun B, Chen S, Zhan S, Le W, Krahl SE. Subthalamic nucleus stimulation for primary dystonia and tardive dystonia. Acta Neurochir Suppl. 2007;97(Pt 2):207-14.
90. Vidailhet M, Vercueil L, Houeto JL, Krystkowiak P, Lagrange C, Yelnik J, et al. Bilateral, pallidal, deep-brain stimulation in primary generalised dystonia: a prospective 3 year follow-up study. Lancet Neurol. 2007;6(3):223-9.
91. Freund HJ, Barnikol UB, Nolte D, Treuer H, Auburger G, Tass PA, et al. Subthalamic-thalamic DBS in a case with spinocerebellar ataxia type 2 and severe tremor-A unusual clinical benefit. Mov Disord. 2007;22(5):732-5.
92. Slavin KV, Thulborn KR, Wess C, Nersesyan H. Direct visualization of the human subthalamic nucleus with 3T MR imaging. AJNR Am J Neuroradiol. 2006;27(1):80-4.
93. Liu X, Rowe J, Nandi D, Hayward G, Parkin S, Stein J, et al. Localisation of the subthalamic nucleus using Radionics Image Fusion and Stereoplan combined with field potential recording. A technical note. Stereotact Funct Neurosurg. 2001;76(2):63-73.
94. Ostergaard K, Sunde N, Dupont E. Effects of bilateral stimulation of the subthalamic nucleus in patients with severe Parkinson's disease and motor fluctuations. Mov Disord. 2002;17(4):693-700.
95. Valldeoriola F, Pilleri M, Tolosa E, Molinuevo JL, Rumià J, Ferrer E. Bilateral subthalamic stimulation monotherapy in advanced Parkinson's disease: long-term follow-up of patients. Mov Disord. 2002;17(1):125-32.
96. Chen SY, Tsai ST, Lin SH. (2011). Controversial Issues in Deep Brain Stimulation in Parkinson's Disease. Towards New Therapies for Parkinson's Disease. [online] Available from https://www.researchgate.net/publication/221918993_Controversial_Issues_in_Deep_Brain_Stimulation_in_Parkinson's_Disease [Last accessed March, 2023].
97. Starr PA, Vitek JL, DeLong M, Bakay RA. Magnetic resonance imaging-based stereotactic localization of the globus pallidus and subthalamic nucleus. Neurosurgery. 1999;44(2):303-13.
98. Gasparotti R, Pinelli L, Liserre R. New MR sequences in daily practice: susceptibility weighted imaging. A pictorial essay. Insights Imaging. 2011;2(3):335-47.

99. Pinsker MO, Volkmann J, Falk D, Herzog J, Alfke K, Steigerwald F, et al. Electrode implantation for deep brain stimulation in dystonia: a fast spin-echo inversion-recovery sequence technique for direct stereotactic targeting of the GPI. Zentralbl Neurochir. 2008;69(2):71-5.
100. Ishimori T, Nakano S, Mori Y, Seo R, Togami T, Masada T, et al. Preoperative identification of subthalamic nucleus for deep brain stimulation using three-dimensional phase sensitive inversion recovery technique. Magn Reson Med Sci. 2007;6(4):225-9.
101. Sudhyadhom A, Haq IU, Foote KD, Okun MS, Bova FJ. A high resolution and high contrast MRI for differentiation of subcortical structures for DBS targeting: the Fast Gray Matter Acquisition T1 Inversion Recovery (FGATIR). Neuroimage. 2009;47:T44-T52.
102. Bot M, Bour L, de Bie RM, Contarino MF, Schuurman PR, van den Munckhof P. Can We Rely on Susceptibility-Weighted Imaging for Subthalamic Nucleus Identification in Deep Brain Stimulation Surgery? Neurosurgery. 2016;78(3):353-60.
103. Laitinen LV. Brain targets in surgery for Parkinson's disease. Results of a survey of neurosurgeons. J Neurosurg. 1985;62(3):349-51.
104. Alho EJL, Grinberg L, Heinsen H, Fonoff ET. Review of printed and electronic stereotactic atlases of the human brain. INTECH Open Access Publisher. 2011.
105. Sudhyadhom A, Okun MS, Foote KD, Rahman M, Bova FJ. A Three-dimensional Deformable Brain Atlas for DBS Targeting. I. Methodology for Atlas Creation and Artifact Reduction. Open Neuroimag J. 2012;6:92-8.
106. Nestor KA, Jones JD, Butson CR, Morishita T, Jacobson 4th CE, Peace DA, et al., Coordinate-based lead location does not predict Parkinson's disease deep brain stimulation outcome. PLoS One. 2014;9(4):e93524.
107. Anthofer J, Steib K, Fellner C, Lange M, Brawanski A, Schlaier J. The variability of atlas-based targets in relation to surrounding major fibre tracts in thalamic deep brain stimulation. Acta neurochirurgica. 2014;156(8):1497-504.
108. Maiti TK, Konar S, Bir S, Kalakoti P, Nanda A. Intra-operative microelectrode recording in functional neurosurgery: Past, present, future. J Clin Neurosci. 2016;32:166-72.
109. D'Haese PF, Pallavaram S, Li R, Remple MS, Kao C, Neimat JS, et al. Cranial Vault and its CRAVE tools: a clinical computer assistance system for deep brain stimulation (DBS) therapy. Med Image Anal. 2012;16(3):744-53.
110. Machado A, Rezai AR, Kopell BH, Gross RE, Sharan AD, Benabid AL. Deep brain stimulation for Parkinson's disease: Surgical technique and perioperative management. Mov Disord. 2006;21(S14):S247-S258.
111. Sharma M, Deogaonkar M. Accuracy and safety of targeting using intraoperative "O-arm" during placement of deep brain stimulation electrodes without electrophysiological recordings. J Clin Neurosci. 2016;27:80-6.
112. Larson PS, Starr PA, Bates G, Tansey L, Richardson RM, Martin AJ. An Optimized System for Interventional MRI Guided Stereotactic Surgery: Preliminary Evaluation of Targeting Accuracy. Neurosurgery. 2012;70(Operative):95-103.
113. Brodsky M, et al. Clinical Outcomes in Parkinson's Disease for Asleep Deep Brain Stimulation with Electrodes Placed using Intraoperative Imaging versus Awake Deep Brain Stimulation with Microelectrode Recording (S40.003). Neurology. 2016;86 (Supplement):16.
114. Ostrem JL, Galifianakis NB, Markun LC, Grace JK, Martin AJ, Starr PA, et al. Clinical outcomes of PD patients having bilateral STN DBS using high-field interventional MR-imaging for lead placement. Clini Neurol Neurosurg. 2013;115(6):708-12.
115. Milian M, Tatagiba M, Feigl GC. Patient response to awake craniotomy: a summary overview. Acta Neurochir (Wien). 2014;156(6):1063-70.
116. Sammartino F, Krishna V, King NKK, Bruno V, Kalia S, Hodaie M, et al. Sequence of electrode implantation and outcome of deep brain stimulation for Parkinson's disease. J Neurol Neurosurg Psychiatry. 2016;87(8):859-63.
117. Metman LV, Pilitsis JG, Stebbins GT, Bot M, Bakay RAE. Intraoperative X-ray to measure distance between DBS leads: A reliability study. Mov Disord. 2012;27(8):1056-9.
118. Holloway K, Docef A. A quantitative assessment of the accuracy and reliability of O-arm images for deep brain stimulation surgery. Neurosurgery. 2013;72(1 Suppl Operative):47-57.
119. Servello D, Zekaj E, Saleh C, Pacchetti C, Porta M. The pros and cons of intraoperative CT scan in evaluation of deep brain stimulation lead implantation: A retrospective study. Surg Neurol Int. 2016;7(Suppl 19):S551-6.
120. Gross RE, Krack P, Rodriguez-Oroz MC, Rezai AR, Benabid AL. Electrophysiological mapping for the implantation of deep brain stimulators for Parkinson's disease and tremor. Mov Disord. 2006;21 (Suppl 14):S259-83.
121. Hubel D. Tungsten microelectrode from recording from single units. Science. 1957;125:549-50.
122. Lenz FA, Dostrovsky JO, Kwan HC, Tasker RR, Yamashiro K, Murphy JT. Methods for microstimulation and recording of single neurons and evoked potentials in the human central nervous system. J Neurosurg. 1988;68(4):630-4.
123. Ondo WG, Bronte-Stewart H. The North American survey of placement and adjustment strategies for deep brain stimulation. Stereotact Funct Neurosurg. 2005;83(4):142-7.
124. Bejjani BP, Dormont D, Pidoux B, Yelnik J, Damier P, Arnulf I, et al. Bilateral subthalamic stimulation for Parkinson's disease by using three-dimensional stereotactic magnetic resonance imaging and electrophysiological guidance. J Neurosurg. 2000;92(4):615-25.
125. Benabid AL, Krack PP, Benazzouz A, Limousin P, Koudsie A, Pollak P. Deep brain stimulation of the subthalamic nucleus for Parkinson's disease: methodologic aspects and clinical criteria. Neurology. 2000;55(12 Suppl 6): S40-4.
126. Vitek JL, Bakay RA, Hashimoto T, Kaneoke Y, Mewes K, Zhang JY, et al. Microelectrode-guided pallidotomy: technical approach and its application in medically intractable Parkinson's disease. J Neurosurg. 1998;88(6):1027-43.
127. Hariz M, Fodstad H. Do Microelectrode Techniques Increase Accuracy or Decrease risks in pallidotomy and Deep Brain Stimulation. Stereotact Funct Neurosurg. 1999;72:157-69.
128. Garonzik IM, Hua SE, Ohara S, Lenz FA. Intraoperative microelectrode and semi-microelectrode recording during the physiological localization of the thalamic nucleus ventral intermediate. Mov Disord. 2002;17 (Suppl 3):S135-44.
129. Yokoyama T, Sugiyama K, Nishizawa S, Yokota N, Ohta S, Uemura K. Subthalamic nucleus stimulation for gait disturbance in Parkinson's disease. Neurosurgery. 1999;45(1):41-7.
130. Saint-Cyr JA, Hoque T, Pereira LCM, Dostrovsky JO, Hutchison WD, Mikulis DJ, et al. Localization of clinically effective stimulating electrodes in the human subthalamic nucleus on magnetic resonance imaging. J Neurosurg. 2002;97(5):1152-66.
131. Herzog J, Fietzek U, Hamel W, Morsnowski A, Steigerwald F, Schrader B, et al. Most effective stimulation site in subthalamic deep brain stimulation for Parkinson's disease. Mov Disord. 2004;19(9):1050-4.
132. Deuschl G, Paschen S, Witt K. Clinical outcome of deep brain stimulation for Parkinson's disease. Handb Clin Neurol. 2013;116:107-28.
133. Bjerknes S, Skogseid IM, Sæhle T, Dietrichs E, Toft M. Surgical Site Infections after Deep Brain Stimulation Surgery: Frequency, Characteristics and Management in a 10-Year Period. PLOS One. 2014;9(8):e105288.
134. Woloszko JA, Hendriks M, Cahalan PT, Verhoeven MLP, Cahalan LL, Camps ANJ. (1998). Intramuscular stimulation lead with enhanced infection resistance. [online] Available from https://patents.google.com/patent/US5755758A/en [Last accessed, 2023].

135. Byrd DL, Marks Jr WJ, Starr PA. Deep brain stimulation for advanced Parkinson's disease. AORN J. 2000;72(3):387-90.
136. Kleiner-Fisman G, Fisman DN, Sime E, Saint-Cyr JA, Lozano AM, Lang AE. Long-term follow up of bilateral deep brain stimulation of the subthalamic nucleus in patients with advanced Parkinson disease. J Neurosurg. 2003;99(3):489-95.
137. Volkmann J, Moro E, Pahwa R. Basic algorithms for the programming of deep brain stimulation in Parkinson's disease. Mov Disord. 2006;21 (Suppl 14):S284-9.
138. Picillo M, Lozano AM, Kou N, Munhoz RP, Fasano A. Programming Deep Brain Stimulation for Parkinson's Disease: The Toronto Western Hospital Algorithms. Brain Stimul. 2016;9(3):425-37.
139. Tsuboi T, Watanabe H, Tanaka Y, Ohdake R, Yoneyama N, Hara K. Distinct phenotypes of speech and voice disorders in Parkinson's disease after subthalamic nucleus deep brain stimulation. J Neurol Neurosurg Psychiatry. 2015;86(8):856-64.
140. Moro E, Lozano AM, Pollak P, Agid Y, Rehncrona S, Volkmann J, et al. Long-term results of a multicenter study on subthalamic and pallidal stimulation in Parkinson's disease. Mov Disord. 2010;25(5):578-86.
141. Krack P, Pollak P, Limousin P, Benazzouz A, Deuschl G, Benabid AL. From off-period dystonia to peak-dose chorea. The clinical spectrum of varying subthalamic nucleus activity. Brain. 1999;122 (Pt 6):1133-46.
142. Deuschl G, Herzog J, Kleiner-Fisman G, Kubu C, Lozano AM, Lyons KE, et al. Deep brain stimulation: postoperative issues. Mov Disord. 2006;21 (Suppl 14):S219-37.
143. St George RJ, Nutt JG, Burchiel KJ, Horak FB. A meta-regression of the long-term effects of deep brain stimulation on balance and gait in PD. Neurology. 2010;75(14):1292-9.
144. Deogaonkar M, Rezai A. Deep Brain Stimulation for Movement Disorders and Mood Disorders, in Atlas of Neurosurgical Techniques: Brain. 2015.
145. Pilitsis JG, Rezai AR, Boulis NM, Henderson JM, Busch RM, Kubu CS. A preliminary study of transient confusional states following bilateral subthalamic stimulation for Parkinson's disease. Stereotact Funct Neurosurg. 2005;83(2-3):67-70.
146. Krack P, Batir A, Blercom NV, Chabardes S, Fraix V, Ardouin C, et al. Five-year follow-up of bilateral stimulation of the subthalamic nucleus in advanced Parkinson's disease. N Engl J Med. 2003;349(20):1925-34.
147. Krause M, Fogel W, Heck A, Hacke W, Bonsanto M, Trenkwalder C, et al. Deep brain stimulation for the treatment of Parkinson's disease: subthalamic nucleus versus globus pallidus internus. J Neurol Neurosurg Psychiatry. 2001;70(4):464-70.